BSAVA Manual of Wildlife Casualties
second edition

T0329652

Editors:

Elizabeth Mullineaux
BVM&S DVM&S CertSHP MRCVS
RCVS Recognised Specialist in Wildlife Medicine (Mammalian)
Secret World Wildlife Rescue, New Road,
Highbridge, Somerset TA9 3PZ, UK

Emma Keeble
BVSc DZooMed (Mammalian) MRCVS
RCVS Recognised Specialist in Zoo and Wildlife Medicine
Royal (Dick) School of Veterinary Studies, The University of Edinburgh,
Easter Bush Campus, Midlothian EH25 9RG, UK

Published by:

British Small Animal Veterinary Association
Woodrow House, 1 Telford Way,
Waterwells Business Park, Quedgeley,
Gloucester GL2 2AB

A Company Limited by Guarantee in England
Registered Company No. 2837793
Registered as a Charity

ISBN 978 1 905319 80 0

The publishers, editors and contributors cannot take responsibility for information provided on dosages and methods of application of drugs mentioned or referred to in this publication. Details of this kind must be verified in each case by individual users from up to date literature published by the manufacturers or suppliers of those drugs. Veterinary surgeons are reminded that in each case they must follow all appropriate national legislation and regulations (for example, in the United Kingdom, the prescribing cascade) from time to time in force.

Printed in the UK by Hobbs the Printers Ltd, Totton SO40 3WX

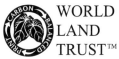

WORLD LAND TRUST™
www.carbonbalancedprint.com
CBP2250

Carbon Balancing is delivered by World Land Trust, an international conservation charity, who protects the world's most biologically important and threatened habitats acre by acre. Their Carbon Balanced Programme offsets emissions through the purchase and preservation of high conservation value forests.

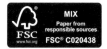

MIX
Paper from responsible sources
FSC® C020438

19437PUBS24

Titles in the BSAVA Manuals series

For further information on these and all BSAVA publications, please visit our website: **www.bsava.com**

Contents

Contributors

James Barnett
BVSc(Hons) BSc MRCVS
British Divers Marine Life Rescue,
c/o Bohortha, Holywell Road,
Playing Place, Truro, Cornwall TR3 6EP, UK

Michelle Barrows
BSc BVMS DZooMed (Avian) MRCVS
Veterinary Department,
Bristol Zoo Gardens,
Clifton, Bristol BS8 3HA, UK

Dick Best
BVSc MSc
Quantock View Farmhouse,
Steart, Somerset TA5 2PX, UK

Steve Bexton
BVMS CertZooMed MRCVS
RSPCA East Winch Wildlife Centre,
Station Road, East Winch,
King's Lynn, Norfolk PE32 1NR, UK

Tiffany Blackett
BVetMed MRCVS

Debra Bourne
MA VetMB PhD MRCVS
Beckenham, Kent, UK

John Chitty
BVetMed CertZooMed CBiol MSB MRCVS
Anton Vets,
Unit 11, Anton Mill Road,
Andover, Hampshire SP10 2NJ, UK

John E. Cooper
DTVM FRCPath FRSB CBiol FRCVS
Wildlife Health, Forensic and Comparative Pathology
Services (UK) and DICE, The University of Kent,
Canterbury, Kent CT2 7NZ, UK

Margaret E. Cooper
LLB FLS
Wildlife Health, Forensic and Comparative Pathology
Services (UK) and DICE, The University of Kent,
Canterbury, Kent CT2 7NZ, UK

David Couper
BVMS MSc MRCVS
RSPCA West Hatch Wildlife Centre,
West Hatch, Taunton,
Somerset TA3 5RT, UK

Sara Cowen
RVN

Neil A. Forbes
BVetMed DipECZM (Avian) FRCVS
Great Western Exotics at Vets Now Referrals,
Unit 10 Berkshire House, County Business Park,
Shrivenham Road, Swindon SN1 2NR, UK

Sally Goulden
BVetMed MRCVS
51 Dorset Road, Ashford,
Middlesex TW15 3BZ, UK

Adam Grogan
BSc MCIEEM
RSPCA Horsham,
Wilberforce Way, Southwater,
West Sussex RH13 9RS, UK

Joanna Hedley
BVM&S DZooMed (Reptilian) DipECZM (Herpetology) MRCVS
RVC Exotics Service,
Royal Veterinary College,
Royal College Street,
London NW1 0TU, UK

Emma Keeble
BVSc DZooMed (Mammalian) MRCVS
Royal (Dick) School of Veterinary Studies,
The University of Edinburgh,
Easter Bush Campus,
Midlothian EH25 9RG, UK

Andrew Kelly
PhD
Chief Executive Officer,
Irish Society for the Prevention of Cruelty to Animals,
ISPCA HQ, Derryglogher Lodge,
Keenagh, Co. Longford,
Republic of Ireland

Becki Lawson
MA VetMB MSc PhD DipECZM (Wildlife Population Health) MRCVS
Institute of Zoology,
Zoological Society of London,
Regent's Park, London NW1 4RY, UK

Anna Meredith
MA VetMB PhD CertLAS DZooMed DipECZM MRCVS
Royal (Dick) School of Veterinary Studies,
The University of Edinburgh,
Easter Bush Campus,
Midlothian EH25 9RG, UK

Elizabeth Mullineaux
BVM&S DVM&S CertSHP MCRVS
Secret World Wildlife Rescue,
New Road, Highbridge,
Somerset TA9 3PZ, UK

Ranald Munro
BVMS MSc DVM Dip Forensic Medicine MRCVS
Honorary Fellow,
Royal (Dick) School of Veterinary Studies,
The University of Edinburgh,
Easter Bush Campus,
Midlothian EH25 9RG, UK

Romain Pizzi
BVSc MSc DZooMed DipECZM MACVSc(surg) FRES FRSB FRGS MRCVS
Scottish SPCA,
National Wildlife Rescue Centre, Fishcross,
Clackmannanshire FK10 3AN, UK
and
Royal Zoological Society,
Costorphine Road,
Edinburgh EH12 6TS, UK
and
University of Nottingham,
School of Veterinary Medicine and Science,
Sutton Bonington Campus,
Leicestershire LE12 5RD, UK

Jenna Richardson
BVMS MRCVS
Royal (Dick) School of Veterinary Studies,
The University of Edinburgh,
Easter Bush Campus,
Midlothian EH25 9RG, UK

Richard Saunders
BSc(Hons) BVSc FRSB CBiol CertZooMed DZooMed (Mammalian) MRCVS
Veterinary Services and Conservation Medicine,
Bristol Zoological Society,
Clifton, Bristol BS8 3HA, UK

Colin Seddon
Scottish SPCA,
National Wildlife Rescue Centre, Fishcross,
Clackmannanshire FK10 3AN, UK

Guy Shorrock
BVSc(Hons)
Senior Investigations Officer,
RSPB UK Headquarters,
The Lodge, Sandy,
Bedfordshire SG19 2DL, UK

Victor Simpson
BVSc DTVM CBiol FRSB HonFRCVS
Wildlife Veterinary Investigation Centre,
Little Jollys Bottom Farm,
Chacewater, Truro,
Cornwall TR4 8PB, UK

Steve Smith
BVetMed(Hons) CertZooMed DipECZM (Avian) MRCVS
Tiggywinkles Wildlife Hospital,
Aston Road, Haddenham,
Aylesbury, Buckinghamshire HP17 8AF, UK

Alexandra Tomlinson
MA VetMB MSc PhD DipECZM (Wildlife Population Health) MRCVS
The Paddock, Newtown,
Longnor, Buxton,
Derbyshire SK17 0NE, UK

Molly Varga
BVetMed CertZooMed DZooMed (Mammalian) MRCVS
Rutland House Veterinary Hospital,
Abbotsfield Road, St Helens,
Merseyside WA9 4HU, UK
and
Manor Vets Edgbaston,
371–373 Hagley Road,
Birmingham B17 8DL, UK

Foreword

The handling of wildlife casualties is a very broad subject covering a range of disciplines including veterinary science and ecology, ethics and legislation, and is often surrounded by controversy. Attitudes to the treatment and rehabilitation of individual wild animals vary from those who regard it as an act of compassion to those who regard it as an irrelevance or even an act of cruelty. However, the decision to intervene is always a welfare issue, rarely one of conservation, and is very popular with a large section of the general public. With increasing public awareness, there is more likely to be intervention when orphaned or injured wildlife casualties are seen.

In the first edition of this manual the BSAVA broke new ground by providing an introduction to the subject in a British context. The aim of its editors at that time was to produce a practical guide to the handling, treatment and natural history of the species that are likely to be presented to those working in veterinary practice. It described the need for high standards of care with the aim of returning each wildlife casualty back to the wild 100% fit: able to hunt, fulfil natural behaviours and survive. It emphasized the need to understand that housing and care of wildlife casualties are very different from the requirements of farm, exotic or domestic animals. Since the first edition was published in 2003, it has proven to be very popular and obviously filled a gap in the literature for the veterinary profession and for those involved directly with wildlife casualties or in education.

This second edition follows the same principles as a manual and a reference text, but advances in techniques in exotic veterinary medicine and surgery, and in knowledge of the natural history of British fauna, have spilled over into realms of wildlife rehabilitation bringing this volume up to date and creating a valuable guide for all those involved in this field.

The BSAVA is to be congratulated on producing this valuable contemporary manual.

Pauline Kidner and Dick Best
July 2016

Preface

The first edition of the *BSAVA Manual of Wildlife Casualties*, published in 2003, was a ground-breaking resource for those working in general veterinary practice. Prior to this, despite an RCVS requirement for all vet surgeons to provide emergency care to all animal species, there was no readily available information for those presented with British wildlife casualties. In the first edition subjects such as ethics, basic wildlife care and clinical pathology were introduced and followed by species-specific chapters covering all common British wildlife species.

Over the following decade the disciplines of wildlife medicine and rehabilitation have vastly expanded, with specialization occurring within these fields and increased research output providing a strong evidence-based information source. In this brand new edition we have been privileged to work with some of these experts and specialists to bring together new scientific evidence and combine it with a broad spectrum of practical knowledge and experience.

This second edition of the *BSAVA Manual of Wildlife Casualties* has allowed us to expand subject areas such as the ethics of wildlife intervention, legislation, clinical pathology and rehabilitation and release and also add brand new chapters including triage and decision-making, first aid and emergency care, anaesthesia and wildlife crime. Following on from these general chapters are species-specific chapters, which follow the same user-friendly format as the previous edition, with greatly expanded content and references.

It has been a great privilege to work with the chapter authors, bringing together individuals from many different organizations to collaborate on this book. We are indebted to our authors for their contributions, time and patience during the production of the book. We would like to thank Pauline Kinder and Dick Best for writing the foreword; they have both been an inspiration to us over the years. We would also like to thank BSAVA for making this second edition possible. This book would never have been published without the support and patience of our families and in particular we would like to thank Phil, Mat, Adam, Rosie and Charlie.

Elizabeth Mullineaux and Emma Keeble
August 2016

Chapter 1

Wildlife casualties and the veterinary surgeon

Alexandra Tomlinson

A casualty is defined by the Oxford English Dictionary as 'a person or thing badly affected by an event or a situation'. In this context, the 'thing' in question is a wild animal. This manual brings together expertise on how to handle and treat a broad range of casualty wildlife, including mammals, birds, reptiles and amphibians. Despite the enormous diversity in the biology and ecology of these species, there is one thing they all have in common: they are free-living and wild. Unlike our pets, livestock and zoo animals, they are neither domesticated nor captive.

Their very 'wildness' is central to our goals in their treatment. Understanding what it means to be 'free-living and wild' forms the focus of this chapter. Despite use of the phrase 'free-living and wild', it is hard to envisage a setting in the United Kingdom where there is not some element of habitat or species management that influences this status. As a result, any wildlife intervention may well be complicated by issues pertaining to land and/or animal ownership, and will regularly trigger heated debate. It is vitally important for the profession that veterinary surgeons (veterinarians) involved in wildlife work address issues honestly and fully in order to take seriously the responsibility associated with the treatment of injured wildlife, and to retain public and stakeholder trust.

Ethical issues associated with wildlife casualty management

Veterinary surgeons are accustomed to making ethical judgements in clinical practice. Deciding when and how to intervene in the discipline of wildlife casualty management is no different in this regard, although there may be greater inherent complexity due to the wide range of animals and people potentially involved. Where there are clear anthropogenic causal factors giving rise to wildlife casualties, and/or where there is severe animal suffering, there are few who would argue against intervention. Examples might include oil spills, road traffic casualties, or the consequences of human conflict – in these instances the decision to intervene to alleviate suffering and/or to prevent further losses is likely to have widespread, even universal support. There may however be less clear cut cases, in which the nature of intervention, and/or the decision to intervene in the first instance, are more likely to be challenged. Examples might include cases where stakeholder opinions on euthanasia criteria diverge, or scenarios where

veterinary opinions are sought on wildlife health and disease issues perhaps without the direct presentation of individual casualty animals. It is not the purpose of this chapter to be prescriptive about such decisions; rather to emphasize that there are grey areas and that we need to consider all the issues and form our own defendable opinions. Factors to be considered in addition to the primary concern of the welfare of the individual(s), include welfare concerns for other animals (free-living wildlife, captive wildlife and domesticated animals) and humans; species conservation status; the nature of the relationship between the species and a variety of stakeholders; and practical and legal aspects (see Chapters 2 and 4).

Specific detailed criteria have intentionally not been categorized, since to do so is highly subjective and opinions will vary even amongst veterinary surgeons. By being involved in wildlife work veterinary surgeons are assuming a degree of responsibility, but the responsibility for wild animals and indeed the whole ecosystem in which they live is a collective responsibility with many interested parties. It is little wonder then that wildlife intervention debates can become heated and polarized. It is rarely possible to satisfy everyone in these situations, but open, honest and proactive discussion will reduce the likelihood of conflict between parties.

The wildlife casualty – its niche in the ecosystem

The wildlife casualty is not an isolated entity. It is part of a complex ecosystem that incorporates the casualty's own parasites (be they pathogenic or non-pathogenic), other members of its species (conspecifics), other wildlife species, domesticated animals, humans and the environment (Figure 1.1). This conceptual image of the niche each individual wildlife casualty occupies is an important framework, and undertaking wildlife casualty work on this basis should ensure that the approach used is truly holistic. This conceptual model also embraces the 'One Health' principles of integrating human, animal and environmental health. Adoption of such an approach should ensure that the veterinary profession retains its reputation as a caring, intelligent, progressive and trustworthy profession.

The following sections consider the major issues that are likely to arise in wildlife casualty management, firstly with regard to the health and welfare of the individual

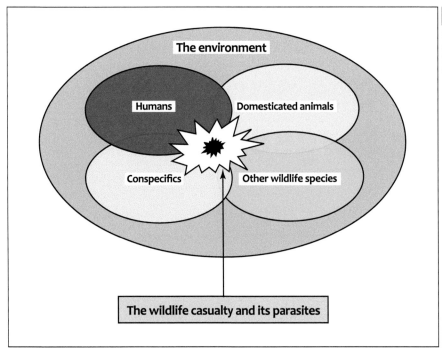

1.1 Conceptual framework for a holistic approach to the management of an individual wildlife casualty, incorporating the casualty's own parasites, its conspecifics, other wildlife, domesticated animals, humans and the environment.

casualty, and secondly with regard to conspecifics, other wildlife, domesticated animals, humans and the environment. A working knowledge of wildlife biology and ecology is essential to address all these issues successfully throughout the period during which the veterinary surgeon is responsible for the wildlife casualty. The definition of such a 'responsibility period' is both crucial and difficult. It is not just the period of captivity but the period of time from initial presentation of the casualty to the veterinary surgeon (which may be notification rather than actual presentation) right through to the point at which the individual has re-established, or is likely to have re-established, itself successfully in the wild. This endpoint is not easy to define, but it has been deliberately chosen instead of the 'point of release'. It is important to understand that the actions of the veterinary surgeon during the captive period can affect events beyond the point of release and that there are considerable practical limitations to what can be achieved once a wild animal has been released.

Health and welfare of the individual wildlife casualty

Primary considerations in all cases are the health and welfare of the casualty. It is incumbent on the veterinary surgeon to do as much as is practically possible to safeguard health and welfare throughout the wildlife rescue and rehabilitation process. Indeed, the RCVS Code of Professional Conduct makes it very clear that 'veterinary surgeons must make animal health and welfare their first consideration when attending to animals'. Figure 1.2 outlines the flow of events from initial presentation to release and indicates the key points at which the veterinary surgeon should take responsibility.

Primary decision-making

Primary decision-making can be divided into the initial decision about whether intervention is indicated at all (an ethical judgement), progressing to a decision about whether the veterinary surgeon is equipped (both in terms of facilities and expertise) to treat a wildlife casualty beyond the provision of immediate first aid, culminating in the decision to treat or to euthanase (see Chapter 4). Since the goal of wildlife casualty treatment is a successful return to the wild within a short timeframe, an honest assessment following the initial examination is important to determine the likelihood of this being achieved. Prompt euthanasia may be indicated in some cases and should not necessarily be viewed as a failure. Conservation status of the casualty may be a factor to consider in such decision-making, but the individual's welfare should always be the primary consideration. If the decision is made to treat, it is important to draft and regularly review a realistic treatment plan, repeating the assessment of likely success at defined intervals.

Managing the captive period

The wildlife casualty is likely to be in pain, therefore adequate analgesia is indicated (see Chapters 5 and 6). Veterinary surgeons are familiar with the variety of pain indicators in domesticated animals, in particular the quiet unresponsive signs, and analgesia for the wildlife casualty must be similarly addressed.

It is also likely that the entire process, from initial presentation right up to release, will trigger a stress response in the wildlife casualty due to human proximity, proximity of other animals, handling, transportation and an unfamiliar environment. Such stress can be minimized by, for example, quiet and calm handling, minimizing auditory and visual stimulation, and providing appropriate housing and nutrition, but the captive period should always be as short as possible.

To minimize the likelihood of the casualty acquiring novel infections from other animals, humans or the environment, good hygiene and biosecurity practices should be observed during the captive period (see Chapter 7). Clearly a shorter time period in captivity equates to fewer transmission opportunities. Acquiring a novel infection

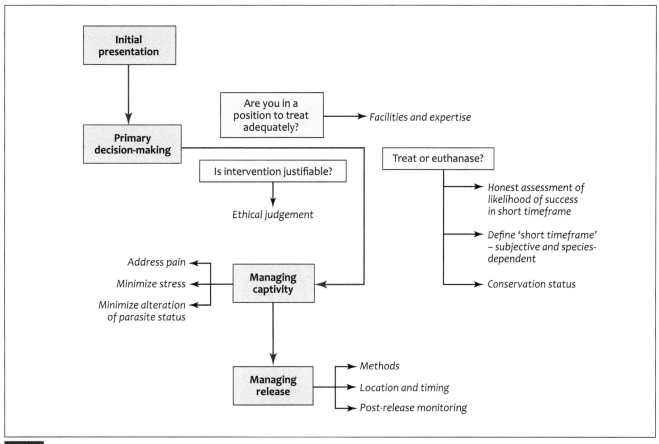

1.2 Flowchart indicating the critical points of veterinary responsibility for wildlife casualty health and welfare from initial notification to release.

may have direct consequences for the health of the casualty; for example, parvovirus enteritis in young badgers (*Meles meles*) (Barlow *et al.*, 2012) or Tyzzer's disease in otters (Simpson *et al.*, 2008). Alternatively, acquired agents may not affect the health of the casualty at all, but the consequences of subsequent release of an animal with an altered parasite status may extend to other wildlife, domesticated animals and humans. One final consideration is the alteration of the casualty's parasite burden during the captive period; for example, by the administration of anthelmintics (see Chapter 7). Such action may improve the individual's health in order to aid recovery but altering the balance of parasites may have unpredictable effects on infections acquired post-release. An important element of pre-release management is, therefore, the screening of casualties for specific parasites and adopting a risk-based approach to select specific tests (see Chapters 9 and 10).

There are other potentially negative welfare consequences for the casualty relating to the time spent in captivity. The longer an animal is dependent on its carers, the more attention needs to be given to appropriate preparation for release to ensure, for example, that it is able to forage or hunt successfully in the wild. In addition, for social species, extended time in captivity can have deleterious effects on acceptance by conspecifics upon release.

Managing release

Following successful treatment, attention turns to the release of the animal. The natural world is an uncompromising and competitive environment for wildlife. Fitness to survive and thrive (e.g. reproduce successfully) is a step up from fitness to be returned to the care of an owner, as is the case with domesticated species. Working knowledge of the biology and ecology of the species will underpin preparation and assessment of fitness for release. An honest appraisal of an individual's ability to thrive in the wild is essential for successful and humane completion of management of the casualty. Key issues to consider include:

- Release methods
- Release location and timing
- Post-release monitoring.

Release methods range from 'hard', an 'open the door, let it go' type of approach, through to 'soft', which involves more of an acclimatization period with access to food and shelter (see Chapter 9). The latter might be particularly pertinent if animals have been housed in a hospital setting that differs in temperature, lighting and humidity from their natural environment. Experience and familiarity with the available literature will assist with method selection.

The ideal release site for an adult wildlife casualty is within its home range (with the caveat that any potential threats that may have resulted in the casualty event in the first instance have been addressed). It can rarely be known with certainty that the site where the casualty was found is within its home range, but it is the usual choice for release in the absence of any other information. In the case of very young casualties, for example orphans arising from fatal injuries to the dam, release is only considered once the animal has been reared to an independent state. This presents a particular problem since the now independent animal should be released at a location not only in a suitable habitat but also where it is unlikely to come into immediate conflict with conspecifics (e.g. through competition for resources) or with other species (wildlife, domesticated animals or humans). Release into a novel environment may also carry disease risks for the casualty, relating, for example, to parasites to which it has not previously been exposed. Other concerns at the ecosystem level, extending beyond those of the wildlife casualty, are addressed in a later section.

Timing of release should take into account the biology and ecology of the casualty species, including its age, sex and reproductive status. For example, release at a time when natural food sources are scarce, or release of a reproductively mature animal at a time of year when competition for mates is at its peak, may not be in the best interests of the casualty. Rehabilitated wildlife should be permanently identifiable, for example with a microchip, and attempts made to determine the outcome following release. Monitoring may be achievable for some species using simple observation, or by attaching tracking devices such as radio or global positioning system (GPS) collars or harnesses (see Chapter 9). In some cases, however, monitoring may be very challenging. Advances in the methodologies used for monitoring continue apace and it is important that wildlife rehabilitators are up to date with current research in this area. Whether post-release monitoring is feasible or not, it is vital that the veterinary profession acknowledges its responsibility in this field. Information gathered post-release should be analysed, recorded and disseminated in order to continually update, modify and improve practices and methods.

Robust primary decision-making, adopting a well thought-out treatment and management plan during captivity, accurately assessing fitness prior to release, and planning release will all help to reduce the likelihood of post-release problems for the casualty. Despite the practical difficulties associated with post-release monitoring and intervention, 'out of sight, out of mind' is an indefensible stance for the veterinary professional to take.

The impact of wildlife casualty release

The impact of actions taken during the management of the wildlife casualty will not be restricted to the treated individual alone. This does not differ from the treatment of domesticated species, particularly livestock, but is easy to ignore if the casualty is viewed in isolation and not as part of a population and, indeed, of an ecosystem (see Figure 1.1). There are likely to be additional consequences for wild animals of the same and different species, domesticated animals, humans and the environment following release of the casualty. Key points to consider in this regard are the length of time the casualty has been in captivity, its parasite status on release, the site and timing of its release, its niche in the ecosystem and its conservation status.

It is vital for the veterinary surgeon to acknowledge the interests of other stakeholders, including landowners, farmers and local residents, when casualty wildlife work is undertaken. There are two important questions the veterinary surgeon should address specifically prior to release:

- Has the parasite status of the casualty animal been significantly altered?
- Is the casualty being released at a location remote from its original home range?

If the answer to either of these questions is 'yes', then there exists the potential for changing the status quo within the ecosystem. It is such changes, which are difficult to predict and even more difficult to reverse, that can be the most contentious for the veterinary surgeon involved in the rescue and rehabilitation of casualty wildlife (Figure 1.3). It is worth noting that there may be no consequences at all, but, due to the complexity of the whole ecosystem, it would be very hard to predict this with any certainty.

Effects on conspecifics

Fluidity of social structure and competition for mates and resources mean that the longer a wild animal is absent from its population, the more difficult it may be for it to re-establish. For social species, this can result in aggressive encounters or even social exclusion from the reintroduced animal's original social group. In addition, if a wildlife casualty is released at a location remote from its original home range, there is an increased likelihood of aggressive encounters between it and those members of the species established in that home range, or similarly social exclusion.

Parasites acquired by the casualty during captivity may be transmitted to conspecifics following release. Pathogenic organisms are an obvious concern, but any novel agent may alter the parasite status of the wild population with unpredictable and, most significantly, often irreversible consequences. Infection of the wild population with a novel agent may also arise without the need for acquisition by the casualty in captivity. This can occur if a casualty animal, infected prior to its captivity with a geographically restricted parasite, is released into a previously uninfected population remote from the casualty's original home range. This scenario may particularly apply to orphan animals reared in captivity and released in sites some distance from where they were found. As previously discussed, a risk-based approach to health screening for specific parasites prior to release may be indicated.

Effects on other wildlife, domesticated animals, humans and the environment

In common with the consequences for conspecifics, ecosystem level consequences for other wildlife, domesticated animals, humans and the environment are likely to centre around either the physical presence of the casualty and/or onward transmission of parasites carried by the casualty (see Figures 1.3 and 1.4).

Effects arising from the physical presence of a casualty include species interactions (e.g. competition, predator–prey relationships), habitat modification and clashes with humans. The onward transmission of parasites carried by the casualty is influenced by many factors, such as the ability of the parasite to cross species barriers, its routes of transmission (direct and/or indirect) and the interactions (direct and/or indirect) between the casualty and other wildlife, domesticated animals or humans. A few examples of parasites that may have ecosystem consequences are given in Figure 1.4. However, it must be stressed that there are many unknowns in these scenarios; the transmissibility and species-dependent pathogenicity of all parasites cannot be predicted with certainty. This reiterates the necessity for a risk-based approach relating to casualty release.

One final consideration in this web of complexity is the conservation status of not only the species of the casualty being released but of other wildlife species in

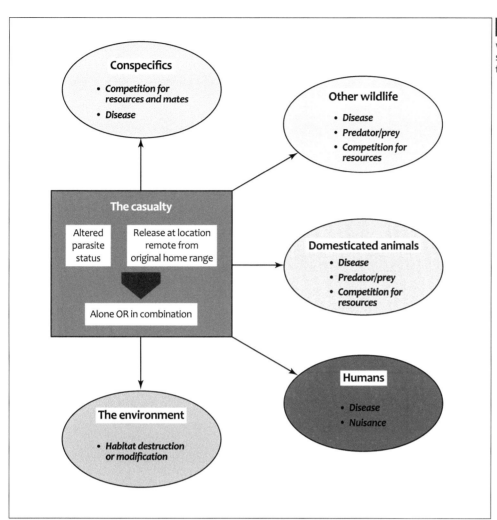

1.3 Potential consequences following the release of a wildlife casualty with altered parasite status and/or in a location remote from its original home range.

Wildlife casualty species	Considerations at the ecosystem level		
	Physical presence	*Parasites carried by the casualty*	
		Example pathogens	*Other species which may be susceptible*
Natterjack toad (*Epidalea* (formerly *Bufo*) *calamita*)[ab]	Competitor species with common frog (*Rana temporaria*) Predated by rats and gulls	*Batrachochytrium dendrobatidis* (chytridiomycosis)	Other amphibian species
Red fox (*Vulpes vulpes*)[cd]	Predator (e.g. lagomorphs, pheasants, domesticated poultry and lambs) Raids domestic rubbish bins	*Angiostrongylus vasorum*	Domestic dogs
Roe deer (*Capreolus capreolus*)[ef]	Damage to cereal crops and saplings in forestry plantations	*Mycobacterium avium paratuberculosis*	Domesticated livestock (e.g. cattle)
European badger (*Meles meles*)[g]	Crop damage, and undermining of buildings and domestic gardens	*Mycobacterium bovis*	Domesticated livestock (e.g. cattle)

1.4 Examples of ecosystem considerations in wildlife casualty management, relating to both the physical presence of the casualty and the parasites it may carry.

([a]Beebee and Denton, 1996; [b]Cunningham and Minting, 2008; [c]Baker and Harris, 2008; [d]Taylor *et al.*, 2007; [e]Hewison and Staines, 2008; [f]Böhm *et al.*, 2007; [g]Delahay *et al.*, 2008)

the ecosystem. For example, if the species of casualty is highly abundant, there may be less sympathy amongst stakeholders for release at locations remote from where the animal was found, particularly if the casualty species is a competitor or predator of other less abundant wildlife species. Conversely, if the casualty species is endangered there may be stronger arguments for release of reared orphans outside their original home range. These considerations are in addition to the legal requirements that govern non-native and other species (see Chapter 2).

This section has been purposefully provocative. This is not with a view to saying what is right or wrong but simply to highlight some of the critical issues that should be addressed, and the importance of a truly holistic approach to the entire process of wildlife rescue and rehabilitation.

Conclusion

The aim of this chapter is to encourage the reader to take a holistic view of the individual wildlife casualty in the context of the ecosystem from which it originated. This begins with the initial decision to intervene in the first instance, a decision which may raise complex ethical questions. During any intervention, the health and welfare of the individual are primary concerns, which are complicated by the 'wild nature' of the animal. Finally, due consideration should be given to the impact of intervention, specifically the release of a rehabilitated casualty, on members of the same species, other wildlife species, domesticated animals, humans and the environment.

The following questions serve as a useful *aide memoire* in all cases, and seem a fitting way to end this chapter and set the scene for the wealth of information to follow on best management practices for wildlife casualties.

- Can you defend and justify the initial intervention?
- Have you safeguarded the health and welfare of the individual wildlife casualty?
- Have you considered the health and welfare of all elements of the ecosystem (conspecifics, domesticated animals, humans and the environment) into which you are releasing the rehabilitated casualty?

References and further reading

Baker PA and Harris S (2008) Family Canidae. Fox. In: *Mammals of the British Isles, 4th edn*, ed. S Harris and DW Yalden, pp. 407–422. The Mammal Society, Southampton

Barlow AM, Schock A, Bradshaw J *et al.* (2012) Parvovirus enteritis in Eurasian badgers (*Meles meles*). *Veterinary Record* **170**, 416

Beebee T and Denton J (1996) *IN291: The Natterjack Toad Conservation Handbook*. English Nature, Peterborough

Böhm M, White PC, Chambers J *et al.* (2007) Wild deer as a source of infection for livestock and humans in the UK. *The Veterinary Journal* **174**, 260–276

Cunningham A and Minting P (2008) *National Survey of Batrachochytrium dendrobatidis infection in UK Amphibians*. Zoological Society of London, London

Delahay RJ, Wilson G, Harris S *et al.* (2008) Genus *Meles*. In: *Mammals of the British Isles, 4th edn*, ed. S Harris and DW Yalden, pp. 425–436. The Mammal Society, Southampton

Hewison AJM and Staines BW (2008) Genus *Capreolus*. In: *Mammals of the British Isles, 4th edn*, ed. S Harris and DW Yalden, pp. 605–617. The Mammal Society, Southampton

Simpson VR, Hargreaves J, Birtles RJ *et al.* (2008) Tyzzer's disease in a Eurasian otter (*Lutra lutra*) in Scotland. *Veterinary Record* **163**, 539–543

Taylor MA, Coop RL and Wall RL (2007) *Veterinary Parasitology, 3rd edn*. Wiley-Blackwell, Oxford

Chapter 2

Law affecting British wildlife casualties

Margaret E. Cooper

The care and treatment of wildlife casualties presents special challenges to the veterinary surgeon (veterinarian), not only in terms of unusual species and their lack of habituation to captivity, but also in respect of the legislation that applies to the rescue of sick and injured wild animals and their rehabilitation and release. Whilst a veterinary surgeon is well aware of the day-to-day legal requirements of veterinary practice, the special circumstances of wildlife rehabilitation raises new questions of how that law is to be applied. Rehabilitation also operates within the framework of wildlife laws and these may be unfamiliar to those who practise mainly with domesticated or captive exotic species. The purpose of this chapter is to point to the areas of law that are particularly relevant to wildlife rehabilitation and which may be useful to those who work in this field.

Key websites for information regarding the law relating to British wildlife casualties are summarized in Figure 2.1 at the end of this chapter.

UK legislation

The legislation discussed in this chapter is that which applies to the United Kingdom (UK). There are core aspects that are similar in countries outside the UK, but there are also some fundamental differences, such as the ownership of wildlife, as well as many variations of detail. It is important to ascertain the exact law applicable to any particular situation and country, preferably by taking professional advice.

The UK consists of England (E), Wales (W) and Scotland (S) (together known as Great Britain (GB)) and Northern Ireland (NI). Whilst there is substantial similarity in the legal provisions and some shared legislation within the UK, devolution (i.e. the power of the National Assembly for Wales, the Scottish Parliament and the Northern Ireland Assembly to make their own laws in certain spheres) means that there is also some legislation that applies to one country only or, quite often, to England and Wales together, whilst Northern Ireland, and to some extent Scotland, have their own comparable legal provisions. It is therefore important to check carefully how the legislation in force in the UK applies to its component countries. The primary internet source for all current legislation in the UK is www.legislation.gov.uk. On this website, shared legislation is annotated to show which provisions apply to a particular country. Likewise, consolidated legislation indicates amendments and the impact of subsidiary legislation (i.e. statutory instruments, mainly 'Orders'). The key Acts and some Orders are cited in this chapter, but it should be generally assumed that, in most cases, there may have been some amendments or supplementation by subsidiary legislation.

European and international legislation

UK wildlife law implements the relevant European Union (EU) Regulations and Directives and the **Council of Europe (CoE) Convention on the Conservation of European Wildlife and Natural Habitats**. This legislation can be found at the EUR-Lex and the CoE Treaty Office websites.

EU Regulations apply directly to all Member States with no further legislation at the national level than provisions for enforcement and stricter measures. Directives are given effect in national laws. See the EU Environment website for further information.

The UK also implements many international conventions that affect wildlife, particularly the **Convention on International Trade in Endangered Species of Wild Fauna and Flora (CITES)**. A guide to the EU CITES legislation is provided on the EU Environment website. Information on the CITES controls and enforcement within the UK can be found online at the Department for Environment, Food and Rural Affairs (Defra) and Animal and Plant Health Agency (APHA) websites.

Information on law relevant to wildlife rehabilitation

It is important to keep up to date with developments in the law, since it is often subject to change. Those using this chapter must also apprise themselves independently of the current state of the law. A number of organizations committed to wildlife conservation and animal welfare are very well informed and closely follow developments in legislation relating to species in which they specialize. It is therefore worth referring to their relevant literature, often available online, or consulting their staff directly.

Books on animal law, together with publications on rehabilitation or related subjects that also cover the law relevant to wildlife, provide further information (see 'References and further reading'). For current information on wildlife law, see the Joint Nature Conservation Committee (JNCC) website and for wildlife offences (E and W) see the Crown Prosecution Service website. The British Wildlife Rehabilitation Council (BWRC) provides comprehensive information on the legislation, ethics and guidance applicable to wildlife rehabilitation, as does Raptor Rescue. For contact details of these organizations, see Figure 2.1.

The law discussed in this chapter has been selected for its relevance to veterinary surgeons dealing with wildlife casualties and rehabilitation facilities. It has been summarized as simply as possible and forms a pointer towards the detailed provisions that are to be found in the actual legislation, relevant guidance and other literature. The reader must refer to this material to understand the full effect of the law.

The process of rehabilitation falls into three stages: rescue, rehabilitation and release. Each of these stages is affected by legislation.

Rescue

Access to the casualty

The land

A wildlife casualty may be found in a place that is readily accessible to the public; however, if it is discovered on private land, the landowner's permission to go on to the land should be obtained, to avoid trespassing and as a matter of good practice. Access to a protected area such as a national park or nature reserve may require a permit from the appropriate authority.

The animal (ownership)

- In the UK, normally a free-living wild animal does not belong to anyone until it is 'reduced into possession', i.e. someone takes it into captivity. It then belongs to the person who takes it. There are a few exceptions to this principle; for example, young animals that are not yet independent belong to the landowner, and the law on taking game species that is based on the issue of poaching (see 'Species protection'). The position may be very different in the countries outside the UK that consider that free-living wildlife belongs to the state.
- Once a free-living wild animal has been taken into captivity, it has the same status in law as other property. To steal it is an offence under the **Theft Act 1968**. Also, it becomes the property of the owner, whose consent must be obtained if the animal is to undergo treatment or to be disposed of in any way. For this reason, consent at the point of admission to a veterinary practice or wildlife centre is important (see Chapter 3). The finder can keep the animal, provided that the acquisition was in conformity with relevant wildlife legislation. The scope of any treatment given must comply with the **Veterinary Surgeons Act 1966** (VSA) (see 'Veterinary aspects of wildlife rehabilitation'). If the animal is taken to a rehabilitator for attention, the latter should obtain ownership from the finder so that the relevant provisions regarding treatment by non-veterinary surgeons are applicable and the rehabilitator, as the owner, can authorize a veterinary surgeon to treat the animal.

- A rehabilitator is strongly advised to obtain a history of the casualty and a written agreement to transfer the ownership, signed by the finder (see Chapter 3). This should form part of the rehabilitator's records that can be used to demonstrate compliance with the wildlife and other legislation.

Taking the casualty

- Wildlife and Countryside Act 1981 (WCA) (E, W and S)
- The Conservation of Habitats and Species Regulations 2010 (E, W and S)
- The Conservation (Natural Habitats, etc.) Regulations 1994 (S)
- Wildlife and Natural Environment (Scotland) Act 2011 (S)
- The Wildlife (Northern Ireland) Order 1985 (TW(NI) O) (NI)
- Wildlife and Natural Environment Act (Northern Ireland) 2011 (NI)
- The Conservation (Natural Habitats, etc.) Regulations (Northern Ireland) 1995 (NI)

- Wildlife legislation permits the taking from the wild of a sick or injured wild bird or other creature (including protected species) for the purpose of tending it until it is fit to be released.
- Specific legislation regarding deer, badgers and seals (see 'Species protection') has similar provisions.
- The right to keep a disabled protected species lasts only until it is no longer disabled. It should not be kept in a manner that would inhibit its capacity to return to the wild (e.g. by deliberate imprinting) (see Chapter 9).
- The WCA/TW(NI)O Schedule 4 (birds) lists nine species of birds of prey, including the golden eagle (*Aquila chrysaetos*), goshawk (*Accipiter gentilis*), merlin (*Falco columbarius*) and peregrine (*F. peregrinus*) that must be ringed and registered if they are taken into care (see 'Species protection'). In Northern Ireland, any bird of prey in captivity must be registered (see Department of the Environment Northern Ireland/Northern Ireland Environment Agency (DOENI/NIEA) website).
- Some methods of taking an animal (such as by nets or traps) are illegal, restricted or require a licence from Natural England (NE) or its counterpart elsewhere.

Species protection

The wildlife rehabilitator needs to know the general principles of species protection. The wildlife legislation listed above provides various degrees of protection for wild birds and some other animals, as summarized below:

- All wild birds are protected. The legislation defines a 'wild bird' as 'any bird of a species that is ordinarily resident in or is a visitor to any European territory of any member State in a wild state'. It does not include poultry or gamebirds (i.e. 'any pheasant, partridge, grouse (or moor game), black (or heath) game or ptarmigan'), but see 'Species-specific legislation'
- The wildlife legislation does not apply to a bird that has been bred in captivity (i.e. both its parents were lawfully in captivity when the egg was laid)
- Mammals, reptiles, amphibians and invertebrates that are listed in Schedule 5 of the WCA/TW(NI)O (or

comparable legislation) are also protected. The Schedule is amended from time to time and a current list can be obtained from the JNCC. All reptiles and amphibians have some level of protection (e.g. the grass snake (*Natrix natrix*) and common toad (*Bufo bufo*) can be taken and kept in captivity, but not sold) and rare species, such as the natterjack toad (*Epidalea colamita*) and great crested newt (*Triturus cristatus*), are fully protected. Badgers (*Meles meles*) are covered by specific legislation (see 'Species-specific information' and Chapter 17).

The basic protection that is given to wild birds and WCA Schedule 5 animals (together referred to as 'protected species') can be summarized as follows:

- It is an offence to:
  - Take, injure, kill or sell a protected species
  - Disturb a protected species in its nest or place of shelter
  - Possess a protected species
  - Release certain species into the wild without the authorization of a licence
  - Deliberately release or allow to escape into the wild any non-indigenous species or a species (already established in the wild) that is listed on Schedule 9 WCA/TW(NI)O (e.g. the grey squirrel (*Sciurus carolinensis*), edible frog (*Pelophylax kl. esculentus*), African clawed frog (*Xenopus laevis*), Canadian goose (*Branta canadensis*), Egyptian goose (*Alopochen aegyptiaca*), chukar partridge (*Alectoris chukar*) and muntjac deer (*Muntiacus reevesi*) except under licence from NE, Natural Resources Wales (NRW), Scottish National Heritage (SNH), or DOENI/NIEA, as appropriate.
- There are various additional forms of protection. These include:
  - Close seasons for listed gamebirds (see Chapter 27)
  - Special penalties in respect of offences involving rare birds listed on Schedule 1 of the WCA/TW(NI)O or equivalent legislation
  - Provisions for ringing and registration of the nine diurnal birds of prey listed on Schedule 4 (see 'Taking the casualty')
  - Special provisions to protect bats and bat roosts from damage (see also Chapter 15).
- Methods such as nets and traps for taking animals from the wild are either prohibited (in respect of birds and Schedule 6 animals) or restricted, as are certain hunting methods (such as specified firearms and pursuit with vehicles)
- The use of self-locking snares is also illegal; see references for the distinction between these and permitted free-running snares
- Many activities that are *prima facie* prohibited can be authorized by the grant of a licence from the appropriate authority (NE, SNH, Marine Scotland or NRW) if they are for specified purposes, such as scientific studies, aviculture or crop protection
- A number of species (such as bats (Chiroptera), dormice (*Muscardinus avellanarius*), otters, marine turtles, wildcats and natterjack toads) are also protected under the **Conservation of Habitats and Species Regulations 2010** as 'European protected species'.

Further information on wild bird law is available from the Royal Society for the Protection of Birds (RSPB) and in the references.

Species-specific legislation

Badgers:

- Protection of Badgers Act 1992 (E, W and S)
- The Wildlife (Northern Ireland) Order 1985 (NI)
- Wildlife and Natural Environment (Northern Ireland) Act 2011 (NI)

- Badgers are given protection comparable to that for WCA/TW(NI)O Schedule 5 species (see above) together with additional provisions relating to cruelty and protection of their setts (see Chapter 17).
- The restriction on methods of killing or taking wild animals (see 'Taking the casualty') also applies to badgers, as this species is included in Schedule 6 of the WCA/TW(NI)O.
- The law on badgers is set out on the NE website and on the websites of the Badger Trust, Scottish Badgers and the Northern Ireland Badger Group.
- For current information on the law on badger control and bovine tuberculosis (TB) in England, see the NE and Defra websites.

Close season legislation

Deer:

- Deer Act 1991 (E and W)
- Regulatory Reform (Deer) (England and Wales) Order 2007 (E and W)
- Wildlife and Natural Environment (Scotland) Act 2011 (S)
- The Wildlife (Northern Ireland) Order 1985 (NI)
- Wildlife and Natural Environment (Northern Ireland) Act 2011 (NI)

Marine mammals:

- Conservation of Seals Act 1970 (E and W)
- Marine (Scotland) Act 2010 (S)
- The Wildlife (Northern Ireland) Order 1985 (NI)

Game:

- Game Acts (various) (rabbits (*Oryctolagus cuniculus*), hares (*Lepus* spp., gamebirds)
- The Regulatory Reform (Game) Order 2007 (E and W)
- Wildlife and Natural Environment (Scotland) Act 2011 (S)
- Game Preservation (Northern Ireland) Act 1928 (NI)
- Game Preservation (Amendment) Act (Northern Ireland) Act 1928 (NI)

- Animals such as gamebirds (see Chapter 27), deer (red (*Cervus delphus*), fallow (*Dama dama*), roe (*Capreolus capreolus*), sika (*Cervus nippon*) and Chinese water deer (*Hydropotes inermis*); see also Chapter 22) and seals (see also Chapter 23) are protected during a specified close season (and on Sundays and Christmas Day) and by the fact that certain methods of capture and killing are prohibited by the relevant legislation.
- There are provisions for deer and seals comparable to those in the WCA, whereby disabled animals may be taken for rehabilitation or may be killed if so seriously injured that they have no reasonable likelihood of recovering.

- Gamebirds are not protected by the WCA apart from the provisions relating to methods of killing and taking from the wild (see 'Taking the casualty').
- In common law, free-living wild game (including gamebirds that have been reared and released into the wild) that is not enclosed or captive does not belong to anyone until a person takes or kills it. Taking and killing are regulated by the game laws. The legal right to take the game must be obtained (usually given or assigned by the landowner or tenant) and legal access to the land where the game is situated must be granted. Killing or taking in other circumstances may constitute poaching, for example when trespass or taking at night is involved.

Further information can be found in the listed references.

Unprotected species

- Many species of wild mammal are not protected by the WCA (e.g. European hedgehogs (*Erinaceus europaeus*), foxes (*Vulpes vulpes*) and weasels (*Mustela nivalis*)) other than by various restrictions on the use of traps, snares and poison.
- The **Animal Welfare Acts**, which make causing unnecessary suffering an offence (see 'Welfare'), do not apply to free-living wildlife, but are applicable once an animal is under the control, permanent or temporary, of a person.
- The **Wild Mammals (Protection) Act 1996** provides some protection against specified forms of inhumane treatment in respect of wild mammals.
- Various laws, including the **Pests Act 1954** and the **Spring Traps Approval Orders for E, W, S, and NI** permit the use of specified kinds of traps to deal with pest animals. There are requirements that apply to the placing and checking of traps and snares. The British Association for Shooting and Conservation (BASC) Codes of Practice on trapping pest birds and mammals and the snaring of foxes are useful guides.
- The poisoning of animals is an offence under various Acts but certain kinds of poison may be used in specified ways to control pest animals under the **Control of Pesticides Regulations 1986 (E and W)** and the **Control of Pesticides Regulations (Northern Ireland) 1987 (NI)** as amended.
- Certain sporting and other activities can be carried out, but:
  - There are limits on the type and use of firearms and other methods of taking and killing (see 'Taking the casualty')
  - In England, Wales and Scotland, falconry as a sport and as a method of preparing a casualty bird for return to the wild is not regulated, although compliance with other laws relating to the provenance of the bird, taking of certain species as quarry, and access to land, is necessary. In Northern Ireland, a licence is required to keep a bird of prey or to keep one for the purposes of falconry, captive breeding or display
  - Hunting of wild mammals with a dog is prohibited in England and Wales (**Hunting Act 2004**) and in Scotland (**Protection of Wild Mammals (Scotland) Act 2002**). There are numerous exceptions to this principle including (subject to detailed conditions) the rescue of an injured mammal with the intent to relieve its suffering. See the relevant Acts and the Crown Prosecution Service (CPS) website. Hare

coursing is illegal throughout the UK under the WCA (E and W), under the **Protection of Wild Mammals (Scotland) Act 2002 (S)** and the **Wildlife and Natural Environment Act 2011 (NI)**.

Further information can be found in the listed references and relevant websites.

Emergency care of the casualty
Veterinary law

Any person may give emergency first aid to an animal for the purpose of saving life and relieving suffering. The owner of an animal may give minor medical treatment. Otherwise veterinary treatment must be carried out by a registered veterinary surgeon or, in some respects, by a registered veterinary nurse, student veterinary surgeon, or student veterinary nurse (see 'Veterinary aspects of wildlife rehabilitation').

Ownership

If it is obvious that a 'wild' animal has an owner, that person's consent should be obtained before treatment is carried out by someone else. Hence, a rehabilitator who accepts a wild animal should ensure that ownership is transferred at the same time (see Chapter 3).

Rehabilitation
Right to keep the animal
Ownership

This is discussed above under 'Rescue'.

Wildlife law aspects

- The wildlife legislation provides that a casualty of a species protected by that Act may be kept only for the purpose of tending it and until it is no longer disabled. A casualty that is so severely disabled that there is no reasonable chance of recovery may be killed.
- Schedule 4 WCA/TW(NI)O birds (see 'Taking the casualty') that have been taken for rehabilitation must be ringed or microchipped, or have a licence to be kept unringed and registered with the appropriate authority (see the APHA and SNH websites).
- General licences issued by NE provide that immediate registration is not required as follows:
  - A veterinary surgeon may keep, for up to 6 weeks without registration, any Schedule 4 bird that is receiving professional veterinary treatment. After this time the bird should be registered with the APHA. The veterinary surgeon must keep records of treatment for each bird for 2 years. Licence conditions in respect of rescued wild birds specify, *inter alia*, that every effort must be made to avoid imprinting or impairing a bird's fitness for release (see Chapter 9). The bird must be released near the place where it was taken and the landowner's permission obtained
  - Royal Society for the Prevention of Cruelty to Animals (RSPCA) inspectors, RSPB officials and authorized keepers of registered Schedule 4 disabled wild birds may keep disabled wild-bred Schedule 4 birds for up

to 15 days for rehabilitation provided that they notify APHA within 4 days of receipt and keep specified records. Thereafter they must release the bird, pass it to a veterinary surgeon or register it. Records must be kept for 2 years. The conditions regarding release are as for the veterinary licence

- Comparable general licences are issued by NRW for Wales and by SNH for Scotland but the terms are slightly different. In Northern Ireland a licence is required to keep any disabled bird of prey
- Animal Health and Veterinary Laboratories Agency (AHVLA) Guidance Note 6 sets out the requirements for keeping Schedule 4 birds that cannot be released.
- The WCA and equivalent legislation does not apply to captive-bred animals (see 'Taking the casualty').
- A few species listed on Schedule 3 Part I, such as blackbird (*Turdus merula*), barn owl (*Tyto alba*), magpie (*Pica pica*) and chaffinch (*Fringilla coelebs*), can be sold or exhibited if they have been captive-bred and ringed.
- Anyone in possession of an animal protected by the WCA/(TW(NI)O must be able to prove that he/she is legally in possession of it – for example, that the animal is captive-bred, or has been imported, sold or taken in accordance with the Act (e.g. as a casualty) or is held under a licence. The burden of proof falls on the person (including any wildlife rehabilitator) who has such an animal in his/her possession. It is therefore essential to keep good records of any animals that are acquired, including their provenance. This point also applies to parts and derivatives of a protected species, such as bones or feathers that are retained for reference, research or education, diagnosis or sentimental purposes.
- If CITES species are kept for display or other purposes that include some commercial use, an Article 10 licence should be obtained from APHA.
- Keeping certain pest species, such as mink (*Mustela (Neovison) vison*), grey squirrel (*Sciurus carolinensis*) or rabbits (other than European rabbit), requires a licence under the **Destructive Imported Animals Act 1932**.

CITES

- Convention on International Trade in Endangered Species of Wild Fauna and Flora (CITES) (conservation controls)
- Council Regulation (EC) No. 338/97 (and 792/2012) (CITES provisions)
- Commission Regulation (EC) No. 750/2013 (Annexes A,B,C,D)
- Commission Regulation (EC) No. 865/2006 (consolidated) (implementation)
- Regulation (EC) No. 578/2013 (suspension of import of certain species)
- Commission Recommendation No. 2007/425/EC (enforcement recommendations)
- Control of Trade in Endangered Species (Enforcement) Regulations 1997 (as amended) (UK enforcement provisions)

- The CITES legislation covers the whole of the UK. The management authority is Defra and APHA is responsible for issuing CITES permits and certificates throughout the UK.
- The many species that are listed in Annexes A to D of Regulation 338/97 are subject to import and export controls.

- The EU CITES Regulation also requires the sale, display, captive breeding or other commercial use of CITES Annex A species, including all European birds of prey and owls, to be authorized by an Article 10 certificate. This provision also applies to parts and derivatives of all Annex A species.
- Zoos must hold an Article 60 certificate to authorize the commercial display or trade between Article 60 holders of CITES-listed animals.
- An Article 10 certificate is not needed where there is no commercial element, for example, a gift.
- Annex A species in commercial use must be permanently marked with a microchip or, for birds, where possible, with a closed ring. It is also good practice to identify individually all animals in permanent captivity so that they can be identified for the purpose of record keeping or in case an animal is stolen.
- These and other provisions are described in Guidance Notes issued by AHVLA.

The regulation of keeping animals in captivity

- Dangerous Wild Animals Act 1976 (DWAA) (E, W and S; NI (S7))
- The Dangerous Wild Animals Act 1976 (Modification) Order 2007) (E, W)
- The Dangerous Wild Animals Act 1976 (Modification) (Scotland) Order 2008 (S)
- The Dangerous Wild Animals (Northern Ireland) Order 2004 (NI)
- The Dangerous Wild Animals (Northern Ireland) Order 2004 (Modification) Order (Northern Ireland) 2010 (NI)

The wildcat (*Felis silvestris*), adder (*Vipera berus*), grey wolf (*Canis lupus*) and wild boar (*Sus scrofa*) are designated as 'dangerous wild animals' and if a wildlife rescue facility accepts such species, it should be licensed by the local authority. This is not necessary if the facility is already registered as a zoo or pet shop. There is no provision in the Act for short-term accommodation for such animals and it may take some weeks to obtain a licence.

- Zoo Licensing Act 1981 (E, W and S)
- Zoo Licensing Act 1981 (Amendment) (England and Wales) Regulations 2002 (E and W)
- The Zoo Licensing Act 1981 Amendment (Scotland) Regulations 2003 (S)
- The Zoo Licensing Act 1981 (Amendment) (Wales) Regulations 2003 (W)
- The Zoos Licensing Regulations (Northern Ireland) 2003 (NI)
- Council Directive EC No. 22/1999

- The Zoo Licensing Act applies to all collections of non-domesticated animals that are open (whether or not for a fee) to the public on 7 or more days in any 12-month period.
- If a wildlife rehabilitation facility is open to the public, it is likely to require a licence (issued by the local authority) and inspection as a zoo unless it qualifies for an exemption on account of its small size or the species that are kept.
- The Regulations extend zoos' responsibilities in conservation and public education, and for the

- behavioural needs of their animals, good animal husbandry, veterinary care and record keeping.
- If CITES species (e.g. birds of prey) are kept for display or for captive breeding with a commercial element, CITES Article 10 or 60 certificates are likely to be needed.
- The British and Irish Association of Zoos and Aquariums (BIAZA) and Defra websites provide additional information.

Veterinary aspects of wildlife rehabilitation
Veterinary legislation and guidance

- Veterinary Surgeons Act 1966 (VSA) (and supplementary legislation) (UK)
- The Veterinary Surgeons Act 1966 (Schedule 3 Amendment) Orders 1980–2002 (UK)

- Only veterinary surgeons registered with the Royal College of Veterinary Surgeons (RCVS) have the right to practise veterinary surgery (i.e. diagnosis, treatment and surgery, and advice based thereon) in respect of mammals (including marine mammals), birds and reptiles.
- There are several exceptions to this general rule whereby other people may carry out certain levels of treatment (Schedule 3 VSA):
  - Anyone may treat fish, invertebrates and possibly amphibians, since they are not mentioned in the VSA. Any treatment given is nevertheless subject to the provisions of the Animal Welfare Act 2006 (see 'Welfare')
  - Anyone may give first aid in an emergency to save life or alleviate suffering. This term has not been legally defined but some people use it as a guide to the provision of care until a veterinary surgeon can attend to the animal
  - Owners of animals (and their employees and families) may give minor medical treatment
  - Registered veterinary nurses (RVNs) may carry out medical treatment and minor surgery not involving entry into a body cavity; both RVNs and student veterinary nurses (SVNs) may give such levels of care to any category of animal, provided that they act under the conditions and levels of supervision laid down in the amendment to Schedule 3
  - Veterinary students may perform diagnostic tests, treatment and surgery under specified levels of supervision
  - Detailed information on this topic is available from the RCVS website.
- Collecting data from wildlife casualties:
  - In research that involves wildlife casualties, care must be taken to consider whether this should be licensed under the **Animal (Scientific Procedures) Act (ASPA) 1986** (as amended). If any pain, suffering, distress or lasting harm is likely to be caused the research must be authorized under the Act
  - The Home Office has a specific advice note dealing with ASPA and work with wild animals
  - The Act does not apply to 'non-experimental veterinary practices'. Nor does it apply to certain procedures that only cause momentary pain, suffering or distress, or none at all

- The RCVS website provides guidance on the line between veterinary practice and research and indicates that it is necessary to ask whether the primary purpose of the proposed procedures form part of normal veterinary practice or constitute scientific research and also whether the person is acting as a veterinary surgeon in practice or as a research scientist. Careful attention should be given to the full RCVS advice.
- The RCVS advises that implanting a microchip subcutaneously, or by ear-tagging or bolus, may be carried out by a person who is not a veterinary surgeon. However, any other method is considered to be veterinary practice, as is usually the repair or closure of the entry site or when sedation or anaesthesia is used or the risk to the health of the animal requires it.
- The rules for the supply and prescribing of the various categories of veterinary medicinal products should also be carefully followed (see RCVS, Veterinary Medicines Directorate (VMD) and British Veterinary Zoological Society (BVZS) advice).
- Relatively few drugs are licensed for wildlife species although where they have a domesticated counterpart (e.g. rabbits or pigeons) the species may appear on the data sheet. The 'cascade' should therefore be followed when prescribing outside the terms of the marketing authorization for a drug and the client's informed consent should be obtained.
- Further information is available on the websites of the British Veterinary Association (BVA), British Small Animal Veterinary Association (BSAVA), BVZS, RCVS and VMD.

Drug-dart weapons

- Possession of any firearms or weapons, such as a dart gun, crossbow or blowpipe that can be used to discharge tranquillizing drugs, must be authorized by a Firearms Certificate issued by the police. Firearms must be stored securely so that no unauthorized person can access them. During transport they must be kept safely so far as is reasonably possible.
- The use of a crossbow (with or without drugs) for wild animals requires a licence under the WCA.
- For further information on other aspects of gun and shooting law, see the website of the National Gamekeepers' Organisation (NGO) and referenced guidance (NGO, 2010).

Animal health

- Animal Health Act 1981 (E, W and S)
- Diseases of Animals (Northern Ireland) Order 1981 (NI)

These Acts, together with extensive subsidiary legislation, regulate the control and prevention of spread of notifiable diseases. This primarily applies to domesticated animals but when restrictions are in force, the movement of wildlife casualties may be restricted.

A person who finds an animal that is suspected of having a disease (such as tuberculosis, Newcastle Disease, avian influenza, foot-and-mouth disease, anthrax or rabies) that is notifiable under an Order made under the **Animal Health Act 1981** must isolate the animal and report the fact to the police and to the local APHA office (E and W), Divisional Veterinary Manager (S) or Divisional Veterinary Office (NI).

Animal by-products

- Regulation (EC) 1069/2009 and accompanying implementing Regulation (EC) 142/2011, Regulation (EC)/2009 laying down health rules as regards animal by-products and derived products not intended for human consumption and its accompanying implementing Regulation (EC) 142/2011 (as amended)
- Animal By-Products (Enforcement) (England) Regulations 2013 (E)
- Animal By-Products (Enforcement) (Wales) Regulations 2014 (W)
- Animal By-Products (Enforcement) (Scotland) Regulations 2013 (S)
- Animal By-Products (Enforcement) Regulations (Northern Ireland) 2011 (NI)

The animal by-products laws regulate the handling, use, transport and disposal of animal by-products including carcasses and other animal products not destined for human consumption. This applies to pets, zoo and research animals and also to wildlife that is suspected of having a disease communicable to humans or other animals (see UK and Scottish Government, and Department of Agriculture and Rural Development (NI) websites).

Civil law responsibility for damage caused by non-domesticated animals

- Animals Act 1971 (E and W)
- Animals (Scotland) Act 1987
- Animals (Northern Ireland) Order 1976

- The keeper (whether or not the owner) of non-domesticated animals is responsible for any damage that the animals may cause (see website of the Chartered Institute of Loss Adjusters).
- Liability for death, personal injury or damage to property can give rise to claims for compensation in civil law under the heads of negligence and other forms of civil liability, such as nuisance (e.g. excessive noise or smell), trespass, or the escape of animals.
- This responsibility is distinct from the health and safety legislation and it is important to insure adequately against liability.

Health and safety

- Health and Safety at Work etc. Act 1974 (E, W and S)
- Health and Safety at Work (Northern Ireland) Order 1978 (NI)

- The **Health and Safety Act (E, W and S)** and the **Order (NI)** together with extensive subsidiary legislation regulates the provision of a safe work environment for employees, including volunteers and visitors to the premises.
- Rehabilitation and rescue centres should make risk assessments of their work and develop appropriate codes of practice. This may also include the provision of specialized guidance, training and working procedures. Attention should be given to matters such as the need to adapt existing items (e.g. nebulizers and facemasks), or to provide specialized equipment, facilities and protective clothing. It is also necessary to address the hazards involved in catching, handling and the treatment of various species of animal and the risk of zoonoses associated with wildlife (see also Chapters 3 and 7).
- Risk assessments and guidelines should be reviewed and revised regularly in order to provide for new or changed risks.
- Further information, including the specific code of practice for zoos, is given by the Health and Safety Executive (HSE) and Health and Safety Executive Northern Ireland (HSENI).

Welfare

- Animal Welfare Act 2006 (E and W)
- The Mutilations (Permitted Procedures) (England) Regulations 2007 (as amended) (E)
- The Mutilations (Permitted Procedures) (Wales) Regulations 2007 (as amended) (W)
- Animal Health and Welfare (Scotland) Act 2006 (S)
- Welfare of Animals Act (Northern Ireland) 2011 (NI)
- The Welfare of Animals (Permitted Procedures by Lay Persons) Regulations (Northern Ireland) 2012 (NI)

- The Acts apply to domesticated and captive vertebrate animals. They also apply to free-living animals once they are brought under permanent or temporary control.
- It is an offence to cause such animals any unnecessary suffering.
- The owner and any person responsible for such animals has a duty of care to provide for their welfare in terms of suitable environment, diet, expression of normal behaviour patterns, housing alone or with other animals and protection from pain, suffering, injury and diseases in accordance with good practice. Some compromise may be necessary when balanced with the need for treatment and rehabilitation of a casualty, and the Acts recognize this in requiring that the steps taken to care for the animal are 'reasonable in all the circumstances'. It is important to keep records and to develop and follow standards and guidelines for the care and management of casualties so that compliance with the duty of care can be demonstrated. The failure to comply with the duty of care can be prosecuted even if there is no unnecessary suffering involved.
- Killing an animal in an appropriate and humane manner is not an offence under these Acts.
- There are also provisions relating to poisoning and animal fighting.
- See RSPCA and OneKind websites for further information.

- Wild Mammals (Protection) Act 1996 (E, W, S)

This Act provides that it is an offence to carry out specified acts that cause suffering, such as kicking, beating, burning or drowning a wild mammal, with the intent to inflict unnecessary suffering.

Captive birds

- Wildlife and Countryside Act 1981 (E, W, S)
- The Wildlife (Northern Ireland) Order 1985 (NI)

- These Acts provide that it is an offence to keep *any* bird in a cage that is not large enough to allow the bird to stretch its wings freely.
- A smaller cage is permitted for use only whilst transporting or exhibiting a bird or whilst it is 'undergoing examination or treatment by a veterinary surgeon'. Consequently, a rehabilitator who considers it appropriate to use a hospital cage that does not comply with Section 8 should ensure that the casualty is under the care of a veterinary surgeon, although the bird does not have to be kept at the veterinary surgery. The animal welfare requirements should be observed too.

Welfare during transportation

- Council Regulation (EC) No. 1/2005 on the protection of animals during transport and related operations
- The Welfare of Animals (Transport) (England) Order 2006 (E)
- The Welfare of Animals (Transport) (Wales) Order 2007 (W)
- The Welfare of Animals (Transport) (Scotland) Regulations 2006 (S)
- The Welfare of Animals (Transport) Order (Northern Ireland) 1997 (NI)

- Animals of any sort, including invertebrates, must not be transported in any way that causes or is likely to cause them injury or unnecessary suffering. They must be fit to travel.
- In the case of commercial or non-private transportation of vertebrate animals, additional requirements apply to the provision of suitable containers and vehicles, food, water, ventilation, temperature and attendance for the animals.

For further information see specific guidance documents on the Government services and information website (gov.uk).

- Additional provisions on transport and movement:
  - Public road and rail carriers may also have their own requirements or may decline to transport animals
  - The International Air Transport Association (IATA) Live Animals Regulations specify standards for the transport of many species by aeroplane (IATA, annual)
  - The CITES Secretariat has issued guidance (2013) for the transportation other than by air of CITES species
  - The Transport Orders (above) makes it a legal requirement to comply with the IATA Regulations
  - The postal service forbids the transport by post of living animals, apart from a few species of invertebrate, such as bees, crickets and mealworms.
- There are also precise requirements for the carriage of biological samples either within Great Britain or internationally, including special packaging and labelling (see APHA website).

Codes of practice for wildlife rehabilitation

In addition to the legal requirements of the animal welfare law, there are voluntary guides and codes that promote good practice, animal welfare and the responsible care and management of animals that are prepared by many organizations that specialize in particular species or activities, including the BVZS, BWRC, Bat Conservation Trust (BCT), Raptor Rescue and RSPCA.

Release

Wildlife law

The rehabilitator is obliged by the wildlife legislation to return a casualty to the wild as soon as it is no longer disabled. There is no specific provision in the legislation to authorize the keeping of an animal that is not fit for release and if investigated, however, this is usually accepted when there is supporting evidence for the decision not to release.

Stricter requirements regarding Schedule 4 birds (see 'Taking the casualty') have been imposed by APHA. These birds must be registered, actively rehabilitated and released as soon as possible. Rehabilitators may be inspected to ensure rehabilitation is proceeding and that they have the skills required to achieve a successful release. If a bird is not likely to be releasable, the keeper must consult the appropriate licensing authority. It may be possible to obtain a WCA licence to keep the bird, but Article 10 certificates for commercial use (such as captive breeding for sale or display) will only be available when there are genuine conservation benefits to the species. Note that in Northern Ireland any captive bird of prey must be licensed (see 'Taking the casualty').

Welfare law

It is necessary to strike a balance between the obligations under the wildlife legislation to release a wildlife casualty and the duty to avoid unnecessary suffering and to provide for an animal's needs under the **Animal Welfare Act 2006**. Any pre-release assessment should be made (and recorded) with both in mind. Sometimes a veterinary surgeon is asked to provide an assessment, particularly in the case of Schedule 4 birds, to support a decision to release or retain in captivity.

If animals are not released, they should always be kept in compliance with the laws relating to welfare and wildlife discussed above, together with documentary records of their provenance, history and care.

Non-indigenous and pest species

- Non-indigenous species may not be deliberately released to the wild; nor may those listed in Schedule 9 Part 1 WCA/TW(NI)O. Many of the latter are non-indigenous animals that are already established in the UK, such as the grey squirrel and muntjac deer (see also Chapters 9, 13, 22 and 29). A licence (from NE, NRW, SNH or the Northern Ireland Environment Agency (NIEA)) is required to release these species into the wild. Schedule 9 is being amended to enable the control of non-native invasive species by the **Infrastructure Act 2015, Part 4 (E and W)**.

- Destructive Imported Animals Act 1932 (E, W and S)
- Destructive Imported Animals Act (Northern Ireland) 1933 (NI)

- It is illegal to keep or release mink, grey squirrels, rabbits (other than the European rabbit) and coypu (*Myocastor coypus*) without a licence (see also Chapters 13 and 19).
- Consideration should also be given to the effect of releasing species that are or will become a pest in the area. Owners and occupiers of land can be required under various laws to control a variety of wildlife (e.g. rabbits, deer or wild birds) if they become pests (see 'References and further reading').

Guidelines

There are international guidelines relating to the translocation and reintroduction of endangered species that may provide useful advice in planning the release of a wildlife casualty (see the International Union for Conservation of Nature (IUCN) website).

Conclusion

The aim of this chapter has been to provide veterinary surgeons with a summary of the UK law that is particularly relevant to wildlife rehabilitation (Figure 2.1). It is hoped that it will be a useful guide to the legislation that is generally applicable to the veterinary care of wildlife and that it will help veterinary surgeons to protect themselves and rehabilitators from finding themselves in breach of the law. It will also add a further dimension to the service that they provide for their clients and those who are active in wildlife rehabilitation.

Organization	Homepage	Useful contents
Animal and Plant Health Agency	www.gov.uk/government/organisations/animal-and-plant-health-agency	Registration of Schedule 4 birds (England) CITES permits and guidance Animal by-products Carriage of biological samples Animal health
Badger Trust	www.badgertrust.org.uk	Badger law in England and Wales
Bat Conservation Trust	www.bats.org.uk	Bat law and information
British and Irish Association of Zoos and Aquariums	www.biaza.org.uk	Zoo legislation and other information
British Association for Shooting and Conservation	www.basc.org.uk	Information on traps and snares
British Small Animal Veterinary Association	www.bsava.com	Medicines guidance Darting Manual
British Veterinary Association	www.bva.co.uk	RSPCA Memorandum of understanding Medicines guidance
British Veterinary Zoological Society	www.bvzs.org	Guidelines for the prescription, supply and control of POM-Vs in zoological collections and wildlife rescue centres Good practice guidelines for wildlife centres
British Wildlife Rehabilitation Council	www.bwrc.org.uk	Legislation, ethics and guidance applicable to wildlife rehabilitation Voluntary codes of conduct
Chartered Institute of Loss Adjusters	www.cila.co.uk	Paper on liability for animals
Convention on International Trade in Endangered Species of Wild Fauna and Flora	www.cites.org	CITES species Documentation information Transport guidelines 2013
Council of Europe Treaty Office	www.conventions.coe.int	CoE Conventions EU wildlife regulations and directives
Crown Prosecution Service	www.cps.gov.uk	Wildlife offences in England and Wales
Department of Agriculture and Rural Development (Northern Ireland)	www.dardni.gov.uk	Animal by-products laws
Department for Environment, Food and Rural Affairs	www.gov.uk/government/organisations/department-for-environment-food-rural-affairs	Wildlife licensing (with Natural England) Animal welfare Zoo licensing, guides and standards Carriage of biological samples guidance Animal health Badger control and bovine TB (England) Animal by-products Transportation of animals
Department of the Environment Northern Ireland Environment Agency	www.doeni.gov.uk/niea	Licenses for keeping birds of prey in captivity NI wildlife law Badger law (NI)
European Commission – Environment	www.ec.europa.eu/environment	EU CITES legislation information Reference Guide to EU Wildlife Trade Regulations Birds Directive information Habitats Directive information

2.1 Law relating to British wildlife casualties – useful websites. (continues) ▶

Organization	Homepage	Useful contents
EUR-Lex (Access to European Union law)	eur-lex.europa.eu/collection/eu-law.html	CITES Regulations Birds and Habitats Directives All other EU law
Health and Safety Executive	www.hse.gov.uk	Health and safety law and information Guidance for zoos
Health and Safety Executive Northern Ireland	www.hseni.gov.uk	Health and safety law and information (NI)
Home Office	www.gov.uk/government/organisations/home-office	Firearms law and guides Advice note on ASPA and working with wild animals
International Air Transport Association	www.iata.org	Live Animals Regulations
International Union for Conservation of Nature	www.iucn.org	Guidelines for translocation and release of endangered species
Joint Nature Conservation Committee	jncc.defra.gov.uk	Wildlife law
Legislation.gov.uk	www.legislation.gov.uk	All UK statutes and subsidiary legislation
National Gamekeepers' Organisation	www.nationalgamekeepers.org.uk	Gun and shooting law
Natural England	www.gov.uk/government/organisations/natural-england	Wildlife licensing (with Defra) General licences to keep disabled Schedule 4 wild birds in captivity for rehabilitation Badger law (England)
Natural Resources Wales	nationalresources.wales	Wildlife licensing General licences to keep disabled Schedule 4 wild birds in captivity for rehabilitation Schedule 9 release licences (Wales)
Northern Ireland Badger Group	www.badgersni.org.uk	Badger law (NI)
OneKind	www.onekind.org	Animal Welfare in Scotland – a review of legislation, enforcement and delivery
Raptor Rescue	www.raptorrescue.org.uk	Rehabilitation Handbook and Code of Practice
Royal College of Veterinary Surgeons	www.rcvs.org.uk	Veterinary legislation Codes of Professional Conduct Medicines guidance Microchipping Research
Royal Society for the Prevention of Cruelty to Animals	www.rspca.org.uk	Animal welfare law (England and Wales) Guidance for rehabilitators
Royal Society for the Protection of Birds	www.rspb.org.uk	Wild bird law guides (England and Wales; Scotland)
Scottish Badgers	www.scottishbadgers.org.uk	Badger law (Scotland)
Scottish Government	www.gov.scot	Scottish wildlife legislation and guidance
Scottish National Heritage	www.snh.gov.uk	Scottish wildlife law Wildlife licensing General licences to keep disabled Schedule 4 wild birds in captivity for rehabilitation Schedule 9 release licences
Scottish Society for the Prevention of Cruelty to Animals	www.scottishspca.org	Animal welfare law (Scotland)
UK Government portal	www.gov.uk	Public general information
Veterinary Medicines Directorate	www.gov.uk/government/organisations/veterinary-medicines-directorate	Medicines guidance

2.1 (continued) Law relating to British wildlife casualties – useful websites.

References and further reading

Cooper ME (2007) Importance and application of animal law. In: *Introduction to Veterinary and Comparative Forensic Medicine*, ed. JE Cooper and ME Cooper. Blackwell Publishing, Oxford

Cooper ME (2013) Legislation. In: *Wildlife Forensic Investigation: Principles and Practice*, ed. JE Cooper and ME Cooper. CRC Press, Boca Raton

Frost D (2011) *Sporting shooting and the law : a user's guide to the firearms acts 1968-1997 and other legislation affecting sporting shooting*. National Gamekeepers' Organisation, Darlington

NGO (2010) *Gamekeepers and the Law: Guidance for the Police*. National Gamekeepers' Organisation, Darlington

Palmer J (2001) *Animal Law: a Concise Guide to the Law Relating to Animals*, 3rd edn. Shaw, Crayford

Parkes C and Thornley J (1997) *Fair Game, 3rd edn*. Pelham, London

Parkes C and Thornley J (2009) *Deer: Law and Liabilities, 2nd edn* (revised). Quiller Publishing, Shrewsbury

Rees PA (2008) *Urban Environments and Wildlife Law. A Manual for Sustainable Development*. Wiley, Oxford

Robertson I (2014) *Animal Law and Welfare: Fundamental Principles*. Routledge, Oxford

RSPB (2010) *Wild Birds and the Law: England and Wales*. RSPB, Bedfordshire: www.rspb.org.uk/Images/WBATL_tcm9-132998.pdf

RSPB Scotland (2008) *Wild Birds and the Law: Scotland*. RSPB, Edinburgh: www.rspb.org.uk/Images/WbatlScotland_tcm9-202599.pdf

RSPCA (2007) *Animal Welfare Act 2006 Guidance for Wildlife Rehabilitators*. RSPCA, Horsham

Stewart A (2012) *Wildlife and the Law. A Field Guide to Recognising, Reporting and Investigating Wildlife Crime in Scotland*, Update supplement 2014. Argyll Publishing, Argyll

Chapter 3

Principles of capture, handling and transportation

Steve Smith

Members of the public are often responsible for discovering, reporting and attempting to intervene with wildlife casualties. Although there are many excellent wildlife care centres and animal welfare organizations, the local veterinary practice is frequently the point of initial contact. Rescuers often have variable wild animal awareness and experience; they may have already taken action or they may be seeking specific guidance, so veterinary practice staff should be prepared to give general advice on the best way to manage wildlife casualties.

Telephone advice to the general public

Whether or not a veterinary practice is experienced in treating wildlife casualties, there is an expectation and a responsibility (moral and legal) to provide good and accurate advice, administer first aid and assist in involving a more appropriate care provider.

Staff who answer the phone will invariably be the initial point of contact with concerned members of the public. It is, therefore, necessary to ensure that all staff, including receptionists and veterinary nurses, are aware of the appropriate course of action; training should be given in basic steps, and calls warranting further advice passed to more experienced staff members. A client record should be created for 'wildlife' and each call recorded as a separate patient to ensure that advice given to the public is recorded and retained in the event of subsequent complications or complaints. This also allows clinical records to be made if the animal is brought to the surgery.

All members of the public asking for advice on rescuing a wildlife casualty should be warned of handling risks, such as bites and scratches, even from apparently tame or lifeless animals (see Figure 3.1). They should also be made aware of zoonotic disease risks (see Figure 7.4) from wild animals and advised to take precautions to protect their hands and practice good hygiene during and after a rescue.

Orphaned animals

The most common wildlife-related calls to the veterinary practice concern apparently 'orphaned' or 'abandoned' young animals. The majority of these calls involve fledgling birds, but people will phone about young foxes, badgers, otters, bats, hedgehogs, rabbits, deer and seals. If the young animal is clearly injured or in immediate danger, then it is likely to need rescuing. However, if it is simply in an unusual spot, it may have just wandered from its parents. In many cases, a parent will be watching nearby, so the caller should initially be advised to observe from a distance.

Advice should be sought from local wildlife specialist centres on the best way to deal with different orphans in different situations (see Chapter 8). Often, the parent will return to recover its young or continue feeding it where it is. If, after 24 hours, the young animal is still present and there is no sign of a parent, then it may be a candidate for rescue and rehabilitation.

The prognosis for rescued orphans in captivity is not always positive. They are time- and resource-consuming and require specialist care facilities. Furthermore, they are especially susceptible to disease and other captivity-related problems, and it may be difficult to find them a suitable release site.

- Adult bats are sometimes mistaken for pups, due to the very small size of some species, such as the common pipistrelle bat (*Pipistrellus pipistrellus*), which weighs just 3–7 g. Local bat specialists can be contacted through the Bat Conservation Trust (BCT) to give the rescuer appropriate advice (see Chapter 15 for contact details).
- Fawns and leverets (see Chapters 22 and 16, respectively) are normally left alone from an early age for long periods of time, but the mother will return to feed them, usually around dusk. These animals should be observed from a distance prior to being taken into captivity.
- Rabbits (*Oryctolagus cuniculus*) keep their kits in a burrow, returning to nurse once daily. Kits start to emerge from the burrow at around 18 days old, when they will look like miniature adults. If they are found above ground with their eyes still closed, they are too young to survive, and should be rescued.
- In April and May it is common to see 1-month-old red fox (*Vulpes vulpes*) cubs above ground during the day, playing and developing survival skills. Adults are usually watching nearby. Cubs seen above ground may also just be waiting for their mothers; when vixens feel their dens have been disturbed, they move their young one by one. Fox cubs are best left alone unless they are in immediate danger, obviously injured or their eyes

are still closed. If after 24 hours they are still around and apparently alone, then some puppy food and water or puppy milk can be left nearby. It is preferable to offer orphaned cubs supplementary resources and leave them in the wild than take them into captivity (see Chapters 8 and 21).

- Juvenile hedgehogs (*Erinaceus europaeus*), also known as hoglets, born late in the season may be found in autumn with insufficient fat reserves to survive the winter, and may be in need of assistance (see Chapter 12). If in immediate danger, the mother has been killed or its eyes are still closed, the hoglet should be taken into captivity. If its eyes are open and there is no imminent danger, it can be offered some food. Suitable foods include dog or cat food (not fish-based), minced liver or mealworms. **Never** give cow's milk to hedgehogs as it causes diarrhoea. If the hoglet accepts the food, it is probably weaned and should be able to survive. If it does not eat the food or does not move on after a few days, it should be taken into captivity.

- Seal pups are often seen alone as they are weaned and left to fend for themselves at 3–4 weeks of age. They should be monitored and only rescued if clearly injured, obviously underweight, showing signs of disease or are in imminent danger (e.g. dog attack). Occasionally, very young pups can be separated from their mother during a storm or some weaned pups may fail to thrive; these pups will need help. Expert handling will be required for rescue and specialist marine mammal organizations should be contacted in the first instance (see Appendix 1 and Chapter 23).

- In spring, telephone calls about baby birds are frequently received in most small animal practices. If the bird has most of its feathers, then it is probably a fledgling and should be left alone as it is likely that the parents will be nearby; fledglings have a much better chance of survival in the wild than in captivity. Tawny owlets (*Strix aluco*), for example, can climb back up a tree to the nest if they fall out. If there is immediate danger, such as cats or traffic, then the fledgling can be moved to a nearby sheltered spot. They should not be returned to the nest as this may disturb other chicks and disturbing a nest whilst 'in use' is an offence according to the Wildlife and Countryside Act 1981. If the bird is a nestling (no feathers) or appears to be genuinely orphaned, then it may be appropriate to recommend rescue.

Wildlife capture and handling

Figure 3.1 provides a starting point for veterinary practice staff giving advice to the general public about the handling and capture of a wildlife casualty. If an animal is encountered that requires assistance then, where safe to do so, attempts should be made to capture it or prevent escape until help arrives. The specific action taken will depend on the species and situation encountered, and there must be consideration about how to proceed without causing excessive distress or further injury to the animal. Ensuring the safety of the rescuers, helpers and onlookers is paramount; the risk to human health must be assessed prior to attempting rescue. The exact location and time of the rescue should be recorded for use when preparing the animal for release, which is the ultimate aim of any intervention.

> **PRACTICAL TIP**
>
> It is useful for the veterinary surgeon (veterinarian) to have a ready-prepared wildlife rescue kit for attending casualties away from the surgery. This should include:
>
> - Wire basket with secure lid (or crush cage)
> - Grasper
> - Dog catcher
> - Landing net
> - Selection of blankets/towels
> - Waterproof sheet/tarpaulin
> - Gauntlets
> - Wire cutters/pliers
> - Pig board
> - Latex gloves
> - Facemask
> - Immobilization drugs
> - Head torch
> - Binoculars
> - Reflective jacket
> - Warning triangle

Small mammals

Capture methods and equipment

Small rodents (e.g. mice, voles and shrews) can usually be lifted by the base of the tail, by covering them with a cloth and scooping them up, or by the scruff of the neck. Use of nets may also be beneficial. Small mammals may attempt to bite and, although the injury is usually only minor, there is still a risk of zoonotic disease transmission.

Larger rodents (e.g. rats and squirrels) and smaller mustelids (e.g. stoats and weasels) should be handled with more caution, as the risk of a significant bite is greater, as well as the risks of zoonoses. Larger rodents should be captured using nets or large towels/blankets, and then picked up with thick leather gloves, taking care not to harm them in the process.

Capturing hedgehogs is fairly straightforward; they can simply be picked up using thick gloves or a thick towel to prevent injury from spines and transmission of ringworm infection to the handler. Given the nature of the locations where hedgehogs often become trapped, it is useful to have wire cutters and pliers available to assist in their release (see Chapter 12).

Wild hares (*Lepus europaeus*) and rabbits are quick to escape if they are not injured, so nets and cage traps are recommended. Less mobile rabbits can be wrapped in a towel or blanket, which helps to reduce stress by minimizing noise and stimulation. Stress is a major problem in wild lagomorphs and can lead to heart failure, oliguric renal failure and reduced gut motility, the latter of which can alter the gut microflora and lead to enterotoxaemia or secondary hepatic lipidosis.

Handling

Many small mammal casualties will require general anaesthesia for adequate examination. This reduces stress caused to the animal, minimizes the risk of bites and allows first aid to be administered (see Chapter 6). Small mammals may be placed in clear plastic containers to allow observation and assessment without the stress of handling.

Animal group	Risk/danger*	Capture advice	Transport
Small garden birds	• Minimal • Death of casualty due to shock of handling • Damage to feathers, wings and limbs	• Wrap or scoop in cloth/towel • Small net	• Secure dark box with air holes • Pillowcase
Medium birds (pigeons, crows)	• Scratches and bites • Damage to feathers, wings and limbs	• Wrap or scoop in cloth/towel • Small net	• Secure dark box or pet carrier with air holes • Soft bedding • Can be kept restrained in towel for short journeys
Water birds	• Bites • Gannets and herons stab at face • Swans strike with wings • Damage to feathers, wings and limbs	• Prevent re-entry to water (if on water seek expert advice) • Cover with large towel/blanket and wrap up body; immobilize head and legs to prevent injury	• Restrain in towel/blanket • Swan bag if available • Can also use a secure dark box or pet carrier with air holes
Birds of prey (falcons, hawks, owls)	• Bites and grabbing with sharp talons on feet • Damage to feathers, wings and limbs	• Wrap in towel/blanket; restrain feet initially to prevent 'footing' and then restrain head; can allow talons to grip something	• Secure dark box or pet carrier with air holes • Can be kept in towel for short journeys with feet/legs held
Small rodents	• Bites • Degloving injury to tail	• Wrap or scoop in cloth/towel or carefully use thick gloves	• Secure dark plastic box with air holes
Bats	• Bites	• Wear gloves; scoop in cloth/towel	• Secure dark box with air holes • Pillowcase
Rabbits and hares	• Bites and scratches	• Wrap in cloth/towel; support back legs	• Secure dark box or pet carrier with air holes • Soft bedding
Hedgehogs	• Injury from spines	• Wrap in cloth/towel or carefully use thick gloves	• Secure dark box with air holes
Squirrels and small mustelids	• Bites and scratches • Degloving injury to tail (squirrels)	• Net or carefully use thick gloves (may still bite through these)	• Secure dark box or plastic pet carrier with air holes
Foxes	• Bites and scratches	• Approach with care • May appear tame but will readily bite • Best handled by experts	• Dustbin with lid or thick sack • Wire crush cage
Badgers	• Bites and scratches	• Approach with care • May appear tame but will readily bite and scratch • Best handled by experts	• Dustbin with lid or thick sack • Wire crush cage
Deer	• Injury from antlers, teeth and hooves	• If small and not avoiding capture approach with care and cover head, legs and feet • Seek expert advice if larger or ambulatory	• Do not transport without expert assistance, may require sedation
Reptiles and amphibians	• Bites (adder) • Damage to amphibian's skin • Loss of tail • Bufotoxin (toads)	• Lizards: catch or scoop with gloved hands • Snakes: snake hook; species ID is essential	• Cloth bag or pillowcase secured in ventilated container • Moisture for amphibians
Marine mammals	• Bites (seals)	• Seek expert advice	• Do not transport without expert assistance

3.1 General advice for the public, when rescuing wildlife casualties. *For all species zoonotic infections are a potential risk (see Figure 7.4).

Hedgehogs may need to be anaesthetized for examination if they curl up into a tight ball. Gloves should be worn to prevent transmission of ringworm to the handler. Hedgehogs can be encouraged to uncurl by leaving them to relax for a few minutes or by gently bouncing them in cupped hands. Stroking the spines firmly from neck to rump may also work. Once uncurled, the hindlimbs can be grasped from underneath and held higher than the forelimbs to keep the hedgehog in a wheelbarrow position (see Chapter 12).

Rabbits can be handled by grasping the scruff and supporting the hindlegs and back with a hand or arm underneath the rabbit, which should reduce the risk of the animal kicking out and potentially fracturing their spine. They should not be grasped by the ears. At all times during lifting and carrying, the spine and hindlegs should be supported. Rabbits do not commonly bite, but often kick and scratch with their back feet, which can quickly cause significant wounds to the handler. It should be borne in mind that they will often be very still prior to making a sudden and vigorous escape. Holding a rabbit on its back ('trancing') is generally considered to be a prey animal stress response, causing immobility whilst maintaining awareness of external stimuli, and should not be used in handling rabbits (see Chapter 16).

Transportation

Small mammals generally only require a secure darkened wooden or plastic box with small air holes for transportation. Cardboard boxes may be used for short periods of transport; however, these may be chewed through, allowing the animal to escape. Ideally, a non-slippery floor with bedding such as newspaper, shredded paper, straw or hay to hide in should be provided.

Bats

The Microchiropteran bat families found in the UK are vesper bats and horseshoe bats, with the most widespread species being the common pipistrelle. Rabies viruses (specifically the European Bat Lyssavirus 2 (EBLV-2) in the UK) are a concern and, whilst infection is rarely reported, it has been detected in healthy bats (Whitby *et al.*, 2000; Fooks *et al.*, 2002; Johnson *et al.*, 2002). Rabies vaccinations are recommended for anyone in regular contact with bats, particularly ill or debilitated bats (see Chapter 15).

Capturing a grounded bat requires no direct contact, it can simply be scooped up in a towel and then placed in a small escape-proof ventilated container (e.g. a taped-shut shoebox with air holes). During handling, latex gloves (as a minimum) should be worn, or light leather gloves for larger bats. Anyone bitten or scratched by a bat should immediately wash the wound well and seek medical advice, regardless of their vaccination status. A veterinary surgeon should always see a bat that has been caught by a cat, as there is a high risk of septicaemia from bite wounds, which can be fatal within 48 hours (see Chapter 15).

Larger mammals

Capture methods and equipment

Larger mammals, such as foxes, deer and badgers, should be approached with caution. They may appear comatose or very calm, but can attack or bite suddenly in defense, or attempt to flee.

Foxes: Foxes are more likely to bite without warning, and, if the casualty is not recumbent, it will be able to outrun the handler. Equipment used is similar to that for handling an aggressive dog. A secure wire-mesh carrying basket, ideally with a crush facility, should be available, open and ready to place the fox into. Using one or more long-handled nets and corralling the fox into an escape route where it is then allowed to run into another net is often effective, although foxes can jump over 2 m high. Once in the net, the head can be pinned down with a soft broom and the scruff grabbed. Alternatively, if the fox is not mobile (Figure 3.2), or is in a confined space, a dog catcher pole with a quick-release noose or a rope can be used. Loop the noose around the neck with just enough

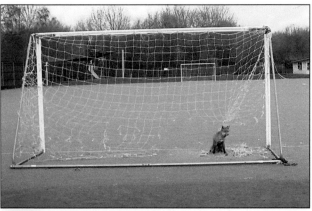

3.2 Fox trapped in goal netting.
(Courtesy of D Lovell)

pressure for adequate restraint and then pull the fox into an area where the scruff can be grasped. Scruffing an otherwise unrestrained fox should not be attempted. Once scruffed, the fox can be picked up, with its bodyweight supported by a hand under the back end, and placed in the available carrier (see Chapter 21).

Badgers: Badgers (*Meles meles*) are large and very powerful mustelids. Carrying baskets must be robust (Figure 3.3) and ideally include a crush facility to allow sedatives to be given by injection. Leather gloves provide poor protection against a badger's strong bite, so are not useful in these situations; however, latex gloves should be used to prevent disease transmission. Nets are also ineffective. On approaching an injured badger, it is essential to determine the animal's level of consciousness before attempting to handle it. Touching the badger lightly on the head with a pole and assessing its reaction is a good starting point. If little or no response occurs, the animal may be scruffed, fitted with a muzzle and lifted, supporting its rear, to be placed in the carrier. Otherwise, a dog catcher pole may be used around the badger's neck to achieve restraint, and the animal lifted into the carrier, supporting its rump. Pig boards may be useful to encourage badgers to move in a desired direction. Baited traps can be used for casualties known to visit a site regularly.

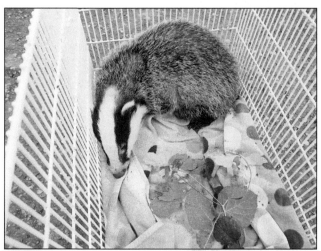

3.3 Badger in a strong white wire crate.
(Courtesy of D Lovell)

Deer: There are six species of deer found in Britain and each one can be a danger to handlers (see Chapter 22). The larger deer species (e.g. red (*Cervus elaphus*), sika (*Cervus nippon*) and fallow (*Dama dama*)) are very strong; male red deer can weigh up to 250 kg. Deer will often panic when faced with human contact, becoming stressed and frantic, which can lead to the infliction of significant injuries with their antlers, hooves and overall strength. Smaller deer are also violently averse to human contact and will struggle, rear and strike out to avoid being restrained. The teeth and hooves of muntjac (*Muntiacus reevesi*) are well known in veterinary practice for inflicting deep flesh wounds in dogs. Proper planning and preparation is required to prevent injury to handlers or the casualty, including remote immobilization if necessary (e.g. using a dart gun; Figure 3.4) (see also Cracknell, 2014).

Before approaching the animal, inspection from a distance (with binoculars and a torch, if required) is vital. It is important to consider the safety of bystanders and helpers at all times, particularly if the deer might suddenly bolt.

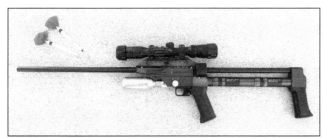

3.4 Carbon dioxide powered dart gun for remote delivery of sedative or anaesthetic drugs.

Smaller deer can usually be corralled using soft netting and a combination of thick towels, blankets and sheets to cover the head and help restrain and protect flailing limbs. Hobbling the legs may help prevent injury and covering the head and eyes has a calming effect. Larger deer may need to be sedated, with drugs administered via a dart gun, blowpipe or pole syringe (see Chapters 6 and 22).

Most deer will flee from a scene unless trapped (Figure 3.5) or severely injured, especially when approached by humans. If the deer is not trapped and does not flee (Figure 3.6), this carries a poor prognosis, especially if found in lateral recumbency. If the deer is mobile and active, the stress of capture, handling, confinement and treatment may be counterproductive (e.g. leading to capture myopathy) and not in the welfare interests of the animal. Many deer will cope very well with minor injuries, so careful assessment should be carried out before deciding to capture a potential casualty. Injuries not consistent with survival in the wild include deer with extensive injuries caught in wire or other material, those with mandibular or facial injuries that prevent feeding, pelvic fractures, spinal trauma and those with multiple limb fractures.

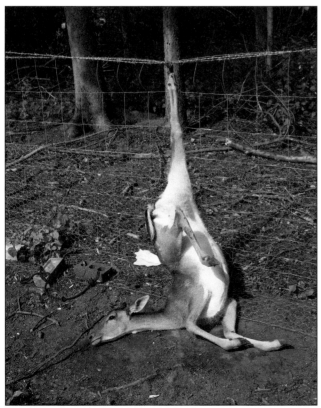

3.5 Fallow deer trapped in stock fencing.
(Courtesy of Les Stocker MBE)

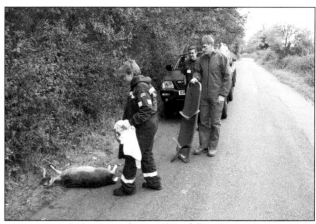

3.6 Roadside rescue of a recumbent fallow deer.
(Courtesy of Les Stocker MBE)

Handling

Foxes: Foxes should be handled similarly to a fractious cat or dog, as they will snap, bite and are very mobile. Gauntlets can be used, but they interfere with effective scruffing and rarely protect adequately from a significant bite. If the fox is scruffed, a muzzle can be placed over the mouth and nose (Figure 3.7) and the body wrapped in a towel or blanket for examination. This is really only effective in debilitated foxes, so usually sedation or general anaesthesia should be used to reduce stress and increase handler safety (see Chapter 6).

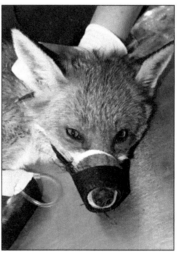

3.7 Fox with tape muzzle and Mikki® muzzle applied.
(Courtesy of Les Stocker MBE)

Badgers: Young badger cubs and moribund adult badgers will usually allow safe examination with little restraint other than a Baskerville™ muzzle to prevent biting. Most other badger casualties will require sedation or anaesthesia to prevent injury from biting or scratching.

Deer: Small deer (that are recumbent) can be approached from behind and quickly covered with a blanket and the head placed in a hessian sac or hood. Large deer that can be approached easily or lying quietly in the back of a car are candidates for euthanasia unless the reason for their compliance is obvious and carries a good prognosis. Full clinical examination in conscious deer is difficult and stressful, and physiological parameters are abnormally elevated, so sedation or anaesthesia is invariably preferable (see Chapter 6).

Transportation

Foxes and badgers should be moved in a robust and secure covered carrier. A wire crush cage is the most effective option as it allows easier administration of a sedative by injection if needed for handling and examination at a later stage. Thick sacks or dustbins with secure lids have also been used to good effect. Cages should be covered with a blanket to minimize noise and disturbance and maintain insulation. Carrying baskets should ideally be placed on a polythene sheet in a tray in the transport vehicle to prevent contamination of the vehicle with faeces and urine. Moving larger mammals, especially deer, can be dangerous and is best left to experienced handlers. If they are settled, smaller deer can be wrapped tightly in a large cloth with their head covered and be transported whilst being held; this is often how members of the public present them to veterinary surgeries. Legs can be hobbled or folded underneath (with the animal in a small cage) to minimize the risk of injury.

Marine mammals

Marine mammals are divided into two groups: cetaceans (whales, porpoises and dolphins) and pinnipeds (seals, sea lions and walruses). Most veterinary surgeons in general practice will not see cetaceans or pinnipeds. The resident seal populations in Britain are the grey seal (*Halichoerus grypus*) and common seal (*Phoca vitulina*). Marine mammal rescue organizations should be involved in the capture and transport of these types of casualties. See Chapter 23 for more detailed information and useful contacts.

Birds

Capture methods and equipment

Birds with minor injuries (Figure 3.8) can often fly away and it may be impossible to catch them. Many avian casualties will be weak, trapped or badly injured and will be unable to fly, although they can often still run fast! If the casualty is still mobile, a short pursuit into a corner or enclosed space will normally enable capture. Waterfowl and sea birds must be directed away from water, as if they make it back on to a lake or river they become very hard to catch, usually requiring expert assistance and equipment (Figure 3.9).

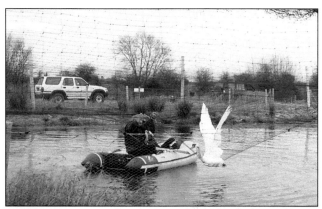

3.9 Water rescue of a swan trapped in netting. Buoyancy aids should be worn when working on or near to water.
(Courtesy of Les Stocker MBE)

The difficulty, stress and risks associated with catching a bird will depend on the size and species encountered. For the majority, capture is best performed by covering and completely enclosing the bird with a cloth, blanket, towel or coat. Once enclosed in this way, the wings and legs are held close to the body and head covered, which will usually relax the bird and stop it struggling. Rapid capture and immobilization of birds with leg or wing fractures is vital to prevent further trauma to the animal from flapping and struggling.

Larger birds, such as swans and geese, are best caught by the neck using hands or a swan hook. The body, wings and legs can then be restrained with a large blanket, sack or 'swan bag' (Figure 3.10; see Chapter 26). Care should be taken to quickly immobilize the wings as they can strike out and cause injury (Figure 3.11). Pointed beaks in herons, cranes and seabirds can cause serious eye and facial injuries and goggles should always be worn when handling these animals (see Chapters 24 and 25).

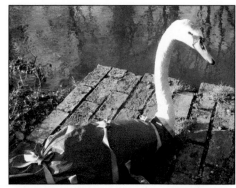

3.10 Mute swan (*Cygnus olor*) restrained in a 'swan bag' enclosing and immobilizing the wings and legs.
(Courtesy of D Lovell)

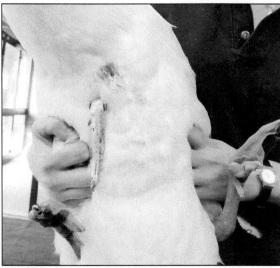

3.8 Fishing spinner attached to a goose casualty.
(Courtesy of D Lovell)

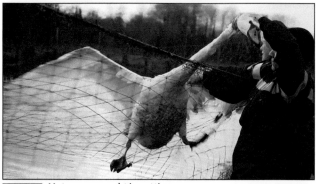

3.11 Mute swan caught in netting.
(Courtesy of Les Stocker MBE)

Birds of prey require slightly different handling. The talons on the feet will normally pose the greatest danger, as well as the beak, which, in larger species, can give a nasty bite. A net or towel can be used to drop on to the bird and capture it. A towel or blanket is then used to wrap the bird, restraining the wings and feet, and covering the head and eyes. When wrapping, the legs should be restrained by hand or within a towel (see Chapter 29).

Diurnal species are easier to catch in darkness, and this is useful in certain circumstances, such as a bird trapped in a building or an injured raptor roosting in a tree. Lengths of mist netting (fine nylon mesh nets used to trap wild birds for ringing) can be used to catch birds trapped in large buildings, or long lengths of coarser netting may be used across open ground or water to catch larger flightless birds. Birds of prey, when chasing quarry, can become trapped inside large buildings. The majority of such birds will eventually escape through an open door if left undisturbed; attempts to catch them should only be mounted if they are causing a problem or are clearly injured. A veterinary surgeon should always see a bird that has been caught by a cat as there is a high risk of septicaemia from bite wounds, which can be fatal within 48 hours (see Chapter 30).

Handling

If possible, birds should be examined at a distance (in the carrier), as their behaviour and vital parameters will change once handled. Any physical examination should be performed efficiently and safely to minimize stress to the bird, and should be carried out in a darkened quiet room. General anaesthesia can be considered if the bird is very stressed and unlikely to tolerate a conscious examination.

Small passerines can be held using the 'ringer's grip' (Figure 3.12a), where the neck is held between the first two fingers and the body held in the palm of the hand. Pigeons can be held using the 'pigeon fancier's grip' (Figure 3.12b), where the body is supported in the palm of the hand and the legs held behind the bird between the fingers. Larger birds should be wrapped in a towel or blanket (Figure 3.12c), by placing a hand over each wing and wrapping the blanket under the bird to ensure immobilization of the wings and legs. This will prevent further injury to the bird and to the handler. The head should be restrained by holding the neck or by covering with a towel; this is especially important in birds of prey that can inflict injury with the beak (Figure 3.12d). The handler should also have a very strong grip on the feet and over the talons. Handling of all birds should be firm but gentle.

Transportation

Over short distances, most birds can be moved safely whilst wrapped in a blanket, towel or other cloth. The main consideration is overheating, which can occur if wrapped tightly for extended periods, especially if the head is covered.

Small birds will tend to lie calmly in dark cloth bags or pillowcases without damaging themselves. Most small- to medium-sized birds (e.g. pigeons, crows, seabirds and birds of prey) can be transported in secure and darkened boxes or carriers with air holes. The door should be covered with a towel to prevent startling and further damage to the casualty. Carpet or paper can be provided in the bottom of the carrier to reduce slipping. Ideally, birds with wing or leg injuries should not be transported

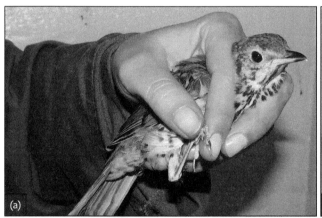
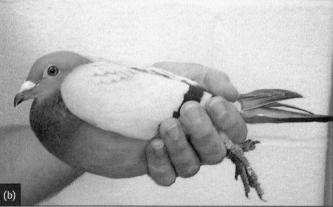
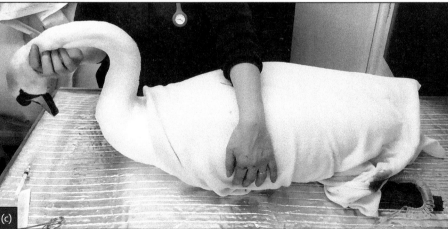
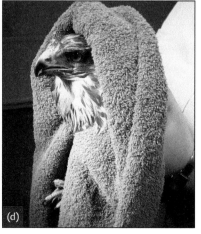

3.12 Handling birds: (a) ringer's grip; (b) pigeon fancier's grip; (c) mute swan wrapped in blanket; (d) holding a bird of prey.

unless the affected limb is immobilized. Where specific immobilization methods are not practical (or known by the rescuer), it may be advisable to transport casualties with fractures wrapped in a blanket as above. The feet of birds of prey should be included in the wrapping to prevent injury. Large waterfowl are best transported with their bodies restrained in a swan bag (see Figure 3.10), which restrains the legs and wings safely, leaving the head and neck free. The same effect can similarly be achieved with a blanket tightly wrapped around the legs, wings and body (see Figure 3.12c). Birds transported in this way may overheat and can become stiff, resulting in a transient lameness if transportation is prolonged. Long-legged birds, such as waders, should be transported in a box or crate tall enough for them to stand. Restraining the legs underneath can lead to circulatory compromise and leg paralysis. If the bird is unable to travel in a standing position, its legs should be held caudally and transport time kept to a minimum.

Reptiles and amphibians

There are only a few reptile and amphibian species that are indigenous to the UK (see Chapter 31). Of these, only the adder (*Vipera berus*) is venomous, with a bite capable of causing death in the young, old or debilitated, although this is reportedly extremely rare (Reid, 1976).

When considering capture, handling and transport of reptiles and amphibians, it is important to remember that they cannot control their temperature internally and require exogenous sources of heat. The skin of amphibians is vulnerable to desiccation and damage, and rough handling will cause damage to the mucus layer; moistened gloves should be worn, where possible, when handling these species. Extreme care should be taken when handling adders due to their bite. Specialist equipment, such as snake hooks, may be required for handling snakes, unless the handler is experienced. Most lizards can be caught and held in the hands for transfer to their transport container, but they may bite. All British lizard species can autotomize their tails; therefore restraint should be kept to a minimum to avoid this.

Reptiles can be transported in a cloth bag or pillowcase, or secured in a ventilated container for longer journeys. Amphibians can be transported similarly, but ensure damp vegetation is placed inside the bag or box to keep the environment moist.

Health and safety

Rehabilitation centres, rescue centres and veterinary practices that take in wildlife casualties must develop risk assessments and appropriate codes of practice for their work. These assessments should be reviewed and revised regularly, depending on the evolving nature of cases seen and turnover of staff. All staff should be included in health and safety protocols and be fully aware of any revisions that are made to them. Protocols should be readily available to staff at all times. Wildlife casualties will often try to escape, especially as they start to recover, and are likely to bite, peck, scratch and kick at handlers. Consideration should be given to the equipment required, facilities available, personal protective equipment and hazards that may occur during handling, including zoonoses, for the wide range of species encountered.

Zoonoses

There is a moderately long list of possible zoonotic infections that can be transmitted by British wildlife, but the actual risk to those handling wildlife casualties appears to be low, with the majority of handlers and rescuers having little or no experience of confirmed zoonotic infections (Best and Mullineaux, 2003). Most of the zoonotic diseases are covered in Chapter 7 and discussed in more detail in species-specific chapters. It is important that those who handle wildlife casualties are made aware of the potential hazards, and that health and safety risk assessments are made within veterinary practices and rehabilitation units.

There are no vaccines for the majority of the potential zoonotic infections. Veterinary staff involved in wildlife handling should ensure they are up to date with tetanus boosters, and those handling bats should maintain current rabies vaccination. Bacillus Calmette–Guérin (BCG) vaccination against tuberculosis may be appropriate for some individuals.

Infection with pathogens usually arises from a limited number of routes and awareness of these allows precautions to be taken (Figure 3.13).

Routes of infection
• Direct skin contact (e.g. fleas, lice, ringworm)
• Direct contact with faeces, blood, urine or other secretions
• Respiratory aerosol exposure
• Trauma from bites and scratches with possible inoculation of pathogens

Protection strategies to minimize zoonotic disease risk
• Putting in place appropriate risk assessments (tailored to commonly seen wildlife species and their potential zoonotic infections)
• Regular staff training in handling techniques
• Provision of suitable handling equipment and training in use
• Use of gloves (latex), protective clothing and masks as necessary
• Suitable hygiene precautions before and after handling
• Protective clothing, appropriate hygiene and minimal exposure to other staff when carrying out post-mortem examinations
• Vaccination of staff involved in handling (e.g. rabies and BCG vaccination)
• Rapid and appropriate medical attention when incidents occur

3.13 Routes of zoonotic infection risk from wildlife and strategies to minimize these.

Legal considerations

Provisions of the Wildlife and Countryside Act 1981 make the rescuer of a wild animal its legal owner since they have 'taken it into possession'; therefore, strictly speaking, the rescuer's permission and informed consent is required to carry out any tests, treatments or euthanasia, and they are financially responsible for work done (see Chapter 2). The simplest way to avoid difficulties is to have the rescuer sign ownership of the animal over to the veterinary practice or rehabilitation centre on admission. This removes financial responsibility from the rescuer and allows the veterinary practice or rescue centre to make treatment decisions in the interest of the animal without needing to seek informed consent. The consent form in Figure 3.14 requires the rescuer to fill in various sections so that as much information as possible is obtained. The rescuer is given options about signing over the animal, whether they are interested in contributing to the cost of treatment or would like to be involved

Name of rescuer: ....

Date presented: .... Time: ....

Address of rescuer: ....

Contact number/s: ....

Type of animal: **Bird**   **Reptile**   **Small/large mammal**   **Other**
(circle as appropriate)

                Species: ....

                Age: .... Sex: ....

                Colour: ....

                Other ID: ....

Where found: ....

....

....

.... Date and time: ....

Injuries present: ....

....

....

....

Food given: ....
(including amount, date and time)

....

....

....

Treatment given: ....
(including amount, date and time)

....

....

....

Other information: ....

....

....

....

According to the Wildlife and Countryside Act 1981, when a wild animal is 'rescued' and taken into captivity the rescuer becomes the ***legal owner*** of that animal and becomes responsible for ongoing care. As a veterinary surgery, we do have some responsibilities to offer first aid to injured wildlife. To simplify the process we ask that ownership of the animal is signed over to (***insert name of veterinary practice and/or rescue centre***) so that we may make decisions regarding the most appropriate first aid treatment (including euthanasia if needed) and ongoing care, rehabilitation and release. With this in mind, please complete (circle as appropriate) and sign the following:

I, the rescuer named above:

- **transfer/do not transfer** ownership of the animal detailed above to (***insert name of veterinary practice***) and (***insert name of rescue centre***)
- **wish/do not wish** to be notified of the eventual outcome, and
- **wish/do not wish** to contribute financially to the treatment of this animal, and
- **wish/do not wish** to be involved in rehabilitation and/or release of this animal where appropriate.

Signed: .... Print name: ....

Date: ....

3.14 Suggested wildlife admission form (used at the author's practice).

in rehabilitation (if deemed competent by the veterinary surgeon to do so).

Registered veterinary surgeons in the UK are obliged by the Royal College of Veterinary Surgeon's Code of Professional Conduct (RCVS, 2015) to provide first aid and pain relief for any animal of a species treated by the practice during normal working hours. A veterinary surgeon on call should not unreasonably refuse to provide first aid and facilitate the provision of pain relief for all other species until such time as a more appropriate emergency veterinary service accepts responsibility for the animal. This applies to wildlife casualties as well as pets.

There is also a Memorandum of Understanding (MoU) between the British Veterinary Association (BVA) and the Royal Society for the Prevention of Cruelty to Animals (RSPCA), which covers England and Wales and was first entered into in 1939 (revised in 2001) and has been under review since 2010 (BVA, 2014). With respect to wildlife casualties, the MoU covers emergency treatment of sick or injured wildlife (and strays), and establishes an agreement between the RSPCA and BVA on the level of RSPCA financial contribution to the initial emergency treatment (IET) carried out by veterinary surgeons. Its purpose is to ensure that appropriate professional treatment is available for all injured or sick animals. Currently, according to the MoU, any small wild mammal or wild bird presented to a veterinary surgeon during normal working hours should be provided first aid (which can include euthanasia) free of charge. Technically, as the agreement is between the BVA (which also endorses the views of BSAVA) and the RSPCA, then the veterinary surgeon is only obliged to provide free services if they are a member of the BVA/BSAVA, although most practices will endeavor to provide this first aid regardless. If larger animals (e.g. deer) are presented, the veterinary surgeon has to visit the scene of an accident, or small mammals or birds are presented out of hours, then the RSPCA will contribute funds for the IET providing specific criteria are met. For further information regarding the specific conditions of the MoU and provision of IET, visit the RSPCA website (www.rspca.org.uk) or BVA (www.bva.co.uk) website. For up to date information on the legal aspects of veterinary care of wildlife casualties, see Chapter 2.

References and further reading

Best D and Mullineaux E (2003) Basic Principles of treating wildlife casualties. In: *BSAVA Manual of Wildlife Casualties*, ed. E Mullineaux, D Best and J Cooper, pp. 6–28. BSAVA Publications, Gloucester

British Veterinary Association (2014) *RSPCA Memorandum of Understanding*. Available at: www.bva.co.uk

Dmytryk R (2012) *Wildlife Search and Rescue: A guide for First Responders*, Wiley-Blackwell

Cracknell J (2014) *Darting Manual*. Available at: www.bsava.com

Fooks AR, Finnegan C, Johnson N *et al.* (2002) Human case of EBL type 2 following exposure to bats in Angus, Scotland. *Veterinary Record* **151**, 679

Girling SJ (2013) *Nursing of Exotic Pets 2nd edn.* Wiley-Blackwell, Chichester

Johnson N, Seldon D, Parsons G *et al.* (2002) European bat lyssavirus type 2 in a bat found in Lancashire. *Veterinary Record* **151**, 455–456

Reid HA (1976) Adder bites in Britain. *British Medical Journal* **2**(6028), 153–156

Royal College of Veterinary Surgeons (2015) *Code of Professional Conduct for Veterinary Surgeons*. Available at: www.rcvs.org.uk

Stocker L (2005) *Practical Wildlife Care, 2nd edn.* Wiley-Blackwell, Chichester

Whitby JE, Heaton PR, Black EM *et al.* (2000) First isolation of rabies-related virus from a Daubenton's bat in the United Kingdom. *Veterinary Record* **147**, 385–388

Chapter 4

Wildlife triage and decision-making

Anna Meredith

When an injured or orphaned wild animal is presented to a veterinary surgeon (veterinarian), rapid and important assessments and decisions have to be made, primarily to prevent suffering, but also in relation to staff health and safety and legislative requirements.

Triage is the process of prioritizing patients based on the severity of their condition, so as to treat as many as possible when resources are insufficient for all to be treated immediately. The term comes from the French verb *trier*, meaning 'to sort, sift or select'. True triage in this sense can be applicable to wildlife casualty situations where large numbers are involved, such as mass cetacean strandings or oiling incidents, but more frequently the practitioner is faced with a single individual animal, for which 'triage' has come to refer to the process of decision-making in terms of **whether to treat or to euthanase**; however, the process of assessment and decision-making is essentially similar in both situations.

It is important that everyone involved with wildlife casualty work has a clear idea of what they are trying to achieve and why. There are complex moral and ethical issues to be addressed regarding if and when intervention is justified, and different people will have differing opinions on what is acceptable (see Chapter 1). However, in practice the most common scenario is that of being presented with an injured wild animal for treatment, and so the intervention process has already begun.

The process of dealing with a wildlife casualty can be divided into six stages (Best and Mullineaux, 2003):

1. Initial location, capture and translocation.
2. Examination and assessment for rehabilitation.
3. First aid and stabilization.
4. Treatment.
5. Recuperation and rehabilitation.
6. Release.

Capture, handling and translocation have already been discussed in Chapter 3. This chapter will discuss the second stage of the process, that of triage, which entails examination and assessment for successful rehabilitation. Decisions based on the triage process must always be undertaken as quickly as possible, and at the most within 48 hours of admission (Kelly *et al.*, 2011), in order to minimize any unnecessary suffering associated with the injury or disease itself, or the stress of captivity. Triage decisions should involve the veterinary surgeon and a clinical examination wherever possible, but agreed protocols and decision-making schemes (preferably written) may be put in place in wildlife hospitals that allow non-veterinary trained staff to undertake the triage process and carry out euthanasia, or this may also take place in the field at the point of capture or retrieval. It should be noted that euthanasia is not, in law, an act of veterinary surgery, and may be carried out by anyone provided that it is carried out humanely (see Chapter 2). However, as noted in the Royal College of Veterinary Surgeons' Code of Professional Conduct, generally only veterinary surgeons, and veterinary nurses acting under their direction, will have access to the controlled drugs used to carry out euthanasia of animals, such as pentobarbital. One exception to this is that pentobarbital may be used by Royal Society for the Prevention of Cruelty to Animals (RSPCA) Inspectors in England and Wales and Scottish Society for the Prevention of Cruelty to Animals (SSPCA) Inspectors in Scotland for the euthanasia of wild animals. A veterinary surgeon may additionally make provision for small quantities of pentobarbital to be made available to wildlife centres for use in animals under that veterinary surgeon's care and following appropriate triage (BVZS, 2014).

Wildlife rehabilitation in the UK

Wildlife rehabilitation is defined by the International Wildlife Rehabilitation Council (IWRC) as: 'the treatment and temporary care of injured, diseased, and displaced indigenous animals and the subsequent release of healthy animals to appropriate habitats in the wild' (Miller, 2012).

In the United Kingdom there are an estimated 80 wildlife rescue centres (Mullineaux and Kidner, 2011), although there may be many more. A 2007 study indicated that they deal with approximately 30–40,000 animals per year, although a more recent study has indicated that the true figure is likely to be at least double this (Grogan and Kelly, 2013). Wildlife rescue centres can vary from fully appointed professional hospital set-ups with excellent housing and veterinary facilities for wildlife, to small-scale volunteer arrangements run by well meaning and enthusiastic members of the public, with no specific training, in private houses or gardens. Therefore standards of care and welfare can vary widely, and there is no current regulatory framework specifically for wildlife rehabilitation centres in place in the UK (Mullineaux, 2014). Recently published information on the reasons for admission of wildlife casualties is lacking, but the British Wildlife Rehabilitation Council (BWRC) operated a Wildlife Casualty Recording

Scheme from 1993–2000 using a quarterly return sheet. However, only small numbers of rehabilitation units were known to regularly submit returns (Kirkwood and Best, 1998). Statistics from these returns for the year 2000, indicated that approximately 67% of casualties were birds, and 32% mammals, with only very small numbers of reptiles and amphibians (Kirkwood, 2003). Of these, five common species predominated, with hedgehogs (*Erinaceus europaeus*), pigeons (feral and racing pigeons (*Columba livia*) and wood pigeons (*Columba palumbus*)), blackbirds (*Turdus merula*) and collared doves (*Streptopelia decaocto*) accounting for over 40% of admissions. Approximately 50% of animals in the BWRC survey were immature animals (50% of birds and 54% of mammals). Where the reason for admission was known (Figure 4.1), 27% of mammals and 32% of birds were considered orphans, with no injuries or disease (Kirkwood, 2003). For individual species in the UK, other studies have found that 65% of polecat (*Mustela putorius*) (Kelly *et al.*, 2010) and 68% of wood pigeon (Kelly *et al.*, 2011) admissions were juveniles. Elsewhere, studies also show a large proportion of juvenile animals being admitted; for example, 53% of little owls (*Athene noctua*) (Molina-Lopez and Darwich, 2011) and 32% of raptors in Spain were juvenile admissions (Molina-Lopez *et al.*, 2011).

Trauma, particularly due to road traffic accidents (RTAs), is a major reason for admission, accounting for 39% of all UK admissions (Kirkwood, 2003). For badgers (*Meles meles*), one study showed that 28% of badger admissions to wildlife hospitals were due to RTAs (Mullineaux and Kidner, 2011), but trauma due to 'territorial' (conspecific) wounds was also found in 58% of all badgers admitted. In another study on hedgehogs, 40% of admissions were due to trauma (Reeve and Huijser, 1999). Incidences of trauma, such as RTAs and window collisions, are also high in birds, accounting for 30% of bird admissions (Kirkwood, 2003). For example, a study of Eurasian sparrowhawks (*Accipiter nisus*) found that 70% of admissions were due to trauma (Kelly and Bland, 2006). Predation by domestic cats as a cause of trauma is also common, affecting mammals, birds, reptiles and amphibians. For example, in a study on wood pigeons, 21% of adults and 16% of juveniles admitted were injured by cats (Kelly *et al.*, 2011). In other European countries, bats are a common victim of cats, with 29% of bat admissions in Italy (Ancillotto *et al.*, 2013) and approximately 50% of deaths in free-ranging bats in Germany (Mühldorfer *et al.*, 2011) caused by cat predation.

The decision-making process

The primary aim of wildlife rehabilitation must always be to return an animal successfully to the wild, as rapidly as possible and with minimal adverse effects on its welfare. To do this the animal must be released with a chance of survival at least equivalent to that of other free-living members of its species, and this will depend on it being both physically and behaviourally fit to cope normally with a free-living existence. The alternatives are permanent captivity, which is rarely acceptable on welfare grounds, or euthanasia, which must always be considered at every stage of the assessment and treatment process (Figure 4.2).

The conservation status of the animal should not, in principle, be a factor in the triage process as individual animal welfare is the main consideration. However, in reality, pragmatic factors and value judgements are often brought into play, and when faced with a conservation-sensitive or endangered species, this can and does affect decisions over the degree of effort and resources allocated to that animal when compared to a very common species, or one that might be considered a pest species or vermin. It is absolutely vital that these conservation-based decisions must never be at the expense of any compromise to animal welfare.

Assessment must be carried out on an individual case basis and will depend on many factors. Setting aside any fundamental moral or ethical arguments or considerations (see Chapter 1), a practical approach to the decision-making or triage process is to consider the following questions:

- Is it possible to treat the injury or disease in this animal?
- What species is it and what is its natural history and behaviour in the wild?
- What is the age and sex of the animal?
- How long will the animal have to be in captivity and how often will it have to be handled for treatment?
- Does the time of the year have an impact?
- Are suitable veterinary facilities available?
- Are rehabilitation facilities available?
- Are suitable release sites available?
- What are the risks to personnel?
- Will rehabilitation of the animal pose any risks to free-living species or livestock?
- Are there any legislative requirements?

Is it possible to treat the injury or disease in this animal?

The severity of the injury or disease has been found to be the most important factor that can be used to predict whether or not a wildlife casualty will eventually be released (Moloney *et al.*, 2007). Consider if the veterinary skills and equipment are available to deal with the injury/disease in this species. If treatment would require referral to a more specialist practice or centre, can the stress and delay of transfer be justified? Most importantly, is the disease or injury treatable, such that recovery will not lead to permanent disability (see 'Clinical examination').

Species	Injury[a]	Poison	Abandoned	Natural	Cat injury	Other	Total
Birds	3058 (30%)	254 (3%)	3310 (32%)	409 (4%)	1373 (13%)	1857 (18%)	10,261 (67%)
Mammals	1201 (25%)	73 (2%)	1305 (27%)	690 (14%)	264 (5%)	1300 (27%)	4833 (32%)
Amphibians and reptiles	24 (34%)	0	0	4 (5%)	17 (24%)	26 (37%)	71 (<1%)
Total	4283 (28%)	327 (3%)	4615 (30%)	1103 (7%)	1654 (11%)	3183 (21%)	15,165

4.1 British Wildlife Casualty Recording Scheme: summary of reason for admission of casualties (approximate %) during the year 2000.
[a] Injuries caused by unnatural (anthropogenic) agency.
(Adapted from Kirkwood, 2003)

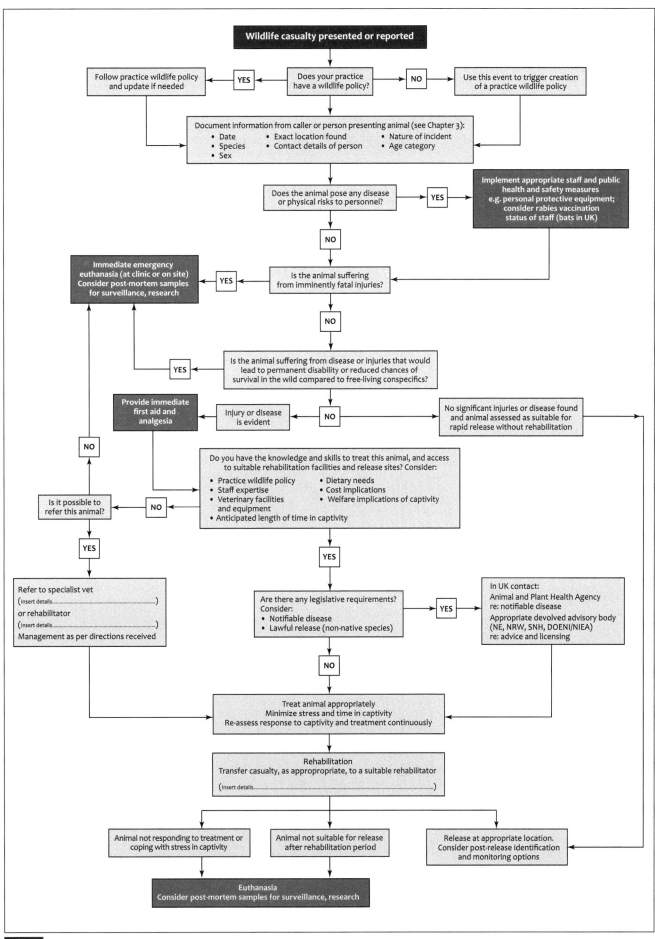

4.2 Triage decision tree to guide the veterinary decision-making process for an adult wildlife casualty.

For example, an open fracture with necrotic bone may require amputation of the affected limb, which would not be suitable for a wild animal (Figure 4.3). It is unlikely to be possible to repair an eye that has been pecked by crows or gulls. If an animal is emaciated and collapsed, it is likely to have severe chronic underlying disease.

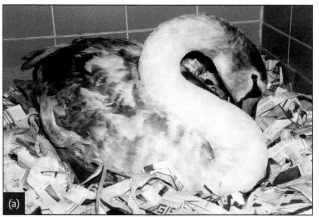

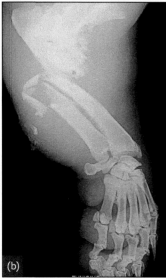

4.3 (a) Cygnet with lead toxicity. This animal is a good candidate for treatment and rehabilitation as the condition generally responds well to therapy and swans cope well with periods of captivity. (b) Radiograph of a badger with a comminuted and open fracture of the radius and ulna. This animal should be euthanased due to the severity of the injury and the poor prognosis for a successful outcome.
(© Elizabeth Mullineaux)

What species is it and what is its natural history and behaviour in the wild?

For a wild animal to be released back to the wild with a chance of survival equivalent to that of other free-living members of its species means different things for different species; for example, birds of prey need to be 100% fit with their full capability of flight, sight and grasping for hunting, whilst small passerines only need to be able to fly from bush to bush to forage and escape from predators, and so an injury that affects wing function will have different implications. Accurate species identification is very important, to enable assessment of conservation status, dietary and behavioural requirements, and any legal implications for keeping it in captivity or its release. It is also very important to know if the species is migratory, if it lives in family groups, or if it is highly territorial.

What is the age and sex of the animal?

Orphaned animals are often not true orphans. Many are uninjured and healthy and should not have been taken from the wild (see Chapter 3). It is essential that the animal does not become imprinted on humans (see Chapter 9). Some species are more prone to this than others, for example fox cubs, owl chicks, and deer fawns. Conversely, a very aged animal is likely to be at the end of its natural lifespan and is presented as a casualty because it cannot compete successfully for resources. A young adult may be being ousted by conspecifics and needs to find new territory. It is also very important, though not always immediately obvious, to determine the sex of the animal. For example, a female bird or mammal that has a displaced pelvic fracture should not be released, as this could lead to egg binding or dystocia in the future, and the sex of a juvenile animal may be important in determining its ability to be integrated into a group for release.

How long will the animal have to be in captivity and how often will it have to be handled for treatment?

It is very important to appreciate that the animal is wild; it is not used to being handled or surrounded by humans or other pet animals. The stress associated with this situation must always be a major factor for consideration in terms of the animal's welfare and there are significant species differences in how wild species 'cope' with captivity. For example, some will not feed well, such as woodcock (*Scolopax rusticola*) and nightjars (*Caprimulgus europaeus*); some birds of prey and pheasant species frequently do not survive in captivity for longer than 1–2 days due to the stress of captivity; and foxes (*Vulpes vulpes*) and deer frequently exhibit behavioural problems that lead to self-trauma. Even if the disease or injury is treatable, for example a repairable fracture, if the treatment requires long periods of captivity and/or immobility the adverse effects on welfare due to the stress involved in some species may outweigh the opportunity for eventual recovery and release. Long periods of time in captivity may also result in loss of a territory, which may impair successful return. Cost/benefit assessments in these situations are undoubtedly largely subjective and may depend on factors such as personnel experience and facilities available.

Does the time of the year have an impact?

Time of year is especially important in species that migrate or hibernate, and may mean either rapid release is required, or prolonged captivity will be necessary before release if the time window for successful migration or hibernation is missed. Food resources may also be variable depending on time of year. If it is the breeding season, consider if the animal is likely to have a bonded mate or dependent offspring, which requires rapid return to the wild or a search instigated in the locality where the casualty was found to locate the offspring (e.g. a lactating female deer). Territorial issues may be encountered in some species if a male is released during the period of the breeding season where territories are being or have been established.

Are suitable veterinary facilities available?

Before admitting the animal, the necessary facilities to handle, house and look after the animal must be available; at the very least a small area or room away from domestic animals, as wild and domestic species should never be mixed. Large animals such as deer will need appropriate accommodation such as a stable, or large isolated pen/walk-in kennel. Consider if the staff have sufficient knowledge of the biology and natural history of the animal to cater for its needs, are experienced at handling the animal and have the time available for nursing care. The cost of treatment and who will fund it is also a necessary consideration.

Are rehabilitation facilities available?

A good working relationship with rehabilitators, ecologists and naturalists is essential for successful rehabilitation (Miller, 2012). Some species (e.g. badger cubs) need highly specialized long-term care and socialization before release and this is not widely available. Establishing contact with local wildlife groups, charities and rehabilitation units with local knowledge and resources is vital. Releasing an animal back to the wild after the stress of captivity and treatment without any consideration for its habitat and resource requirements, or social structure, could have very serious implications for its welfare and survival, despite the 'feel-good' factor for the personnel involved.

A current list of UK rehabilitators is held by the British Wildlife Rehabilitation Council and can be found at www. bwrc.org.uk.

Are suitable release sites available?

As the primary aim of wildlife rehabilitation is to return an animal successfully to the wild, the availability of a suitable release site is essential and should be established early on in the decision-making process. Information on the initial capture site will inform decisions, and consultation and collaboration with rehabilitation staff or local wildlife groups may be necessary. In many situations the release site should be the same as the capture site, but in some instances this may not be suitable, for example where there is poor food supply, a risk of recurrent injury, or where the wild animal is causing a nuisance. For some species, such as juvenile foxes and badgers, identification of a release site where there will not be territorial issues from resident conspecifics can also be a challenge. Further information is given in Chapter 9.

What are the risks to personnel?

It is necessary to have an appreciation of whether the animal is likely to have a zoonotic disease and measures in place to minimize this risk to staff. Examples include: the risk of rabies from bats and the recommendation that any bat handler is vaccinated; badgers and tuberculosis; and hedgehogs and dermatophytosis. Significant zoonotic infections of British wildlife are summarized in Chapter 7.

All staff dealing with wildlife must be trained in how to handle the animal without getting injured (see Chapter 3) – for example, herons and many seabirds are likely to stab at the face of the handler with their sharp beaks (see species-specific chapters for details). In the UK the only venomous wild species is the adder (*Vipera berus*).

Will rehabilitation of the animal pose any risks to free-living species or livestock?

Disease transmission must always be considered, for example, badger cubs should be screened for tuberculosis (Mullineaux and Kidner, 2011). If animals are translocated as part of the rehabilitation process, comprehensive pathogen screening may be indicated, in accordance with International Union for the Conservation of Nature Guidelines (IUCN/Species Survival Commission, 2013) to ensure any risk of introduction of pathogens is assessed. Other considerations, such as competition for resources or the possibility of genetic differences may also be a factor in some situations (see Chapter 1).

Are there any legislative requirements?

It is vital that veterinary surgeons dealing with wildlife have a clear working knowledge of relevant wildlife legislation, as this may have an immediate impact on the decision-making process in terms of options for release (see Chapter 2). Although many species are protected under the Wildlife and Countryside Act (WCA) 1981, veterinary surgeons are legally allowed to take them into captivity for the purposes of treatment until no longer disabled. Under the Destructive Imported Animals Act 1932, it is an offence to keep non-native species in captivity or release them back to the wild; this includes grey squirrels (*Sciurus carolinensis*) and mink (*Mustela (Neovison) vison*). Similarly, under the WCA it is illegal to release Schedule 9 species, such as sika (*Cervus nippon*) and muntjac deer (*Muntiacus reevesi*) and ruddy duck (*Oxyura jamaicensis*). If there is any doubt about the ability to retain or release a certain species, the relevant governmental bodies can be contacted for guidance (e.g. Natural England (NE), Scottish Natural Heritage (SNH), Natural Resources Wales (NRW) or Department of the Environment Northern Ireland/Northern Ireland Environment Agency (DOENI/NIEA) in the UK).

Continuous reassessment is an essential part of the decision-making and rehabilitation process (see Figure 4.2), and should be undertaken even through the relatively rapid process of initial triage, to ensure that any unnecessary suffering is always minimized and euthanasia is undertaken if necessary.

Initial assessment and clinical examination

As much information as possible should be obtained prior to examination of the animal, such as where it was found, what clinical signs were noticed and what, if any, treatment or first aid has already been administered by the first people on the scene. Precise details of the geographical location where the casualty was found should be recorded and kept with the animal throughout any treatment and rehabilitation process. For many casualties, release back at the site of capture will be essential in order for rehabilitation back into the wild to be successful. Information from the site of capture can also be useful, for example blood on the road as evidence of trauma, or faecal soiling, indicating the animal has been lying in one place for some time. As is often the case with wildlife, this information may not be readily available.

Brief examination at a distance allows respiratory rate and character, faeces, urine, blood in the transport carrier, lameness and limb or wing position (Figure 4.4) to be evaluated. First aid (see Chapter 5) or euthanasia may be indicated at this stage; however, if not immediately indicated, the animal should be left in the carrier and placed in a warm dark environment for a short period of time prior to restraint and direct examination.

In some situations this initial process may need to take place in the field rather than at a clinic or hospital, for example if called out to an RTA or stranding incident.

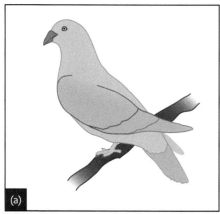 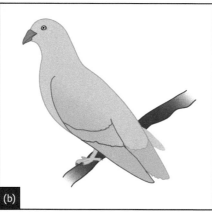 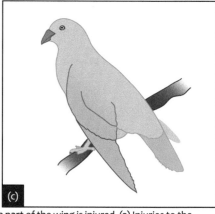

(a)   (b)   (c)

4.4 Observation from a distance of wing position in birds may be useful to help determine which part of the wing is injured. (a) Injuries to the shoulder or coracoid bone result in skewing of the affected wing upwards such that the primary feather tips are held higher than those of the unaffected wing opposite. (b) Injuries to the elbow or humerus result in the wing being held away from the body and slightly dropped, but the primary wing feathers are not dropped. (c) Injuries involving the carpal joint, ulna, radius or distal to the carpus result in the wing tip dropping and the primary feathers trailing.

Capture and handling

The safety and health of all personnel involved – laypeople and staff – must be paramount. The risk of physical injury and zoonotic disease must always be considered. In general, members of the public should be discouraged from handling most wildlife casualties, and they should contact professional organizations such as the RSPCA or SSPCA, or local wildlife rescue centres that have trained staff. It is a good idea to have a practice protocol and details of who to contact drawn up to be able to advise members of the public appropriately (see also Chapter 3).

Details of capture and handling are covered in Chapter 3. Any capture method must ensure that the casualty does not injure itself further or escape. Appropriate equipment and transport facilities for the species will need to be available – this is often easily achieved for small species such as hedgehogs where gloves and a simple box will suffice, but is more complex for larger species such as deer, or potentially dangerous carnivores such as foxes, otters (*Lutra lutra*) and badgers where nets, blankets, dog catcher poles and strong containers may be necessary. More often than not wildlife is presented to the veterinary surgeon already captured, but this can often be in inappropriate containers or even in some cases loose in the back of a car, so great care must be taken when retrieving the animal for assessment. If dealing with a field casualty, sedation or anaesthesia should never be attempted without prior restraint, as the animal may easily get away and become a danger to the public, traffic, or injure itself further, especially if it goes into a body of water.

Whatever method is used to catch an animal, the aim should always be to minimize further stress by acting quickly, subduing light, minimizing noise and restricting movement.

Clinical examination

In highly stressed animals, those with severe injuries or dangerous animals, general anaesthesia may aid clinical examination. Body condition of the animal should be assessed and wherever possible an accurate bodyweight should be determined early in the assessment process, as it is essential as a guide to health status and for calculation of therapeutic doses. Average adult bodyweight ranges of selected British wildlife species are given in Appendix 2.

Clinical examination should be carried out systematically, starting with the head and working caudally, as for other animal species. Important body systems to consider and parameters to assess are given in Figure 4.5. All

Body system	Parameters assessed
Primary survey	
Cardiovascular	• Heart rate • Pulse quality and any pulse deficits • Mucous membrane colour • Capillary refill time • Cardiac auscultation • Evidence of severe (arterial) haemorrhage
Respiratory	• Rate • Effort • Mucous membrane colour • Thoracic auscultation • Thoracic wall injuries
Neurological	• Consciousness • Mentation • Gait/movement • Cranial nerve responses
Secondary survey	
Head and neck	• Head position • Eye position and general ocular examination • Ears • Jaw (crepitus, malalignment, asymmetry) • Teeth (wear, fractures, missing) • Beak (apposition, length, wear)
Abdominal/coelomic	• Body wall trauma (bites, punctures) • Distension • Herniation • Abdominocentesis as required (consider any infection risks)
Genitourinary	• Cloaca (birds, reptiles) • Palpation of kidneys and bladder • Vulva • Anus • Mammary glands • Prepuce • Scrotum

4.5 Clinical assessment of the emergency wildlife patient. The procedure should be as stress-free as possible for the animal. It is also essential to ensure the safety and health of all personnel involved and the risk of physical injury and zoonotic disease must always be considered beforehand. (continues) ▶

Body system	Parameters assessed
Secondary survey continued	
Musculoskeletal	• Palpate length of limbs or wings • Palpate tail • Manipulate all joints
Skin and integument	• Epidermis • Feathers • Coat/fur/spines • Scales • Nails • Evidence of bruising, bleeding, wounds, etc.
Lymphatic system	• Palpate superficial lymph nodes, where appropriate
Additional observations	
Hydration status Temperature Pain	See Figure 5.2 See Figure 5.12 See Chapters 5 and 6

4.5 (continued) Clinical assessment of the emergency wildlife patient. The procedure should be as stress-free as possible for the animal. It is also essential to ensure the safety and health of all personnel involved and the risk of physical injury and zoonotic disease must always be considered beforehand.

animals should be scanned to check for the presence of a microchip as part of a routine examination; these will typically have been placed between the scapulae in mammals and in the pectoral muscles of birds. Areas of the clinical examination that may be of particular relevance when assessing the suitability of a wild animal for treatment and rehabilitation include:

- Assessment of the oral cavity (mucous membrane colour, presence of fishing hooks or lines, dentition)
- Ocular examination, especially for intraocular haemorrhage (retina or pecten)
- Thoracic auscultation (e.g. pulmonary haemorrhage may occur following RTA in mammals)
- Assessment of body condition. In birds this is achieved by pectoral muscle mass palpation and prominence of the keel bone (Figure 4.6). In mammals, reptiles and amphibians, palpation of fat cover and bony prominence of the spine, ribs and pelvic bones, and assessment of hindlimb muscle mass is used as for domestic species. Animals that are thin and underweight may have a reduced post-release survival rate. For example, seabirds that are underweight often have systemic disease or heavy endoparasite burdens. It should be remembered that at certain times of the year (e.g. the moulting season for seabirds), some wild animals are more likely to be in poor body condition
- Assessment of feathers/fur/spines condition. Ectoparasites are common in debilitated animals and indicate a lack of grooming or preening; traumatic fight wounds are common in badgers and otters, and subcutaneous abscesses and ringworm are common in hedgehogs
- Thorough palpation of wings and legs for fractures or luxations, which are common findings in debilitated wild animals following trauma; manipulation of joints for swellings and degree of movement
- Thorough assessment for wounds or evidence of subcutaneous emphysema; puncture wounds (e.g. cat bites) or ballistic entry and exit wounds, which can be difficult to detect and may be easily missed.

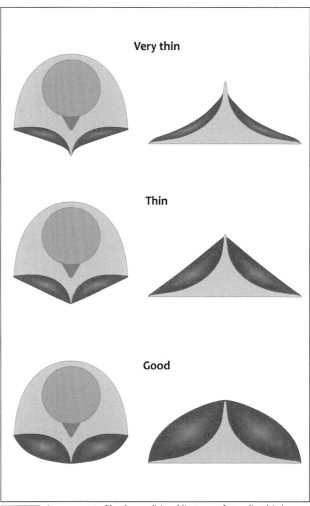

4.6 Assessment of body condition (diagram of standing bird viewed from above (left) and skyline view of keel with bird lying on its back (right)). In birds this is achieved by pectoral muscle mass palpation and prominence of the keel bone. Red shaded area = pectoral muscle mass, ranging from very thin (top), thin (middle) to good (bottom).

Following clinical examination (and further diagnostic tests carried out before or after first aid (see Chapter 5), such as radiography if appropriate), the decision whether to treat or euthanase should be made. Poor prognostic indicators, which are commonly identified in wild animals, are emaciation, heavy ectoparasite burden and fractures. Wing and limb fractures, particularly if open fractures or situated close to a joint, may also be poor prognostic indicators. Staff at wildlife centres should be given veterinary instruction on how to recognize these common conditions, which are associated with an extremely poor prognosis, and learn to recognize when euthanasia is likely to be required (Figure 4.7).

It is essential that any animal, once released into the wild, is able to function normally in order to catch food and survive. Fracture repair for most species, particularly predators, needs to be 100% effective to ensure that this is the case. Opinions may vary, but in general animals should not be released with any orthopaedic implants in place, due to the possible future risk of loosening or infection (see Chapter 5).

Condition / reason	Justification	Training required for non-veterinary personnel
Animal *in extremis* where death is obviously imminent	Patient is already beyond help and dying; euthanasia required to end suffering	Recognition of the signs of imminent death (including typical body postures, behaviour, and breathing pattern) and ability to recognize pain and distress in different species
Severe, deep or extensive injuries, especially where large areas of tissue are damaged (cases needing euthanasia usually obvious – often caused by vehicle collisions)	Severe traumatic injuries carry a poor prognosis, especially where multiple sites affected	Recognition and assessment of critical injuries (especially wounds and traumatic injuries) and ability to grade severity to determine whether recovery is likely
Severe emaciation associated with debilitating injury or disease	Problem likely to be longstanding with resultant starvation or cachexia, therefore limited or no chance of recovery	Ability to assess body condition in different species
Open (compound) fractures, i.e. where the skin is broken at the fracture site exposing bone (exceptions may be made if the injury is recent and uncontaminated)	Exposed bone likely to be contaminated with high risk of infection and subsequent failure of bone healing and other complications	Ability to recognize obvious fractures (especially of long bones) and to differentiate whether open or closed
Prolapse or rupture of tissues with exposure of deeper structures or organs, especially if contaminated, e.g. exposed abdominal contents	Such injuries usually carry a grave prognosis due to the risk of infection and are also often associated with multiple injuries	Ability to recognize and judge the severity of such lesions
Severe myiasis (flystrike) with deep invasion of tissues or multiple sites affected especially when maggots are large and have therefore been present longer; however, many cases of myiasis can be successfully treated depending on the species, duration and underlying problems	Presence of maggots associated with toxin production, tissue damage and toxic shock Additionally, flystrike is often secondary to other pre-existing disease or injury or abnormal behaviour patterns, e.g. orphan hedgehogs lying out during the day	Ability to make a subjective assessment based on a number of prognostic factors
Blind and naked neonates	Very young juveniles have poor survival chances because they are more difficult to rear They need constant care, with usually round-the-clock one-to-one attention They have poor thermoregulation and immunity, associated with a high risk of digestive disorders Aspiration pneumonia is a common complication in weak hand-reared animals	Determination of approximate age in a variety of species
Permanent disability, e.g. limb amputees, joint disorders or bone malformation	Disabilities can significantly affect survival chances, especially the ability to find food, cope with adverse weather and avoid or escape from predators or conspecifics	Recognition of common conditions such as missing limbs, angular wing deformities, metabolic bone disease, etc. Careful assessment is essential to decide whether the disability is compromising welfare and survival
Untreatable systemic disease, e.g. myxomatosis in rabbits	Affected animals are unlikely to recover as the disease is difficult to treat, and may also be very contagious; some wild animals pose a zoonotic risk to human health; there is no effective treatment	Recognition of typical signs of such disease
Legal reasons	Certain species cannot be released back into the wild unless a licence can be obtained from the relevant authority (NE, SNH, NRW, DOENI/NIEA) You may also need a licence to keep some species in captivity	If licences cannot be obtained and the animal's welfare in captivity is compromised then it should be euthanased
Lack of release sites	If there are no available or suitable release sites for the animal, then euthanasia must be considered as early in the rehabilitation process as possible	Lack of sites could be due to lack of compliance from landowners in areas with suitable habitat

4.7 Reasons for euthanasia of wild animal casualties, their justification and training required for non-veterinary professionals.

Euthanasia

Euthanasia (from the Greek *euthanatos* meaning 'easy death') can be defined as the killing of an animal with the minimum of physical and mental suffering (Best and Mullineaux, 2003). Euthanasia, performed correctly, is therefore not a welfare issue in itself and it is often better to euthanase quickly and eliminate the possibility of further suffering than to hold a wild animal captive and attempt treatment. Although members of the public frequently find this upsetting or unacceptable, it is an important educational opportunity to explain the reasons for any decision. Methods of euthanasia are given in Figure 4.8.

Under some circumstances, such as emergencies in the field where suitable chemical methods are not available, physical methods of euthanasia may be the most humane option. Where at all possible, euthanasia techniques should concur with the *American Veterinary Medical*

Group	Chemical methods*	Emergency physical methods
Small birds (up to crow size, approx. 500 g)	Inhalation anaesthesia followed by suitable physical method or lethal injection Lethal injection: intrahepatic, intravenous, intraosseous	Dislocation of cervical vertebrae* Skull crush*
Large birds	Lethal injection: intravenous, intracardiac, intrahepatic, intraosseous	Skull crush*
Small mammals (up to juvenile rabbit)	Inhalation anaesthesia followed by suitable physical method or lethal injection Lethal injection: intravenous, intracardiac, intrahepatic, intrarenal, intraosseous	Skull crush* Dislocation of cervical vertebrae*
Medium-sized mammals (adult rabbit)	Lethal injection, preferably pre-sedate: intravenous, intracardiac, intrahepatic, intrarenal, intraosseous	Skull crush*
Large mammals (fox, badger, deer)	Lethal injection, preferably with pre-sedation: intravenous, intracardiac	Firearms, headshot
Reptiles and amphibians	Lethal injection, usually without pre-sedation: intravenous or intracardiac	Skull crush* Do not use decapitation alone Special care must be taken to ensure animal is indeed dead

4.8 Methods of euthanasia for wildlife casualties. *For use only by trained and competent personnel.

Association Guidelines for the Euthanasia of Animals. Physical methods of euthanasia must ensure immediate loss of consciousness and must only be performed by trained and competent personnel. Any hesitation or lack of confidence can have serious welfare consequences for the animal. Many people, including veterinary surgeons and nurses, find physical methods unpleasant and are reluctant to use them.

On some occasions, the situation may dictate that euthanasia using physical methods by members of the public or non-trained emergency service personnel is the most humane option, for example when giving telephone advice for a remote event where it is not possible to attend quickly or move the animal, or when the situation means that the public are in danger.

In all species, intraperitoneal or intracoelomic injection of barbiturate may be slow in onset of action and cause pain, and so should be avoided.

The preferred method of euthanasia for birds is intravenous barbiturate injection using the medial metatarsal vein. Alternative venous access sites in birds include the right jugular and the ulnar vein (see Chapter 5). General anaesthesia may be indicated prior to injection. In avian species intrahepatic injection of barbiturate is indicated where peripheral circulation is compromised. The caudal border of the sternum is palpated and the needle introduced cranially at a 45-degree angle, to enter the liver.

In large mammals (e.g. deer, fox, badger, otter) the author prefers to induce heavy sedation or general anaesthesia via the intramuscular route (e.g. medetomidine 0.05 mg/kg and ketamine 5 mg/kg is suitable for most species), followed by intravenous barbiturate injection using the cephalic or jugular vein. In seals, an intravenous barbiturate injection into the extradural intervertebral vein should be used (see Chapter 23). Shooting by a suitably qualified and licensed person is an alternative option in deer and cetaceans up to 3 m (see Chapters 22 and 23).

In small mammals (e.g. hedgehog, rabbit, rodents, bats), induction of general anaesthesia in a chamber using isoflurane or sevoflurane (the latter being less irritant to the mucous membranes) followed by intravenous or intracardiac barbiturate injection is a reliable method. Gaseous anaesthesia may only be administered by a veterinary surgeon.

Permanent captivity

In general, retention of a wild animal in permanent captivity can rarely be justified on welfare grounds, and should be strongly discouraged. For most wild animals, freedom to express most normal patterns of behaviour, and freedom from fear, enshrined in the 'five freedoms' of animal welfare (Farm Animal Welfare Council, 2009), cannot be provided in captivity with close proximity to humans. Occasional justifications for keeping permanently disabled wild animals in captivity include for captive breeding programmes of rare or endangered species, for educational purposes, or use as imprint models for young animals of the same species to allow rearing without imprinting on humans. Individual animal welfare must always remain the primary concern and sound justification sought on a case by case basis, with veterinary input into any decision-making process.

Acknowledgements

With thanks to Maria Parga and Emma Keeble for student wildlife lecture notes that were used as the basis for some parts of this chapter, Liz Mullineaux for the provision of Figure 4.5 and Andrew Kelly, Adam Grogan, David Couper and Steve Bexton for the provision of Figure 4.7.

References and further reading

American Veterinary Medical Association (2013) *AVMA Guidelines for the Euthanasia of Animals: 2013 edition.* www.avma.org/KB/Policies/Documents/euthanasia.pdf

Ancillotto L, Serangeli MT and Russo D (2013) Curiosity killed the bat: Domestic cats as bat predators. *Mammalian Biology* **78**, 369–373

Best D and Mullineaux E (2003) Basic principles of treating wildlife casualties. In: *BSAVA Manual of Wildlife Casualties*, ed. E Mullineaux *et al.*, pp. 6–28. BSAVA Publications, Gloucester

British Veterinary Zoological Society (2014) *Guidelines for the prescription, supply and control of prescription only veterinary medicines (POMs) in zoological collections and wildlife rescue centres.* BVZS, London

Farm Animal Welfare Council (2009) *Farm Animal Welfare in Great Britain: Past, Present and Future.* FAWC, London

Grogan A and Kelly A (2013) A review of RSPCA research into wildlife rehabilitation. *Veterinary Record* **172**, 211–215

International Union for the Conservation of Species/Species Survival Commission (2013) *Guidelines for Reintroductions and Other Conservation Translocations, Version 1.0*. IUCN Species Survival Commission, Switzerland

Kelly A and Bland M (2006) Admission, diagnoses, and outcomes for Eurasian Sparrowhawks (*Accipiter nisus*) brought to a wildlife rehabilitation centre in England. *Journal of Raptor Research* **40**, 231–235

Kelly A, Halstead C, Hunter D *et al.* (2011) Factors affecting the likelihood of release of injured and orphaned woodpigeons (*Columba palumbus*). *Animal Welfare* **20**, 523–534

Kelly A, Scrivens R and Grogan A (2010) Post release survival of orphaned wild-born polecats (*Mustela putorius)* reared in captivity at a wildlife rehabilitation centre in England. *Endangered Species Research* **12**, 107–115

Kirkwood JK (2003) Introduction: wildlife casualties and the veterinary surgeon. In: *BSAVA Manual of Wildlife Casualties*, ed. E Mullineaux *et al.*, pp. 1–5. BSAVA Publications, Gloucester

Kirkwood JK and Best R (1998) Treatment and rehabilitation of wildlife casualties: legal and ethical aspects. *In Practice* **20**, 214–216

Miller EA (2012) *Minimum Standards for Wildlife Rehabilitation, 4th edn*. National Wildlife Rehabilitators Association and International Wildlife Rehabilitation Council, St Cloud, Minnesota

Molina-López RA, Casal J and Darwich L (2011) Causes of morbidity in wild raptor populations admitted at a wildlife rehabilitation centre in Spain from 1995–2007: A long term retrospective study. *PLoS ONE* **6**, 24603

Molina-López RA and Darwich L (2011) Causes of admission of little owl (*Athene noctua*) at a wildlife rehabilitation centre in Catalonia (Spain) from 1995 to 2010. *Animal Biodiversity and Conservation* **34**, 401–405

Molony SE, Baker PJ, Garland L, Cuthill IC and Harris S (2007) Factors that can be used to predict release rates for wildlife casualties. *Animal Welfare* **16**, 361–367

Mühldorfer K, Speck S and Wibbelt G (2011) Diseases in free-ranging bats from Germany. *BMC Veterinary Research* **7**, 61

Mullineaux E (2014) Veterinary treatment and rehabilitation of indigenous wildlife. *Journal of Small Animal Practice* **55(6)**, 293–300

Mullineaux E and Kidner P (2011) Managing public demand for badger rehabilitation in an area of England with endemic tuberculosis. *Veterinary Microbiology* **151**, 205–208

Reeve NJ and Huijser MP (1999) Mortality factors affecting wild hedgehogs: A study of records from wildlife rescue centres. *Lutra* **42**, 7–24

Specialist organizations and useful contacts

See Appendix 1.

Chapter 5

First aid and emergency care

Elizabeth Mullineaux and Emma Keeble

Unlike domestic animal patients, wildlife casualties usually come with limited short-term history (e.g. found at the road-side) and with no longer-term history (e.g. how long the animal has been injured or unwell). 'Clients' presenting wildlife to the veterinary surgeon (veterinarian) can, how-ever, often provide useful information on things observed at the time the casualty was found, such as mobility, level of consciousness, behaviour, haemorrhage and obvious injuries. An attempt should therefore be made to take a thorough history. Some casualties will be otherwise healthy animals with acute trauma. Many others will have been dis-abled for a while before they are found and brought into captivity. During this time they are often unable to obtain food and water and may have become dehydrated and cachectic. Other cases will have primary medical reasons for dehydration and weight loss.

This chapter provides information on appropriate first aid and emergency care for most wildlife species in the United Kingdom. Some aspects of critical care that are included in domestic small animal emergency texts (e.g. transfusion medicine, cardiopulmonary resusci-tation) have been intentionally left out as these are rarely applied to wildlife cases and, with limited references for their use, would be directly extrapolated from care of domestic species.

Primary assessment and treatment of wildlife casualties

The primary assessment of the wildlife casualty should include as full a clinical examination as is possible with the animal conscious, whilst minimizing both human risk and unnecessary stress to the patient (see Figure 4.5). At the same time, assessment should be made of the casual-ty's hydration status, body temperature and any evidence of pain, all of which are covered in more detail below.

Assessment and treatment of shock

Evaluation of the cardiovascular system in the primary survey provides information on the animal's systemic per-fusion, as well as identifying any cardiac abnormalities. Hypoperfusion will ultimately lead to organ failure if left untreated. Hypovolaemic shock is common in wildlife casualties, often following acute haemorrhage secondary to trauma. Systemic inflammatory response syndrome

(SIRS), anaphylaxis, cardiogenic and obstructive causes of shock may all occur but these usually carry a poor prognosis due to their underlying causes. The degree of shock can be established using the cardiovascular parameters assessed in the primary survey (see Figure 4.5). In all species, as shock worsens, heart rate and capillary refill time increase, and peripheral pulses decrease both in amplitude and duration.

Emergency treatment of dyspnoea

Many wildlife casualties are tachypnoeic as a result of pain and stress. These cases will respond to appropriate systemic analgesia and a period of time in a dark quiet environment. True dyspnoea can be diagnosed by consid-eration of respiratory rate alongside respiratory effort, pattern of respiratory movements and presence of abnor-mal sounds on thoracic auscultation. Care should be taken to avoid making the dyspnoea worse through excessive handling and so detailed examination, such as thoracic auscultation, may be best delayed until the patient is more stable. Treatment should include:

- **Provision of a small, darkened quiet space**; to minimize stress for the casualty
- **Provision of oxygen**; an oxygen cage is most appropriate (e.g. Buster ICU Cage®). The patient's box or cage can be placed within the oxygen cage if necessary to reduce the need for handling. For small mammals and birds, incubators (e.g. Brinsea® TLC-40, R-COM Bird Pavillion®) can be used and oxygen piped into them. Alternatively, a clean pet travel carrier with a bin liner secured around it will suffice. In larger mammals with reduced mentation, anaesthetic circuits and masks can be used to provide flow-by oxygen without excessive handling. In birds, air sac cannulation (see Chapter 6) can be used to administer emergency oxygen, particularly in cases with suspected upper airway obstruction. In all cases, supplementary oxygen should be administered until breathing rate and effort return to normal and then be slowly reduced whilst the patient continues to be observed. Oxygen should ideally be humidified by, for example, bubble-type humidifiers
- **Appropriate patient positioning**; in most cases, if the patient is recumbent and can be handled, it should be supported in sternal recumbency. For avian patients that are unable to perch, to facilitate respiration and

maintain an upright posture, a doughnut-shaped 'towel nest' can be fashioned from rolled towels on the floor of the enclosure. This will avoid sternal weight-bearing in recumbent avian patients, which impedes respiratory sternal movements (Figure 5.1). Care should be taken to protect the tail feathers, for example by use of a tail guard (see Chapter 29).

Ideally, once the patient's condition is stable, the cause of dyspnoea should be established. In some cases appropriate medication (e.g. analgesics, bronchodilators, mucolytics, nebulization) may be given according to the species involved and common respiratory conditions occurring in those species (see species-specific chapters). A full clinical examination should be performed, using sedation as appropriate, including the oral cavity and upper airways, which may become obstructed by parasites or other disease processes, especially in birds (see bird-specific chapters). The external thorax should be carefully checked for evidence of bite or gunshot wounds and other signs of trauma penetrating the lungs or air sacs. Thoracic auscultation should be performed, together with imaging as necessary (see 'Thoracic and abdominal injuries').

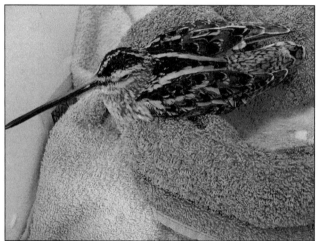

5.1 A collapsed adult snipe (*Gallinago gallinago*) that has been placed in an incubator with a doughnut-shaped 'towel nest' to prevent it from falling to one side and to aid respiration.

Emergency treatment of neurological signs

Some casualties will present with acute neurological signs, such as seizures. These may occur for a variety of reasons including hypoglycaemia, other metabolic imbalances (e.g. hypocalcaemia), inflammatory and infectious causes, systemic disease processes, head trauma and toxicity (see 'Poisoning'). Clinical examination and laboratory tests can provide additional information on the cause of the clinical signs. Emergency treatment should include fluid therapy with appropriate supplementation to correct any metabolic disturbances (see 'Fluid therapy') and anticonvulsant drugs such as diazepam (mammals: 0.2–0.5 mg/kg i.v. or 1–5 mg/kg i.m. or 0.5–1 mg/kg rectally; birds: 0.5–1 mg/kg i.v. or i.m. Intravenous doses can be repeated two or three times at 5–10 minute intervals if required) or phenobarbital (mammals: 12 mg/kg i.v., allowing up to 30 minutes for this dose to achieve central nervous system (CNS) levels; further doses of 4–6 mg/kg i.v. may be given at 30-minute intervals on two occasions if necessary).

Wildlife casualties that are poorly responsive to such treatment and/or have significant underlying problems should be euthanased.

Assessment of hydration

Wildlife patients are very often dehydrated as a result of a failure to eat and drink normally prior to presentation, or as a result of systemic disease causing water and electrolyte loss. In dehydration, unlike hypovolaemia, fluid is lost from the intracellular and interstitial spaces as well as the intravascular space.

Methods of hydration assessment are similar to those employed in domestic species, although some species-specific considerations are necessary (Figure 5.2). Assessment of dehydration is very subjective. Laboratory tests can provide additional information on hydration status.

Assessment of body temperature

On admission the cloacal/rectal temperature should be obtained in all collapsed animals, and routinely where possible (see Figure 5.13). If hypothermia is diagnosed or suspected, thermotherapy should be immediately instigated (see 'Maintenance of optimal temperature').

Assessment of pain

The casualty should be assessed for evidence of pain and appropriate analgesia must be provided (see 'Analgesia' and Chapter 6). Prey species may mask signs of pain as a normal response to a stressful situation. Consequently, any wildlife casualty with a condition that would be likely to result in pain in domestic animals should receive appropriate analgesia, regardless of the clinical signs observed in that individual.

Emergency diagnostic tests

The same diagnostic tests can be used in wildlife casualties as in domestic species, including radiography, ultrasonography, endoscopy and blood and urine analysis, as well as more advanced techniques such as magnetic resonance imaging (MRI) and computed tomography (CT). When deciding to use a diagnostic test, the following should be considered:

- How appropriate is the test? What is the cost/benefit to the animal? Will the test result change the prognosis, case management or treatment plan? Is the expense justified?
- Is the equipment available suitable for the casualty? For example, most in-practice haematology machines will not be suitable for wildlife blood samples; most biochemistry machines will be, but reference ranges may not be available for interpretation
- Can zoonotic infection risks be controlled? For example, urine samples from badgers (*Meles meles*) may carry a risk to the handler of infection with bovine tuberculosis (*Mycobacterium bovis*)
- Can contamination risks be controlled? For example, endoscopy of an infectious case (e.g. a badger *M. bovis* case) may risk transfer of infection to subsequent cases and adequate disinfection of the endoscope to alleviate these concerns may be practically difficult.

Reference ranges for common blood tests in specific species are given, where available, in the chapters that follow. In reality, full blood profiles are unlikely to change a triage outcome based upon careful clinical examination; however, a simple emergency database may provide useful information prior to fluid therapy.

Parameter	Degree of dehydration					Comments
	<5%	5–6%	7–9%	10–12%	12–15%	
Skin turgor	No clear evidence of loss of skin elasticity or skin tenting	Slight loss of skin elasticity and slight skin tenting	Significant loss of skin elasticity and notable skin tenting	Complete loss of skin elasticity and marked skin tenting	Complete loss of skin elasticity and marked skin tenting	• Very variable; greater elasticity in younger and fatter animals and in mammals compared with birds and reptiles • Best assessed over the pectoral muscles in birds and the scruff of the neck of most mammals
Mucous membranes	Minimal loss of moisture	Slightly tacky	Tacky	Dry	Dry	• May be practicably difficult to assess in many wildlife species
Capillary refill time (CRT) (gum – mammals)	<2 seconds	<2 seconds	>2 seconds	>3 seconds	>3 seconds	• May be practicably difficult to assess in many wildlife species • Difficult in birds (see below) and species with pigmented mucous membranes
Venous refill time (superficial ulnar vein – birds)	<2 seconds	<2 seconds	>2 seconds	>3 seconds	>3 seconds	• In birds the venous refill time and turgidity of the superficial ulnar vein (see Figure 5.6b) can be used as an alternative to CRT (Rupley, 1998)
Eyes	Normal	Normal	Slightly sunken	Noticeably sunken	Markedly sunken	• Not a very accurate assessment • Varies with species and bodyweight; less noticeable in fatter animals • Dehydrated seals lack a tear film
General clinical condition associated with hydration status	Appears well	Normal	Mild changes in mentation	Signs of mild shock Marked changes in mentation	Signs of moderate shock Moribund	• Variable between species • May be difficult to assess 'normal' mentation in wild animals as stress response to captivity occurs • Often compounded by other medical problems

5.2 Assessment of hydration status in wildlife casualties.

Emergency database

An emergency database of laboratory diagnostic tests (Figure 5.3) can be carried out on critical patients. This range of tests relies on only a small blood sample size, taken from a hypodermic needle or intravenous catheter hub directly into a microhaematocrit tube (for packed cell volume, buffy coat and total solids for an estimation of serum proteins) or directly on to test strips (e.g. for urea in mammals), and can be performed in all species. In larger mammals it is useful to complement the database with measurement of urine specific gravity and an estimation of serum electrolyte levels prior to fluid therapy. Care should be taken when handling both blood and urine because of the potential zoonotic risk of disease. Blood collection sites are described below.

Test variable (method)	Increased in	Decreased in	Comments
Packed cell volume (PCV) (microhaematocrit tube)	Dehydration Polycythaemia	Haemorrhage Haemolysis Chronic non-regenerative anaemia	• To aid accuracy of interpretation, PCV should be considered alongside serum total solids
Buffy coat (microhaematocrit tube)	Infection Lymphoproliferative disease	Infection	• Ideally a stained blood smear should also be examined for cytology and a total white blood cell count performed if possible
Serum total solids (TS) (refractometer; measurement of total solids provides an estimation of serum total protein)	Dehydration Hyperglobulinaemia	Haemorrhage Hypoglobulinaemia Protein-losing conditions (enteric, renal, liver disease) Malnutrition/starvation	• To aid accuracy of interpretation, serum total solids should be considered alongside PCV
Blood urea nitrogen (BUN) in mammals (test strip)	Dehydration Advanced renal failure Urinary tract obstruction Shock Association with some natural diets	Malnutrition/starvation Liver disease Some diets	• Should be considered alongside serum total solids, PCV and urine specific gravity if possible • May be elevated if associated with certain natural diets (e.g. earthworms in badgers)
Blood glucose (glucometer)	Stress Endocrine disorders (diabetes mellitus, hyperadrenocorticism) Head trauma Acute pancreatitis	Starvation Sepsis Some types of neoplasia Hypoadrenocorticism End-stage liver disease	• Glucose levels can fall quickly in small mammals and birds with high metabolic rates • Neonates are also especially susceptible to hypoglycaemia • Medical stress and the stress of handling and blood sampling can result in transient hyperglycaemia • The use of some sedative drugs (e.g. ketamine, alpha-2 agonists) pre-sampling may also result in hyperglycaemia
Urine specific gravity (refractometer)	Dehydration	Renal failure	• Care in sampling where potential zoonotic pathogens may occur in urine (e.g. *Mycobacterium bovis* in badgers)

5.3 Emergency diagnostic laboratory database.

Intravenous access

Intravenous access is required both for blood collection and for intravenous fluid therapy (Figure 5.4). The volume of blood collected should be a maximum of 1% of body-weight, preferably less in debilitated or shocked animals. When tests are not performed immediately, suitable anti-coagulants will be required (Figure 5.5).

Intravenous access in birds

Intravenous access sites in birds are summarized in Figure 5.4 and illustrated in Figure 5.6. Intravenous access in birds requires some degree of manual or chemical restraint.

Right jugular vein

In most species, the right jugular vein lies under a feather-less tract of skin on the lateral aspect of the neck directly in line with the external auditory meatus (Figure 5.6a). The vein is superficial but mobile and haematomas can occur with poor sampling technique. Gentle pressure should be applied to the site after sampling; however, care should be taken that this is not excessive as it may result in triggering of a vasovagal reflex and slowing of the heart. A drop of tissue adhesive may aid haemostasis. Occasionally, a full crop or a subcutaneous air sac needs to be pushed caudally to reveal the length of the vein. Some species (e.g. gamebirds) have very dense feathering on the neck, making this site difficult to locate. Pigeons

and doves (Columbidae) have a venous plexus rather than a clearly defined jugular vein, making this site unsuitable for sampling in these species.

Superficial ulnar vein (basilic vein)

The ulnar vein is located on the ventral aspect of the wing (Figure 5.6b). It crosses the radius and ulna just distal to the elbow and then extends proximally along the humerus. The vein is most easily found with the bird restrained in a cloth and held in lateral recumbency (with the head covered and the feet securely held in larger species) and the wing extended. It is a very fragile vein and usually forms a haematoma following venepuncture; manual pressure and/or a drop of tissue adhesive may aid haemostasis. This site can be used in pigeons and gamebirds.

Medial metatarsal vein (caudal tibial vein)

This is accessible in most birds weighing over 100 g (preferably using a 27 G needle). The vein runs medially along the length of the tarsometatarsus and over the cranio-medial aspect of the intertarsal joint (Figure 5.6c). With the bird restrained in a cloth and held in lateral or sternal recumbency, its leg can be extended caudally. The vein will be seen more clearly if the overlying skin is swabbed with surgical spirit. In species with a scaled tarsus, the vein is well supported by the surrounding connective tissue and will allow repeated venepuncture. This is the preferred site in waterfowl, grey herons (*Ardea cinerea*), waders and seabirds.

Species	Suggested sites	Comments
Birds (all species)	Right jugular vein (see Figure 5.6a) Superficial ulnar vein (see Figure 5.6b) Medial metatarsal vein (see Figure 5.6c)	• Haemostasis may be difficult: digital pressure (with care to avoid a vasovagal reflex when the jugular vein is used) and/or a drop of tissue adhesive may be useful, and careful sampling technique is essential • Right jugular vein preferred in most species • Superficial ulnar vein preferred in pigeons • Medial metatarsal vein preferred in waterfowl, heron, waders and seabirds
Large mammals (e.g. deer, foxes, badgers)	Jugular vein Cephalic vein Lateral saphenous vein	• Chemical restraint will be required in animals that are not very debilitated • Not suitable for marine mammals (see Chapter 23 for blood collection in these species)
Small mammals (e.g. hedgehogs, small mustelids, squirrels, small rodents)	Jugular vein Cephalic vein Cranial vena cava Saphenous vein Femoral vein	• Chemical restraint will be required in animals that are not very debilitated • Cranial vena cava used routinely by the authors for small rodent sampling (see Chapter 14) and is useful in small mustelids where the heart is situated more caudally than other species • Care required in non-mustelid species to avoid the atria when using cranial vena cava venepuncture
Lagomorphs (rabbits and hares)	Marginal ear vein As small mammals	• Marginal ear vein preferred for fluid therapy (see Chapter 16) • Saphenous vein preferred for blood sampling
Reptiles and amphibians	Palatine vein (snakes, not venomous species) Ventral coccygeal vein (reptiles) Cardiocentesis (snakes and amphibians)	• See main text for more detail • Doppler can be used to locate the heart for cardiocentesis • General anaesthesia required in amphibians

5.4 Blood collection and intravenous access sites.

Test to be performed	Suitable sample tube types		
	Mammals	*Birds*	*Reptiles*
Haematology	Ethylenediaminetetraacetic acid (EDTA)	Lithium heparin	Lithium heparin
Biochemistry	Lithium heparin Clotted sample (no anticoagulant)	Lithium heparin Clotted sample (no anticoagulant)	Lithium heparin Clotted sample (no anticoagulant)
Glucose	Fluoride–oxalate	Fluoride–oxalate	Fluoride–oxalate
Serology	Clotted sample (no anticoagulant)	Clotted sample (no anticoagulant)	Clotted sample (no anticoagulant)
Clotting studies	Citrate	Citrate	Citrate

5.5 Anticoagulants for blood collection in wildlife species. For advice on sample tube types for other specific laboratory tests, the relevant diagnostic laboratory should be contacted.

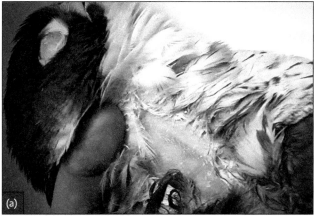

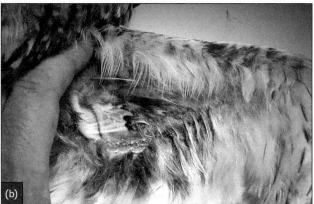

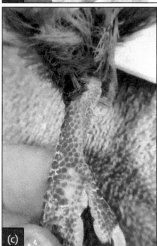

5.6 Venepuncture sites in birds. (a) Right jugular vein (peregrine falcon (*Falco peregrinus*), anaesthetized). (b) Superficial ulnar vein (tawny owl (*Strix aluco*)). (c) Medial metatarsal vein (pigeon (*Columba livia domestica*)).

Intravenous access in mammals

Intravenous access sites in mammals are summarized in Figure 5.4. Chemical restraint will be required to handle and gain intravenous access in all but the most debilitated of mammals.

Intravenous access in reptiles and amphibians

Intravenous access in wild reptiles and amphibians is likely to be limited to blood sampling (see Figure 5.4). In snakes, the palatine vein (not venomous species), ventral coccygeal vein or cardiocentesis are most commonly used.

Additional information on sampling of these species can be found in appropriate texts (e.g. Girling and Raiti, 2004) and other sources (e.g. publications of the US National Wildlife Health Centre, www.nwhc.usgs.gov).

Ventral coccygeal vein access in snakes

Identify the ventrally-located cloaca and swab the site with surgical spirit. Insert the needle distal to the cloaca into the tail along the midline at a 45–90-degree angle. In male animals, care must be taken to avoid the hemipenes; the needle is placed distal to these structures (usually at least six scales distal to the cloaca). Advance the needle to touch the vertebrae, then aspirate whilst slowly withdrawing. The vessel is just ventral to the vertebrae. Use a 1–2 ml syringe with a 23–25 G needle, depending on the size of the animal.

The ventral coccygeal vein may also be used to obtain a blood sample from **lizards**, with careful handling to avoid tail autonomy.

Cardiocentesis in snakes

Palpate or visualize the beating heart on the ventrum of the animal, approximately a third of the way along the length of the snake from the head. Alternatively, locate the heart using a Doppler probe. Stabilize the area with finger and thumb, and swab the area with surgical spirit. Slide a 23–25 G needle on a 1–2 ml syringe (dependent on the size of the animal) under the ventral scale and aspirate using the syringe. If only clear fluid is withdrawn, this is pericardial fluid. The needle should be withdrawn, replaced and the insertion position shifted.

In **amphibians**, cardiocentesis may also be used to collect a blood sample, but should be performed under general anaesthesia.

Fluid therapy

The two primary reasons for using fluids in wildlife casualties are: to correct dehydration and electrolyte imbalances; and to correct hypovolaemia. It is important to ask:

- Does the patient need fluid therapy?
- How will the fluid be given?
- Which fluid type is most appropriate?
- At what rate will the fluid be given and for how long?
- How will the 'success' of fluid therapy be determined and monitored?
- Are there possible adverse effects of fluid therapy and how will these be monitored?

These are obviously the same questions that should be asked for domestic species. In wildlife casualties, however, the answers are often less straightforward as the ability to administer fluid, maintain intravenous lines for any length of time, and carry out any direct monitoring may be limited. Remember that excessive use of fluid therapy, especially intravenous or intraosseous, can be as dangerous as underuse.

The choice of a suitable route for administration of fluid therapy is dictated by the species of animal, the degree of debilitation, the nature of any injuries and the facilities available. Severely debilitated, hypovolaemic and dehydrated animals will have a poor blood supply to peripheral tissues and the gastrointestinal tract, making oral and subcutaneous administration of fluids less effective than using intravenous or intraosseous routes. Suggested routes of administration and emergency volumes to be given are summarized in Figures 5.7 and 5.8. In all cases the fluid should be warmed to the approximate body temperature of the casualty before it is administered (see 'Maintenance of optimal temperature').

Route of administration	Method	Suggested initial emergency volumes[a]
Oral	Unassisted drinking Crop tube (gavage) (see Figures 5.9 and 5.10)	50 ml/kg (see Figure 5.10)
Subcutaneous	Inguinal area (pre-crural fold) Interscapular area Propatagium (wing web) Axilla (see Figure 5.11)	20 ml/kg initially
Intracoelomic	Not recommended in birds due to risk of injection into air sacs	n/a
Intravenous	Right jugular vein (see Figure 5.6a) Superficial ulnar vein (see Figure 5.6b) Medial metatarsal vein (see Figure 5.6c)	10–30 ml/kg as a bolus
Intraosseous	Ulna (proximal or distal) Tibiotarsus (proximal, into the tibial crest) **Do not use in pneumatized bones**	10–30 ml/kg as a bolus

5.7 Summary of emergency fluid administration routes and volumes for avian casualties. [a]See also main text for further information on volumes and rates of fluid administration.

Route of administration	Method	Suggested initial emergency volumes[a]
Oral	Unassisted drinking Syringe directly into mouth Gavage into stomach Nasogastric tube Pharyngostomy tube	50 ml/kg
Subcutaneous	Loose skin over scruff of the neck or over the shoulders 'Skirt' area in hedgehogs	20 ml/kg
Intraperitoneal	May be useful in very small mammals Administer just behind the umbilicus, angled cranially and parallel to the body wall, in a patient supported vertically	20 ml/kg at a time
Intravenous	Jugular vein Cephalic vein Lateral saphenous vein Marginal ear vein (lagomorphs)	10–20 ml/kg as an initial bolus
Intraosseous	Very useful in small mammals (see main text)	10–20 ml/kg as an initial bolus

5.8 Summary of emergency fluid administration routes and volumes for mammalian casualties. [a]See also main text for further information on volumes and rates of fluid administration.

Fluid administration in birds

Crop tubing (gavaging)

All native British birds have a buccal cavity with a simple anatomy (Figure 5.9), which facilitates the passage of a gavage tube into the pharynx and down the oesophagus to the crop, or to the proximal portion of the cervical oesophagus (at the level of the thoracic inlet) in those species that do not have a well-developed crop (e.g. owls, gulls). Rigid gavage tubes are available commercially in several sizes and are suitable for most avian species (e.g. metal crop tubes from Harrison Bird Foods®). Semi-rigid tubes can be made from cut-down urinary catheters, care being taken to round off the cut edges over a flame to

prevent damage to the oesophageal mucosa. Alternatively, domestic animal feeding tubes (e.g. lamb, dog/cat) can be used appropriate to the size of bird.

This technique is suitable for demonstration to lay workers as a standard first aid procedure:

- The tube and syringe are preloaded with oral fluids prior to administration to minimize handling time
- The bird is suitably restrained by an assistant, usually by wrapping in a towel, and its mouth is opened using one hand
- The tube is introduced laterally into the mouth to avoid the central glottis (Figure 5.9a), then advanced caudolaterally along the pharynx, into the oesophagus and then into the crop
- In larger birds the beak is most easily, and safely, kept open with a finger inserted in the commissure of the mouth (Figure 5.9b)
- The progress of the tube can be checked by palpation and observation of the right side of the neck
- The correct position is identified when the tip of the tube is at the thoracic inlet
- During administration of fluids, the oropharynx should be monitored in case any regurgitation occurs. If this happens stop gavaging immediately, remove the tube and tilt the head of the bird downwards to avoid aspiration of fluid
- The bird is then placed immediately back in its cage to recover and observed for a few minutes for any signs of stress or regurgitation.

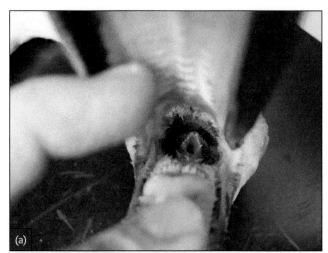
(a)

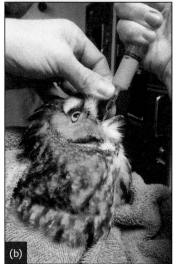
(b)

5.9 (a) The glottis lies centrally within the buccal cavity in all bird species and is easily avoided when passing a gavage tube. (b) Gavage is well tolerated by birds, such as this short-eared owl (*Asio flammeus*), and can be performed quickly to reduce stress.

Approximate volumes of fluid that can safely be deposited at one time into the crop or proximal cervical oesophagus of fully grown common birds are given in Figures 5.7 and 5.10. As a general rule, crop volume is calculated as 5% of bodyweight and volumes of 50 ml/kg can be tolerated at each feed. However, in the debilitated patient or one with a history of regurgitation, administer one-third to one-half of the estimated volume for the first feed and then increase the volume over two or three feeds. In neonatal birds (see Chapter 8), larger volumes may be given as crop volume may be up to 10% of bodyweight.

Species	Approximate volume of liquid to be given by single gavage administration (ml)
Robin (*Erithacus rubecula*)	1
Blackbird (*Turdus merula*)	2
Feral pigeon (*Columba livia domestica*)	5
Carrion crow (*Corvus corone*)	10
Common buzzard (*Buteo buteo*)	30
Grey heron (*Ardea cinerea*)	100
Mute swan (*Cygnus olor*)	500

5.10 Approximate volume of fluid to be given by single gavage administration to some common species of British birds.

Subcutaneous injection

Sites for subcutaneous fluid administration in birds are illustrated in Figure 5.11. The preferred site is the loose skin on the medial aspect of the thigh in the groin (inguinal or precrural fold), which appears to cause little discomfort to the patient. Layworkers may be taught this technique for use in emergency situations. The bird is restrained in lateral recumbency, with the leg extended. The site is disinfected and at the same time made more visible by swabbing the feathers with a small amount of surgical spirit. Injections can be made bilaterally and the use of a small needle (25 or 27 G) will reduce the amount of fluid leaking through the needle puncture in the thin, inelastic skin.

Alternative sites include the propatagium (wing web), axilla and interscapular area (see Figure 5.11). Avoid injections at the base of the neck as the cervicocephalic air sac is located here in some species.

The maximum volume of warmed fluid to be injected at each site varies with the size of the bird: typically a volume of approximately 20 ml/kg is used, although volumes of up to 50 ml/kg are quoted in some texts. If the patient is warmed (see 'Maintenance of optimal temperature'), the fluid is absorbed quickly from the site and may have disappeared within 30–60 minutes. Hyaluronidase may be used in most species, added to sterile crystalloid fluids at a dilution of 1500 IU/l fluid to increase the absorption rate and dispersion of subcutaneous fluids (Thomas *et al.*, 2008).

Intravenous injection

This is the preferred route in a severely debilitated and dehydrated patient requiring rapid correction of circulating fluid volume and electrolyte balance. Intravenous access sites are as described previously and in Figure 5.4. Fluids can be administered either as an intravenous bolus or by continuous infusion. Continuous infusion is through an indwelling intravenous catheter and can usually only be carried out in a debilitated sedentary bird or sedated patient. The exception to this are large water birds, such

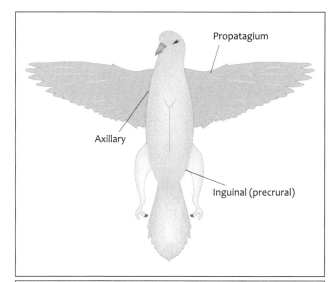

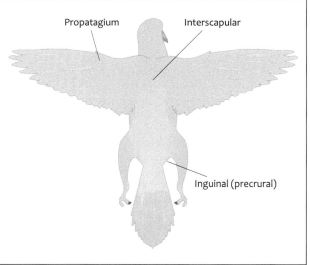

5.11 Sites for subcutaneous fluid therapy administration in birds.

as swans, that appear to tolerate intravenous lines well. In very debilitated birds with poor peripheral circulation, intravenous access may be difficult. In these cases, intraosseous or subcutaneous fluids with added hyaluronidase should first be administered to increase peripheral circulation in order to enable intravenous access. Fluid rates are given below (see 'Fluid administration rates') and summarized in Figure 5.7.

Intraosseous injection

This is possibly the most useful route in severely debilitated birds with poor peripheral circulation. A non-pneumatized long bone must be used: the most commonly selected are the ulna (proximal or distal) and tibiotarsus (proximal into the tibial crest). The procedure should be carried out aseptically under general anaesthesia. Intraosseous needles with stylettes are available, but in most birds an 18 or 20 G hypodermic needle attached to a syringe can be driven through the cortex and into the medulla. Once the correct placement and patency of the needle have been confirmed by flushing with a small volume of heparinized saline, it can then be connected to a delivery system and infusion performed in a similar manner to that used with intravenous catheters. Fluid volumes and rates are described below (see 'Fluid administration rates') and summarized in Figure 5.7.

Fluid administration in mammals

Oral fluids

Successful passage of a stomach tube in conscious mammals is generally difficult (with the exception of marine mammals, see Chapter 23). Laypeople frequently attempt this technique, but there is a real risk of the tube being chewed or fluids being inadvertently administered into the trachea. Nasogastric tubes may be placed in some species under light sedation and local anaesthesia, but these are rarely tolerated for long in unsupervised mammals. Very few casualties will drink readily when first admitted. However, some species (e.g. hedgehogs (*Erinaceus europaeus*), rabbits (*Oryctolagus cuniculus*), badgers and foxes (*Vulpes vulpes*)) will lap if offered fluids from a syringe dripped slowly on to the gum or into the mouth. Care should be taken to avoid aspiration of fluids using this technique in debilitated animals. The handler must also be aware of safe handling practice (see Chapter 3).

Subcutaneous injection

This may be used where the animal is mildly hypovolaemic and oral or intravenous administration of fluid is not possible. Laypeople can easily be taught the technique. Fluids should be sterile, isotonic and warmed to body temperature. Only small volumes of fluid should be given at one site (up to 20 ml/kg). Suitable sites in most species are the scruff of the neck or over the shoulders. The casualty should be warmed slowly, to encourage peripheral vasodilation. Care should be taken with repeat administration of fluids to monitor for local tissue necrosis, although this is rarely encountered, even with large fluid volumes. Hyaluronidase may be used in most species, added to sterile crystalloid fluids at a dilution of 1500 IU/l, to increase the absorption rate and dispersion of subcutaneous fluids.

Intraperitoneal injection

Intraperitoneal injections may have an increased absorption rate over subcutaneous injections for fluid therapy, but are still only suitable for mildly hypovolaemic patients where oral fluids cannot be administered. Warmed sterile crystalloid fluids should be used. Volumes of around 20 ml/kg at a time are suitable, although larger volumes can be given. The patient should be kept warm to encourage vasodilation and fluid uptake. The technique may be taught to laypeople for emergency situations, but care should be taken to make them aware of the risks of infection and organ damage. The standard technique of passing the needle through the body wall just caudal to the umbilicus, angled cranially and parallel to the body wall, in a patient supported vertically, is appropriate in most cases. Aseptic technique is required.

Intravenous injection

This is the preferred route for administration of fluids in moderate to severely hypovolaemic or dehydrated mammalian casualties. Intravenous access sites are as described in Figure 5.4. Over-the-needle catheters are the most appropriate type for most species. Catheters are usually well tolerated in animals requiring fluid therapy. Baskerville™-type muzzles can be placed on larger mammals, or light sedation used, to prevent chewing of drip lines. Fluid volumes and rates are described below (see 'Fluid administration rates') and summarized in Figure 5.8.

Intraosseous injection

This is the preferred method of fluid administration in moderate to severely hypovolaemic mammals where intravenous access is not possible, for example in smaller species. The humerus, tibia and femur are all possible sites for administration; the most practical is usually the trochanteric fossa of the femur. General or local anaesthesia is administered and the site of penetration should be clipped as necessary and surgically prepared. Small volumes of local anaesthetic should be used to infiltrate the local tissues and periosteum. The density of mammalian bone means that spinal or intraosseous needles are the most suitable for these procedures, but hypodermic needles of an appropriate size (usually 18–20 G) can be used in smaller species. Needles require initial and periodic flushing with heparinized saline. This technique is further described in Chapter 16. Fluid volumes and rates are described below (see 'Fluid administration rates') and summarized in Figure 5.8.

Use of supplementary equipment

Drip pumps, syringe drivers, drip warmers, coiled drip lines, t-ports, 3-way taps and other ancillary equipment are especially useful in wildlife patients where there may be practical issues with fluid administration. Gravity-fed drip sets are difficult and unreliable to use as they frequently become obstructed and the very slow delivery rates required for some patients mean that overhydration is a real risk. Syringe drivers and drip pumps, especially those in which the delivery rate can be set as low as 1 ml/hr, are the preferred method for intravenous and intraosseous infusion of fluid.

Types of fluid

The choice of an appropriate fluid for a particular wildlife case is often complicated by the lack of an accurate clinical history. Careful clinical examination and blood tests where possible will assist with the choice of fluid as well as its route and rate of administration. An ideal fluid would replace the fluid deficit, maintain intravascular volume and homeostasis of body fluid spaces, and possibly provide an immediate source of energy. The choice of fluid in individual situations will vary and change over time.

Oral fluids

Proprietary hypotonic oral rehydration electrolyte and glucose mixtures should be used. The glucose content of these is variable when used as directed by the manufacturers. Ideally the glucose content of the fluid should be appropriately chosen to correct diagnosed deficits. Where the blood glucose level is not known, it is better in most instances to use solutions containing higher glucose concentrations, and in an emergency, a freshly prepared 5% glucose solution can be used.

Parenteral fluids

Crystalloid solutions: Fluids for injection via the intravenous, intraosseous, intraperitonal or subcutaneous routes are usually **isotonic crystalloid solutions**. The solutions must be sterile and ideally warmed to the normal body temperature of the animal (see Figure 5.13) prior to use using a water bath set to the required temperature. Crystalloid fluids can be used at low rates via all parenteral routes to treat dehydration or provide maintenance fluids, and at high rates intravenously or intraosseously to treat hypovolaemia. The most commonly used crystalloid fluids are buffered solutions (lactated Ringer's solution, Hartmann's solution, compound sodium lactate) or 0.9% sodium chloride (normal strength or physiological saline). Ideally the choice of fluid should be based upon diagnosed acid–base and electrolyte imbalances.

For maintenance, **hypotonic crystalloid solutions** may be used (e.g. 0.45% sodium chloride + 2.5% dextrose (glucose) + appropriate potassium supplementation), although fluid administration in wildlife casualties is rarely maintained for long periods via parenteral routes and instead oral routes are used once the patient is more stable.

Hypertonic crystalloid solutions can be used intravenously or intraosseously to treat shock, but this effect is transient when these solutions are used alone and the authors' preference would be to use rapid rates of isotonic solutions or colloids for the treatment of hypovolaemia in wildlife.

Colloid solutions: All types of colloid solution used in veterinary medicine can be used in wildlife casualties. These include:

- **Gelatin solutions** (e.g. Gelofusine®, Haemaccel®). These are veterinary licensed products and remain in the circulation for about 10 hours
- **Hydroxyethyl starches** (including a variety of products with a wide range of molecular weights, e.g. tetrastarch (Voluven®), pentastarch, hetastarch). These products may last longer in the circulation than gelatins (e.g. hetastarch up to 24 hours), which can be an advantage in wildlife species. At the time of writing, concerns have been raised regarding the use of these products in humans and this has affected their availability
- **Haemoglobin-based oxygen carriers (HBOCs)** (e.g. Oxyglobin®). These provide oxygen-carrying capacity as well as colloid effects and may be useful in wildlife species as an alternative to blood transfusion (see 'Blood products') as they allow for cross-species use without the risk of disease transmission. HBOCs remain effective in the circulation for around 24 hours.

Colloids are used intravenously or intraosseously; in both cases care must be taken to ensure needle or catheter placement is correct (flush with a small volume of saline first) and that fluid administration is not subcutaneous. Colloids must always be warmed carefully in a water bath and not a microwave.

Colloid solutions are especially useful in the treatment of large mammals (e.g. fox, badger, deer (Cervidae)) following trauma such as road traffic accidents where rapid correction of hypovolaemia is required. There is, however, little evidence to suggest that their effect is any better than that achieved with rapid administration of crystalloids and colloids are not without potential side effects (e.g. coagulopathies).

Blood products: Species-specific blood products are not available for wildlife. There is little indication for the use of blood transfusions in British wildlife casualties. If blood transfusions are to be considered, then these should be homologous, cross-matched and screened for disease.

Fluid administration rates

Emergency fluid administration rates are summarized in Figures 5.7 and 5.8.

Birds

Maintenance fluid requirements for birds vary with size, with birds weighing above 100 g requiring 5% of their body mass in fluids per day (50 ml/kg/day), rising to 50% of the body mass (500 ml/kg/day) for small birds weighing 10–20 g (Sturkie, 2000). An average daily maintenance fluid volume of 100 ml/kg/day (4 ml/kg/hr) is commonly used when calculating fluid requirements for birds. In cases of **dehydration**, it is safe to assume that a casualty bird in a debilitated state will have lost at least 10–15% of total body fluids and this deficit should be replaced at a steady rate over the first 48 hours of hospitalization in addition to the animal's calculated daily fluid maintenance requirement. Clinical assessment and reassessment is the key to ensuring that adequate hydration is provided.

Example calculation for a 1 kg bird with 10% dehydration

Deficit = 1000 g x 0.1 = 100 ml

Daily maintenance requirements = 100 ml/kg/day

Give 150 ml in first 24 hours (maintenance plus half deficit) and 150 ml over next 24 hours

Can be divided into 5 x 30 ml boluses given every 5 hours throughout the 24 hour period, or given as a continuous infusion at 6 ml/hr (150 ml divided by 24 hours)

In clinically shocked (**hypovolaemic**) birds, intravenous fluid boluses of isotonic crystalloid fluids of at least 10–30 ml/kg should be used, ideally administered over a 5–10-minute period, followed by clinical reassessment and repeat administration as necessary up to a total maximum volume of 90 ml/kg/hr. Use of intravenous colloids at a rate of 5–10 ml/kg as a slow intravenous bolus, followed by maintenance crystalloid fluid therapy (10 ml/kg bolus) is an alternative approach and may reduce the risk of hypervolaemia.

Mammals

As in birds, the **maintenance fluid requirements** for mammals vary with the body mass of the animal: it is lower for larger animals and higher for smaller ones (Kirkwood, 1983b), increasing considerably in very small animals. For larger mammals (e.g. deer, fox, badger, otter (*Lutra lutra*)), maintenance requirements are usually assumed to be similar to dogs and cats (50 ml/kg/24h). For smaller mammals, larger volumes are required; for example, in domestic rabbits, maintenance requirements are considered to be 100 ml/kg/24h. For practical reasons, as in birds, an assumption can be made of 10–15% dehydration on presentation (see example calculation above). Once again, good clinical assessment and repeated reassessment is key to ensuring that rehydration is successful.

In **hypovolaemic** patients, boluses of isotonic crystalloid products at rates of 10–20 ml/kg should be administered and the animal reassessed after 30 minutes; boluses are repeated as necessary up to a maximum volume of 60–90 ml/kg/hr. 'Shock' boluses of colloid products at rates of 10–20 ml/kg can be used as an alternative to rapid-rate boluses of crystalloids. These products, particularly those with a longer half-life, are especially useful where the animal is unlikely to tolerate the maintenance of an intravenous line for very long. If intravenous lines can be maintained, crystalloid fluid therapy should be used in all cases; alternative routes of fluid therapy may also be employed (see above).

Provision of nutritional support

Many small animals have a high metabolic rate and once dehydration and hypovolaemia have been corrected, appropriate 'energy', usually in the form of fluids containing glucose (see 'Fluid therapy') or more ideally appropriate food and water, must be provided. The daily energy requirements vary with the bodyweight of the animal. Larger birds can survive without food for many days; for example, common buzzards (1100 g) (*Buteo buteo*) might lose 15% of their bodyweight after 7 days of starvation, whilst the smaller common kestrels (250 g) (*Falco tinnunculus*) might lose 12% of their bodyweight in only 3 days of starvation (Kirkwood, 1981). Small passerines such as blue tits (*Cyanistes caeruleus*) may not survive for more than 48–72 hours without food (Perrins, 1979), and this is also the case in many small mammals.

A diet should be provided that most closely resembles the wild diet of the casualty as this will be most readily accepted and is less likely to result in gastrointestinal upset. In the short term, clinical recovery diets (e.g. Reanimyl®; Hill's Prescription Diet a/d®) can be used in most mammalian carnivorous species. There are several commercially available 'exotic pet' recovery diets that may be administered initially by crop tube to birds and by syringe or free access to mammals: these include Harrison's Recovery Formula® (birds), Vetark Critical Care Formula® (all species), Oxbow Carnivore Critical Care Formula® (carnivores), Oxbow Critical Care Formula® (herbivores) and Lafeber's Emeraid® Nutritional Care system (avian and mammalian, omnivore, carnivore, herbivore and piscivore formulations).

Enteral feeding requirements should ideally be calculated based on the individual animal's calorific requirement and divided into two to four feeds per day. Most manufacturers of recovery diets provide information about the calorific content of the diet. However, the following formula can also be used (after Kirkwood, 1991) to calculate resting energy rate (RER):

Resting energy rate (RER) kcal/day = K x BWt$^{0.75}$

K = kcal/kg/day constant (placental mammal = 70, non-passerine bird = 78, passerine bird = 129)
BWt = bodyweight (kg)

RER is the amount of energy required for maintaining homeostasis whilst the animal rests quietly in a stress-free, non-fasted, thermoneutral environment. Once the casualty is exercising normally, maintenance energy requirements (MER) (approximately 1.5 x RER) should be provided.

Neonates require special feeding and this is discussed in Chapter 8. For more information on feeding adult casualties in captivity, see Chapter 7 and the species-specific chapters.

Maintenance of optimal temperature

Many casualties, especially those that are debilitated, will be hypothermic. All mammalian and avian casualties benefit from being kept at an environmental temperature that lies within their thermoneutral range (the range of environmental temperatures within which an animal needs to expend no energy, in addition to its maintenance requirements, to maintain a stable body temperature) (Figure 5.12). For most mammals, this is 15–24°C. For birds, the optimal temperature varies with their body mass. Reptiles and amphibians are ectothermic ('cold-blooded'). There is a range of natural temperatures known as the **activity temperature range** (ATR; this term may also be referred to as the Preferred Optimal Temperature Zone (POTZ), but ATR is preferred as it is less anthropomorphic and does not convey a sense of choice), within which the reptile can thermoregulate and actively control its body

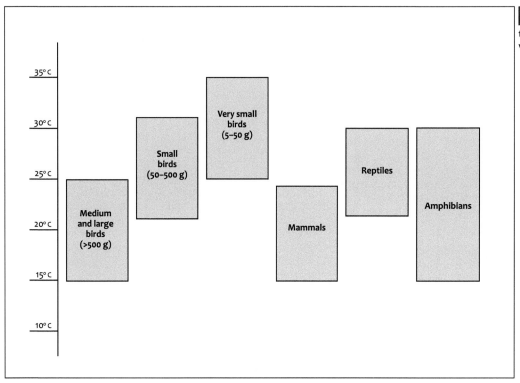

5.12 Thermoneutral ranges and activity temperature ranges for British wild animals.

temperature. At extremes of temperature, the reptile is unable to do this and the critical maximum and minimum temperatures define this. For most British reptiles, the ATR is 22–30°C and for amphibians, 15–30°C.

A range of thermometers and thermal probes are available and less invasive techniques for recording body temperature may be useful in wildlife casualties, such as infrared laser thermometry. Cetaceans require specialist equipment for this procedure (see Chapter 23). Reference ranges for normal body temperature in British wildlife species are given in Figure 5.13.

Species	Body temperature °C (°F)
Hedgehogs[e]	35.4–37 (95.7–98.6)
Other small mammals[e]	36.5–38.5 (97.7–101)
Rabbits and hares	38.5–40 (101–104)
Wildcats	37.5–39.2 (99.5–102.5)
Badgers[b]	36–38 (96.8–100.4)
Otters[c]	35.9–40.4 (96.6–104.7)
Small mustelids[e]	37.8–40 (100–104)
Foxes[d]	39–40.5 (102–104.9)
Deer[a]	38.6–39.3 (101.5–102.7)
Seals	36–38.5 (96.8–101.3)
Cetaceans	36–37.5 (96.8–97.7)
Birds	41–44 (105.8–111.2)

5.13 Reference ranges for normal body temperature in common British non-poikilothermic wildlife species.

Note: Temperature will be influenced by environmental temperature, time of year, stress during capture and clinical condition; these effects will frequently be more significant than in comparable domestic species.

([a]Demaris et al., 1986; [b]Bevanger and Brøseth, 1998; [c]Kruuk et al., 2009; [d]Kreeger et al., 1989; [e]Carpenter, 2013 (based upon similar domestic species). For additional sources of information, see the species-specific chapters.)

The first stage of treating hypothermia is to prevent further loss of heat by wrapping the casualty in insulating materials such as blankets, bubble wrap or silver foil. Fluid therapy should be provided (with warmed fluids) and then the patient should be slowly warmed to its optimal temperature. All the usual warming methods used in small animal practice can be used with wildlife casualties, provided damage to equipment and iatrogenic trauma to the casualty can be avoided.

- Hot water bottles and microwave-heated plastic or wheat/cherry stone/grain bags may be useful as a temporary source of heat in an emergency, but their use needs to be closely monitored: they cool rapidly and can then draw warmth from the patient. Many of these heat sources are also easily chewed.
- Electric heat pads are helpful for immobile mammals but, with some types, need to be covered to prevent the risk of overheating (or even burning) of the animal through direct contact with the pad; the pads may also need protection to prevent damage from being chewed. They are of limited use in smaller animals as many are activated by the weight of the animal on the pad.
- Water-circulating heat mats can be thermostatically controlled and used in patients of all sizes.
- Heat lamps and electric heaters can be suspended within walk-in pens, or over cages, or attached to the outside of smaller cages. They are ideal for mobile

patients, as they create a heat gradient that allows the animal to select its preferred temperature. Care must be taken when positioning a heat lamp to ensure that the patient is not overheated and cannot entangle itself in any wires. Some heat lamps can be controlled with a thermostat. These forms of heating can cause desiccation of wounds.
- Hospital cages, incubators and brooders, with built-in thermostatically controlled heating, are commercially available and are suitable for small mammals and small to medium-sized birds.
- Warm air blanket systems (e.g. Bair Hugger®; Figure 5.14).
- Heaters and fans to maintain general room temperature.

With all forms of heated accommodation, the provision of a thermometer (preferably a maximum/minimum one) to measure the temperature within the immediate environment of the patient is valuable. Where possible the body temperature (see Figure 5.13) of the patient should also be recorded on a regular basis.

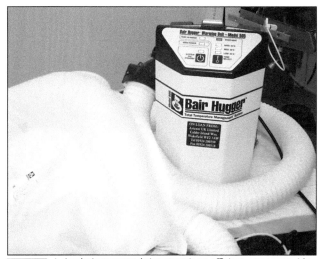

5.14 A circulating warmed air system is an efficient way to provide supplementary warmth.

(Reproduced from the BSAVA Textbook of Veterinary Nursing, 5th edition)

Emergency medication

Analgesia

The provision of pain relief is an essential part of first aid for an injured casualty. Analgesics increase the comfort of the casualty, reduce the amount of stress suffered by the animal, reduce self-trauma and improve recovery time. Analgesics are discussed in Chapter 6. Emergency analgesic drugs are summarized in Figure 5.15. In general, the same classes of analgesic drugs that are used in domestic animals can be used in wildlife medicine and doses are extrapolated from domestic species.

Corticosteroids

In the past, corticosteroids were used in first aid in both people and animals to treat shock. In human medicine and domestic small animal medicine, this has largely stopped apart from in the very small number of cases where steroid use is appropriate.

Drug	Species									
	Hedgehogs	Other small mammals	Rabbits and hares	Wild cats	Badgers, otters and foxes	Deer	Seals	Cetaceans	Birds[a]	Reptiles
Non-steroidal anti-inflammatory drugs (NSAIDs)										
Meloxicam	0.5 mg/kg s.c.	0.5–2 mg/kg s.c.	0.3–0.6 mg/kg s.c.	0.2 mg/kg s.c.	0.2 mg/kg s.c.	0.5 mg/kg i.v., s.c.	0.1 mg/kg i.m.	0.2 mg/kg i.m.	0.5–2 mg/kg i.m., orally	0.1–0.5 mg/kg i.m.
Carprofen	5–10 mg/kg i.v., i.m., s.c.	2–5 mg/kg i.v., i.m., s.c.	2–4 mg/kg s.c.	4 mg/kg i.v., s.c.	4 mg/kg i.v., s.c.	1 mg/kg i.v., s.c.	4 mg/kg i.m.	4 mg/kg i.m., orally	1–5 mg/kg i.v., i.m., s.c.	1–4 mg/kg i.m., s.c.
Ketoprofen	4 mg/kg i.v., i.m., s.c.	1–3 mg/kg i.m., s.c.	1–3 mg/kg i.m., s.c.	2 mg/kg i.v., i.m., s.c.	2 mg/kg i.v., i.m., s.c.	3 mg/kg i.v., i.m.	1 mg/kg i.m.	Not suggested for use in these species	1–5 mg/kg i.m.	Not suggested for use in these species
Flunixin	Not suggested for use in this species	Not suggested for use in these species	Not suggested for use in these species	Not suggested for use in this species	Not suggested for use in these species	2 mg/kg i.v.	Not suggested for use in these species	1 mg/kg i.v., i.m.	Not suggested for use in these species	Not suggested for use in these species
Opioid drugs										
Morphine	Not suggested for use in this species	2–5 mg/kg i.m., s.c.	2–5 mg/kg i.m., s.c.	0.1–0.4 mg/kg i.v., i.m.	0.5 mg/kg i.v., i.m.	Not suggested for use in these species	Not suggested for use in these species	Not suggested for use in these species	Not suggested for use in these species	1–4 mg/kg i.m.[b]
Buprenorphine	0.02–0.05 mg/kg i.v., i.m., s.c.	0.05 mg/kg i.m., s.c.	0.01–0.05 mg/kg i.v., i.m., s.c.	0.02 mg/kg i.v., i.m., s.c.	0.02 mg/kg i.v., i.m., s.c.	Not suggested for use in these species	0.01–0.02 mg/kg i.m.	Not suggested for use in these species	0.01–0.05 mg/kg i.v., i.m.	0.01–0.02 mg/kg i.m.[c]
Butorphanol	0.2–0.4 mg/kg s.c.	2 mg/kg s.c.	0.1–0.5 mg/kg s.c.	0.2–0.5 mg/kg i.v., i.m., s.c.	0.2–0.5 mg/kg i.v., i.m., s.c.	Not suggested for use in these species	0.2 mg/kg i.m.	Not suggested for use in these species	0.5–4 mg/kg i.v., i.m.	0.5–2.0 mg/kg i.m.[c]

5.15 Emergency analgesic drugs for use in wildlife. Note: Drugs are not licensed for use in wildlife species but, where possible, drugs that are licensed in 'similar' domestic species are suggested (Carpenter, 2013; Ramsey, 2014). For additional sources of data relating to dose, suggested frequency and duration of administration, see the individual species chapters and Chapter 6. Doses are for initial administration via parenteral routes for emergency and preoperative use; drugs may also be used orally in some species as outlined in the species-specific chapters. Where appropriate, multimodal analgesia should be used (e.g. NSAID plus opioid). Other drugs used for sedation and anaesthesia also have analgesic properties (see Chapter 6). [a] In birds, the higher end of the dose range should be chosen in the small species and the lower end of the dose range in the larger species. [b] May not be effective in snakes. Morphine is suggested at doses of 1–4 mg/kg (Meredith, 2015), although higher doses (1–10 mg/kg) have also been suggested (Sladky, 2014). Higher doses may cause significant respiratory depression. [c] Butorphanol and buprenorphine have been shown to have no effect in some species, even at higher doses (Sladky and Mans, 2012).

Evidence in humans, dogs and cats (Cornin *et al.*, 1995; Dewey, 2000; Adamantos and Corr, 2007) has shown:

- There are no benefits to steroid use in shock
- Mortality rates are higher where steroids are used
- In central nervous system (CNS) trauma, prognosis is worse in almost all cases where steroids are used
- Fluid therapy is key to treating shock and CNS trauma by correcting hypovolaemia and maintaining tissue perfusion.

Despite this strong evidence base, there still appears to be excessive steroid usage in some areas of wildlife medicine. As well as the reasoning above, steroid usage is additionally not recommended in wildlife because:

- The immunosuppressive effects of corticosteroids are likely to be magnified by the effects of stress due to captivity
- Captivity may expose wildlife casualties to novel infections
- Shedding of certain infectious agents (e.g. salmonellae, mycobacteria) are increased in immunosuppressed people and animals. This may result in problems for not only the individual casualty, but also for the staff handling the animal and the veterinary practice and/or wildlife centre
- Steroid usage limits the subsequent use of non-steroidal anti-inflammatory drugs for analgesia (see Chapter 6) and increases the risk of gut, liver and renal compromise.

Antibacterial agents

In common with their use in other species, antibacterial drugs should only be administered to wildlife casualties where there is a clear indication for their use and ideally where causal agents and antibiotic sensitivity can be established (see Chapters 7 and 10). The excessive use of antibacterials by some wildlife centres must be strongly discouraged. In an emergency situation, antibacterials (preferably broad-spectrum intravenous drugs) should be administered as part of first aid treatment where there is evidence of a penetrating injury, the patient is febrile and/or blood samples suggest infection.

Management of traumatic injuries

The majority of injuries sustained by wildlife in the UK are caused either by human activity, as a result of attack by predators, or from conspecifics in territorial disputes. Many of these are considered in more detail in the species-specific chapters.

Soft tissue injuries

Wildlife casualties frequently suffer from wounding as a result of, for example, road traffic accidents, collisions with power lines or windows, entrapment in netting, and firearm and trapping injuries. Wounds originating from such incidents may include abrasions, avulsions, lacerations, burns (both chemical and thermal), contusions, crushing injuries, penetrating and puncture wounds and gunshot wounds. The medical management of these differs little from that in domestic species; however, the practical management of wounds in wildlife may require some degree of ingenuity.

Wound evaluation

Careful evaluation of wounds is necessary to understand the extent of damage present and this should be part of the triage process (see Chapter 4). Recent burns should be especially carefully evaluated as they are often more extensive than they appear and may change over subsequent days. Injury from snares and power cables may also suffer delayed ischaemic necrosis and this should be considered both in triage and prior to any excessive debridement and treatment.

Wound management

Cleaning and preparation: Analgesia should be used appropriately for all patients prior to wound care, even in emergency situations and regardless of the requirement for general anaesthesia. Haemostasis should be achieved using direct pressure. Using an aseptic technique where possible, a water-soluble gel (e.g. Intrasite®) should be applied to the wound before hair or feather removal to prevent further contamination. A minimal amount of hair should be clipped or feathers plucked, as if this is excessive it may delay the ultimate release of the casualty. A large volume of fluid should be used to flush and clean the wound thoroughly. The use of warmed fluid helps prevent excessive cooling of small patients, although attention should still be given to heat loss (see 'Maintenance of optimal temperature'). Sterile phosphate-buffered saline or lactated Ringer's solution are both suitable for use in wounds in all species. A 0.05% solution of chlorhexidine (1 in 40 dilution of most products) may be used as an alternative in all species, except amphibians.

Treatment: Many simple soft tissue injuries, such as abrasions from entangled netting, may require only first aid and topical treatment. For more severe wounds, standard procedures of management (i.e. debridement, drainage and closure) are appropriate; ideally, subsequent nursing should involve minimal handling. If wounds are surgically closed, monofilament absorbable sutures and an intradermal suture pattern should be used. Closure of wounds may not be possible or appropriate as bacterial contamination is commonly evident on initial examination; topical dressings and bandages may be more appropriate, but will require subsequent nursing care.

Dressings and bandages: Wound dressings can be applied using the same products and techniques as in other species. Movement and self-trauma following dressing application may be an increased problem in wildlife compared to most domestic species. Well managed dressings and bandages reduce pain (less friction) and speed wound healing by preventing further contamination and desiccation, whilst at the same time aiding debridement and reducing bacterial proliferation. Badly managed dressings are however, in most cases, worse than no dressing at all.

Keeping dressings as small and light as possible is essential especially in small mammals and birds. Topical wound products such as hydrocolloid gels (e.g. Intrasite®), silver products (e.g. Flamazine®) and more novel products such as sterile honey, can all be used in wildlife casualties. In some instances topical cleaning followed by application of these products is adequate with no need for bandaging. Adhesive dressings (e.g. Allevyn® Thin; Opsite® Flexigrid®) are especially useful in this role. Suture loops, into skin or around feathers, may also be used to hold in place primary dressing layers, reducing the need for heavy secondary and tertiary layers. Care must be taken with adhesive tape, especially in birds, where the adhesive may damage feathers. In birds, dressings are best held in place using cohesive bandages or medical tape (e.g. Leukoplast® Sleek®) the adhesive of which will not damage the plumage.

Consideration must be given to how frequently dressings will need to be changed, especially if general anaesthesia or sedation is needed. This will have both welfare and cost implications and these should be established at the triage stage (see Chapter 4). Dressings must not be left on too long as a compromise to avoid frequent changes; a wound care plan involving leaving the wound open may be preferred in these cases, or alternatively euthanasia may be considered.

Self-trauma to wounds or interference with dressings may be controlled with collars or muzzles. Some birds will tolerate either Elizabethan collars, made to measure from plastic sheeting or radiographic film, or available commercially, or neck braces, made from lengths of plastic-foam water-pipe cladding. Such collars and braces can be very stressful and should be used only in wild birds in exceptional circumstances and tolerant individuals. Most mammals tolerate Elizabethan collars poorly, but they may be useful in some individuals.

Orthopaedic injuries

Fractures of long bones, especially wing bones in birds, are very common disabilities and present many problems with their management and treatment. Assessment of the significance of a fracture requires an accurate diagnosis of its site and nature, the extent of soft tissue damage and the risk of infection. Deciding the general suitability of an individual case for treatment is discussed in Chapter 4; considerations relating directly to fractures are summarized in Figure 5.16. Postoperative rehabilitation, including adequate facilities for a full return to fitness, must be provided (see Chapter 9).

Fractures of long bones require some form of immediate immobilization of the fracture or patient to minimize further soft tissue damage. The emergency care of these fractures is detailed below. Fractures may often be associated with other injuries (see 'Thoracic and abdominal injuries') and care must be taken to attend to such potentially life-threatening damage as well.

Consideration	Comments
Species and ecology	• Many predatory species (e.g. raptors) rely on speed and agility to hunt and must have a fully functional musculoskeletal system to do this; any persistent abnormality of the axial skeleton or limbs will prejudice this • Many prey species (e.g. lagomorphs) rely on speed to escape predators and require a fully functional skeletal system to do this • Small mammals such as hedgehogs or a small species of waterfowl may survive adequately in the wild with a less than perfectly functioning limb; however, the possibility of chronic pain should be considered
Age of animal	• Young animals generally heal more quickly than older animals • Young animals may need a period of time in captivity for rearing so a healing fracture will not necessarily delay release • Young animals appear to tolerate dressings, external fixators, etc. better than adult animals • Adult animals may need a prolonged period of hospitalization for fracture healing and this may not be possible for territorial or seasonal reasons
Sex of animal	• Poorly aligned fractures of the limbs and pelvis may affect copulation or result in dystocia
Site of fracture	• Uncomplicated fractures of some bones may heal spontaneously, requiring only restricted activity (e.g. fractured digits and ribs, some coracoid fractures in birds) • Other fractures may require only minimal support (e.g. fractures of the avian ulna with an intact radius (see Figure 5.17a), fractures of distal limb bones in passerine fledglings (see Figure 5.18), or small immature rodents) • Fractures of limb bones require the greatest care with assessment and repair as these fractures are most significant • The prognosis is generally better with a mid-shaft fracture than one adjacent to a joint • Surgical fixation is often simpler in a long bone with a straight shaft than one with a curved shape, notably the 'S'-shaped avian humerus • Beak and jaw fractures need to heal with good alignment to allow normal feeding, preening and defending of territory
Type of fracture (e.g. open/closed, simple/comminuted)	• Simple closed fractures present no additional complications • In wildlife casualties the fractures are frequently old, comminuted, open and infected • Fractures of the limb bones in birds, especially the pneumatized bones (the humerus and, in some species, the femur), frequently involve shattering of the cortex, producing a severely comminuted fracture that is often beyond satisfactory repair • Many fractures (especially those in birds described above) have extensive soft tissue damage, carrying a poor prognosis
Type of fracture repair required	• Techniques for fixation must be carefully and appropriately selected • The techniques used should be chosen so as to ensure the best prognosis in the shortest possible time • Some species (such as foxes) commonly interfere with dressings and external fixators • Most birds appear to tolerate dressings and external fixators well • Ideally all metal implants should be removed before the casualty is released
Complications of fracture repair	• Nonunion • Malunion • Infection (especially with compound fractures) • Avascular bone sequestra (especially in comminuted fractures in birds) • Callus formation interfering with soft tissue (especially in birds) • Ankylosis of joints (especially in birds)
Time in captivity	• Fractures in small birds heal quickly, usually within 10–14 days • Fractures in small mammals typically heal within 20–30 days • Fractures in the larger mammals (badgers, foxes) typically take at least 4–6 weeks to heal • Animals should not be released until fully fit and this will take additional time (see Chapter 9)
Skills and costs	• Good surgical skills must be ensured • Good surgical facilities must be available • Financial support must be available for both equipment and professional time

5.16 Considerations when assessing wildlife fracture cases. Both general triage of the casualty (see Chapter 4) and the availability of suitable postoperative rehabilitation facilities to allow the casualty to return to full fitness (see Chapter 9) must also be considered.

Following stabilization of the patient, general anaesthesia is required to more fully assess the fracture site, with the use of multiple radiographic views, including the joints proximal and distal to the fracture site. The orthopaedic techniques used in wild mammals and birds are not different to those used in similar domestic species, provided specific considerations are observed (Figure 5.16). Some specific techniques applicable to avian casualties are outlined in Chapter 29.

Emergency care of wing fractures in birds

Immobilization of the fractured wing is imperative, especially in cases involving the humerus. This bone is pneumatized (the medulla contains an extension of an air sac) with thin cortices, and a fracture invariably results in the formation of long sharp fragments of bone that may puncture the skin and cause soft tissue damage as the bird flaps its injured wing. Immobilization of the wing must take place as soon as possible. Depending on the site and nature of the fracture, which can often be assessed by the wing position (see Figure 4.4), various emergency bandaging methods can be employed:

• Fractures of the manus or fractures of either the radius or ulna alone may need only simple support of the wing by using medical tape (e.g. Leukoplast® Sleek®) to tape together the primaries of the closed wing (Figure 5.17a)
• Fractures of the radius and the ulna can be supported with a 'figure-of-eight' dressing, using a conforming bandage, which will hold the ulna and radius against the humerus for support (Figure 5.17b). The carpal and elbow joints are flexed but the shoulder maintains movement and the other wing is left free

- Fractures of the humerus must be held against the body to give temporary immobilization and this can be achieved with a 'figure-of-eight' dressing, again using a conforming bandage that includes the body but leaves the opposite wing free (Figure 5.17c). Care should be taken that this is not so tight that it impedes movement of the sternum for normal respiration
- Fractures of the bones of the pectoral girdle, commonly the coracoid, may result in a wing that is tilted or 'dropped' (see Figure 4.4). Suitable bandaging, as above, should be employed to hold the wing in a normal position and prevent further trauma.

It should be noted that these techniques are for emergency immobilization of the wing and such dressings should not be left in place for more than 2–3 days initially, as the joints of the avian wing stiffen when held in flexion. It is unusual to need to strap wings for more than a total time of 7–10 days, with regular (every 2–3 days) bandage changes and wing manipulation to ensure joint mobility.

Protection of wing and tail feathers in birds, especially birds of prey, is a key part of their management in captivity and is discussed in Chapter 29.

Emergency care of leg fractures in birds

Fractures of the leg in birds must be immobilized temporarily to prevent further damage prior to fixation, especially in active larger birds that are free to jump and struggle inside an inappropriate container.

- Fractures of the tarsometatarsus in larger birds can be splinted using suitable rigid materials held with tape. In passerines, the use of an Altman splint formed from medical or masking tape, to include the intertarsal joint, is tolerated extremely well (Figure 5.18).
- Fractures of the tibiotarsus in larger species can be supported with Robert Jones dressings. Femoral fractures are usually well supported by the surrounding muscle mass, although strapping of the leg to the body will offer additional short-term support.
- Fractures of the toes in perching birds can be immobilized using a 'ball' bandage made by placing a firm ball of cotton wool within the grasp of the foot and taping the toes to the ball with conforming tape (Figure 5.19).

Emergency care of limb fractures in mammals

In mammals, fractures are usually best left unsupported at the first aid stage because:

- Good splinting and bandaging is usually impossible without sedation or general anaesthesia and these should not be carried out until the patient is stable
- Few fractures suffer further trauma provided the patient is kept restricted and as undisturbed as possible. Small boxes, cages, tea chests, etc. are suitable for this purpose
- Incorrect splinting is as likely to make things worse as better, e.g. forcing bone through soft tissue and making a closed fracture open.

If immobilization is required, then the standard methods used in domestic species are employed: modified Robert Jones dressing or splinted bandages, applied in a sedated or anaesthetized animal. In many cases, if the casualty and fracture is considered suitable, then rapidly proceeding to surgical fixation is preferred.

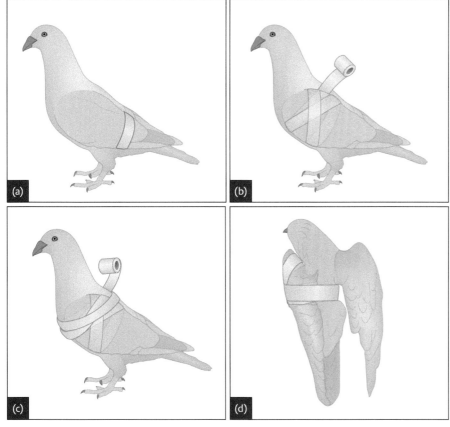

5.17 Wing bandaging technique. (a) Medical tape can be used to hold the primary feathers to the tertiary feathers in a closed wing. This is suitable for fractures of the manus or simple fractures of the radius or ulna alone. (b) Conforming bandage can be used to produce a 'figure-of-eight' dressing to support fractures of the radius and ulna. The radius and ulna are held against the humerus, the carpal and elbow joints are held flexed but the shoulder maintains movement. The wing is not strapped to the body and the opposite wing remains free. (c) Conforming bandage can also be used to produce a 'figure-of-eight' dressing to support the humerus. In this case the body of the bird is included in the dressing to restrict movement at the shoulder as well as the elbow and carpus. Care should be taken not to make the dressing too tight and so impede normal respiration. (d) The opposite wing remains free. In all cases strapping should be removed and the wing reassessed after 2–3 days in order to help prevent the risk of joint stiffness.

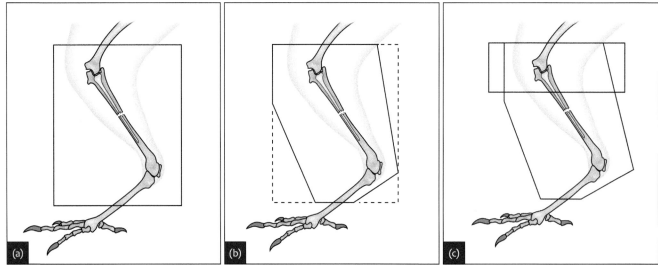

5.18 Altman splint. (a) Two pieces of medical or masking tape are applied either side of the leg and pressed firmly together to form the splint. For effective immobilization, the resulting splint must include as much as possible of the limb above and below the fracture site. (b) Excess tape is cut away from the splint to reduce size and weight. The splint is very well tolerated by most patients. (c) Pieces of tape can be added to the splint around the stifle joint to give added stability. Simple fractures will have formed a callus and immobilized themselves within 2–3 weeks, after which the splint can be removed to allow the bird to regain limb function.

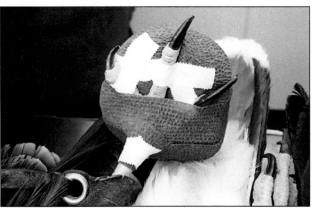

5.19 'Ball bandage' of foot used to immobilize the toes of a raptor. (© Kevin Eatwell)

Traumatic thoracic and abdominal injuries

Birds

The most common reason for thoracic and abdominal injuries in small birds and mammals, as well as some reptiles and amphibians, is cat predation (Woods *et al.*, 2003). Penetrating cat injuries are often much more extensive than external examination may suggest and are frequently contaminated with *Pasteurella multocida* (Müldorfer *et al.*, 2011) and other bacteria. Fluid therapy, broad-spectrum systemic antibacterials, analgesia and treatment of dyspnoea, as well as wound management, as previously described, are all required in these cases. In cases with extensive damage, euthanasia is indicated.

Thoracic and abdominal trauma may also occur in birds as a result of collision with vehicles or windows. Injuries are more severe in larger birds and may be accompanied by fractures of long bones (vehicle collisions) and coracoids and clavicles (window collisions) (Cousins *et al.*, 2012). Air sacs may suffer blunt trauma and/or penetration by bone fragments in these cases. Birds may present with dyspnoea and blood may be evident at the glottis, which is associated with fractures of pneumatized bones. Head trauma is also commonly associated with these collisions and a full neurological examination should be carried out.

An ophthalmological examination should be performed to rule out intraocular haemorrhage (see 'Ocular trauma'). Supportive treatment (as above) including fracture support (and potentially repair) is indicated.

Mammals

Small mammals frequently present with thoracic and abdominal injuries from cat predation, as described in birds. In larger mammals, thoracic and abdominal trauma is usually associated with road traffic collisions or gunshot wounds and sometimes with snares. Careful assessment of the casualty for other injuries and general suitability for release must be made before surgery is carried out (see Chapter 4). Good surgical skills and time will be required and some expense incurred; if these are not available, euthanasia is the preferred option. Consideration should be given to the potential zoonotic infection risks of surgical procedures (e.g. mycobacteria).

Thoracic injuries in mammals: Mammalian casualties may present with a range of traumatic thoracic injuries similar to those seen in domestic species. These commonly include rupture of the diaphragm, lung contusions, pneumothorax and haemothorax. These can be confirmed using a combination of radiography, ultrasonography and chest drainage. Drainage of air from the chest cavity can easily be carried out under appropriate sedation and/or local anaesthesia using a needle, syringe and three-way tap or an appropriately sized chest drain. Most species will not tolerate chest drains left *in situ* and any cases requiring repeated drainage are best euthanased. Diaphragmatic ruptures may be repaired in the standard way in mammals that are large enough to be ventilated during surgery (e.g. foxes and badgers). The chest should be drained, as previously described, at the end of surgery.

Abdominal injuries in mammals: Common traumatic abdominal injuries in mammals are abdominal wall rupture (with or without prolapse of abdominal contents through the skin) and haemoperitoneum. Animals with prolapsed abdominal contents require immediate first aid (protection of the prolapsed material, analgesics, systemic antibiosis and fluids), followed by general anaesthesia and surgery.

The abdominal wound should be opened to allow examination of all the structures involved. If there is any chance of loss of tissue vitality or contamination with gut contents or external debris, the patient should be euthanased. Bleeding into the abdomen can be diagnosed from radiographs, ultrasonography and a peritoneal tap. Abdominal wrapping may be used to control bleeding in some cases; however, this does not allow for assessment of abdominal contents for future release. Where bleeding is significant, therefore, patients should be stabilized and exploratory surgery performed. Bleeding from minor organs can be surgically controlled. Euthanasia is preferred where there is damage to vital organs. Splenectomy in wild mammals is easily performed but has unknown long-term immunological consequences.

Ocular trauma

Eye abnormalities or trauma can be a significant influencing factor in triage decisions in wildlife casualties (see Chapter 4). It is especially important, and difficult, to examine the eyes of raptors and this is discussed further in Chapter 29. Seals (Phocidae) have especially vulnerable eyes requiring protection (see Chapter 23). Eyes should be examined fully and very carefully in all animals, which may require sedation. In the short term, the eyes of mammals and birds should be protected using an ocular lubricant. The decision to enucleate an eye (or leave an animal blind in one eye) is dependent upon species-specific ecology and more information is given in the chapters that follow. An animal with vision compromised in both eyes should be euthanased.

Poisoning

Generally, wild animals have an innate ability to avoid most natural toxic substances, due to the evolution of selective feeding habits; however, they cannot avoid toxins introduced accidentally or intentionally into their environment by human activity. Individual animals may be affected or large groups involved. Where criminal activity is suspected and/or environmental damage has taken place, this should be reported to the appropriate authorities (see Chapters 2 and 11).

Classification of wildlife poisoning

Poisoning incidents in wildlife can be classified as follows:

- **Natural** toxins are released by naturally occurring microorganisms, such as *Clostridium botulinum* (botulism) (see Chapter 26), blue-green algae, dinoflagellates ('red tides') (see Chapter 24), mycotoxins (fungi) and venom from higher vertebrates and invertebrates
- **Accidental** poisoning involves spillage, mishandling or poor storage of pesticides, herbicides and rodenticides; industrial and marine accidents leading to pollution (see Chapter 24).
- **Intentional** poisoning can be associated with legitimate use in controlled pest control schemes (e.g. anticoagulant rodenticides, see Chapters 12 and 14) and illegitimate use (e.g. carbamate insecticides) (see Chapter 29), mostly in attempts to destroy (protected) predators on shooting estates or destructive pest species. See also Chapter 11 for information on common toxic agents used in intentional wildlife poisoning cases.

Diagnosis of poisoning

A diagnosis of poisoning is difficult even in a domestic animal situation, where clinical signs of intoxication may be correlated with changes in environment or exposure to chemicals, medications, known household toxins, etc. In wildlife, where history is unknown and there are often rapidly dying casualties, diagnosis can be almost impossible. Often immediate assistance is limited to symptomatic and supportive treatment of the less severely affected cases and euthanasia of the hopeless ones. An accurate diagnosis of poisoning requires the following:

- A suggestive history – for example, several dead raptors, crows (Corvidae) or foxes found in the same vicinity might indicate the illegal use of pesticides
- Suggestive clinical signs – for example, dead or paralysed waterfowl on a shallow pond during hot weather might suggest botulism
- Detection of the toxic agent – for example, elevated blood lead levels and/or radiographic evidence of lead in the gizzard of a mute swan showing weakness and loss of weight
- Specific pathological signs at post-mortem examination and/or detection of the toxin in tissue samples post-mortem (see Chapters 10 and 11).

Treatment of poisoning

Acute poisoning is always an emergency, with no time to wait for laboratory investigations. Treatment can be considered in three stages:

1. Prevent further absorption of the poison.
2. Treat acute clinical signs and provide supportive care.
3. Give specific antidotes.

Prevention of further absorption

Most poisons that are likely to affect wildlife are taken by mouth, either through direct ingestion of the toxin or secondary to grooming a contaminated pelage. Prevention of further absorption requires removal from the alimentary canal, which in cases treated early, means removal from the stomach of mammals and the crop or proventriculus/ventriculus of birds. However, more often than not, by the time a casualty has been captured, any ingested material will have already moved from the stomach into the small intestines, where it is absorbed.

Topical decontamination: In casualties with chemical or oil pollution of the coat or plumage, it is important to remove as much of the contaminant as possible to prevent local damage to the skin and to minimize the amount swallowed when the animal licks or preens itself. Paper towels are often best used in the first instance to brush or wipe away excessive contamination. Water-soluble products are most easily removed using a good quality household washing-up liquid. Oil-based products can also be removed using washing-up liquid. Vegetable-based margarine has also been suggested as a useful degreasing product prior to using washing-up liquid in bats (see Chapter 15). Special attention should be given to removing contamination from the eyes and other orifices. Eyes should be further protected using an ocular lubricant. See Chapter 24 for more information on treatment of oiling in seabirds.

Emetics: In mammals that can vomit (i.e. carnivores and omnivores with a simple single stomach), the use of oral emetics (syrup of ipecacuanha, 3% hydrogen peroxide, washing soda (sodium carbonate) crystals) or parenteral emetics (apomorphine) may be helpful in the first few hours following ingestion. Doses of emetics should be extrapolated from a small animal formulary. The benefits of emesis should be considered alongside the possible detriments (further fluid loss, dangers of inhalation of vomit) and the clinical condition of the animal before emetics are used. Irrigation of the stomach under sedation or general anaesthesia is an alternative to the use of emetics and may be more appropriate in many cases.

Crop washing: In birds with a full crop it is possible, with care, to manipulate and expel the contents through the mouth in a conscious patient. Take care that the bird does not aspirate during this process or become dyspnoeic as crop material compresses the trachea/glottis as it is expelled. The crop and proventriculus can be irrigated, preferably in an anaesthetized and intubated bird, using a wide-bore rubber or plastic tube (as wide a tube as possible) passed down the oesophagus. Warm water is repeatedly run in through the tube, agitated and then removed by lowering the bird's head to allow it to run out by gravity.

Adsorbents and cathartics: Once a poison has entered the small intestine, it is possible to attempt to limit further absorption into the body by the use of adsorbents and cathartics. The use of adsorbents may be as useful as gastric evacuation in mild to moderate poisoning. Activated charcoal is the most commonly used adsorbent in small animal practice and is therefore likely to be the most easily available for treatment of wildlife. Kaolin (natural aluminium silicate as a very fine powder) and bismuth salts are also used as adsorbents. Fuller's earth (bentonite clay) is used as a specific binding agent for paraquat and diquat poisoning.

Cathartics increase the elimination of toxins via the gut. Several cathartics are available containing sodium or magnesium sulphate or sorbitol. These are given orally, usually on a single occasion to prevent side effects, and may be combined with activated charcoal.

In wildlife casualties, the practical administration of oral adsorbents and cathartics can be very difficult. Birds can be gavaged (see 'Fluid administration in birds') and mammals syringed, or the medications mixed into food. In many cases, the clinical condition of the animal makes any form of oral dosing impossible.

Lipophilic toxins (e.g. avermectins) can be treated using intravenous lipid infusions (e.g. Intralipid®). Although there is information regarding the use of these products in dogs and cats, the authors are unaware of them having been used in wildlife.

Treatment of acute signs and supportive care

If the casualty is suffering from acute poisoning, the cause of which is unknown, symptomatic treatment and supportive care may be all that is possible whilst the poison is being excreted. The clinical condition of the animal may also mean that the use of emetics, or oral adsorbents and cathartics, is inappropriate.

The cinical signs displayed by an acutely poisoned animal are typically gastrointestinal (vomiting or regurgitation, with or without diarrhoea) and neurological. Renal and hepatic damage may also occur. Supportive treatment includes fluid therapy, correction of acid–base and electrolyte imbalances, treatment of seizures, and maintenance of body temperature. These have all been described previously in this chapter.

Specific antidotes

Specific antidotes are available for some poisons (Figure 5.20) and these must be given as early as possible in the treatment of the patient. Supportive treatment, as described above, must be used alongside these medications.

Toxin	Specific antidote	Dosage	Wildlife-specific comments
Anticoagulant rodenticides	Vitamin K1	• 2.5 mg/kg (second generation anticoagulants require higher doses of 5 mg/kg initially) s.c. q6–12h for 5–7 days, followed by oral doses of 1–2.5 mg/kg for 1–3 weeks • Dose and duration of treatment depends on severity of clinical signs and clotting times	• Accidental or intentional poisoning of mammals
Ethylene glycol	Ethanol (20%) Fomepizole	• Ethanol (20%): 5.5 ml/kg slow i.v. infusion q4h for 5 treatments, then q6h for 4 treatments • Fomepizole: 20 mg/kg diluted in 0.9% saline infused i.v. over 30 minutes, followed by 15 mg/kg infusion 12 and 24 hours later, then 5 mg/kg q12h until clinical recovery or until serum levels are negligible	• Usually accidental in mammals • Doses given are those used in dogs • Fomepizole may be less effective in other species (e.g. cats) • Few data in wildlife species
Organophosphate and carbamate insecticides	Pralidoxime Atropine sulphate	• Pralidoxime: 10–20 mg/kg i.m. or slow i.v.; repeat after 8 hours • Atropine sulphate: 0.2–0.5 mg/kg; a quarter of the dose is given i.v., the remainder i.m. or s.c.; repeat as necessary (typically 3–6hrs)	• Frequently used in illegal poisoning of birds of prey (see Chapter 29)
Paracetamol	N-acetylcysteine	• 150 mg/kg i.v. diluted with an equal volume of 5% glucose solution given over 15 minutes, followed by 50 mg/kg as a 10% solution in 5% glucose over the next 20 hours	• Has been used in illegal poisoning of species such as badgers
Lead	Edetate calcium disodium (CaEDTA)	• Mammals 25 mg/kg, birds 30–50 mg/kg, swans 62.5 mg/kg, reptiles 10–40 mg/kg i.m. or s.c. q12h for 5 days or until clinical signs and blood lead levels reduce	• Common in waterfowl, especially swans, following ingestion of lead shot and angling weights (see Chapter 26) • CaEDTA should be diluted 1:4 with sterile water or saline

5.20 Common toxins and their management in wildlife.

Emergency hospitalization, monitoring and record-keeping

Veterinary practices are generally not appropriate places to keep wild animals, even in emergency situations, and appropriate facilities must be provided. The emergency wildlife patient should be continually discreetly observed and where possible (e.g. unconscious or easily handled patients), basic parameters such as temperature, pulse and respiration rates should be measured at regular intervals. Appropriate records must be kept (see Chapter 7).

Acknowledgements

Acknowledgements are due to Dick Best for his contribution to similar information in the previous edition of this book.

References and further reading

Adamantos S and Corr S (2007) Emergency care of the cat with multi-trauma. *In Practice* **29**, 388–396

Bevanger K and Brøseth H (1998) Body temperature changes in wild-living badgers *Meles meles* through the winter. *Wildlife Biology* **4**, 97–101

Carpenter JW (2012) *Exotic Animal Formulary, 4th edn.* Elsevier Saunders, Missouri

Cornin L, Cook DJ, Carlet J *et al.* (1995) Corticosteroid treatment for sepsis: a critical appraisal and meta-analysis of the literature. *Critical Care Medicine* **23**, 1430–1439

Cousins RA, Battley PF, Gartrell BD and Powlesland RG (2012) Impact injuries and probability of survival in a large semiurban endemic pigeon in New Zealand, *Hemiphaga novaeseelandiae*. *Journal of Wildlife Diseases* **48**, 567–574

Demarais S, Fuquay JW and Jacobson HA (1986) Rectal temperatures of white-tailed deer in Mississippi. *The Journal of Wildlife Management* **50**, 702–705

Dewey CW (2000) Emergency management of the head trauma patient, principles and practice. *Veterinary Clinics of North America: Small Animal Practice* **30**, 207–225

Girling S and Raiti P (2004) *BSAVA Manual of Reptiles, 2nd edn.* BSAVA Publications, Gloucester

King LG and Boag A (2007) *BSAVA Manual of Canine and Feline Emergency and Critical Care, 2nd edn.* BSAVA Publications, Gloucester

Kirkwood JK (1981) Maintenance energy requirements and rates of weight loss during starvation in birds of prey. In: *Recent Advances in the Study of Raptor Diseases*, ed. JE Cooper and AG Greenwood. Chiron Publications, Keighley

Kirkwood JK (1983a) Dosing exotic species. *Veterinary Record* **112**, 486

Kirkwood JK (1983b) Influence of body size on health and disease. *Veterinary Record* **113**, 287

Kirkwood JK (1991) Energy requirements for maintenance and growth of wild mammals, birds and reptiles in captivity. *Journal of Nutrition* **121(11 suppl)**, S29–S34

Kreeger TJ, Monson D, Kuechle VB, Seal US and Tester JR (1989) Monitoring heart rate and body temperature in red foxes (*Vulpes vulpes*). *Canadian Journal of Zoology* **67**, 2455–2458

Kruuk H, Taylor PT and Mom GAT (2009) Body temperature and foraging behaviour of the Eurasian otter (*Lutra lutra*), in relation to water temperature. *Journal of Zoology* **241**, 689–697

Meredith A (2015) *BSAVA Small Animal Formulary 9th edn – Part B: Exotic Pets.* BSAVA Publications, Gloucester

Mühldorfer K, Speck S and Wibbelt G (2011) Diseases in free-ranging bats from Germany. *BMC Veterinary Research* **7**, 61

Perrins C (1979) *British Tits.* Collins, London

Ramsey I (2014) *BSAVA Small Animal Formulary, 8th edn.* BSAVA Publications, Gloucester

Rupley AE (1998) Critical care of pet birds, procedures, therapeutics and patient support. *Veterinary Clinics of North America: Exotic Animals Practice.* **1**, 11–41

Sladky K (2014) Analgesia. In: *Current Therapy in Reptile Medicine and Surgery*, ed. D Mader and S Divers, pp. 217–228. Elsevier Saunders, St Louis

Sladky K and Mans C (2012) Clinical analgesia in reptiles. *Journal of Exotic Pet Medicine* **21**, 158–167

Sturkie PD (ed) (2000) *Avian Physiology, 5th edn.* Academic Press, San Diego, California

Thomas JR, Yocum RC, Haller MF and von Gunten CF (2008) Assessing the role of human recombinant hyaluronidase in gravity-driven subcutaneous hydration: the INFUSE-LR study. *Journal of Palliative Medicine* **10(6)**,1312–1320

Varga M, Lumbis R and Gott L (2012) *BSAVA Manual of Exotic Pet and Wildlife Nursing.* BSAVA Publications, Gloucester

Woods M, McDonald RA and Harris S (2003) Predation of wildlife by domestic cats *Felis catus* in Great Britain. *Mammal Review* **33**, 174

Chapter 6

Basic principles of wildlife anaesthesia

Michelle Barrows

Anaesthesia of wildlife casualties can be challenging. Many patients suffer stress, related not only to disease or injury, but also to confinement in captivity. This is exacerbated by restraint and handling and often necessitates the use of sedation or anaesthesia for thorough examination of even small and relatively easily handled species. It is important that the basic principles of good anaesthesia are applied, that the patient and equipment are prepared correctly and that appropriate methods of chemical restraint are chosen.

Equipment required for wildlife anaesthesia

As wildlife anaesthesia can be especially unpredictable, it is essential to have all the equipment that might be required available in advance (Figure 6.1).

Equipment	Comments
Anaesthetic machine; vaporizer(s); volatile anaesthetic agent(s); circuits; oxygen cylinders; reservoir bags; appropriate scavenging	• Non-rebreathing systems are used most often as they offer low resistance with minimal dead space and allow for rapid changes in depth of anaesthesia (for animals <10 kg, O_2 rate of at least 500 ml/kg/minute required) • Rebreathing systems (e.g. circle, to-and-fro) are recommended for animals ≥10 kg as they have low gas flow requirements and low anaesthetic consumption, making them economical. The systems can be run open or closed; expired moisture and heat are also conserved
Induction chamber (see Figure 6.4)	• Partitions allow subdivision so that smaller patients can be induced more rapidly • There should be a port for gas inflow at the bottom and another for the exhaust pipe at the top (connected to the scavenger). If gas is removed from the bottom of the chamber, this will increase induction time because isoflurane and sevoflurane are denser than air • High fresh gas flow rates should be used • Avoid operator exposure by flushing the chamber well before opening the lid to remove the patient
Facemasks	• A range of sizes should be available and these can be adapted from other equipment, e.g. syringe cases or plastic bottles for birds with long beaks (see Figure 6.3) • There should be a tight seal and the smallest facemask available should be used to reduce unnecessary dead space • Operator exposure to anaesthetic gas is greater than when animal is intubated
Endotracheal tubes and stylets	• A range of sizes, down to 1 mm and 1.5 mm, should be available (uncuffed and short for small animals to minimize dead space, e.g. Portex® or SurgiVet®) • Smaller endotracheal tubes can be made from intravenous catheters connected to the nozzle of a 2 ml syringe, which is cut off and attached to an 8 mm endotracheal tube connector
Lidocaine spray	• Used in medium to small animals, especially cats, prior to intubation to prevent laryngospasm
Mouth gags and/or specula	• Smith–Baxter or standard; rodent/rabbit mouth gags
Laryngoscope	• Long and short blades; paediatric
Ophthalmic lubricant	• Used during anaesthesia to protect the cornea when the blink reflex is lost • Paraffin ointment (e.g. Lacri-Lube®); carbomer gel (e.g. Optixcare®)
Monitoring equipment (e.g. stethoscope; thermometer; records)	• Paediatric and oesophageal stethoscopes are useful • Body temperature can be measured with electronic thermometers or flexible temperature probes placed into the rectum, cloaca or oesophagus • Other useful monitoring equipment includes: electrocardiogram; Doppler ultrasound monitor; pulse oximeter; blood pressure monitor; capnograph
Heat source	• Warm air blanket (e.g. Bair Hugger®) (see Figure 6.6); electrical or microwaveable heat pad; circulating warm water blankets; radiant heat source; conductive fabric warming system

6.1 Equipment required for wildlife anaesthesia. (continues) ▶

Equipment	Comments
Fluid therapy equipment	• Including: intravenous catheters; paediatric and adult fluid administration sets; fluids (small bags are useful for small patients); fluid infusion pumps or syringe drivers; heparinized saline; swabs, spirit, tape, bandage and three-way tap
Small animal ventilator	• Very useful for consistent intermittent positive pressure ventilation (IPPV)
Anaesthetic emergency kit	• Emergency drugs and dose charts for patients of different species and sizes
Remote chemical injection delivery system	• For example: dart gun; darts; flights and caps; needles; sealing sleeves; pressurizing adaptor; CO_2 canisters; venting pin; range finder; pole syringe with syringes and needles. Firearms licence and secure locked storage required

6.1 (continued) Equipment required for wildlife anaesthesia.

Pre-anaesthetic considerations and assessment

Wildlife casualties are often high-risk patients for anaesthesia as a result of acute trauma, dehydration or nutritional compromise. A complete pre-anaesthetic assessment is, however, not always possible due to the stress of handling and the fact that, in certain species, anaesthesia may be required to allow safe handling in the first instance (see Chapter 3). Often the risks of anaesthesia are fewer than those of manual restraint and examination of a stressed and/or ill or potentially dangerous patient. Nevertheless, an attempt should be made to assess the patient visually and, where possible, to stabilize its condition prior to anaesthesia (Figure 6.2 and Chapter 5). Advance planning, with consideration of actual and potential problems, as well as ensuring that all equipment needed for examination, diagnostics and treatment is available (see Figure 6.1), will minimize anaesthetic time and risk.

Pre-anaesthetic consideration	Comments
Fasting	• Fasting is recommended prior to anaesthesia in most mammals except rodents and lagomorphs, but should not be prolonged in animals weighing <5 kg • Birds should be fasted long enough to allow the crop to empty, which may be less than an hour for small passerines, 3–12 hours for waterfowl, or over 24 hours for large raptors and waterfowl; debilitated and emaciated birds should not be fasted • Snakes should be fasted (for up to 48 hours) to avoid lung compression by a full stomach and prevent regurgitation • If fasting is not possible due to the emergency nature of a procedure, the patient should be intubated and positioned with the head and neck elevated to minimize the likelihood of regurgitation and aspiration
Weight; sex; physiological state	• These ideally need to be determined prior to anaesthesia if injectable agents are being used; a stag in rut, for example, will require higher anaesthetic doses than at other times of the year
Visual assessment	• Visual assessment before handling or otherwise disturbing the patient; note attitude/demeanour, awareness of surroundings, activity, respiratory rate and effort, passage of faeces and urine/urates and presence of obvious injuries
Physical examination	• Brief physical examination to assess body condition and hydration status, measure heart rate and rhythm, assess capillary refill time, measure respiratory rate and body temperature and examine relevant organ systems
Fluid and electrolyte deficiencies	• Shock, fluid, electrolyte and glucose imbalances are common in all wildlife patients and should ideally be assessed and corrected before anaesthesia
Body temperature	• Hypothermia or hyperthermia should be addressed prior to anaesthesia • When treating hypothermia, the aim is to gradually re-warm the animal's core; rapid surface re-warming of small patients can result in rapid peripheral vasodilation and subsequent hypotensive crisis; hypothermic birds and small mammals will rapidly become hypoglycaemic • Reptiles must be warmed to a temperature within their activity temperature range before anaesthesia
Trauma patients	• Anaesthesia should ideally be postponed until the animal is stable; this may involve circulatory support in the form of aggressive fluid therapy to address hypotension, improve circulation and preserve tissue perfusion, oxygen therapy or haemostasis
Biochemistry and haematology	• Basic parameters including packed cell volume (PCV), total protein (or total solids) and blood glucose provide a useful minimum database prior to anaesthesia
Pre-anaesthetic medications	• These are not used as frequently in wildlife as in domestic animals, but should be considered in order to reduce the amount of anaesthetic agent required and minimize the stress of induction; adverse side effects such as cardiovascular depression are also reduced • For animals undergoing surgery, an analgesic plan is necessary; pre-emptive analgesia aims to minimize sensitization of central nociceptive pathways and amplification of pain and should be provided for all surgical patients along with intra- and postoperative pain relief
Capture myopathy	• Take precautions to prevent this in susceptible species (e.g. deer, cranes); avoid prolonged restraint, either manually or in traps; minimize stress, for example by the use of blindfolds, and use capture drugs that minimize induction and recovery times and promote physiological stability; avoid prolonged chases before chemical capture and avoid capture when ambient temperatures are high (>25°C) • Treat hyperthermia immediately; consider vitamin E supplementation prior to capture if possible

6.2 Pre-anaesthetic considerations and assessment of wildlife casualties. For additional information on many of these considerations, see Chapters 4 and 5.

Analgesia

Many wildlife species mask signs of pain or show withdrawal responses such as immobility, making pain hard to recognize. Signs of pain may also be less obvious in neonates than adults of the same species, and in nocturnal species observed during the day. Analgesia should therefore be appropriately provided for all wildlife species, regardless of obvious signs of pain. Where possible, analgesia should be pre-emptive and multimodal analgesia (using several classes of drugs to provide optimal pain control) should be considered. Neuroleptanalgesia (combining a neuroleptic drug such as a sedative with an analgesic) can reduce fear and anxiety as well as pain. Figure 5.15 provides a summary of doses for emergency analgesic drugs in wildlife.

Local anaesthetics

Local anaesthetics are useful components of multimodal analgesia. These may be used topically, for example on the cornea; via local infiltration or splash block at a surgical site; or for local nerve blockade. Either lidocaine, which lasts 2–3 hours, or bupivacaine, which lasts 6–8 hours, can be used. Suggested dose rates are 1–4 mg/kg for lidocaine and 1–2 mg/kg for bupivacaine. Local anaesthetic drugs may need to be diluted to allow accurate dosing. Care must be taken and the lower end of these ranges should be used in birds, which are more sensitive to local anaesthetic toxicity than mammals due to rapid systemic uptake.

Opioids

Opioids are potent analgesics and useful drugs in wildlife medicine (see Figure 5.15). They may be used alone or synergistically with sedative drugs (see 'Sedation'), allowing reduction in doses of other anaesthetic agents. Injectable opioids useful in mammals include buprenorphine (0.01–0.05 mg/kg i.v., i.m., s.c. q6–12h), butorphanol (0.1–2 mg/kg i.v., i.m., s.c. q2–6h) and morphine (0.1–5 mg/kg i.v., i.m., s.c. q2–4h). Most research into avian analgesia has been carried out on parrots and chickens and, based on this, butorphanol (1–4 mg/kg i.v., i.m.) is considered to be a better choice than buprenorphine (0.01–0.05 mg/kg i.v., i.m.) in birds, although duration is unlikely to be more than 2–4 hours (Paul-Murphy and Hawkins, 2012). Research into reptile analgesia has shown considerable variability between snakes, lizards and chelonians in their response to opioid administration, indicating differences in the types of endogenous opioid receptors they possess (Duncan, 2012). This makes general recommendations for the best type of opioid to use in reptiles difficult; however, morphine and tramadol (5–10 mg/kg orally q48–72h) are likely to be more effective analgesics than butorphanol (0.5–2.0 mg/kg i.m.) or buprenorphine (0.01–0.02 mg/kg i.m.) (Sladky, 2014). Morphine is suggested at doses of 1–4 mg/kg i.m. (Meredith, 2014), although higher doses (1–10 mg/kg i.m.) have also been suggested (Sladky, 2014); higher doses may cause significant respiratory depression.

Non-steroidal anti-inflammatory drugs

Non-steroidal anti-inflammatory drugs (NSAIDs) are commonly used in mammals, reptiles and birds. Care should be taken with patients of unknown clinical status because NSAIDs are contraindicated in patients with dehydration, hypotension or shock, and those with haemorrhage, due to anti-thromboxane activity reducing platelet plug formation and potential renal impairment. Carprofen and meloxicam have minimal anti-thromboxane activity and are unlikely to affect haemostasis. Meloxicam doses start at 0.1 mg/kg but up to 1–2 mg/kg (i.m., s.c., orally) every 12 hours may be necessary in birds and small mammals (see Figure 5.15). Glucocorticoids are contraindicated for use as analgesics in all species (see Chapter 5).

Options for chemical restraint

Sedation

All types of sedation cause some degree of central nervous system depression, resulting in decreased perception and reaction times. Sedative drugs in veterinary medicine include phenothiazines (e.g. acepromazine), alpha-2 adrenoreceptor agonists (e.g. medetomidine), benzodiazepines (e.g. diazepam) and opioids (e.g. morphine). Short-acting or reversible drugs, such as alpha-2 adrenoreceptor agonists and benzodiazepines, are preferred for wildlife casualties. Opioids may be used concurrently for analgesia and as anaesthetic agents. Sedation may allow animals to be examined, treated or undergo diagnostic procedures without the need for general anaesthesia and may be safer than anaesthesia for shocked, old or otherwise compromised patients. Animals should be monitored whilst sedatives are taking effect. The depth of sedation is usually dose dependent and many sedatives can be combined with other agents to further increase the sedative depth, eventually producing surgical anaesthesia in some species. Concurrent use of local anaesthesia may allow minor surgical procedures to be carried out using sedatives alone.

Alpha-2 adrenoreceptor agonists

Alpha-2 adrenoreceptor agonists such as medetomidine, dexmedetomidine and xylazine provide good muscle relaxation, sedation and analgesia, and are antagonized by atipamezole and yohimbine to allow rapid recovery. Alpha-2 adrenoreceptor agonists cause cardiopulmonary depression and are best combined with synergistic agents such as ketamine, allowing a reduction in effective dose and inducing general anaesthesia at higher doses. It is important to leave the patient undisturbed in a quiet and dark location after injection to encourage rapid, smooth induction. Provision of oxygen to the sedated patient may help reduce the effects of cardiopulmonary depression. See species-specific chapters for dose ranges.

Benzodiazepines

Benzodiazepines include midazolam, zolazepam and diazepam. They provide muscle relaxation and sedation with minimal cardiovascular effects, making them useful for debilitated and critical patients, and are also anxiolytic. Midazolam is soluble in water and can be given intranasally or by intramuscular injection. Benzodiazepines are antagonized by flumazenil (0.01–0.2 mg/kg i.m.), and may be combined with other agents such as ketamine and tiletamine to produce deep sedation and anaesthesia in some species. See species-specific chapters for dose ranges.

Other drugs

Some drugs, often referred to as 'tranquillizers', can be used to modify behaviour with minimal sedation and reduce aggression, anxiety and stress (Ebedes and Raath, 1999). Short-acting tranquillizers, such as the butyrophenones haloperidol (8–12 hours) and azaperone (2–4 hours), can be useful for transportation or initial adaptation to a new environment. Longer-acting neuroleptics such as perphenazine (lasts 7–10 days) and zuclopenthixol acetate (lasts 2–3 days) can greatly facilitate hospitalization of wildlife and have been used in species as diverse as deer (Cervidae) (Caulkett and Haigh, 2007) and cranes (Gruidae) by the author.

General anaesthesia and routes of administration

General anaesthesia is a reversible state of unconsciousness, along with muscle relaxation and ideally analgesia, sufficient to allow surgery and other painful or stressful procedures. Choice of general anaesthetic technique depends on the facilities and equipment available and the species, age and health status of the patient, as well as the experience and preference of the anaesthetist. Towels, brooms, herding boards, nets and crush cages may all be useful for restraint to allow safe delivery of injectable agents. Appropriate health and safety precautions and personal protective equipment (PPE) must be used. Maintaining venous access during anaesthesia is important, though not always easy in smaller patients. Placement of intravenous catheters should be routine where possible, as should provision of appropriate fluid therapy during anaesthesia (see Chapter 5).

Inhalant anaesthetics

The inhalant anaesthetic agents isoflurane and sevoflurane are commonly used for both induction and maintenance of anaesthesia in British wildlife patients, particularly birds, small mammals and the small native reptile species. They allow rapid induction and recovery, as well as good control of anaesthetic depth. Inhalant anaesthetics are primarily eliminated by the lungs, have fewer side effects than injectable agents and high safety margins, making them a good choice for compromised patients. Respiratory and myocardial depression are common, but the latter is offset by vasodilation and decreased afterload. Induction of anaesthesia by inhalation via facemask (Figure 6.3) or induction chamber (Figure 6.4) can be used in amphibians, snakes, lizards, birds and small mammals. Snakes and lizards can also be intubated while conscious and anaesthesia induced with intermittent positive pressure ventilation (IPPV). Alternative methods of reptile and amphibian anaesthesia are given in the sections below.

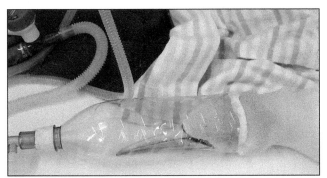

6.3 Mask induction of anaesthesia in a gannet (*Morus bassanus*) using a mask adapted from a plastic bottle to accommodate the elongated bill. The smallest container possible should ideally be used to avoid increasing dead space unnecessarily.
(© Richard Saunders)

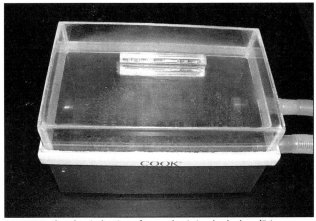

6.4 Chamber induction of anaesthesia in a hedgehog (*Erinaceus europaeus*).
(© Richard Saunders)

Sevoflurane has a lower blood/gas partition coefficient than isoflurane, leading to a faster increase in alveolar anaesthetic concentration and faster induction and recovery, but it also has a higher minimum alveolar concentration (MAC), so higher concentrations are needed. Typically with isoflurane, 5% is used for induction and 2–3% for maintenance of anaesthesia, *versus* 6–8% for induction and 3–4% for maintenance of anaesthesia with sevoflurane. Low-to-high protocols, where the concentration is increased slowly, may be appropriate for very debilitated patients, reducing the risk of overdose and apnoea. Sevoflurane is less irritating to mucous membranes than isoflurane, so breath-holding is less likely and induction less stressful for the patient. Ophthalmic lubricant (see Figure 6.1) should be applied to reduce the irritant effect on the conjunctivae, if possible prior to induction of anaesthesia or alternatively immediately after, when using these anaesthetics.

Dissociative anaesthetics

Ketamine: Ketamine is a dissociative anaesthetic and also provides good analgesia. It causes minimal cardiorespiratory depression, but does not provide good muscle relaxation and can cause muscle tremors and seizures if used alone. Although it has a high safety margin in most mammals, fatal complications have occurred when used on its own in some species such as North American river otters (*Lontra canadensis*) (Spelman, 1999). In order to negate the effects on muscle tone, it is most often combined with sedative drugs (see 'Sedation'). Ketamine, and ketamine combinations, can be given by several routes. Duration of anaesthesia and recovery are longer if given intramuscularly than if given intravenously. Ophthalmic lubricant should be applied to prevent corneal damage due to loss of blink reflexes. Self-mutilation has been reported after intramuscular injection, which can be irritant and painful. Reversing alpha-2 adrenoreceptor agonists is not recommended within 30 minutes of giving ketamine, due to the undesirable effects of ketamine alone. Recovery from ketamine anaesthesia should ideally take place in a quiet, darkened environment.

Tiletamine: Tiletamine is chemically related to ketamine, with a longer duration of action. It is available as a commercial product in combination with the benzodiazepine zolazepam (Zoletil 100®; Telazol®). These products result in anaesthesia, requiring the same considerations as those including ketamine.

Other injectable agents

Alfaxalone: Alfaxalone is a short-acting steroid anaesthetic that can be given by intramuscular as well as intravenous injection and results in smooth, rapid induction of anaesthesia. It causes dose-dependent cardiorespiratory depression.

Propofol: Propofol, a short-acting non-barbiturate anaesthetic, is used less commonly than other injectable agents in wildlife due to the requirement for intravascular administration, but results in smooth, rapid induction of anaesthesia and good muscle relaxation. Apnoea is common, especially when propofol is given rapidly. It can be used by continuous infusion to maintain anaesthesia.

Etorphine: Etorphine is a potent opioid agonist, used mainly in large deer or for euthanasia of cetaceans (see Chapter 23). At the time of writing, etorphine is only available in the UK as M99® (9.8 mg/ml etorphine), imported from South Africa (see also Chapter 23). Etorphine is a thousand times more potent than morphine and extremely dangerous to humans if absorbed via mucous membranes or through open wounds. It is antagonized in patients by diprenorphine, which is usually given intravenously at 2–3 mg per mg of etorphine. It should only be used by a veterinary surgeon (veterinarian) if the human antidote naloxone is available. Etorphine, in common with morphine and ketamine, is a Schedule 2 Controlled Drug that must be kept in a locked cabinet, and recorded in the Controlled Drugs Register.

Field anaesthesia

Field anaesthesia may be necessary to safely immobilize a wildlife patient for treatment, transportation or euthanasia. Typically injectable agents are used, delivered either remotely via a dart rifle or pole-syringe (see 'Mammalian anaesthesia') or injected by hand. For useful guidance on maintaining and preparing darting equipment, see Cracknell (2014). Wildlife biologists may also use mobile inhalant anaesthetic equipment, which allow, greater flexibility in anaesthetic depth and, in birds in particular, are usually the safest choice. Standard vaporizers must always be emptied for transport to avoid dangerous levels of anaesthetic gas delivery that can result if they are tilted when full (Heath, 2007). Lewis (2004) gives examples of several circuit configurations used with a simple, lightweight isoflurane and air anaesthetic machine in clinically normal mammals and birds under field conditions. Specific post-anaesthesia considerations must be made.

Anaesthetic monitoring techniques

Vigilant monitoring of respiratory and cardiovascular function, along with body temperature, is important in all anaesthetized animals. Monitoring respiratory rate and depth, colour of mucous membranes, capillary refill time, heart and peripheral pulse rate (in larger species) and body temperature are the basic priorities. A good, appropriately trained anaesthetist and the use of suitable anaesthetic monitoring forms are as essential as any monitoring equipment.

Monitoring anaesthetic depth

In domestic mammals, ocular reflexes, jaw and anal tone, and pedal reflexes are commonly used to assess depth of anaesthesia and these are applicable to mammalian wildlife casualties. In birds, the position of the eye does not change during anaesthesia and the most useful reflex is the corneal reflex, which should remain during surgical anaesthesia; the palpebral reflex is unreliable in birds. In lizards, toe pinch withdrawal, righting, corneal and palpebral reflexes are useful, as is cloacal tone; the corneal reflex should remain during surgical anaesthesia. In snakes, which do not have moveable eyelids, tongue flick and righting reflexes, as well as tail pinch reflexes, can be used. Corneal, righting and limb withdrawal reflexes are useful in amphibians.

Monitoring cardiovascular parameters

Stress prior to anaesthesia, such as that caused by handling, can induce cardiovascular complications such as arrhythmia and hypertension. In larger species, a stethoscope or oesophageal stethoscope can be used (Figure 6.5). Heart rate monitors for smaller species should be capable of registering heart rates of at least 350–400 bpm.

Doppler ultrasonography

Doppler ultrasonography is a very useful cardiac monitoring technique, allowing changes in heart rate and rhythm to be easily heard. Probes can be placed over the heart in amphibians, snakes, some lizards and small mammals or over a peripheral artery such as the brachial, ulnar or metatarsal artery in birds (Figure 6.6) or the saphenous artery in small mammals.

Electrocardiography

Electrocardiography (ECG) is useful for detecting dysrhythmias, but machines must be able to monitor high heart rates for use with birds or small mammals and slower (temperature-dependent) heart rates in reptiles and amphibians. ECG clips can be connected to hypodermic needles to avoid trauma from alligator clips in small

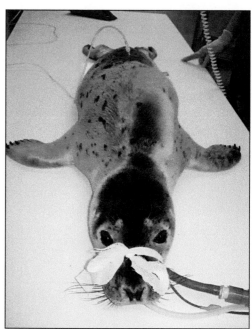

6.5 Anaesthetized grey seal (*Halichoerus grypus*) with oesophageal stethoscope and catheterized extradural intravertebral vein.
(© Richard Saunders)

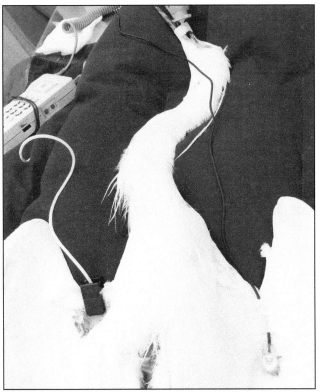

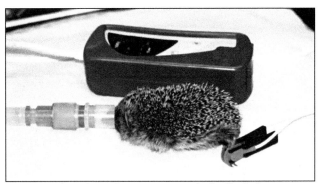

6.7 Pulse oximetry in use on an anaesthetized hedgehog.
(© Elizabeth Mullineaux)

6.6 Pulse oximetry and Doppler ultrasound probe in use on an anaesthetized little egret (*Egretta garzetta*). A Bair Hugger® forced-air warming device is also in use.

patients, or to penetrate the skin between scales in reptiles. Sticky ECG pads can also be used, although these pose practical difficulties in the smaller species.

Arterial blood pressure monitoring

Arterial blood pressure monitoring is a useful measure of cardiovascular function. In wildlife it is usually more practical to use indirect techniques, based on occlusion of blood flow to an extremity by inflation of a cuff. Pulsatile blood flow is detected either by sensors in the cuff itself (oscillometric) or by placement of a Doppler ultrasound probe over an artery distal to the cuff. The cuff is inflated until all flow through the artery ceases and then deflated slowly until the first flow is detected. The pressure (read from a manometer) at which blood flow recommences is systolic blood pressure. As the cuff is deflated further, diastolic blood pressure is measured. In birds, the cuff can be placed on the metatarsal region. In reptiles, the cuff can be placed over the brachial artery of a forelimb or the caudal tail artery. Reptiles have lower systemic arterial blood pressures than mammals as well as deep-lying vessels, which mean that indirect blood pressure measurement may be less reliable.

Pulse oximetry

Pulse oximetry measures percentage oxygen saturation in arterial blood (S_pO_2). Values are calibrated based on the oxygen–haemoglobin dissociation curve of mammals, so, in non-mammalian species especially, trends may be more useful than individual values. Transmittance probes can be clipped on non-pigmented mucous membranes including oral, cloacal or vaginal mucosa or on thin areas of skin such as ear, interdigital skin or wing web (see Figures 6.6 and 6.7). Heavily pigmented or furred areas may not work

and the probe may slip off the tongue in small mammals. Flat reflectance probes can be placed into the oesophagus, cloaca or rectum.

Monitoring respiratory parameters

Respiratory monitors for use in smaller wildlife casualties should be able to detect small tidal volumes. Patient positioning can have an impact upon respiratory parameters (see species-specific information).

Capnography

Capnography detects carbon dioxide (CO_2) concentration in expired gases and allows assessment of ventilation. Since alveolar gas is equilibrated with arterial blood, end-tidal gas concentrations should reflect arterial gas concentrations. This relationship has not been validated in birds and is complicated in reptiles by the presence of cardiac shunts that allow pulmonary bypass; however, trends may still be useful. Measurements can be made either on the gas stream as it flows into the endotracheal tube (mainstream) or by removing a continuous sample of gas for analysis inside the monitor (sidestream) (Figure 6.8). Both types may be inaccurate in small patients, however, due to the extra dead space in mainstream units and relatively high sampling rates in some sidestream capnography units.

Blood gas analysis

Blood gas analysis has not, to date, been commonly used in anaesthetized wildlife patients. Point-of-care analysers that require very small amounts of arterial or venous blood (e.g. 0.1 ml) are now more widely available.

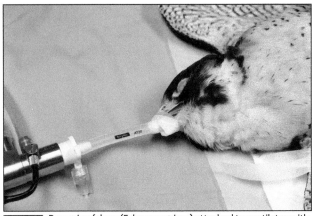

6.8 Peregrine falcon (*Falco peregrinus*) attached to ventilator with sidestream capnography.
(© Jenna Richardson)

Reference values for some avian and other wildlife patients are reported (Harms and Harms, 2012) (see also species-specific chapters), making evaluation of ventilation and acid–base status possible in these species.

Monitoring body temperature

Small animals with a high surface area to volume ratio will lose heat rapidly during anaesthesia unless precautions are taken to address this. Examples of equipment used to maintain body temperature are given in Figure 6.1 and in the mammal-specific information later in this chapter. Normal ranges of body temperature in British wildlife species are given in Figure 5.13. Hyperthermia may also be an issue, as anaesthetic drugs interfere with normal thermoregulation, and this is seen most often in some mammalian species.

Post-anaesthetic considerations

Hypothermia is common in small patients post-anaesthesia and will prolong recovery due to decreased respiration and slower elimination of volatile anaesthetics; it also causes hypotension. Heated recovery cages or incubators are useful for small birds and mammals as well as reptiles. The position of the patient should be changed frequently if recovery is prolonged in order to prevent uneven heating as well as hypostatic congestion.

The endotracheal tube, if used, should be removed once protective laryngeal reflexes have returned. The patient should be allowed to recover in a quiet, dark place. The recovery area should be padded for deer. Birds can be lightly wrapped in a towel to prevent them flapping around and sustaining injuries during recovery.

Continue monitoring the patient at least until it can maintain sternal recumbency (mammal) or stand (bird). Small animals with high metabolic rates such as small birds and rodents, as well as lagomorphs and neonates, should return to feeding soon after anaesthesia. Effective analgesia is important to promote this (see 'Analgesia' and Chapter 5). If birds less than 100 g have not fed within 30 minutes of full recovery from anaesthesia, they should be fed using a crop tube (see Chapter 5).

Care must be taken when releasing animals after sedation or general anaesthesia in the field. Disorientation and stress can result in released animals running into hazards such as fences and water bodies or across roads. If it is safe to do so, they should be released where they were found or in a nearby familiar location (see Chapter 9). It may be advisable to confine smaller animals in a secure container until they appear to be fully recovered and the time is appropriate for release (e.g. dusk for nocturnal species).

Species-specific considerations

Mammalian anaesthesia

Although a wide variety of species may present to the wildlife anaesthetist, many are similar in anatomy and physiology to domestic animals and basic principles of mammalian anaesthesia should be adhered to. Further information on anaesthesia in individual mammalian species is given in the chapters that follow.

Hypothermia

Hypothermia is common, particularly in small species with a large surface area to volume ratio, such as rodents, insectivores and microchiropteran bats. Care should be taken to minimize heat loss during anaesthesia, for example by minimizing anaesthetic and surgical time, avoiding exposure to cold surfaces, maintaining warm ambient temperature, minimizing radiant and evaporative heat losses and using warm fluids. Warm air blankets (e.g. Bair Hugger®) (see Figures 5.14 and 6.6) circulating warm water blankets, conductive fabric warming systems (e.g. Hot Dog®) and radiant heat sources above the patient are most useful. Care must be taken with heat mats to prevent thermal injuries. Aluminium foil or bubble wrap can be used for insulation. Hot water bottles and microwaveable grain bags have the potential to cause significant thermal injury, as well as diverting heat away from the casualty as they cool, making them unsuitable heat sources.

Hyperthermia

Hyperthermia is common in some species (e.g. pinnipeds, otters and cervids). If body temperature exceeds 41°C, active cooling is necessary, for example by administering cold water enemas or use of ice packs (e.g. on the flippers of seals). Since hyperthermia increases oxygen demand, supplemental oxygen should be provided. Consideration should be given to reversing the anaesthesia if severe hyperthermia occurs. Hyperthermia may predispose to capture myopathy, which may be acute, subacute or chronic, and is often fatal.

Neonatal mammals

Neonatal mammals have increased tissue oxygen demand compared to adults and their small airways are at greater risk of obstruction, resulting in increased likelihood of hypoxia under anaesthesia. IPPV should be considered in these patients. Liver glycogen storage is minimal and pre-anaesthetic fasting can result in hypoglycaemia. Neonates are also predisposed to developing hypothermia due to reduced thermoregulatory ability, increased surface area to volume ratio and lower fat reserves than adults. Appropriate precautions and treatments should be used to avoid hypothermia and hypoglycaemia (administer glucose (see Chapter 5) and feed as soon as fully recovered from anaesthesia).

Dive response in seals

Phocid seals may develop bradycardia, peripheral vasoconstriction and apnoea due to their dive response, which conserves oxygen for vital organs such as the brain and heart. Intubation is recommended to allow IPPV if necessary, although this can be challenging due to spongy peripharyngeal tissue and a flaccid soft palate (Lynch and Bodley, 2007) (see Chapter 23).

Remote delivery of anaesthetic agents in mammals

Remote delivery of anaesthetic agents may be necessary in larger mammals; for example, for roadside sedation of deer prior to transport. Options include pole syringes, blowpipes and dart rifles (Figure 6.9). A firearms license is required to use any remote chemical injection delivery system. These are obtained from the firearms licensing units of the local police force (see 'Specialist organizations and

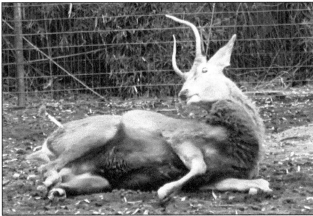

6.9 Remote delivery of etorphine in a red deer (*Cervus elaphus*) using a dart rifle to project a 3 ml dart into the gluteal muscles.

useful contacts'). Dart placement sites include the muscle mass of the hindlimbs or gluteal area (Figure 6.9), the shoulder (triceps muscle) and the neck.

Positioning of deer

Like other ruminants, deer are at risk of regurgitation of rumen contents under anaesthesia. Sternal recumbency with the head elevated and the nose pointing downwards minimizes this risk. If lateral recumbency is necessary, intubate and place the deer in right rather than left recumbency to minimize pressure on the rumen. Since fermentation of rumen contents continues, bloat can develop during prolonged anaesthesia and is an emergency, requiring prompt decompression and/or reversal of anaesthesia (see also Chapter 22).

Avian anaesthesia

The avian respiratory system is much more efficient than that of mammals, with several fundamental differences.

- The glottis is at the base of the tongue. Endotracheal intubation is straightforward in most birds and is recommended for all other than very brief procedures. Gently pulling the tongue forward with forceps or fingers can improve visualization (Figure 6.10). In small species (<100 g), tubes may become easily blocked with mucoid secretions and must be closely monitored. Apnoea is common in anaesthetized birds and intubation allows IPPV and prevents aspiration if regurgitation occurs. IPPV should be carried out at 10–12 bpm in the apnoeic bird.
- Avian tracheal volume and functional dead space is larger than that of mammals and there are complete tracheal rings. Uncuffed endotracheal tubes should be used to prevent pressure necrosis. The avian trachea shows a lot of variation, with some species having elaborate coils or loops, whilst in some Procellariiformes, the trachea is partially divided by a cartilaginous septum. The trachea divides at the level of the syrinx into the primary bronchi. In many ducks the male has a syringeal bulla, which is obvious on radiographs. The bronchi divide into secondary and then tertiary bronchi, otherwise known as parabronchi and the site of gas exchange. A countercurrent system in the parabronchi and a thinner blood–air barrier than mammals enables very efficient oxygen extraction, but also makes birds at greater risk of suffering adverse consequences of overdose with gaseous anaesthetics.

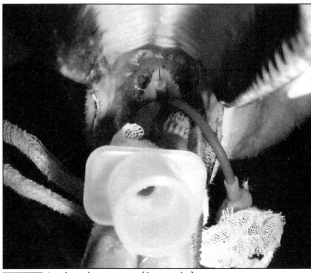

6.10 Intubated mute swan (*Cygnus olor*).
(© Richard Saunders)

- The air sacs, with diverticulae extending into bones often including the femur and humerus, account for up to 80% of respiratory capacity but are not involved in gas exchange. Air sacs act as bellows to ventilate the lungs. The presence of pneumatized bones means that it may be difficult to maintain a stable plane of inhalational anaesthesia when an open fracture is present. Birds have no diaphragm and it is movement of the sternum that creates negative pressure to draw air into the respiratory tract. Inspiration and expiration are both active processes. When handling birds, it is vital not to restrict these sternal movements by exerting pressure on the pectoral region. If there is deliberate or inadvertent surgical entry into air sacs, for example during coeliotomy, then maintaining an appropriate plane of gaseous anaesthesia may become more difficult and risk of staff exposure to the anaesthetic agent increases.

Birds are susceptible to hypercapnia and should receive assisted ventilation and ideally be monitored using a capnograph. Although use of capnography is poorly validated in birds, trends can be observed. Reduction in core body temperature occurs within 20 minutes of induction, increasing cardiovascular instability and making provision of thermal support essential (see 'Mammalian anaesthesia' and Figure 6.6). Most birds are best placed in lateral recumbency during anaesthesia. Dorsal and sternal recumbency can reduce ventilation, due to the coelomic viscera compressing the air sacs and impairment of movement of the sternum respectively. In waterfowl, the use of a facemask for induction may cause apnoea due to stimulation of trigeminal receptors around the beak and nares, which is a stress response often called the 'dive reflex'. Some practitioners use injectable agents such as medetomidine and ketamine, alfaxalone or propofol in waterfowl for this reason; however, an alternative is to intubate and start IPPV.

Air sac cannulation of birds

Air sac cannulation (Heatley, 2008) allows maintenance of anaesthesia in cases of tracheal obstruction or where surgical access to the head or oral cavity is needed (Korbel, 2000), and can also be life-saving in cases of obstructive dyspnoea. Commercial air sac tubes are available, or they can be made from cuffed endotracheal tubes or pieces of sterile drip tubing with holes in the sides as well as the end. Sutures should be preplaced so that the tube can be easily fixed to the skin and underlying musculature once in position. Tubes may be placed into the caudal thoracic air sac (Figure 6.11) either just caudal to the last rib, or between the last two ribs, or alternatively into the abdominal air sac just caudal to the thigh muscles. The left side is preferred to avoid the larger right liver lobe. A short incision is made through the skin and then small haemostats are pushed through the musculature into the air sac. A popping sound should be heard. The haemostats are then opened and the prepared tube pushed through into the air sac. Condensation on the inside of the tube indicates correct positioning. Care should be taken in birds with full gizzards or hepatomegaly, as these structures could inadvertently be damaged on surgically entering the coelomic cavity. Enlargement of these organs can be confirmed radiographically if necessary prior to tube placement. Use in ascitic birds is contraindicated. A fresh gas flow of 0.5–1 litres/minute is usually sufficient to maintain adequate ventilation. On tube removal the incision is closed with one or two sutures, through skin and muscle. Tubes are well tolerated and may be left *in situ* for 3–4 weeks if necessary.

Further information on anaesthesia in specific avian species is given in the chapters that follow.

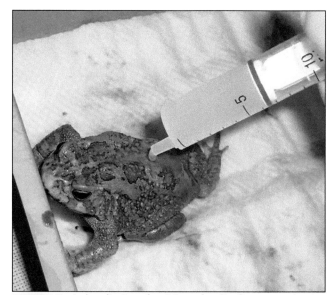

6.12 Topical application of a mixture of 3 ml isoflurane, 1.5 ml water and 3.5 ml KY Jelly® to induce anaesthesia in a guttural toad (*Amietophrynus gutturalis*) given to effect.

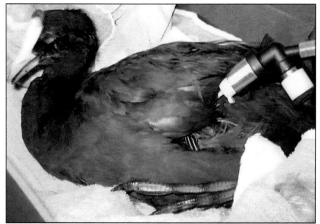

6.11 Coot (*Fulica atra*) with air sac tube *in situ* in the left caudal thoracic air sac.

Amphibian anaesthesia

Powder-free wetted latex gloves should always be used when handling amphibians to avoid damaging the delicate amphibian dermis. Respiration in amphibians can occur via gills or lungs and also passively through the skin. Cutaneous respiration is sufficient to prevent hypoxia during anaesthesia as long as the skin is kept moist. The most commonly used anaesthetic is tricaine methane sulphonate (MS-222) buffered with sodium bicarbonate, via immersion in a water bath. Terrestrial anurans (frogs and toads) typically require 2–3 g MS-222 per litre of well oxygenated, dechlorinated water, which should cover the ventrum but allow them to hold their head out of the water. Aquatic amphibians require lower doses, typically 1–2 g per litre. Benzocaine may be used as an alternative to MS-222; it must be dissolved in ethanol first and then buffered. Isoflurane can also be used via immersion in a bath, mixed with KY Jelly® (3 ml isoflurane mixed with 1.5 ml water and 3.5 ml KY Jelly®) and applied topically to effect (Figure 6.12), or by inhalation in an induction chamber followed by intubation and maintenance using IPPV.

Reptile anaesthesia

Reptiles are ectotherms and their metabolic rate and other physiological processes, including immune function, are optimal within a species-specific temperature range, known as their activity temperature range (ATR) (see Chapter 5). Reptilian cardiorespiratory anatomical and physiological features that have relevance to anaesthesia include the following:

- The glottis is located at the base of the tongue and opened only during active respiration. In snakes and lizards, the trachea has incomplete cartilage rings to allow partial collapse during ingestion of food. Uncuffed endotracheal tubes are generally used
- There is no diaphragm. Inspiration and expiration are both active processes, requiring expansion of the coelomic cavity using intrapulmonary and intercostal muscles in snakes and lizards. Anaesthesia causes relaxation of these muscles and so reptiles are usually apnoeic and require intubation and IPPV during anaesthesia. One to four breaths per minute is usually adequate (Bertelsen, 2007), but this may need to be adjusted for individual patients, for example if capnography indicates hypoventilation
- Reptile lungs are sac-like structures with a honeycomb network of alveoli. Although lung volume is larger, the gas exchange surface is much smaller than in mammals. Tidal volume is variable and affected by factors such as gut fill and the presence of eggs or follicles, as well as temperature. Positioning in dorsal recumbency can reduce the tidal volume due to the weight of the viscera on the respiratory system
- Reptiles can survive on anaerobic metabolism and can hold their breath for long periods. In lizards and snakes, the cardiac ventricle is a single chamber which, during periods of apnoea, allows shunting of blood to the systemic circulation, bypassing the lungs. This makes induction with volatile anaesthetics slow. Mask or chamber induction can be used in small lizards and snakes, for example by placing them in small plastic bags filled with isoflurane or sevoflurane in oxygen.

Injectable options for induction of anaesthesia include propofol (5–10 mg/kg slowly i.v.), alfaxalone (10 mg/kg i.v. or 10–20 mg/kg i.m.) or ketamine and medetomidine (10 mg/kg ketamine with 0.1–0.3 mg/kg medetomidine i.m.). Injectable anaesthetic agents may be given to snakes and lizards by intramuscular injection into the paravertebral muscles, intravenously into the ventral tail vein or intracardiac (snakes only). Snakes and lizards can also be intubated whilst conscious and anaesthesia induced using IPPV, but this is not recommended in venomous species and may be difficult in small British species.

Injectable drugs in reptiles, including anaesthetics, should ideally be given into the cranial half of the body if it is safe to do so. Although pharmacokinetic studies have only been carried out in a few species with a limited number of drugs, it seems that hepatic first-pass extraction may reduce plasma levels and efficacy of some drugs if given into the caudal half of the body (Kummrow *et al.*, 2008; Lahner *et al.*, 2011). Similar concerns about the effect of the renal portal system probably have more theoretical than practical relevance (Holz, 1999).

Recovery from anaesthesia in reptiles can sometimes be prolonged, especially after non-reversible injectable agents have been used. IPPV must be continued until spontaneous respiration resumes but over-ventilation is counterproductive, since high oxygen tension decreases respiratory rate. Using room air rather than oxygen, for example by using an Ambu-bag®, may speed up recovery; 2 bpm is usually appropriate. It is essential to maintain the animal in its ATR.

References and further reading

Bertelsen M (2007) Squamates (Snakes and Lizards). In: *Zoo Animal and Wildlife Immobilization and Anaesthesia*, ed. G West, D Heard and N Caulkett, pp. 233–243. Blackwell Publishing, Iowa

Caulkett N and Haigh J (2007) Deer (Cervids). In: *Zoo Animal and Wildlife Immobilization and Anaesthesia*, ed. G West, D Heard and N Caulkett, pp. 607–612. Blackwell Publishing, Iowa

Cracknell J (2013) Remote chemical injection: darting in practice. *In Practice* **35**, 17–23

Cracknell J (2014) *Darting Manual*. Available at: www.bsava.com

Duncan A (2012) Reptile and Amphibian Analgesia. In: *Fowler's Zoo and Wild Animal Medicine Current Therapy*, ed. R Miller and M Fowler, pp. 247–253. Elsevier Saunders, Missouri

Ebedes H and Raath J (1999) Use of Tranquilisers in Wild Herbivores. In: *Zoo and Wild Animal Medicine Current Therapy 4*, ed. M Fowler and R Miller, pp. 575–585. WB Saunders, Philadelphia

Edling T (2006) Updates in anaesthesia and monitoring. In: *Clinical Avian Medicine*, ed. G Harrison and T Lightfoot, pp. 747–760. Spix Publishing, Palm Beach

Grint N (2013) Anaesthesia. In: *BSAVA Manual of Rabbit Surgery, Dentistry and Imaging*, ed. F Harcourt-Brown and J Chitty, pp. 1–25. BSAVA Publications, Gloucester

Harms C and Harms R (2012) Venous blood gas and lactate values of mourning doves (*Zenaida macroura*), boat-tailed grackles (*Quiscalus major*) and house sparrows (*Passer domesticus*) after capture by mist net, banding and venepuncture. *Journal of Zoo and Wildlife Medicine* **43(1)**, 77–84

Heard D (2007) Monitoring. In: *Zoo Animal and Wildlife Immobilization and Anaesthesia*, ed. G West, D Heard and N Caulkett, pp. 83–91. Blackwell Publishing, Iowa

Heath B (2007) Mobile inhalant anaesthesia techniques. In: *Zoo Animal and Wildlife Immobilization and Anaesthesia*, ed. G West, D Heard and N Caulkett, pp. 75–80. Blackwell Publishing, Iowa

Heatley J (2008) Anaesthesia and analgesia. In: *BSAVA Manual of Raptors, Pigeons and Passerine Birds*, ed. J Chitty and M Lierz, pp. 97–113. BSAVA Publications, Gloucester

Holz P (1999) The reptilian renal portal system: influence on therapy. In: *Zoo and Wild Animal Medicine Current Therapy 4*, ed. M Fowler and R Miller, pp. 249–252. WB Saunders, Philadelphia

Isaza R (2007) Remote Drug Delivery. In: *Zoo Animal and Wildlife Immobilization and Anaesthesia*, ed. G West, D Heard and N Caulkett, pp. 61–74. Blackwell Publishing, Iowa

Kock M and Burroughs R (2012) *Chemical and Physical Restraint of Wild Animals. A Training and Field Manual for African Species*. International Wildlife Veterinary Services, Greyton, South Africa

Korbel R (2000) Disorders of the posterior eye segment in raptors – examination procedures and findings. In: *Raptor Biomedicine III*, ed. J Lumeij, D Remple, P Redig *et al.*, pp. 179–193. Zoological Education Network

Kummrow M, Tseng F, Hesse L *et al.* (2008) Pharmacokinetics of buprenorphine after single-dose subcutaneous administration in red-eared sliders (*Trachemys scripta elegans*). *Journal of Zoo and Wildlife Medicine* **39(4)**, 590–595

Lahner L, Mans C and Sladky K (2011) Comparison of anaesthetic induction and recovery times after intramuscular, subcutaneous or intranasal dexmedetomidine-ketamine administration in red-eared slider turtles (*Trachemys scripta elegans*). *Proceedings of American Association of Zoo Veterinarians Conference 2011*, p.136

Lewis J (2004) Field use of isoflurane and air anaesthetic equipment in wildlife. *Journal of Zoo and Wildlife Medicine* **35(3)**, 303–311

Lynch M and Bodley K (2007) Phocid seals. In: *Zoo Animal and Wildlife Immobilization and Anaesthesia*, ed. G West, D Heard and N Caulkett, pp. 459–468. Blackwell Publishing, Iowa

Machin K (2007) Wildlife Analgesia. In: *Zoo Animal and Wildlife Immobilization and Anaesthesia*, ed. G West, D Heard and N Caulkett, pp. 43–59. Blackwell Publishing, Iowa

Montesinos A and Ardiaca M (2013) Acid–base status in the avian patient using a portable point-of-care analyzer. *Veterinary Clinics of North America: Exotic Animal Practice* **16**, 47–69

Murray M (2006) Cardiopulmonary Anatomy and Physiology. In: *Reptile Medicine and Surgery*, ed. D Mader, pp. 124–134. Saunders Elsevier, St Louis

Norton T and Walsh M (2012) Sea Turtle Rehabilitation. In: *Fowler's Zoo and Wild Animal Medicine Current Therapy*, ed. R Miller and M Fowler, pp. 239–246. Elsevier Saunders, Missouri

Paul-Murphy J and Hawkins M (2012) Avian Analgesia. In: *Fowler's Zoo and Wild Animal Medicine Current Therapy*, ed. R Miller and M Fowler, pp. 312–323. Elsevier Saunders, Missouri

Redrobe S (2004) Anaesthesia and analgesia. In: *BSAVA Manual of Reptiles, 2nd edn*, ed. S Girling and P Raiti, pp. 131–146. BSAVA Publications, Gloucester

Richardson C and Flecknell P (2009) Rodents: anaesthesia and analgesia. In: *BSAVA Manual of Rodents and Ferrets*, ed. E Keeble and A Meredith, pp. 63–72. BSAVA Publications, Gloucester

Schumacher J and Mans C (2014) Anaesthesia. In: *Current Therapy in Reptile Medicine and Surgery*, ed. D Mader and S Divers, pp. 134–153. Elsevier Saunders, St Louis

Sladky K (2014) Analgesia In: *Current Therapy in Reptile Medicine and Surgery*, ed. D Mader and S Divers, pp. 217–228. Elsevier Saunders, St Louis

Spelman L (1999) Otter Anaesthesia. In: *Zoo and Wild Animal Medicine Current Therapy 4*, ed. M Fowler and R Miller, pp. 436–443. WB Saunders, Philadelphia

Stetter M (2007) Amphibians. In: *Zoo Animal and Wildlife Immobilization and Anaesthesia*, ed. G West, D Heard and N Caulkett, pp. 205–209. Blackwell Publishing, Iowa

Wright K (2001) Restraint techniques and euthanasia. In: *Amphibian Medicine and Captive Husbandry*, ed. K Wright and B Whitaker, pp. 111–112. Krieger Publishing Company, Florida

Specialist organizations and useful contacts

See also Appendix 1

Firearms resources – UK Government
www.gov.uk/government/collections/firearms

Chapter 7

Initial management in captivity

Joanna Hedley

Unlike companion animals, wildlife casualties generally arrive at the veterinary clinic or wildlife hospital with little or no prior warning. Consequently, ideal accommodation, food and other resources may not be immediately available for every species. However, all veterinary clinics, even if they do not have specialized facilities, should have the basic equipment, drugs, fluids and nutrition required to stabilize a wildlife casualty and indeed have a legal and ethical responsibility to do so (see Chapters 1 and 2). In-house enclosures such as dog kennels or small mammal cages may be adapted to provide temporary accommodation (Figure 7.1). For longer-term treatment and rehabilitation, patients will usually need to be transferred to a wildlife hospital where there are more appropriate facilities and personnel with the knowledge and resources to deal with these animals (see Chapter 9). It is important to have good links with local wildlife hospitals that can provide help and advice, especially with unfamiliar species. Certain species such as deer (Cervidae), otters (Lutrinae) and seals (Phocidae) require particularly specialized facilities for rehabilitation and their needs can rarely be met for any length of time in a veterinary clinic. Some animals, such as an adult grey seal (*Halichoerus grypus*) or a wild boar (*Sus scrofa*), will not be safe to confine in a veterinary clinic at all, so should be redirected to more appropriate facilities following initial triage (e.g. at the roadside or on the beach). After triage (see Chapter 4) all these species should be transferred to a wildlife hospital with suitable facilities (see Chapter 9).

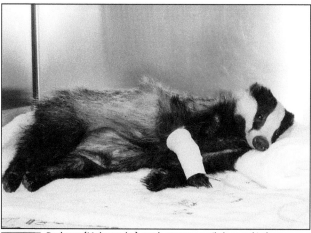

7.1 Badgers (*Meles meles*) can be temporarily housed in large secure dog kennels for initial treatment, but will need to be moved to larger pens for longer-term hospitalization.

Hospitalization

Accommodation

On initial admission, the wildlife casualty is likely to be extremely stressed and, after assessment and first aid (see Chapters 4 and 5), handling should be minimized and the animal allowed time to adjust to its new environment. Appropriate types of accommodation will vary between species and with the severity of the animal's condition, but the following principles apply to all.

Enclosure considerations

Quiet and secluded from predators: Animals should always be housed away from sights, sounds and, ideally, smells of domestic animals, especially from potential predators such as dogs and cats. In a busy veterinary clinic this may be difficult to achieve for any length of time and isolation facilities or a quieter area of the clinic may need to be used. Secure outbuildings, if available, may be especially useful. Both human and animal traffic passing the enclosure should be minimized, especially for easily stressed species such as deer. Predator and prey species should be housed in separate areas. A natural photoperiod for the species should be provided, but bright lights should be avoided to reduce stress.

Suitable size: The hospital enclosure should be of sufficient size to allow the animal to fully stretch out, stand up and turn around. The nature of its injuries and temperament may limit how much opportunity for exercise is initially given. Deer, for example, should be confined on arrival in a relatively small area to minimize opportunities for self-trauma and to allow easy capture for examination and treatment.

Suitable design: Whilst wildlife hospitals may have enclosures specifically designed for one species, most veterinary clinics will need to adapt enclosures designed for domestic animals. The enclosure should ideally be set up so that food and water can be changed without disturbing the animal. It should be easy to observe the animal discreetly, for example by use of a spyhole for walk-in enclosures or by placing a blanket partially over the door of a regular kennel so that the animal feels secure but can still be observed. Animals will also need to be able to be caught easily from the enclosure so access should be unobstructed. It should be remembered that a wild animal casualty placed in an enclosure sedated or moribund may be a very different animal to handle once recovered and enclosures should be chosen with this in mind.

Secure: Wild animals will often escape from poorly constructed enclosures designed for domestic animals. For example, foxes (*Vulpes vulpes*) and rodents will chew their way out, whilst hedgehogs (*Erinaceus europeaus*) display an impressive ability for climbing. In addition to the inconvenience and potential danger of having a sick or injured wild animal loose in the clinic, animals may damage both themselves and their enclosure. Significant dental and limb injuries may result from attempted escape. Care should therefore be taken to ensure that enclosures are sturdy and secure. Bars or mesh should be small enough to prevent the animal partially or completely squeezing through. Restraint equipment, including nets for birds, should be at hand when opening the enclosure and an ability to dim the lights of the room is useful in the event of an escape.

Temperature and humidity: Animals should be kept warm until they are able to thermoregulate, but should be given the option to move away from any focal heat source if desired. Recommended environmental temperatures for mammals range from 15–24°C, whereas small birds may require temperatures of 25–30°C in order to maintain body temperature whilst expending minimal energy (see also Figure 5.12). Once initial shock has been treated and the animal's condition has been stabilized, the environmental temperature may be slowly reduced, except for young animals, which may continue to need an additional source of warmth (see also Chapters 5 and 8). Reptiles and amphibians are ectothermic, relying completely on an external heat source to maintain their body temperature. It is therefore important to provide an appropriate range of temperatures within their enclosure (dependent on species). Environmental humidity should also be considered for those animals closely associated with water, especially amphibians, and frequent spraying of the enclosure may be necessary to maintain appropriate humidity levels.

Cage furniture: All animals should be given a hide area. This may be as simple as a cardboard box for a small rodent or a towel for a hedgehog. It should, however, be possible to retrieve the animal from the hide quickly if necessary, so solid wooden boxes are not advised unless the top can be removed for easy access. Most birds will feel more secure at a height and should also be given the opportunity to perch. The perch should be placed within the enclosure in such a way that it can be easily used and at such a height off the floor that feather damage may be avoided. They should, however, not be placed above food and water bowls as these may quickly become contaminated with droppings. Perches may be natural branches if available or rolled up newspapers or towels can be used as a temporary measure. For debilitated birds that cannot perch, towels can be used to create a nest in which the bird can sit in order to avoid keel damage (Figure 7.2). Cages for short-term hospitalization should not be overfilled with excessive numbers of hides, perches or other cage furniture as initial observation and capture may be limited by these. However, for longer-term use, a more varied naturalistic environment with enrichment and opportunities to bathe if appropriate is important for rehabilitation of wildlife casualties (see Chapter 9).

Substrate and bedding: Substrate should be non-toxic, non-slip, easy to clean and unlikely to cause impaction if ingested. Initially most animals can be housed on newspaper or towels, which can be easily replaced when

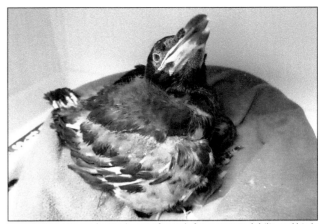

7.2 Nests can be made out of towels for young or debilitated birds such as this fledgling raven (*Corvus corax*).
(© Jenna Richardson)

soiled. Light-coloured towels or paper are recommended so that any bleeding or discharges can be easily observed. Over a longer time period, straw, hay, shavings or shredded paper may be used. Any sharp edges or corners of the enclosure should be well padded to avoid trauma and extra bedding will be required for recumbent animals. Suitable padding should be provided to prevent keel damage in water birds (see Chapters 24, 25 and 26); in the short term, use can be made of blankets and other bedding (Figure 7.3).

Hygiene and infection control

As with domestic species, there are many infectious diseases carried by wildlife casualties, including those that can potentially affect humans (Figures 7.4, 7.5 and 7.6) (Simpson, 2008). Consequently, good hygiene and barrier nursing are vital to prevent transmission of infections both to people and to other animals within the clinic. One study performed in two Californian wildlife hospitals identified potentially zoonotic *Campylobacter, Vibrio, Salmonella, Giardia* or *Cryptosporidium* species in 31% of faecal samples from their wildlife casualties (Siembieda *et al.*, 2011). Conversely, some diseases carried by domestic animals may be of increased clinical significance in a wildlife casualty. For example, wildcats (*Felis silvestris*) are thought to be susceptible to diseases

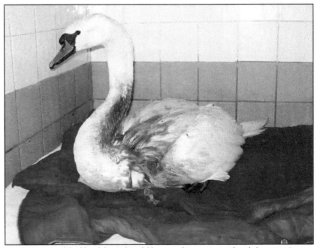

7.3 Padded bedding should be used to prevent keel damage in recumbent patients such as this mute swan (*Cygnus olor*).
(© Secret World Wildlife Rescue)

Zoonotic disease	Species commonly affected	Common routes of zoonotic infection
Viral infections		
Avian influenza	Birds	Aerosol
Parvovirus infection	Most species	Faecal–oral
Rabies (lyssaviruses)	Bats, foxes	Bites, saliva contamination of wounds
Seal pox (poxvirus)	Seals	Skin contact
West Nile virus (flavivirus)	Birds	Insect (mosquito) bites, aerosol
Bacterial infections		
Campylobacteriosis (*Campylobacter* spp.)	Most species, especially birds	Faecal–oral
Chlamydiosis (Ornithosis) (*Chlamydia psittaci*)	Pigeons and other birds	Aerosol
Coliform infections (*Escherichia coli* and others)	Most species	Faecal–oral
Leptospirosis (*Leptospira* spp.)	Rodents, foxes	Urine contamination
Lyme disease (*Borrelia burgdorferi*)	Deer, foxes	Tick bites
Mycoplasmosis ('seal finger') (*Mycoplasma* spp.)	Seals	Skin contact
Salmonellosis (*Salmonella* spp.)	Most species	Faecal–oral
Tuberculosis (*Mycobacterium bovis, M. avium*)	Badgers, deer	Aerosol, post-mortem examination
Fungal infections		
Dermatophytosis (ringworm) (*Trichophyton erinacei, Microsporum*, other *Trichophyton* spp.)	Hedgehogs (see Figure 7.6), foxes	Skin contact (especially via spines of hedgehogs)
Protozoal infections		
Cryptosporidiosis (*Cryptosporidia* spp.)	Most species	Faecal–oral
Giardiasis (*Giardia* spp.)	Most species	Faecal–oral
Ectoparasitic infections		
Sarcoptic mange (*Sarcoptes scabiei*)	Foxes (see Figure 7.5)	Skin contact

7.4 Examples of zoonotic infections that may be carried by British wildlife casualties.

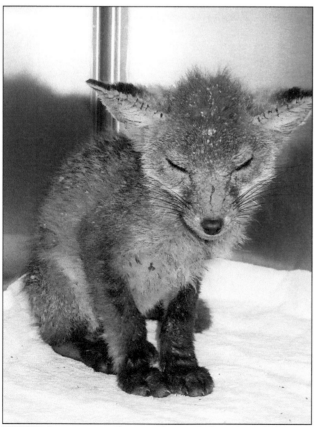

7.5 Foxes can carry the zoonotic parasite *Sarcoptes scabiei*, as shown in this cub with patchy alopecia, scaling and crusting.

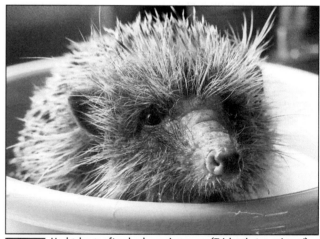

7.6 Hedgehogs often harbour ringworm (*Trichophyton erinacei*) with alopecia and crusty lesions typically around the face, as shown here.

of the domestic cat with infections potentially spreading rapidly through populations (McOrist, 1992) (see also Chapter 20). In wildlife hospital situations, examples of suspected nosocomial infections include Tyzzer's disease in a young European otter (*Lutra lutra*) (Simpson *et al.*, 2008) and parvovirus in badger cubs (Barlow *et al.*, 2012) (see also Chapter 17).

All practices should have appropriate written health and safety risk assessments in place for dealing with wildlife casualties, as well as an in-house policy for both disease control and disease investigation.

With the exception of young animals being hand-reared (see Chapter 8), all patients should be isolated initially, both for assessment and to prevent spread of disease. Ideally separate overalls, footwear and equipment should be used for dealing with animals in quarantine facilities. Some patients may require strict isolation throughout their stay in hospital to reduce stress, potential imprinting or disease. Others, particularly young animals, should be kept with companions of the same species and age group to ensure socialization, and may need to be transferred to an appropriate wildlife facility quickly to ensure this can occur. Badger cubs are a classic example of young animals that need to be kept with others and which can become rapidly imprinted on humans with excessive contact (see Chapters 9 and 17).

The level of hygiene considered appropriate will depend on the species involved and the disease risk posed. Many practices will opt to barrier nurse these patients as their disease status is unknown. Enclosures should at minimum be spot-cleaned daily and completely cleaned and disinfected as often as practical. For patients with potentially infectious diseases, barrier nursing may be required, including wearing latex gloves and disposable plastic aprons or overalls to prevent spread of dermal infections. Masks should be worn when patients are presented with clinical signs suspicious of airborne zoonotic diseases (e.g. avian chlamydiosis). Hands should be washed and surfaces, equipment and scales disinfected after handling each patient or diagnostic samples. When wildlife casualties leave the veterinary practice, enclosures should be thoroughly cleaned using disinfectant agents appropriate to the disease risks, at appropriate concentrations and for the correct contact time.

All staff should be aware of the potential risk for zoonoses when dealing with wildlife casualties and only staff vaccinated for rabies should routinely handle bats (Bat Conservation Trust, 2008). Further information for health and safety considerations when handling different wildlife casualties can be found in Chapter 3 and the individual species chapters.

Initial diet

On admission many wildlife casualties will be dehydrated and malnourished. Fluid deficits should be corrected (see Chapter 5) and appropriate nutritional support provided. This may be by offering food that can be eaten voluntarily, or by tube feeding if the patient is debilitated. Enteral feeding requirements should ideally be calculated based on the individual animal's caloric requirement and divided into 2–4 feeds per day (see Chapter 5). There are a variety of complete liquid diets readily available for herbivores (e.g. Oxbow Critical Care®; Supreme Science Recovery), carnivores (e.g. Oxbow Carnivore Care®), and granivores (e.g. Harrison's Bird Foods® Recovery Formula™). Omnivore diets are also available (e.g. Emeraid® Omnivore), but if these are not in stock, combinations of other formulas may be adapted taking into consideration the animal's natural diet. Birds and young mammals such as seal pups will often need repeated tube feeding until eating voluntarily, whilst neonatal mammals and birds may need hand-rearing for several weeks to months and will need more specialized formulas (see Chapter 8).

Once the patient is eating by itself, a suitable diet should be provided (Figures 7.7, 7.8 and 7.9; see also species-specific chapters). Bill shape can be used to help establish the type of food naturally eaten in small bird species (see Figure 30.3). In the long term it is important to try to replicate the wildlife casualty's natural diet, but for the first few days this may be unavailable or, due to the debilitated condition of the patient, it may not be appropriate. As well as the main diet, additional highly palatable 'treats' may also be used to stimulate appetite, but animals should be weaned on to a more balanced diet as soon as appetite returns. The diets suggested in Figure 7.7 are only suitable for short-term use; details of longer-term appropriate diets for each species are given in the chapters that follow.

The amount and type of food required will vary depending on the age, activity level and health status of the animal and should be adjusted for the individual based on amount eaten, with the aim to either maintain or

Species	Natural dietary preference	Food that could be used for short-term feeding (see also species-specific chapters)
Fox	Omnivore	Dog food: 350–550 g/day (tinned plus a handful of dry biscuits)
Badger	Omnivore	Dog food: 550–750 g/day (tinned plus a handful of dry biscuits)
Hedgehog	Insectivore	Dog or cat food: approximately 80 g/day (tinned plus a handful of dry biscuits) (see Figure 7.8)
Bat	Insectivore	Mealworms or jelly from wet cat food if no mealworms available
Deer	Herbivore	Fresh browse (e.g. hawthorn, willow, rose), hay, small amount of sheep or goat concentrates
Otter	Piscivore	Whole fish with vitamin supplementation
Rabbit	Herbivore	Grass, hay, rabbit pellets, leafy greens
Small rodents	Omnivore	Grass, hay, seeds, commercial pet rodent feeds
Small garden birds	Insectivore (e.g. blackbird)	Cat food, mealworms, waxworms
	Granivore (e.g. greenfinch)	Mixed grain (wild bird seed mixes, breakfast cereal mixes)
Pigeon	Granivore	Mixed grain or corn, wild bird seed mixes, breakfast cereal mixes
Swan, duck, goose	Herbivore	Chopped leafy greens, herbivore pellets or grain from deep water-filled bowl
Raptors	Carnivore	Day-old chicks (see Figure 7.9), mice, avian carnivore diet, strips of meat
Seabirds	Omnivore	Whole fish with vitamin supplementation Tinned dog or cat food for gulls

7.7 Examples of food that may be offered on admission to wildlife casualties for short-term feeding. Please note that these are for short-term feeding only and may not be nutritionally suitable for long-term feeding. In some cases alternative items are suggested as overnight substitutes, where a more appropriate diet may not be readily available in the veterinary practice.

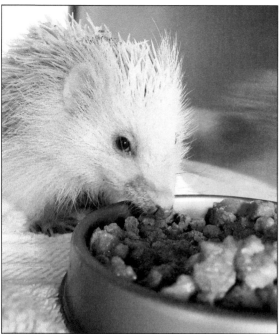

7.8 Hedgehogs should be offered dog or cat food for short-term feeding. This is a leucistic individual, which is a rare colour variation in the UK and would be particularly susceptible to predation.

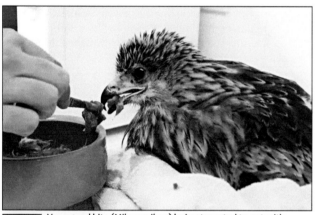

7.9 Young red kite (*Milvus milvus*) being tempted to eat with chopped up day-old chicks.

increase weight. Obesity and dental disease are rarely concerns in the first few days' treatment of wildlife casualties, although may occur in patients hospitalized for longer (e.g. overwintered juvenile hedgehogs). Consideration should be given to how often the species usually eats and at which time of day; for example, nocturnal animals such as hedgehogs should be fed in the evenings to encourage more natural behaviour and avoid food spoilage. Certain species such as woodcocks (*Scolopax rusticola*) and nightjars (*Caprimulgus europaeus*) will often not voluntarily eat at all in captivity and are highly stressed, whereas others, such as swifts (*Apus apus*), will only feed 'on the wing' and therefore have to be hand-fed, and some aquatic birds will only eat food from the water. Some birds that have more specialized ways of feeding, such as woodpeckers (Picidae) and kingfishers (*Alcedo atthis*), will only feed if food items are presented in a more natural form, for example by placing insectivorous diet or mealworms on the bark of a log for woodpeckers and injecting air into fish so that they float for kingfishers. For some of these patients assisted feeding may be required and their stay in captivity should be minimized.

Water should always be freely available for all species. Containers should be used which cannot be easily tipped over and in which the animal has no possibility of injury or drowning; young animals are more susceptible to hypothermia should they become soaked by water. Water should be changed daily or more frequently if necessary.

Therapeutics

Principles of first aid and emergency care have already been detailed earlier (see Chapter 5) but consideration should also be given to the administration of longer-term therapeutics. For example, drug choice may be influenced by frequency and route of administration and any available data on drug use in that species. Ideally, drugs licensed for a specific condition in that species should be prescribed but as very few drugs are licensed for use in wildlife, those authorized for use in a different species will generally have to be considered in accordance with the prescribing cascade. If likely to enter the human food chain, drug withdrawal periods for food-producing species must be observed (see Chapter 22). All treatments and procedures should be timed to occur together and all medication and equipment prepared beforehand to minimize length and frequency of handling.

Routes of medication
Oral

Animals being tube fed may have oral medications mixed in with the liquid food and administered at the same time. Small amounts of oral suspensions can also be administered to bats with a dropper, pipette or cut-off intravenous cannula sleeve attached to a 1 ml syringe. For most other animals, restraint for direct oral administration of drugs via syringe or tablet is stressful and often unsuccessful. In-food medications can be useful for animals that are eating, but rely on the entire meal or treat being eaten and the animal having a functional gastrointestinal system for absorption of the drug. Many species, such as badgers and hedgehogs, also have a well developed sense of smell, so will easily detect and avoid in-food medication, although some of the 'palatable' formulations of canine medications may help overcome this. In-water medication is similarly unreliable as water intake is variable. Consequently, the oral route is not ideal for initial treatment of the wildlife casualty.

Parenteral

Administering medications via the parenteral route ensures that the complete dose of medication is received but requires restraint, so longer-acting drugs should ideally be selected to minimize frequency of handling. This is both from the viewpoint of reducing stress for the animal and reducing the risk of human injuries if handling more dangerous species. Subcutaneous and intramuscular injections may be administered relatively easily to most animals. Intravenous injections, however, will often require sedation unless the patient is extremely debilitated, so are not usually given except in emergency situations.

Topical

Topical medications may be used for the treatment of wounds and skin disease, or in amphibians for systemic disease. Regular application may be limited by the need to handle and restrain the patient. Most wild animals will not tolerate bandages or collars and ointments may be rapidly licked off so patient compliance may limit the use of this route. For animals with respiratory disease, especially smaller species such as hedgehogs, administration of drugs by nebulization can also be a useful route in conjunction with systemic therapy.

Dose rates

Drug doses for wildlife species have rarely been established by scientific trials and are instead based on experience and extrapolated from similar domestic animals. For example, drug doses used in foxes may be based on those used in the domestic dog. For smaller animals, direct scaling of drug dosages may not be appropriate as their metabolic rate will be much higher. Allometric scaling may be indicated in these situations using formulae to calculate more appropriate dose rates. These calculations, however, do not take into account the variations in pharmacokinetics for different drugs in different species so, if possible, information should be found regarding drug use in the individual species (Hunter and Isaza, 2008). Suggested doses for common drugs are given in the species-specific chapters that follow. Other resources available include the *BSAVA Small Animal Formulary* (Ramsey, 2014), *BSAVA Small Animal Formulary Part B: Exotic Pets* (Meredith, 2015), *Exotic Animal Formulary* (Carpenter, 2013) and Wildpro® resources provided by the Wildlife Information Network (see Appendix 1).

Prophylactic treatment

Parasite treatment

Many wild animals naturally live with a parasite burden. For example, foxes and hedgehogs may live with fleas and swans with lice. In a healthy wild animal the host–parasite relationship is usually balanced so that parasite numbers do not become excessive or cause any obvious clinical effects to the host (see Chapter 1). In a debilitated animal, especially one confined in captivity, parasite numbers may rapidly increase and result in significant pathological effects. Juvenile animals may also carry large parasite burdens, which, as well as being debilitating for the casualty, can also be problematic when handling the animal for feeding and other care. Wildlife casualties may therefore need to be treated for parasites at an early stage to prevent numbers escalating. Treatment should ideally be based on the type and number of parasites found, with the aim being not to completely eliminate parasites but simply to reduce levels. In some situations, treatment protocols may be designed based not specifically on the parasites detected from one individual, but on knowledge of a likely parasite burden in a geographical area or in a specific casualty group, for example lungworm in young hedgehogs in the autumn. Alternatively, parasite treatment may be indicated for those animals kept in a ward with others to prevent parasite transmission either to other animals or humans. Examples include treatment of a fox for sarcoptic mange (see Figure 7.5) or a hedgehog for fleas and ticks (Figure 7.10). Specific treatments for these and other parasitic infections are given in the species-specific chapters that follow.

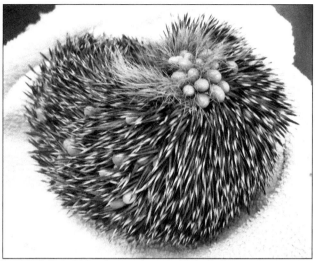

7.10 High tick burdens, as shown in this hedgehog, are not uncommon, especially in debilitated animals.

Vaccination

Vaccination of wildlife casualties is rarely indicated except in situations where there is already a disease outbreak in the local area. Examples include distemper in common seals (*Phoca vitulina*) (Visser *et al.*, 1992) (see Chapter 23), myxomatosis in rabbits (Guitton *et al.*, 2008) (see Chapter 16) and tuberculosis and parvovirus in badgers (see Chapter 17). Vaccination should not replace strict quarantine protocols in a disease outbreak and euthanasia of infected animals may need to be considered to reduce the spread of disease.

Patient monitoring and record-keeping

Record-keeping is vital to monitor the progress of individual animals, especially in wildlife hospitals receiving large numbers of admissions and in those situations where care of the animal is performed by multiple individuals. Records can also be used to review admissions over a period of time and provide evidence of which protocols are successful and which need further modification. Records are also essential for the development of a scientific evidence base for the treatment and rehabilitation of wildlife and knowledge of outcomes following release (Mullineaux, 2014).

Animals should be visually checked daily and basic parameters should be recorded as for domestic animal patients. Minimal information should include amount and type of food eaten, water drunk, urine or faeces passed and any abnormal behaviour noticed. A daily record should be kept of any treatments or medications that the animal has received, with dose rates, route of administration and frequency noted. Weight (Figure 7.11) and body condition (see Chapter 4) should be measured and recorded on admission and then at regular intervals during the individual's period in hospital. Weight measurement is essential for accurate dosage of medication, especially for small animals, which may be easily over- or under-dosed. Animals should always be weighed at the same time of day consistently before or after feeding to avoid too much variation. Frequency of weighing will depend on the species and stress of handling.

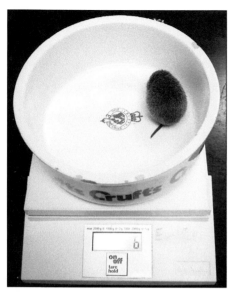

7.11

All patients should be weighed on admission and at regular intervals throughout their time in hospital. Small digital scales may be required, as for this immature field vole (*Microtus agrestis*).

Acknowledgements

Thanks to Sue Schwar and all at South Essex Wildlife Hospital for providing photographs and their help with this chapter. Thanks also to Steve Smith for his contributions to Figure 7.4.

References and further reading

Barlow AM, Schock A, Bradshaw J *et al.* (2012) Parvovirus enteritis in Eurasian badgers (*Meles meles*). *Veterinary Record* **170(16)**, 416

Bat Conservation Trust (2008) *Bat care guidelines: a guide to bat care for rehabilitators.* Bat Conservation Trust, London

Carpenter JW (2013) *Exotic Animal Formulary, 4th edn.* Elsevier Saunders, Missouri

Guitton JS, Devillard S, Guénézan M *et al.* (2008) Vaccination of free-living juvenile wild rabbits (*Oryctolagus cuniculus*) against myxomatosis improved their survival. *Preventative Veterinary Medicine.* **84(1–2)**, 1–10

Hunter RP and Isaza R (2008) Concepts and issues with interspecies scaling in zoological pharmacology. *Journal of Zoo and Wildlife Medicine* **39(4)**, 517–526

Meredith A (2015) *BSAVA Small Animal Formulary, 9th edn. Part B: Exotic Pets.* BSAVA Publications, Gloucester

McOrist S (1992) Diseases of the European wildcat (*Felis silvestris Schreber, 1777*) in Great Britain. *Revue Scientifique et Technique* **11(4)**, 1143–1149

Mullineaux E (2014) Veterinary treatment and rehabilitation of indigenous wildlife. *Journal of Small Animal Practice.* **50**, 293–300

Ramsey I (2014) *BSAVA Small Animal Formulary, 8th edn.* BSAVA Publications, Gloucester

Siembieda JI, Miller WA, Byrne BA *et al.* (2011) Zoonotic pathogens isolated from wild animals and environmental samples at two California wildlife hospitals. *Journal of the American Veterinary Medical Association* **238(6)**, 773–783

Simpson V (2008) Wildlife as reservoirs of zoonotic diseases in the UK. *In Practice* **30**, 486–494

Simpson VR, Hargreaves J, Birtles RJ *et al.* (2008) Tyzzer's disease in a Eurasian otter (*Lutra lutra*) in Scotland. *Veterinary Record* **163(18)**, 539–543

Stocker L (2005) *Practical Wildlife Care, 2nd edn.* Blackwell Publishing Ltd, Oxford

Visser IK, Vedder E, Van De Bildt MW *et al.* (1992) Canine distemper virus ISCOMs induce protection in harbour seals (*Phoca vitulina*) against phocid distemper but still allow subsequent infection with phocid distemper virus-1. *Vaccine* **10**, 435–438

Chapter 8

Care and hand-rearing of young wild animals

Sara Cowen

Working with wildlife casualties can be varied and extremely busy, especially during the period of March through until October, when large numbers of 'orphaned' animals may be seen. In the author's experience, approximately 80% of these will be juvenile birds, with only 20% juvenile mammals. This chapter will discuss the principles of rearing orphaned wildlife; further species-specific information is given in the chapters that follow. Where the author has found specific products to be useful in her experience in rearing, the product name has been included for further information.

Juvenile wildlife casualties may be admitted for a number of reasons including abandonment, accidental disturbance and, very commonly, cat attack. They will often require care for an appreciable amount of time. The process of hand-rearing, weaning and rehabilitation varies with each species; for birds this may be as little as 3–4 weeks, whilst some mammals, for example fox (*Vulpes vulpes*) and badger (*Meles meles*) cubs, may take anything up to 8 months to rear, rehabilitate and release at an appropriate available site and time of year (see Chapter 9).

There are many considerations that must be explored before even attempting to rear juvenile wildlife species. These include housing, time and resources available and, in particular, consideration of potential malprinting and the knock-on effects this will have on release options and survival rates (see Chapter 9).

Although in principle working with orphaned mammals involves the same level of care and responsibility as for domestic neonates such as puppies or kittens, it should always be borne in mind that these animals are not domesticated and, as such, handling may be stressful and should be restricted where possible.

Where neonatal wildlife casualties are admitted to a general veterinary practice, this can lead to potential pitfalls and problems. Generally the practice is not the ideal place for any wild animal as many are prey species, so coming into contact with predators such as cats and dogs can cause considerable stress just by being in the same locality. Wildlife casualties can also carry diseases and parasites, which may affect in-contact domestic animals or be zoonotic (see Chapter 7). It is vital to triage all wildlife cases, regardless of age, at the point of first contact (see Chapter 4) and always consider the long-term plan and possibility of moving the animal on to specialized centres with species-specific facilities (see Chapter 9).

When treating and rehabilitating wildlife casualties, either short or long term, the most important consideration at all times is the welfare of the animal as some species do not tolerate captivity well and are easily stressed.

Considerations for rearing wildlife casualties

Housing and equipment

In preparation for looking after juvenile animals, it is advisable to have a number of basic pieces of equipment in the veterinary practice/rehabilitation centre.

Incubators are vital, especially for very young birds and mammals, as these are less able to maintain their own body temperature and are usually featherless or hairless when newly hatched/born (Figure 8.1). As alternative heat sources, electric heat pads, hot water bottles, microwaveable heat pads or wheat bags can be used (see Chapter 5). Particular care should be taken with neonatal animals as they are less able to regulate their temperature. Heat sources should always be covered, for example with a towel, to avoid the possibility of burns. Environmental temperature should be measured regularly to ensure neonatal animals are being kept at an appropriate thermoneutral range (see Figure 5.12). Once over 2 weeks of age, most young animals are more able to regulate their own body temperature so a direct heat source that they can choose to move away from can be safely used.

Keeping a variety of different sized feeding bottles, syringes, teats, tweezers, paintbrushes, pipettes and feeding tubes in stock is also important, as each orphan species may require a different type of equipment for feeding (Figure 8.2).

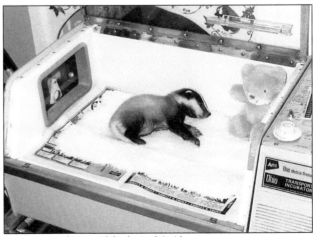

8.1 Incubator with badger cub inside.
(© Secret World Wildlife Rescue)

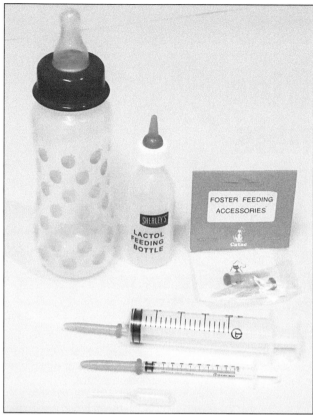

8.2 It is essential to have a variety of different-sized feeding bottles, syringes, teats and pipettes in stock, as each orphan species may require a different type of equipment for feeding.
(© Secret World Wildlife Rescue)

In addition it is vital to stock the correct milk replacement product for each species encountered, such as Esbilac®, goat milk and various commercial veterinary canine or feline milk replacement products. A well stocked supply of towels, fleeces and cotton wool is also essential.

All equipment should be thoroughly cleaned after each feed and placed in sterilizing fluid for disinfection to limit the risk of disease transfer between juvenile animals. Ideally separate utensils are allocated to each individual to be used only on that animal; even so, cleaning and disinfection should still be carried out. It is essential to maintain excellent standards of hygiene as juvenile animals, especially neonates, are highly susceptible to disease. Mammals may have compromised immunity due to lack of maternal antibodies that are normally derived from colostrum.

Wildlife may carry zoonotic diseases and thus also pose a disease risk to humans (see Chapter 7), so it is vital to ensure high levels of personal hygiene and biosecurity, and wear protective clothing such as aprons, masks and gloves. Health and safety assessments should be made and standard operating procedures adhered to.

Casualty-specific considerations

Initial assessment of the casualty should consider the following questions:

- **What is it?** Wildlife species, especially birds, are often misidentified. It is extremely important to ensure the species is correctly identified so that an appropriate diet is used. Advice should be sought from specialists if unsure. There are also useful fledgling identification guides available online (see 'Specialist organizations and useful contacts')

- **How old is it?** It is important to assess the stage of development of the orphaned animal to ensure correct feeding amounts and intervals are applied
- **What should it be fed?** Once the species has been established, then all the dietary requirements and needs for that animal can be provided. For mammals, this also includes determining the weaning status to ascertain whether the patient requires hand-feeding or is self-feeding, and whether it requires milk replacements or can go straight on to solid food
- **Will it need toileting?** In the wild, the majority of juvenile mammals will be stimulated by the parent to defecate and urinate. This can be replicated in captivity by gently wiping the anogenital area with damp cotton wool before and after each feed. Juvenile birds toilet automatically after being fed, depositing a sac containing faeces and urates over the side of the nest
- **What are the possible complications?** Juvenile animals may suffer from nutritional diarrhoea, constipation, bloating and other gastrointestinal problems following dietary changeover; any changes to faecal output should be monitored closely and treated immediately to prevent further problems developing.

Avoiding malprinting and habituation

Imprinting is age-dependent learning, which in the case of neonates happens quickly after birth or hatching and includes behaviour such as the young following the first moving thing they see. If the natural parent is not present, **malprinting** may occur, especially in altricial species, in which the animal rapidly establishes behaviour recognition and attraction to another animal, person or thing and sees them as a parent, learning behaviour from that individual. Malprinting is a huge concern in juvenile rearing as the animal risks the real possibility of becoming too 'tame' to be released. **Habituation** is the process in which an animal stops responding to a specific stimulus as a result of over familiarization; in the case of hand-reared neonates, this can result in them losing their natural 'flight' responses to humans (see also Chapter 9). Most mammals and birds are fairly robust and relatively easy to rear; however, the individual animal's welfare must be the priority and this requires careful management. Handling of wildlife casualties must be kept to an absolute minimum if they are to have any hope of returning to the wild.

To avoid malprinting and habituation, the following steps should be considered:

- Ensure that the time spent with orphans is limited to essential feeding and cleaning out
- Ensure that only a limited number of essential staff deal with the orphans to avoid them becoming confident around all humans
- Keep noise and interaction to the lowest levels possible
- If possible, place individuals with other orphans of the same species to ensure interactive play and other activities are with another animal
- Once weaned, place the animal into an environment where it can be stimulated with natural activities that would take place in the wild
- Provide ample opportunity for exercise and enrich the enclosure with objects that will encourage natural behaviour, such as hunting, foraging and areas to hide
- At the later stage of rearing, all human activity should be kept to a minimum and if possible the animals should be shut away during feeding and cleaning so there is no association with humans.

Considerations for release

All wildlife must be 100% fit for survival in the wild and independent of humans before release can be considered. Pre- and ideally post-release monitoring of behaviour is especially vital in the case of hand-reared animals (see Chapter 9). Most juveniles will require a 'soft' release with initial support feeding. Suitable habitats and release sites should be carefully surveyed and will require the landowner's permission for use (see also Chapters 2 and 9). Some species, such as grey squirrels (*Sciurus carolinensis*), require specific licences for keeping and releasing them and their rehabilitation should not be undertaken without these in place. General advice and licences are available from Natural England, Natural Resources Wales and Scottish Natural Heritage (see also Appendix 1 and Chapter 2).

Rearing juvenile mammals

The following procedures should be followed for mammalian casualties:

- On arrival identify the species, weigh and sex the orphan and record this information on an individual patient record card. Note the animal's size, weight, whether the eyes are open or not and other relevant characteristics; assess its age and base feeding amounts and intervals on this information
- 'Toilet' the juvenile animal (stimulate it to urinate and defecate by wiping the perineal region with damp cotton wool), as it may have been separated from its parent several hours before and need relieving. This will need to be continued until the animal is approximately 3 weeks of age
- Place the animal in an incubator set at a temperature range of 28–30°C
- If there is more than one animal in a litter, identify the orphans individually with a differently placed small mark using, for example, correction fluid, or clipping a small area of fur (Figure 8.3)
- If weak, unable to lift the head and there is no swallow reflex, do not be tempted to feed the orphan, as there is a risk of aspiration of fluids. In this instance, parenteral fluid therapy should be instigated, blood glucose should be measured and supportive care provided (see Chapter 5)
- Once more responsive and able to swallow, the juvenile mammal should be offered a feed. A good indication that the juvenile animal is hungry is that it is vocalizing and moving around in search of food
- The first feed should consist of an electrolyte replacement fluid (e.g. Vetark® Critical Care Formula) to rehydrate the animal and limit potential damage if accidentally aspirated, until the animal is used to taking fluids from a bottle or teat
- Subsequent feeds should consist of the appropriate milk feed for the species with the volume and frequency calculated according to the age of the animal (see Figure 8.4 and species-specific information)
- Always record the individual feed amounts taken and work out the total daily volume fed to ensure there is a daily increase in volume ingested
- Feed between 6am and midnight; only newborns (e.g. mammals with the umbilical cord still attached) will require feeding through the night

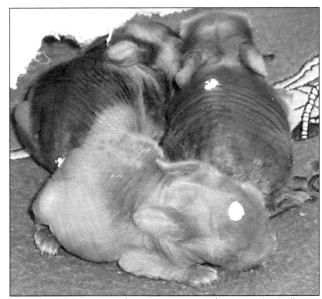

8.3 Juvenile rabbits (*Oryctolagus cuniculus*) can be individually identified using, for example, correction fluid.
(© Secret World Wildlife Rescue)

Age	Frequency of milk feeding
1–2 weeks old	2 hourly
3 weeks old	3 hourly
4 weeks old	4 hourly
At 4–6 weeks begin weaning process	4 hourly but reducing as weaning progresses

8.4 General guidelines for the frequency of milk feeding of juvenile mammals.

- Milk must be fed warm to the touch (as a general guide, the temperature should be tested before each feed on the wrist). If a baby mammal is reluctant to feed or stops feeding halfway through a feed, in the author's experience this is usually a result of the milk being too cold
- If tiny or not sucking, feed initially using teats or intravenous catheter sleeves and syringes and later move on to a baby bottle of an appropriate size (Figure 8.5). The juvenile animal should be fed in a natural position and winded after feeding. This is performed by carefully placing the young animal on a towel and gently rubbing the shoulder areas and back

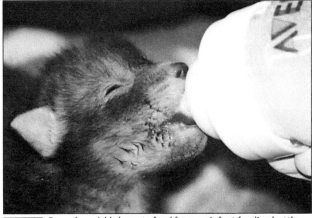

8.5 Fox cubs quickly learn to feed from an infant feeding bottle and teat.
(© Secret World Wildlife Rescue)

- The weaning process may take time and should be done gradually to prevent complications such as nutritional diarrhoea due to dietary change, bloating, or gut stasis/dysbiosis
- Introduce new dietary items slowly. The diet should be as near to a natural diet as possible.

Rearing neonatal badgers, foxes, squirrels and hedgehogs

Feeding guidelines are given for neonatal badgers (Figure 8.6), foxes (Figure 8.7), squirrels (Figure 8.8) and hedgehogs (*Erinaceus europaeus*) (Figure 8.9). Hoglets (young hedgehogs) will initially learn to feed from a syringe with a teat attached (Figure 8.10), but will progress to lapping milk from a bowl when older (Figure 8.11).

Rearing neonatal deer

Guidelines for feeding neonatal deer fawn (calves or kids) are given in Figure 8.12. Exact volumes and frequency will depend on the species, strength and feeding interest of the fawn. (For more information, see Figure 22.23.) Once sucking, they will regulate their own food intake, usually

Age (days)	Frequency of milk feeding	Approx. amount per feed (ml)*
1–3	2 hourly	1–2
3–7	3 hourly	1–2
8–14	3 hourly	2–3
15–21	4 hourly	3–5
22–28	4 hourly; begin to wean, lap from bowl	5–6
20–27	5 hourly; begin weaning on to solid meat	7–10
28	Provide water, cat food and invertebrates	Leave milk in bowl
Up to 8 weeks	Fully weaned	Phase out milk

8.9 Feeding guidelines for hoglets. *Esbilac® puppy replacement milk.

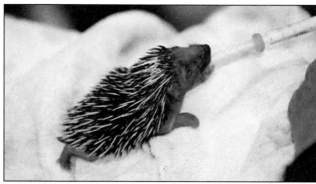

8.10 Hoglets will initially learn to feed from a syringe with a teat attached.
(© Secret World Wildlife Rescue)

Age (weeks)	Frequency of milk feeding	Approx. amount per feed (ml)*
0–1	2 hourly	3–5
1–2	2–3 hourly	5–10
2–3	3–4 hourly	10–20
3–4	4 hourly	20–40
4–7	4–5 feeds daily	40–100
7–12	3–4 feeds daily; begin weaning	100–250

8.6 Feeding guidelines for badger cubs. *Esbilac® milk replacement (ml) and 1 drop of Abidec® multivitamins.

Age (weeks)	Frequency of milk feeding	Approx. amount per feed (ml)*
0–1	2 hourly	5–10
1–2	2–3 hourly	10–20
2–3	3–4 hourly	20–30
3–4	4 hourly; begin weaning	40
4–5	4 feeds daily; reduce as weaning progresses	50

8.7 Feeding guidelines for fox cubs. *Puppy replacement milk.

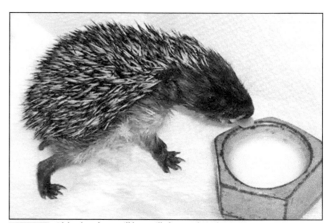

8.11 Older hoglets will lap milk from a bowl.
(© Secret World Wildlife Rescue)

Age (weeks)	Frequency of milk feeding	Approx. amount (ml)*
0–1	2 hourly	0.5–1
1–2	2–3 hourly	1–2
2–3	3 hourly	2–4
3–4	3–4 hourly	4–6
4–5	4 hourly; begin weaning	6–8
5–6	5 hourly; reduce as weaning progresses	8–10
7–8	3 feeds a day; reduce as weaning progresses	10–14

8.8 Feeding guidelines for squirrel kits. *Kitten replacement milk/goat milk.

Age (weeks)	Frequency of milk feeding	Approx. amount per feed (ml)* (dependent on species)
0–1	2 hourly	20–40
1–2	2–3 hourly	40–80
2–3	3–4 hourly	80–120
3–4	4 hourly	120–200
4–7	4–5 feeds daily	200–500
7–12	3–4 feeds daily; begin weaning	500
Up to 7 months	1 feed daily; continue weaning	500

8.12 Feeding guidelines for fawns (calves and kids). *Goat milk/lamb replacement milk.

with a fairly frenzied rapid sucking. If not sucking within 24 hours, stomach tubing should be considered. Deer wean very late and it is important to remember that they will still take a bowl of milk daily, in some species, up to 7 months of age. Fawns should be given access to soil and browse to eat from day 3 in addition to milk (Figure 8.13).

If there is a problem getting a fawn to feed using a bottle, milk should be offered instead from a bowl and, if accepted, this method of feeding is less labour intensive. If bottle-fed initially, introduce feeding from a bowl as soon as the fawn begins drinking water. At the same time, gradually reduce bottle feeds. Weaning will usually begin when the fawn is approximately 2 months old.

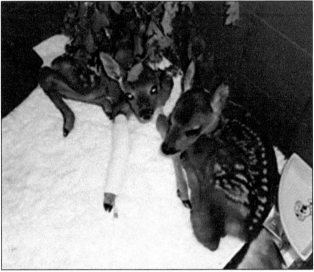

8.13 Deer fawns should also be offered browse from an early age. (© Secret World Wildlife Rescue)

Rearing neonatal bats

Young bats should be placed inside a tightly closed plastic vivarium set partly on top of a heat mat, with a towel draped inside for the bat to hang on to (Figure 8.14). Bats should be fed milk replacement, such as Esbilac®, and will suck from a paintbrush, small pipette or 1 ml syringe attached to an intravenous catheter sleeve. The amount taken is difficult to measure with the former two methods and will differ with each species. Milk feeds should be

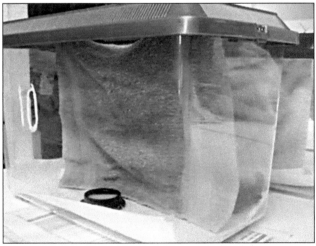

8.14 Juvenile bats can be housed in a tightly closed plastic vivarium with a towel draped inside for the bat to hang on to. (© Secret World Wildlife Rescue)

continued for up to 6 weeks, reducing their frequency and offering mealworms with their heads removed to wean. A small amount of water or milk should be placed in a shallow container to lap from. Specialist help will be required for release and should be sought from local bat groups (via the Bat Conservation Trust, see Appendix 1 and Chapter 15).

Rearing neonatal rabbits and leverets

Rabbits are notoriously difficult to hand-rear and need to be kept warm and have a minimum of 5 feeds per day (see also Chapter 16 for feed volumes and frequency). Goat milk, Esbilac® or Cimicat™ milk replacer should be used, supplemented with vitamins (e.g. Abidec®) and probiotics (e.g. Avipro® Plus; Bio-Lapis®; Fibreplex™) to assist in maintaining a stable gut flora. A 1 or 2 ml syringe and small teat should be used to administer the milk. Although in the wild kits are often only fed once daily by the mother, as rabbit's milk is higher in protein and fat than most other species, in captivity they require more regular feeds to reduce the incidence of bloat and provide adequate calories. Weaning should be gradual in this species to avoid gastrointestinal upsets such as gastric or caecal tympany or intestinal bacterial overgrowth, which are common potentially fatal consequences associated with too rapid weaning. Handling should be kept to a minimum to reduce stress and strict hygiene should be maintained. Prokinetic drugs such as metoclopramide, ranitidine and cisapride should be considered prophylactically around the time of weaning to encourage normal gut motility. For more information see Chapter 16. Hay, dried grass and fresh grass should be offered daily as a source of fibre and is vital to encourage normal gut motility and function.

Rearing neonatal dormice and mice

Small rodent species should be fed 2 hourly with Esbilac® using a small pipette or a cut-down intravenous catheter sleeve to administer the milk. They need toileting and should be kept warm and dry at all times. When the eyes open they need to be weaned and at this stage a very shallow dish with water can be left in with them.

Rearing neonatal birds

On arrival, firstly check the bird has no injuries, as many young birds will be victims of cat attack and have puncture wounds, tears to the skin or subcutaneous emphysema. These animals will require systemic antibiotics (e.g. enrofloxacin 10 mg/kg orally q12h) and analgesia (e.g. meloxicam 0.1–0.5 mg/kg orally q12h), which is easy to administer orally in young birds with a gape reflex (see Figure 8.15c and also Chapter 30).

Weigh the bird and record the result on the animal's individual admittance form, as this will enable daily changes in weight to be monitored and help assess the bird's rate of growth. Identify what species of bird it is so that the correct diet can be fed (Figure 8.15). For example, young pigeons are often misidentified by members of the public as raptors or herons (Figure 8.15a).

Place the bird in an incubator at a temperature of 28–30°C. A false nest can be fashioned out of a wicker basket or plastic dish the correct size for the patient and this can be lined with paper towelling (Figure 8.16). The nest will keep the bird warm, clean and prevent growth

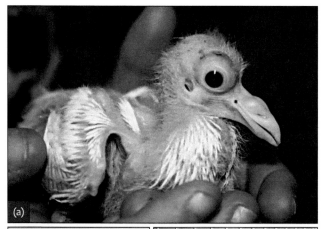

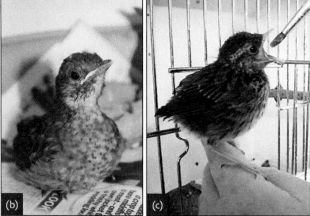

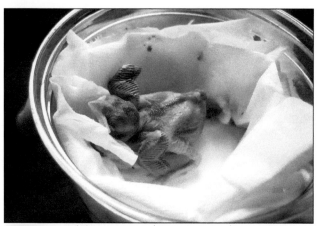

8.15 (a) Juvenile pigeons (*Columba* spp.) are often misidentified by members of the public as raptors or herons. (b) Juvenile blackbird (*Turdus merula*). (c) Juvenile robin (*Erithacus rubecula*).
(© Secret World Wildlife Rescue)

8.16 Juvenile house sparrow (*Passer domesticus*) housed in an artificial nest made from a plastic tub and lined with paper towels.
(Courtesy of Emma Keeble)

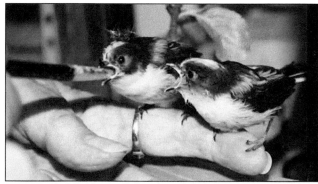

8.17 Fledgling long-tailed tits (*Aegithalos caudatus*) showing the gape reflex whilst being fed using a fine paintbrush.
(© Secret World Wildlife Rescue)

paintbrush (Figure 8.17) or a pair of plastic tweezers (Figure 8.18). Very small species may need feeding half hourly. They will usually produce a faecal sac (containing both faeces and urates) after the first mouthful of each feed, and failure to do so, or straining, may indicate dehydration or an impaction. Water should therefore always be given at the end of every feed from a paintbrush, to reduce the risk of dehydration or impaction. Most birds self-regulate the amount they ingest per feed and will stop gaping once full, after a few mouthfuls. If the bird is not gaping, gently tapping the side of the beak will encourage this reflex. Aquatic birds usually self-feed from an early age, and appropriate food and water should be provided at all times. To stimulate feeding and pecking behaviour, the food can be sprinkled into the enclosure from a height, as the movement will provoke the bird's interest in the food. Sprinkling food on the animal's back will also encourage preening and secondary food ingestion.

Young birds should be handled as little as possible to avoid stress and malprinting. The bird should ideally be fed inside the incubator, as opposed to getting each individual animal out to feed, as this will avoid the bird becoming chilled. Individual animals should be weighed daily when young; however, when they have fledged and begin to fly this procedure becomes less practical and weights may be recorded less frequently.

Squabs (juvenile pigeons) and doves will require tube feeding (gavaging, see below) when young until they are self-feeding.

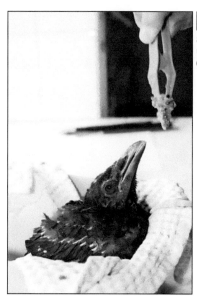

8.18 Juvenile crow (*Corvus corone*) in an artificial nest being fed using tweezers.
(© Secret World Wildlife Rescue)

abnormalities, particularly involving the legs. If the bird is a very young nestling, placing bubble wrap gently on top of it will help keep it warm and insulated.

The first feed should be given if the bird looks reasonably alert, with a gape reflex present. If hypothermic and collapsed, enteral feeding should be avoided as there is a risk of aspiration and also food may accumulate in the crop and ferment, resulting in a crop infection (sour crop). In this instance parenteral fluid therapy and supportive care should be instigated (see Chapter 5). Most birds will need feeding hourly and will gape for their food (Figure 8.17). Place small amounts in their mouth using a

Diets for juvenile birds

Birds are usually easier and much quicker than mammals to rear from nestling to fledgling and can be fully fledged in as little as 21 days. Amounts fed are difficult to monitor accurately, but birds will regulate the amount they ingest at each feed. Once they are self-feeding at approximately 2–3 weeks old assessment is more difficult, so it is important to ensure that food is available at all times. Nestlings should be fed hourly and once fledging starts, the feeds are decreased to 2 hourly and solid food is provided to stimulate self-feeding. Once birds are eating on their own, food can just be topped up through the day. Once flying, birds can be moved to aviaries for flight practice and eventually released, with support feeding provided on bird tables nearby.

The main basic diet for the majority of young birds encountered will be 80% meat-based (wet cat/dog food), mashed with 20% avian insectivorous diet (e.g. Bogena Dried Insect Food; Orlux Insect Mix) and water. This is referred to as 'fledgling mix'. Feeding guidelines for common juvenile bird species are given in Figure 8.19.

For tiny newly hatched birds a liquid feed should be given, as solids are difficult to digest and these individuals often require an easily assimilated food with increased levels of nutrition (e.g. Harrison's Bird Foods® Neonate Formula™).

Avian vitamin and mineral supplements can be added to the feed to assist in growth and feather development and prevent nutritional deficiencies, such as nutritional secondary hyperparathyroidism, which is seen in juvenile birds of prey fed solely on day-old chicks.

Feeding live food is more ideal, but expensive. Waxworms (Pyralidae) or mealworms (*Tenebrio molitor*) can be offered, although maggots (Diptera) or earthworms (Annelida) can be used as an alternative and are naturally readily available.

Feeding juvenile birds of prey

Feeding guidelines for juvenile birds of prey are given in Figure 8.20 (also see Chapter 29). Initially, hand feeding is required (Figure 8.21).

Species	Recommended diet (plus avian vitamin/mineral supplement)
Blackbirds, thrushes, starlings	Fledgling mix, waxworms, mealworms, wild bird seed
Robins, wrens	Fledgling mix, mealworms, earthworms
Sparrows, finches	Fledgling mix, millet, wild bird seed
Crows, magpies, jackdaws	Fledgling mix, chopped day-old chick, beef mince
Tits, housemartins, swallows	Waxworms, mealworms, maggots
Woodpeckers	Fledgling mix, mealworms, earthworms
Owls, kestrels, sparrowhawks, buzzards	Chopped adult mice, chopped day-old chick (with beak and yolk sac removed) – add avian vitamin/mineral supplement if solely feeding day-old chicks
Coots, moorhens	Mealworms, avian insectivorous diet, maggots, whole whitebait
Ducklings, cygnets, goslings	Chick crumbs, bread, millet, lettuce or watercress in water, or commercially available waterfowl pellets
Gulls, terns	Cat/dog food, chopped day-old chick, whole whitebait

8.19 Fledgling bird diets. NB 'Fledgling mix' consists of 80% meat base (wet cat/dog food) mashed with 20% of an avian insectivorous diet (e.g. Bogena Dried Insect Food; Orlux Insect Mix) and water.

Age (weeks)	Frequency of feeding
0–1	2 hourly, meat only, no fur or bones
1–2	2–3 hourly, meat only
2–3	3–4 hourly, add small amount of bones and feathers
3–4	4 hourly, increase the amount of bones
4–5	4 feeds daily, chick chopped into small pieces
5–6	3 feeds daily, larger pieces
7–8	2–3 feeds daily, chicks halved or whole

8.20 Feeding guidelines for juvenile birds of prey.

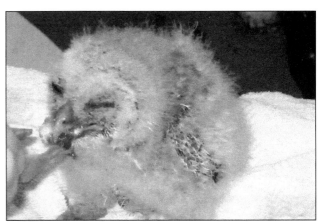

8.21 Tawny owl (*Strix aluco*) chick being hand fed. This species may overfeed if offered food *ad libitum*.
(© Secret World Wildlife Rescue)

Feeding juvenile pigeons and doves

Juvenile pigeons and doves (*Columba* spp., *Streptopelia* spp.), flamingos (*Phoenicopteridae*) and emperor penguins (*Aptenoclytes forsteri*) are fed a liquid secretion called crop milk produced by the parents and fed from mouth to mouth. For this reason, in captivity, juvenile pigeons and doves should be tube-fed liquid food (e.g. Exact® Hand Feeding Formula; Nutri-Start® Baby Bird Formula). A suggested method for crop tubing is as follows (see also Chapter 5):

- Check the crop is empty. Do not proceed with the feed if the crop is still full
- Use a 5–20 ml syringe (dependent on age and size of bird), attach to this a small soft tube, about 7 cm long, and preload the syringe and tube with feeding formula
- Hold the bird's head in one hand and use a finger as a gag to open the beak
- With the other hand, advance the crop tube into the left side of bird's mouth
- Advance the tube to the right and over the back of the tongue
- Pass the tube down the bird's oesophagus to the crop (avoiding the glottis, located centrally at the base of the tongue)
- Confirm correct placement by palpation of the end of the tube in the crop and slowly administer the feed, checking the oropharynx for regurgitation of food. Stop if this occurs
- Feed until there is a visible, nicely rounded full crop
- Feed 2 hourly if very young
- Feed from dawn till dusk to mimic the natural feeding pattern in the wild.

The amounts being fed and intervals between feeds will be gradually increased as the bird gets older. Once pigeons and doves are approximately 3 weeks old, pellets should be fed made from soaked chick crumb with a little grain added, and these should be alternated with gavaged feeds. Leave the pelleted mix in the cage to encourage self-feeding. Pigeons and doves are weaned on to millet or a general wild bird seed mix once self-feeding (see also Chapter 28 for pigeon and dove-rearing formulae).

References and further reading

Best D (1999) BWRC Wildlife Casualty Recording Scheme – The First Five Years. *The Rehabilitator*, **28**, 2–3

Cooper B, Mullineaux E and Turner L (2011) *BSAVA Textbook of Veterinary Nursing, 5th edn*. BSAVA Publications, Gloucester

Gosden C (2004) *Exotics and Wildlife: A Manual of Veterinary Nursing Care*. Butterworth-Heinemann, Edinburgh

Ruth I (1997) *First Aid for Wildlife (Basic Care for Birds and Mammals)*. Bick Publishing House, Connecticut

Stocker L (2005) *Practical Wildlife Care, 2nd edn*. Blackwell Publishing Ltd, Oxford

Varga M, Lumbis R and Gott L (2012) *BSAVA Manual of Exotic Pet and Wildlife Nursing*. BSAVA Publications, Gloucester

Specialist organizations and useful contacts

See also Appendix 1 and species-specific chapters.

Alpha Laboratories Ltd (Stockists of small pipettes)
www.alphalabs.co.uk

Bedfordshire Wildlife Rescue (Fledgling identification guide)
www.wildlife-rescue.org.uk

Brinsea Products Ltd (Incubator manufacturer)
www.brinsea.co.uk

Catac Products UK Ltd (Equipment suppliers)
www.catac.co.uk

Chapter 9

Rehabilitation and release

Adam Grogan and Andrew Kelly

The aim of this chapter is to set out the criteria by which rehabilitated wild animals may be assessed prior to release and to discuss some of the methods for release and post-release monitoring so that questions regarding the effectiveness of the rehabilitation and release process can be addressed. Reviewing these processes is an essential component of wildlife veterinary medicine and rehabilitation. Only through such assessment can important questions regarding animal welfare and the costs and/or benefits of the rehabilitation process be truly assessed.

As has been described in Chapter 4, adequate triage of casualties must take place before treatment and rehabilitation is attempted in order to ensure, as far as is possible at that stage, that the animal is a suitable candidate for rehabilitation and eventual release back to the wild. Such triage should ideally involve a veterinary examination, but may often be carried out by lay rehabilitators. Adequate training of those undertaking triage is required (see Figure 4.7). Wild animals tend to be less tolerant of treatment regimens and protracted periods in captivity than their domestic counterparts. They may be stressed in captivity (which may slow the healing process), may not adapt to being in captivity and are not usually readmitted for reassessment once they have been released. Rehabilitators and veterinary surgeons (veterinarians) have legal and ethical responsibilities to ensure that wildlife casualties are not exposed to unnecessary suffering, are capable of surviving once released and that they will not have a detrimental impact on the environment post-release (see also Chapters 1, 2 and 4).

It must be recognized that the wild is a challenging environment and rehabilitated animals must be as fit as their wild conspecifics in order to:

- Locate food sources, forage and/or hunt successfully
- Avoid predators
- Avoid human–animal conflict
- Compete for resources with their conspecifics and other species
- Defend and maintain territories
- Adapt to variations in temperature and weather conditions
- Have the ability to reproduce successfully
- Hibernate or migrate successfully.

Wild animals reared in captivity may additionally lack some of the necessary skills for survival, as not all such skills are innate and may need to be learned from parents or other individuals. As rehabilitated orphaned juvenile animals are not able to do this, some substitution may be required to stimulate learning (Llewellyn, 1987; Spencer et al., 2007).

Management during rehabilitation

Housing

Ideally, the casualty should be kept in an environment that fulfils all its needs throughout the rehabilitation period, although during veterinary treatment it may be necessary to keep the animal in controlled accommodation so it can be closely observed and handled easily for treatment (see Chapter 7). When the casualty no longer needs to be handled regularly for treatment or rearing, it should be placed in a suitable environment to improve its fitness and to exercise more natural behaviours. Some standards for housing are available (e.g. Miller, 2012), but it must be remembered that these are minimum standards, which can often be improved upon. Examples of different types of enclosure are provided in Figures 9.1, 9.2 and 9.3. Figure 9.1 shows an aviary that is suitable for passerines, or larger birds if scaled up in size. Birds can be housed here; they will have space to exercise and can also be released through a hatch (see Figure 9.8). Figure 9.2 shows an enclosure suitable for water birds or species such as otters (Lutra lutra). Figure 9.3 shows a terrarium that could be used for reptiles and amphibians.

Enclosures must:

- Be of adequate size (both in height and length) for the species concerned; for large raptors this could be an aviary that allows for full flight, or for juvenile badgers (Meles meles) enough space for them to explore and forage
- Contain suitable substrates and environmental enrichment such as perches, pools or branches, as appropriate for the species concerned, that allow the animal(s) to express normal behaviours such as climbing, swimming, flying and digging (Young, 2003)
- Be constructed of suitable materials to prevent escape, to stop predators getting in, be easily cleaned and disinfected and not pose a hazard to animals or people
- Include other precautions to prevent escape, for example double doors of an airlock-type design and sunken fences to prevent mammals digging underneath

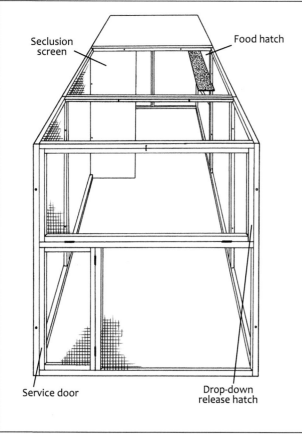

9.1 Sectional rehabilitation and release flight cage with solid back and sides. Dimensions, mesh size and furniture will depend on the species being housed.

- Include somewhere for the animal to hide from observers (to reduce stress) and to shelter from adverse weather; this could be a kennel or similar for foxes (*Vulpes vulpes*) or badgers, or a partitioned area of an aviary that has been roofed over
- Include facilities for patients to be observed. Peepholes are standard practice; however, the animal is usually aware that a human is nearby and so will not behave naturally. Remote observation using CCTV systems inside enclosures can improve the assessment of the normal behaviour of casualties (see below)
- If the enclosure is to be used for soft-release (see 'Release methods'), it must have a means of exit and entry for the animals (see below and Figure 9.8).

Care should be taken not to overstock enclosures. A maximum number of individuals that can be kept in the enclosure without affecting their welfare should be determined and this number should not be exceeded. Even when normally sociable young animals like fox cubs are kept in high numbers, they may become stressed, causing developmental problems (such as poor weight gain). This may occur even if the animals are spread out among individual adjoining pens (Robertson and Harris, 1995a). Infectious disease may also be more common and more difficult to control at high stocking densities. Some animals (e.g. hedgehogs (*Erinaceus europaeus*)) may also injure others during aggressive encounters when housed together in high stocking densities (Bullen, 2002).

Predator and prey species must be kept separate from each other so that they cannot see, hear or smell each other (see Chapter 7). Predators may be stressed if they can detect the presence of prey species but cannot

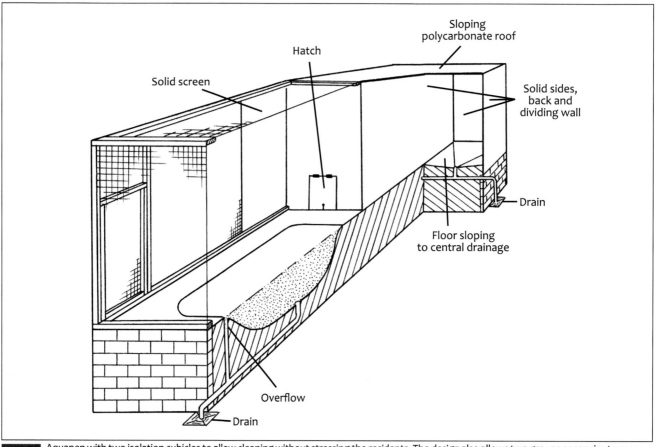

9.2 Aquapen with two isolation cubicles to allow cleaning without stressing the residents. The design also allows two groups or species to access the water independently.

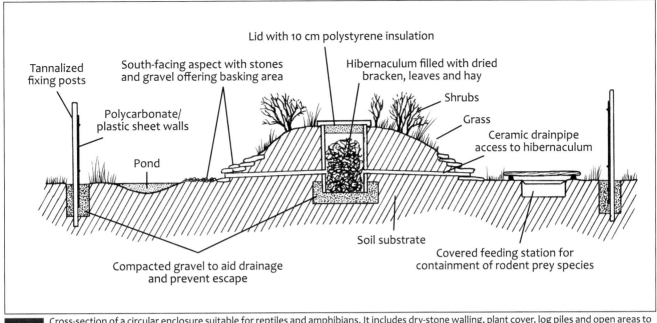

9.3 Cross-section of a circular enclosure suitable for reptiles and amphibians. It includes dry-stone walling, plant cover, log piles and open areas to maximize foraging potential and temperature gradients for recovering casualties.

access them, and prey species may be stressed if they can detect predators but cannot escape or hide.

Feeding

Prior to release, it is essential that casualties move on to more natural types of food compared to those that may have been fed during initial captivity (see Chapter 7). Provision of a natural food source involves consideration of both the type of food and how it is presented to the animal (Figure 9.4).

Flight cages

Some species will require more room in order to exercise before being released. Such large enclosures also allow veterinary surgeons and rehabilitators to assess the animal's fitness prior to release, especially if used in conjunction with remote video surveillance systems. Flight cages are an example of such enclosures (see Figure 9.1). Large flight cages can be used to exercise birds of prey and other large birds such as grey heron (*Ardea cinerea*). These can be constructed of timber, often with

Dietary grouping	Food items	Source	Enrichment/comments
Carnivorous animals (e.g. badgers, foxes, polecats, birds of prey)	Bird and mammal prey items	Road kill 'Healthy' (non-diseased and unmedicated) 'recycled' casualties	Offer whole if possible Care must be taken to ensure cause of death is known and food sources are as free from disease, toxins and parasites as is possible
Piscivorous animals (e.g. otters, most seabirds)	Whole fish	Good wholesalers	Offered whole if possible Vitamin supplement required if fish were frozen (e.g. Mazuri® Fish Eater Tablets)
Ground-living insectivores (e.g. hedgehogs, blackbirds)	Mealworms, waxworms, slugs, snails, earthworms, crickets	Good wholesalers Worm farms	Provide trays with bark/earth and sprinkle prey on tray so animals can forage naturally Supplement with vitamins and minerals, as necessary
Flying insectivores (e.g. bats, hirundines, passerines)	Mealworms, waxworms, wild insects, earthworms, flies	Good wholesalers Worm farms	Mealworms can be provided on aerial feeders hung from posts or ceilings Flight cages can be designed to allow access into the cage for flying insects
Herbivores (e.g. rabbits, deer, waterfowl)	Favoured vegetation depending on species (e.g. roe deer – browse including leaves of hazel, bramble, ivy in winter; rabbits – grass; swans – leaves of submerged or emergent plants favoured such as water crowfoot or duckweed); suitable alternatives in captivity include chopped greens, kale, cabbage	Suitable material (pesticide and disease-free) can be collected from suitable habitats	Provide handfuls in pen or allow a mixture of vegetation to grow in outdoor enclosures
Reptiles and amphibians (e.g. common lizard)	Mealworms, waxworms, earthworms, flies	Good wholesalers Worm farms	Provide trays with bark/earth and sprinkle prey on tray so animals can forage naturally

9.4 Natural feeding in preparation for release.

overlapping slatted walls to allow light in, but not enough space between the slats to allow the birds to get out or provide a direct line of sight with the outside. One design used at Royal Society for the Prevention of Cruelty to Animals (RSPCA) East Winch Wildlife Centre has a hooped tarpaulin roof and timber-framed walls. More specialized flight cages, constructed from a converted salmon farming cage, have been used to test the fitness of rehabilitated oiled seabirds. Flight cages have also been developed for bats (Figure 9.5). These have an external wire mesh so predators cannot get in and an internal plastic mesh to prevent the bats from damaging themselves on the internal walls. Such flight cages may have baffles and internal doors that allow the size and shape of the internal area to be changed, creating different challenges for the occupants.

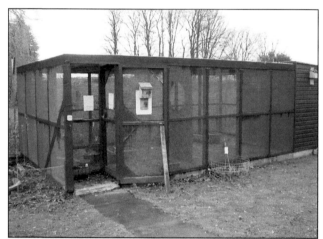

9.5 Bat flight cage. This allows bats to fly free and forage on wild prey before release. The mesh allows for small insect prey (e.g. midges) to enter and the cage contains items to attract insects, such as water and vegetation. When ready for release, the bat boxes used by the bats for roosting are placed outside the cage.
(© RSPCA Photolibrary)

Training and conditioning
Birds of prey
Some species of birds of prey may benefit from training using falconry techniques such as a creance (a long tether used for flying birds of prey during training) (Holz *et al.*, 2006). However, this is a time-consuming technique and requires particular handler skills. Rehabilitators may consider an arrangement with a local falconer or organizations such as the Hawk Conservancy Trust. As yet, there are few data to determine for which species such training is necessary, but one study indicates that free-flight training may be better than exercise in an aviary alone (Holz *et al.*, 2006). However, some species, such as kestrels (*Falco tinnunculus*), appear to survive well post-release without free-flight training (RSPCA, unpublished data). See also Chapter 29.

Other species
For other species, preparing animals for release by stimulating expression of normal behaviours, such as foraging, can also improve general fitness levels and increase the likelihood of survival after release (Kelly *et al.*, 2008). This can be achieved by doing something as simple as scattering food items around the animal's enclosure, rather than providing food from a bowl, or hiding food items so that animals have to actively search for them. Plastic trays can be used for this; for example, a tray can be filled with leaf litter and sprinkled with mealworms and other food items for animals such as hedgehogs, badgers or even blackbirds (*Turdus merula*) to forage in as natural a way as possible (see Figure 9.4).

Pre-release assessment
Health assessment
Prior to release, all casualties must undergo an assessment of their health. This should ideally include a full veterinary examination and appropriate diagnostic screening tests (see Chapters 4 and 10). In certain situations, such as translocation or reintroduction of a species to a new area, screening for known or potential diseases may form part of this assessment to avoid the transmission of any novel pathogens or parasites to wild populations upon release (IUCN, 2012) (see also Chapter 1). Screening tests are also useful to determine the health status of the wildlife casualty prior to release, for example faecal parasitology for lungworm (Strongylida) in hedgehogs. Screening tests should always be interpreted with care, as they may indicate previous exposure to a pathogen rather than a current active infection (see Chapter 10).

Body condition
Any wild animal undergoing rehabilitation may lose general condition whilst in captivity. Although it may be possible to return the animal to a reasonable pre-release weight (see Appendix 2), the animal may not have the correct muscle to fat ratio required for survival (Fox, 1995). Animals that have been kept in rehabilitation for long periods may be suffering from muscle atrophy due to their clinical condition and lack of exercise during rehabilitation. Trends in an individual's body condition (see Chapter 4) can be a more useful measurement than body mass in this instance. An animal released at a good bodyweight, but without a high level of fitness and stamina, may be at a disadvantage in terms of hunting for food or avoiding predators. This may be overcome with appropriate housing or training (see 'Training and conditioning'), but it may be difficult to provide the necessary conditions for the animal to improve its physical fitness in captivity.

Behaviour
Veterinary surgeons and rehabilitators must also have an understanding of the natural behaviour of healthy individuals of the species they treat, rehabilitate and release. This can be difficult when the animals most commonly seen are unhealthy. Knowledge of wild animals' postures, movements and feeding behaviours are essential if casualties are to be assessed correctly prior to release. Armed with this knowledge an assessment of animals' psychological and behavioural fitness can be made. CCTV cameras can be especially useful in monitoring behaviour (see 'Post-release monitoring').

Problems associated with human contact
Malprinting occurs when an animal becomes attached to its carer and as a result it lacks the correct response to humans (see Chapter 8). This is a problem often observed in rehabilitated wildlife casualties. Malprinting is more likely in altricial animals – those that have a greater dependency on their parents early in their development – and can lead

to permanent psychological damage. Experienced rehabilitators avoid developing a bond between themselves and the animals in their care by minimizing human contact. Less experienced rehabilitators often make the mistake of spending too much time with wild patients, resulting in an animal that is used to being with humans. In this case the animal may be unlikely to survive in the wild, and may even be a risk to humans if it does not respond to humans in the same way as one of its wild conspecifics (Cooper and Gibson, 1980; Wimberger and Downs, 2010).

Whittaker and Knight (1998) define three forms of wild animal response to humans; attraction (of which malprinting is one extreme form), habituation and avoidance. Habituation is said to have occurred when repeated presentations of the stimulus by itself (in this case proximity to humans) cause a decrease in the behavioural response, the simplest form of learning.

Malprinting can be avoided by taking the following measures:

- Returning the animal to its parents if possible – many animals are brought into rehabilitation unnecessarily and would probably thrive if returned to where they were found (Robertson and Harris, 1995a)
- Mixing the young animal with others of its own species, if this is appropriate
- Fostering to an appropriate parent (but not cross-fostering to different species (Bird *et al.*, 1985))
- Exposing the animal to appropriate sounds (e.g. birdsong for passerines (Spencer *et al.*, 2007))
- Minimizing the exposure to people, such as by weaning young animals quickly, but at an appropriate stage for that species.

Release

Choice of release site

Adult animals

Most adult casualties should be returned to exactly where they were found. Not all animals are territorial, but almost all have home ranges in which individuals know where to find resources like food and shelter. By returning an adult or independent juvenile animal to the area it came from, this knowledge does not need to be relearnt (depending on species and time in care) and so the animal should be at less of a disadvantage. For animals that are territorial and/or social (e.g. badgers), it is even more important to return them to the correct area. Wild animals may, however, lose their territory during rehabilitation; how long a territory may be vacant before a new animal moves in depends on the time of year, the population density of that species in the area and other possible threats such as disease. Even in these circumstances it is still better for that animal to be returned to a familiar area where it has the knowledge to find food and shelter, rather than to release it in a location where it does not know where to find these resources. If, for some reason, the original site is not considered suitable due to persecution or wounding by conspecifics, or if no information is known about the location where the animal was found, then an alternative strategy is required. This will depend on species and available resources, but the likely outcomes are euthanasia or a prolonged rehabilitation/translocation process such as would be undertaken for a juvenile animal (Brown and Cheeseman, 1996; Molony *et al.*, 2006).

Juvenile animals

For juvenile animals that have been raised in captivity with little or no experience of life in the wild, a suitable site must be found for their release. For commonly encountered species this is relatively easy, as their habitat requirements are well known. In these situations released animals can integrate easily with the wild population, especially if supplementary feeding is available. For other animals, there may be limitations on where animals can be released. These limitations can be imposed by:

- Species ecology: for instance, badgers are social and territorial and so it can be very difficult to find areas that are suitable for hand-reared cubs due to the density of the existing population in many areas
- Disease: badgers can be carriers of bovine tuberculosis (*Mycobacterium bovis*) and so finding landowners that are willing to accept them can be difficult
- Human/wildlife conflict: agencies working to conserve otters may be unwilling to allow the release of rehabilitated otters into new areas due to the potential conflicts with fishing interests.

When assessing potential release sites, the following need to be considered:

- The habitat needs to be suitable for the species concerned; capable of providing shelter, water and suitable food sources or prey
- The local population of the species being released – are conspecifics present and if not, why not? If the species is already present, is there capacity for more in terms of food and resource availability, or will introducing more animals increase stress?
- The site needs to be secure from human interference – particularly important for soft-release
- The site needs to be away from potential hazards, such as major roads, or possible areas of conflict (e.g. fisheries if releasing otters)
- The rehabilitator must have a legal right of access to the land used and authorization from the landowner to do so (see Chapter 2). Ideally neighbouring landowners' permissions should also be sought.

The first two points above create a dilemma; if the habitat appears to be suitable and the species is not present, why is this the case? There may be good reasons for this, but it may take time to determine them. It may be easier, and better for the animal, to use sites where the species is known to be present, and accept that the animal will have to adapt to the new environment and compete with conspecifics as any wild-reared juvenile animal would.

Rehabilitators should have a number of release sites on standby so that animals are not left in captivity for an unnecessary amount of time whilst waiting for a release site to become available. If suitable release sites cannot be identified, the animals may need to be euthanased, as releasing them in unsuitable sites may impact directly on their welfare.

Release methods

There are two basic methods for releasing rehabilitated wildlife: hard-release (where the animal is released without support feeding or other resource provision) and soft-release (where the animal is released using an enclosure that allows it to acclimatize to its new environment). The method chosen for release will depend on:

- Species
- Age of the animal
- Length of time the animal has been in captivity
- Location chosen for release
- Resources available for release (location, time and cost involved)
- Experience of the rehabilitator.

Hard-release

Adults or independent juveniles can usually be hard-released back to where they were found, ideally within a relatively short period of time following capture. As these animals do not need to acclimatize to the area or surroundings, they can be released directly into the environment. Supplementary food may be given if a feeding station can be provided and maintained easily. Hard-releases are less labour intensive and so are easier to plan and less costly, but their success depend on a number of factors:

- Timing: animals should be released at a time that is appropriate for them; for example, badgers should be released during the hours of darkness as they are nocturnal; diurnal birds of prey should be released early in the morning to give them time to hunt and feed during the day they are released
- Weather conditions: animals should not be released if the weather is adverse or extreme (e.g. strong winds or heavy rain). Ideally the weather forecast for the next few days should be consulted prior to release
- Other animals: presence of other animals that may cause problems; for example, released birds of prey may be mobbed by crows (Corvidae).

Soft-release

Soft-release provides an opportunity for animals to become acclimatized to the environment into which they are to be released and so should be used for naïve animals, such as hand-reared juveniles (Kelly *et al.*, 2010) or animals that may have been moved from another location (Molony *et al.*, 2006). It could also be used for animals that have had a prolonged period of rehabilitation. Acclimatization occurs in an enclosure suitable for that species, such as an aviary for passerines or a pen for foxes. The enclosure should have features similar to those found in the animals' enclosure at the rehabilitation centre. Materials from their rehabilitation enclosure can be used in the soft-release enclosure to provide a familiar habitat and scent during the acclimatization process. The animals are kept in the enclosure for a period of time, depending on their species and age. Release occurs by opening a door or hatch, so the inhabitants can leave the enclosure when they are confident enough and ready to do so. The enclosure then stays on site, allowing the animals to return if necessary; it also provides a focus for supplementary feeding, although this is not always required; for example, Griffiths *et al.* (2010) found that tawny owls (*Strix aluco*) did not return to the soft-release pen to collect food after they had been released.

The disadvantages of soft-releases are that they can be expensive and time-consuming; a suitable site needs to be identified, with the correct habitat and cooperative landowners; a suitable enclosure needs to be constructed;

then the animal(s) need to be cared for whilst in the enclosure before release. For example, the otter pen in Figure 9.6 took 2 days to construct, with costs related to both manpower and building materials. Careful planning and design and reuse of materials can reduce some of these costs. For instance, the enclosure for polecats (*Mustela putorius*) in Figures 9.7 is constructed from metal panels that can be moved to and constructed on site. This has the advantage of allowing the pen to be used year after year at different sites. Similar 'flat-pack' methods can be used for aviaries and other enclosures. For other species, the same site can be used repeatedly, so aviaries, such as the one in Figure 9.8, can be built *in situ*. However, despite the expense, soft release has been demonstrated as a necessary requirement for species such as juvenile foxes (Robertson and Harris, 1995b) and otters (Woodroffe, 1997).

Animals in soft-release enclosures should be fed by distributing the food around the enclosure, ideally hiding it under logs and stones. A good release site should also allow an element of natural foraging; for instance, badgers should be able to access earthworms and other invertebrates in the enclosure. Human contact should be kept to a minimum and feeding times should be irregular so that the animals do not become accustomed to a regular feeding time.

It is rare for adult animals to be released using soft-release methods, although there are exceptions. It will usually be juvenile animals of similar ages that will require this extra investment in the release process. If mixed age groups are being released – then care needs to be taken to

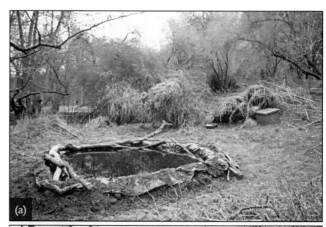

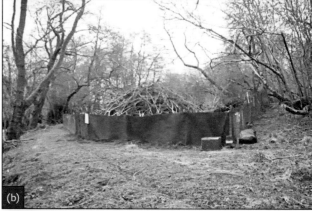

9.6 Soft-release enclosure for otters. (a) Construction of the pool and artificial holt. (b) The fence used for the enclosure. The fence comprises an electric mesh fence (such as that used for chickens) with a plastic windbreak on the outside, so that the otter cannot see outside the pen.
(© RSPCA)

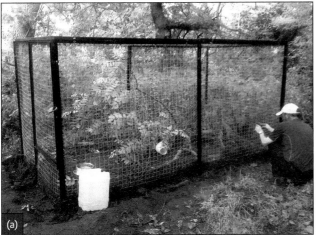
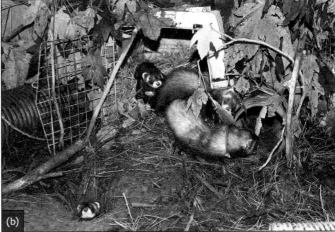

9.7 Preparing a soft-release cage for polecats. (a) The wire mesh cage is transported to the site in sections. The cage contains cut vegetation and other items such as plastic pipes and logs for enrichment. (b) Food can be left in the pipes or hollow logs to reduce the chances of attracting corvids or other scavengers. These animals have been fitted with collars with very high frequency (VHF) radio transmitters attached.
(© RSPCA)

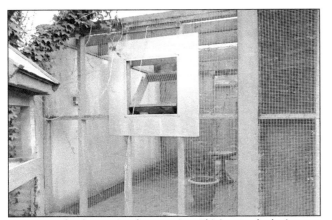

9.8 Soft-release aviary for passerines. This is a standard aviary used for passerines. The aviary should contain a number of natural perches constructed from branches and cut vegetation. The hatch is opened when the birds are ready for release.
(© RSPCA)

ensure that, if the young animals are 'dependent' on the older ones, the older animals do not disperse and so effectively abandon the younger animals.

As with hard-release, weather and time of day for release are factors that should also be considered when opening the soft-release enclosure.

Timing of releases

Consideration must also be given to the timing of releases. The aim should be to release rehabilitated adult animals as soon as possible after treatment, although severe weather may postpone such releases. Migratory animals need to be released in plenty of time to allow them to regain fitness before migration. If this is not possible, overwintering is a possibility, but this comes with its own problems, so euthanasia should also be considered. Hibernating animals need to have time to be able to find suitable hibernacula and releasing them at a good weight will certainly provide a cushion to help them during this period.

Juvenile animals should be released when wild-reared juveniles of their species are naturally dispersing. Reproducing the dispersal behaviours of a wild juvenile animal can be problematic (Robertson and Harris, 1995b), especially when for some species, like badgers, such dispersal is limited (Macdonald et al., 2008).

Post-release monitoring

The aim of wildlife rehabilitation is to release the rehabilitated animal back into the wild, where it will be able to survive and become integrated with the wild population. This can only be determined if the fate of the animal is known. Therefore, some form of post-release monitoring is required along with good record-keeping of admissions, releases, and the treatment and management of casualties in captivity (see Chapter 7).

The aims of such monitoring are to:

- Determine survival rates and survival times post-release
- Determine if the animal's behaviour is typical of a wild animal of the same species/age/sex
- Determine if poor survival was due to inadequacies in the triage and rehabilitation process
- Improve assessment techniques, rehabilitation procedures and decision-making
- Prevent suffering of rehabilitated wildlife casualties as a result of poor or unsuitable case selection
- Monitor behavioural interactions between rehabilitated and wild animals and other animals (including humans)
- Assess the ecological impacts of releases (see Chapter 1).

Post-release monitoring should not be seen as optional and should instead be viewed as an essential part of the treatment, rehabilitation and release of wildlife casualties. All wildlife rehabilitators should assume that rehabilitation is unsuccessful unless they can demonstrate that the released animals survive for a minimum period. Clearly, if rehabilitated animals die of malnutrition very quickly after release, the rehabilitation process should be reviewed; where possible this must also be considered alongside natural mortality rates under the same circumstances.

Despite the importance of this stage of the process, literature relating to post-release monitoring and survival rates of wildlife casualties is sparse. The available literature also tends to concentrate on juvenile groups of casualties rather than individual adult animals. Reviews of the available literature have been published (Grogan and Kelly, 2013; Mullineaux, 2014).

Methods of post-release monitoring

There is a variety of methods for marking and tracking animals following release and these are summarized in Figure 9.9.

It should be remembered that the attachment of any leg ring or band, telemetry device or other equipment to the animal can have a detrimental effect upon it (Wilson, 2011). Monitoring systems may have an effect upon the animal's behaviour and activity (Vandenabeele et al., 2012; 2014), and in the worst situations may cause trauma (Peniche et al., 2011; Michael et al., 2012). Rehabilitators have an advantage over most wildlife biologists in that they have the animal in captivity for a period of time, so devices or rings can be fitted to the animal prior to release and assessed to ensure that they are not causing the animal any discomfort (Kelly et al., 2008). Rehabilitators should also refer to the available scientific literature to determine which form of monitoring is best suited for each species.

It is recommended that any device fitted to an animal should weigh less than 5% of the animal's mass (3% for collars, 5% for harnesses and 1–2% for tags glued to the fur/feathers; Kenward, 2000), although there are very few studies that have tested these recommendations (Vandenabeele et al., 2012). Some species require licences to mark them in certain ways prior to release (see Chapter 2 and species-specific chapters).

	Advantages	Disadvantages
Methods of marking animals		
Rings or bands	• Relatively cheap but require specialized training and permits	• Standard metal rings have low return rate; more visible plastic rings better, but more cumbersome for animal
Other tags (ear, flipper)	• Relatively cheap but require training and licenses	• Returns limited but tags are visible to casual observer, unlike microchips or tattoos • Cause animal pain on placement • Can tear through and be lost
Tattoos	• Relatively cheap but require training and licenses	• Returns limited and tattoos may fade over time • Cause animal pain on placement and require sedation/anaesthesia
Microchips (passive integrated transponders (PIT) or radiofrequency identification (RFID) tags)	• Relatively cheap	• Returns limited as animal needs to be 'scanned' • Chips may also migrate and can eventually fail • Placement may be painful
Fur clips and dye	• Relatively cheap	• Temporary – most clip marks and dyes are only used for temporary marking
Natural markings	• Cheap	• Requires good photographs and/or video footage along with pattern recognition software
Genetic profiling	• Can identify individuals or family groups • Costs of DNA sampling are becoming cheaper	• Currently expensive • Can be difficult to narrow down to individuals • Some sampling techniques (e.g. blood collection) are invasive
Methods for tracking animals		
Direct observation	• Cheap	• Time intensive; subject to vagaries in weather
Camera traps	• Getting cheaper; easy to set up	• Can produce multiple images and/or video that then require a lot of time for viewing and analysis
Microchips (PIT or RFID)	• Chips are relatively cheap and do not usually cause any problems for the animal	• Most readers are hand-held although remote reader technology is increasingly available; larger chips have greater range
Radio tracking	• Transmitters and attachments reasonably cheap • Location can be accurately determined by trained people and certain behaviours can be observed	• Manpower intensive • Possible health and safety issues related to tracking especially at night
Satellite tracking using Argos system	• Accurate to around 100 m • Transmitters as light as 5 g	• Transmitters are expensive and are usually lost
Global positioning system (GPS) tracking	• Accurate to less than 5 m • GPS receiver is light	• Transmitters are expensive • Data must be retrieved from the device – additional devices required to access data increase the weight
Geolocation	• Devices are relatively cheap and are very light • Good for migratory species	• Not very accurate • Must be retrieved to obtain the data so not usually suitable for rehabilitation projects
DNA collection	• As for genetic profiling • DNA can be retrieved from faeces (certainly in mammals) • Hair samples can also be collected (e.g. using barbed wire traps)	• Requires careful handling of samples • May not always be able to identify individuals

9.9 Methods for marking and tracking wild animals.

Direct observation at the release site

The easiest way to monitor the animals that have been released is to observe them at the release site, either directly or indirectly using cameras recording either stills or video (see 'Use of CCTV systems in wildlife observation'). This is most useful at soft- release sites where, hopefully, the animals will not disperse too quickly, allowing observations to be made. Animals can be encouraged to stay through the use of feeding stations and these also provide a target area for observers/cameras. It is, however, difficult to identify individual animals unless they have been marked in some way (see 'Capture-mark-recapture'). This may not be important if there are no other animals of that species present in the area, or you do not need to identify individual animals in a group. However, the ability of different individuals in a group to survive will vary and some form of individual marking is recommended.

Capture-mark-recapture

The simplest method for obtaining information on a wildlife casualty in the longer term is to mark it in some way before it is released. If it is subsequently found dead or observed alive, the information gathered will be very useful. This technique, known as capture-mark-recapture (CMR), has been used for many years, although methods of marking and 'capturing' have changed. Note that some species require licences to mark them in certain ways (e.g. the use of tattoos in badgers); see Chapter 2 for further details.

Animals can be identified using:

- Rings (also known as bands) for birds (see Figure 9.10a) and bats (see Figure 9.10b)
- Ear tags (e.g. for foxes; Baker *et al.*, 1998), patagial tags (e.g. for birds of prey), web tags for waterfowl, or flipper tags for seals
- Tattoos (e.g. in badgers, see Chapter 17)
- Microchips (passive integrated transponders (PIT) or radiofrequency identification (RFID) tags)
- Fur clips and dye (e.g. clipping away badger guard hairs allows the pale fur underneath to show well on

images captured by infrared cameras (Stewart and Macdonald, 1997))
- Natural patterns of colouring or other features (e.g. patterns on the bills of Bewick's swans (*Cygnus columbianus bewickii*; Evans, 1977)
- Genetic profiling (e.g. from hair or faecal samples).

Methods of 'recapture' include:

- Conventional live capture in a trap (note, some species require licences to trap, e.g. badgers)
- Found dead (e.g. road traffic accidents)
- Live sightings
- Photographs from public
- Photographs from camera trap
- Remote monitoring of microchips
- Radio tracking or satellite tracking fixes
- DNA samples from hair (e.g. using barbed wire traps) or faeces.

Ringing: The most easily recognized form of CMR is ringing (or leg banding), commonly used on birds, but also on some other species too, such as pipistrelle bats (*Pipistrellus pipistrellus*) (Kelly *et al.*, 2012). The British Trust for Ornithology (BTO) has been coordinating a ringing programme in the UK for over 100 years, with over 900,000 birds ringed each year by 2600 ringers (BTO, 2013). The standard ring is aluminium and inscribed with a unique number that allows the bird to be reported (referred to as a control), should that bird/ring be found or read in the field. This can provide useful information for the rehabilitator (Martell *et al.*, 2000; Leighton *et al.*, 2008). Reading these rings in the field is difficult, so other more visible rings (e.g. Darvic rings, Figure 9.10a) are available. These are large plastic rings, which can be easily read by an observer at a distance and then reported to the BTO. Darvic rings have been used in bird species such as herring gulls (*Larus argentatus*) (Figure 9.10a), mute swans (*Cygnus olor*) and Canada geese (*Branta canadensis*). The use of such rings can greatly improve data collection and so survival estimates. For example, a study using Darvic rings on rehabilitated herring gulls demonstrated a much better survival rate than had been previously estimated

---

Use of closed circuit television (CCTV) systems in wildlife observation

- CCTV systems have developed a great deal in recent years. The range of cameras and other equipment has advanced so that some cameras are small and easy to install and conceal in enclosures, whilst computer systems and software allow the user to record, review and analyse footage with comparative ease. Modern wireless systems also mean that there is no need for installation of extensive cabling.
- Camera systems can be used to assess an animal's injury; how it is adapting to captivity; how it is adapting to a ring or tag; or how it behaves naturally. Such systems provide a great advantage in that there is no unnecessary disturbance to the animal and so their behaviour is much more natural than it would be if being directly observed by a human.
- CCTV cameras can also be used for education and fundraising purposes. CCTV footage of animals in rehabilitation centres allows members of the public to view the animals without disturbing them, which is much less stressful for the animals.
- There are two main camera types: those connected to a computer or a recording device via cables or over local area wireless networks, and those that are self-contained units, like stealth cams. The former are better for recording animals in a facility as a direct connection to a computer makes it easier to observe the footage in real time and it also allows for several cameras, possibly set up in several areas of housing, to be connected to the same computer.
- Self-contained systems like stealth cams are useful for filming animals outdoors, but the disadvantage is that the film needs to be retrieved from the camera and cannot be viewed in real time.
- Cameras can be set up to record images at set times using a timer or can be activated using a trigger. These triggers are often based on movement, possibly using motion detectors that can be set using 'frames' that can be viewed through the screen, or using passive-infrared (PIR) detectors that detect the energy given off by an animal when it passes within range. Modern stealth cameras often have timers and triggers built in to provide a versatile range of operation.

using data from standard aluminium rings recovered from dead birds (Thompson, 2013).

In bats, aluminium rings fitted to the forearm of rehabilitated pipistrelles (Figure 9.10b) have allowed identification of released animals for up to 4 years post-release (Kelly *et al.*, 2012).

Radiofrequency identification: Radiofrequency identification (RFID) transponders or passive integrated transponder (PIT) tags use wireless radio communications

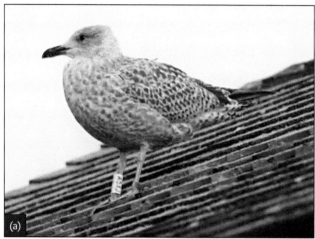

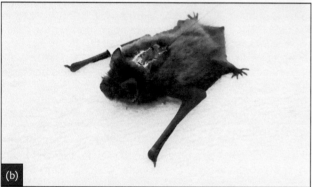

9.10 (a) Juvenile herring gull with aluminium BTO ring and plastic Darvic ring. (b) Pipistrelle bat with aluminium ring and very high frequency (VHF) radio transmitter.
(© RSPCA)

(radiofrequency electromagnetic fields) to uniquely identify objects, animals or people. Unlike simple barcoding (e.g. used to mark items in supermarkets), RFID does not rely on a direct line of sight and can cope with the dust and dirt of a wild environment. Transponders placed subcutaneously (e.g. microchips) or as tags (e.g. ear tags or collars) are used to identify individual animals. The simplest form is the use of a standard pet microchip, which can be very small and light, allowing its use in a variety of species.

A RFID reader has an attached antenna, which is used to both transmit and receive the radiofrequency signal. Tags can be of several types; some require no battery and are read at short ranges via magnetic fields (electromagnetic induction), while others use a local power source and emit radio waves (electromagnetic radiation at radio frequencies) over larger distances. Readers can be placed to identify animals moving through feeding tubes or shelter openings (Griffiths *et al.*, 2010; Rigby *et al.*, 2012).

DNA sampling: The ability to sequence the DNA of many species and individual animals has provided new techniques for monitoring animals in the wild, although this is

not without problems. The techniques can be largely non-invasive, although the best results are obtained when a reference tissue or blood sample is taken from the animal (under licence or for clinical reasons) prior to release. When the animal has been released, surveys of the area should be undertaken to look for fresh faeces from that species or individual. These can be collected and then examined for epithelial cells from the gut, which can be analysed for DNA (Dallas, 2003). Alternatively, traps such as barbed wire can be used to take hair from the animal; this can then be collected and analysed (Mullins *et al.*, 2010). The margins of error in the collection and analysis of DNA samples, especially from faeces, means that the detection of individuals is not guaranteed and finding samples that are suitable for analysis can be difficult. The analysis of samples is currently carried out by only a few laboratories in the UK and so can be expensive. Costs can be reduced by increasing batch size or by collaborating in a larger project in which samples of the species concerned are being collected and analysed for another purpose.

Radio tracking

Radio tracking uses small transmitters, or tags, that emit a very high frequency (VHF) signal on a specific frequency that can be detected by a specialist receiver (Kenward, 2000). The transmitter is attached to the animal, which can then be followed by a trained operator equipped with a suitable receiver and antenna. The range and lifespan of the transmitter is dictated by its battery pack and this in turn determines the transmitter size and weight. As described above, the total weight should not exceed 5% of bodyweight (Kenward, 2000), so a compromise has to be reached over how the battery power available is used; transmitters requiring a greater range will require more power and will not last as long as a similar-sized transmitter with a shorter range. For small species like bats (see Figure 9.10b), transmitters weighing 0.35 g can be used, but have a battery life of only up to 14 days (Kelly *et al.*, 2008). For larger animals like badgers, transmitters working over short ranges can last over a year (Tuyttens *et al.*, 2002). The devices can be attached using collars for mammals such as polecats (Figure 9.11) (Kelly *et al.*, 2010) and foxes (Robertson and Harris, 1995b), harnesses (Walls *et al.*, 2005), tail or leg mounts for birds of prey and other bird species (O'Doherty, 2013), or just glued to the skin of hedgehogs (Morris *et al.*, 1993, Morris and Warwick, 1994) or fur of bats (Kelly *et al.*, 2008; 2012).

Rehabilitators should take into account the resources required for these methods both in terms of financial cost and observer effort. The equipment for radio tracking is

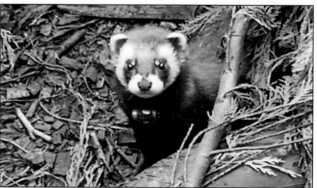

9.11 Polecat with very high frequency (VHF) transmitter on collar.
(© RSPCA)

relatively cheap, with transmitters varying in cost depending on species. Receivers are more specialized and so can be expensive and antennae designed for radio tracking are also required. However, the biggest cost is labour; radio tracking is very labour intensive and to get the most out of the study, people will need to track the animals for a number of hours each day and over several weeks, if not months, depending on species. Volunteers can be used but need to be trained, not only in radio tracking, but also in the hazards that may exist in the area where the study is being conducted. Health and safety risks can be considerable. Those radio tracking animals should also consider the observer effect, where their presence may influence the animal's behaviour. Project design is important to ensure that enough data is collected both on sufficient numbers of animals and on each animal.

Some projects have used radio transmitters to collect data remotely; for example the recording of individual common guillemots (*Uria aalge*) coming and going from a nesting colony (Hamel *et al.*, 2004). However, these data can only be considered as CMR data as there is no information recorded on the animals' movements away from the colony.

Satellite tracking

Satellites can be used to track animals in two ways. In the first option a satellite tag is attached to the animal, much like a conventional radio transmitter. These tags emit a signal that is received by a satellite system called Argos (see 'Specialist organizations and useful contacts'). The satellites hold the data and this can be downloaded to a computer at the operator's convenience. The advantages of these systems are that there is no need to follow the animal in the wild, so there is a considerable saving on observer time, effort and costs. There are also no negative effects associated with direct observation of the animal. Animals can be tracked over much great distances, including at sea (Figure 9.12). Morrison *et al.* (2011) used this system to follow rehabilitated common seals (*Phoca vitulina*) and found that their survival and behaviour was comparable with wild seals tracked over the same period of time.

The development of small solar-powered tags means that many species can be tracked using this method, for example cuckoos (*Cuculus canorus*) (BTO, 2014). The main disadvantage of satellite tags is that they are expensive and are usually lost once they fall off the animal. Attachment to the animal can be problematic. Satellite tags may also have negative effects on the animal. The accuracy of most satellite systems is about 100 m, which is good for tracking migratory birds but not for other applications where more detail is required.

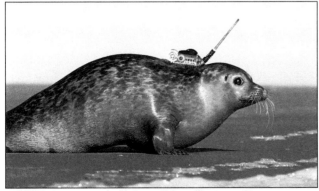

9.12 Common seal with Argos CLS satellite transmitter.
(© RSPCA)

The second option of monitoring using satellite technology is to use global positioning systems (GPS). The animal is fitted with a GPS receiver weighing as little as 1 g, which records the animal's movement by recording signals from satellites over time. This provides detailed temporospatial data with minimal manpower costs. The main disadvantage of this system, apart from cost, is that data needs to be retrieved from the device. This can be done by:

- Trapping the animal, removing the device and downloading the data
- Downloading the data remotely over a radio or short message service (SMS)
- For mammals only: programming the device to drop off, either at a set time, or by remote control when the animal is in view so it can be retrieved.

Unfortunately, all the last two methods add physical weight to the system, in addition to that of the actual receiver, which limits the use of GPS equipment to larger species.

Geolocation

Geolocation uses small photosensitive detectors, called archival light loggers or geolocators, to measure day length as well as record sunrise and sunset times. This allows location to be determined – latitude by length of day (for that time of year) and longitude by sunrise and sunset times. This is a relatively crude method to determine an animal's location (accuracy is at best 1 degree = 180 km), but the big advantage is that the geolocation devices are extremely light (weighing as little as 1 g) and can be fitted to existing devices, such as rings on birds' legs. Their use for rehabilitation is very limited as the device needs to be retrieved to download the data, but they have been used extensively in birds that migrate or forage over long distances (Guildford *et al.*, 2009; Harris *et al.*, 2010).

Licences for releases and post-release monitoring

Some species are covered by legislation restricting their rehabilitation and these require a specific licence to keep them (e.g. grey squirrels (*Sciurus carolinensis*)) and release them (e.g. grey squirrels and muntjac deer (*Muntiacus reevesi*)). Certain birds of prey may need to be registered if kept in care for more than 6 weeks by a qualified veterinary surgeon (15 days for a rehabilitator) and other native species of bird need to be released under a general licence (e.g. red kites (*Milvus milvus*) (England) or barn owls (*Tyto alba*) (England and Wales)) (see Chapter 2).

When considering marking a wild animal for a post-release study, rehabilitators and veterinary surgeons need to be aware of any relevant legislation. National guidelines that may apply should also be followed; for example in the UK, bird ringing is administered by the BTO and they have a special category for recording rehabilitated birds that are ringed under their scheme. If marking or attaching tracking devices to animals, there may be legislation regulating this; for instance, a licence is required under the Protection of Badgers Act 1992 to mark or collar badgers, or to trap them for collar removal, or to place an RFID system on a badger sett.

Although many of the techniques discussed have had no observed effect on the animals' welfare, it may be prudent to discuss plans with other researchers who are working on that species so to learn from their experiences, and with the Home Office as a licence will be required for procedures falling under the Animals (Scientific Procedures) Act 1986 (ASPA) (see also Chapter 2).

Acknowledgements

The editors would like to acknowledge Paul Llewellyn for the use of figures from his chapter in the previous edition of this manual.

References and further reading

Baker PJ, Robertson CPJ, Funk SM and Harris S (1998) Potential fitness benefits of group living in the red fox (*Vulpes vulpes*). *Animal Behaviour* **56**, 1411–1424

Bird DM, Burnham W and Fyfe RW (1985) A review of cross-fostering in birds of prey. *ICBP Technical Publication* **5**, 433–438

Brown JA and Cheeseman CL (1996) The effect of translocation on a social group of badgers (*Meles meles*). *Animal Welfare* **5**, 289–309

BTO (2013) About ringing. www.bto.org/volunteer-surveys/ringing/about

BTO (2014) Tracking cuckoos to Africa. www.bto.org/cuckoos

Bullen K (2002) *Hedgehog rehabilitation*. British Hedgehog Preservation Society, Ludlow, Shropshire

Cooper JE and Gibson L (1980) The assessment of health in casualty birds of prey intended for release. *Veterinary Record* **10**, 340–341

Dallas JF, Coxon KE, Sykes T *et al.* (2003) Similar estimates of population genetic composition and sex ratio derived from carcasses and faeces of Eurasian otter (*Lutra lutra*). *Molecular Ecology* **12**, 275–282

Evans ME (1977) Recognizing individual Bewick's Swans by bill pattern. *Wildfowl* **28**, 153–158

Fox N (1995) *Understanding the Bird of Prey*. Hancock House Publishers, Surrey

Griffiths R, Murn C and Clubb R (2010) Survivorship of rehabilitated juvenile tawny owls (*Strix aluco*) released without support food, a radio tracking study. *Avian Biology Research* **3**, 1–6

Grogan A and Kelly A (2013) A review of RSPCA research into wildlife rehabilitation. *Veterinary Record* **172(8)**, 21 doi: 10.1136/vr.101139

Guildford T, Meade J, Willis J *et al.* (2009) Migration and stopover in a small pelagic seabird, the Manx shearwater (*Puffinus puffinus*): insights from machine learning. *Proceedings of the Royal Society B*. doi:10.1098/rspb.2008.1577

Hamel NJ, Parrish JK and Conquest LL (2004) Effects of tagging on behavior, provisioning and reproduction in the common murre (*Uria aalge*). *The Auk* **121**, 1161–1171

Harris MP, Daunt F, Newell M, Phillips RA and Wanless S (2010) Wintering areas of adult Atlantic puffins (*Fratercula arctica*) from a North Sea colony as revealed by geolocation technology. *Marine Biology* doi: 10.1007/s00227–009–1365–0

Holz PH, Nasbitt R and Mansell P (2006) Fitness level as a determining factor in the survival of rehabilitated peregrine falcons (*Falco peregrinus*) and brown goshawks (*Accipiter fasciatus*) released back into the wild. *Journal of Avian Medicine and Surgery* **20**, 15–20

IUCN Species Survival Commission (2012) *IUCN Guidelines for Reintroductions and Other Conservation Translocations*. www.iucn.org

Kelly A, Goodwin S, Grogan A and Mathews F (2008) Post-release survival of hand-reared pipistrelle bats (*Pipistrellus* spp.). *Animal Welfare* **17**, 375–382

Kelly A, Goodwin S, Grogan A and Mathews F (2012) Further evidence for the post-release survival of hand-reared, orphaned bats based on radio-tracking and ring-return data. *Animal Welfare* **21**, 27–31

Kelly A, Scivens R and Grogan A (2010) Post-release survival of orphaned wild-born polecats (*Mustela putorius*) reared in captivity at a wildlife rehabilitation centre in England. *Endangered Species Research* **12**, 107–115

Kenward R (2000) *A Manual of Wildlife Radio Tagging, 2nd edn*. Academic Press, London

Leighton K, Chilvers D, Charles A and Kelly A (2008) Post-release survival of hand-reared tawny owls (*Strix aluco*) based on radio-tracking and leg-band return data. *Animal Welfare* **17**, 207–214

Llewellyn P (1987) Assessing conditions prior to raptor release. In: *Breeding and Management in Birds of Prey: Proceedings of the Conference held at the University of Bristol, January 24–26, 1987*, ed. DJ Hill, pp. 103–119

Macdonald DW, Newman C, Bueshing CD and Johnson PJ (2008) Male-biased movement in a high-density population of the Eurasian badger (*Meles meles*). *Journal of Mammalogy* **89**, 1077–1086

Martell M, Goggin J and Redig P (2000) Assessing rehabilitation success of raptors through band returns. In: *Raptor Biomedicine III, including bibliography*

of diseases of birds of prey, ed. JT Lumeij *et al.*, pp. 327–334. Zoological Education Network, Lake Worth, FL

Michael S, Gartrell B, Hunter S and Morgan K (2012) Wing injury caused by backpack harnesses for radio transmitters in takahe (*Porphyrio hochstetteir*). *Proceedings of the joint 61st WDA/10th biennial EWDA conference 'Convergence in wildlife heath' Lyon 23–27 July 2012*, p304

Miller EA (2012) *Minimum Standards for Wildlife Rehabilitation, 4th edn*, International Rehabilitation Council National Wildlife Rehabilitators Association, p116

Molony SE, Baker PJ, Garland L, Cuthill IC and Harris S (2007) Factors that can be used to predict release rates for wildlife casualties. *Animal Welfare* **16**, 361–376

Molony SE, Dowding CV, Baker PJ, Cuthill IC and Harris S (2006) The effect of translocation and temporary captivity on wildlife rehabilitation success: an experimental study using European hedgehogs (*Erinaceus europaeus*) *Biological Conservation* **130**, 530–537

Morris PA, Meakin K and Sharafi S (1993) The behaviour and survival of rehabilitated hedgehogs (*Erinaceus europaeus*). *Animal Welfare* **2**, 53–66

Morris PA and Warwick H (1994) A study of rehabilitated juvenile hedgehogs after release into the wild. *Animal Welfare* **3**, 163–177

Morrison C, Sparling C, Sadler L *et al.* (2011) Post-release dive ability in rehabilitated harbor seals. *Marine Mammal Science* **14**, E110–E123

Mullineaux E (2014) Veterinary treatment and rehabilitation of indigenous wildlife. *Journal of Small Animal Practice* **50**, 293–300

Mullins J, Statham MJ, Roche T, Turner PD and O'Reilly C (2010) Remotely plucked hair genotyping: a reliable and non-invasive method for censusing pine marten (*Martes martes* L 1758) populations. *European Journal of Wildlife Research* **56**, 443–453

O'Doherty J (2013) An analysis of common buzzard (*Buteo buteo*) admissions into RSPCA wildlife rehabilitation centres and an investigation into their post release survival. MSc thesis, University of Birmingham

Peniche G, Vaughn-Higgins R, Carter I *et al.* (2011) Long term health effects of harness-mounted radio transmitters in red kites (*Milvus milvus*) in England. *Veterinary Record* **169(12)**, 311

Rigby EL, Aegerter J, Brash M and Altringham JD (2012) Impact of PIT tagging on recapture rates, body condition and reproductive success of wild Daubenton's bats (*Myotis daubentonii*). *Veterinary Record* **170**, 101–106

Robertson CPJ and Harris S (1995a) The condition and survival after release of captive-reared fox cubs. *Animal Welfare* **4**, 281–294

Robertson CPJ and Harris S (1995b) The behaviour after release of captive-reared fox cubs. *Animal Welfare* **4**, 295–306

Spencer KA, Harris S, Baker PJ and Cuthill IC (2007) Song development in birds: the role of early experience and its potential effect on rehabilitation success. *Animal Welfare* **16**, 1–13

Stewart PD and Macdonald DW (1997) Age, sex and condition as predictors of moult and the efficiency of a novel fur-clip technique for individual marking of European badger (*Meles meles*). *Journal of Zoology* **241**, 543–550

Thompson R (2013) Factors influencing the admission of urban nesting herring gulls (*Larus argentatus*) into a rehabilitation centre and post release survival in comparison with wild counterparts. Masters Thesis, University of Sussex

Tuyttens FAM, Macdonald DW and Roddam AW (2002) Effects of radio-collars on European badgers (*Meles meles*). *Journal of Zoology* **257**, 37–42

Vandenabeele SP, Grundy E, Friswell MI *et al.* (2014) Excess baggage for birds: inappropriate placement of tags on gannets changes flight patterns. *PLOS One* **9(3)**, e2657

Vandenabeele SP, Shepard EL, Grogan A and Wilson RP (2012) When three per cent may not be three per cent; device-equipped seabirds experience variable flight constraints. *Marine Biology* **159(1)** 1–14

Walls SS, Kenward RE and Holloway GJ (2005) Weather to disperse? Evidence that climatic conditions influence vertebrate dispersal. *Journal of Animal Ecology* **74**, 190–197

Whittaker D and Knight RL (1998) Understanding wildlife response to humans. *Wildlife Society Bulletin* **26(2)**, 312–317

Wilson R (2011) The price tag. *Nature* **469**, 164–165

Wimberger K and Downs CT (2010) Annual intake trends of a large urban animal rehabilitation centre in South Africa: a case study. *Animal Welfare* **19**, 501–513

Woodroffe G (1997) *Reinforcing the Otter Population in the Yorkshire Derwent, 1990–1997*. Unpublished report, University of York.

Young RJ (2003) *Environmental Enrichment for Captive Animals*. UFAW Animal Welfare Series, Blackwells, Oxford

Specialist organizations and useful contacts

See also Appendix 1

Argos (Worldwide tracking and environmental monitoring by satellite) www.argos-system.org

Biotrack (Animal monitoring equipment) Biotrack Ltd, 52 Furzebrook Road, Wareham, Dorset BH20 5AX, UK Tel: 01929 552 992 www.biotrack.co.uk

The Hawk Conservancy Trust Sarson Lane, Weyhill, Andover, Hampshire SP11 8DY, UK Tel: 01264 773773 www.hawk-conservancy.org

Chapter 10

Clinical pathology, post-mortem examinations and disease surveillance

John E. Cooper

Over the past decade, since the first edition of the *BSAVA Manual of Wildlife Casualties* was published, there has been a notable increase in interest amongst veterinary surgeons (veterinarians) in the health and diseases of British wildlife. Much of this has been driven by naturalists and concerned members of the public – now sometimes called 'citizen scientists' – who are not necessarily professional biologists or scientists. An example of one particular area to which such people have contributed substantially is the 'Garden Bird Health initiative' (Lawson *et al.*, 2012a; 2012b; Toms, 2012) now part of Garden Wildlife Health (see 'Specialist organizations and useful contacts').

Reports by members of the public and concerned naturalists/biologists of unexpected or unexplained mortality ('die-offs') or of wildlife showing signs of ill health or behaving abnormally can sometimes be a useful early warning system, but need to be backed by clinical and pathological examination if appropriate action is to be taken.

Alongside a general interest in wildlife health there has been an encouraging growth of input by professional veterinary bodies, such as (in England and Wales) the wildlife team of the Animal and Plant Health Agency (APHA), who run a wildlife disease monitoring programme that aims to detect reservoirs of potential zoonoses, diseases of livestock, and new pathogens and environmental pollutants (Duff, 2003; Duff *et al.*, 2010). As a result, incidents and diseases involving free-living animals are now more likely to be properly investigated and studied than they might have been in the past.

Current concerns over emerging diseases (e.g. Paul, 2012) emphasize the need for surveillance. This may be 'risk-based' where there is a danger of spread of an infectious agent to domestic stock or humans. Such was the case, for example, when a new highly virulent H5N1 strain of avian influenza emerged and spread into South East Asia, Africa and Eastern Europe (Snow *et al.*, 2007). This example highlighted the importance in surveillance of interdisciplinary studies. Following the deaths of six people in Hong Kong from infection with influenza A H5N1 strain, a debate surfaced centring on the relative roles of wild birds and domestic poultry in the spread of the virus. Professional ornithologists played an important role in countering claims made by the media and others that wild birds were largely responsible (Feare, 2007; Gauthier-Clerc *et al.*, 2007).

Clinical ability and acumen play an essential role in the diagnosis and treatment of disease in wildlife casualties. Detailed examination is often hampered, however, by difficulties of handling (see Chapter 3) or the undesirability of using chemical restraint (see Chapter 6). There are, therefore, limitations on the amount of information that can be gained from clinical investigation alone. Aids to examination, such as endoscopy and radiography, can provide additional data but in order to make a diagnosis there is often a need to obtain laboratory-generated parameters. This is not always easy, especially when dealing with free-living wildlife in the field (Cooper, 2002a; 2013).

Laboratory investigations may be restricted to examination of samples from live animals, or involve post-mortem examination (necropsy) of casualties that fail to survive or have to be euthanased. Whatever the origin of the sample, laboratory tests have an important role to play in providing data on the causes of morbidity and mortality of wild animals and in the assessment and treatment of individual casualties, which can be of great value prior to release or if animals are found or recaptured afterwards (Sainsbury *et al.*, 1996). They can also generate information about potential zoonoses and those infectious agents that may present a threat to domesticated livestock.

Post-mortem examination of a wild animal may help to determine the cause of death, shed light on the cause of an injury, or reveal factors that could have contributed to its being presented as a casualty. It can, in addition, provide information about zoonoses, as shown in the post-mortem survey of British hedgehogs (*Erinaceus europaeus*) by Keymer *et al.* (1991), which highlighted, amongst others, the presence in some animals of *Salmonella* spp., *Trichophyton erinacei* and *Yersinia pseudotuberculosis*. It can also allow the detection of parasites and/or changes in organs and thus provide background information about the health of that individual, or the group or population from which it came, or its species (Cooper, 1989; 2002a).

Many biologists bemoan the fact that so little scientific information about British wildlife emanates from rehabilitation centres or from the numerous veterinary practices where casualty animals are seen. If this situation is to be rectified, those involved in wildlife care, both veterinary surgeons and rehabilitators, should endeavour to ensure that data are collected. In the context of this chapter, this means that, whenever it is feasible, practicable and safe, a gross post-mortem examination should be carried out on each animal that dies or has to be euthanased.

As the value of disease surveillance has become better recognized and its practice more systematic and precise, laboratory investigations too have become more sophisticated and sensitive. For instance, whilst bacteriological and mycological culture and virus isolation still have an important part to play in the diagnosis of infectious diseases, other procedures are often needed. Thus, for example, Davison et al. (2010) used a combination of biochemical, molecular and serological techniques, in addition to culture, to identify a host-adapted group B Salmonella enterica in harbour porpoises (Phocoena phocoena).

Laboratory investigations on live animals

General considerations

Although the examination of blood and other samples from casualty animals can provide a great deal of valuable information, this must be balanced against the stress that can be caused to a casualty through restraint and sampling. Whenever possible, a non-invasive or minimally invasive technique should be used (Cooper, 1998). The financial costs of tests should also be considered. A careful cost/benefit analysis of all aspects of each case is essential.

Even when a relatively invasive method (such as the taking of a biopsy sample) is deemed necessary, every effort should be made to reduce the adverse effect of this on the animal, whilst still obtaining optimal results. Ways of so doing include the following:

- There should be prior discussion with the pathologist or laboratory staff regarding appropriate sample collection techniques and how the specimen is best presented to the laboratory
- All the equipment that is likely to be needed for sampling should be available before the animal is restrained
- The duration of handling must be minimized; prolonged restraint for sample-taking can be stressful and adversely influence some laboratory tests (see 'Sampling methods')
- The correct samples must be taken and they should be transported and processed promptly, safely and proficiently.

Sampling methods

A sample can be defined as a 'representative portion of the original' and this definition is a reminder that any sample should reflect, as closely as possible, the material or site from which it came. A sample has to be collected, transported to the laboratory and there it has to be examined. Errors can occur at each of these stages and, as a result, the findings and conclusion may not accurately reflect the situation in the live or dead animal. Therefore, standard techniques should be used and reliable equipment employed (Cooper and Cooper, 2013). The main sampling methods that are likely to be employed in wildlife casualties are described in Figure 10.1.

Sample	Collection	Storage	Investigations/tests	Relevant health and safety considerations
Faeces	• Freshly voided faeces or collection of material from the rectum or cloaca	• Chilled (4°C) for up to 10 days, then may need freezing • Fixed faeces are of some value	• Gross examination and use of hand lens • Record of colour, consistency and smell • Contents: food remnants and abnormalities, such as free blood or excessive undigested food (e.g. starch or fat) • Direct examination: wet preparations in saline should be examined first, followed by flotation methods and smears • Presence/absence and numbers of endoparasites (see Figure 10.9) • Aerobic (sometimes anaerobic) bacteriological examination • Other microbiological investigations	• Various zoonotic or opportunistic organisms (e.g. Salmonella spp., Pseudomonas spp.) • Do not pipette samples by mouth • Wear gloves • A risk assessment is always necessary
Blood	• Taking blood samples with a needle and syringe (or perhaps a 'vacutainer') from a vein or occasionally from an artery or a sinus • Taking smaller samples of blood from a vessel by pricking with a needle, or (with care, depending upon the species) by pricking the skin elsewhere, e.g. for blood glucose levels using a glucometer • See Chapter 5 for sites for blood sampling collection and appropriate anticoagulants	• Chilled (4°C) until processed	• Packed cell volume (PCV) and smears (for differential blood cell counts and parasitological examination) • Other haematological investigations (where practicable) • Biochemical estimations, including enzymes • Serology	• Some zoonotic or opportunistic organisms if the animal has a blood-borne infection or the sample is contaminated • Do not pipette samples by mouth • Wear gloves • A risk assessment is always necessary

10.1 Main sampling methods and important diagnostic tests employed in wildlife. (continues) ▶

Sample	Collection	Storage	Investigations/tests	Relevant health and safety considerations
Urine and urates	• Similar procedures are used for mammalian samples as for dogs and cats • Bird and reptile samples usually comprise urates; interpretation of results is not always easy	• Chilled (4°C) until processed	• Gross examination and use of hand lens • Record of colour, consistency (urates) and smell • Standard 'dip-stick' investigations • Specific gravity (using refractometer) • Centrifugation and cytological examination of deposit	• Some zoonotic or opportunistic organisms if the animal has a urinary infection or the sample is contaminated • Do not pipette by mouth • Wear gloves • A risk assessment is always necessary
Skin, including hair, feather and scale samples (see Figure 10.2)	• Skin scrapings and impression smears • Collecting hair, feather, scales or shed skin (sloughs) (see Figure 10.3) and plucking hair, feather and scales • Plucked feathers of birds, scales of reptiles and skin mucus of amphibians or fish often give good results	• Chilled (4°C) until processed initially • Should not be frozen unless long-term reference material (e.g. for DNA studies) • Hairs, feathers and scales can be stored dry in paper	• Gross examination and use of hand lens • Parasitological (see Figure 10.4), microbiological, cytological and histopathological examination	• Some zoonotic or opportunistic organisms if the animal has a skin infection (including dermatophytes) or the sample is contaminated • Wear gloves • A risk assessment is always necessary
Swabs from various sites (including orifices)	• Swabs for bacteriology, mycology, cytology, etc.	• Chilled (4°C) until processed	• Record of colour, consistency and smell • Cytology • Aerobic (sometimes anaerobic) bacteriological examination • Other microbiological investigations	• Some zoonotic or opportunistic organisms if the animal has an infection or the sample is contaminated • Wear gloves • A risk assessment is always necessary
Biopsies, either external (e.g. skin) or internal (via endoscopic laparoscopy/ coelioscopy or laparotomy/coeliotomy)	• Excised tissue from a live animal • See text	• Fixed immediately and/or chilled (4°C) until processed • See text	• Cytology • Histology • Aerobic (sometimes anaerobic) bacteriological examination	• Some zoonotic or opportunistic organisms if the animal has an infection or the sample is contaminated • Wear gloves • A risk assessment is always necessary
Post-mortem samples, including many of the above	• Various • See text and Figures 10.7 and 10.17	• Chilled (4°C) until processed • See text	• Various • See text and Figures 10.7 and 10.17	• Some zoonotic or opportunistic organisms if the animal has an infection or the sample is contaminated • Wear gloves • A risk assessment is always necessary

10.1 (continued) Main sampling methods and important diagnostic tests employed in wildlife.

Samples from wildlife casualties can present special problems. First of all, they are often taken under difficult circumstances, for example from a wild animal that from the start is struggling, stressed and not amenable to restraint. Casualties may require chemical restraint to allow handling, which may also have an effect upon the specimens collected. Handling and associated stressors can alter the haematological and clinical chemical parameters of some species and sedation (depending on the agent(s) used) may also adversely affect biological parameters. An often overlooked effect of handling some species, such as rodents, is stress-associated hyperthermia (Dallmann et al., 2006), which could have a significant effect on a sick or injured animal. Some specimens from wild animals are taken in the field, where conditions are unpredictable, facilities are limited and improvisation is often necessary (Cooper, 2002a; 2013).

Samples are taken in a similar way as for domestic animals. Where differences exist, these are referred to and described in more detail in the relevant species-specific chapter in this book. It is often good practice to perfect a technique first on either a domesticated species or a dead wild animal before attempting to do so on a frightened and stressed living casualty.

Laboratory investigations should always be preceded by gross, or hand lens, examination of the sample (see Figure 10.1). In a few cases there are reliable published data on normal and abnormal features – of the faeces of hedgehogs, for example (Bunnell, 2001) – and these are further described in the species-specific chapters of this book.

Precautions must always be taken to minimize pain and distress to the animal by using appropriate handling techniques as well as anaesthesia and analgesia where this is indicated (see Chapter 6). Care must also be taken to reduce the risk of injury or spread of organisms to humans or other patients (see Figure 10.1, Chapter 7 and species-specific chapters). In the UK and some other countries, there are legal implications associated with sample collection from live animals when material is not collected solely for diagnostic purposes (see Chapter 2).

Processing of samples

The movement (transportation) of samples can have adverse effects on certain laboratory results. Some tests, such as the measurement of packed cell volume (PCV), may be best performed *in situ* if sending the blood elsewhere is likely to result in haemolysis.

Methods of processing samples from wildlife casualties are briefly described in Figure 10.1 and further described in the sections below. These are not significantly different from those used for comparable material from domestic animals or captive 'exotic' species. Some reference data are available in textbooks and scientific papers: see, for example, information on microbiological isolates from birds and reptiles in Cooper (1999a; 1999b).

Types of investigation
Specific samples

Skin, hair, feathers and scales: Skin and hair of wild mammals can be examined in a similar way to integumentary samples from domesticated animals. Some methods suitable for use in wildlife are given in Figure 10.2.

- **Simple magnification**
  - Hand lens
  - Otoscopy
  - Wood's lamp
- **Brushings**
  - Sample collection
    - The coat of mammals may be brushed to collect surface debris for closer examination using a flea comb or stiff plastic hairbrush into a petri dish for examination under a microscope or hand lens
  - Wet paper test
    - Debris from the coat is brushed on to a piece of dampened white paper; the faeces of fleas that have fed stain the damp paper reddish-brown, because of the presence of blood
  - Mackenzie toothbrush technique
    - This employs a small brush which, following brushing of the animal's coat, is used to inoculate a fungal culture medium
- **Samples for direct microscopy**
  - Hair or feather pluckings or pieces of scale
  - Adhesive (sticky) tape impressions (see Figure 10.4)
  - Smears of expressed follicular contents (see Figure 10.11)
  - Smear of aural wax/exudate (see Figure 10.11)
  - Skin scrapings (see Figure 10.4)
  - Stained smears from pustules and other lesions (see Figure 10.11)
  - Fine needle aspirates

10.2 Examination and sampling of the skin and hair of wild animals.

Examination of feathers was discussed in detail by Cooper (2002b); it can shed much light on causes of feather and skin disease and help in the assessment of plumage prior to the release of casualty birds. It should be coupled with gross and, if necessary, microscopic investigation of the preen gland and its oily secretion.

Sloughed skins of reptiles can be examined with a hand lens (Figure 10.3a) and/or microscope (Figure 10.3b) and can be cultured for bacteria and fungi. Useful information can also be obtained from preparations of the keratinous 'sloughs' from the skin of amphibians. Hair, feathers and scales can also be analysed for heavy metals.

Ectoparasites from the skin (and sometimes the environment) of a wild animal can often provide valuable diagnostic, epidemiological or forensic information. The correct collection of such specimens is therefore

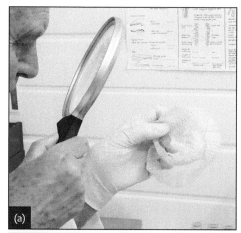

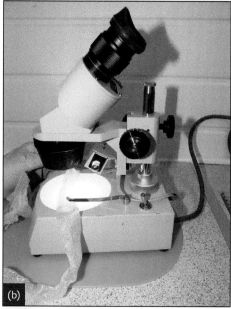

10.3 Investigation of the shed skin ('slough') of snakes requires careful handling and examination using (a) a hand lens and (b) a dissecting microscope. Examination using a dissecting microscope should include use of both transmitted and reflected light.

vital (Figure 10.4). Methods for the preservation and transportation of arthropods are described in Figure 10.5 and for mounting for identification in Figure 10.6.

Biopsies: Biopsies from live animals can provide very useful information but, in the case of non-domesticated species, must be very carefully selected, sampled and processed (Cooper, 1994) (Figure 10.7). Examination of a biopsy sample should always be considered, despite the costs involved and the fact that it is a relatively invasive procedure. A rapid diagnosis using biopsy is often pref-erable to drawn-out investigations on, for example, skin scrapings, as it can reduce the total amount of stress and pain caused to a wild animal casualty and accelerate its return to the wild. Biopsy specimens are best transported fixed (Figure 10.7), but if there is sufficient tissue available, a portion should also be retained 'fresh' (unfixed) so that microbiological and other investigations can be performed.

Faeces: Investigation of faeces will involve various types of investigation (see Figure 10.1), not just parasitological examination (Figures 10.8 and 10.9). Familiarity with the normal appearance of the faeces of wild animals is important.

Technique	Equipment	Methods	Advantages	Disadvantages	Comments
Direct examination of ectoparasites					
Direct isolation and removal from animals	Suitable source of illumination; hand lens or dissecting loupe; forceps; swab sticks; dissecting needles; parasiticidal aerosol spray (mammals); comb; large sheet of plastic or paper; aspirator ('pooter')	Search coat using comb or fingers to turn back hair. On sighting ectoparasites either with the naked eye or aided by a lens, remove parasite manually or with an aspirator (fleas), forceps (lice and lice eggs), moistened swab stick or dissecting needle (forage mites, harvest mites, *Otodectes*)	Rapid method for heavy infestations (lice, *Otodectes*, harvest mites)	Difficult and laborious in light infestations. Recovery of fleas may be improved by prior use of a suitable parasiticidal aerosol in mammals or by placing the mammal or bird in a plastic bag with its head protruding and introducing a parasiticidal or anaesthetic agent into the bag	A standard technique for domesticated animals that can be used successfully in wildlife
Combing and grooming mammals	Quill fashion comb or fine toothed metal comb; large sheet of plastic or paper; mild parasiticidal aerosol spray	Place subject on large sheet of plastic or paper and apply adequate restraint. Groom thoroughly and collect all debris that falls on to sheeting. In suspected flea infestations, spray subject with suitable parasiticidal aerosol spray prior to grooming	Rapid. Valuable in cases of low infestation and for the collection of flea debris	Necessary to separate skin debris from hair, grit and to sort manually prior to laboratory examination	A standard technique for domesticated animals that can be used successfully in wildlife
Examination of material containing ectoparasites					
Direct examination using dissecting microscope	Plastic petri dishes; dissecting needles; warming plate (45°C)	Place debris to be examined in petri dish. Leave for 12–24 hours, then transfer petri dish and contents on to warming plate for 10 minutes. Observe under microscope for movement and subsequent identification of parasites	Useful for the examination of skin debris and vacuum sweepings. Can be used for identification of lice and larger ectoparasites	Little value for detection of parasites in old samples	A standard technique for domesticated animals that can be used successfully in wildlife. Often applicable in forensic cases (see Chapter 11)
Direct microscope examination	Plain or hollowed microscope slides; coverslips; dissecting needles; mounting fluid; microscope; source of heat	Place selected ectoparasite, together with drop of mounting fluid, on either a plain or hollowed microscope slide. Examine under low power objective. Gently lower coverslip on to preparation. Samples of scale and debris may be mounted on a microscope slide with either potassium hydroxide or lactic acid and covered with either a second slide or a coverslip. Gently warm or leave the preparation to clear. Adjust the microscope condenser and diaphragm to provide an evenly distributed, but relatively low, light intensity. Examine the material on the slide methodically. This may be followed by a more detailed study of an individual organism under higher power if a coverslip has been used during preparation	Routine method of study of individually mounted ectoparasites. Rapid technique for routine screening of small amounts of skin debris or scrapings	There may be some difficulty adequately clearing material containing heavily pigmented epithelial debris. Time-consuming if large amounts of skin debris require examination	A standard technique for domesticated animals that can be used successfully in wildlife. Often applicable in forensic cases (see Chapter 11).
Examination following sedimentation	Test tube; 10% potassium hydroxide; source of heat; pipette; centrifuge; slides; coverslips	Place skin debris or scrapings into test tube. Boil gently until all debris has dissolved. Allow sedimentation or spin down. Pipette off supernatant fluid. Use deposit to make smears. Examine with microscope	Valuable when larger amount of material requires examination	Ectoparasites may be damaged or destroyed if boiled excessively. Time-consuming. Not satisfactory for permanent mounting	A standard technique for domesticated animals that can be used successfully in wildlife. Often applicable in forensic cases (see Chapter 11)
Sugar flotation modification	As above but using saturated sucrose solution	As above but after removal of supernatant, half-fill test tube with water and then complete filling using saturated sugar solution. Centrifuge (1000 rpm) for 1 minute. Remove parasites from the surface film using a slide or cover slip. Examine under the microscope	Valuable for screening large amounts of material and for the diagnosis of mite infestations	Ectoparasites may be damaged or destroyed if boiled excessively. Time-consuming. Not satisfactory for permanent mounting	A standard technique for domesticated animals that can be used successfully in wildlife. Often applicable in forensic cases (see Chapter 11)

10.4 Collection and examination of ectoparasites from wild animals. (continues) ▶

Technique	Equipment	Methods	Advantages	Disadvantages	Comments
Examination of material containing ectoparasites (continued)					
Collection of material using 'sticky' tape	Tape; scissors or clippers; microscope slide	Select area to be sampled. Remove hair. Press tape firmly on to skin and then remove and mount on microscope slide with or without potassium hydroxide.	Rapid Valuable as a research method and for the detection of *Cheyletiella* and, on occasions, *Demodex* infestations	Only possible to collect a limited amount of material Mites may be obscured by debris Unsatisfactory for *Sarcoptes* Necessary to remove hair	A standard technique for domesticated animals that can be used successfully in wildlife
Collection of hair by skin scraping	Scalpel blade; scissors; microscope slides; light lubricating oil or 10% potassium hydroxide	Select area to be sampled (lesions). Clip away hair. Pinch up skin into fold. Moisten with a drop of oil or potassium hydroxide. Scrape skin several times in one direction. Transfer any scale that collects on blade on to microscope slide. Repeat process until small amount of bleeding noted	Possible to take deep skin samples When oil is used, specimens remain fresh for several days	Animal/operator may be injured if the animal moves unexpectedly Time-consuming when large amount of material is required Impossible to clear specimens once oil has been used Parasites may be damaged during collection	A standard technique for domesticated animals that can be used successfully in wildlife Often applicable in forensic cases (see Chapter 11)
Collection of material from habitat	Vacuum cleaner; large sheet of plastic or paper	Material may be collected from flooring, sometimes undergrowth	Particularly valuable for assessing infestations of environment in flea infestations Often essential in *Dermanyssus* infestations	Laboratory examination of material is time-consuming	Particularly useful in forensic cases (see Chapter 11)

10.4 (continued) Collection and examination of ectoparasites from wild animals.

- In sealed plastic bags
  - Essential to remove air before sealing
  - Specimens remain in satisfactory condition for several days, so long as they were not obtained from suppurating or exuding lesions and have not been dampened with either water or potassium hydroxide (KOH)
- In mineral oils
  - Keep well for several days
  - Very difficult to clear material during subsequent laboratory examination
- In surgical spirit (70% ethyl alcohol)
  - Shrinkage of parasites may occur
- In Oudeman's solution
  - Formula:
    - Ethyl alcohol (70%) 87 parts
    - Glycerine 5 parts
    - Glacial acetic acid 8 parts
  - Valuable for short-term preservation of mites, but not all ectoparasites

10.5 Preservation and transportation of ectoparasites and other arthropods.

Mounting medium	Notes
Water	- Used only when nothing else is available - Unsatisfactory when clearing or the preparation needs to be retained
Normal saline	- Reduces damage to specimens and can prolong longevity of some species
Glycerine and glycerine jelly	- A useful temporary mount when clearing of preparation not required

10.6 Mounting of ectoparasites and other arthropods for identification. (continues) ▶

Mounting medium	Notes
Potassium hydroxide (KOH) (10 or 20%)	- Useful for initial examination - Possible to clear specimens either by gentle heating (the light microscope may help to do this) or leaving overnight in a moist container
Light lubricating oil	- Useful when no clearing or preparation required - Will preserve parasite for several days
Lactic acid	- Will clear preparations when warmed gently - Only useful as a temporary mount

Lactophenol	- Helpful for clearing specimens but can cause shrinkage of soft-bodied invertebrates
	- Formulation:
	  • Phenol 20g
	  • Lactic acid 16.5 ml
	  • Glycerol 32 ml
	  • Distilled water 20 ml

Permanent mounting medium	- Little shrinkage
	- Preserves specimens for several years
	- Formulation:
	  • Methocellulose 5 g
	  • Ethyl alcohol (95%) 25 ml
	  • Carbowax 2 g
	  • Diethyglycol 1 ml
	  • Lactic acid 100 ml
	  • Distilled water 75 ml
	- Method:
	  • Mix methocellulose and alcohol
	  • Add remainder
	  • Filter through glass wool
	  • Mature by incubating for 5 days at 40°C

10.6 (continued) Mounting of ectoparasites and other arthropods for identification.

- Histological sections of high quality demand good preservation of structure. This implies that samples should be taken and fixed as soon as possible – in the case of post-mortem material, speed is particularly important when handling such tissues as the nervous system, eye, pancreas, stomach and intestines. Correct and rapid fixation is also essential (see below).
- Tissues should be sampled at the edge of a lesion and include a small rim of adjacent apparently normal tissue. If there is more than one lesion, or if the lesions vary in appearance, samples should be obtained from multiple sites.
- Every effort should be made to avoid crushing or distorting the tissues during sampling. This can be a particular hazard when small biopsy specimens are removed from poorly accessible sites.
- As stressed above, tissues should be fixed as soon as possible after death or removal from a live animal. They should be placed in wide-necked (preferably plastic) containers containing a large volume of fixative in relation to the volume of the tissue (a ratio of at least 10:1).
- The penetration of fixative into a large piece of tissue is slow. Large portions of friable tissue may be fixed for 24 hours and then cut into smaller pieces. Central nervous tissue should be fixed in this way for at least 96 hours before it is further cut.
- Peripheral nerve and skeletal muscle will become contracted and distorted if simply immersed in fixative. They should be gently pressed on to a piece of cardboard, which is then placed in the fixative.
- Large samples of intestinal tract are often best fixed by tying off both ends of a small loop of intestine, which is then injected with fixative and immersed *in toto* in the formalin. Smaller samples can be placed or pinned on card as above.
- The most commonly used fixative is formalin (a solution of formaldehyde gas in water). Commercially available solutions are normally 40% formaldehyde (equivalent to 100% formalin). 10% formalin is usually used for fixation, thus requiring a 1 in 10 dilution of the concentrated (40% formaldehyde) solution. Formalin becomes acidic if left for any period of time and this produces unwanted pigment in the tissues. This can be prevented by a few chips of calcium carbonate in the bottom of the container or dilution of the concentrated solution in neutral phosphate buffer rather than water alone.
- Formalin presents health hazards and appropriate precautions should be taken and standard operating procedures followed.
- Other fixatives may be required for specific purposes (e.g. for fixation of eyes or nervous tissue).

10.7 Selection and fixation of tissues from wild animals for histological examination.

Environmental water samples: Water analysis may assist in the diagnosis of disease or the detection of environmental problems and can prove particularly helpful when dealing with amphibians and aquatic birds and mammals. The results usually need to be linked with clinical or pathological findings – for instance, as in Baker's (1989a) detection of uterine lesions in grey seals (*Halichoerus grypus*) in a location where polychlorinated biphenyl (PCB) values were known to be high.

Food samples: The examination of the food that animals are eating may reveal, for example, the presence of chemicals, such as herbicides, or of potentially pathogenic organisms such as *Aspergillus fumigatus* (see Figure 10.10).

Specific types of investigation

Microbiological examination: Microbiological (bacteriological and mycological) examination is of great value when dealing with wild animal casualties, especially when it is linked with antimicrobial sensitivity tests. Ideally, both aerobic and anaerobic culture for bacteria should be performed; where this is not feasible, perhaps on the grounds of cost, aerobic culture can be coupled with cytological examination of the lesion – which may reveal anaerobes as well as providing information on cellular changes. Samples that can usefully be examined microbiologically include those in Figure 10.1 and Figure 10.17.

Culture can be for bacteria, for fungi (e.g. using Sabouraud's agar) or for certain other organisms, such as *Trichomonas* spp.

Special stains have an important initial role to play in confirming or refuting the involvement of certain organisms in lesions in wildlife. Examples include the Ziehl–Neelsen (acid-fast) stain for mycobacteria and periodic acid–Schiff (PAS) or silver stains for *Aspergillus* and other fungi (Figure 10.10).

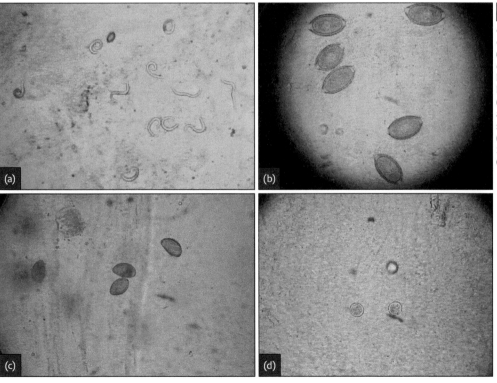

10.8 Common endoparasites of hedgehogs seen during direct microscopic examination of faecal smears. (a) *Crenosoma striatum* larvae; often highly motile approx. 300 μm long. (b) *Capillaria* spp. eggs; bipolar, approx. 50–60 μm long. (c) *Brachylaemus erinacei* eggs; asymmetry of sides, operculated, small, approx. 30 μm long. (d) Coccidial oocysts; small, approx. 20 μm in diameter. (© Steve Bexton)

Technique	Equipment	Method	Advantages	Disadvantages	Comments[a]
Direct smear method (e.g. see Figure 10.8)	Slides; coverslips; microscope	1. Place a few drops of normal saline or water on a slide 2. Add a little faeces with spatula (a plastic coffee stirrer is ideal) 3. Attach coverslip and examine microscopically. Screen under 10 or 25x objective	Ease of preparation, not costly Provides an opportunity to examine other material in the faeces, not just parasites (see Figure 10.1)	Purely qualitative May not detect light infections	A standard technique for domesticated animals An important initial 'screen' when working with wildlife
Flotation methods	Slides; coverslips (22 mm square); 15 ml flat-bottomed test tubes; tea strainer; bowl; microscope; if possible, a centrifuge Flotation solutions are used at saturation or near saturation. Use either: • Saturated sodium chloride (SG 1.2) • Zinc sulphate (SG 1.33) • Magnesium sulphate (SG 1.35) • Sugar (SG 1.35)	**Technique – without centrifugation** 1. Mix 3–4 g of faeces with 50 ml water 2. Pour mixture through 100 mesh sieve (e.g. a tea strainer) into a bowl 3. Rotate bowl and tip filtrate into two test tubes and allow to sediment for 5 minutes 4. Remove supernatant and mix sediment with enough flotation solution to ensure a distinct meniscus at top of the tube 5. Place coverslips on tubes and allow to stand for 15 minutes 6. Remove coverslips from each tube in one motion and examine microscopically. Use 25x objective to screen for helminth eggs, coccidial oocysts or larvae. A higher magnification is better **Technique – with centrifugation** As above except that both the faecal suspension in saline water and that in flotation fluid should be spun at 1500 rpm for 3 minutes in lieu of a standing period	Clear preparation	Qualitative Does not permit examination of other, non-parasitic material in the faeces	A standard technique for domesticated animals All applicable to wildlife but care has to be taken in interpretation when working with birds and reptiles, where urates will be present All techniques may be needed in forensic cases
Modified McMaster method	Balance; beakers; 15 ml flat-bottomed test tubes; strainer; bowl; centrifuge; Pasteur pipettes; microscope; McMaster slides; solution – usually saturated salt (NaCl)	1. Thoroughly mix 3 g of faeces with 42 ml of water (a mechanical stirrer is an advantage) 2. Pour mixture through 100 mesh sieve or strainer into bowl 3. Tip filtrate into a 15 ml test tube and centrifuge for 3 minutes at 1500 rpm 4. Discard supernatant, agitate sediment and fill test tube with salt solution 5. Invert or shake tube several times and withdraw sufficient fluid into Pasteur pipette to fill one chamber of the McMaster slide (0.15 ml) 6. Repeat and fill other chamber (it helps to wet the slide prior to filling) 7. Examine McMaster slide using the 4x objective of the microscope. Count the total eggs within lined areas of both chambers. The number of eggs per gram (epg) is obtained by multiplying the total number of eggs by 50 (3 g of faeces gave 45 ml suspension and 2 x 0.15 ml fluid in chamber, i.e. 0.3 ml are examined)	Quantitative	More costly. Detailed identification of small organisms, such as coccidial oocysts or larvae, is difficult Does not permit examination of other, non-parasitic material in the faeces	As in domesticated animals
Simple Baermann method for recovery of larvae from faeces	Beaker; muslin; test tubes; Pasteur pipettes; coverslips; slides	1. Take 10 g of faeces and wrap in muslin 2. Suspend muslin bag containing faeces in a beaker of warm water and leave overnight 3. Siphon or pour off most of supernatant and pour remaining sediment into test tube 4. Allow to stand for 2 hours and pour off supernatant 5. Add a few drops of clean water to sediment, agitate and pipette on to slides 6. Place coverslips and examine with 40x or 100x objective	Detects low numbers of first-stage larvae of (e.g. Oslerus osleri, Angiostrongylus and Aelurostrongylus spp.)	Time-consuming – not always practicable in a busy practice	As in domesticated animals
Modified Baermann method	Filter paper (17 cm); retort stand; filter funnel; rubber tubing and clip; sieve; beaker; test tubes; slides; coverslips; microscope	1. Spread 10 g of faeces thinly on 17 cm filter paper 2. Place sieve in contact with warm water in funnel with rubber hose and clip 3. Reverse filter paper and place on sieve 4. Leave overnight 5. Release clip and run off water from bottom of funnel into beaker 6. Pour into test tube and screen sediment on slides under 40x objective 7. If larvae are present, use 100x objective for species identification	As above. Can detect first-stage larvae	Less time-consuming than simple method but still not always practicable in a busy practice	As in domesticated animals

10.9 Collection and examination techniques for identification of endoparasites in the faeces of wild animals. [a] In all investigations that involve handling faeces from wild animals attention should be paid to health and safety, including possible infectious risks from zoonotic organisms and physical risks from, for example, spicules of bones that may be present in the gastrointestinal tract of carnivores.

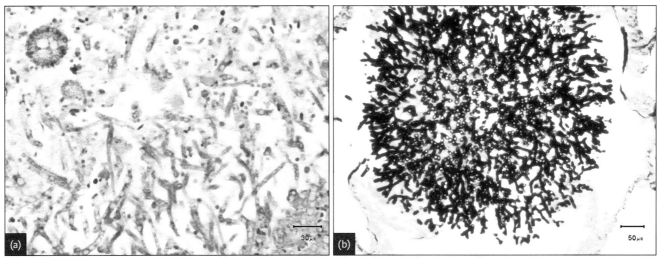

10.10 *Aspergillus* special staining techniques. (a) Aspergillosis in a bullfinch (*Pyrrhula pyrrhula*). The affected lung shows damage to parenchyma and extensive septate fungal hyphae, characteristic of *A. fumigatus*. Stained with periodic acid–Schiff (PAS). (b) An early *Aspergillus* lesion in the lung of a mammal. Branching fungal hyphae are beginning to invade adjacent alveoli. Stained with Grocott.

Haematological and biochemical investigations: Information on blood sampling is briefly summarized in Figure 10.1 and sampling sites and anticoagulants are described in Chapter 5. Sampling of some species, reptiles and amphibians for instance (Eatwell *et al.*, 2014), require special techniques. These tests can provide valuable data, although (in common with other types of test) there is a paucity of information on 'normal' reference ranges for interpretation, as emphasized by Lewis *et al.* (2002) in their study of blood samples from hedgehogs. Where reference ranges are available, examples of these are given in the species-specific chapters that follow. The effect on results of stressors such as handling and anaesthesia was discussed earlier.

Urinalysis: This has the same application in casualty mammals as it does in domesticated mammals (Ristić and Skeldon, 2011). It can also be used, to a certain extent, to examine the 'urinary' (renal) urate component of droppings of birds, reptiles and amphibians (see Figure 10.1). Urine can also be used to detect certain poisons. Familiarity with the normal appearance of the urine and urates of wild animals is important.

Parasitology: A wide variety of investigations can be performed to detect parasites, ranging from the examination of blood or urine to the investigation of regurgitated food, pellets (castings) from birds (Cooper and Cooper, 2013) or faeces (e.g. Figure 10.8). Some methods suitable for work with casualties are given in Figures 10.1, 10.4, 10.5, 10.6 and 10.9.

Cytology: Cytological examination of lesions (Figure 10.11), especially the use of 'impression smears' or 'touch preparations', is of great value in domesticated animals (Freeman and Farr, 2014) and should be routine in wild animal work but it is often forgotten or poorly practised. It can yield valuable results, rapidly and inexpensively. Cytological examination can be carried out using samples from either live or dead wild animals. In the case of the latter it can, amongst other things, help to distinguish bacteria that were present before death (intracellular) from those that were probably post-mortem contaminants (free organisms, often variable appearances/species).

One good example of the value of cytological examination, applicable when working with casualty birds, is the taking and staining of swabs from buccal cavity lesions, especially when trichomonosis is amongst the differential diagnoses (Figure 10.12).

Histology: This is a valuable tool in the investigation of both live and dead casualties (see Figure 10.1). It is, however, a specialized subject and cannot be discussed in detail here. Methods of fixation and other advice for the practitioner are provided in Figure 10.7.

Molecular techniques: One of the most important molecular diagnostic tests, applicable to various types of sample, is the polymerase chain reaction (PCR). This can be used to advantage in wild animal casualties (e.g. in the rapid detection of *Mycobacterium* and *Leptospira* spp.) and in the monitoring of spread of pathogenic organisms in the environment. PCR is not, however, a panacea. It often does not work as well as some other techniques, for example when searching for such intestinal organisms as *Giardia* spp., probably because of the presence of PCR inhibitors in faeces.

PCR offers the following advantages over traditional methods of identifying bacteria and other organisms:

- **Specificity:** this can be at the genus, species, serotype, or strain level
- **Speed:** whilst at least a day of culture is needed in order to obtain one colony on an agar plate, a comparable level of amplification can be reached in 1 or 2 hours with PCR. This is even more significant if the organism in question cannot be easily be cultured or takes a long time to grow or multiply, such as some mycobacteria and some viruses
- **Sensitivity:** one DNA molecule alone can be amplified and detected in a PCR well
- **Simplicity:** ready-to-use assays and methods are becoming widely available and the results can be analysed automatically
- **Stability:** PCR reagents are now extremely stable and can be transported at room temperature or kept at 2–8°C.

Types of cytology

- Fluid – blood, other tissue fluids, pus, exudates, transudates, aspirates, urine, bile, semen, washings
- Solid – tissue biopsy samples, pus, scrapings, brushings, washings, swabs

Advantages of cytology

- Rapid, cheap, simple and samples are relatively easy to take (surface access)
- Applicable in the field where facilities may be limited
- Detection of organisms (e.g. anaerobes or protozoa) that may be missed on culture
- Less invasive than biopsy and often provides information over a wider area (e.g. tracheal wash *versus* lung biopsy)

Disadvantages of cytology

- Exfoliated cells may not be typical of the whole lesion
- Concurrent histological examination should be performed where expenses and facilities permit

Collecting the sample

- Methods – impression smears (touch preparations) including sticky tape, swabs, scrapings, brushings, washings, fluid aspiration, lavage and fine-needle aspiration (FNA)
- Many errors are possible, including those relating to variation in technique, intermittent shedding of cells, excess blood and circadian or other variations (e.g. microfilariae in blood or lymph)
- Samples on at least two slides (preferably three) should be taken from each lesion. Frosted glass slides should be used and labelled using a pencil. The slides should be cleaned and polished
- Health and safety precautions – zoonotic infection, toxicity from stains and other reagents

Transporting the sample to the laboratory

- Many errors are possible, including those relating to delay, desiccation and deterioration. Unfixed samples are particularly vulnerable. Care should be taken with fixatives and anticoagulants as they can cause artefacts. Samples should be prepared *in situ*. Standardized packing and transportation should be used
- Submission of duplicate (or more) samples is always advisable
- Labelling – the slides should be labelled, on the correct side of the slide, with the vital patient information
- Supporting data and records (e.g. paperwork, computerized records, tape recordings) should be submitted with samples
- Ensure 'chain of custody' if it is likely to be a legal case (see Chapter 11)

Processing the sample

Preparation
- Fluids – dried smears are best. Haematological (thin smear) techniques should be used. Slides should be cleaned first and then a concentration of low cellularity fluids (centrifugation, sedimentation, filtration) can be added to the slide. High-viscosity fluids present problems (e.g. clumps of cells, poor spreading)
- Solids – imprints ('touch preparations' or 'impression smears'), crushing and scraping techniques ± saline
- Too thick *versus* too thin preparations. The aim of cytology, as with haematology, is to produce slides where the cells:
  - Are well spread
  - Exhibit detail of cytoplasm
  - Contain the nucleus and nucleoli

Fixation
- Fixation with methanol or ethanol will make staining with, for example, Gram stain difficult and the findings may be erroneous. Traditionally, ethanol fixation preceded Papanicolaou staining, whilst air-drying preceded May–Grünwald–Giesma staining. Air-drying can cause crenation in blood smears
- If in doubt, 100% methanol or a commercial fixative should be used. Buffered formalin (10%) can be employed (and will kill most pathogens) but stained cells become rather blue in colour

Staining
- Many standard stains can be used, but direct wet mounts can also be useful. In avian, reptilian or amphibian work, the following stains are particularly valuable:
  - Romanowsky stains (e.g. Wright's, Giemsa, Wright–Giesma, May–Grünwald–Giemsa) are used for routine cytology
  - Commercial stains (Diff-Quik, Avicolor) are easy and rapid to use
  - Giemsa stain is used for the detection and preliminary classification of certain microorganisms
  - Ziehl–Neelsen stain is used for acid-fast organisms
  - Macchiavello stain is used for *Chlamydia* (and *Mycoplasma* spp.)
  - Sudan stains or oil red O stain are used for the detection of fat (also visible as 'holes' in the sample). A fat stain should always be considered when a smear appears to be 'greasy'
  - New methylene blue (NMB) stain is used for the detection of fungal hyphae and fibrin. It can be combined with other stains (such as eosin)
- Variations in staining results may be related to:
  - Quality of the preparation
  - Age and quality of the stains
  - Experience and technique of the person performing the staining
  - Deterioration (old preparation)
- Quality control is important. Quality control consists of procedures that provide for a continual check on the accuracy of testing methods, equipment, reagents and working practices

Interpretation of the results

What is needed for the interpretation of findings?
- A sound knowledge of normal host cell morphology and normal appearance of microorganisms and metazoan parasites
- An understanding of pathological changes, especially at the cellular level (e.g. pyknosis, karyorrhexis, inclusion body formation)
- An appreciation of the limitations of cytological techniques and of our poorly developed understanding of the relevance of changes, especially in non-mammalian species

10.11 Cytological examination of material from wild animals. (continues) ▶

Interpretation of the results (*continued*)

On what is the interpretation based?
- Clinical or post-mortem examination
- Analysis of cytological findings on microscopy (NB low power first)
  - Normal host cells – may show an increase in numbers (e.g. lymphoid hyperplasia of the spleen, proliferation of the epithelium) or be present in abnormal sites (e.g. heterophilic infiltration of the liver)
  - Abnormal host cells – may be indicative of pathology but may also be artefacts due to poor sample collection, transportation or processing
  - Pathological host cells – may show discrete individual changes (e.g. degeneration, vacuolation, metaplasia, neoplasia) or be part of a pattern involving different types of cell. The size of cells may be important (should be measured with graticule or compared with cells of known size, e.g. erythrocytes)
  - Extrinsic cells – these are cells that are not derived from the host (patient) but may be relevant to diagnosis (e.g. parasites, inhaled material, foreign bodies)
  - Contaminants – be aware of plant and other contaminants (e.g. pollen, talc), especially when working in the field or when several samples are being collected or processed at the same time (i.e. to prevent the transfer of cells)

Types of cytological response
- Important pathological changes that may require examination of many fields under the microscope and involve several cell types. These include those associated with:
  - Acute inflammation
  - Chronic inflammation
  - Non-malignant proliferation
  - Malignant proliferation (neoplasia)
- Inflammatory (acute and chronic) responses can sometimes be confused with neoplastic responses. Cells seen with inflammation include:
  - Neutrophils/heterophils (normal alone) – acute inflammation
  - Neutrophils/heterophils (degenerate) – infection (usually bacterial)
  - Mixed population (neutrophils/heterophils, lymphocytes, etc.) – chronic or subacute infection
  - Macrophages in abundance, sometimes giant cells – fungal infection, Mycobacterium infection or foreign body reactions
- General features of neoplasia are populations of similar cells with individual differences, including a variable nucleus:cytoplasm ration, prominent nuclei and nucleoli, and sometimes abnormal and/or multiple nuclei. An increase in the mitotic index is also seen. Specific examples include:
  - Spindle-shaped cells that exfoliate poorly – sarcoma
  - Round/oval cells, often in patterns – carcinoma
  - Round/oval cells, lymphoblast-like – lymphoid tissue (e.g. leukaemia)
  - Mixed cells (with neoplastic features) – poorly differentiated neoplasm
  - Squamous epithelial cells in large numbers – papilloma (or tissue hyperplasia) but few features of neoplasia

Possible errors in interpretation
- Buccal cavity or oesophagus – with Gram stain, red blood cell nuclei can be mistaken for yeasts and keratinized debris can be confused with cocci
- Alimentary tract and faeces – yeasts and parasites (e.g. mites, nematode eggs) may be ingested with food and not be relevant to the casualty animal's problem
- Contaminants (e.g. bacteria on the slide, from the clinician's hands or in the fixative) may be detected and erroneously thought to be significant. This possibility should be considered when there are organisms detected on the slide but no cells. Artefacts associated with preparation include 'smudge cells' (damaged mononuclear cells) and 'basket cells' (damaged granulocytes). These artefacts should be recorded but not taken into consideration during the interpretation of the findings
- Large numbers of blood cells (red and white) may be indicative of poor preparation and can mask important findings (e.g. inflammatory cells). Touch preparations should be as free of blood as possible (dab repeatedly on filter paper beforehand to remove excess blood)

10.11 (continued) Cytological examination of material from wild animals.

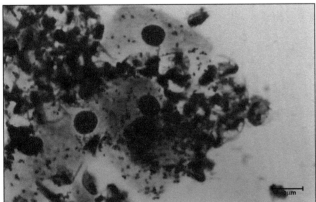

10.12 Cytological preparation of a buccal cavity swab taken from a bird of prey with a stomatitis. There are clusters of *Trichomonas gallinae*, recognizable by their distinct flagella, against a background of large squamous epithelial cells with abundant cytoplasm and scattered bacteria (Quick stain).

Another molecular technique that can be used to advantage in work with wildlife is immunohistochemistry, which – in addition to its established role in the differentiation of neoplasms in conventional veterinary practice – permits the detection of infectious agents in tissues (e.g. the diagnosis of canine distemper).

Serology: Various serological tests are available and these may indicate previous exposure to an organism or antigen or demonstrate a protective antibody response (using paired samples).

Toxicology: Some casualties will have been exposed to toxic chemicals (see Chapters 5 and 11 and species-specific chapters). These may be the cause of death or could have contributed to the animal's ill health, either directly or by increasing its susceptibility to infectious disease. It is important that samples from casualties are taken routinely for toxicological analysis; this not only assists with diagnosis but also contributes to scientific study and understanding of environmental pollution. Examples include the testing of tissues from marine mammals for polychlorinated biphenyls (PCBs), of seabirds for heavy metals and metallothionein, and of reptiles for zinc. Similar tests can be performed on apparently healthy wild animals as part of diagnostic health monitoring – for instance, the analysis of urine of different species for evidence of rodenticides, which may not have caused clinical signs but are still detectable in the animal and thereby give an indication of exposure. This area of study of wildlife warrants more attention. Data are especially needed in respect of chemicals that are increasingly being utilized on a large scale in agriculture, but about which relatively little is known in terms of side effects on vertebrate and invertebrate animals – for example, the broad-spectrum systemic herbicide glyphosate, which is widely used to kill weeds, especially those known to compete with commercial crops.

Even if poisoning is suspected in a wild animal casualty, confirmation is not easy. Trying to identify a specific toxicant is at best difficult. In wild animals, the problem is exacerbated because of the marked variation in pharmacokinetics exhibited by different poisons in disparate species. Likewise, there are no hard-and-fast rules insofar as the choice of samples for laboratory investigation is concerned. A useful, but very general, guide if poisoning is suspected is always to take blood, urine and faeces from a live animal and samples of liver and kidney plus urine, stomach contents and faeces if it has died. If more than one dead animal is available for investigation and the carcasses are not too large, they can be frozen *in toto* pending proper investigation. Rotstein (2008) gives useful information on the taking of samples from wild animals for toxicological analysis.

Perhaps the best advice to those dealing with a casualty where poisoning is suspected is to seek advice at an early stage from a toxicologist or experienced laboratory. The Wildlife Incident Unit (WIU) of the Food and Environment Research Agency (Fera) considers poisoning cases where pesticides are suspected, working closely with the Science and Advice for Scottish Agriculture (SASA). The APHA also investigates incidences through their GB Wildlife Disease Surveillance Partnership. In addition, practitioners should consider subscribing to the Veterinary Poisons Information Service (VPIS), which, although primarily concerned with toxicoses of domesticated animals, is able to provide valuable advice about current usage of potentially toxic substances and the prevalence and distribution of poisoning incidents in dogs and cats (see Appendix 1). Finally, the veterinary practice should have to hand the BSAVA/VPIS *Guide to Common Canine and Feline Poisons,* which provides information on many different poisons and, particularly useful in a busy practice, a 'traffic light' system indicating the level of necessary concern and urgency.

Other investigations

Collection of samples for other investigations may or may not be feasible. If there is a suspicion of a particular disease (e.g. a viral infection), appropriate specimens (which, depending upon the circumstances, could range from faeces to pieces of liver or brain) should be collected so that the relevant examination can be carried out. Virological techniques are often specialized and cannot be discussed in detail here; laboratory advice should be sought at an early stage.

The selection, collection, transportation and appropriate processing of any sample require careful coordination between the rehabilitator, the veterinary surgeon and the laboratory.

Additional considerations when sampling wildlife casualties

Sampling for legal cases

Legal cases relating to wildlife require a special focus on such matters as the maintenance of an intact 'chain of custody' and tests should be performed following recognized forensic procedures (see Chapter 11 and standard textbooks – e.g. Cooper and Cooper, 2007; 2013).

Health monitoring (screening)

Opinions differ as to which parameters are most important in assessing health and there are strong constraints (financial, legal and practical) on carrying out too many tests. Nevertheless, the 'screening' of wildlife prior to release or translocation is now a well established procedure and there is strong pressure (sometimes legal, always moral) on those involved in rehabilitation to follow established guidelines (Woodford, 2001; IUCN, 2013) in the interests of both the animal to be released and the population that it is to join (see Chapters 1 and 9). Important investigations, relevant to health monitoring as well as to the diagnosis of disease, are listed in Figure 10.1.

Interpretation of laboratory findings

As stressed earlier, in most cases there are few, if any, reference values for 'healthy' wildlife, although examples are given where possible in the chapters of this Manual. The collation of such data is most important, but care has to be taken that the procedures used for data collection are in accordance with the law (see Chapter 2). Pre-anaesthetic screening of animals can provide useful samples but they may not be 'normal'. Therefore extrapolation from other species, preferably those that are closely related to the one under investigation, is often necessary.

Interpretation of results is not easy (Fudge, 2000). They should be analysed in discussion with colleagues, in the light of the particular animal and the plans for its future treatment and release (see Chapters 4 and 9). Some 'abnormalities' may be considered acceptable; the presence of small numbers of intestinal nematodes may not be a reason for declining to release a patient if those same parasites are present in the free-living population (see Chapter 7).

Whenever possible, findings using one diagnostic procedure should be correlated with other results – for example, the concurrent use of histological and faecal examination for the study of lungworms in hedgehogs (Majeed *et al.*, 1989).

It is important that the veterinary surgeon who is working with wildlife builds up a close relationship with a laboratory that has an interest in non-domesticated species. Consultation *before* taking and submitting samples is always wise. In the UK, quite apart from the government and universities, there are several commercial laboratories that will accept samples from wild animals (see 'Specialist organizations and useful contacts' and Appendix 1).

Recording and dissemination of results

A vital part of laboratory testing is to ensure that findings are recorded, stored and – whenever possible – published or otherwise made available to interested people. There is an acute shortage of reliable information on laboratory values of wild animals that might aid rehabilitators and others. The overall value of having such data and making information available cannot be overemphasized.

Recognition and reporting of notifiable diseases is important (Cooper, 2002a) and may require the input of a specialist pathologist – as in the case with avian influenza, for example, that can affect free-living and captive birds as well as poultry (Irvine, 2013).

The retention of records is particularly important in legal ('forensic') cases (Cooper and Cooper, 2007; 2013) (see also Chapter 11).

Post-mortem examinations

Post-mortem examination is a very useful and important way of building up information on wild animal casualties and obtaining data on the causes of morbidity, mortality and failure to thrive. However, such data are really only of long-term value if the examination is carried out in a systematic way and the findings are properly recorded.

Ideally a post-mortem examination should be carried out on every wild animal casualty that dies or has to be euthanased (Figure 10.13). In addition, full supporting laboratory tests should be performed and material such as serum and tissues retained for reference. In practice, because of the constraints of time and money and sometimes health and safety considerations (see 'Procedures'), this approach is rarely feasible. It is usually necessary to restrict the examination to a gross necropsy with retention of some specimens in case they are needed at a later date.

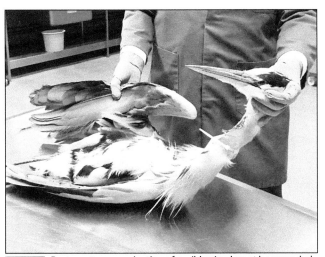

10.13 Post-mortem examination of a wild animal must be preceded by careful external examination, paying particular attention to the morphological features of the species in question – in this case, the beak and feet of this heron (*Ardea cinerea*).

Some necropsies need to be performed in an appropriate (biological) safety cabinet because of the possible risks to human health. Examples relevant to wildlife casualties include cases where chlamydiosis or tuberculosis is suspected. The classification of biological safety cabinets is shown in Figure 10.14.

Classification	Biosafety levels	Application	Examples of use, with particular reference to wildlife
Class I	1, 2, 3	Low-risk work with normally non-hazardous Hazard Group 1 biological agents	*Lactobacillus* species, *Citrobacter* species
Class II	1, 2, 3	Medium-risk work with Hazard Group 2 biological agents	Distemper/measles viruses, morbilliviruses, *Chlamydia psittaci*
Class III	4	High-risk work with Hazard Group 3 biological agents	*Mycobacterium tuberculosis*, *Yersinia pestis*

10.14 Classification of biological safety cabinets.

Procedures

The post-mortem examination itself should follow standard procedures (Woodford, 2000; Cooper and Cooper, 2013), which often do not differ greatly from those used for domestic animals. Where unusual species are involved (e.g. marine mammals), it may be wise to seek specialist help in the form of Royal College of Veterinary Surgeons or European College of Zoological Medicine Specialists and/or a specialist laboratory (see 'Specialist organizations and useful contacts'). Some special features relevant to different groups of wildlife are listed in Figure 10.15.

Health and safety is an important consideration, as dead wild animals may be a source of infectious organisms (see Chapters 2 and 7) (Cooper, 1990; Palmer *et al.*, 1998). As a general rule, it should be assumed that a carcass is dangerous and, following a risk assessment (see Chapter 2), standard precautions (as practised by veterinary surgeons when dealing with domesticated

Group	Special features	Relevance to post-mortem examination
Mammals	• Many variations in external and internal anatomy (e.g. presence or absence of tail, structure of gastrointestinal tract) • All mammals have mammary glands and some hair	• Careful attention should be paid to special structures, such as the patagium of bats and the blowhole of cetaceans
Birds	• Variations in external and internal anatomy (e.g. presence or absence of preen (uropygial) gland, crop, caeca) • Certain specialized features (e.g. modified syrinx in male duck) • All birds have feathers • All are oviparous	• Plumage and preen gland should be checked at the outset • All orifices, including the auditory canal, require careful investigation, where appropriate using an otoscope
Reptiles	• Much anatomical variation but lizards and snakes essentially very similar • All reptiles have scaled skin • Most are oviparous; some are viviparous • All have a cloaca • Melanin often abundant in internal organs	• The scalation, dorsal and ventral, must be checked carefully for lesions and parasites • Apparent discoloration (usually darkening) of internal organs may be due to melanin
Amphibians	• Marked distinction in most species between immature (larval/tadpole) stage with gills and other modifications to aquatic lifestyle, and mature (adult) with lungs and terrestrial lifestyle • All amphibians have unscaled mucous skin • Melanin often abundant in internal organs	• Dead amphibians rapidly decompose: therefore the necropsy should be performed as soon as possible • Sensitive external tissues (skin and gills) begin to dry soon after death: they (or the whole carcass) should be kept moist • Apparent discoloration (usually darkening) of internal organs may be due to melanin

10.15 Special features relevant to post-mortem examination of wildlife.

animals) should be taken. Some species, such as bats (see Chapter 15), require special precautions and should be submitted to a specialist laboratory, such as APHA, and not examined under practice conditions.

Whatever the type of animal to be examined, the following general rules apply:

- As full a history as possible should be obtained
- Whenever feasible, the environment from which the animal came and (where applicable) the management to which it was subjected should be evaluated
- If several animals are available for post-mortem examination, particularly if there may be a common aetiology for the deaths, a series of examinations comparing and contrasting the findings is necessary; a pattern may emerge. Such necropsies may need to be coupled with microbiological and chemical investigation of, say, water samples (see 'Environmental water samples')
- The circumstances of death, including the method of euthanasia, must be ascertained and taken into account
- Biological data must be obtained.

Even basic information such as measurements and bodyweight (mass) (see Appendix 2) are of value to biologists and others who are studying the species. At the same time, those data can be of assistance in assessing the health of the animal. Recording only the bodyweight (mass) of the animal is, however, not satisfactory: it gives no indication of condition, size or configuration. Standard measurements that are used by field biologists should be utilized whenever feasible; the key ones are listed in Figure 10.16.

Body condition (see Chapter 4) should also be recorded. How this is assessed will vary with species and even, sometimes, with the time of the year because it relates to the demands facing that individual at a particular time (Sears, 1988).

Examination and description of the contents of the alimentary tract is always important in wild species as this provides information on whether or not the animal has been feeding, the type of ingesta and any lesions or abnormalities of the gastrointestinal tract.

Wild animals will sometimes ingest unusual dietary items or foreign material, especially when there is a shortage of natural food: for example, Hogg *et al.* (2010)

described mass mortalities in gulls (*Larus* spp.) associated with eating livestock fodder.

Certain taxa may warrant special investigation and recording of data. For instance, the thickness (depth) of blubber is important when examining dead seals and cetaceans (Baker, 1989b). Bats should be tested for lyssavirus (see Chapter 15) and, in view of the paucity of biomedical data on many chiropteran species, their parasites collected and properly identified, as emphasized by Barlow *et al.* (2013) and Simpson (2013).

Many wild animal casualties are small (e.g. rodents, nestling birds, lizards, frogs) and it can be difficult to carry out a meaningful necropsy. A useful approach here is to perform a 'mini necropsy' using a magnifying lens or loupe and microsurgical instruments and, if histological examination is to be carried out, to fix (see Figure 10.7) and embed in paraffin the whole specimen and then examine serial or step sections (Cooper and Cooper, 2007).

The post-mortem examination of eggs and embryos is discussed in some detail by Cooper (2002b; 2007); it will not be discussed here as it is of limited importance in work with wildlife casualties.

The most important samples that may be taken from post-mortem cases are listed in Figure 10.17.

Group	Standard measurements
Mammals	Bodyweight (mass) Crown–rump length Specific measurements (e.g. wings and digits of bats)
Birds	Bodyweight (mass) Tarsal length (measure length of the tarsometatarsal bone) Carpal length (measure from distal carpus to tip of longest primary feather)
Reptiles	Bodyweight (mass) Snout–vent (SV) (rostrum–cloaca) Vent–tail tip (VT)
Amphibians: tailed (Caudata)	Bodyweight (mass) Snout–vent (SV) (rostrum–cloaca) Vent–tail tip (VT)
Amphibians: tailless (Urodela)	Bodyweight (mass) Snout to end of body

10.16 Standard measurements when examining live or dead wildlife casualties.

Samples	Comments
Tissues in 10% formalin for histology (see Figure 10.7)	• Have the advantage that they can be stored indefinitely and examined at a later stage • General rule should be to take lung, liver and kidney (LLK), plus any organs that show abnormalities or are considered important because they may provide information about the animal's health or biology (e.g. bursa of Fabricius of young birds can yield data on immune status) • Small carcasses can be fixed whole, following opening of the body cavity to allow penetration of formalin
Cytological preparations (see Figures 10.11 and 10.12)	• Easy to take, cheap to process (readily carried out in veterinary practice or in the field) and produce rapid results • Usually consist of touch preparations or impression smears, which can provide valuable information within a few minutes • Should be retained after examination in case they are needed later • As with formalin-fixed samples, should be taken and stored even if there is no immediate prospect of their being analysed.
Swabs, organ/tissue samples and other specimens for microbiological and other investigations	• Usually comprise swabs, portions of tissue or exudates/transudates • If culture proves impossible for financial or other reasons, impression smears stained with Gram or other stains often provide some useful information
Tissues for toxicological examination	• Need to be taken routinely from casualties • Usually frozen and can be analysed at a later date • As with formalin-fixed samples, should be taken and stored even if there is no immediate prospect of their being analysed

10.17 Samples from post-mortem cases.

Retention of material

An important rule (often overlooked) is to retain as much material as possible after the post-mortem examination. The reason for not discarding material immediately after necropsy is that the veterinary surgeon can return to the material later if necessary – for example, if further tests are needed or if samples are required for forensic (legal) purposes (Cooper and Cooper, 2007; 2013) (see also Chapter 11).

A whole carcass can be kept for up to 7 days at 4°C. After this time it is wiser to freeze it at as low a temperature as possible (at least -20°C and ideally as low as -70°C), even though this can result in tissue damage that will hamper histological investigations. If it is not realistic to retain the whole carcass frozen, selected tissues or all the viscera can be kept.

Quite apart from the point made above, those who examine dead wild animals should not discard carcasses and tissues too hastily. Such material is part of the database for that individual and for that species, which can contribute substantially to our knowledge of wildlife health and disease.

Sometimes, especially if the animal examined is of a rare species, a museum may ask to have the whole body, the skin or representative portions of the carcass. It is important to ascertain whether this is likely to be the case before the necropsy is carried out, because it may influence how the examination is performed – for example, how much damage is done to the skull. In some such cases it may be wise to have the examination carried out by a specialist pathologist (Cooper and Cooper, 2007).

It is always good practice to offer material from wildlife cases to museums (another part of building bridges with non-veterinary scientists). The establishment of reference collections, which can be used by the veterinary profession and others in retrospective and research studies, should also be considered, especially in the case of rare or declining species (Cooper et al., 1998; Cooper and Cooper, 2007). Retention of skins, bones and soft tissues from animals that are protected by law is unlikely to require a licence (see Chapter 2) but the veterinary surgeon who carries out a post-mortem examination and stores material is well advised to keep a written record of origin and to provide notice of this to anyone who receives any of it, for whatever purpose.

Disposal of carcasses and other material

There are important legal restrictions in the UK governing the disposal of carcasses and these are relevant to work with wildlife casualties. Waste contractors employed by veterinary surgeries and wildlife rehabilitation centres must be appropriately licensed to deal with these products.

The British Veterinary Association (www.bva.co.uk) provides useful current guidance for the disposal of veterinary waste. The British Government website (www.gov.uk) has additional information specifically on dealing with animal by-products.

References and further reading

Baker JR (1989a) Pollution-associated uterine lesions in grey seals from the Liverpool Bay area of the Irish Sea. *Veterinary Record* **125**, 303

Baker JR (1989b) Natural causes of death in non-suckling grey seals (*Halichoerus grypus*). *Veterinary Record* **125**, 500–503

Barlow A, Wills D and Harris E (2013) Enteric nematodes and *Sarcina*-like bacteria in a brown long-eared bat. *Veterinary Record* **172**, 508

BSAVA (2012) *BSAVA/VPIS Guide to Common Canine and Feline Poisons.* British Small Animal Veterinary Association, Gloucester

Bunnell T (2001) The importance of faecal indices in assessing gastrointestinal parasite infestation and bacterial infection in the hedgehog (*Erinaceus europaeus*). *Journal of Wildlife Rehabilitation* **24(2)**, 13–17

Cooper JE (1989) *Disease and Threatened Birds.* Technical Publication No. 10. International Council for Bird Preservation (now Bird Life International), Cambridge

Cooper JE (1990) Birds and zoonoses. *Ibis* **132**, 181–191

Cooper JE (1994) Biopsy techniques. *Seminars in Avian and Exotic Pet Medicine* **3**, 161–165

Cooper JE (1998) Minimally invasive health monitoring of wildlife. *Animal Welfare* **7**, 35–44

Cooper JE (1999a) Avian microbiology. In: *Laboratory Medicine Avian and Exotic Pets,* ed. AM Fudge. WB Saunders, Philadelphia and London

Cooper JE (1999b) Reptilian microbiology. In: *Laboratory Medicine Avian and Exotic Pets,* ed. AM Fudge. WB Saunders, Philadelphia and London

Cooper JE (2002a) Diagnostic pathology of selected diseases in wildlife. *Revue Scientifique et Technique de L'Office International des Epizooties* **21(1)**, 77–89

Cooper JE (2002b) *Birds of Prey: Health and Disease.* Blackwell Science, Oxford

Cooper JE (2007) Pathology A. Disease. In *Raptor Research and Management Techniques,* ed. DM Bird and KL Bildstein. Hancock, Canada

Cooper JE (2013) Field Techniques in Exotic Animal Medicine. *Journal of Exotic and Pet Medicine* **22(1)** 4–6

Cooper JE and Cooper ME (2007) *Introduction to Veterinary and Comparative Forensic Medicine.* Blackwell, Oxford

Cooper JE and Cooper ME (2013) *Wildlife Forensic Investigation: Principles and Practice.* CRC Press, Taylor and Francis Group, Florida

Cooper JE, Dutton CJ and Allchurch AF (1998) Reference collections in zoo management and conservation. *Dodo* **34**, 159–166

Dallmann R, Steinlechner S, von Hörsten, S and Karl T (2006) Stress-induced hyperthermia in the rat: comparison of classical and novel recording methods. *Laboratory Animals* **40**, 186–193

Davison NJ, Simpson VR, Chappell S *et al.* (2010) Prevalence of host-adapted group B (*Salmonella phocoena*) from the south-west coast of England. *Veterinary Record* **167(5)**, 173–176

Duff JP (2003) Wildlife disease surveillance by the Veterinary Laboratories Agency. *Microbiology Today* **30**, 157–159

Duff JP (2013) Mass mortality of starlings roosting by a roadside. *Veterinary Record* **173**, 613–614

Duff JP, Harris MP and Turner DM (2013) Mass mortality of puffins, linked to starvation. *Veterinary Record* **173**, 224

Duff JP, Holmes JP and Barlow AM (2010) Surveillance turns to wildlife. *Veterinary Record* **167**, 154–156

Eatwell K, Hedley J and Barron R (2014) Reptile haematology and biochemistry. *In Practice* **36**, 34–42

Feare CJ (2007) The spread of avian influenza. *Ibis* **149**, 424–425

Freeman K and Farr A (2014) Collection, handling and staining of veterinary cytologic specimens. *Veterinary Practice Today, Spring 2014,* 10–14

Fudge AM (2000) Laboratory Medicine. *Avian and Exotic Pets.* WB Saunders, Philadelphia

Gauthier-Clerc M, Lebrarbenchon C and Thomas F (2007) Recent expansion of highly pathogenic avian influenza H5N1: a critical review. *Ibis* **149**, 202–214

Hogg R, Whitaker K and Duff JP (2010) Mass mortalities in gulls associated with eating livestock fodder. *Veterinary Record* **167(5)**, 183

Irvine RM (2013) Recognising avian notifiable diseases 1. Avian influenza. *In Practice* **35**, 426–437

IUCN (2013) *Guidelines for Reintroductions and Other Conservation Translocations.* IUCN, Switzerland. https://portals.iucn.org/library/efiles/documents/2013-009.pdf

Keymer IF, Gibson EA and Reynolds DJ (1991) Zoonoses and other findings in hedgehogs (*Erinaceus europaeus*): a survey of mortality and review of the literature. *Veterinary Record* **128(11)**, 245–249

Lawson B, Lachish S, Colvile KM *et al.* (2012a) Emergence of a novel avian pox disease in British tit species. *Plos ONE* e40176

Lawson B, Robinson RA, Colvile KM *et al.* (2012b) The emergence and spread of finch trichomonosis in the British Isles. *Philosophical Transactions of the Royal Society B* **367**, 2852–2863

Lewis JCM, Norcott MR, Frost LM and Cusdin P (2002) Normal haematological values of European hedgehogs (*Erinaceus europaeus*) from an English rehabilitation centre. *Veterinary Record* **151**, 567–569

Mader DM and Divers SJ (2014) *Current Therapy in Reptile Medicine and Surgery.* Elsevier Saunders, Missouri, USA

Majeed SK, Morris PA and Cooper JE (1989) Occurrence of the lungworms *Capillaria* and *Crenosoma* spp. in British hedgehogs (*Erinaceus europaeus*). *Journal of Comparative Pathology* **100**, 27–36

Palmer SR, Soulsby EJL and Simpson DIH (1998) *Zoonoses.* Oxford University Press, Oxford

Paul E (2012) *Emerging Avian Disease (Studies in Avian Biology) no. 42.* University of California Press, Berkeley and Los Angeles

Ristić J and Skeldon N (2011) Urinalysis in practice – an update. *In Practice* **33**, 12–19

Rotstein D S (2008) How to perform a necropsy if a toxin is suspected. *Journal of Exotic Pet Medicine* **17(1)**, 39–43

Sainsbury AW, Cunningham AA, Morris PA, Kirkwood JK and Macgregor SK (1996) Health and welfare of rehabilitated juvenile hedgehogs (*Erinaceus europaeus*) before and after release into the wild. *Veterinary Record* **138**, 61–65

Sears J (1988) Assessment of body condition in live birds; measurement of protein and fat reserves in the mute swan, *Cygnus olor*. *Journal of Zoology London* **216**, 295–308

Simpson V (2013) Nematodes in brown-eared bats. *Veterinary Record* **172**, 535

Snow LC, Newson SE, Musgrove AJ *et al.* (2007) Risk-based surveillance for H5N1 avian influenza virus in wild birds in Great Britain. *Veterinary Record* **161**, 775–781

Toms M (2012) The spread of avian pox. *BTO News* Winter 2012, 19

Woodford MH (2000) *Post-mortem Procedures for Wildlife Veterinarians and Field Biologists*. Office International des Epizooties, Paris

Woodford MH (2001) *Quarantine and Health Screening Protocols for Wildlife Prior to Translocation and Release into the Wild*. OIE, VSG/IUCN, Care for the Wild International and EAZWV, Paris

Specialist organizations and useful contacts

Laboratories in Britain that accept material from wild animals:

Animal and Plant Health Agency (APHA, see Appendix 1)

Greendale Veterinary Diagnostics
Lansbury Estate, Knaphill, Woking GU21 2EW, UK
Tel: 01483 797707; Fax: 01483 797552
www.greendale.co.uk

International Zoo Veterinary Group LLP
Station House, Parkwood Street, Keighley BD21 4NQ, UK
Tel: 01535 692000; Fax: 01535 690433
www.izvg.co.uk

Pinmoore Animal Laboratory Services (PALS) Limited
The Coach House, Town House Barn, Clotton,
Cheshire CW6 0EG, UK
Tel: 01829 781855; Fax: 0870 7583638
www.palsvetlab.co.uk

Scotland's Rural College SRUC
Analytic Services, Allan Watt Building,
Bush Estate, Penicuik EH26 0PH, UK
Tel: 0131 5353170
www.sruc.ac.uk

Wildlife Health Services
www.wildlifehealthservices.com

Other useful contacts:

Garden Wildlife Health
www.gardenwildlifehealth.org

Wildlife Incident Investigation Scheme (WIIS)
Freephone: 0800 321600

Also in Scotland see:
www.sasa.gov.uk/wildlife-environment/wildlife-incident-investigation-scheme-wiis

Wildlife Incident Unit (WIU)
http://fera.co.uk/ccss/WIIS.cfm

Chapter 11

Investigating wildlife crime

Ranald Munro and Guy Shorrock

The veterinary surgeon's (veterinarian's) role in the investigation of wildlife crime falls within the developing specialist area of forensic veterinary medicine. Although veterinary surgeons have long been involved in these types of cases, the standard of investigation and reporting of alleged wildlife crime has improved markedly in recent times. Consequently, investigators (whether they belong to the police or other agencies) have high expectations of the potential depth and quality of evidence that might be provided by the veterinary profession.

In the UK, the police have the primary lead on the investigation of wildlife crime and may be assisted by a number of statutory and non-government agencies. Police forces have one or more Wildlife Crime Officers (WCOs) who have experience and knowledge of wildlife crime issues. Many welfare and cruelty-related cases are investigated by agencies, such as the Royal Society for the Prevention of Cruelty to Animals (RSPCA) and Scottish SPCA. The level of expertise in wildlife matters varies dramatically amongst individuals in these agencies and considerable guidance from veterinary surgeons may be needed in some instances. Scenarios might include: firearms injuries; suspected poisoning; blunt injuries; alleged drowning; trap and snare injuries or trauma associated with dog bites. The animals may be alive or deceased or, in cases where there are multiple victims, a mix of cadavers and survivors. In all cases involving live animals, the welfare needs of the injured animal are paramount. Administration of appropriate emergency treatment and care takes precedence over other considerations and should not be delayed (see Chapter 5). However, as much forensic evidence as possible should be preserved (e.g. by taking photographs before surgery).

Typically, a wildlife crime investigator may want to know:

- Has an offence been committed?
- What was the cause of injury or death of an animal?
- What species are involved?
- Are there any witnesses to the incident or the finding of the animal(s)?
- Is any evidence securely stored and identifiable?
- Are any further tests or examinations likely to be of benefit?

Fundamentals of veterinary forensic medicine

The major difference between veterinary and human forensic medicine stems from the wide variety of species that the veterinary surgeon may be asked to examine. Although veterinary surgeons are required to provide emergency treatment for all animals, it is recognized that no one person can be knowledgeable about all species. In forensic practice, it is extremely important that clinicians recognize the limits of their expertise and avoid the ever-present danger of straying beyond the limits of their professional competence. At the beginning of every potential forensic case it is important to ask: 'Am I the right person to examine and report upon this case?' For example, where an initial examination or radiograph suggests an animal has received unlawful injuries, a necropsy may be required. Veterinary surgeons should consider the implications of undertaking such work and whether it would be better if it were performed by a specialist (e.g. veterinary pathologist). Wildlife crime investigators will be looking to gather the best evidence, which is accurate, reliable and able to withstand potential challenges during criminal proceedings.

Three important rules in forensic cases are:

- Objectivity
- Meticulous record-keeping
- Maintenance of the chain of evidence.

It is also important to recognize that the veterinary surgeon's report forms only part of the wider evidence that is drawn together by the legal teams. The veterinary practitioner is relieved of the responsibility of 'proving a case'; it is for the courts to make such decisions. However, the courts require the expertise of the veterinary profession to describe and explain what has happened to the animal and to identify any suffering involved.

Investigation of wildlife crime may include examination of the scene where the alleged incident took place or of paraphernalia associated with particular crimes (e.g. badger baiting or trapping wild birds). The animal, although part of the overall crime scene, is usually processed as a crime scene in its own right. Veterinary surgeons may also be asked to interpret or pass comment on video evidence and photographs. In all cases, veterinary surgeons should be prepared to examine the animal (or other evidence), document the findings in detail and prepare a report giving a balanced interpretation of the facts in plain English. The primary purpose of the report is to guide and inform the legal teams. A report in 'medical speak' is unhelpful since it will have to be translated into plain English before it can be understood by others. Much better is for the report to present the findings in layman's language. If necessary, anatomical terms (e.g. tibiotarsal bone), can be placed in brackets after the plain English version to ensure accuracy.

Many wildlife crime investigations will rely on evidence from professional or expert witnesses. In the UK, there is no definitive legal definition of an expert. For example, the Crown Prosecution Service (England and Wales) defines an expert as:

'A person whose evidence is intended to be tendered before a court and who has relevant skill or knowledge achieved through research, experience or professional application within a specific field sufficient to entitle them to give evidence of their opinion and upon which the court may require independent, impartial assistance'.

The court, however, will decide whether a person is to be classed as an expert witness. The expert's primary responsibility is to assist the court; even if called and paid for by one of the parties to the case, the expert must remain independent of that party's vested interest. The various UK prosecuting agencies have issued guidance for expert witnesses, stressing the requirement for sound, current and practical knowledge of the subject matter, based on actual clinical or practical experience, and for the expert witness to have the ability to provide accurate and robust evidence that can withstand challenges that may be made in court.

A 'professional witness' is a witness of fact, who by reason of some direct professional involvement in the facts of a case, is able to give an account of those facts to the court. However, this can be a 'grey area' because the professional witness, in the course of carrying out their role, may have formed an opinion based on the observed facts. Consequently, there may be occasions when a professional witness will be asked to explain their findings, and this may lead them into expert witness territory.

First contact and instructions

First contact with the forensic case is usually through a telephone call, but the police or other investigating agency may arrive, unannounced, with an animal for examination. It is essential that certain information is gathered at this time (Figure 11.1) and contemporaneous notes made. Every contact, treatment, sample taken,

Information	Comments
Who?	Name and contact details of person submitting case/specimen With wildlife, ownership is not usually an issue but it is necessary that someone takes responsibility for the patient (see Chapters 2 and 3)
When?	Date and time that the veterinary surgeon is first contacted regarding the case This information is crucial for the chain of evidence
Where?	Record where the animal was found, remembering that the animal or bird may have moved (or been moved) from the place where the incident occurred
What?	Brief details of animal/photographs/other evidence presented
Why?	Outline of what is expected of you. What are you being asked to do? For example, a full examination and report or radiography only?
Which?	Record case numbers/log references or other identifying marks on the patient at the time of first presentation
Write	List other information you require, but which is not immediately available from the person making the contact; this might include details of the investigating officer or a police reference number

11.1 Initial information to be gathered when dealing with a forensic wildlife case.

procedure undertaken, decision made and test result should be documented, dated and signed. The better the notes, the easier it will be to write the report, and to talk confidently about the case, weeks or months later.

Chain of evidence (chain of custody)

Courts are obliged to make decisions on the evidence that is presented to them. If doubts are raised over the identity of an animal, or whether some change has taken place in this animal between discovery and subsequent examinations, the court may consider that any evidence based on this animal is unsound.

In effect, the chain of evidence is a 'trail' showing how the evidence was handled from the time it was recovered until its introduction to the court. It shows how the item was recovered, where it was between the time of recovery and the time of trial, who handled it, and where it was stored.

A full chain of custody consists of three elements:

* Testimony that the evidence is what it says it is (e.g. four tail feathers from a hen harrier (*Circus cyaneus*))
* Testimony of continuous possession by each individual who has had possession of the evidence from the time it was gathered to presentation in court
* Testimony of each individual who has had possession of the evidence that such evidence has remained in substantially the same condition from the moment one person took possession until it was released into the custody of another person.

This last requirement does not mean that a veterinary surgeon cannot change the condition of the animal through surgery or medical treatment. All that is required is for the veterinary evidence, in the form of contemporaneous notes and photographs, to record the need for treatment, the treatment given and the progress following treatment. Figure 11.2 sets out the types of documentation that might be useful.

One roe deer (*Capreolus capreolus*) may look very much like another roe deer to people unfamiliar with this species. Consequently, labels/tags/collars bearing the case number or logbook reference must be attached securely to the animal and this identification label/tag should remain attached to the animal throughout transportation, examination, treatment and, if necessary, storage.

Evidence	Documentation required
Notes and lists	• Contemporaneous notes including initial contact details • List of items collected during examination (including samples taken) • Log giving details of where and under what conditions evidential items are stored and of samples sent for laboratory examination • Log of telephone calls or other contacts with crime investigator
Photography	• Log of photographs, video taken and radiographic images • Contemporaneous notes related to photography
Sketches or diagrams	• Body outlines/templates may be used to record wounds • Sketches can be valuable when the position of one object relative to another is recorded • Measurements can be marked on the templates and sketches

11.2 Documentation of evidence.

When dealing with specimens or derivatives it may be advisable to avoid recording species at this time, unless absolutely certain of the identification. This prevents potential confusion if definitive identification of a specimen is made later by an expert. It is sufficient, in the beginning, if the specimen is labelled simply, for example, 'Owl species Ref AB1' or 'Animal hairs Ref CD2'.

If suitable procedures are in place, maintenance of the chain of evidence is straightforward. Preparation of standard operating procedures (SOPs) helps make chain of evidence processes easy to follow. SOPs can be written to cover receipt of specimens, photography, clinical examination and treatment, sample collection/storage and laboratory testing and report writing. Once drafted, they should be updated annually or when procedures change. Although SOPs may sound bothersome, they make life much simpler.

All information gathered during an enquiry should be retained and the wildlife crime investigator made aware of what material is held. Ensure all records and information are securely and safely held. With electronic records, information should be password protected and a backup system should be in place. All photographs should be retained and not deleted, renamed or altered in any way.

Sampling equipment

Having the appropriate clinical equipment to hand greatly simplifies the sampling procedures. Examples of the measuring scales, evidence bags and types of sealing tape and labels that support good forensic practice are shown in Figures 11.3, 11.4 and 11.5. Other items often required include weighing scales, tape measures, various sizes of sample bottles, and still and video cameras.

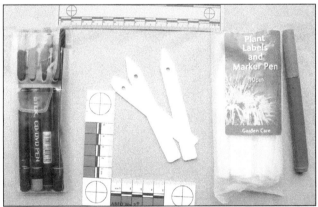

11.3 Forensic examination equipment essentials: pens; labels; ruler; photographic scales.
(© Simon Newbery)

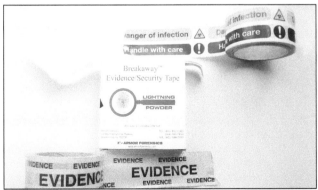

11.4 Various tapes are available for the identification of potential biohazards, highlighting evidential material or for sealing evidence containers.
(© Simon Newbery)

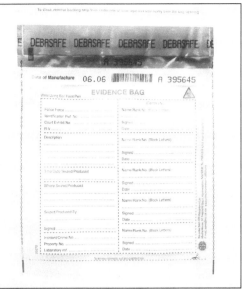

11.5 Evidence bags are convenient, provide space for recording details and are readily sealed and resealed.
(© Simon Newbery)

Firearms injuries

Veterinary surgeons are, not infrequently, asked to examine birds and mammals that may have been shot. Various scenarios include accidental shooting, incidents where the public may have been endangered, poaching, out-of-season shooting and firearms injuries in protected species.

To provide reliable evidence that enhances an understanding of what might have happened, the veterinary surgeon should have a basic knowledge of the weapons commonly used and the characteristic injuries caused by the various projectiles.

Air rifles

Possibly the most common firearms injuries in garden birds, waterfowl visiting urban ponds and small mammals (e.g. squirrels (*Sciurus* spp.)) are caused by air rifle pellets. Many of these pellets are constructed of soft lead. However, others have a compound construction consisting of a metal head and a nylon or plastic jacket. On penetration of the tissues, the radiodense head may become separated from the radiolucent jacket. This can make location of the jacket problematic. Both parts of the pellet may be of evidential value and should be recovered if possible. Successful healing of the wound tract may also depend on removal of the radiolucent jacket.

Although air rifle pellets may cause rapidly fatal injury to small mammals and birds, they frequently result in non-fatal wounding of larger creatures. For example, swans subjected to airgun attacks may have been shot on previous occasions and care needs to be taken to distinguish old pellet wounds (in which the pellet is partially or completely encapsulated by fibrous tissue) from recent injuries.

Shotguns

Shotgun cartridges contain numerous small round metal pellets. All the pellets in a specific cartridge are of a certain size, which is marked on the outside of the cartridge. Small pellets are used to shoot game birds, for example, whilst foxes (*Vulpes vulpes*) may be killed with larger pellets. Pellets recovered during surgery may be important evidentially, and these pellets should be handled and stored with care (see Figure 11.9) before being submitted to a ballistics expert.

In cases of shotgun wounding, the question often asked is 'How far was the shooter from the animal when the shot was discharged?' Many attempts have been made over the years to devise a formula to calculate this distance accurately. Usually, however, there is insufficient information available to allow a refined answer. The best that can be offered is 'close', ranging from a few centimetres to 1–2 metres (Figure 11.6), and 'distant' where the spread of pellets over the body, wings and legs is much wider (Figure 11.7). This difference in pattern can be of some value as it may provide information that either confirms or casts doubt on witness evidence or the history provided by the accused. However, considerable caution is advocated when pressed by investigators or legal representatives to make a statement on the discharge distance.

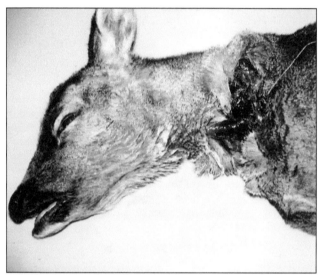

11.6 Roe deer shot in the neck with a 12-bore shotgun from a distance of a few metres. Large numbers of shotgun pellets were found clustered within the wound.

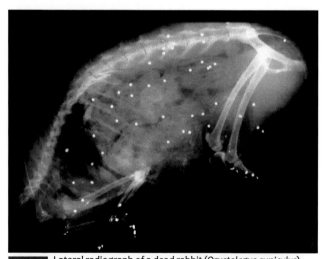

11.7 Lateral radiograph of a dead rabbit (*Oryctolagus cuniculus*) struck by shotgun pellets from a 12-bore shotgun. The distribution of pellets throughout the body indicates that the shooter was at a considerable distance from the rabbit. It is worth noting that many of the shotgun pellets would have passed above, below and to the sides of this rabbit.

Rifles

Basically, rifle bullets may be classified as low velocity (less than 2000 feet/610 metres per second) or high velocity. The injuries caused, and the forensic evidence left, by these two types are substantially different. Radiography plays a crucial role in the detection of the bullet track and in determining which type of bullet was involved.

When low-velocity bullets strike bone they become deformed and shed variously sized fragments of metal. These fragments of bullet and splintered bone are readily identified by radiography. Fragmentation of a high-velocity bullet is usually characterized by a pattern of fine radiopaque particles (derived from the lead core of the bullet) along the bullet track, accompanied by a number of 'flying seagull' shaped slivers of the copper jacket that partially covers this type of bullet (Figure 11.8)

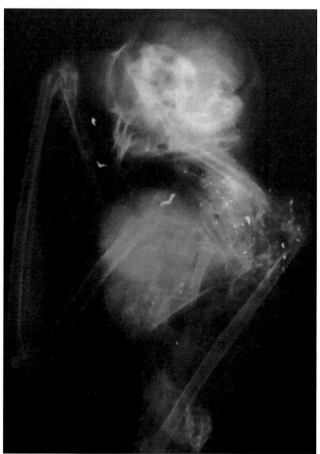

11.8 Radiograph of a tawny owl (*Strix aluco*) showing the characteristic fragmentation pattern of a high-velocity rifle bullet. The radiodense 'flying seagull' shapes are fragments of the copper jacket.

Handling of pellets or bullets recovered during surgery

Rifling marks on bullets and air rifle pellets can, in some circumstances, assist in linking a particular rifle to a shooting incident. Determination of the size and composition of shotgun pellets also falls within the remit of the ballistics expert. However, careless handling of pellets or bullets when they are recovered by the veterinary surgeon can obscure vital marks and so reduce the value of these pieces of evidence. Figure 11.9 sets out a procedure for handling bullets and pellets.

- Carefully separate the soft tissues surrounding the pellet or bullet.
- Using fingers or plastic forceps, remove the pellet and place gently in a plastic bowl.
- Remove adherent blood and strands of tissue by washing gently in water.
- After removal from the water, dip the bullet in 70% alcohol to dispel remaining water droplets.
- Air dry and wrap in bubble wrap or similar transparent soft material. Avoid using cotton wool or paper tissues which can become snagged on the irregular surface of the projectile.
- Place the wrapped specimen in a clear plastic container with sufficient wrapping to prevent the bullet rattling about inside.
- Seal the top, mark the container with the reference number and nature of contents, sign and date.
- Dispatch to ballistic laboratory for examination.

11.9 Procedure for handling bullets or pellets recovered at surgery.

Poisoning

The UK Wildlife Incident Investigation Scheme (WIIS) makes enquiries into suspected pesticide poisoning. Cases accepted for investigation usually fall into one of three main categories of pesticide use: approved use; misuse; or abuse. Establishing contact with the relevant laboratory is important as it ensures that up-to-date advice on sampling, handling, storage and transportation of specimens is received. A Freephone number for reporting suspected wildlife poisoning incidents is given in 'Specialist organizations and useful contacts'.

The identification of poisons in wildlife incidents is a highly skilled and demanding task. It may begin when a substance (powder, granule, pellet or liquid) is found at a suspected crime scene or in the premises of a suspect. Although the physical appearance of the compound provides clues to its identity, this can be misleading because of the similarities amongst the products (Figure 11.10). In other cases, confirmation depends on detection of poisons in tissue samples or gut contents of victims. Validated toxicological analyses are required, in every case, to confirm the nature and concentration of the substance. Figure 11.11 lists some of the more commonly used compounds in wildlife poisoning incidents. The illegal use of pesticides usually involves them being applied to a carrion bait, such as a rabbit carcass. The bait is usually cut open to make it more attractive to a potential predator. Meat or other food items may also be used (Figure 11.12). Solid pesticides are usually sprinkled over

Compound	Comments
Aldicarb	Potent inhibitor of acetylcholinesterase activity
Bendiocarb	Potent inhibitor of acetylcholinesterase activity
Carbofuran	Potent inhibitor of acetylcholinesterase activity
Carbosulfan	Potent inhibitor of acetylcholinesterase activity
Chloralose	Narcotic plus interference of temperature regulation
Isofenphos	Cholinesterase inhibitor
Metaldehyde	Metabolized to acetaldehyde Neurological signs, respiratory and liver failure Over 150 products currently approved
Methiocarb	Molluscicide Inhibitor of acetylcholinesterase activity
Mevinphos	Organophosphorus compound Inhibitor of acetylcholinesterase activity Highly toxic Absorbed through skin Vapour is hazardous Liquid concentrates were marketed as Phosdrin® and Phosdrin® 24 Extreme care should be exercised
Sodium cyanide	Hydrolysed to hydrogen cyanide Interferes with cytochrome oxidase and inhibits cellular respiration Death occurs during asphyxial convulsions Highly toxic by inhalation but also absorbed through skin and eyes
Strychnine hydrochloride	Alkaloid Tetanic spasms with severe extensor rigidity Death through hypoxia during seizures

11.11 List of compounds commonly associated with wildlife poisoning incidents.

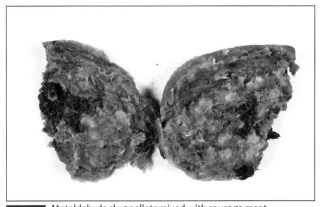

11.12 Metaldehyde slug pellets mixed with sausage meat.
(SASA © Crown Copyright)

the food item; liquid pesticides may be poured on to the food item or injected into items such as eggs.

Although it is possible that live intoxicated animals may be presented for examination (see Chapter 5), it is more probable that suspected poisoning cases will be dead on arrival. Veterinary advice may be sought to eliminate other causes of death or to estimate the time since death. Radiography can be enormously helpful in these cases by clearly identifying whether the animals have been shot or suffered bone fractures. Radiographs may also be helpful in identifying, before necropsy, whether a bird has recently eaten (Figure 11.13), thereby raising suspicion of poisoning. Radiographs showing shotgun pellets in the gullet or gizzard of a bird whose cause of death is unknown may indicate an illegal poisoning incident in which shot animals were used to prepare poisoned baits.

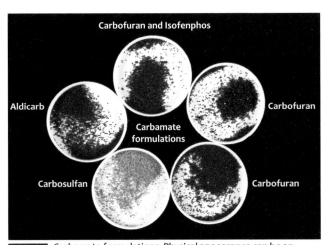

11.10 Carbamate formulations. Physical appearance can be an unreliable guide to the identity of specific compounds.
(SASA © Crown Copyright)

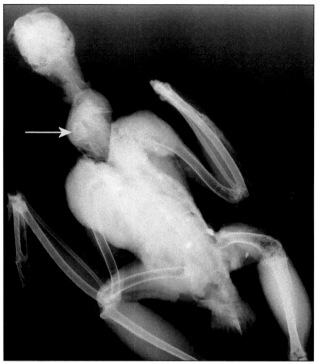

11.13 Ventrodorsal radiograph of a dead goshawk (*Accipiter gentilis*) with food in the crop (arrowed), but no signs of trauma or firearm injury. The radiodense objects scattered through the radiograph are pieces of stone/grit in the feathers. This goshawk was in good body condition and toxicology under the WIIS confirmed illegal poisoning in this bird and four other raptors.
(© RSPB)

Any disgorged material or faeces passed by suspect poisoning cases should be collected into separate containers. Fresh gloves should be worn for each sample to prevent cross-contamination. It is also important from a health and safety perspective to wear suitable gloves and protective clothing when investigating suspected poisoning cases. Many of the compounds used are very hazardous to human health and care needs to be exercised when handling live animals, cadavers, suspect samples or paraphernalia related to the incident.

Traps and snares

The main questions in trapping cases often hinge on legal issues concerned with proper use or misuse of traps. Fortunately for the veterinary surgeon, the investigating officer deals with the legal aspects. As a general rule an offence is committed if, when using a trap or snare, an operator:

- Fails to check traps or snares as and when required
- Sets traps or snares on land without the land manager/owner's permission
- Sets traps or snares in a way that is likely to cause unnecessary suffering
- Sets traps or snares in situations where protected species are likely to be caught
- Sets traps or snares in breach of the conditions set out in the relevant legislation or licences.

Figure 11.14 shows an illegal pole trap. Further examples of traps and their uses can be accessed via the websites in 'Specialist organizations and useful

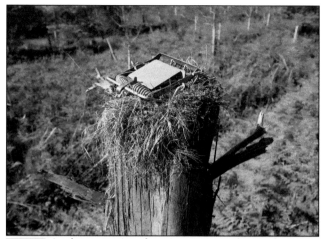

11.14 A pole trap consists of a spring trap set on the top of a post for the purpose of trapping any raptor that alights on it. They are often set near pheasant-rearing pens.
(© G Shorrock, RSPB)

contacts' at the end of this chapter. However, care needs to be taken because legislation varies in the different parts of the UK.

Veterinary surgeons may be asked to examine trapped animals and give appropriate treatment, describe the injuries and provide an estimate of how long the animal had been held in the trap. This estimate is usually based on the nature of any injuries, damage to feathers/teeth/claws, assessment of body condition and degree of hydration. Depending on the circumstances, charges related to unnecessary suffering may be considered by the prosecutor on the basis that, once trapped, wildlife may be classified as 'captive' with ensuing welfare responsibilities for the person setting the trap.

Photographic evidence that details injuries relating to the trap or snare is crucial (Figure 11.15). Although the animal may have been released from the trap or snare before clinical examination, any injuries found should be considered, objectively, in the light of the type of trap used. Could these injuries have been caused by the trap? Could these injuries have been caused in some other way? Could the animal have been injured before being trapped?

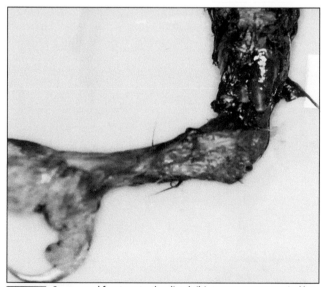

11.15 Compound fracture to the distal tibiotarsus, accompanied by considerable tearing and laceration of the skin, in a long-eared owl (*Asio otus*). This is a common type of injury in birds caught in spring traps.

Aids to diagnosis

Radiography

Digital radiography offers a number of advantages over conventional radiography systems, including dispensing with radiographic films, darkroom and film storage facilities. There are two systems for digital radiography: computed radiography and direct digital radiography. However, both systems store image data as DICOM (Digital Imaging and Communications in Medicine) files. These files are designed to store, in addition to the image information, other relevant data such as reference number, date and time of acquisition, patient details and acquisition parameters. These data are entered into the system before capturing the images and they form an integral part of the file. This information can be evidentially important and the DICOM file format is legally recognized. A further advantage of digital radiography is the wide range of tissue thicknesses and physical densities for which the computer can compensate. This allows all parts of the image to be assessed and can simplify explanation of the image to the court.

Some cadavers are, at the time of presentation, soiled with earth and vegetation. Particles of this surface contamination may show up on radiography, causing difficulties when deciding whether the animal has been shot (see Figure 11.13). To overcome this problem it is tempting to dust off the body before radiography. Normally this should be avoided because pellets and even low-velocity .22 bullets may be lodged in the coat or feathers. If much grit appears to be present on the surface, enclose the body in a polythene evidence bag, shake the material from the surface, remove the body for radiography and seal/label the bag containing the dislodged material. This material, which may contain shotgun pellets or bullet fragments, forms part of the overall evidence.

Entomology

Establishment of the time at which colonization by immature arthropods occurred can help to determine the minimum post-mortem interval (PMI). However, because development rates vary amongst arthropod species, it is essential that identification of these immature forms is accurate. Arthropod succession patterns also need to be considered. A natural progression occurs whereby the species colonizing a cadaver change as the state of decomposition develops. Further complications may arise through variations in temperature and weather conditions, and the predilection of some species of arthropods for sunny locations whilst others prefer the shade.

Maggots around the mouth and nostrils are readily seen, but careful examination of the ears, axilla and snares or other ligatures may uncover further sites of colonization. Fly eggs are usually laid in clumps. They can be found in wounds or natural orifices, but may also be laid in the coat or around traps or ligatures (Figure 11.16). Eggs are especially important when maggots or later insect stages are absent. The time at which they hatch is vital. Collaboration with an entomologist with forensic experience is essential for the development of a specimen handling SOP (see 'Specialist organizations and useful contacts').

DNA evidence

This has increasingly been used in wildlife crime investigations and can assist in a number of areas:

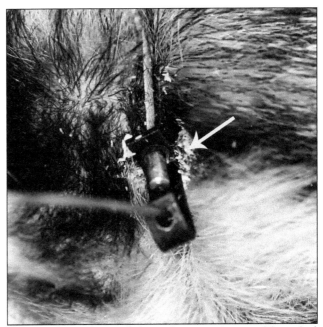

11.16 Fly eggs (arrowed) clustered on snare wire around the neck of a badger (*Meles meles*). Eggs are collected with a damp paintbrush or forceps. Half are preserved in alcohol and half are collected alive.

- Parentage tests to establish whether captive breeding claims are correct
- Identification (e.g. blood or tissue samples from clothing, tools or illegal traps)
- Linking to particular animals (e.g. DNA from dog saliva recovered from a hare (*Lepus europaeus*) after a coursing incident).

There are express sampling powers included in the legislation to allow statutory agencies to gather DNA evidence. With live animals, these require that the samples are taken by a veterinary surgeon, who must be satisfied that no lasting harm will be caused to the animal. Such cases usually relate to checks on paternity, and blood samples or buccal swabs are normally taken (Figure 11.17). The wildlife crime investigator should provide the necessary guidance on what type of samples would be most suitable in a particular case. Guidance on collection and storage of samples is provided in the Partnership for Action against Wildlife Crime (PAW) Forensic Working Group website and through the Animal and Plant Health

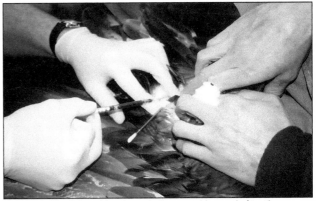

11.17 Obtaining a blood sample from a golden eagle (*Aquila chrysaetos*) for DNA analysis. If blood samples from a live animal or bird are required, regulations require that these samples are collected by a veterinary surgeon.
(© G Shorrock, RSPB)

Agency (APHA) (see 'Specialist organizations and of useful contacts' and Appendix 1). Sampling is not technically difficult but it is important to comply with the sampling procedure and to complete the paperwork as required. Samples may be taken from animals brought by prior arrangement to a practice. On other occasions, a veterinary surgeon may be asked to be present during a search undertaken by the statutory agencies.

References and further reading

British Association for Shooting and Conservation (BASC) http://basc.org.uk/shooting/pest-and-predator-control/

Cooper JE and Cooper ME (2013) *Wildlife Forensic Investigation: Principles and Practice*. CRC Press, Boca Raton

Di Maio VJM (1999) *Gunshot Wounds: Practical aspects of firearms, ballistics, and forensic techniques*. CRC Press, Boca Raton

Hall M, Whitaker A and Richards C (2012) Forensic entomology. In: *Forensic Ecology Handbook: From Crime Scene to Court*, ed. N Márquez-Grant and J Roberts, pp. 11–140. Wiley-Blackwell, West Sussex

Huffman JE and Wallace JR (2012) *Wildlife Forensics: Methods and applications*. John Wiley and Sons Ltd, West Sussex

Munro R and Munro H (2008) *Animal Abuse and Unlawful Killing; Forensic Veterinary Pathology*. Saunders Elsevier, Edinburgh

Newbery S and Munro R (2011) Forensic veterinary medicine 1. Investigation involving live animals. *In Practice* **33**, 220–227

PAW Forensic Working Group (2014) *Wildlife Crime. A guide to the use of forensic and specialist techniques in the investigation of wildlife crime*. http://

www.tracenetwork.org/wp-content/uploads/2012/08/Wildlife-Crime-use-of-forensics-FWG-April-2014.pdf

PAW Scotland (2013) http://www.scotland.gov.uk/Topics/Environment/Wildlife-Habitats/paw-scotland/types-of-crime/Trappingsnaring

Robertson I and Thrall D (2013) Digital radiographic imaging. In: *Textbook of Veterinary Diagnostic Radiology, 6th edn*, ed. DE Thrall, pp. 22–27. Saunders Elsevier, St Louis

Specialist organizations and useful contacts

See also Appendix 1

National Ballistics Intelligence Service (NABIS)
c/o West Midlands Police Headquarters, Force Intelligence,
PO Box 52, Lloyd House, Colmore Circus, Queensway,
Birmingham B4 6NQ, UK
Tel: 0121 626 7114
Email: nabis@west-midlands.police.uk
www.nabis.police.uk

National Wildlife Crime Unit
www.nwcu.police.uk

Natural History Museum Forensic Consulting
www.nhm.ac.uk/business-services/consulting/science-technical-services/forensic-consulting.html

Partnership for Action against Wildlife Crime (PAW)
www.gov.uk/government/groups/partnership-for-action-against-wildlife-crime

Partnership for Action against Wildlife Crime (PAW) Scotland
www.gov.scot/Topics/Environment/Wildlife-Habitats/paw-scotland

TRACE Wildlife Forensics Network including PAW Forensic Working Group
www.tracenetwork.org

Wildlife Incident Investigation Scheme (WIIS)
Freephone: 0800 321600
Also in Scotland:
www.sasa.gov.uk/wildlife-environment/wildlife-incident-investigation-scheme-wiis

Chapter 12

Hedgehogs

Steve Bexton

There are 14 species of spiny hedgehog worldwide, with some, for example the African pygmy hedgehog (*Atelerix albiventris*), kept as pets. The only species native to the British Isles is the (Western) European hedgehog (*Erinaceus europaeus*), which is found throughout the UK and Ireland in suitable habitat, usually up to the treeline (Churchfield, 2008). Hedgehogs are easily recognized by their distinctive spines and are familiar to most people as they often inhabit parks and gardens near to human habitation. Their popularity, relative abundance and easy capture make them one of the most common wildlife patients presented for veterinary attention, with thousands taken into care annually (Morris, 1998). Recent studies suggest that the UK population of hedgehogs has been declining for many years; at present, the reasons are poorly understood but are most likely related to habitat changes (Hof, 2009; Roos *et al.*, 2012).

Ecology and biology

Hedgehogs are found in many habitats including parks, gardens, cemeteries, waste ground and farmland. They generally prefer woodland edges, scrubland, grassland and hedgerows, and tend not to inhabit intensively farmed arable land, large coniferous forests, moorland or mountainous terrain.

They are solitary for most of the year, and have a social structure based on mutual avoidance, except during courtship and breeding or when exploiting a particularly rich food source (Morris, 1969, cited in Reeve, 1994). Each hedgehog occupies a 'home range', which is usually established when youngsters first disperse. Home ranges vary in size according to the habitat type and food availability, but generally cover 10–30 hectares. Males tend to have larger ranges than females, and rural home ranges tend to be larger than urban ones (Reeve, 1982; Morris, 1986). Hedgehogs are not territorial and the home ranges of different individuals often overlap. In the wild, aggression is rare, even between males, and fight wounds are rarely sustained.

Hedgehogs are nocturnal, therefore diurnal activity (other than at dawn and dusk) is usually a sign of injury, disease or food shortage (with the exception of nursing mothers that sometimes leave their offspring in the nest for short periods during the day in order to forage for food). Generally, hedgehogs rest during the day in nests constructed from vegetation (especially leaf litter) under the cover of hedges or shrubs. Their choice of nesting site can expose them to anthropogenic hazards such as the lighting of bonfires, grass cutting, or compost heaps being forked through.

During the night hedgehogs forage for food using their keen sense of smell to locate beetles (Coleoptera), caterpillars (Lepidoptera), earthworms (Annelida), slugs (Gastropoda) and other invertebrates. They are primarily insectivorous but are also opportunistic omnivores and will occasionally consume small vertebrates and carrion. Activity continues throughout the night as they meander around sniffing for prey, sometimes travelling a mile or two in the process.

During the winter hedgehogs hibernate so are rarely seen unless they are disturbed, although they may wake periodically to forage or move nest. Hibernation is the single greatest mortality factor for the species and up to 70% of young hedgehogs can die in their first winter. In springtime, they emerge from hibernation and begin to disperse, putting them at risk of traumatic injury especially from vehicle collisions. Males account for most of these casualties as they wake first and typically range further than females. Gardening activities also pose a common hazard to hedgehogs, especially mowing and strimming, and warm weather increases the risk of myiasis, which is a common secondary finding. Abandoned juveniles are generally found in the summer, usually as a result of nest disturbance or maternal mortality. During the autumn, large numbers of juveniles, especially those from late-born litters, are forced to forage during the daytime as food becomes scarce and they need to build up sufficient fat reserves to survive the winter. Most of these animals have significant parasite burdens, particularly parasitic bronchopneumonia, which contributes to their morbidity and mortality.

The major natural cause of mortality in hedgehogs is during their first winter when many fail to make it through hibernation. Litters born late in the season are under the greatest pressure as they have less time in which to build up the necessary energy reserves. Recently weaned animals are at the greatest risk of traumatic injury, illness and predation (Reeve, 1994). Their main natural predator is the badger (*Meles meles*).

Biological data are given in Figure 12.1.

Hibernation

In the UK, the onset and duration of the hibernation period is variable, but typically lasts from November/December to March. The main trigger for hibernation is prolonged

Parameter	Comments
Weight	Average adult 800–1200 g (fluctuates seasonally) Peak weight by 3 years of age Males generally larger than females
Sexing (see Figure 12.3)	Male: preputial opening usually mid-ventral abdomen Female: vulva and anus short distance apart
Teats	5 pairs
Oestrus	Normally polyoestrous
Breeding season	April/May to September/October
Gestation	35 ± 4 days
Litter size	3–5
Number of litters	1 or 2 per year
Birthweight	8–25 g
Sexual maturity	8–10 months
Lifespan	Average 2 years (Morris, 1983) Maximum 6–8 years in wild, 10 years in captivity (Reeve, 1994)
Diet	Primarily insectivorous (beetles, caterpillars, slugs and other invertebrates) Also opportunistic omnivores (small vertebrates, carrion)
Respiration	Normal resting rate 20–25 breaths per minute
Heart rate	200–280 beats per minute
Temperature	Normal (non-hibernating) rectal temperature 33.5–36.8°C

12.1 Biological data for hedgehogs.

ambient temperatures below 8°C but other factors such as photoperiod, food availability and accumulation of sufficient fat reserves may also be involved (Reeve, 1994). A specialized sturdy nest called a hibernaculum is constructed prior to hibernation. Hibernation is normally punctuated by periodic bouts of arousal, when animals may change nests. During hibernation, the hedgehog's body temperature falls to below 10°C, and the heart and respiratory rates slow dramatically to as low as 2–12 beats per minute and 13 breaths per minute, respectively, at 4°C (Reeve, 1994).

Anatomy and physiology

Hedgehogs are adapted to foraging in the undergrowth in low light conditions, using their keen sense of smell and sensitive hearing to detect invertebrates. Their eyesight is comparatively poor and of lesser importance. The vomeronasal organ, situated at the base of the nasal cavity, is involved in olfaction, pheromone detection and initiation of the peculiar natural activity of self-anointing, where they flick saliva over their bodies in response to certain smells and tastes.

The spines which cover the dorsum are in fact modified hairs and number approximately 5,000 on an adult hedgehog (Morris, 1983), their pointed tips acting as a defence against predators. When threatened, the hedgehog rolls into a ball using powerful muscles; the panniculus carnosus covers the dorsum and flanks and the orbicularis is a 'purse-string' muscle that encircles the 'skirt' (the junction between spined and haired skin). At the same time, the spines are erected, presenting the attacker with a tight ball of spines. The internal

structure of the spines also makes them efficient shock-absorbers, which cushion the impact if the hedgehog falls.

The rest of the body is covered in normal hairs. Both hairs and spines are continuously shed and regrow throughout the year. Coat colour is generally brown or grey, although individuals with abnormal pigmentation may occasionally be encountered (particularly albinism and leucism, Figure 12.2). Hedgehogs lacking pigment are more susceptible to predation but can thrive where predators are scarce, such as Alderney in the Channel Islands, which supports a small population of leucistic (blond) hedgehogs (Morris and Tutt, 2009).

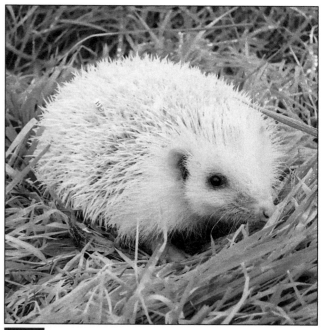

12.2 Leucistic hedgehog.

The hedgehog has seven cervical vertebrae in a short, strong neck. Each foot has five toes and the gait is plantigrade. There are 36 teeth in the adult. The molars are cusped for crushing insects and the first upper molar is four-sided. The dental formula is shown below (temporary dentition in parentheses).

$$2 \times \left\{ I \; \frac{3\,(3)}{2\,(1)} \; C \; \frac{1\,(1)}{1\,(1)} \; P \; \frac{3\,(3)}{2\,(2)} \; M \; \frac{3\,(0)}{3\,(0)} \right\} = 36\,(22)$$

The timing of tooth eruption is variable and therefore an unreliable method of ageing hedgehogs (Reeve, 1994). The degree of tooth wear and tartar build-up give a rough guide to the age of adult animals, but this is variable and dependent on diet and other factors.

Males are generally slightly larger than females, although bodyweights can fluctuate seasonally. Sex determination is possible once the hedgehog has been uncurled by observing the anogenital distance, which is greater in males (Figure 12.3a); additionally, the appearance of the external genitalia is slightly different, with a round preputial opening in the male and a slit-like vulva in the female (Figure 12.3ab). The scrotal pouches may also be visible in mature males, especially during the breeding season. Although sexing is relatively straightforward in uncurled adults, the difference is often less distinct in baby hedgehogs ('hoglets'). Both sexes have five pairs of teats. Male hedgehogs have enlarged internal accessory sex glands during the breeding season (Figure 12.3c).

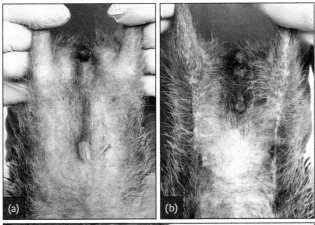

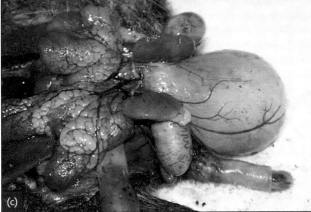

12.3 (a) Male and (b) female hedgehogs showing difference in external genitalia including anogenital distance. (c) Enlarged internal accessory sex glands during the breeding season in male hedgehogs are usually obvious on post-mortem examination or exploratory laparotomy.
(c, Courtesy of S Cowen)

The breeding season commences after arousal from hibernation, and courtship is often prolonged and noisy. Hoglets are born after a 5-week gestation period. It is thought that hedgehog milk contains maternal antibodies for the entire lactation period (Morris and Steel, 1964). If disturbed during the early nursing period, the female will often kill and eat her offspring. The timing of spine emergence, eye and ear opening and the ability to curl up can be used to age hoglets (Figure 12.4). Hedgehogs less than 18 months of age can also be aged by the radiographic appearance of the growth plates and sesamoids involving the bones of the forelimbs (Figure 12.4). After weaning, the juveniles disperse to new areas to feed and lay down fat reserves in preparation for hibernation.

Capture, handling and transportation

Hedgehogs are relatively easy to capture because their defence tactics are passive and they seldom attempt to flee or attack. Most will curl up instinctively when approached and no special equipment is needed to handle them, other than gloves (e.g. rubber gardening gloves) or a towel to protect the hands against the spines and reduce the risk of disease transmission. Although they can bite, this is very unusual; however, some individuals react to being touched by making sudden upward jumps in a bid to stab the assailant with their spines.

When threatened, some hedgehogs snort noisily, which can be mistaken for a sign of respiratory disease. Rarely, an individual hedgehog will emit a shrill warning cry in response to being handled. Hoglets will often make high-pitched 'peeping' sounds when they are hungry and these vocalizations can be misinterpreted as a sign of pain.

Age	Spines	Eyes and ears	Teeth	Comments
At birth	Hairless with small pink pimples along back;	Closed	Absent	Umbilical remnant present
24 hours	First spines appear from pimples: white, bristly but flexible	Closed	Absent	Unable to roll up
2 days	First appearance of second-generation spines: stouter and brown	Closed	Absent	Unable to roll up
2 weeks	White and brown spines of equal length	Begin to open (complete by 17 days)	Deciduous teeth begin to erupt	Able to roll up partially
3 weeks	White spines completely obscured by brown	Open	Deciduous teeth at various stages of eruption	Begin to follow mother on short foraging trips
4 weeks	Brown spines	Open	Deciduous teeth at various stages of eruption	Able to roll up fully
5–6 weeks	Brown spines	Open	Deciduous teeth at various stages of eruption	Weaned, fully independent
2–3 months	Brown spines	Open	Deciduous teeth at various stages of eruption	Metacarpal and phalangeal epiphyses visible on radiograph of forefoot
3–4 months	Brown spines	Open	Deciduous teeth replaced by adult teeth	
12 months	Brown spines	Open	Full adult dentition (Morris, 1983)	Sexually mature
18 months	Brown spines	Open	Full adult dentition	Only distal radial and ulnar epiphyses incompletely fused; sesamoids radiodense (Morris, 1971)

12.4 Development of hoglets and determination of their age.

Once captured, the hedgehog should be placed in a sturdy cardboard box or similar container (such as a pet carrier) with holes for ventilation and a secure lid to prevent escape. Dry leaves, newspaper or a towel should be used as a substrate to provide a non-slip surface, some insulation, and something for the hedgehog to hide beneath.

Zoonoses

The two main zoonotic concerns from hedgehogs are salmonellosis and dermatophytosis (ringworm). Ringworm is probably the most common zoonosis reported in wildlife rehabilitators, producing uncomfortable progressive scaly lesions on human skin. Infection is carried by up to a quarter of hedgehogs (Morris and English, 1969), but as most infections are subclinical, detection is difficult. As a precaution, gloves should always be worn when handling hedgehogs or their bedding.

Hedgehog faeces are a potential source of several enterobacteriaceae, including *Salmonella* spp., *Escherichia coli*, *Klebsiella* spp. and *Proteus* spp., all of which are capable of causing human infection. Some cases of human salmonellosis have been linked to contact with hedgehogs (Nauerby *et al.*, 2000; Handeland *et al.*, 2002; Riley and Chomel, 2005) and it is advisable to wear disposable gloves and follow general hygiene precautions when in contact with hedgehogs and their environment.

In addition, hedgehogs are a potential source of many other zoonotic infections, including leptospirosis, sarcoptic mange, toxoplasmosis, *Cryptosporidium*, *Giardia*, *Capillaria aerophila* and *Campylobacter* (Riley and Chomel, 2005), but the risk of human infection is considered to be low (see 'Infectious diseases' and Chapter 7).

Examination and clinical assessment for rehabilitation

On initial presentation, it is important to ascertain the reason for intervention and to derive a full history from the finder (see Chapter 4). This should include the circumstances in which the animal was found (e.g. whether the animal was trapped, picked up by a dog, found by the roadside) and any other relevant information such as recent gardening activities (e.g. strimming, bonfires) or pesticide use. The location where the animal was found should be recorded for subsequent release. The time of year and weather conditions should always be considered, as many of the problems and diseases of hedgehogs show a seasonal pattern. The animal should be signed over from the finder into the veterinary surgeon's (veterinarian's) care (see Chapters 2 and 3).

Most hedgehogs are taken into care because they have been found out during daylight, which is usually an indication that they are suffering from disease, injury or food shortage; the only major exceptions being when a sleeping animal has been disturbed or when a nursing mother temporarily leaves the nest to forage alone.

If a hibernating hedgehog is accidentally disturbed, it should be left alone as it is not unusual for them to wake periodically during the winter anyhow. However, a hedgehog found active during the daytime in winter has probably emerged early from hibernation because of disease or starvation, and is likely to be in need of assistance.

Clinical examination

Before starting the clinical examination, the casualty should be observed at a distance in a quiet environment with minimal disturbance, to assess its behaviour, coordination and gait. Weakness and debility typically cause a staggering gait and muscle tremors. The character and rate of respiration should also be observed before the animal is disturbed. The normal resting respiratory rate is 20–25 breaths per minute, but this is increased by handling and stress. Increased respiratory effort causes exaggerated flank movements and dyspnoea often manifests as open-mouth breathing or gasping in severe cases. Respiratory disorders can also cause increased respiratory sounds such as loud wheezing, and a moist cough is a frequent finding in hedgehogs with lungworm. A mild serous nasal discharge is normal. The carrying box can be examined for the presence of faeces, dropped spines, maggots, ectoparasites, blood and other discharges.

The body condition is visually assessed, and this can be a good guide to the chronicity of the problem; thin hedgehogs have sunken flanks, a prominent spine and a bony pelvis (Figure 12.5). Many juveniles found in the autumn will be suffering primarily from reduced food availability and will be visibly underweight. All hedgehog casualties should be weighed routinely. The age (adult or juvenile) can be determined based on body size, weight and time of year (Haigh *et al.*, 2014).

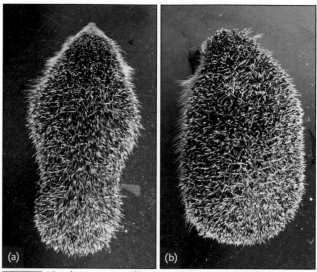

12.5 Visual assessment of body condition is possible. (a) Thin hedgehogs have sunken flanks, a prominent ridged spine and a bony pelvis. (b) Animals in good body condition have a rounded appearance.

If the hedgehog is curled up, it is possible to check if any limbs or the head are protruding, which could indicate injury such as a fracture or luxation. The dorsum can be examined for skin lesions and ectoparasites. Whilst a modest parasite burden is a normal finding in healthy animals, increased numbers of ticks and fleas are usually indicative of an underlying problem. Dehydration and hypothermia are very common and, in many instances, it is necessary to administer first aid (see 'First aid' and Chapter 5) and make a more detailed examination once the patient is more stable. For a thorough examination, the hedgehog needs to be uncurled, and reluctance or inability to roll up when touched is usually a sign of weakness, traumatic injury or ill-health.

Hedgehogs should be thoroughly examined for myiasis, which is common in this species, especially during the warmer months. Predilection sites include the orifices (anus, genitals, oral cavity, under the eyelids and in/around the pinnae) and in association with wounds or faecal soiling.

The buccal cavity should be inspected to assess the condition of the teeth and palate. Tartar build-up and periodontal disease are common in both wild and captive hedgehogs (see 'Dental disease'). Traumatic injuries of the snout can occur, including fractures of the nasomaxillary, mandibular and palatine bones.

Uncurling the hedgehog

Gloves should be worn when handling hedgehogs to reduce the risk of zoonotic infection. There are many techniques for uncurling the conscious hedgehog, but the general principles include avoiding noise, clumsy handling and touching the face, whiskers or belly, as these will stimulate it to curl up. Some hedgehogs will unroll spontaneously if simply left undisturbed for a few minutes. Some handlers gently bounce a rolled-up hedgehog between cupped hands. Another effective method is to stroke the spines firmly from the neck to the rump.

Once uncurled, the hindlimbs can be grasped by sliding the fingers underneath. Then, by extending the hindlimbs and raising them upwards to arch the back, the hedgehog can be restrained in a 'wheelbarrow' position (Figure 12.6) and is unlikely to curl up again. Held this way, it is possible to visually inspect the ventrum, limbs and face, although anaesthesia is required for a thorough examination of the mouth and palpation of the limbs and abdomen. The animal should also be sexed at this stage (see 'Anatomy and physiology'). Some juveniles, especially young hoglets, can alternatively be gently scruffed to prevent them rolling up. Immersion in water is not a suitable method of uncurling a hedgehog due to the risk of water inhalation.

Clinical assessment for rehabilitation and pre-release considerations

Hedgehog casualties must be fully fit and able to survive independently before release. An early decision about their prospects for a full recovery should be made, and individuals unlikely to recover should be euthanased immediately to prevent unnecessary suffering (see 'Euthanasia'

and Chapter 4). In some situations a sheltered environment, for example a walled garden, with supplementary feeding may be an acceptable alternative to euthanasia. If maintained in permanent captivity the animal's 'five freedoms' (see Chapter 4) must be fulfilled and be able to be monitored for the rest of the animal's life.

Important considerations for the species include:

- Hedgehogs must be able to fully curl up for protection from predators; obesity should be avoided as this reduces their ability to curl up tightly
- Olfaction is their primary sense and hedgehogs with nasal damage are unlikely to be able to forage efficiently
- The prognosis for dyspnoeic hedgehogs is poor; most have severe damage to the upper and lower respiratory tract and should generally be euthanased to prevent further suffering
- Chronic dental disease is common and extreme cases are unlikely to be able to survive in the wild; many are probably also at the end of their natural lifespan
- Emaciated hedgehogs may be suffering from chronic debilitating disease such as permanent end-stage lung damage and often have little chance of recovery
- One-eyed individuals appear to cope well, however, blind hedgehogs (e.g. with bilateral cataracts) should not be released
- Three-legged hedgehogs can thrive (hindlimb amputees only), although they have increased susceptibility to external parasites due to reduced grooming ability and reduced ability to climb so are prone to becoming trapped. They should therefore not be returned back to the wild and the decision whether to keep in captivity or euthanase should be made on an individual case basis.

Diagnostic techniques

The gross appearance of the faeces (colour, volume and consistency) can provide useful information. Normal droppings are brown and well formed; endoparasitism commonly results in green mucoid faeces (Figure 12.7a), and the presence of blood or pus can indicate enteric infection such as salmonellosis (Figure 12.7b). Direct microscopic examination of wet faecal smears is useful to detect endoparasites and should form part of the routine case work-up (see Chapter 10).

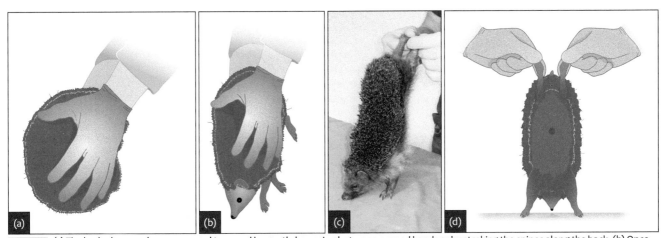

12.6 (a) The hedgehog can be encouraged to uncurl by gently bouncing between cupped hands or by stroking the spines along the back. (b) Once uncurled, the hindlimbs are grasped by sliding the fingers underneath. (c–d) The hindquarters are then elevated, with the forelimbs resting on the surface ('wheelbarrow' restraint).

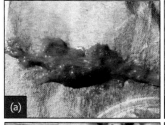
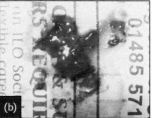
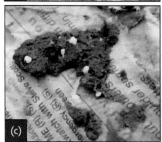

12.7 Gross faecal appearance suggestive of certain diseases. (a) Soft green faeces streaked with mucus typical of endoparasitism. (b) Green diarrhoea with fresh blood is typical of salmonellosis. (c) Cestode proglottids in faeces. Laboratory tests should be carried out to further investigate the causal agents.

Radiography is a useful diagnostic technique (see Figure 12.13b), especially in hedgehogs with suspected traumatic injuries. The best results are usually achieved with fine detail mammography films or digital radiography, although the spines can obscure soft tissue structures. On lateral views, the spines can be taped dorsally out of the way.

Blood collection is possible in hedgehogs, although intravenous access requires anaesthesia and can be difficult, especially in small individuals. The medial and lateral saphenous veins, cranial vena cava and jugular vein have all been used for blood collection (Lewis *et al.*, 2002). Intravenous access to the jugular is hampered by the relatively short neck and the overlying fat and fascia in this species.

Some suggested reference ranges for blood chemistry and haematology in hedgehogs are given in Figure 12.8; however, caution is advised when interpreting results as marked differences can occur between males and females, juveniles and adults, and under different environmental conditions. Seasonal variations in the haemogram are also well recognized and even the time of day can affect the results (Lewis *et al.*, 2002).

Variable (units)	Reference interval
Haematology	
Red blood cell (RBC) count (x 10¹²/l)	4.5–10[ab]
Haemoglobin (g/dl)	10–16[bc]
Packed cell volume (PCV) (l/l)	0.30–0.45[a]
Mean corpuscular haemoglobin (MCH) (pg)	14–18.2[abc]
Mean corpuscular volume (MCV) (fl)	35–50[abd]
Mean corpuscular haemoglobin concentration (MCHC) (g/dl)	33–42[ab]
Reticulocytes (x 10⁹/l)	<0.8[a]
White blood cell (WBC) count (x 10⁹/l)	3–15[ab]
Neutrophils (x 10⁹/l)	1.43–11.7[a]
Lymphocytes (x 10⁹/l)	0.8–5.5[ab]
Monocytes (x 10⁹/l)	0.06–0.58[a]
Eosinophils (x 10⁹/l)	0.05–1.87[ab]
Basophils (x 10⁹/l)	0.07–0.69[a]
Thrombocytes (x 10⁹/l)	230–430[ac]

12.8 Suggested reference ranges for haematology and blood biochemistry in the European hedgehog. (continues) ▶

([a] Jamie MacDonald, personal communication; [b] Lewis *et al.*, 2002; [c] Isenbügel and Frank 1985)

Variable (units)	Reference interval
Biochemistry	
Calcium (mmol/l)	1.45–2.55[a]
Phosphorus (mmol/l)	1.07–2.17[a]
Sodium (mmol/l)	121–141[a]
Potassium (mmol/l)	3–6[a]
Chloride (mmol/l)	90–106[a]
Creatinine (µmol/l)	0–71[ab]
Urea (mmol/l)	2.9–12.7[ab]
Total bilirubin (µmol/l)	<7[a]
Glucose (mmol/l)	2.9–5.9[ab]
Cholesterol (mmol/l)	2.7–3.9[a]
Creatine kinase (CK) (IU/l)	<360[a]
Lactate dehydrogenase (LDH) (IU/l)	<490[a]
Alkaline phosphatase (ALP) (IU/l)	20–80[ab]
Alanine aminotransferase (ALT) (IU/l)	22–70[a]
Aspartate aminotransferase (AST) (IU/l)	1–79[a]
Amylase (IU/l)	<1500[a]
Total protein (g/l)	44–62[a]
Globulin (g/l)	16–32[a]
Albumin (g/l)	21–31[a]

12.8 (continued) Suggested reference ranges for haematology and blood biochemistry in the European hedgehog.

([a] Jamie MacDonald, personal communication; [b] Lewis *et al.*, 2002; [c] Isenbügel and Frank 1985)

Euthanasia

The most suitable technique for euthanasia is by the intrahepatic injection of pentobarbital with the animal under deep sedation or anaesthesia. The liver of the hedgehog is relatively large and an easy target if the operator has some knowledge of internal anatomy. The onset of action is usually rapid. Alternatively, intracardiac or intravenous administration is also possible (with the animal under anaesthesia) (see 'First aid' for sites). There are no physical euthanasia techniques suitable for hedgehogs.

First aid and short-term hospitalization

First aid

Many hedgehog casualties will benefit from the immediate provision of warmth and fluid therapy when first received. In moribund or severely shocked animals, further procedures such as diagnostic tests, surgical procedures or treatments should be delayed until the animal is stabilized.

Hypothermia is common, especially in small, young and thin individuals. The normal rectal temperature of the hedgehog is 33.5–36.8°C (Herter, 1965, cited in Reeve, 1994) (see Figure 12.1), although the use of a rectal thermometer is not possible in animals capable of rolling up. Hypothermic animals feel noticeably cold to the touch. Supplementary heat can be provided using a warm air incubator, radiant heat lamp, electric heat mat, covered hot water bottle, microwaveable heat pad/bag or circulating warm air or water blanket. Regular monitoring and provision of appropriate fluid therapy are essential with the use of all heat sources as hyperthermia and dehydration can occur.

Dehydration can be detected by testing the skin turgor along the dorsum using the skin tent test as in other species. Fluids are administered subcutaneously along the dorsum or skirt. The skin should be elevated with the fingers or forceps to facilitate the injection and the needle inserted between the spines. Hedgehogs have a relatively large subcutaneous space; large volumes of fluid should be divided between multiple sites to aid absorption. Keeping the hedgehog warm is important, and the addition of hyaluronidase to subcutaneous fluids also improves their uptake (see Chapter 5).

The subcutaneous route is used for most injections. Intravenous access is possible, but venepuncture can be difficult especially in small or fat animals, and general anaesthesia is required to prevent animals from curling up. Intravenous fluid therapy is not a practical option due to poor vein access and the difficulty in keeping the catheter *in situ*. Where rapid fluid absorption is essential, warmed fluids can be given by the intraosseous route (into the proximal femur) or intraperitoneally.

For intramuscular injections, the orbicularis muscle (deep in the skirt) is generally utilized as it is accessible even in a rolled-up hedgehog. The gluteal mass can also be used if the hindlimb is accessible.

Short-term hospitalization

Individual hedgehogs can be kept overnight in a secure cardboard box or plastic tub. Newspaper, shavings or (non-frayed) towelling can be used as bedding material. In the short-term, adult hedgehogs can be fed on tinned or dry dog or cat food. For further details see 'Management in captivity'.

Anaesthesia and analgesia

Inhalational anaesthesia using a volatile agent such as isoflurane or sevoflurane is the most convenient and effective method of anaesthetizing the hedgehog, with relatively rapid induction and recovery times. If the hedgehog is not curled up, induction is relatively straightforward by placing a facemask or simply the connector of the circuit directly over the nose. For hedgehogs that are rolled up, an induction chamber is most useful or, alternatively, by placing the anaesthetic connector near the face it should relax sufficiently to enable better access to the face, so that a facemask can then be applied. Maintenance can be provided via a facemask or via endotracheal intubation (only usually possible in larger individuals); endotracheal tube placement is facilitated by the use of a stylette and a small laryngoscope. Animals should not be fed immediately before a planned anaesthesia, although this is rarely a concern as hedgehogs are nocturnal and eat mostly at night. Regurgitation can be a problem in hoglets that are on milk feeds, and therefore these must not be fed directly prior to anaesthesia.

Injectable anaesthetic agents can be used (Figure 12.9), but relative overdose and prolonged recovery are common problems, especially in debilitated individuals. Animals should consequently be weighed before doses are calculated.

Analgesia, if required, should be given as early as possible and preferably pre-emptively. Both opiates and non-steroidal anti-inflammatory drugs (NSAIDs) can be used (Figure 12.9).

Drug	Dosage	Some indications
Anaesthetics		
Medetomidine	0.1 mg/kg i.m.	Can be used on its own for light sedation or combined with ketamine for anaesthesia Variable effects, sometimes prolonged recovery Reverse with atipamezole
Ketamine	10–20 mg/kg i.m.	In combination with medetomidine for anaesthesia Variable effects; sometimes prolonged recovery
Atipamezole	0.5–1.0 mg/kg i.m., s.c.	Reversal of medetomidine (equal volume)
Diazepam	1.0–3.0 mg/kg i.v., i.m.	Sedative and anticonvulsant (higher dose) Can also be combined with ketamine for anaesthesia
Analgesics		
Buprenorphine	0.02–0.05 mg/kg i.m., s.c. q8h	For moderate/severe pain (e.g. traumatic injuries and postoperative analgesia)
Butorphanol	0.2–0.4 mg/kg i.m., s.c. q6-8h	For moderate/severe pain (e.g. traumatic injuries and postoperative analgesia)
Carprofen	5–10 mg/kg s.c. q24h, orally q12h	Analgesic and anti-inflammatory
Ketoprofen	4 mg/kg i.m., s.c., orally q24h	Analgesic and anti-inflammatory
Meloxicam	0.5 mg/kg s.c., orally q24h	Analgesic and anti-inflammatory

12.9 Anaesthetic and analgesic dose rates for use in hedgehogs.

Specific conditions

Trauma

Entrapment

Hedgehogs often inhabit suburban areas, putting them at increased risk of injury from man-made hazards. They are prone to falling into open drains, cattle grids and garden ponds, from which they often struggle to escape. Entanglement in netting (e.g. garden and sports nets) is also a relatively common problem (Figure 12.10). Hedgehogs can also become trapped in rodent traps and entangled in litter such as plastic ring binders, and sometimes get their head stuck in empty tin cans and plastic pots. Once trapped, they often instinctively roll up, making matters worse. They can usually be freed (under anaesthesia) without long-term harmful effects, although they are often dehydrated at presentation, and may have wounds and/or secondary myiasis, depending on how long they have been trapped. They should always be monitored in captivity for a few days for signs of pressure necrosis and wound infection.

Skin wounds

Common causes of skin wounds in hedgehogs include injuries from garden machinery, such as strimmers (Figure 12.11) and mowers, entanglement, dog bites and road vehicle collisions. With all wounds, it is important to check thoroughly for fly eggs and maggots. Bite wounds can

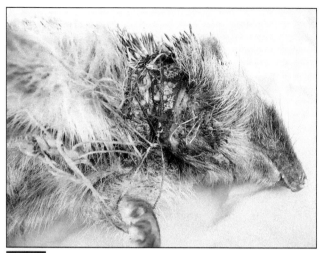

12.10 Netting entanglement in a hedgehog with secondary myiasis.

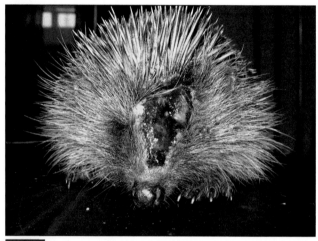

12.11 Strimmer laceration in a hedgehog.

penetrate deeply and are often difficult to find between the spines. Fresh lacerations (e.g. strimmer wounds) can be cleaned and sutured, but the majority of wounds are contaminated and should be allowed to heal by second intention. The area around the wound is clipped to allow access and prevent further wound contamination, but cutting too many spines should be avoided as they are needed for protection against predators. Simple wounds can be flushed copiously with sterile saline or dilute (1:40 in water) chlorhexidine solution. De-sloughing agents are useful for removing the necrotic tissue of chronic contaminated wounds. Topical hydrogel products can also be useful in the management of wounds to encourage granulation. Antibacterial therapy is always necessary due to the high risk of secondary infection; amoxicillin/clavulanate (co-amoxiclav), enrofloxacin, cefalexin or clindamycin are suitable (see Figure 12.20). Fluid therapy and NSAIDs may also be indicated. Regular cleaning and treatment are necessary but hedgehog skin heals well, albeit relatively slowly. In order to be released, the hedgehog must be able to fully curl up and the skin should be fully healed with no reduction in spine coverage.

Road traffic accidents

Hedgehogs rarely forage by the roadside and naturally tend to avoid roads at busy times (Dowding *et al.*, 2010a); however, tens of thousands of hedgehogs are still killed on the roads every year (Reeve, 1994). Most are killed outright, but sometimes injured individuals are found by the roadside or nearby with injuries consistent with being struck by a vehicle.

- Limb fractures are often compound with a poor chance of healing. Crush injuries to the feet are fairly common, but are often chronic and infected by the time they are seen, and most cannot be salvaged. In these cases euthanasia is indicated.
- Pelvic fractures are of particular importance in female animals and, if there is any narrowing of the pelvic canal, they should be euthanased as there is a significant risk of subsequent dystocia. Sciatic nerve damage often accompanies pelvic injury.
- Spinal fractures and spinal cord injury can be detected by the panniculus reflex cut-off, whereby the bristling and erection of spines is absent caudal to the lesion. This is usually accompanied by hindlimb paresis or paralysis, so that the legs are left protruding when the animal tries to curl (Figure 12.12), and urinary incontinence. Radiographic assessment is helpful, and hedgehogs with confirmed spinal injury should be euthanased.

Eye prolapse and globe rupture can occur. Enucleation may be necessary in acute proptosis, but in many cases the damaged eye has already fibrosed causing no long-term problems. Blind or partially-sighted hedgehogs can cope if kept in permanent captivity in a sheltered environment where they can be monitored and given supplementary food. Suitability for permanent captivity should be judged on an individual case basis and if maintained in permanent captivity the animal's 'five freedoms' (see Chapter 4) must be fulfilled and be able to be monitored for the rest of the animal's life.

- Rupture and herniation of the abdominal muscles, diaphragmatic rupture and traumatic rectal prolapse can also occur during vehicle collisions.

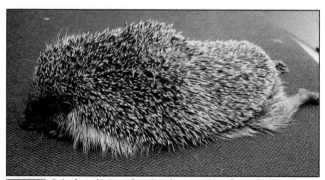

12.12 Spinal cord injury showing demarcation of panniculus (indicated by flattened spines caudally) and hindlimb paralysis.

Limb fractures

The management of fractures in hedgehogs is similar to other small mammals, except in two important respects:

- The hedgehog's defence mechanism of rolling up, with the limbs tucked inside, means that fixators and dressings are more likely to become dislodged or loosened, or may impede this mechanism
- Many fractures are compound, contaminated or infected by the time the hedgehog is found, and so internal fixation techniques are often contraindicated.

Coaptation splints and casts (Plaster of Paris, synthetic lightweight casting material and rigid splints) can be used to support distal limb fractures, especially of the radius, ulna, tibia, metatarsals and metacarpals. Dressings should be kept clean and dry by the use of absorbent bedding material and regularly cleaning out the accommodation. External fixator systems are useful for lower limb (radius/ulna and tibia/fibula) fractures. Intramedullary pinning is suitable for some fractures of the femur and humerus. Fractures must be healed and the implants removed before animals are released.

Naturally healed fractures are occasionally noticed as an incidental finding in hedgehogs; some also result in malunion and limb distortion. Limb amputation can be an option, but three-legged animals should not be released back to the wild. Hindlimb amputees can cope in captivity, but have increased risk of ectoparasitism and skin disease on the affected side due to reduced ability to groom. Amputation of a forelimb is not recommended as mobility is severely compromised.

Orbicularis muscle prolapse

The orbicularis ('purse-string') muscle is a ring-shaped muscle deep within the skirt that encircles the body and enables the hedgehog to roll up. Muscle prolapse is possible, usually as a result of extreme muscle exertion, such as entanglement in netting or vehicle collision. This causes it to slip over the pelvis and go into spasm. The affected hedgehog is unable to roll up and the dorsal skin is twisted over the back, with the legs and pelvis visible. Colloquially, the condition is termed 'pop-off syndrome'. Anaesthesia is required to relax the muscle, which can then be gently eased back into place. Analgesia is necessary, and animals usually make a full recovery.

Subcutaneous emphysema

Another peculiar presentation seen in the hedgehog is 'balloon syndrome', where the body is grossly inflated by subcutaneous emphysema (Figure 12.13). This is usually a sequel to traumatic injury to the mediastinum or ribcage, typically from a road accident, or rarely from a deep sub-cutaneous gas-forming infection. The subcutaneous space over the hedgehog's dorsum is comparatively large and the skin loosely attached, which enables the animal to roll up. This creates a large potential space for gas collection, which results in the striking appearance of these cases.

Treatment involves deflation via a skin incision or needle aspiration, but this usually needs to be repeated several times as gas reappears. Broad-spectrum anti-biotics and analgesia are indicated. The prognosis depends on the severity and extent of the underlying injuries, and concurrent haemorrhage and pulmonary emphysema are common complications.

Nasal trauma

Injuries to the snout are commonly seen in hedgehogs; most are traumatic in origin from being struck by a road vehicle. Inspection of the mouth and nose should form part of the clinical examination of all injured animals, especially when there are signs of respiratory distress or facial injury (see Chapter 4). Nasomaxillary and palatal fractures usually cause dyspnoea and carry a grave prognosis; most animals require immediate euthanasia. Simple fractures can be surgically stabilized, but most have concurrent damage to other structures within the nasal cavity and are

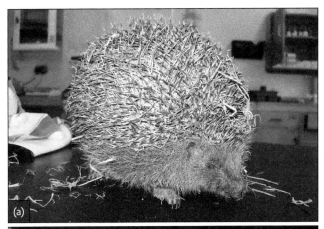

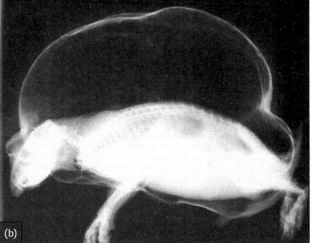

12.13 (a) Subcutaneous emphysema ('balloon syndrome') in a hedgehog. (b) Radiographic appearance.

unlikely to recover. Permanent damage to the nasal cavity reduces survival by interfering with respiration, olfaction and foraging ability.

Burns

The hedgehog's habit of nesting in log and leaf piles and unlit bonfires is well known and gardeners are advised to check bonfires for sleeping animals or rebuild the pile immediately before it is lit. Hedgehogs that manage to escape from fires have charred spines (Figure 12.14) and burns to the skin, which can slough later on. Smoke

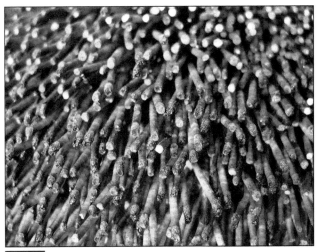

12.14 Charred spines from fire damage.

inhalation can cause lung damage, and corneal irritation is also common. Oxygen therapy, fluid therapy, ocular medication and analgesia, including anti-inflammatory treatment, should be commenced as soon as possible. Parenteral antibacterials are needed to control secondary infections, and skin burns can be treated with topical silver sulfadiazine cream. However, the prognosis for recovery is generally guarded, and an early decision should be made to euthanase if the survival prospects are poor.

Poisoning

Hedgehogs are unlikely to be a target for deliberate poisoning as they rarely come into conflict with human interests. However, their close association with human habitation, especially gardens, potentially exposes them to a variety of toxins. Accidental poisoning is possible during rodent control, vegetation clearance and gardening activities. Cases of poisoning are probably underdiagnosed due to the non-specific nature of the clinical signs and the difficulty and expense of laboratory confirmation, unless exposure to a known poison occurs or can be proven.

There is little specific information about the effects of many toxins in the hedgehog, and the long-term effects of poisons (including chronic exposure) such as changes in behaviour, fertility, growth and immunity have received little attention (Reeve, 1994). For general information about poisoning in wildlife see Chapters 2 and 11, and for further advice on treatment see Chapter 5.

Molluscicides (slug pellets)

The widespread use of molluscicides in gardens and agriculture has prompted concerns that hedgehogs may be at risk of poisoning, either by direct consumption or by the ingestion of poisoned slugs (Reeve, 1994). Metaldehyde slug pellets are widely used by gardeners, and hedgehogs are known to ingest them (Keymer et al., 1991), however, the toxicity risk to hedgehogs is considered to be low (Bunner, 2002). Hedgehogs would need to consume a huge amount of slug pellets or poisoned slugs to receive a toxic dose, which is considered to be very unlikely (Gemmeke, 1999).

Slug pellets that contain carbamates, such as methiocarb, are thought to pose a much greater risk as they are more palatable and toxic to hedgehogs (Bunner, 2002). They also have a wider spectrum of activity as pesticides, potentially making secondary poisoning more likely. Signs of toxicity include salivation, incoordination, tremors, vomiting (which may be blue-tinged), miosis and possibly seizures. Carbamates inhibit cholinesterase activity, so the treatment is atropine (0.2–0.5 mg/kg s.c. or i.m, with ¼ dose i.v if possible) and supportive care with warmth, fluids and oxygen if there is respiratory compromise. The laboratory measurement of red blood cell cholinesterase activity or response to atropine injections can be used to confirm the diagnosis.

Anticoagulant rodenticides

Exposure of hedgehogs to anticoagulant rodenticides, especially second-generation products such as bromadiolone and difenacoum, is common (Dowding et al., 2010b). Hedgehogs are thought to acquire the toxin through the ingestion of invertebrates that have fed directly on the bait or on poisoned carcasses. The effects of chronic exposure in the hedgehog are unknown. Acute toxicity could occur if a hedgehog consumed sufficient contaminated invertebrates, scavenged a poisoned carcass or had direct access to unprotected bait. Signs of acute poisoning include weakness, pallor and haemorrhage such as epistaxis. In cases of known or suspected exposure, individuals can be treated with vitamin K injections (2.5–5 mg/kg s.c.; see also Figure 5.20), along with supportive care including minimizing trauma and fluid therapy. Ideally coagulation status should be monitored but this is not easily achieved in hedgehogs due to the stress to the animal of repeat sampling and the costs involved.

Other poisons

- Fatal paraquat poisoning has been reported in a number of wildlife species including hedgehogs after herbicide spraying (van Oers et al., 2005). Its use is now banned.
- Organophosphate and alphachloralose poisoning have been reported (Robinson and Routh, 1999) but are probably rare.

Infectious diseases

Viral diseases

Foot-and-mouth disease (FMD): Natural infection of hedgehogs with FMD virus was reported during an outbreak in cattle in 1947 (McLaughlan and Henderson, 1947). Some hedgehogs were asymptomatic but in others the disease was fatal. Hedgehogs were very susceptible to infection, and clinical signs included daytime activity, anorexia, sneezing, hypersalivation, and erythema and vesicles on the feet, tongue, snout, lip margins and perineum.

It is theoretically possible for the virus to overwinter in hedgehogs during hibernation and be reintroduced to livestock the following spring, but the role of hedgehogs in the spread of FMD is probably insignificant (Hulse and Edwards, 1937). To reduce disease spread during the 2001 FMD outbreak in the UK, movement restrictions were placed on all susceptible species, including captive hedgehogs, although no cases were reported.

Morbillivirus: Infection with morbillivirus is possibly not uncommon in free-living hedgehogs. The virus has been isolated from healthy individuals, as well as from the faeces and lungs of sick animals (Visozo and Thomas, 1981). Clinical signs are predominantly associated with the nervous system, including circling, running, hypermetria, incoordination, hindlimb paresis and paralysis, diurnal activity, inappetance and weight loss. There may also be oculonasal discharge and blindness, and the footpads may be swollen and ulcerated or hyperkeratotic. Symptomatic treatment involves fluid therapy and antibiotics to control secondary infections. Supplementary B vitamins may also help. Typical post-mortem findings include bronchopneumonia and neurohistopathological lesions resembling those of canine distemper.

Bacterial diseases

Salmonellosis:

Epidemiology: Salmonellosis is endemic in hedgehog populations (Keymer et al., 1991; Robinson and Routh, 1999). Sporadic disease occurs in the wild, and acute outbreaks are common within rehabilitation facilities, especially affecting juvenile animals. Several *Salmonella* enterica subsp. *enterica* serovars infect hedgehogs. *S.* Enteritidis (PT11) is isolated from most cases, but *S.* Brancaster and *S.* Typhimurium are also occasionally recovered (Keymer *et al.*, 1991). Transmission is by the faeco–oral route, with symptomless carriers the most likely source of infection. Transmission can also occur via ingestion of carrion and invertebrates (e.g. carabid beetles (Carabidae) and maggots (Diptera)). Outbreaks are most common during the summer. Once present within a facility, disease spreads rapidly and the mortality rate can be very high, especially in juveniles. Immunosuppression and stress may be important factors in the pathogenesis of the disease. *Klebsiella* spp. can cause a similar disease; all such infections are potentially zoonotic.

Signs and diagnosis: In most cases, *Salmonella* causes enteritis, with anorexia, weight loss and diarrhoea (which is characteristically green and mucoid and often contains fresh blood, see Figure 12.7b). Regurgitation and vomiting can also be a problem, especially in hoglets that are being hand-reared. Occasional individuals have rectal prolapse due to tenesmus, and intussusception is sometimes found on post-mortem. Disease can also manifest as septicaemia with neurological signs, tachypnoea and collapse. Peracute cases present as sudden death.

Direct microscopy of faecal samples can be useful to eliminate gastrointestinal parasitism as a diagnosis, although animals with salmonellosis can have concurrent parasite burdens. Attempts can be made to culture the organism from faecal samples. Enrichment techniques and prompt culture increase the likelihood of *Salmonella* being isolated, as it is often overgrown by other enteric bacteria. If possible, a whole fresh carcass should be submitted to a suitable laboratory for direct culture from the gut and liver.

Post-mortem findings include mucohaemorrhagic enteritis with congestion of the intestinal mucosa and green gut contents. A common finding is hepatosplenomegaly, especially in septicaemic animals, along with focal pneumonia, which may be catarrhal or purulent.

Treatment: Strict barrier nursing is essential, and quarantine with extra hygiene precautions is necessary to reduce the risk of disease transfer to humans and other animals. High-dose antibacterials (e.g. amoxicillin) are effective in many cases, but there is a risk that treatment may promote a carrier status and lead to prolonged shedding of bacteria. In most cases fluid therapy and the provision of warmth are beneficial, and antidiarrhoeals such as kaolin may provide some symptomatic relief. Severely ill animals rarely recover and should be euthanased to prevent unnecessary suffering and reduce the risk of further disease transmission.

Bordetellosis: *Bordetella bronchiseptica* causes a contagious respiratory disease with tracheitis and catarrhal rhinitis that may progress to bronchopneumonia. Infection often accompanies lungworm infestation (see 'Endoparasites' below), and other opportunistic pathogens are often also involved, including *Pasteurella multocida*, other *Pasteurella* spp., and haemolytic streptococci (Saupe and Poduschka, 1995).

Clinical signs include hyperpnoea, dyspnoea, wheezy respiratory noises and nasal discharge. Suitable antibacterials include oxytetracycline, amoxicillin, enrofloxacin or cefalexin (see Figure 12.20). NSAIDs, mucolytics and bronchodilators are also helpful in many cases, either by parenteral administration or nebulization. The prognosis depends on the severity of the disease, but individuals with severe dyspnoea are unlikely to recover and should be euthanased.

Leptospirosis: Leptospirosis is probably of little clinical significance in hedgehogs, but is zoonotic and therefore an important consideration for hedgehog carers. *Leptospira interrogans* serovar *Bratislava* has been isolated from hedgehogs, which may act as a reservoir in the wild (Twigg *et al.*, 1968).

Yersiniosis: This is a rare disease, usually of juvenile hedgehogs, causing hindlimb weakness, chronic weight loss and sometimes diarrhoea. The pathology is typical of pseudotuberculosis, with white-grey caseous granulomatous lesions in the liver, spleen and mesentery, and mesenteric lymphadenopathy (Keymer *et al.*, 1991; Saupe and Poduschka, 1995). *Mycobacterium avium* and other mycobacteria have also been isolated from the mesenteric lymph nodes of hedgehogs (Smith, 1968; Matthews and McDiarmid, 1977).

Pyoderma and abscessation: Exudative dermatitis is occasionally encountered, especially on the ventrum. It is usually associated with staphylococci, particularly coagulase-positive *Staphylococcus aureus*, which should be treated appropriately (see Figure 12.20). Bacterial pyoderma is also a common secondary complication in cases of ringworm and mange (see 'Fungal diseases'). Abscesses are common anywhere on the body, with many possible pathogens isolated, especially staphylococci, *Escherichia coli* and *Pseudomonas* spp.

Neonatal enteritis: Hoglets can develop pale green sticky diarrhoea (see Figure 12.7) due to enteric infection that can rapidly progress to dehydration and death. *Salmonella* spp., *E. coli* (notably serotypes 078 and 055) and *Proteus* spp. have been implicated in outbreaks of disease (Smith, 1968). Haemolytic *E. coli* infection (colibacillosis) can also result in faeces streaked with mucus and blood, or containing bright green jelly or pus. Morbidity and mortality can be very high; treatment includes high-dose antibacterial agents, fluid therapy and warmth, and control involves good hygiene, barrier nursing and sterilization of equipment.

Tick-borne diseases: Q fever, a rickettsial disease caused by *Coxiella burnetii*, has been reported in hedgehogs but its clinical significance is unknown. Infection in other species has been associated with influenza-like disease. It is zoonotic and can be transmitted by inhalation of dust or droplets of urine or faeces containing rickettsiae (Smith, 1968).

Borrelia burgdorferi, which can cause Lyme disease, has been isolated from hedgehogs and hedgehog ticks, but there have been no reports of clinical disease associated with infection. Transmission can be via the ticks *Ixodes ricinus* and *I. hexagonus*, and hedgehogs could act as a wildlife reservoir of infection (Couper *et al.*, 2010).

Fungal diseases

Ringworm:
Epidemiology: Ringworm is a common skin disease, usually caused by *Trichophyton erinacei* (*T. mentagrophytes* var. *erinacei*), which is endemic in the hedgehog population. *Microsporum* spp. have also occasionally been isolated. Dermatophytes are carried by up to 25% of

hedgehogs, often as a subclinical infection (Morris and English, 1969). Transmission can be by direct contact, and ringworm is more common in suburban hedgehogs where the population density is greatest. Fungal spores persist in dry nests (English and Morris, 1969), and transmission may also occur during nest sharing. Some studies indicate that the disease is more common in males as these tend to use more nests and also have more social interactions with other hedgehogs (Morris and English, 1969; 1973). Mites, specifically *Caparinia tripilis*, may be a concurrent infection and have also been implicated in disease spread; dermatophytes have been recovered from their faeces (Smith and Marples, 1963).

Signs and diagnosis: Infection does not always result in skin lesions and it is possible that some degree of immunosuppression (e.g. due to stress, malnutrition or underlying parasitism) is required for clinical disease to develop. Disease is most commonly seen in juvenile hedgehogs undergoing rehabilitation. Localized lesions are also occasionally encountered in geriatric animals; mostly with other underlying problems, such as dental disease and starvation.

Clinical disease typically causes alopecia with cutaneous crusts and scabs; any part of the body can be affected (Figure 12.15). Lesions on the dorsum and flanks result in scurf and spine loss, which can be localized or generalized. Dropped spines are usually obvious in the animal's environment, and may have crusts and scale around their base. Lesions of the skirt (the margin between spines and fur) usually cause crusting and matting, with scabs that bleed when removed. Lesions on the head (typically affecting the snout and crown) consist of crusts and hair loss, and in chronic cases the pinnae can become encrusted and thickened. Some cases present as ventral alopecia with matted hairs and little else. Generally, lesions cause little irritation and pruritis is unusual. Most animals continue to thrive, even with extensive lesions. Concurrent mite infestation and secondary bacterial pyoderma are often present and these may lead to pruritis.

Although the lesion appearance and distribution is often highly suggestive, fungal culture on Sabouraud's agar is required to confirm the diagnosis. Fungi can also be demonstrated on biopsy specimens. Direct microscopy of skin scrapes and hair plucks is less reliable and *T. erinacei* does not fluoresce under a Wood's lamp. Concurrent mite infestation should be investigated by the microscopic examination of skin scrapes and acetate tape strips.

Treatment: Without treatment, ringworm lesions are progressive, and spontaneous recovery has not been recorded in hedgehogs during rehabilitation. However, the widespread occurrence of subclinical infection in the population and relatively low pathogenicity suggests that lesions could resolve with time. Treatment of affected animals in captivity is necessary because it is contagious and zoonotic, and adequate precautions need to be taken to reduce the risks of disease transmission. Affected animals should be isolated and their cage and any utensils thoroughly cleaned and disinfected daily to prevent constant reinfection from infective skin and hair in the environment. Concurrent disease such as lungworm, mite infestation and pyoderma should also be treated.

Topical antifungal treatment, for example repeated washes with enilconazole, may be sufficient for localized accessible lesions. More severe or generalized cases respond better to a prolonged course of parenteral antifungal therapy, for example with itraconazole or terbinafine (see Figure 12.20). Recovery and regeneration of spines and hair can take several weeks, depending on the severity of disease. Resolution of lesions is adequate basis on which to stop treatment, but negative fungal cultures are considered confirmatory.

T. erinacei is probably the most common zoonotic infection of wildlife rehabilitators. Cutaneous lesions in humans are not typical of ringworm and may not be recognized as such. Lesions are progressive, initially vesicular and erythematous with pruritis, becoming increasingly scaly with thickening of the epidermis. If zoonotic infection is suspected consult a doctor for diagnosis and treatment. All veterinary practices and wildlife centres should have appropriate, written health and safety risk assessments in place for dealing with hedgehogs, as well as in-house policy for disease diagnosis and control.

T. erinacei can also cause lesions on the lips and muzzle of dogs from picking up and investigating affected hedgehogs.

Parasites

Ectoparasites:
Fleas: Most hedgehogs have fleas, which are easily visible due to the hedgehog's relatively sparse spine and hair. A small number of fleas are well tolerated and cause little problem to the host unless it is already debilitated. Large flea burdens can indicate more serious problems, and can cause anaemia. The most common species is the hedgehog flea *Archaeopsylla erinacei*, which, unlike

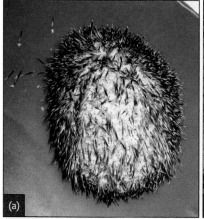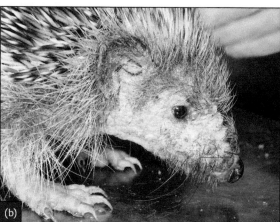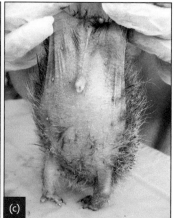

12.15 Dermatophytosis: (a) dorsal spine loss and crusting, (b) facial hair loss and crusting, (c) alopecia of the ventrum.

other species, has a dorsoventrally flattened body to facilitate its passage between the spines. Flea eggs are laid in the nest, and the hatched larvae feed on detritus. These then infest any hedgehog visiting or inhabiting the nest. Various treatments have been used successfully including topical pyrethrum, permethrin and fipronil, but generally only heavy burdens need treating (see Figure 12.20).

Ticks: Low to moderate numbers of ticks are found on most hedgehogs, especially around the ears, on the hindlimbs and skirt. Species include the hedgehog tick *Ixodes hexagonus*, the sheep tick *I. ricinus* and occasionally the shrew tick *I. trianguliceps*. Large burdens can cause anaemia, and are usually indicative of other more serious problems. Tick bites occasionally cause localized inflammation, and they are potential vectors of Lyme disease, Q fever, tick-borne encephalitis and tick paralysis. The incidence of tick-borne diseases in the hedgehog has been little studied. Ticks can be removed using a commercial tick remover. Topical acaricides such as ivermectin (and fipronil) are also effective (see Figure 12.20). Dressing the tick with olive oil or alcohol is not recommended as it can cause the ticks to regurgitate potentially infective material into the host's skin.

Mites: Caparinia tripilis is a non-burrowing mite of hedgehogs that can cause hair loss, scurf, scale and pruritis (Figure 12.16). The mites are just visible to the naked eye as motile powdery skin deposits, often around the face, head and ears. Occasionally, they cause a more generalized infestation over the whole body. Diagnosis is by the demonstration of mites using a hand lens or microscopic examination of skin debris. Topical avermectins are the treatment of choice (see Figure 12.20). Capariniosis can also occur synergistically with dermatophytosis (see 'Ringworm').

Sarcoptic mange is less common in the hedgehog, but occasional cases are seen. It typically affects young animals, causing generalized erythema and alopecia. Diagnosis is by demonstration of the burrowing mites on deep skin scrapings taken from several sites. Treatment is with injectable or spot-on ivermectin or amitraz washes, repeated after 7 and 14 days.

Demodex erinacei can cause follicular mange with raised papules and crusty skin lesions, but is rare in hedgehogs. The distinctive mites can be seen on deep skin scrapes within the sebaceous glands of haired skin. Amitraz can be used topically for treatment.

Other mites, including *Notoedres cati* and *Otodectes cynotis* are occasionally isolated from hedgehogs, and are probably acquired as a result of contact with domestic cats. Experience is needed to identify the mites from hedgehogs as the larval and nymphal forms of different species can look similar. Treatment is with ivermectin as above.

Harvest (trombiculid) mites are not uncommon in hedgehogs, usually appearing as tiny orange clusters on the face, axillae, pinnae, ventrum and interdigital area. They are probably of little clinical significance (Figure 12.17).

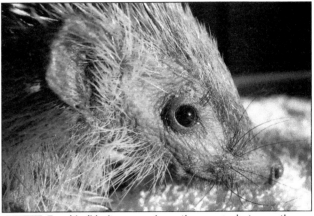

12.17 Trombiculid mites appearing as tiny orange clusters on the face of a hedgehog.

Myiasis: Flystrike can be a particular problem of hedgehogs during warm weather, and is most commonly caused by *Lucilia* spp. and *Calliphora* spp. Weak and debilitated animals attract flies and are most at risk of primary myiasis. Eggs are laid around body orifices (eyes, ears, mouth, nares, anus and genitals) and a thorough inspection of these sites is important as part of the clinical examination of hedgehog casualties. Secondary cutaneous myiasis is usually associated with wounds (see Figure 12.10) or diarrhoea on the skin. Maggots can cause considerable tissue damage and produce toxins, which can be rapidly fatal.

Treatment involves brushing the fly eggs away with a toothbrush or clipping the fur to remove clumps of eggs. Topical application of cyromazine helps prevent any remaining eggs from developing. Maggots can be removed manually using forceps. Maggots under the eyelids can be squeezed out and a viscous eye ointment (e.g. chloramphenicol eye ointment) applied to smother any that remain.

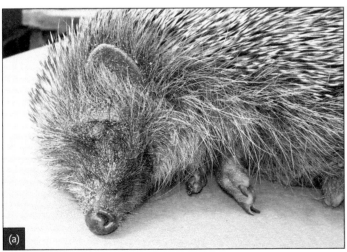

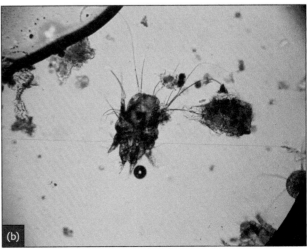

12.16 (a) Capariniosis of the face. (b) *Caparinia* mite seen on microscopy of a skin scrape. Magnification X40.

The ears can be cleaned using cotton buds, and then instilled with insecticidal ear drops. Dental irrigators can also be useful for flushing maggots from wounds.

Topical spot-on preparations (e.g. permethrin, ivermectin) or injectable ivermectin are effective insecticides for any undiscovered maggots. Most cases will need additional fluids and warmth, systemic antibacterial cover and NSAID therapy for antitoxic and analgesic effects. Myiasis in hedgehogs is often a very serious and painful condition and many individuals will be in an advanced stage of disease when presented and need immediate euthanasia on humane grounds.

Endoparasites:

Hedgehog lungworm: Adult and larval nematodes (*Crenosoma striatum*) are commonly present in the lumen of the trachea, bronchi, bronchioles and alveolar ducts (Majeed *et al.*, 1989). First-stage larvae are coughed up from the respiratory tract, swallowed, and passed in faeces. The intermediate hosts are slugs and snails, in which they develop to the infective stage. After ingestion by the hedgehog, the mollusc is digested, and the larvae migrate from the gut to the airways. Direct transmission may also occur, since worms are sometimes found in the lungs of pre-weaned animals (Majeed *et al.*, 1989). Lungworm contributes significantly to the syndrome colloquially known as 'autumn juveniles', where a combination of late-born litters, reduced food availability and parasitism can result in large numbers of underweight juvenile hedgehogs struggling to survive. Some immunity against lungworm may develop in older animals.

Significant clinical disease is principally seen in juvenile hedgehogs, especially during autumn, when the incidence of parasitic bronchopneumonia reportedly approaches 100% in some areas (Robinson and Routh, 1999; Gaglio *et al.*, 2010). The most consistent clinical sign is a distinctive moist cough (which is virtually pathognomonic), often accompanied by weakness and weight loss. Many animals have a secondary bacterial pneumonia, which can produce rattling respiration, hyperpnoea and sometimes nasal discharge and faecal abnormalities. Severe cases may present with dyspnoea, cyanosis, pulmonary emphysema and circulatory failure. The mortality rate can be high, especially in chronic cases.

Diagnosis is confirmed by finding motile larvae (approx. 300 μm in length) on direct microscopy of fresh faecal wet preparations (or expectorated tracheal mucus or sputum) (see Figure 10.8a). Larvae are not passed continuously in faeces and one-off faecal examination may pick up only about a quarter of cases, so repeat faecal examinations are recommended.

Lungworm is so common in some areas, especially in first-year weaned hedgehogs, that it may be advisable for treatment in these individuals to be undertaken routinely. Waiting for microscopic confirmation can lead to unnecessary delays in treatment and the possibility of false negatives. The need for prophylactic worming should be determined in consultation between veterinary staff and rehabilitators and an appropriate therapeutic regime instigated, which should ideally be reviewed on a regular basis. Survival rates are improved when treatment is started early; the anthelmintic of choice is levamisole because it has a relatively rapid onset of therapeutic effects. Repeat treatments are needed, and these are generally given at 48-hour intervals to reduce the risk of side effects. The risk of anaphylaxis or airway occlusion by dead worms can be reduced by the concurrent use of a corticosteroid (e.g. dexamethasone) or NSAID (see Figure 12.20), which will also reduce lung inflammation. Broad-spectrum antibacterial therapy is required due to secondary bacterial infections (see Figure 12.20). A reduction in airway exudate and expulsion of dead lungworms can be helped by the use of mucolytics and bronchodilators (see Figure 12.20). Hedgehogs often cough more whilst undergoing treatment as dead lungworms are being expelled.

Nebulization can be a useful adjunct to other therapy in hedgehogs with respiratory disorders and is relatively easily performed using a human asthma nebulizer or custom-built chamber. Bronchodilators, mucolytics and antibacterials (e.g. gentamicin or F10) are suitable for nebulization. Health and safety considerations apply to avoid inhalation by operators.

Pulmonary capillariasis: Adult lungworms of *Capillaria aerophila* 10–13 mm long can be present in the respiratory epithelium and lumen, especially within the bronchi and bronchioles. Worms can also be present in the tracheal mucosa, causing tracheitis and granulomas (Majeed and Cooper, 1984). *Capillaria aerophila* is often associated with *Crenosoma striatum* and mixed lung infestations are very common.

The lifecycle is direct, with eggs coughed up and passed in the faeces. The eggs may also be ingested by transport hosts such as earthworms and possibly beetles (Majeed *et al.*, 1989).

Diagnosis is confirmed by the demonstration of oval bipolar eggs in fresh faeces (or tracheal washes) (see Figure 10.8b), but repeat examinations may be necessary as they are often intermittently shed. Clinical disease and treatment are the same as for *Crenosoma* spp. (see above). Levamisole may have slightly less activity against *Capillaria* spp. but follow-up treatment with ivermectin or fenbendazole is generally effective in cases refractory to levamisole (see Figure 12.20).

Capillaria aerophila is capable of infecting numerous species of mammals including cats and dogs, and also has zoonotic potential so adequate precautions must be taken (see 'Zoonoses').

Intestinal capillariasis: Intestinal capillariasis (*C. erinacei* and *C. ovoreticulata*) is very common and a significant cause of morbidity in hedgehogs (Gaglio *et al.*, 2010; Pfäffle, 2010). The bipolar eggs are passed in faeces, but it can be difficult to differentiate these from *C. aerophila*. Heavy burdens of intestinal *Capillaria* spp. produce green mucoid diarrhoea (see Figure 12.7a), lethargy, restlessness and weight loss. The intermediate hosts are earthworms, although direct transmission may also occur. See Figure 12.20 for recommended anthelmintics.

Intestinal trematodes: The intestinal trematode, *Brachylaemus erinacei*, can cause fatal haemorrhagic enteritis in severe cases. Currently, the incidence of disease is relatively low, and the parasite appears to be restricted to certain regions of the UK, but infestation may become more common and widespread. Trematodes are often present concurrently with other endoparasites, in particular *Capillaria* spp.

The adult fluke is 5–10 mm in length, 1–2 mm in thickness and lancet-shaped. The eggs are unipolar and slightly asymmetrical, and measure approximately 20 x 30 μm (see Figure 10.8c). They are demonstrable on direct microscopic examination of wet faecal smears, but are small and usually present in small numbers and therefore easily missed. Flotation techniques can be used to improve the chances of detection.

The metacercariae develop in slug and snail intermediate hosts (Keymer *et al.*, 1991; Saupe and Poduschka, 1995). Adult flukes can be present in the intestine and bile ducts of hedgehogs, causing weight loss, inappetance, melaena, diarrhoea, or mucoid slimy faeces. Characteristically, affected animals are restless and hyperactive during the daytime, and will often climb and scratch at their enclosure walls. Infestation can be fatal, especially with large burdens, severe diarrhoea, or flukes in bile ducts. Treatment is with praziquantel (see Figure 12.20).

Cestodes: Tapeworm segments are usually seen in hedgehog faeces as an incidental finding, although large burdens can be clinically significant, especially in debilitated animals or those with concurrent disease. *Hymenolepis erinacei* is probably the most common species encountered. There may be geographical variations in the prevalence of hedgehog tapeworms in the UK. Adult cestodes can be up to 80 mm long and live within the intestines. The proglottids (3 x 1 mm) are passed in faeces (see Figure 12.7c) and are ingested by the intermediate hosts, which are arthropods (chiefly beetles). The proglottids and eggs (with characteristic internal oncosphere hooks) are occasionally seen in faecal smears. Treatment is with praziquantel (see Figure 12.20).

Acanthocephala: Thorny-headed worms are often discovered attached to the intestinal wall, omentum and mesentery (Figure 12.18) during post-mortem examination or intra-abdominal surgery of hedgehogs. In some cases they are an incidental finding, but when present in large numbers they can cause ulceration of the gut wall and peritonitis, especially in juveniles. Most species are probably the avian acanthocephalan *Plagiorhynchus cylindraceus*, which hedgehogs acquire by eating woodlice (Oniscidea) (Skuballa *et al.*, 2010). Hedgehogs are an aberrant (paratenic) host, which leads to the parasites invading the peritoneum and migrating within the abdominal cavity. The diagnosis can be challenging because the clinical signs are non-specific (weight loss, diarrhoea, abdominal discomfort), and eggs are not passed in faeces. Occasionally the faeces contain adult acanthocephalans, which are visible to the naked eye, resembling small seed-like structures. Praziquantel and levamisole have been used as treatment (see Figure 12.20).

Other species of acanthocephalan have also been identified from hedgehogs including *Moniliformis* spp. and *Echinorhynchus/Prosthorhynchus* spp. (Smith, 1968; Keymer *et al.*, 1991; Gaglio *et al.*, 2010), but their significance is unknown.

Coccidiosis: Coccidial oocysts (see Figure 10.8d) are sometimes seen in small numbers in faecal smears or flotation as an incidental finding. Clinical disease is usually associated with large numbers of oocysts in the faeces and may be more common where there is overcrowding and poor hygiene. Clinical signs include inappetance, weight loss, and haemorrhagic diarrhoea. The pathogenic species are *Isospora rastegaiev*, *I. erinacei* and possibly some *Eimeria* spp. (Saupe and Poduschka, 1995). Treatment with sulphonamides or toltrazuril is effective (see Figure 12.20).

Other endoparasites: Toxoplasma gondii has been recorded in hedgehogs, but the significance of infection is unknown (Smith, 1968). *Giardia*, *Cryptosporidium* and other intestinal protozoans may occasionally be encountered, although their importance is currently poorly understood.

Other nematodes have been recorded, but they seem to be of low pathogenicity and of little significance. These include *Physaloptera clausa* (oesophagus and stomach), *Gongylonema mucronatum*, ascarids, *Strongyloides* spp. and *Trichinella* spp. (Saupe and Poduschka, 1995).

Other conditions

Dental disease

Dental disease is common in captive hedgehogs, especially when fed exclusively on soft food, but it is also surprisingly common in free-living hedgehogs. Tartar aggregations can lead to gingivitis, gum recession, periodontal disease and pyorrhoea (Figure 12.19). Affected animals are often severely underweight due to an inability to feed. After initial stabilization with fluid therapy, antibacterial and anti-inflammatory medication, dentistry techniques including extractions and descaling can be useful in uncomplicated cases. However, many hedgehogs with dental disease are elderly animals with other problems such as osteoarthrosis, chronic lung pathology, submandibular lymphadenopathy, cataracts, and/or ringworm, and carry a grave prognosis.

Whilst hedgehogs are being kept in captivity, hard foods can be added to the diet, such as cat biscuits or insect chitin exoskeleton (e.g. mealworms or commercial insectivorous diets) to reduce tartar formation.

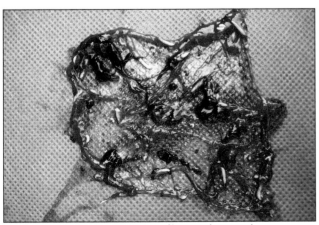

12.18 Post-mortem appearance of haemorrhages and acanthocephalae in the omentum of a hedgehog.

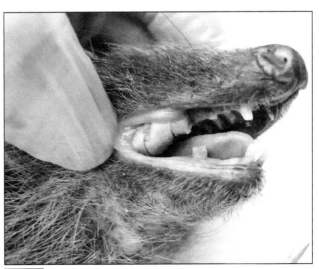

12.19 Tartar aggregations in an aged hedgehog.

Nutritional diseases

Obesity: The most common nutritional disease of hedgehogs in captivity is obesity, which can have serious health effects, including cardiovascular compromise and fatty liver degeneration. Obesity also interferes with the ability to curl up tightly, which puts individuals at increased risk of predation after release.

Dietary deficiencies: Vitamin and trace element deficiencies (e.g. zinc) can occasionally cause spine loss. Rickets can occur if homemade diets containing inadequate calcium or vitamin D are fed. Nutritional secondary hyperparathyroidism and hypervitaminosis A and D should also be considered, as in other species. For these reasons, it is preferable to feed a nutritionally balanced commercial dog/cat or specific hedgehog food to hedgehogs whilst in captivity.

Hindlimb paresis and paralysis and splayed legs in hand-reared hoglets less than 4 weeks of age have been reported. Some respond to vitamin B1 therapy, and in these cases the cause is presumed to be reduced thiamine absorption due to digestive disturbances.

Underweight autumn juveniles: Late litters, especially those born in September and October due to late conception in repeat breeders or second litters, often have insufficient time in which to lay down the necessary fat reserves to survive hibernation. In order to have a favourable chance of surviving an average British winter, hedgehogs should have a minimum bodyweight of 550 g by November (Morris, 1984). As autumnal temperatures drop, the amount of natural prey declines and young hedgehogs are forced to forage in the daytime in a bid to meet their nutritional needs. Many are found wandering around in daylight in autumn and taken into care. The majority of these also have significant endoparasite burdens, especially lungworm, and anthelmintic treatment is essential (see 'Endoparasites' and Figure 12.20). They should be kept in captivity until they have sufficient fat reserves to be released (sometimes this involves keeping them for the whole winter). With warmth and access to food, they will not hibernate. Most rehabilitators choose to release hedgehogs slightly heavier than the 550 g minimum to allow for some weight loss after release. Once up to release weight, they can be returned to the wild (even during winter as long as the weather is relatively mild).

Other conditions

- Otitis externa is not uncommon, especially in association with blowfly contamination of the external ear canal. Treatment is possible with antibacterial and antiparasitic ear drops, but daily application can be problematic as hedgehogs usually curl up in response to the ears being touched.

- End-stage lung disease (e.g. pulmonary emphysema and consolidation), which may be accompanied by secondary cardiac failure, is a common finding in hedgehogs. Clinically, they have noisy wheezy respiration and hyperpnoea, and most are also in a poor nutritional state. Some animals improve with antibacterial and anti-inflammatory therapy, but full recovery is rare and these animals should be euthanased at an early stage. The underlying cause is rarely established, but severe lungworm infestation, pneumonia, or smoke damage is often suspected.

- Neoplasia, including mammary carcinoma and squamous cell carcinoma, are occasionally seen, usually in old individuals that should be euthanased.

- Paraphimosis is seen occasionally in males following trauma.

- Circling behaviour is occasionally seen in hedgehogs. Typically, they obsessively run around in the same direction, and there is usually an absence of other neurological signs such as head tilt and ataxia. Most have unilateral ocular lesions and clinical signs are probably related to head trauma, but middle ear infection and other neurological disorders could be involved in some cases. A proportion of animals recover with time.

- Wobbly hedgehog syndrome is an idiopathic neurodegenerative disease of captive African pygmy hedgehogs. A similar disease has been reported affecting European hedgehogs in a wildlife rescue centre (Palmer *et al*, 1998).

Therapeutics

In hedgehogs, the parenteral administration of drugs is preferred over the oral route because dosing is more precise and better tolerated. Subcutaneous injection can be given with minimal disturbance to the animal (even when it is rolled up), and is generally the method of choice for most drugs. Intravenous injection is not possible in the hedgehog without anaesthesia and is seldom used. For details about injection techniques, see 'First aid'.

Oral medications can be mixed with a small amount of food, but appetites and therefore drug intake are often unpredictable, making oral dosing less accurate. In compliant individuals (especially hoglets), it may be possible to administer oral liquids directly per os.

Topical cutaneous treatments, including spray, powder and spot-on preparations are also useful.

A drug formulary for hedgehogs is given in Figure 12.20. Drug doses are derived from allometric principles, published references and the author's experience. It should be noted that the effective doses of many drugs in hedgehogs are comparatively high. The cascade system should always be followed.

Drug	Dosage	Comments
Antibacterials		
Ampicillin	20–30 mg/kg s.c., orally q12h	Broad-spectrum bactericidal
Amoxicillin/clavulanate (co-amoxiclav)	30–50 mg/kg i.m., s.c., orally q12h	Broad-spectrum bactericidal, useful for infections of respiratory tract, skin and soft tissue (including abscesses) and enteritis
Amoxicillin LA	50–150 mg/kg s.c. q24h or q48h	A useful first choice broad-spectrum bactericidal used every 48h for most infections (e.g. for secondary bacterial pneumonia associated with lungworm). Higher doses (up to 150 mg/kg) and increased frequency (24h) may, in the author's experience, be effective for more severe infections particularly salmonellosis

12.20 Drug formulary for hedgehogs. (continues)
(Unpublished data; Robinson and Routh, 1999; Carpenter, 2005)

Drug	Dosage	Comments
Antibacterials continued		
Cefalexin	30 mg/kg i.m., s.c., orally q24h or q12h	In the author's experience, dosing every 24h is effective for most soft tissue infections but more severe infections (abscesses and pyodermas) require more frequent (12h) dosing.
Clindamycin	10–20 mg/kg orally q12h	Anaerobic infections, including wounds, abscesses and dental infections; also useful for infections involving bones and joints
Enrofloxacin	10–20 mg/kg i.m., s.c., orally q12h	Broad-spectrum bactericidal, useful for respiratory infections, enteritis and skin wounds Avoid use in young growing animals as potentially causes abnormalities of cartilage
Marbofloxacin	8–10 mg/kg s.c. q24h	Broad-spectrum bactericidal. Avoid use in young growing animals as potentially causes abnormalities of cartilage
Metronidazole	20–40 mg/kg orally q12h	Anaerobic infections
Oxytetracycline	50 mg/kg i.m., s.c., orally q12h	Broad-spectrum bacteriostatic
Antifungals		
Enilconazole	0.2% dilution, applied topically every 3 days for 4–6 applications	Topical antifungal treatment for ringworm applied as a wash or spray. After treatment, keep hedgehogs warm to prevent hypothermia, especially in small juveniles
Itraconazole	10–15 mg/kg orally q12h	Parenteral antifungal treatment for ringworm, treat for 2–4 weeks then re-sample
Terbinafine	50–100 mg/kg orally q24h or q12h	Parenteral antifungal treatment for ringworm, treat for 2–4 weeks then re-sample. Calculated dosing frequency is every 12h, but in the author's experience it is as effective when administered every 24h (especially in larger animals)
Antiparasitic agents		
Amitraz	1:400 dilution applied topically to skin as a wash every 7 days	Demodicosis and sarcoptic mange. Essential to change bedding and clean out cage during treatment. Repeated examinations of skin scrapes are needed to monitor effect; generally 3–6 treatments are required
Cypermethrin	Topical spray applied sparingly to affected skin	A pyrethroid insecticide combined with the antimicrobial F10 in a wound spray useful for treating myiasis and as a fly repellent
Cyromazine	Topical application to wet the affected area	An insect growth inhibitor useful for preventing hatching and development of blow fly larvae Can be used in combination with an insecticide to kill existing maggots Easier to apply, especially between the spines, if used as a spray Beware cooling effect: do not use in hypothermic animals
Fenbendazole	100 mg/kg orally q24h for 5 days	Useful as in-feed treatment against nematodes, and may have some effect against cestodes in hedgehogs
Fipronil	0.25% spray used sparingly or spot-on application 7.5–15 mg/kg	Fleas and ticks Always ensure good ventilation during and after treatment Beware cooling effect: do not use in hypothermic animals
Ivermectin injectable	0.5–3.0 mg/kg s.c.	Good activity against most parasites of hedgehogs Repeat treatment every 7–10 days if necessary
Ivermectin topical	0.2–0.5 mg/kg spot-on application	Fleas, ticks and mites. Repeat treatment after 10 days
Levamisole	27 mg/kg s.c. q48h	Treatment of choice for lungworm; 3 injections given at 48 hour intervals (other dose regimes can be employed)
Mebendazole	50–100 mg/kg orally q24h for 5 days	Nematodes and cestodes
Permethrin	Light topical application of powder to skin or spot-on application 250–350 mg/kg	Fleas, ticks and myiasis
Praziquantel	10–20 mg/kg i.m., s.c., orally once or 30 mg/kg topical spot-on application	Cestodes and trematodes
Pyrethrum	Light topical application of powder to skin	Ectoparasites, especially fleas. Use very sparingly
Sulphadimidine	200 mg/kg s.c. q24h for 3 days	Coccidiosis
Sulfadoxine/trimethoprim	50 mg/kg i.m., s.c. q24h for 5 days	Coccidiosis
Toltrazuril	25–50 mg/kg orally once, repeated if necessary.	Coccidiosis
Miscellaneous		
Bromhexine	1 pinch of powder orally q12h (3 mg/kg q24h)	Mucolytic; aids expectoration of mucus in parasitic bronchopneumonia
Clenbuterol	1 pinch of powder orally q12h	Bronchodilator; relieves bronchospasm and assists mucociliary clearance in respiratory disease
Dexamethasone	1–5 mg/kg i.v. i.m., s.c.,	Corticosteroid may be useful in parasitic bronchopneumonia
Etamiphylline	30 mg/kg i.m., s.c. q12h or q 8h	Cardiorespiratory stimulant; may be useful in parasitic bronchopneumonia
Methylprednisolone	1–6 mg/kg i.m., s.c.	Corticosteroid. Both short- and long-acting preparations are available
Pentobarbital sodium	150–200 mg/kg i.v., intrahepatic or intracardiac	Euthanasia (following gaseous anaesthetic induction); see 'Euthanasia'

12.20 (continued) Drug formulary for hedgehogs.
(Unpublished data; Robinson and Routh, 1999; Carpenter, 2005)

Management in captivity

Housing

Hedgehogs are not naturally gregarious and are best kept singly to reduce the risk of disease transmission. When several animals are kept concurrently, they can be housed in small groups if space is limited provided disease risks are managed. Conspecific aggression is unusual, although occasional bite wounds may be sustained (typically to the flank and upper forelimb) when groups are overwintered together.

Individual hedgehogs can be kept in a cardboard box or plastic tub, allowing approximately 0.5 m² per individual. For longer term and communal housing they should have a larger area allowing approximately 1 m² per animal.

There should be no bars, wire mesh or sharp projections, as hedgehogs often scratch at surfaces and can easily injure their feet. They can climb and dig and a secure lid or door is required to prevent escape. Adequate bedding is needed for insulation and to provide somewhere to hide to make animals feel secure. Newspaper, shavings or (non-frayed) towelling can be used as bedding material; this needs regular replacement as it rapidly becomes soiled with food, water and excreta. Daily monitoring is needed if hay or shredded paper is used as nesting material as these can become twisted around a limb producing a ligature effect. Animals should also be weighed regularly to monitor their progress and their food intake and faecal output recorded daily.

Diet

Adult hedgehogs are relatively easy to feed in captivity and will consume a variety of foods.

- Tinned cat or dog food is satisfactory; approximately 80 g per animal per feed should be given depending on the nutritional content.
- Dried pelleted cat or dog biscuits can be incorporated to reduce the risks of tartar build-up and obesity by encouraging foraging activity if scatter fed.
- Foods for insectivorous birds or proprietary hedgehog foods are available from pet and garden stores and are suitable alternatives.
- Invertebrates such as mealworms (*Tenebrio molitor* larvae) may also be fed and can be used as environmental enrichment with scatter feeding or to stimulate appetite.
- The traditional hedgehog diet of bread and milk is nutritionally unsuitable and tends to cause diarrhoea in adults due to lactose intolerance. It is therefore not recommended.

As hedgehogs are nocturnal, it is more natural to feed them in the evening but, as the majority of hedgehogs taken into care are underweight, they should be offered food twice daily. Adult hedgehogs will often overeat and are prone to obesity if fed *ad libitum*, so adults in good body condition should be fed once a day only and amounts of food carefully controlled.

Drinking water should be provided in a shallow bowl. Drip drinkers can be used, but are generally messier.

General points

- If well fed and kept in a warm environment (18–22°C), overwintered hedgehogs will not hibernate. This is crucial for animals that lack sufficient body reserves for hibernation (see 'Nutritional diseases').
- Unnecessary handling should be discouraged, as hedgehogs can become accustomed to contact and are at increased risk of predation after release if they do not immediately roll up when under threat.
- The claws can become overgrown when hedgehogs are kept for a long time in captivity due to lack of exercise and should be trimmed if necessary.

Rearing of hoglets

Litters (averaging 4–5 hoglets) are generally born from May to October, in a specially constructed breeding nest. Hoglets may be abandoned if the nest is disturbed, for example during gardening, scrub clearance or building work. They can also be orphaned by death of the sow. Deserted hoglets often leave the nest when they get hungry, and usually vocalize, making characteristic whistling and peeping noises. If abandoned hoglets are discovered, a thorough search of the area is essential to ensure none are left behind. Hand-rearing is a time-consuming and difficult task that should not be undertaken lightly (Figure 12.21; see also Chapter 8). Fostering hoglets on to other nursing females has been described as being successful, but is generally not advisable due to the risk of infanticide and cannibalism.

Age	Typical bodyweight (g)	Feeding (milk replacer)
Newborn	12–20	1–2 ml every 2 hours
3 days to 1 week	30–50	2 ml every 2–3 hours
1–2 weeks	50–80	2–5 ml every 3–4 hours
2–3 weeks	80–100	5–10 ml every 4 hours
3–4 weeks	110–170	6 ml every 4 hours Wean on to puppy or cat food Encourage to lap milk from dish
5 weeks	190–220	Weaned on to solid foods

12.21 Suggested feeding regime for hoglets.

Once in care, hoglets need immediate warmth and fluids, and should be checked over for flystrike and any injuries. They should be weighed, and their age estimated based on the characteristics described in Figure 12.4. On arrival, and after every feed, they should be stimulated to defecate and urinate (known as 'toileting'), by gently massaging the anogenital area with a damp cotton bud. The droppings of unweaned juveniles are naturally green, becoming paler with time, until after weaning when they become brown. Hoglets should be routinely weighed every day before the first morning feed to monitor their progress.

The minimum ambient temperature should be 25–30°C. This can be achieved using a heat pad, heat lamp or incubator. A temperature gradient is desirable, so that hoglets can move away from the heat source if they get too hot; thermoregulation is poor in neonates. Newspaper plus a towel is suitable as the substrate.

After arrival, the first feed should be a rehydrating solution. Subsequent feeds should consist of diluted milk substitute given in gradually increasing concentration. Many milk substitutes have been used with success, including goat colostrum, goat milk and proprietary dog and cat milk replacers. Ready-made liquid milk formula may be superior to powdered varieties because inconsistencies in preparation and mixing are avoided. The milk is warmed and fed via a plastic pipette and kitten-size teat (some workers make small teats for very small hoglets by building up layers of modelling latex over a blunted hypodermic needle). See also Chapter 8 for further details.

Individuals that are too weak, or reluctant to suck, can be fed via a stomach tube, but the technique requires experience to avoid milk inhalation. Alternatively, milk can be slowly dripped into the mouth a drop at a time, until the sucking reflex becomes stronger. The main problems seen in hand-reared hoglets are milk aspiration and bloat; the risk of developing these is reduced once they are able to eat for themselves. The ability to self-feed varies greatly between individuals, but all should be encouraged to lap milk from a shallow dish. Once they are doing so, usually at around 3–4 weeks old, solid food (e.g. puppy or cat food; see also 'Diet') can be added gradually. Sometimes, even comparatively small unweaned hoglets will lap milk or milky food from a dish if given the opportunity.

Young hoglets have poorly developed immune systems and rely on maternal antibodies, which are present in milk for the entire lactation period (Morris and Steel, 1964). Without this passive immunity, hoglets have increased susceptibility to infection. Barrier nursing and strict hygiene are therefore very important, especially when large numbers are being reared simultaneously. Overcrowding and mixing hoglets of different ages should be avoided due to the risk of disease spread. Their living quarters should be regularly cleaned out, and a separate set of equipment used for each litter group. Feeding utensils should be sterilized between feeds. Even with such precautions, outbreaks of enteric infection can be a problem.

Release

Most studies (including radio tracking) indicate that rehabilitated hedgehogs released back to the wild generally survive well. Even juvenile animals, despite being raised in artificial conditions in captivity, seem to adapt and thrive once released (Morris *et al.*, 1990, 1993; Morris and Warwick, 1994; Sainsbury *et al.*, 1996; Morris, 1997, 1998; Reeve, 1998; Molony *et al.*, 2006).

Choice of release site

If possible, animals should be returned to where they were found, and released back into a familiar environment. Although translocated hedgehogs appear to adapt well (Molony *et al.*, 2006; Warwick *et al.*, 2006), there is the potential for adverse effects on the existing local population, such as disease introduction (Cunningham, 1996). There are likely to be regional differences in the prevalence of disease (especially parasites) (Gaglio *et al.*, 2010; Pfäffle, 2010; Skuballa *et al.*, 2010; Whiting, 2012) and genetic diversity of hedgehog populations.

If return to the original site is not possible, it is important that hedgehogs are released into a suitable habitat. The presence of other hedgehogs is a good indication that the habitat is appropriate. Generally, hedgehogs favour 'edge habitats' (areas between open land such as grassland and dense vegetation) (Reeve, 1994) (see 'Ecology and biology'). Gardens can be good release sites, especially if they contain shrubs, leaf piles and overgrown areas.

Sites adjacent to busy roads should be avoided if possible, and areas with ground-nesting birds should not be used as release sites (e.g. bird reserves, land managed for gamebirds), because hedgehogs can take eggs and chicks.

Release techniques

Hedgehogs should be released at dusk during periods of fine weather to give them the opportunity to build a nest and find local food sources. Soft release (see Chapter 9) may reduce dispersal and improve survival chances, but hedgehogs rarely return for supplementary feeding after release. Hard release is generally successful.

A period of weight loss usually occurs when rehabilitated hedgehogs are released. Some of this is attributable to the excess weight gained in captivity (Morris, 1998), but some weight loss is probably also due to decreased food intake in the first few days whilst they adapt to their surroundings.

Hedgehogs with sufficient fat reserves can be released in the winter during mild spells, but many hedgehog carers prefer to overwinter such animals in captivity and release them in the spring.

PVC ear tags, clipped spines, glue-on spine tags, colour marking spines, radiofrequency identification (RFID) (using passive integrated transponder (PIT) microchips) and radiotelemetry, have all been used to identify released animals and monitor their post-release survival (see also Chapter 9).

Legal aspects

Hedgehogs have no specific legal protection but are covered by Schedule 6 of the Wildlife and Countryside Act 1981 (amended 1987), which makes it illegal to catch, trap or kill them without a licence. The Wild Mammals (Protection) Act 1996 protects them from cruelty. For general legal considerations, see Chapter 2.

Acknowledgements

The author would like to thank the staff at the Royal Society for the Prevention of Cruelty to Animals (RSPCA) wildlife hospital in Norfolk and Ian Robinson for his contributions to the earlier edition of this chapter and for sharing his expertise over the years.

References and further reading

Best JR (2001) Diagnosis and treatment of poisoning in wildlife – a practical guide for rehabilitators. *Rehabilitator* **31**, 2–7

Bunner J (2002) *The impact of molluscicide application on hedgehog populations: a review.* Mammals Trust UK, London

Carpenter JW (2005) Hedgehogs. In: *Exotic Animal Formulary, 3rd edn*, ed. JW Carpenter, pp. 361–373. Elsevier Saunders, St. Louis

Churchfield S (2008) Insectivores Orders Erinaceomorpha and Soricomorpha. In: *Mammals of the British Isles: Handbook 4th edn*, ed. S Harris and DW Yalden, pp. 241–249. The Mammal Society, Southampton

Couper D, Margos G, Kurtenbach K and Turton S (2010). Prevalence of *Borrelia* infection in ticks from wildlife in south-west England. *Veterinary Record* **167**, 1012–1014

Cunningham AA (1996) Disease risks of wildlife translocations. *Conservation Biology* **10(2)**, 349–353

Dowding CV, Harris S, Poulton S and Baker PJ (2010a) Nocturnal ranging behaviour of urban hedgehogs, *Erinaceus europaeus*, in relation to risk and reward. *Animal Behaviour* **80(1)**, 13–21

Dowding CV, Shore RF, Worgan A, Baker PJ and Harris S (2010b) Rodenticides in a non-target insectivore, the European hedgehog (*Erinaceus europaeus*). *Environmental Pollution* **158(1)**, 161–166

English MP and Morris PA (1969) *Trichophyton mentagrophytes* var. *erinacei* in hedgehog nests. *Sabouraudia* **7**, 118–121

Gaglio G, Allen S, Bowden L, Bryant M and Morgan ER (2010) Parasites of European hedgehogs (*Erinaceus europaeus*) in Britain: epidemiological study and coprological test evaluation. *European Journal of Wildlife Research* **56(6)**, 839–844

Gemmeke H (1999) Untersuchungen zur gefaehrung von igeln durch die bekaempfung mit schneckenkorn (mollusckizide). *Nachrichten des Deutschen Pflanzenschutzdienst* **51**, 245–247

Haigh A, Kelly M, Butler F and O'Riordan RM (2014) Non-invasive methods of separating hedgehog (*Erinaceus europaeus*) age classes and an investigation into the age structure of road kill. *Acta Theriologica* **59(1)**, 165–171

Handeland K, Refsum T, Johansen BS et al. (2002) Prevalence of *Salmonella* Typhimurium infection in Norwegian hedgehog populations associated with two human disease outbreaks. *Epidemiology and Infection* **128(3)**, 523–527

Hof AR (2009) *A study of the current status of the hedgehog (Erinaceus europaeus), and its decline in Great Britain since 1960.* PhD thesis, Royal Holloway, University of London

Hulse EC and Edwards JT (1937) Foot-and-mouth-disease in hibernating hedgehogs. *Journal of Comparative Pathology and Therapeutics* **50**, 421–430

Isenbügel E and Baumgartner RA (1993) Diseases of the hedgehog. In: *Zoo and Wild Animal Medicine – Current Therapy, 3rd edn*, ed. ME Fowler. WB Saunders, Philadelphia

Isenbügel E and Frank W (1985) Kleinsäuger. In: *Heimtierkrankheiten*. Eugen Ulmer, Stuttgart

Keymer IF, Gibson EA and Reynolds DJ (1991) Zoonoses and other findings in hedgehogs (*Erinaceus europaeus*): a survey of mortality and review of the literature. *Veterinary Record* **128**, 245–249

Lewis JCM, Norcott MR, Frost LM and Cusdin P (2002) Normal haematological values of European hedgehogs (*Erinaceus europaeus*) from an English rehabilitation centre. *Veterinary Record* **151**, 567–569

Majeed SK and Cooper JE (1984) Lesions associated with a *Capillaria* infestation in the European hedgehog (*Erinaceus europaeus*). *Journal of Comparative Pathology* **94(4)**, 625–628

Majeed SK, Morris PA and Cooper JE (1989) Occurrence of the lungworms *Capillaria* and *Cremosoma* species in British hedgehogs (*Erinaceus europaeus*). *Journal of Comparative Pathology* **100**, 27–36

Matthews PRJ and McDiarmid A (1977) *Mycobacterium avium* infection in freeliving hedgehogs (*Erinaceus europaeus*). *Research in Veterinary Science* **22**, 388

McLaughlan JD and Henderson WM (1947) The occurrence of foot-and-mouth-disease in the hedgehog under natural conditions. *Journal of Hygiene (Cambridge)* **45**, 474–479

Molony SE, Dowding CV, Baker PJ, Cuthill IC and Harris S (2006) The effect of translocation and temporary captivity on wildlife rehabilitation success: an experimental study using European hedgehogs (*Erinaceus europaeus*). *Biological Conservation* **130(4)**, 530–537

Morris B and Steel ED (1964) The absorption of antibody by young hedgehogs after treatment with cortisone acetate. *Journal of Endocrinology* **30**, 195–203

Morris PA (1971) Epiphyseal fusion in the forefoot as a means of age determination in the hedgehog (*Erinaceus europaeus*). *Journal of Zoology (London)* **164**, 254–259

Morris PA (1983) *Hedgehogs*. Whittet Books, Weybridge

Morris PA (1984) An estimate of the minimum body weight necessary for hedgehogs (*Erinaceus europaeus*) to survive hibernation. *Journal of Zoology (London)* **203**, 291–294

Morris PA (1986) Nightly movements of hedgehogs (*Erinaceus europaeus*) in forest edge habitat. *Mammalia* **50**, 395–398

Morris PA (1997) Released, rehabilitated hedgehogs – a follow-up study in Jersey. *Animal Welfare* **6**, 317–327

Morris PA (1998) Hedgehog rehabilitation in perspective. *Veterinary Record* **143**, 633–636

Morris PA and English MP (1969) *Trichophyton mentagrophytes* var. *erinacei* in British hedgehogs. *Sabouraudia* **7**, 122–128

Morris PA and English MP (1973) Transmission and course of *Trichophyton erinacei* infections in British hedgehogs. *Sabouraudia* **11**, 42–47

Morris PA, Meakin K and Sharafi S (1993) The behaviour and survival of rehabilitated hedgehogs. *Animal Welfare* **2**, 53–66

Morris PA, Munn S and Craig-Wood S (1990) Released hedgehogs – can they cope? In: *Proceedings of the Third Symposium of the British Wildlife Rehabilitation Council*, ed. T Thomas. BWRC, Horsham

Morris PA and Tutt A (2009) Leucistic hedgehogs on the island of Alderney. *Journal of Zoology* **239(2)**, 387–389

Morris PA and Warwick H (1994) A study of rehabilitated juvenile hedgehogs after release into the wild. *Animal Welfare* **3**, 163–177

Nauerby B, Pedersen K, Dietz HH and Madsen M (2000) Comparison of Danish isolates of *Salmonella enterica* serovar enteritidis PT9a and PT11 from hedgehogs (*Erinaceus europaeus*) and humans by plasmid profiling and pulsed-field gel electrophoresis. *Journal of Clinical Microbiology* **38**, 3631–3635

Palmer AC, Blakemore WF, Franklin RJM et al. (1998) Paralysis in hedgehogs (*Erinaceus europaeus*) associated with demyelination. *Veterinary Record* **153**, 550–552

Parkes J (1975) Some aspects of the biology of the hedgehog (*Erinaceus europaeus*) in the Manawatu, New Zealand. New Zealand *Journal of Zoology* **2**, 463–472

Pfäffle MP (2010) *Influence of parasites on fitness parameters of the European hedgehog (Erinaceus europaeus).* PhD thesis, Karlsruhe Institute of Technology (KIT), Karlsruhe, Germany

Reeve NJ (1982) The home range of the hedgehog as revealed by a radiotracking study. *Symposium of the Zoological Society of London* **49**, 207–230

Reeve NJ (1994) *Hedgehogs*. T and AD Poyser, London

Reeve NJ (1998) The survival and welfare of hedgehogs after release back into the wild. *Animal Welfare* **7**, 189–202

Reeve NJ and Huijser MP (1999) Mortality factors affecting wild hedgehogs: a study of records from wildlife rescue centres. *Lutra* **42**, 7–23

Riley PL and Chomel BB (2005) Hedgehog zoonoses. *Emerging Infectious Diseases* **11(1)**, 1–5

Robinson I and Routh A (1999) Veterinary care of the hedgehog. *In Practice*, March, 128–137

Roos S, Johnston A and Noble D (2012) *UK hedgehog datasets and their potential for long-term monitoring*. BTO Research Report 598. British Trust for Ornithology, Thetford

Sainsbury AW, Cunningham AA, Morris PA, Kirkwood JK and Macgregor SK (1996) Health and welfare of rehabilitated juvenile hedgehogs (*Erinaceus europaeus*) before and after release into the wild. *Veterinary Record* **138(3)**, 61–65

Saupe E and Poduschka W (1995) Igel. In: *Krankheiten der Heimtiere, 3rd edn*, ed. K Gabrisch and P Zwart. Schlutessche, Hannover, Germany

Skuballa J, Taraschewski H, Petney TN, Pfäffle M and Smales LR (2010) The avian acanthocephalan *Plagiorhynchus cylindraceus* (Palaeacanthocephala) parasitizing the European hedgehog (*Erinaceus europaeus*) in Europe and New Zealand. *Parasitology Research* **106(2)**, 431–437

Smith JMB (1968) Diseases of hedgehogs. *Veterinary Bulletin* **38**, 425–430

Smith JMB and Marples MJ (1963) *Trichophyton mentagrophytes* var. *erinacei*. *Sabouraudia* **3**, 1–10

Stack MJ, Higgins RJ, Challoner DJ and Gregory MW (1990) Herpesvirus in the liver of a hedgehog (*Erinaceus europaeus*). *Veterinary Record* **127**, 620–621

Twigg GI, Cuerden CM and Hughes DM (1968) Leptospirosis in British wild mammals. *Symposium of the Zoological Society of London* **24**, 75–98

Van Oers L, Tamis W, de Koning A and de Snoo G (2005) *Review of Incidents with Wildlife Related to Paraquat CML Report 165*. Department of Environmental Biology, Institute of Environmental Sciences (CML), Leiden University, Netherlands

Visozo AD and Thomas WE (1981) Paramyxoviruses of the Morbilli group in the wild hedgehog (*Erinaceus europaeus*). *British Journal of Experimental Pathology* **62**, 79–86

Warwick H, Morris P and Walker D (2006) Survival and weight changes of hedgehogs (*Erinaceus europaeus*) translocated from the Hebrides to mainland Scotland. *Lutra* **49(2)**, 89–102

Whiting I (2012) Prevalence of Endoparasites in the European Hedgehog (*Erinaceus Europaeus*) within Regions of the East Midlands. *Reinvention: a Journal of Undergraduate Research*, British Conference of Undergraduate Research www.warwick.ac.uk/go/reinventionjournal/issues/bcur2012specialissue/whiting

Chapter 13

Squirrels

Tiffany Blackett

The Eurasian red squirrel (*Sciurus vulgaris*) (Figure 13.1) and the Eastern grey squirrel (*Sciurus carolinensis*) (Figure 13.2) are tree squirrels. They are both members of the order Rodentia, family Sciuridae, subfamily Sciurinae and genus *Sciurus*. Globally, there are 28 species within the genus *Sciurus* (Bosch and Lurz, 2012). The geographical range of *Sciurus vulgaris* is large, throughout Europe and northern Asia, from the British Isles across continental Europe, to north-eastern China and northern Japan. The range of the North American Eastern grey squirrel has expanded, enabled by its introduction to the UK (see 'Ecology and biology'), Ireland, northern Italy and South Africa.

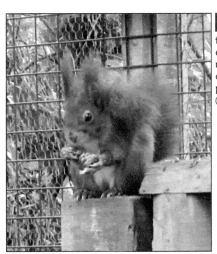

13.1 A red squirrel eating seeds from a pine cone. The ear tufts typical of the red squirrel's winter coat are very prominent.
(© T Blackett)

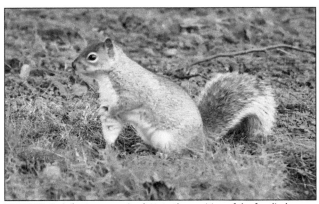

13.2 A vigilant grey squirrel. Note the position of the forelimb, which should not be confused with lameness.
(© T Blackett)

The Eurasian red squirrel is Britain's native squirrel. Both the range and size of the UK red squirrel population has suffered dramatically as a result of a number of introductions of the larger Eastern grey squirrel since 1876. Grey squirrels have increased in number and range, whilst the distribution of red squirrels has become fragmented and their range contracted. The decline of the UK red squirrel population has been attributed to a variety of factors, including habitat loss, habitat fragmentation, competition from the alien grey squirrels and the high mortality rate associated with infection by squirrelpox virus (SQPV). Infection of red squirrels with SQPV is largely fatal (see 'Infectious diseases'). Grey squirrels have been implicated in the transmission of SQPV, which they can carry asymptomatically.

Ecology and biology

Both species can inhabit coniferous and broad-leaved woodlands. The best habitats are large woodlands containing a variety of mature seed-producing trees, as they offer a more reliable source of food. Grey squirrels, however, are better adapted to utilizing oak seed crops (Kenward and Holm, 1993) and can be found at higher densities than red squirrels in deciduous broad-leaved woodlands. Red and grey squirrels may also inhabit urban parks, churchyards and gardens where there is suitable tree cover, hedgerow connectivity and food availability.

Tree seeds are the most important components of the natural diet. Fruits, berries and fungi are other important food items and lichens, tree flowers, shoots and buds are also eaten. Squirrels are opportunistic feeders, hence invertebrates (e.g. caterpillars) and occasionally bird eggs or nestlings may be taken. Food is cached; these small stores are important in times of food shortages or bad weather. Food availability affects bodyweight, reproductive success and, therefore, population numbers. Squirrels may bark-strip to find food or as a result of aggressive interactions (Holm, 1987; Bosch and Lurz, 2012). Both species are diurnal (active during the daytime). They are also active throughout the year and do not hibernate. Most active time is spent foraging. Free-living tree squirrels are generally solitary animals, although nest sharing has been reported in winter. Squirrels may use more than one drey (nest), which helps to reduce ectoparasitic burdens (Holm, 1987). Dominance is related to age and body size. Males are not always dominant and larger dominant individuals often live in better quality home ranges. Home range size may be affected by a number of other factors including food availability, habitat quality, season and squirrel density. Aggressive interactions within a species mostly involve body posturing (e.g. tail flicking) and vocal calls. Interactions can result in chases and some result in injuries, such as bites to the tail, rump, back and ears. Both species scent mark.

Anatomy and physiology

Red and grey squirrel characteristics are described in Figure 13.3. Red and grey squirrels both have long back legs and long flexible hind feet for agility in the tree canopy. Claws are very important for climbing. A squirrel's tail provides balance when running and jumping and plays a role in communication and thermoregulation. Red squirrels are slight of frame and lighter compared to the heavier grey squirrels (Figure 13.3). In both species melanistic individuals can occur. Albino squirrels may also occur but are rare.

Characteristic	Red squirrel (*Sciurus vulgaris*)	Eastern grey squirrel (*Sciurus carolinensis*)
Ear tufts	Prominent in winter, thin or absent during summer	None
Bodyweight	277–303 g[a]	542–659 g[a]
Coat colour	Varies throughout its geographical range Individual coat colour varies with season as the coat moults Colours vary from black, dark brown, to orange/bright red Underside: white or cream	Winter coat: speckled grey, banded tail hairs have a white tip, no ear tufts Summer coat: grey-brown with patches of orange typically over its feet and sides Underside: white or cream
Life span	6–8 years[b]	7–9 years[b]

13.3 Red and grey squirrel characteristics. Bodyweight varies with both time of year and habitat.
([a] Holm, 1987; [b] Gurnell *et al.*, 2012)

Gender determination and ageing

The distance between the genital opening and the anus is considerably greater in males, compared to females. Out of breeding season, testes are withdrawn into the abdomen and not visible in the scrotum, although a darker discolored scrotum may be apparent in males that have previously been reproductively active.

Ageing squirrels can be difficult and involves considering the bodyweight, body condition, dentition and reproductive status. Young squirrels are smaller and, in males that have not yet reached sexual maturity, there will be no scrotal discoloration. In squirrel kittens tooth eruption can be used for ageing (see 'Rearing of squirrel kittens' and Figure 13.14).

Dentition

Squirrels, in common with other rodents, have continuously growing incisors that are maintained at the correct length by wear through accurate occlusion. The molars do not continuously grow (Bosch and Lurz, 2012). The dental formula of both red and grey squirrels is:

$$2 \times \left\{ I \ \frac{1}{1} \ C \ \frac{0}{0} \ P \ \frac{2}{1} \ M \ \frac{3}{3} \right\} = 22$$

The first upper premolar is undeveloped (Lurz *et al.*, 2005). The cheek teeth (molars and premolars) erupt from 7 weeks of age onward and by 10 weeks of age all the cheek teeth are present (Sainsbury *et al.*, 2004). Only the lower and second upper premolars are deciduous and are replaced by permanent dentition at 16 weeks of age (Holm, 1987). The lower jaw muscles enable the lower incisors to move slightly relative to one another, to allow the incisors to grip food items and crack open nuts (Holm, 1987).

Reproduction

The breeding season in both species is largely determined by food availability and climate, but can begin as early as December and continue until August. Females are polyoestrous, with oestrus lasting 24 hours. Availability of food has a great influencing factor on reproduction. Females will only come into oestrus if they are in good body condition (Wauters and Dhondt, 1989). If there are good food resources, females, except yearlings, may have two litters in the year, with the first between February and April and the second between May and August. Once weaned, the longevity of juveniles is largely dependent on food availability and survival during their first winter; between 75–85% of juveniles may die during their first year. Juvenile dispersal of spring- and summer-born litters may occur in June or July and between September and November respectively. Red and grey squirrels do not interbreed (Holm, 1987). Further information on reproductive and developmental characteristics of squirrels is given in Figure 13.14.

Capture, handling and transportation of casualties

Capture

Red squirrels are protected by the Wildlife and Countryside Act (WCA) 1981 and it is forbidden to disturb or capture them without a licence from the relevant government department. Within the WCA, however, there is a provision that allows casualty free-living red squirrels to be captured by hand for necessary veterinary treatment and care prior to their release without a licence; if it is necessary to use a live trap or nets to capture the casualty, a licence is required. Casualty grey squirrels may be transported to a veterinary surgery for euthanasia on welfare grounds without a licence, but housing grey squirrels in captivity, such as during treatment and rehabilitation, requires a licence (see 'Legal aspects' and Chapter 2).

Live traps, pre-baited with food items such as apple, carrot, peanuts, sunflower seeds or hazelnuts, can be used to capture debilitated squirrels that are still mobile. Traps should be placed in an area that the squirrel has been observed to frequent regularly. They should be checked several times a day and include a covered area offering seclusion and protection from the weather. Blackout nets with soft padded rims and of a very fine gauge mesh (to minimize the risk of damaging teeth, claws, feet and legs) may be useful for capturing casualty squirrels in small enclosed areas. Once captured beneath the net the squirrel can be gently, but firmly, restrained through the net material and promptly transferred to an appropriate transport container. Seriously debilitated or unconscious squirrels may be captured by covering with a towel and using this to place the squirrel into a suitable transport container. Never attempt to catch or hold a squirrel by its tail, as this may result in degloving injuries ('tail slip'), with the skin stripping off the tail.

Capture and subsequent handling is a very stressful experience for the squirrel and potentially hazardous for both squirrel and handler. Squirrels can inflict serious deep bites or scratches that may injure the handler, with the potential for transmission of zoonotic agents. There is also a risk of injury to the squirrel from 'tail slip', inadvertent collision with the rim of a net used for capture, injury to teeth, feet or the skin of the face from interaction with the sides of live traps, or entanglement of claws, teeth, or feet in towels or netting material.

Handling

Squirrels are very agile and fast movers. To minimize stress, they should be handled and restrained quietly, carefully and gently, yet firmly, and for the shortest time possible. Red squirrels are very susceptible to stress and can 'breath-hold', becoming immobile when handled with potentially fatal consequences (Sainsbury, 2003). Should breath-holding occur in response to handling, the animal should immediately be placed in an appropriate secure ventilated box in a quiet darkened room and allowed to recover unassisted.

Casualty squirrels may still scratch, bite and move quickly. When handling squirrels, it is important that the handler always wears gloves (e.g. latex) to reduce the risk of zoonotic disease transmission. Leather gloves may also be beneficial, to protect from bites, although thick gloves can decrease dexterity. Towels or cloths of a suitable thickness may be useful for restraint purposes to enable handling, examination and restraint, but care must be taken to prevent serious injury occurring to claws, feet and teeth by their becoming caught in towelling loops. Casualty squirrels can be carefully covered with and enveloped within the suitable towel or cloth, gently but firmly holding the animal around the shoulders in the towel, whilst also supporting the body through the towel. Sections of the towel may then be reflected to reveal different parts of the squirrel's body for examination (see Figure 13.9). Other methods of restraining squirrels include the use of squirrel wire mesh handling cones (commonly used by researchers), padded rimmed nets (see 'Capture'), handling bags (Bosch and Lurz, 2012) or cloth sacks (Sainsbury, 2003).

Transportation

Casualty squirrels should be quietly transported in a secure box that has appropriately sized air holes for ventilation. Suitable bedding such as hay or appropriate cloths or towels should be provided on the floor of the container to prevent the animal slipping during transit and to offer a hiding place. For very short distances cardboard cat carriers may be used; however, the risk of gnawing is considerable and wire cat carriers of small gauge mesh are preferable (see Figure 13.4). Small gauge mesh is essential to reduce the risk of inadvertent injury to the squirrel. A lightweight towel should be draped over the wire carrier, ensuring adequate ventilation, to minimize visual disturbance and provide seclusion thus reducing stress during transportation.

Zoonoses

Squirrels may become infected by various agents which can be transmitted to humans, including *Salmonella* spp., leptospirosis, *Trichophyton* spp., *Borrelia burgdorferi*, *Campylobacter* spp., *Toxoplasma gondii*, *Capillaria* spp., *Yersinia pseudotuberculosis* and *Y. enterocolitica*, *Erysipelothrix rhusiopathiae* and *Francisella tularensis* (Keymer, 1983; Sainsbury, 2003; Simpson, 2008; Bosch and Lurz, 2012; Gurnell *et al.*, 2012) (see also Chapter 7). Gloves should always be worn when handling squirrels and if a squirrel bite is received medical advice as appropriate should be sought. External parasites, such as fleas, may also be transferred from squirrels to handlers, as well as into the captive environment.

For all centres treating casualty squirrels, suitable health and safety risk assessments should be in place alongside suitable staff training, there should be adequate biosecurity arrangements and there should be documented protocols for ready implementation in case staff are injured by a casualty squirrel.

Examination and clinical assessment for rehabilitation

As much information as possible about the circumstances in which the casualty squirrel was found (e.g. on the road, in a private garden, by the cat), when it was found and how long the finder may have had the casualty in their care, should be obtained. Such a submission history can help the interpretation of injuries, aid a presumptive diagnosis and influence the choice of additional diagnostics.

Handling and stress must be minimized. Quiet observation within the transport container may be helpful in some circumstances and provide information (e.g. on posture, respiratory effort, lameness) that may not be apparent when the animal is physically restrained. Knowledge of normal squirrel behaviours and body posturing may help correctly interpret observations (see Figures 13.2 and 13.4). General signs of illness or pain in rodents include a typical hunched posture, immobility, anorexia,

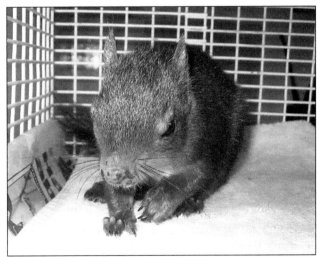

13.4 Sick female Jersey red squirrel, in a small gauge mesh wire carrier, presenting with left forefoot lameness associated with exudative dermatitis lesions. There is a hunched posture and typical fatal exudative dermatitis (FED) lesions are visible on eyes, muzzle and forefeet. Normal vigilance behaviour (see Figure 13.2) should not be confused with lameness.
(© T Blackett)

porphyrin staining around the eyes in rats, and piloerection. Clinical examination should be undertaken in a small quiet secure room, away from domestic animals. Thorough assessment may necessitate a general anaesthetic. Koprowski (1994) notes rectal temperatures of 36.4–38.7°C in grey squirrels and an average heart rate of 259 beats per minute in captive grey squirrels, whilst commenting that heart rates are likely to be lower in free-living animals.

Diagnostic techniques

Once clinically assessed, the casualty should be stabilized using appropriate first aid (see 'First aid and short-term hospitalization'). Radiography and laboratory testing may be required to complete the clinical assessment. Once stabilized and if a favourable tentative prognosis is made (see Chapter 4), a treatment programme for the squirrel can be commenced. The individual animal's welfare must always be a priority.

Blood sampling of squirrels can be difficult and should only be undertaken in an anaesthetized animal. The minimum amount of blood required should be collected. Joslin (2009) suggests a cautious approach, recommending a blood sample volume of 0.8% lean body weight (i.e. 0.8 ml per 100 g bodyweight), whilst also considering size, age and any debility. Blood can be collected from the jugular or femoral vein (Sainsbury, 2003; Wilks, 2008). The cranial vena cava may be used as a blood sampling site in rats under general anaesthesia (Joslin, 2009) and may also be used in anaesthetised squirrels. Pressure should be applied to the vein following sampling to help haemostasis. If blood collection involves the femoral vein great care must be taken to avoid the femoral artery and nerve, which lie adjacent to this. Haematology and biochemistry reference intervals for squirrels are given in Figure 13.5. Squirrels are very susceptible to stress; debilitated squirrels should be carefully monitored before, during and after anaesthesia and blood sample collection.

Variable (units)	Reference interval
Haematology[a]	
Red blood cell (RBC) count (x 10¹²/l)	4.92–8.29 (n=22)
Total haemoglobin (g/dl)	9.9–17.41 (n=22)
Packed cell volume (PCV) (l/l)	30.29–52.62 (n=22)
Mean cell volume (MCV) (fl)	46.63–79.96 (n=22)
Mean cell haemoglobin (MCH) (pg)	14.11–27.76 (n=22)
Mean cell haemoglobin concentration (MCHC) (g/dl)	29.19–36.79 (n=22)
Platelet count (x 10⁹/l)	110.49–708.17 (n=15)
Reticulocytes (% RBC)	0.1–4.6 (n=22)
Heinz bodies (% RBC)	0–0.5 (n=22)
White blood cell (WBC) count (x 10⁹/l)	0–12.28 (n=22)
Neutrophils (x 10⁹/l)	0–6.07 (n=22)
Lymphocytes (x 10⁹/l)	0–6.44 (n=22)
Monocytes (x 10⁹/l)	0–0.43 (n=22)
Eosinophils (x 10⁹/l)	0–0.58 (n=22)
Basophils (x 10⁹/l)	0 (n=22)
Erythrocyte sedimentation rate (mm/h)	0–17 (n=11)
Fibrinogen (g/l)	1.66–3.82 (n=12)

13.5 Haematology reference intervals for squirrels and serum biochemistry reference intervals for red squirrels. (continues) ▶
([a] Zoological Society of London Lynx Reference database; [b] unpublished data, A Meredith and E Milne, Royal (Dick) School of Veterinary Studies, University of Edinburgh)

Variable (units)	Reference interval
Biochemistry[b]	
Calcium (mmol/l)	1.6–2.1 (n=24)
Inorganic phosphate (mmol/l)	0.6–7.7 (n=22)
Sodium (mmol/l)	146.6–160 (n=21)
Potassium (mmol/l)	3.5–9 (n=21)
Chloride (mmol/l)	100.7–110.9 (n=21)
Creatinine (μmol/l)	57.2–116.2 (n=25)
Urea (mmol/l)	4.7–12.7 (n=23)
Bile acids (μmol/l)	20.2–34.9 (n=15)
Bilirubin (μmol/l)	0–3.7 (n=15)
Alkaline phosphatase (ALP) (IU/l)	276.0–975 (n=24)
Alanine aminotransferase (ALT) (IU/l)	6.1–38.3 (n=25)
Total protein (g/l)	50.8–70.1 (n=24)
Albumin (g/l)	25.1–32.8 (n=23)
Globulin (g/l)	18.8–38 (n=23)

13.5 (continued) Haematology reference intervals for squirrels and serum biochemistry reference intervals for red squirrels.
([a] Zoological Society of London Lynx Reference database; [b] unpublished data, A Meredith and E Milne, Royal (Dick) School of Veterinary Studies, University of Edinburgh)

Euthanasia

Euthanasia by pentobarbital injection should be performed in a manner that will cause the least distress to the animal, usually in an anaesthetized animal, by either intravenous injection using the femoral vein or intracardiac injection. Intraperitoneal pentobarbital injection is painful and euthanasia prolonged and is therefore not recommended. Intracardiac injection is only acceptable for anaesthetized animals or animals that are comatose (AVMA, 2013).

First aid and short-term hospitalization

The casualty should be weighed on admission to assist clinical assessment, enable accurate dosing of medication and to aid the monitoring of response to treatment. Where appropriate, keep the casualty warm and prevent further heat loss (see Chapter 5). Supplementary heat that creates a temperature gradient in the squirrel's accommodation may be required and must be provided in a safe, appropriate manner; a casualty squirrel may be unable to move away from the heat source, so careful monitoring is essential to avoid overheating.

Proprietary oral formulations, such as Vetark® Critical Care Formula or Lectade® may be used to offer support and oral rehydration, and oral formulations such as Emeraid® Omnivore can also be used to provide convalescent nutrition for debilitated weaned juveniles and adult animals. Casualty squirrel kittens should be stimulated to urinate/defecate prior to fluid administration. Oral rehydration fluids should be given to abandoned kittens in the first one or two feeds, prior to milk substitutes. See also 'Rearing of squirrel kittens' and Chapter 8.

Intravenous fluid therapy, necessary for collapsed individuals, may be possible via the femoral vein (Sainsbury, 2003) taking great care to avoid the femoral artery and nerve. An intravenous butterfly catheter may be placed. Intravenous injections can be difficult in squirrels and a single bolus of fluid in a collapsed individual is usually most appropriate. Intraosseous fluids may also be used in debilitated animals (see Chapter 5). Intraperitoneal fluids may be given instead or in situations when the veins are inaccessible, although there is a risk of organ damage and infection with this route (see Chapter 5). Subcutaneous fluids are helpful in cases of mild hypovolaemia and, if combined with hyaluronidase, are rapidly absorbed (see Chapter 5). Repeated administration of subcutaneous fluids should be avoided as this may lead to tissue necrosis. Medications, such as antibiotics and analgesia, should be given as appropriate, and their use always recorded. Broad-spectrum antibiotics are essential for victims of cat attacks. Appropriate analgesia can help reduce stress, as well as pain (see 'Anaesthesia and analgesia' and Chapter 5).

As soon as possible, suitable easily digestible foods should be offered to casualties (see 'Diet' and 'Rearing of squirrel kittens').

Anaesthesia and analgesia

There is no need to starve squirrels prior to anaesthesia as they do not vomit (Flecknell, 1996; Sainsbury, 2003). Appropriate steps should be taken to reduce heat loss during both anaesthesia and the recovery period, but overheating may occur and should be avoided, especially in the recovery period. Appropriate fluid therapy during and immediately following anaesthesia should be provided. It is essential to obtain an accurate bodyweight to enable correct dosing of anaesthetic and analgesic drugs.

Inhalational anaesthesia allows for better control of the depth of anaesthesia and recoveries are often more rapid compared to injectable anaesthesia (Orr, 2002). Isoflurane or sevoflurane are the preferred inhalational anaesthetic agents and recovery from these is usually rapid in healthy animals. Maintenance of anaesthesia can be achieved using a suitable facemask. Intubation is difficult in squirrels but, as with other rodents, it should be considered where appropriate and is recommended where possible (Richardson and Flecknell, 2009).

Injectable anaesthesia using a combination of ketamine at 75 mg/kg with medetomidine at 0.5 mg/kg by intramuscular injection has been used in grey squirrels, extrapolated from rat dosages (Sainsbury, 2003; Carpenter, 2013; Figure 13.6). To reduce the risk of muscle pain and necrosis, this combination has been used via the intraperitoneal route in rats (Flecknell, 1996; Orr, 2002; Sainsbury, 2003; Richardson and Flecknell, 2009). However, considerably lower doses have also been reported to be effective with this combination; Meredith (2015) suggests a dose of 5 mg/kg i.m. ketamine with 0.05–0.1 mg/kg i.m. medetomidine (Figure 13.6). Partial reversal of this anaesthesia is possible using atipamezole, although a delay of at least 20 minutes after induction has been recommended in rats to reduce the undesirable effects of ketamine (Sainsbury, 2003). Midazolam can be used as a sedative in rats at a dose of 2.5 mg/kg i.m. (Ramsey, 2014) or intraperitoneal (Orr, 2002; Richardson and Flecknell, 2009) and may be used in squirrels. During injectable anaesthesia or sedation, supplementary oxygen should be provided throughout via a facemask to reduce the risk of hypoxia.

The recovery area should be quiet, warm and darkened and the squirrel's accommodation must be secure. Once the animal has suitably recovered, access to appropriate food and water should be immediately provided.

Pre-emptive analgesia is important to alleviate pain, reduce stress, prevent inappetance caused by pain, and can aid recovery (Figure 13.6).

Specific conditions

Trauma

Squirrels may suffer mortal traumatic injuries as a result of human activities such as road traffic collisions, predation by domestic pets (Figure 13.7) and entrapment injuries (Simpson et al., 2013c). Serious degloving injuries can also occur to the tail of squirrels from inappropriate handling techniques (e.g. trying to catch the squirrel by its tail, see 'Handling'). Degloving tail injuries are painful and can

Drug	Dosage	Suggested route(s)	Frequency / use
Analgesic drugs			
Buprenorphine[a]	0.05 mg/kg	s.c.	q8–12h
Butorphanol[ab]	2 mg/kg	s.c.	q4h
Carprofen[ab]	5 mg/kg	s.c.	q24h
Ketoprofen[b]	1–3 mg/kg	i.m., s.c.	q12–24h
Meloxicam[b]	1–2 mg/kg	s.c. or orally	q24h
Morphine[b]	2.5 mg/kg	i.m., s.c.	q2–4h
Anaesthetic and sedative drugs			
Ketamine (K) + medetomidine (M)	5 mg/kg (K) + 0.05–0.1 mg/kg (M)	i.m.[f]	Relatively low dose rates of this combination of drugs have been reported[f] to produce immobilization in squirrels. Medetomidine may be reversed after 20 minutes using five times the dose (an equal volume of most products) of atipamazole
	75 mg/kg (K) + 0.5 mg/kg (M)	i.p.[acde], i.m.[d]	Much higher dose rates have been used to provide 20–30 minutes surgical anaesthesia[cg]. Individual animal drug responses may vary and therefore suggested dose rates should be used only as a guideline. Medetomidine may be reversed after 20 minutes using five times the dose (an equal volume of most products) of atipamazole
Midazolam	2.5 mg/kg	i.p.[ac], i.m.[b]	Sedation

13.6 Analgesic and anaesthetic agents commonly used in squirrels. The dosages have been extrapolated from data available for rats.
([a]Richardson and Flecknell, 2009; [b]Ramsey, 2014; [c]Orr, 2002; [d]Sainsbury, 2003; [e]Flecknell, 1996; [f]Meredith, 2015; [g]Carpenter, 2013)

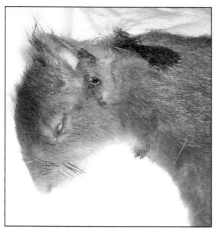

13.7 Subadult male red squirrel with fatal puncture wounds from a predator attack.
(© T Blackett)

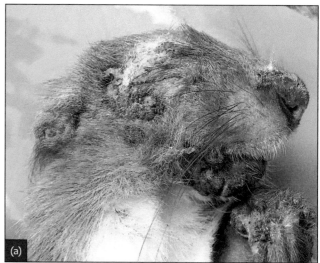

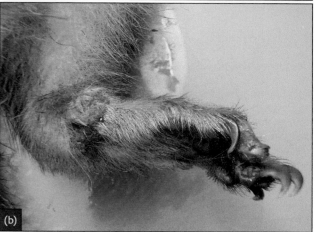

13.8 Typical squirrelpox virus skin lesions (a) on the face and fore foot and (b) on the hind foot of a red squirrel.
(© A Meredith)

result in the loss of skin and underlying soft tissue, exposing the vertebrae and predisposing the animal to infection. Serious degloving tail injuries that have extensive loss of skin and soft tissue may require treatment for shock, in addition to wound management, broad-spectrum antibiotics and analgesia (see Figures 13.6 and 13.13).

Other traumatic injuries include bite wounds from other squirrels. Traumatic injuries in juveniles may be seen resulting from falls out of trees due to poorly developed climbing skills (Stocker, 2005); these casualties, typically 6–7 weeks of age, have often begun the natural weaning process but are not yet fully weaned, so may require some hand-rearing following admission in addition to access to appropriate 'solid' food (see 'Diet' and 'Rearing of squirrel kittens').

The treatment and management of traumatic injuries and wounds is similar to the treatment of such injuries in domestic rodents and small mammals.

Infectious diseases

Viral diseases

Squirrelpox virus: SQPV was previously known as squirrel parapoxvirus (SPPV). The virus is thought to be carried asymptomatically by grey squirrels, which act as a reservoir host, and infection is usually fatal in red squirrels (Sainsbury *et al.*, 1997; Lurz *et al.*, 2005; Sainsbury *et al.*, 2008; Carroll *et al.*, 2009). It remains unclear how the virus is transmitted between squirrels. Recent studies have identified a small number of red squirrels with antibodies to the virus (Sainsbury *et al.*, 2008; Dale *et al.*, 2010).

Early clinical signs of SQPV infection in red squirrels include lethargy and poor coordination. The development of skin lesions follows, characteristically exudative dermatitis lesions on the face (eyes, nose and mouth), feet, genitalia and ventrum (Figure 13.8). There may be a purulent ocular discharge. Secondary bacterial infection of SQPV lesions with *Staphylococcus aureus* has been reported (Sainsbury *et al.*, 1997; Duff *et al.*, 2010). Diagnosis is based on clinical signs and electron microscopy of skin crusts.

If a red squirrel is presented in the early stages of SQPV infection, supportive treatment may be successful. Red squirrels may show a variable immune response to SQPV and some may be able to survive infection (Sainsbury *et al.*, 2008; Dale *et al.*, 2010). Euthanasia on welfare grounds should be considered for squirrels presenting with advanced lesions. Where an informed decision is made to provide supportive treatment, it should involve broad-spectrum antibiotics (see 'Therapeutics' and Figure 13.13), analgesics (see 'Anaesthesia and analgesia' and Figure 13.6) and fluid therapy. Appropriate topical eye medication, such as topical ophthalmic fusidic acid (e.g. Fucithalmic® Vet), may be required, as well as assisted feeding if the squirrel's vision is affected. The use of omega interferon (Virbagen® Omega) has been reported to help reduce mortality rates in red squirrels infected with SQPV (Wilks, 2008; RSNE, 2011a; V Butler, personal communication) (see Figure 13.13). It would also be prudent to appropriately treat any flea burden on the squirrel (see 'Parasites'), as ectoparasites such as fleas may play a role as vectors in the transmission of the disease (Collins *et al.*, 2014).

Adenovirus: Adenovirus, reported both in free-living and captive red squirrels, causes an enteric infection and splenitis commonly associated with sudden death. Diarrhoea and poor body condition may also be observed (Sainsbury *et al.*, 2001; Duff *et al.*, 2007; Everest *et al.*, 2008; 2009b; 2013). Adenovirus infection in red squirrels may be largely asymptomatic (Simpson *et al.*, 2013c), although stress may exacerbate the effects of infection with resultant clinical disease (Martínez-Jiménez *et al.*, 2011; Peters *et al.*, 2011). The mechanism of virus transmission is unclear. Adenovirus has been identified in asymptomatic grey squirrels (Greenwood and Sanchez, 2002; Everest *et al.*, 2009b), but has also recently been confirmed in red squirrels in locations where there are no grey squirrels, such as on the Isle of Wight and Jersey, Channel Islands (Everest *et al.* 2013). It has been suggested that other rodents, such as wood mice (*Apodemus sylvaticus*), may act as a possible reservoir for the virus (Everest *et al.*, 2009b; 2013). Diagnosis of clinical infection is by electron microscopy of intestinal contents. Polymerase chain reaction (PCR) assay of splenic tissue following post-mortem examination may identify clinical and subclinical adenovirus infection (Everest *et al.*, 2012; 2013). Treatment is supportive and should include fluid therapy.

Rotavirus: Rotavirus is an important cause of diarrhoea in many juvenile mammals. Rotavirus infection has been identified in UK red squirrels (Everest *et al.*, 2009a; 2010; 2011) and was reported in two juvenile red squirrels that presented with intussusception and diarrhoea (Everest *et al.*, 2009a). Electron microscopy of faecal samples can be used to aid diagnosis (Everest *et al.*, 2009a; 2011).

Bacterial diseases

Bacterial infections are an important cause of mortality in red squirrels.

Fatal exudative dermatitis: Fatal exudative dermatitis (FED) describes a condition that has caused significant red squirrel mortalities on both the Isle of Wight and Jersey, Channel Islands, areas where there are no grey squirrels. It is characterized by exudative dermatitis lesions associated with *Staphylococcus aureus* infection (Simpson *et al.*, 2010ab; 2013b). Red squirrels with FED lesions may or may not present with concurrent pathology, but there have been no consistent pathological findings, except for the isolation in pure or mixed cultures of moderate to heavy and profuse growths of *S. aureus* from the FED lesions (Simpson *et al.*, 2010a; 2013b). FED skin lesions appear similar to those of SQPV and typically occur on the face and feet (Simpson *et al.*, 2010a; 2013b); however, laboratory testing for SQPV in the cases described proved negative (see Figures 13.4 and 13.9). Affected red squirrels are usually weak, may be in poor body condition, or they are found dead. Whilst the mechanism of this disease is unknown, the condition is normally fatal (Simpson *et al.*, 2013c) and the prognosis is consequently poor. Where an informed decision is made to attempt treatment, it should involve analgesics, antibiotics and appropriate fluid

therapy. Euthanasia on welfare grounds should be considered for red squirrels presenting with advanced lesions and debility. Confirmation of the diagnosis involves electron microscopy of the lesions to examine for virus particles to exclude SQPV, and bacterial culture.

Bacterial bronchopneumonia: In the UK, cases of fatal *Bordetella bronchiseptica* bronchopneumonia have been identified in red squirrels (Simpson *et al.*, 2006; 2013c) and the post-mortem examination of a thin red squirrel with pneumonia recorded *Yersinia enterocolitica* infection (VLA, 2010). *Pasteurella multocida* infection has also been reported in red squirrels (Keymer, 1983; Bosch and Lurz, 2012), as well as inhalational pneumonias with secondary bacterial infection (Simpson *et al.*, 2013c). Treatment should be supportive and should involve broad-spectrum antibiotics, analgesics (see Figures 13.6 and 13.13) and, as appropriate, fluid therapy.

Mycobacterial dermatitis (squirrel leprosy): Since 2006, six Scottish red squirrels have presented with gross lesions of alopecia and marked cutaneous swelling of the muzzle, eyelids, ears and feet (Figure 13.10). Histological examinations of three of these animals revealed granulomatous skin lesions typical of lepromatous leprosy, with Ziehl–Neelsen staining showing colonies of intracellular acid-fast rods; further laboratory testing detected bacteria similar to *Mycobacterium lepromatosis* (Meredith *et al.*, 2014). The condition must be differentiated from SQPV and FED; diagnosis is by histology and PCR analysis.

Bacterial enteritis: Squirrels may suffer from bacterial enteritis. Infection of squirrels with *Salmonella* spp., as well as other types of bacteria that may infect other rodents, is

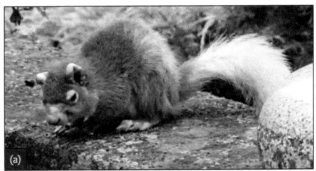

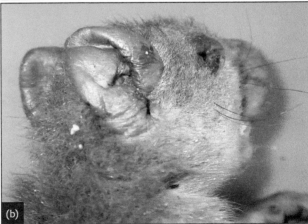

13.9 Sick adult male Jersey red squirrel with skin lesions typical of fatal exudative dermatitis (FED). Lesions can be seen on the eyelids and muzzle. An informed decision was made to euthanase this squirrel on welfare grounds.
(© T Blackett)

13.10 (a) Typical mycobacterial dermatitis (squirrel leprosy) lesions on the muzzle, ears, eyelids and feet of an affected free-living red squirrel and (b) notable cutaneous swelling of the ears and eyelids recorded at post-mortem examination.
(© A Meredith)

possible (Sainsbury, 2003). *Campylobacter* spp. have been recorded in red squirrels (Dipineto, 2009). Diagnosis is by faecal culture. Treatment should be supportive, with appropriate fluid therapy and careful antibiotic usage based on culture and sensitivity results (see 'Therapeutics' and Figure 13.13). Younger animals may be at increased risk of infection and the development of enteritis, particularly during the post-weaning period.

Parasites

Ectoparasites: Debilitated squirrels are more likely to carry greater ectoparasitic burdens than healthy animals and large burdens may further exacerbate the animal's poor health and debility.

- Fleas are commonly found on squirrels in the UK. On red squirrels, *Monopsyllus sciurorum* is the prominent species (Keymer, 1983), although *Taropsylla octodecimdentata* may also be found on red squirrels in Scotland and north-east England (Bosch and Lurz, 2012). *Orchopeas howardi* is the flea commonly found on grey squirrels (Keymer, 1983).
- Ticks (*Ixodes ricinus*) have been recorded on red and grey squirrels in the UK (Keymer, 1983).
- *Neohaematopinus sciuri,* a blood-sucking louse, has been identified on UK red and grey squirrels, although infestations in red squirrels appear to be more typical in Scotland and northern England (Keymer, 1983; Duff *et al.*, 2010; Simpson *et al.*, 2013c); fatal infestations have been reported in juvenile red squirrels (Duff *et al.*, 2010; LaRose *et al.*, 2010). The sucking louse (*Enderleinellus nitzchi*) has also been recorded on red squirrels in Scotland (Simpson *et al.*, 2013c).
- The following mites have been identified on UK red squirrels: *Dermacarus sciurinus*; *Neotrombicula autumnalis*; and *Metalistrophorus pagenstecheri* (Simpson *et al.*, 2010a; 2013c). There are no confirmed records of mange (e.g. *Notoedres* spp.) in UK red squirrels (Keymer, 1983; Sainsbury, 2003). The six-legged larval stage of the harvest mite (*Neotrombicula autumnalis*) is the only parasitic mite form recorded on red squirrels in the UK and light burdens appear to be of little clinical significance (Sainsbury, 2003; Simpson *et al.*, 2010a). *Dermacarus sciurinus* and *Metalistrophorus pagenstecheri* do not appear to be pathogenic on red squirrels (Simpson *et al.*, 2010a). However, heavy *Dermacarus sciurinus* infestations associated with debility may lead to alopecia (Figure 13.11).

Proprietary topical 'spot-on' formulations designed for use on pet rats, such as permethrin (e.g. Xenex® Ultra Spot-On) (Wilks, 2008) and ivermectin (e.g. Xeno 50-mini) may be useful, although accurate topical doses must be applied based on bodyweight (see Figure 13.13). Fipronil spray (e.g. Frontline® spray) can also be used to treat fleas (Sainsbury, 2003). The correctly calculated dose of fipronil spray can be applied to a gloved hand and then wiped over the animal's body, but care should be taken to avoid chilling and ensure good ventilation post-application.

Endoparasites:
Coccidiosis: Coccidiosis (e.g. *Eimeria sciurorum* infection) has been reported as a cause of red squirrel mortality (Keymer, 1983). Although *Eimeria* spp. oocysts may be commonly identified on faecal examination in both red and grey squirrels, the prevalence of associated disease in

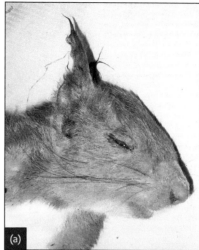
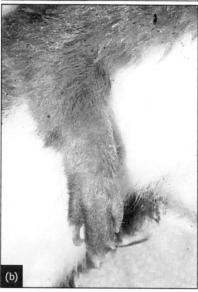

13.11 The post-mortem examination of a thin adult male red squirrel revealed large numbers of *Dermacarus sciurinus* with associated hair loss on (a) the muzzle and (b) the fore feet. This squirrel had concurrent pathology as a consequence of several disease processes.
(© T Blackett)

free-living squirrels is disputed (Sainsbury, 2003; Simpson *et al.*, 2013c). Coccidiosis may be triggered by stressors, or may occur secondary to other diseases or suboptimal husbandry whilst in captivity (Sainsbury, 2003). Faecal examination will aid diagnosis. Treatment should involve appropriate fluid therapy and anticoccidials such as sulphonamides (see Figure 13.13), but it must also include addressing the underlying causes. Toltrazuril has been used in rodents (Carpenter, 2013), but the author has no experience of its use in squirrels.

In general, younger animals are more susceptible to infection and the development of clinical gastrointestinal disease, particularly during the post-weaning period. Post-weaning stress, which can result in immunosuppression, can increase the animal's susceptibility to disease and ill health, typically of gastrointestinal origin. Therefore, when hand-rearing red squirrels, it is important to reduce stress (e.g. minimize handling, provide a quiet, warm environment and use one carer for consistency in handling, feeding and toileting techniques). Good hygiene is important and dietary changes should be made gradually.

Toxoplasmosis: Toxoplasma gondii infection is an important cause of red squirrel mortality (Jokelainen and Nylund, 2012; Simpson *et al.*, 2013c). At histopathology, lesions such as pneumonitis, multifocal splenic necrosis, multifocal hepatocyte necrosis and focal cardiac myopathy have been recorded in affected red squirrels (Simpson et al., 2013c; T Blackett, unpublished data). Diagnosis is usually made at post-mortem examination. Supplementary feeding of red squirrels in private gardens may predispose them to infection.

Hepatozoonosis: Hepatozoon spp. have been recorded in free-living red squirrels and grey squirrels in the UK (Keymer, 1983; Simpson *et al.*, 2006; 2013c). *Hepatozoon* protozoan schizonts may be found in the lung tissue at necropsy. It has been suggested that *Hepatozoon* spp. infection may predispose squirrels to other respiratory infections (Davidson and Calpin, 1976; Simpson *et al.*, 2006), but that *Hepatozoon* spp. infection alone is not a principal cause of death (Simpson *et al.*, 2013c). *Bordetella bronchiseptica* bronchopneumonia has been diagnosed in red squirrels with concurrent *Hepatozoon* spp. infection (Simpson *et al.*, 2006; 2013c).

Helminths: Whilst nematodes have been recorded in both red squirrels (Keymer, 1983; Martínez-Jiménez *et al.*, 2011; Simpson *et al.*, 2013c) and grey squirrels in the UK (Keymer, 1983), and cestodes have been identified in UK grey squirrels (Keymer, 1983), they are generally not thought to cause significant disease (Keymer, 1983). Elsewhere in Europe, cestodes have also been found in red squirrels (Romeo *et al.*, 2013).

Capillaria hepatica can infect a range of species, including humans, but largely occurs in wild rodents (e.g. rats and mice). Mortality as a result of severe *Capillaria hepatica* infection has been recorded in British red squirrels (Simpson *et al.*, 2013c; T Blackett, unpublished data). The extent of infection can vary between individual squirrels, with severe cases involving extensive liver fibrosis (Simpson *et al.*, 2013c; T Blackett, unpublished data). Diagnosis is by post-mortem examination.

Other conditions

Starvation can be the cause of death in many juvenile and adult squirrels (Holm, 1987; LaRose *et al.*, 2010). Possible causes include poor food availability (e.g. poor autumn seed crop, seasonal food shortages), an inability to feed (e.g. secondary to dental problems, trauma, inexperience) or the presence of debilitating disease (e.g. SQPV), although already underweight squirrels may also be more susceptible to disease. Diagnosis requires identification of the underlying causes and is essential to determine the likely prognosis and subsequently the most appropriate course of action.

Examples of other reported conditions in red squirrels include neoplasia, pyometra and intussusception (Everest *et al.*, 2009a; LaRose *et al.*, 2010; Simpson *et al.*, 2013c). Lens opacity has been recorded in dehydrated grey squirrels that resolved with rehydration therapy (Sainsbury, 2003). An encephalomyocarditis virus has been isolated from red squirrels and has been associated with paralysis (Vizoso *et al.*, 1964). On Jersey, Channel Islands, multiple cases of amyloidosis have been identified in free-living red squirrels (Simpson *et al.* 2013a; T Blackett, unpublished data).

Dermatophytosis (ringworm) (*Microsporum cookei* and *Trichophyton* spp.) may also occur in free-living red squirrels (Edwards, 1962; Keymer, 1983; Holm, 1987; Lurz *et al.*, 2005) but infections are uncommon and often self-limiting. Good biosecurity measures and vigilance are recommended when dealing with casualties. Holm (1987) describes 'crusty and flaking ears' on squirrels with *Microsporum cookei* infection.

Dental disease

Incisor malocclusion may arise if teeth are fractured, misaligned, or if there is misalignment of the jaw. It may occur as a consequence of degeneration (e.g. infection), trauma or nutritional problems (Sainsbury, 2003; Sainsbury *et al.*, 2004). Diets low in calcium or with an inverse calcium:phosphorus ratio may result in metabolic bone disease (see 'Nutritional secondary hyperparathyroidism') and deformities of the mandible with resultant incisor malocclusion. Incidences of incisor malocclusion and overgrowth have been recorded in free-living British red squirrels and may result in difficulty eating, starvation and an increased susceptibility to disease (Figure 13.12). Attrition of the cheek teeth has also been recorded in free-living red squirrels (Sainsbury *et al.*, 2004). For squirrels with fractured incisors, analgesia and antibiotics (where there is pulp exposure) should be used where indicated. Fractured incisors will regrow but careful monitoring is required to ensure correct alignment is achieved. A squirrel with incisor malocclusion is not a candidate for release.

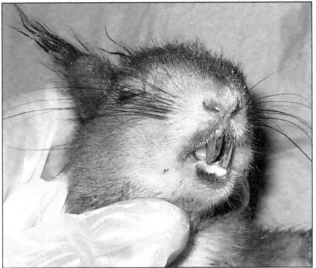

13.12 Incisor malocclusion and overgrowth, associated with an incisor root abscess in an adult male red squirrel found dead.
(© T Blackett)

Nutritional secondary hyperparathyroidism

Nutritional secondary hyperparathyroidism (often referred to as metabolic bone disease (MBD)) may occur in captive squirrels if an inappropriate diet is fed. Foods often fed to squirrels in captivity, such as nuts, can be low in calcium and relatively high in phosphorus. Sunflower seeds and peanuts are high in unsaturated fatty acids that can prevent the effective absorption of calcium (Sainsbury, 2003). MBD has also been reported in a free-living red squirrel possibly associated with supplementary feeding by members of the public at artificial feeding stations (Keymer and Hime, 1977). Signs may include inactivity, weakness, inappetance and weight loss. In severe cases death may occur. Radiography may show reduced bone density especially of the long bone cortices. Fractures or other skeletal deformities may be seen. Careful handling must be employed. If clinical signs are severe, parenteral calcium may be administered once and then followed with oral calcium supplements (Brown and Rosenthal, 1997). Examples of suitable oral calcium supplements include Zolcal-D®, which is a liquid formulation of calcium and vitamin D3 that may be given directly or via drinking water, and Nutrobal®, which is a vitamin/mineral supplement that can be sprinkled on to solid food. Immediately correcting the diet is an important part of treatment (see 'Diet'). The provision of appropriate fluid therapy and analgesia may also be required. During the treatment period it may be beneficial to confine the affected animal to a small suitable cage to limit activity and hence reduce the risk of fractures. Following correction of the diet, pathological fractures as a result of MBD can heal quickly (Brown and Rosenthal, 1997). However, in order to be released, affected free-living red squirrels must be able to regain the necessary level of physical fitness, ability and agility to enable them to survive in the wild. In severe cases of MBD where there are bone deformities due to pathological fractures that are likely to reduce the physical capability of the squirrel, euthanasia should be considered.

Prevention of MBD is by ensuring that a good quality, mixed and balanced diet is offered (see 'Management in captivity'). Squirrels kept in captivity should be given access to shed antlers or cuttlefish bones (Dutton, 2004; RSNE, 2011b). Alternatively, to help ensure adequate calcium intake, suitable oral vitamin/mineral supplements (e.g. Nutrobal®) dusted on to solid food can be beneficial. In general, adequate full-spectrum lighting should be provided where squirrels are housed indoors and do not have access to natural daylight, and should mimic the natural photoperiod (Miller, 2000).

Therapeutics

Obtaining an accurate bodyweight is very important for drug administration in squirrels (see Chapter 7).

Oral dosing can be achieved by offering medication mixed with small amounts of a favoured food. However, careful observation is necessary to ensure the medicated food is eaten and hence the correct dose received. In debilitated animals it may be possible to offer palatable medicines, suitable convalescent nutritional support or oral rehydration fluids through a syringe. For example, on initial presentation, syringe fed proprietary oral rehydration formulations can be useful for debilitated animals, or for abandoned nursing kittens before the introduction of a suitable milk replacer.

Injections, using a 25 G needle, can be given to suitably restrained squirrels. Subcutaneous injections can be given under the skin, either at the scruff over the neck or over the ribs on the dorsolateral thorax. Intramuscular injections can be given into the quadriceps but, because of the small available muscle mass, intramuscular drug administration may cause pain and muscle damage (Orr, 2002). Intramuscular administration, if unavoidable, should involve less than 0.2 ml being given at one site in red squirrels and less than 0.5 ml being given to the larger grey squirrels (Sainsbury, 2003). Intraperitoneal injections should only be performed in an anaesthetized animal or one that is well restrained in dorsal recumbency, as there is a risk of infection and organ puncture. Intravenous injections are difficult in squirrels and should be carried out in an anaesthetized animal (see 'Diagnostic techniques').

The dosages of therapeutic agents for use in squirrels can be inferred from data available for rats (Sainsbury, 2003). Examples of commonly used medications are given in Figure 13.13. When using potentiated sulphonamides, it is recommended to ensure that the animal is kept well hydrated (Ramsey, 2014). All antibiotics should also be used with care to prevent disruption to normal bacterial gut flora and reduce the risk of the development of diarrhoea and fatal enterotoxaemia, the risk of which is greater when antibiotics are given by the oral route (Carpenter, 2013). The use of proprietary formulations of probiotics (e.g. Avipro® Plus; Bio-Lapis) in conjunction with antibiotic therapy may be beneficial. Procaine penicillin and streptomycin medications have been reported to cause direct toxicity in mice and rats and should not be used (Orr, 2002; Carpenter, 2013; Ramsey, 2014).

Drug	Dose	Suggested route(s)	Frequency / use
Antibacterial drugs			
Enrofloxacin[a][b]	10 mg/kg	s.c., orally	q24h
Trimethoprim/ sulphonamide[c]	15–30 mg/kg	i.m., s.c., orally	q12h
Metronidazole[a][b]	20 mg/kg	s.c.	q24h
Antiparasitic drugs			
Permethrin (e.g. Xenex® Ultra Spot-On[d])	Using Xenex® Ultra Spot-On (744 mg permethrin per tube): 50–100 g BW 2 drops 100–200 g BW 3 drops 200–300 g BW 4 drops 300–400 g BW 6 drops Also see drug data sheet for more information	Using Xenex® Ultra Spot-On, topically on the skin between the shoulder blades at the back of the neck	Repeat if necessary at 2 weeks Do not use Xenex® Ultra Spot-On in animals less than 16 weeks of age
Ivermectin (e.g. Xeno 50-mini)	Using Xeno 50-mini (50 µg Ivermectin per pipette) Dose at 200–400 µg/kg: 50–100 g BW 6 drops 100–150 g BW 9 drops 150–200 g BW 12 drops 200–250 g BW 1 pipette 250–500 g BW 2 pipettes Also see drug data sheet for more information	Using Xeno 50-mini, topically on the skin between the shoulder blades at the back of the neck	Repeat at 2 and 4 weeks as necessary

13.13 Therapeutic agents commonly used in squirrels. The dosages have been extrapolated from data available for rats. BW = bodyweight; MU = mega unit. (continues)

(ᵃRamsey, 2014; ᵇOrr, 2002; ᶜCarpenter, 2013; ᵈWilks, 2008; ᵉRSNE, 2011a; ᶠV Butler, personal communication)

Drug	Dose	Suggested route(s)	Frequency / use
Antiparasitic drugs continued			
Fipronil (e.g. Frontline® spray)	Using Frontline® 0.25% cutaneous spray: Apply 3 ml/kg BW (lower end of dose range) Also see drug data sheet for more information	Topically Apply correct dose of spray to a gloved hand and then wipe over animal's body, taking care to avoid chilling	Repeat as necessary at 4 weeks
Toltrazuril [c] 2.5% solution (Baycox®)	10 mg/kg Note the 2.5% solution has a very low pH and should be diluted with equal parts of both water and propylene glycol (1:1:1), there is no need to dilute the 5% solution in this way	Orally	q24h for 3 days, off for 3 days, on for 3 days
Other drugs			
Interferon omega (Virbagen® Omega)	1 MU/kg[e]	s.c.	q24h for 3 consecutive days
	1 MU/squirrel or 2.5 MU/kg[f]	s.c.	This dose is to be repeated after 2–3 days

13.13 (continued) Therapeutic agents commonly used in squirrels. The dosages have been extrapolated from data available for rats. BW = bodyweight; MU = mega unit.

([a] Ramsey, 2014; [b] Orr, 2002; [c] Carpenter, 2013; [d] Wilks, 2008; [e] RSNE, 2011a; [f] V Butler, personal communication)

Management in captivity

Housing

Good husbandry provision depends on understanding the natural biology and behaviours of squirrels. Red and grey squirrels are arboreal (tree-living) rodents that are very agile and excellent climbers. All accommodation must be secure and indestructible as squirrels are fast and can easily gnaw through wood and plastic to escape. Housing should be located away from human activity, noise, domestic animals and out of drafts, but with sufficient ventilation. The type of housing should be appropriate for the age of the casualty squirrel and its health status.

Intensive care and restricted activity

Seriously debilitated squirrels need close monitoring. Narrow gauge wire cat carriers are useful for debilitated squirrels needing short-term intensive care (Bourne, 2002) and may be placed in a quiet warm room, off the floor. The carrier should be suitably lined and hiding places and appropriate bedding should be provided. Placing a light towel over the top of the wire carrier can help minimize visual disturbance and reduce stress. Care should be taken when using towels as bedding (see 'Capture, handling and transportation').

Short- to medium-term housing for hospitalization

Indoor stainless steel aviary type cages that provide adequate vertical height may be used. There should be access to natural daylight or alternatively appropriate full-spectrum lighting must be used. Offer a nest box, along with appropriate bedding (e.g. hay), and branches (that have not been chemically treated) for gnawing and climbing on. Branches from oak, beech, hazel, pine, apple and willow may be suitable, for example (Dutton, 2004). Stress can be reduced by providing visual barriers (e.g. by partially covering an area of the cage with a light towel/cloth). Handling should be kept to a minimum.

Long-term housing for rehabilitation and pre-release

Rehabilitation housing should be larger, more complex and should provide ample opportunity for exercise and foraging. Suitable outdoor aviary-style enclosures that offer protection from the weather, are escape-proof and secure against predators can be used. The wire mesh should be small and narrow enough to exclude rats. A choice of wooden nest boxes, with nesting materials, should be provided. There should be many leafy branches, as well as sturdy branches and logs with intact bark cover to encourage natural behaviours. A double-door entry system is recommended to prevent escapes.

Social grouping

In general, casualty squirrels should be housed singly when accommodated in hospitalization cages to avoid aggressive interactions and stress associated with competition or dominance, and should be kept out of sight of other squirrels (Sainsbury, 2003). Large outside, aviary-style enclosures with sufficient space may be used to accommodate mixed-sex pairs/trios of squirrels, but there must be at least one nest box provided for each squirrel (Sainsbury, 2003; Dutton, 2004) and introductions should be very closely monitored for signs of aggression. Overcrowding can lead to stress. Hand-reared squirrels should generally be housed singly, unless they arrive together in a sibling group. Sufficient nest boxes, at least one per squirrel, and space must be provided as the siblings grow and develop.

Behavioural problems

Free-living squirrels housed in captivity can develop stereotypies (e.g. repetitive to-and-fro movements, circling). To prevent these, limit the time the squirrel is kept in captivity and provide as large an enclosure as possible. The vertical dimension of the enclosure is of paramount importance, as well as providing areas for seclusion and a suitably complex, stimulating and enriched environment.

Diet

A varied balanced diet of a mixture of good quality foods that occur naturally in the wild should be fed to squirrels that are to be released. Many common items fed to captive squirrels have a low calcium:phosphorus ratio (e.g. nuts, maize and fruit), which if fed alone may predispose the animal to nutritional disorders, such as MBD (see 'Nutritional secondary hyperparathyroidism'). It has been suggested that peanuts and sunflower seeds should not be fed to squirrels (Stocker, 2005) as they are high in unsaturated fatty acids which can prevent the effective absorption of calcium (Sainsbury, 2003) and if fed exclusively, will increase the risk of MBD.

Basic items for a red squirrel diet may consist of hazelnuts, walnuts, pine cones containing seeds, and some vegetables, suitable fungi and fruits (Dutton, 2004). Squirrels are known to chew shed antlers in the wild, so access to antlers or cuttlefish bones should be offered as an additional source of calcium (Dutton, 2004; RSNE 2011b). Fresh shoots from native trees and bushes such as beech may be offered (Holm, 1987; Sainsbury, 2003), alongside a variety of vegetables and fruits (e.g. broccoli, spinach, apple, blackberries, pear). However, whilst apple has low calcium levels (Keymer and Hime, 1977), carrots contain an adequate calcium:phosphorus ratio (Sainsbury, 2003) so small pieces of carrot are particularly beneficial food items (Holm, 1987; RSNE 2011b). Hazelnuts should be offered in their shells. Parrot mix has been used as a base for squirrel food, supplemented with various vegetables, fruits and nuts (Sainsbury, 2003; Dutton, 2004). Brazil nuts have been documented as causing health problems (Dutton, 2004) and should be avoided, along with sweet dried foods (e.g. raisins, sultanas), which are low in calcium (Keymer and Hime, 1977; RSNE, 2011b).

A longer-term diet for squirrels should involve the gradual introduction of a proprietary rodent pellet (e.g. Mazuri® Rodent Pellets) that offers a complete diet and can be supplemented with small amounts of a selection of vegetables, fruits and nuts (Sainsbury, 2003; Stocker, 2005). At first there may be some resistance to the pellets, hence the introduction and dietary transition must be made slowly by mixing in with the initial diet, with careful monitoring (Sainsbury, 2003). Access to shed antlers or cuttlefish bones should be routinely provided. Food should be presented in a manner to encourage natural foraging behaviours.

Access to fresh drinking water should always be available and offered in a heavy dish (e.g. ceramic bowl), of appropriate size and depth, which cannot be easily knocked over. For free-living squirrels held in captivity, where stress may be a problem, the provision of appropriate proprietary probiotics may help minimize disturbance to the normal gut flora. If probiotic formulations are offered, a dish of normal fresh drinking water should always be offered as well.

Rearing of squirrel kittens

The approximate age of the squirrel should be established (Figure 13.14). Handling should be kept to a minimum to prevent imprinting and there should be a single carer to ensure consistency and help reduce stress. Basic hand-rearing principles are found in Chapter 8.

The milk of grey squirrels has a high dry matter and fat content, therefore carnivore milk replacers, which have a higher fat percentage, are suitable for hand-rearing squirrels (Sainsbury, 2003). Examples of milk replacers that have been used include Esbilac®, Cimicat™ (Sainsbury, 2003) and Royal Canin® Babycat Milk. Once started, avoid changing the type of milk replacer used. The milk replacer should be introduced gradually, after one or two initial feeds of a proprietary oral rehydration solution. Feeding frequency (see Chapter 8) depends on the age and health status of the squirrel, although when hand-rearing squirrels, feeds can generally be given at a

Characteristic	Description
Gestation period	38 days (red squirrel); 44 days (grey squirrel)[a]
Average litter size	3 kittens[a]
At birth	Blind, hairless, weigh approx. 10–15 g[b]
Age 14–21 days	Thin layer of hair[b]
Age 20–23 days (3 weeks)	Lower incisors erupt[b]
Age 28–35 days (4–5 weeks)	Responsive to sound[c], eyes start to open[b]
Age 5–6 weeks	Upper incisors erupt[c]
Age 42 days (6 weeks)	Increasingly active, begin to leave nest, but stay very close[c]
Age 45–49 days (7 weeks)	Start to eat solid foods and can climb[b] and may venture further from nest[c] Cheek teeth (permanent molars and deciduous premolars) erupt[d]
Age 10–12 weeks	Fully weaned[be]
Sexual maturity	9–11 months[c]

13.14 Reproductive and developmental characteristics of red and grey squirrels.
([a] Holm 1987; [b] Gurnell et al., 2012; [c] Bosch and Lurz, 2012; [d] Sainsbury et al. 2004; [e] Lurz et al., 2005)

suitable frequency from approximately 6am until approximately 11pm (Holm, 1987). Hand-reared juvenile squirrels should be fed slowly (to help avoid aspiration pneumonia) whilst being held in a horizontal position on a flat surface covered with a clean towel (Figure 13.15). The quantities fed will vary according to the age of the animal and also the individual (see Chapter 8). Overfeeding should be avoided as it may lead to lethargy, bloat or a nutritional diarrhoea. Oral rehydration fluids may be required in cases of diarrhoea, and possibly laboratory testing to rule out infectious causes. Strict hygiene is important.

Regularly, before and after each feed, the squirrel kitten should be stimulated to 'toilet' by gently stroking the anogenital area with warm, moistened cotton wool. This is especially important for kittens that still have closed eyes. Once the eyes have opened, continue to stimulate toileting until it is certain that the squirrel is urinating and

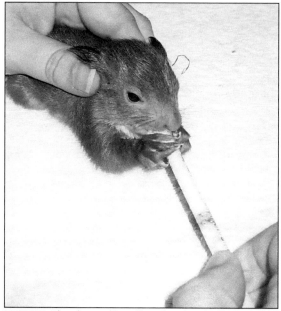

13.15 A hand-reared juvenile male red squirrel being fed using a 1 ml syringe. Note the horizontal position in which the squirrel is held on the towel.
(© T Blackett)

defecating on its own. Penis-sucking behaviour can occur in hand-reared sibling squirrels and if it occurs it may be necessary to separate the squirrels to prevent further trauma (Stocker, 2005).

Once the kitten's eyes have opened (at about 5 weeks of age), appropriate accommodation should include a few suitable branches for play and gnawing, as well as a hiding place/suitable nest box with bedding. As the squirrel grows and develops, the size and furnishings of the cage will need to be appropriately increased. Once fully weaned and independent, the squirrel can be kept in suitable outside rehabilitation accommodation until release. Access to shed antlers or cuttlefish bones should be routinely provided for all weaned juvenile and adult squirrels (see 'Diet').

When the squirrel kittens start nibbling on solids, food items such as rusks (Stocker, 2005) can be offered. Milk replacer still needs to be fed at an appropriate frequency, although the number of feeds should be gradually reduced as the squirrel starts weaning. Soft foods, such as some fruit, or small pieces of rusk soaked in milk replacer, can be initially offered at the start of weaning, followed by a varied and balanced diet, including a mixture of food items such as good quality dry puppy food (Stocker, 2005), carrot, suitable berries and fresh shoots (Holm, 1987), broccoli and shelled hazelnuts and walnuts. Offer as many different natural foods as possible (see 'Diet'). Proprietary rodent pellets should be introduced if the squirrel is to remain in captivity for any length of time. Peanuts and sunflower seeds should not be offered. Fresh clean drinking water should always be available. The frequency of milk feeds should reduce as the solid food intake increases, but bodyweight should be carefully monitored during the weaning process to ensure that the juvenile is eating solids and gaining weight.

Release

All releases of squirrels should be in compliance with national legislation (see 'Legal aspects' and Chapter 2).

To be released, a casualty squirrel must be fully recovered, healthy, physically fit and with no behavioural abnormalities (see Chapter 9). An appropriate assessment and health check should be performed and, with regard to red squirrel reintroduction projects, the necessary blood samples should be taken for disease screening (e.g. SQPV and adenovirus), prior to release.

Where permitted in accordance with national legislation, a squirrel that has only been in captivity for a short time should ideally be released in the same area that it was found as a casualty, away from roads, unless this area is unsuitable. In the UK, red squirrels should not be released into an area 'where grey squirrels are present and are not controlled' (UKRSG, 2004). Diurnal squirrels (including red and grey squirrels) should be released early in the morning and when the weather is advantageous. In the UK, the most ideal time for release may be between August and November, which is a natural time for squirrel dispersal and recruitment and when there should be good tree seed availability (Sainsbury, 2003).

It has been suggested that hand-reared squirrels can be released at 12–14 weeks of age, before imprinting occurs (Sainsbury, 2003). However, hand-reared squirrels must be fully weaned and independent before consideration for release and they must be soft-released. Soft-release (see Chapter 9) allows the squirrel to acclimatize. It is suitable for hand-reared animals, adults that have been in captivity for a long time and adults that cannot be released back into the area where they were found. Suitable housing should be constructed at the release site and it has been suggested that the animals are held in this accommodation for 2–4 weeks (Dutton, 2004; C Shuttleworth, personal communication).

Hard-release is appropriate for adults that have only been held in captivity for a short time, and only if they are to be released in the same area that they were found as casualties.

Small metal ear tags or subcutaneously implanted microchips may be used for post-release monitoring of rehabilitated squirrels. Radio tracking of radio-collared squirrels has also been undertaken for study and research purposes (Bosch and Lurz, 2012). Marking red squirrels prior to release may require a licence, so it is recommended to first seek advice from local government agencies and national licensing bodies (see 'Legal aspects' and Appendix 1).

Legal aspects

See Chapter 2 for general legislation covering squirrels.

Regulated by the Destructive Imported Animals Act 1932 and the 1937 Grey Squirrel (Prohibition of Importation and Keeping) Order, grey squirrels may only be kept in captivity with a licence, meaning that the housing of grey squirrels even if only temporarily, for example if they are injured and receiving treatment, requires a licence; it is an offence under the Wildlife and Countryside Act 1981 (WCA) to release a grey squirrel into the wild without a licence (Natural England, 2008; Gurnell et al., 2009). However, transporting trapped grey squirrels to a veterinary surgery for euthanasia on welfare grounds does not require a licence. Current guidance can be obtained by contacting local government departments.

Licences may be issued for the release of grey squirrels that are rehabilitated casualties taken from the wild for veterinary treatment and care, and such rehabilitated squirrels that are licensed for release must be released at the location of their capture or within 1 km of it (Natural England, 2008). In areas where there are, or may be, red squirrels, licences for the release of grey squirrels will not be issued (Natural England, 2008). The reader is referred to devolved government departments (Natural England, Scottish Natural Heritage, National Resources Wales, Department of the Environment Northern Ireland/Northern Ireland Environment Agency; see Appendix 1) for current guidance, licensing requirements and for information regarding licence applications.

Red squirrels are listed on Appendix III – Bern Convention for Conservation of European Wildlife and Natural Habitats. Red squirrels are fully protected under the WCA; it is an offence to capture, injure or kill them, or disturb, damage or destroy their shelters, dreys or breeding places. It is also an offence to capture free-living red squirrels using certain methods without a licence. However, there is provision within the WCA to allow the capture from the wild of casualty red squirrels to prevent suffering. This provision allows casualty red squirrels to be 'taken' or captured from the wild by hand (Boardman, 2002) for veterinary treatment and care prior to their release, or for euthanasia as a consequence of injuries that would prevent the animal recovering, without a licence. If it is necessary to use a restricted method for capture of the casualty, such as a live trap or nets, a licence from the relevant government department (e.g. NE, SNH, NRW, DOENI/NIEA) is required (Boardman, 2002).

In Britain, licences are required to retain and permanently keep free-living red squirrels in captivity, although captive red squirrels that have been 'legally imported or are captive bred may be sold or possessed without a licence' (UKRSG, 2004). Licences from the relevant government agencies are required for any study or survey that would disturb or interfere with red squirrels or their dreys; licences are needed to capture, handle and trap red squirrels for research and conservation purposes.

In Scotland, the Nature Conservation (Scotland) Act 2004 and Wildlife and Natural Environment (Scotland) Bill 2011 afford the red squirrel additional protection and in Northern Ireland, the applicable legislation is the Wildlife (Northern Ireland) Order 1985 and the Wildlife and Natural Environment Act 2011.

On Jersey, Channel Islands, the red squirrel is protected under the Conservation of Wildlife (Jersey) Law 2000. This Law also prohibits the importation and release of non-native species (e.g. grey squirrels). Contact the local government department (i.e. States of Jersey Environment Department) for licensing requirements and for information regarding licence applications.

Acknowledgements

The author would like to express her sincere gratitude to Vic Simpson for his kind support and advice regarding squirrel pathology over the years and for his helpful comments on an earlier draft of this chapter and Dr Craig Shuttleworth for his helpful comments on an earlier draft of this text. The author would also like to express her sincere thanks to Professor Anna Meredith for the use of the SQPV and squirrel leprosy images and for the use of the red squirrel biochemistry reference intervals.

References and further reading

American Veterinary Medical Association (2013) *AVMA Guidelines for the Euthanasia of Animals: 2013 edition*. www.avma.org/KB/Policies/Documents/euthanasia.pdf

Boardman S (2002) Wildlife Casualty Legislation. In: *Wildlife: first aid and care, Wildpro – the electronic encyclopaedia and library for wildlife*. http://wildpro.twycrosszoo.org/

Bosch S and Lurz PWW (2012) *The Eurasian Red Squirrel*. Westrap Wissenschaften, Germany

Bourne D (2002) Accommodation of casualty squirrels. In: *Wildlife: first aid and care, Wildpro – the electronic encyclopaedia and library for wildlife*. http://wildpro.twycrosszoo.org/

Brown SA and Rosenthal KL (1997) *Self assessment colour review of small mammals*. Manson Publishing Ltd, London

Carpenter JW (2013) *Exotic Animal Formulary, 4th edn*. WB Saunders Company, Pennsylvania

Carroll B, Russell P, Gurnell J, Nettleton P and Sainsbury AW (2009) Epidemics of squirrel poxvirus disease in red squirrels (*Sciurus vulgaris*): temporal and spatial findings. *Epidemiology and Infection* **137**, 247–265

Collins LM, Warnock ND, Tosh DG et al. (2014) Squirrelpox virus: assessing prevalence, transmission and environmental degradation. *PloS One* DOI: 10.1371/journal.pone.0089521

Dale T, Begin M, White S and Chantrey J (2010) Epidemiology of squirrelpox virus in the Eurasian red squirrel (*Sciurus vulgaris*) in the Merseyside area. In: *Proceedings of Disease Invasion, Impacts on Biodiversity and Human Health*, Joint ZSL and Royal Society Symposium, ZSL, London

Davidson WR and Calpin JP (1976) *Hepatozoon griseisciuri* infection in gray squirrels of the southern United States. *Journal of Wildlife Diseases* **12**, 72–76

Dipineto L, Gargiulo A, Cuomo A et al. (2009) *Campylobacter jejuni* in the red squirrel (*Sciurus vulgaris*) population of Southern Italy. *Veterinary Journal* **179**, 149–150

Duff JP, Haley P, Wood R and Higgins RJ (2010) Causes of red squirrel (*Sciurus vulgaris*) mortality in England. *Veterinary Record* **167**, 461

Duff JP, Higgins R and Farrelly S (2007) Enteric adenovirus infection in a red squirrel (*Sciurus vulgaris*). *Veterinary Record* **160**, 384

Dutton JCF (2004) *The Red Squirrel, redressing the wrong*. European Squirrel Initiative, Suffolk

Edwards FB (1962) Red squirrel disease. *Veterinary Record* **74**, 739–741

Everest DJ, Butler H, Blackett T, Simpson VR and Shuttleworth CM (2013) Adenovirus infection in red squirrels in areas free from grey squirrels. *Veterinary Record* **173**, 199

Everest DJ, Dastjerdi A, Gurrala R et al. (2009a) Rotavirus detected in red squirrels from Scotland. *Veterinary Record* **165**, 450

Everest DJ, Duff JP and Higgins RJ (2011) Wildlife: Rotavirus in a wild English red squirrel (*Sciurus vulgaris*) identified by electron microscopy. *Veterinary Record* **169**, 6

Everest DJ, Grierson SS, Stidworthy MF and Shuttleworth CM (2009b) PCR detection of adenovirus in grey squirrels on Anglesey. *Veterinary Record* **165**, 482

Everest DJ, Shuttleworth CM, Grierson SS et al. (2012) Systematic assessment of the impact of adenovirus infection on a captive reintroduction project for red squirrels (*Sciurus vulgaris*). *Veterinary Record* **171**, 176

Everest DJ, Stidworthy MF, Milne EM et al. (2010) Retrospective detection by negative contrast electron microscopy of faecal viral particles in free-living wild red squirrels (*Sciurus vulgaris*) with suspected enteropathy in Great Britain. *Veterinary Record* **167**, 26

Everest, DJ, Stidworthy MF and Shuttleworth C (2008) Adenovirus associated deaths in red squirrels on Anglesey. *Veterinary Record* **163**, 430

Flecknell P (1996) Anaesthesia and analgesia for rodents and rabbits. In: *Handbook of Rodent and Rabbit Medicine*, ed. K Laber-Laird, MM Swindle and P Flecknell, pp. 219–238. Pergamon, Oxford

Greenwood AG and Sanchez S (2002) Serological evidence of murine pathogens on wild grey squirrels (*Sciurus carolinensis*) in North Wales. *The Veterinary Record* **150**, 543–546

Gurnell J, Lurz P, McDonald R and Pepper H (2009) *Practical techniques for surveying and monitoring squirrels practice note*. Forestry Commission. www.forestresearch.gov.uk

Gurnell J, Lurz P and Wauters L (2012) *Squirrels*. Mammal Society, Southampton, UK.

Holm J (1987) *Squirrels*. Whittet Books, London

Jokelainen P and Nylund M (2012) Acute fatal toxoplasmosis in three Eurasian red squirrels (*Sciurus vulgaris*) caused by Genotype II of *Toxoplasma gondii*. *Journal of Wildlife Diseases* **48(2)**, 454–457

Joslin JO (2009) Blood collection techniques in exotic small mammals. *Journal of Exotic Pet Medicine* **22(2)**, 117–139

Kenward RE and Holm JL (1993) On the replacement of the red squirrel in Britain: a phytotoxic explanation. *Proceedings of the Royal Society, Biological Sciences* **251(1332)**, 187–94

Keymer IF (1983) Diseases of squirrels in Britain. *Mammal Review* **13(2–4)**, 155–158

Keymer IF and Hime JM (1977) Nutritional osteodystrophy in a free living red squirrel (*Sciurus vulgaris*). *Veterinary Record* **100**, 31

Koprowski (1994). Mammalian species – *Sciurus carolinensis*. *The American Society of Mammalogists* **480**, 1–9

LaRose JP, Meredith AL, Everest DJ et al. (2010). Epidemiological and post mortem findings in 262 red squirrels (*Sciurus vulgaris*) in Scotland 2005 to 2009. *Veterinary Record* **167(8)**, 297–302

Lurz PWW, Gurnell J, Magris L (2005) *Sciurus vulgaris*. American Society of Mammalogists **769**, 1–10

Martínez-Jiménez D, Graham D, Couper D et al. (2011) Epizootiology and pathologic findings associated with a newly described adenovirus in the red squirrel, *Sciurus vulgaris*. *Journal of Wildlife Diseases* **47(2)**, 442–454

Meredith A (2015) *BSAVA Small Animal Formulary, 9th edition – Part B: Exotic Pets*. BSAVA Publications, Gloucester

Meredith A, Del-Pozo J, Stevenson K et al. (2014) Mycobacterial dermatitis of red squirrels in Scotland: a case series. In: *Proceedings of European Wildlife Disease Association (EWDA) Conference: Conservation Medicine*, 25–29th August 2014, Edinburgh, Scotland

Miller EA (2000) *Minimum standards for wildlife rehabilitation, 3rd edn*. National Wildlife Rehabilitators Association, Minnesota

Natural England (2008) *Wildlife Management & Licensing: Licensing the release of non-native species and species listed in Schedule 9 of the Wildlife & Countryside Act 1981, with particular reference to the Grey Squirrel*. www.gov.uk/government/publications/non-native-species-apply-for-a-licence-to-release-them

Orr HE (2002) Rats and mice. In: *BSAVA Manual of Exotic Pets, 4th edn*, ed. A Meredith and S Redrobe, pp. 13–25. BSAVA Publications, Gloucester

Peters M, Vidovszky MZ, Harrach B et al. (2011) Squirrel adenovirus type 1 in red squirrels (*Sciurus vulgaris*) in Germany. *Veterinary Record* **169**, 182

Ramsey I (2014) *BSAVA Small Animal Formulary, 8th edn*. BSAVA publications, Gloucester

Richardson C and Flecknell P (2009) Rodents: anaesthesia and analgesia. In: *BSAVA Manual of Rodents and Ferrets*, ed. E Keeble and A Meredith, pp. 63–71. BSAVA Publications, Gloucester

Romeo C, Pisanu B, Ferrari N et al. (2013) Macroparasite community of the Eurasian red squirrel (*Sciurus vulgaris*): poor species richness and diversity. *Parasitology Research* **112(10)**, 3527–3536

RSNE (2011a) RSNE Advice Note – *Squirrel poxvirus fact sheet for vets*. Red Squirrels Northern England (RSNE), Carlisle. www.rsne.org.uk

RSNE (2011b) RSNE Advice Note – *Supplementary feeding red squirrels* Northern England (RSNE). www.rsne.org.uk

Sainsbury AW (2003) Squirrels. In: *BSAVA Manual of Wildlife Casualties, 1st edn*, ed. E Mullineaux, D Best and JE Cooper, pp. 66–74. BSAVA Publications, Gloucester

Sainsbury AW, Adair B, Graham D *et al.* (2001) Isolation of a novel adenovirus associated with splenitis, diarrhoea, and mortality in translocated red squirrels, *Sciurus vulgaris*. *Erkrankung der Zootiere* **40**, 265–270

Sainsbury AW, Deaville R, Lawson B *et al.* (2008) Poxviral disease in red squirrels *Sciurus vulgaris* in the UK: spatial and temporal trends of an emerging threat. *Ecohealth* **5(3)**, 305–316

Sainsbury AW and Gurnell J (1995) An investigation into the health and welfare of red squirrels, *Sciurus vulgaris*, involved in reintroduction studies. *The Veterinary Record* **137**, 367–370

Sainsbury AW, Kountouri A, Duboulay G and Kertesz P (2004). Oral disease in free living red squirrels (*Sciurus vulgaris*) in the United Kingdom. *Journal of Wildlife Diseases* **40(2)**, 185–196

Sainsbury AW, Nettleton P and Gurnell J (1997) Recent developments in the study of parapoxvirus in red and grey squirrels. In: *Conservation of red squirrels*, *S vulgaris* L., ed. J Gurnell and PWW Lurz, pp. 105–108. PTES, London

Simpson S, Blampied N, Peniche G *et al.* (2013a) Genetic structure of introduced populations: 120-year-old DNA footprint of historic introduction in an insular small mammal population. *Ecology and Evolution* **3(3)**, 614–628

Simpson VR (2008) Wildlife as reservoirs of zoonotic diseases in the UK. *In Practice* **30**, 486–493

Simpson VR, Birtles RJ, Bown KJ *et al.* (2006) Hepatozoon species infection in wild red squirrels (*Sciurus vulgaris*) on the Isle of Wight. *Veterinary Record* **159**, 202–205

Simpson VR, Davison NJ, Hudson L, Enright M and Whatmore AM (2010b) *Staphylococcus aureus* ST49 infection in red squirrels. *Veterinary Record* **167**, 69

Simpson VR, Davison NJ, Kearns AM *et al.* (2013b) Association of a lukM-positive clone of *Staphylococcus aureus* with fatal exudative dermatitis in red squirrels (*Sciurus vulgaris*). *Veterinary Microbiology* **162**, 987–991

Simpson VR, Hargreaves J, Butler HM, Davison NJ and Everest DJ (2013c) Causes of mortality and pathological lesions observed post-mortem in red squirrels (*Sciurus vulgaris*) in Great Britain. *BioMedCentral Veterinary Research* **9**, 229

Simpson VR, Hargreaves J, Everest DJ *et al.* (2010a) Mortality in red squirrels (*Sciurus vulgaris*) associated with exudative dermatitis. *Veterinary Record* **167**, 59–62

Stocker L (2005) *Practical Wildlife Care, 2nd edn*. Blackwell Publishing Ltd, Oxford

UK Red Squirrel Group (UKRSG) (2004) *Advice Note: Release of red squirrels Sciurus vulgaris into the wild in Britain*. UK Red Squirrel Group, www.forestry.gov.uk/fr/ukrsg

Vizoso AD, Vizoso NR and Hay R (1964) Isolation of a virus resembling encephalomyocarditis from a red squirrel. *Nature* **201**, 849–850

VLA Disease Surveillance Report (2010) Fasciolosis commonly diagnosed in cattle and sheep. *Veterinary Record* **166**, 514–517

Wauters LA and Dhondt AA (1989) Body weight, longevity and reproductive success in red squirrels (*Sciurus vulgaris*). *Journal of Animal Ecology* **58**, 637–651

Wilks K (2008) Red squirrels and the parapoxvirus. *Veterinary Nursing Journal* **23(10)**, 41–42

Specialist organizations and useful contacts

See also Appendix 1 for general contacts

Red Squirrel Survival Trust
Ouston Tower House, Ouston, Whitfield,
Hexham, Northumberland NE47 8DG
Tel: 01434 345 757
www.rsst.org.uk

Red Squirrels Northern England (RSNE)
c/o Northumberland Wildlife Trust,
Garden House, St Nicholas Park,
Jubilee Road, Gosforth, Newcastle upon Tyne NE3 3XT
Tel: 0191 284 6884
www.rsne.org.uk

UK Red Squirrel Group
www.forestry.gov.uk/fr/ukrsg

Chapter 14

Other insectivores and rodents

Richard Saunders

The species included in this chapter (Figure 14.1) are extremely common in terms of numbers but are presented to wildlife centres relatively infrequently: out of 16,639 wild animal admissions to four Royal Society for the Prevention of Cruelty to Animals (RSPCA) wildlife centres in England in 2011, 204 individuals of the species covered in this chapter were admitted, of which 48% were wood mice (A Grogan, personal communication; Grogan and Kelly, 2013). This is probably for the following reasons:

- Their small size makes them less noticeable
- They are usually nocturnal or crepuscular and/or they live underground
- Most diseases or injuries prove rapidly fatal in these species
- They are elusive and can be difficult to catch
- Many people perceive some of the species to be vermin and would not present them for treatment.

These species, however, include many that are under threat or relatively rare due to habitat destruction or fragmentation (e.g. water vole (*Arvicola terrestris*), common dormouse (*Muscardinus avellanarius*)) or are being actively reintroduced into areas of the UK in small numbers (e.g. common dormouse). Other more numerous species are important indicators of environmental change (e.g. mice and voles) and are themselves an important food source for predatory species.

Reasons for admission

The main cause of injury and death in these species is predation. For example, of a year's production of field voles (*Microtus agrestis*), 22% are taken by weasels (*Mustela nivalis*) and 13% by red foxes (*Vulpes vulpes*). They are also the preferred prey of barn owls (*Tyto alba*), especially in winter (The Mammal Society, 2001a), and fluctuations in vole populations can have effects on predator health (Appleby *et al.*, 1999). Other predators include mink (*Mustela (Neovison) vison*), otters (*Lutra lutra*) and other mustelids, herons (Ardeidae), other owl species (Strigiformes), kestrels (*Falco tinnunculus*), buzzards (*Buteo buteo*), shrikes (Laniidae), corvids (Corvidae), predatory reptiles and fish. Victims of these predators are unlikely to be rescued and presented for treatment.

It is estimated that cats kill or bring into the house up to 200 million small mammals per year in Great Britain, of which 65% are rodents and 19% are terrestrial insectivores (Woods *et al.*, 2003). Cats are 'major predators' of some species, with 17% of their prey being wood mice (*Apodemus sylvaticus*) and 14% bank voles (*Myodes glareolus*) (Churcher and Lawton, 1987). In an urban area with a cat population density of 229/km^2, similar prey preferences were recorded (wood mice comprised 62% of their dead prey and 72% of their live prey) (Baker *et al.*, 2005). These figures have been disputed by Nelson (2001) and Tabor

Order and suborder	Family and subfamily	Species	Common name
Order Insectivora	Family Talpidae (moles and desmans)	*Talpa europaea*	European mole
	Family Soricidae (shrews)	*Sorex minutus* *Sorex araneus* *Neomys fodiens* *Crocidura suaveolens** *Crocidura russula**	Pygmy shrew Common shrew Water shrew Lesser white-toothed shrew Greater white-toothed shrew
Order Rodentia Suborder Myomorpha	Family Muridae Subfamily Microtinae (voles and lemmings) Subfamily Murinae (rats and mice)	*Myodes glareolus* *Arvicola terrestris* *Microtus agrestis* *Microtus arvalis** *Rattus norvegicus* *Rattus rattus* *Mus musculus* *Micromys minutus* *Apodemus sylvaticus* *Apodemus flavicollis*	Bank vole Water vole Field or short-tailed vole Common vole Common or brown rat Ship or black rat House mouse Harvest mouse Wood mouse Yellow-necked mouse
	Family Gliridae (dormice)	*Muscardinus avellanarius* *Myoxus (Glis) glis*	Common dormouse Edible or fat dormouse
Suborder Sciuromorpha	Family Castoridae (beavers)	*Castor fiber*	European beaver

14.1 Taxonomy of British insectivores and rodents discussed in this chapter (*Channel Islands and Isles of Scilly only).

(2001), with the latter claiming that the total was nearer 20 million mammals, but there is no doubt that the numbers are significant. Out of 6.3–22.3 billion cat-predated mammals in the US, the majority are killed by unowned cats (Loss *et al.*, 2013). Predation is almost halved in bell-wearing cats (Ruxton *et al.*, 2002). Whilst some of these 'catted' prey are apparently undamaged and are immediately released, many are injured and some are presented for treatment.

Disturbance of nests by predators also leads to orphaned small mammals being discovered by the public. For example, the nests of common dormice, especially those that are near the ground, can be disturbed and the whole litter may be brought in by cats. Juvenile or hibernating dormice are often found after storms: the entire nest might be found blown out of a tree. Both common and edible dormice (*Myoxus (Glis) glis*) are accidentally disturbed in places such as lofts, haystacks, fruit stores and hedges, especially during hibernation (H Ryan, personal communication).

Juvenile animals have a peak incidence of injuries when dispersing from the nest environment. They may also suffer maladaptation problems from choosing unsuitable environments, such as moles (*Talpa europaea*) selecting soil that is too dry or too waterlogged (Corbet and Harris, 1991).

Road traffic accidents are not infrequent (L Garland, personal communication) but such small animals rarely survive to require treatment. Deliberate, accidental or malicious poisoning of most of these species usually results in rapid death (The Mammal Society, 2001a) or the animal dying below ground, so poisoning victims are rarely encountered, though total populations may be adversely affected (Shore *et al.*, 1997). A further hazard is the use of 'glue' traps, which can indiscriminately entrap small rodents and insectivores (Stocker, 2005).

Ecology, biology, anatomy and physiology

Insectivores

The characteristics and biological parameters of the insectivores (moles and shrews) are outlined in Figures 14.2, 14.3 and 14.4.

Moles

The European mole (see Figure 14.2a) is unpopular with groundsmen, gardeners and some farmers, due to its production of soil spoil heaps (molehills). There is also

Parameter	Mole (*Talpa europaea*)
Distribution	Mainland Britain, but not Ireland or Scottish islands
Habitat	Arable, pasture, grassland, woodland (mainly deciduous), gardens, golf courses; avoid very heavy clay and acidic soils or areas liable to waterlogging
Active periods	Day and night, for periods of 4–4.5h, interspersed with sleep periods of 3–4h No hibernation
Food requirements per day (approx. % of bodyweight)	50%
Appearance	Coat black, velvety with coarse and fine hairs; moult three times a year Long tapering mobile snout covered in vibrissae Small deep-set eyes, no external pinnae Short furred tail held erect Broad forelimbs, muscular shoulders, long strong claws; three antebrachial bones, elongated scapula Testes in sac near tail base
Weight	Male <120 g spring/summer, <95 g autumn/winter Female <110 g spring/summer, <75 g autumn/winter
Size	Male <140 mm Female <130 mm
No. of nipples	4 pairs
Senses	Eyesight poor, hearing only moderate, olfactory senses good Main method of food detection via touch and sensitivity to vibration (Eimers organs on vibrissae)
Dentition	$2 \times \left\{ I\frac{3}{3} \ C\frac{1}{1} \ P\frac{4}{4} \ M\frac{3}{3} \right\} = 44$
Breeding season	March–May
Oestrus	Cycle 3–4 days, duration <24h
Gestation	28–30 days
No. of litters per year	Usually 1
Litter size	2–7 (usually 3–4)
Birthweight	3.5 g
Development of young	Furred at 14 days Weigh 60 g at 3 weeks Eyes open 22 days Leave nest at 35 days Share adult tunnels until 10 weeks
Age at weaning	28–35 days
Lifespan	2.5–3 years

14.3 Characteristics and biological parameters of moles.

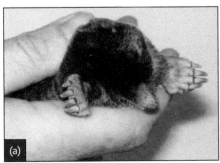
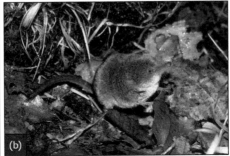
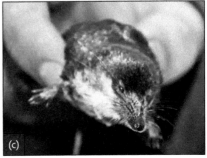

14.2 (a) Mole. (b) Pygmy shrew. (c) Water shrew. It is best practice to wear gloves when handling moles and shrews.
(a, © Richard Saunders; b, Courtesy of Andy Purcell/Conservation Education Consultants, © CEC; c, Courtesy of Lorcan Adrian)

Parameter	Water shrew (*Neomys fodiens*)	Pygmy shrew (*Sorex minutus*)	Common shrew (*Sorex araneus*)	White-toothed shrews (WTS) (*Crocidura* spp.)
Distribution	Sporadically throughout Britain; widespread but not numerous	Mainland Britain, fairly common and widely distributed; only shrew native to Ireland	Lowland mainland Britain, but not in Ireland	Isles of Scilly and Channel Islands only: Sark, Jersey; greater WTS on Alderney, Guernsey, Herm
Habitat	Close to water, living in tunnels along water's edge	Mainly in wooded areas (similar habitats to common shrew)	Rough pasture, woods, hedgerows, dunes, marshes	Wide variety but fairly dry, well vegetated
Active periods	Alternate between periods of activity and rest, approx. every 2–3h. No hibernation	Alternate between periods of activity and rest, approx. every 2–3h. No hibernation	Alternate between periods of activity and rest, approx. every 2–3h. No hibernation	Alternate between periods of activity and rest, approx. every 2–3h. No hibernation
Food requirements per day (approx. % of bodyweight)	Up to 50%	Over 100%	Up to 70%	Up to 55%
Appearance	Fur dark brown/black dorsally (looks silvery in water), silver-grey underside, with sharp demarcation between the two; white patch above eyes; long hairs on toes; hairs on underside of tail form a keel. Fur often short and velvety. Long pointed snouts, small pointed teeth	Fur pale brown on dorsal body, paler underside, fairly sharp dividing line between the two; no eye patch; short hairs fringe toes. Tail is thicker and hairier than common shrew, snout thicker and longer. Skull domed. Fur often short and velvety. Long pointed snouts, small pointed teeth	Fur dark brown dorsally, paler sides and grey-white belly fairly clearly demarcated; no eye patch; short hairs fringe toes. Ears short, covered in fur. Fur often short and velvety. Long pointed snouts, small pointed teeth	Fur reddish-brown. Large ears. Fur often short and velvety. Long pointed snouts, small pointed teeth
Weight	9–16 g	2.5–5 g	7–10 g	Lesser WTS 3–7 g. Greater WTS 4.5–14.5 g
Size	90 mm (+ 60 mm tail)	40–58 mm (+ 40 mm tail)	48–85 mm (+ 24–55 mm tail)	Lesser WTS 50–75 mm (+ 24–44 mm tail). Greater WTS 60–90 mm (+ 33–46 mm tail)
No. of nipples	5 pairs	3 pairs	3 pairs	3 pairs
Senses	Eyesight poor. Prey located by hearing, touch and smell	Eyesight poor. Prey located by hearing, touch and smell	Eyesight poor. Prey located by hearing, touch and smell	Eyesight poor. Prey located by hearing, touch and smell
Dentition	$2 \times \left\{ I\frac{3}{2}\ C\frac{1}{0}\ P\frac{2}{1}\ M\frac{3}{3} \right\} = 30$	$2 \times \left\{ I\frac{3}{1}\ C\frac{1}{1}\ P\frac{3}{1}\ M\frac{3}{3} \right\} = 32$	$2 \times \left\{ I\frac{3}{1}\ C\frac{1}{1}\ P\frac{3}{1}\ M\frac{3}{3} \right\} = 32$	$2 \times \left\{ I\frac{3}{1}\ C\frac{1}{0}\ P\frac{1}{2}\ M\frac{3}{3} \right\} = 28$
Breeding season	March–August	April–October	April–September	March–September
Oestrus	Seasonally polyoestrous. Post-partum oestrus seen	Lactational anoestrus sometimes seen	Post-partum oestrus (<24h) after first litter; later extended by lactation	Polyoestrous, post-partum oestrus; no delayed implantation reported
Gestation	20–24 days	20–21 days	13–19 days	Lesser WTS 24–32 days. Greater WTS 27–33 days
No. of litters per year	2–3	2–3	2–3	Lesser WTS 3–4. Greater WTS multiple
Litter size	3–9	4–7	5–7	Lesser WTS 1–6 (mean 3). Greater WTS 3–11 (mean 3–4)
Birthweight	<1 g	0.25 g	0.5 g	Lesser WTS 0.5–1 g. Greater WTS 0.8–1 g
Development of young	Born naked and blind. Dorsal pigments develop at 4 days. Teeth start to erupt at 10 days. Fur develops at 11 days. First leave nest at 23–25 days	Born naked and blind	Born naked and blind. Soft grey fur at 9 days. Teeth red-tipped 11 days. Weigh 5–7 g by 14 days. Leave nest at 18 days	Born naked and blind. Fur starts growing 7–9 days; fully furred 16 days
Age at weaning	21–25 days	22–25 days	22–25 days	Lesser WTS 17–22 days. Greater WTS 20–22 days
Lifespan	<19 months	<1 year	<1 year	18 months

14.4 Characteristics and biological parameters of shrews.

potential for soil from molehills to contaminate silage production, which may contribute to listeriosis in livestock, and digging by moles raises stones to the surface, which can damage machinery. Molehills covering 7% of the surface area of a single field have been recorded (MacDonald, 1995). Molehills are more common in the spring, when males are looking for females, or in times of food scarcity. Moles may legally be killed by approved traps and gases placed in mole runs but, since 2006, strychnine has no longer been legally permitted for mole control (see 'Legal aspects' and Chapter 2).

Moles are important aerators of soil and also eat large numbers of potentially harmful insect larvae (e.g. wireworms (*Agriotes* spp.)). The tunnel systems form a food trap, which the mole patrols. Moles store food by killing and burying it when plentiful; when food is scarce, the tunnel system is extended in area and the moles tunnel deeper after earthworms (*Lumbricus terrestris*), a major component of their diet. As an alternative to lethal mole control, the number of molehills can be decreased by encouraging increased earthworm numbers – for example, by not liming soil and by encouraging herb-rich swards (Edwards *et al.*, 1999). Reducing the numbers of earthworms and other invertebrates in the soil is another control strategy, as is fencing, which is generally impractical for large areas.

Moles are born naked and blind in a spherical underground nest ('fortress') with vegetation for nesting material. There is no male parental care.

Shrews

There are two broad groups of shrews (see Figure 14.4):

- Red-toothed shrews (*Sorex* and *Neomys* spp.) all have red-tipped teeth, due to iron deposition in the enamel. This group includes the pygmy shrew (*S. minutus*; see Figure 14.2b), common shrew (*S. araneus*) and water shrew (*Neomys fodiens*; see Figure 14.2c)
- White-toothed shrews (*Crocidura* spp.) have no red tips to the teeth.

In areas where one shrew species coexists with other shrew species, the different species are rarely found together at the same time. The common shrew is the second most common mammal in Britain, with an estimated population of 41 million. Pygmy shrews are the smallest mammals in Britain.

Bodies of shrews are frequently found inside discarded bottles, often in large numbers, as one corpse can attract others. They are unpalatable to predators because of their sebaceous skin secretions; thus they are rarely eaten once caught, especially by mammalian predators.

Shrews have a high metabolic rate and must feed regularly, consuming a high percentage of their bodyweight in food daily; even more food is required during lactation. Their prey contains large amounts of water and indigestible chitin. White-toothed shrews add some plant material to the typical insectivore diet of shrews. The bodyweight of shrews varies markedly with season (see Figure 14.4); this is not due solely to food availability, as it applies also to captive shrews.

Shrews are highly territorial, especially the males, and are generally solitary; the white-toothed shrews (*Crocidura suaveolens* and *C. russula*) are solitary but not as aggressive as other species. Shrew territories are marked with sebaceous scent glands and faeces. They are vocal animals, making a series of high shrill squeaks. All species can swim but only the water shrew hunts in water; it swims and dives well.

Only approximately 25% of the juvenile shrew population survive the winter to breed the following spring. Adult shrews usually die in the autumn after their breeding season; only water shrews, which can live for up to 19 months, breed for a second year.

Rodents
Voles

Characteristics and biological parameters of voles are given in Figures 14.5 and 14.6. Voles, which are typically blunt-faced with small eyes, are amongst the most prevalent of British mammals, though the water vole (Figure 14.5c) is relatively scarce and is rapidly declining due to loss and degradation of habitat, pollution and also predation by mink. Water voles swim and dive well; they dive into water if danger threatens and always have at least one underwater burrow entrance.

Lacking the shrews' noxious secretions, voles are eaten by many predators – including stoats (*Mustela erminea*), weasels, polecats (*Mustela putorius*), pine martens (*Martes martes*), wildcats, badgers, foxes, herons, kestrels, buzzards, eagles, harriers and owls. They are commonly brought in by domestic cats, alive or dead. The field or short-tailed vole (Figure 14.5b) is the most common British mammal, with an estimated population of 75 million, but is subject to population fluctuations on a cycle of 3–5 years.

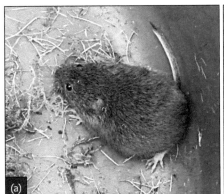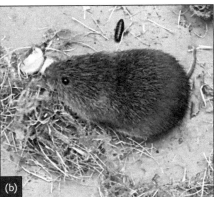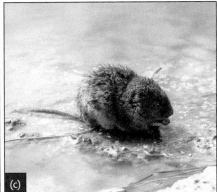

14.5 (a) Bank vole. (b) Field or short-tailed vole. (c) Water vole.
(ab, Courtesy of Kate Long; c, Courtesy of Andy Purcell/Conservation Education Consultants, © CEC)

Parameter	Bank vole (*Myodes glareolus*)	Field or short-tailed vole [a] (*Microtus agrestis*)	Water vole (*Arvicola terrestris*)
Distribution	Mainland Britain and coastal islands	Widespread mainland Britain; absent Ireland, Scilly Isles and northern Scotland	England, Wales, and southern Scotland; absent Ireland
Habitat	Woodland, moist deforested areas, grassland, gardens, hedges	Grassland (creates runs in grass)	Near water; at least one burrow entrance under water
Active periods	Summer day and night Winter mainly diurnal	Cycles (2–2.5 h) of rest and activity; peak activity dawn and dusk More nocturnal summer; more diurnal winter	Active every 2–4 h and for longer in the day than at night Rarely outside in winter
Diet	Leaves, fruits, seeds, fungi, bark, berries	Predominantly grass	Waterside vegetation, 'lawns' of closely cropped grass surrounding burrow entrances; also loose aquatic weeds
Appearance	Fur reddish-brown; blunt muzzle, small ears	Fur grey-brown; very short tail	Fur rich dark brown, occasionally black
Male weight	20–25 g	37 g (20–40 g)	150–300 g
Female weight	15–20 g	30 g (20–40 g)	150–300 g
Size (including tail)	100–110 mm (+ 35–70 mm tail)	100–120 mm (+ 25–44 mm tail)	180–220 mm (+ 55–70 mm tail)
Nipples	4 pairs	4 pairs	4 pairs
Breeding season	April–Sept; can also breed in winter	April–Sept	Spring/summer, starting earliest in warmer years
Oestrus	Induced ovulator	Induced ovulator	Induced ovulator
Gestation	17–22 days	18–20 days	20–22 days
No. of litters per year	Multiple (at least 4)	5–6	1–4
Litter size	3–5	4–6	4–6
Birthweight	2 g (naked and blind)	2 g (naked and blind)	5 g (naked and blind)
Development	Dorsal skin darkens 3 days; coat develops 4–10 days Eyes open 12 days Weaned 17–18 days Thermoregulatory ability develops 16–19 days All molars erupted 28–30 days	21 g by weaning	22 g within 14 days Leave nest around 22 days 160 g within 5 weeks of birth
Age at weaning	14–28 days	14–18 days	14 days
Sexual maturity	Spring following birth (male min. 1.5 months; female min. 2 months)	6 weeks	From 5 weeks
Lifespan	Max. 18 months (mean 4 months)	Max. 18 months	5 months

14.6 Characteristics and biological parameters of voles. [a] The common vole (*Microtus arvalis*) is confined to the Channel Islands and has characteristics and parameters very similar to those of the field vole.

Rats and mice

Characteristics and biological parameters of rats and mice are shown in Figures 14.7 to 14.10.

Rats and mice are found throughout the British Isles (though the yellow-necked mouse (*Apodemus flavicollis*) and the harvest mouse (*Micromys minutus*) have more localized distributions), often in close association with human dwellings and agricultural land. All are largely nocturnal. Mice are important prey species for many animals.

Rats and mice have more pointed muzzles and longer tails than the voles, but shorter muzzles than the shrews. They are anatomically and physiologically similar to their domestic counterparts.

The common or brown rat (*Rattus norvegicus*; Figure 14.7a) and the ship or black rat (*Rattus rattus*; Figure 14.7b) swim well and are often found close to water. Both live in social groups. Brown rats burrow well; black rats are good climbers and rather shy. Rats are able to get through holes no larger than their heads, to walk along narrow paths (e.g. telephone lines), to swim through water traps, to jump up

to 3 feet vertically and 4 feet horizontally and survive falls of up to 50 feet (US Fish and Wildlife Service, 2008). Rat-proofing a facility, either to avoid entry or exit, is therefore a challenge.

House mice (*Mus musculus*) are less common than formerly, due to the improved protection of stored grain, and are less of a pest species than in the past.

Wood mice (Figure 14.9a) are the most common mouse of woods, hedgerows and mature gardens and are an important prey species. They cache food and live in underground burrows and nests of leaves, moss and grass, forming communal nests in winter, but nesting singly to breed. Wood mice undergo torpor if subjected to food deprivation and cold weather.

The yellow-necked mouse was the last small mammal to be recognized as a separate species in Britain, in 1894. They are agile woodland mice and expert climbers. They enter dwellings mainly in autumn and winter months and this is not solely due to cold weather or decreased food availability, though the exact reasons are not fully understood (The Mammal Society, 2001b). They are a species of

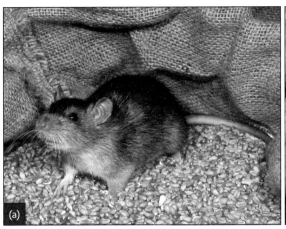 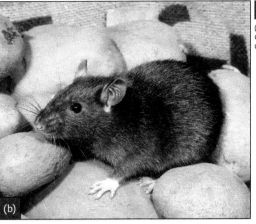

14.7 (a) Brown rat.
(b) Black rat.
(Courtesy of Andy Purcell/
Conservation Education
Consultants, © CEC)

Parameter	Common or brown rat (*Rattus norvegicus*)	Ship or black rat (*Rattus rattus*)
Distribution	Common and widespread	Patchy, now quite rare
Habitat	Towns and agricultural land (especially arable or near food stores); often close to water	Usually near water
Diet	Anything digestible	Omnivorous but more vegetarian than brown rat
Appearance	Fur brown; long naked tail	Fur dark brown to grey/black; slimmer than brown rat
Weight	100–600 g	150–200 g
Head and body length	220–280 mm	200 mm
Tail length	200–220 mm	260 mm
Nipples	6 pairs	5 pairs (variable)
Dentition	$2 \times \left\{ I \frac{1}{1} C \frac{0}{0} P \frac{0}{0} M \frac{3}{3} \right\} = 16$	$2 \times \left\{ I \frac{1}{1} C \frac{0}{0} P \frac{0}{0} M \frac{3}{3} \right\} = 16$
Breeding season	All year if food available	March–November
Oestrus	Post-partum oestrus within 18h of birth; cycle 4–6 days; polyoestrus	Similar to brown rat
Gestation	21–24 days	21–22 days (23–29 if lactating)
No. of litters per year	Up to 5	3–5
Litter size	6–11 (depending on bodyweight of mother)	1–11 (usually 7–8)
Development	Born naked and blind Fully furred and eyes open 15 days	Born naked and blind
Age at weaning	21 days	About 21 days
Sexual maturity (female)	11 weeks; 115 g	3–5 months; 90 g
Lifespan	1–2 years	1 year

14.8 Characteristics and biological parameters of brown and black rats.

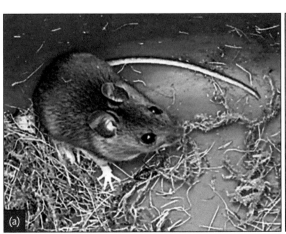 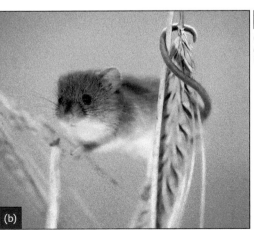

14.9 (a) Wood mouse.
(b) Harvest mouse.
(a, Courtesy of Kate Long;
b, © Secret World Wildlife Rescue)

Parameter	House mouse (*Mus musculus*)	Wood mouse (*Apodemus sylvaticus*)	Yellow-necked mouse (*Apodemus flavicollis*)	Harvest mouse (*Micromys minutus*)
Distribution	Widespread	Throughout mainland Britain and islands	Patchily localized: found only in Wales, central and southern England	Mainly southern and central England; absent from Ireland
Habitat	Usually in association with human habitation or arable land	Commonest mouse of woods, hedgerows, mature gardens; may come inside dwellings in colder weather	Woodland, especially ancient; may enter dwellings in colder months	Stalk zone of reeds, cereal crops, hedgerows, weeds
Nest	Vary from simple pallet to spherical. Any available material used	Underground burrows; nests of leaves, moss, grass (communal in winter; females nest singly to breed)	Extensive burrows and nests	Nest size of tennis ball among plant stems
Diet	Seeds, vegetables, fruit, stored food	Seeds, seedlings, buds, fruit (pips only), nuts, snails, insects, spiders, woodlice, fungi, moss, bark, hips, haws, beetle larvae and adults, caterpillars, grain, grass flowers, weed seeds, earthworms, bulbs, beans, peas, tomatoes	Tree seeds (especially high-energy), fruits, some green plants, invertebrates (caterpillars, other insect larvae, worms)	Cereal grains, seeds, berries, insects, wheat aphids, nectar, moss, roots, fungi
Appearance	Fur greyish-brown dorsally, slightly paler underneath, normally quite greasy	Fur brown dorsally, pale underside	Similar to wood mouse (fur brown dorsally, white underside) but with yellowish collar around throat. Larger than wood mouse	Fur red to golden-brown dorsally, pale underside. Blunt nose; small hairy ears
Weight	12–20 g	13–18 g winter 25–27 g summer	14–45 g	4–6 g
Head and body length	75–100 mm	75–100 mm	95–120 mm	50–70 mm
Tail length	75–100 mm	70–100 mm	75–120 mm	50–70 mm
Nipples	5 pairs	4 pairs	3 or 4 pairs	4 pairs
Dentition	$2 \times \left\{ I\frac{1}{1} \; C\frac{0}{0} \; P\frac{0}{0} \; M\frac{3}{3} \right\} = 16$	As house mouse (molar shape varies between species)	As house mouse (molar shape varies between species)	As house mouse (molar shape varies between species)
Breeding season	April–Sept	February–October	February–October	May–October
Oestrus	Cycle 4–6 days, post-partum oestrus within 24h	Cycle 4–6 days, post-partum oestrus	Cycle 4–6 days, post-partum oestrus	Polyoestrous, post-partum oestrus
Gestation	19–20 days (up to 36 if lactating)	19–20 days (up to 26 when lactating)	23 days	17–19 days
No. of litters per year	Up to 10	Up to 6 (typically 1–2)	Successive Feb–Oct	2–3
Litter size	5–6	2–11 (typically 4–7)	2–11	3–8
Birthweight	1 g (naked and blind)	1–2.5 g (naked and blind)	2.8 g (naked and blind)	0.6–1 g (naked and blind)
Eyes open	2–3 days	16 days	13–16 days	8–9 days
Development	Skin darkens 5–7 days; hair half-grown 8–10 days; hair growth complete and incisors erupted 14 days	Fur appears 6 days, starting on dorsum; incisors erupt 13 days; hind feet darken 14 days; autumn-born young develop more slowly	Juvenile coat developed 14 days; yellow collar visible	Dorsal fur 4 days; ventral fur develops 8–9 days; juvenile grey/brown fur 14 days
Age at weaning	18 days	18–22 days (6–8 g)	21 days	15–16 days
Sexual maturity	5–6 weeks	2 months (male 15 g, female 12 g)	2–3 months (male 20 g, female 10 g)	35–45 days
Lifespan	1–2 years	<1 year	1 year (av. 3–4 months)	<18 months (generally 6 months)

14.10 Characteristics and biological parameters of mice.

ancient woodland (their distribution is similar to that of mistletoe) and feed off tree seeds; they are therefore vulnerable to woodland loss and fragmentation (The Mammal Society, 2001a). They form extensive nests and burrows, some of which are used to cache food.

Harvest mice (*Micromys minutus*; see Figure 14.9b), Britain's smallest rodents, are preyed upon by weasels, stoats, foxes, cats, owls, hawks and crows, and their remains form 1% of barn owl pellets. They are excellent climbers, with prehensile tails almost as long as their bodies. They construct nests the size of tennis balls, among plant stems.

Dormice

Characteristics and biological parameters of the two species of dormice found in the UK are given in Figures 14.11 and 14.12. Both species are largely nocturnal or crepuscular.

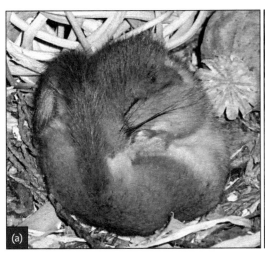
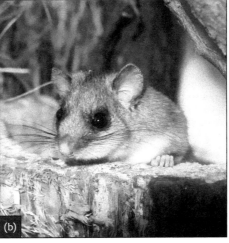

14.11 (a) Common dormouse. (b) Edible dormouse.
(a, © Secret World Wildlife Rescue; b, Courtesy of Andy Purcell/Conservation Education Consultants, © CEC)

Parameter	Common dormouse (*Muscardinus avellanarius*)	Edible (fat) dormouse (*Myoxus (Glis) glis*)
Distribution	Scarce, localized and declining population; isolated colonies Wales and central and southern England	Chilterns
Habitat	Preferably coppiced hazel woodland in trees at approx. 5 m above ground level	Preferably beech woods
Nest	Globular; 7.5 cm diameter (twice as big for breeding); hibernatory nests nearer or on ground	Arboreal, also rock clefts, old woodpecker holes, lofts
Hibernation	October–May	October–April
Diet	Flowers, nuts and fruits, especially honeysuckle and hazel; insects eaten in summer	Fruits and nuts, insects, birds' eggs and young birds, acorns, seeds, buds, bark, fungi
Appearance	Fur reddish; hamster-like appearance but well furred prehensile tail; male longer anogenital distance than female, and small dark-pigmented scrotum in breeding season	Greyish coat with pale underbelly; short muzzle, many whiskers, large eyes and small rounded ears; long furry tail
Weight	15–30 g (upper weight found only immediately prior to hibernation)	85–140 g (can be up to 250 g shortly before hibernation)
Size (head and body length)	80 mm (tail 60 mm)	120–150 mm
Nipples	4 pairs	4–6 pairs
Dentition	$2 \times \left\{ I\,\frac{1}{1}\ C\,\frac{0}{0}\ P\,\frac{0}{0}\ M\,\frac{3}{3} \right\} = 16$	$2 \times \left\{ I\,\frac{1}{1}\ C\,\frac{0}{0}\ P\,\frac{1}{1}\ M\,\frac{3}{3} \right\} = 20$
Breeding season	June to early August	June to early August
Gestation	21–24 days	30–32 days
No. of litters	1–2	1
Litter size (approx.)	4	5
Birthweight	1 g; blind, naked	1–2 g; blind, naked
Development	Grey fur develops at 7 days; coat well developed by 13 days; leave nest at 30 days	Fur developed by 14–16 days
Eyes open	18 days	21–23 days
Age at weaning	Remains with mother until 6–8 weeks old	28–30 days, when leave nest
Sexual maturity	Spring of year after birth	Spring of year after birth (can be following year in late-born young)
Lifespan	Max. 4 years in wild	Up to 6 years

14.12 Characteristics and biological parameters of dormice.

The preferred environment of the common or hazel dormouse (see Figure 14.11a) is coppiced hazel woodland, where it tends to live in trees at about 5 m above ground level. This habitat has been in decline, which both decreases the amount of available habitat and isolates small populations of dormice from each other. However, recently numbers have increased, thanks to conservation efforts, and were estimated to be approximately 45,000 in 2006 (Bright *et al.*, 2006), although it is noted that populations are discontinuous. Dormice can live in commercial coppiced woods and much effort has been made to attempt to render these 'dormouse-friendly' and to release dormice into them, with some success (D Woods, personal communication).

During hibernation, the dormouse body temperature drops to 5°C or lower. Torpid animals may be mistakenly identified as dead or in shock. Hibernating animals may be injured by hedge trimming, predators or other nest disturbance. Animals with insufficient fat stores or interrupted hibernation may present in very poor body condition. Dormice may select inappropriate nesting sites, which lead to disturbance (e.g. man-made objects; H Ryan, personal communication). For much of the rest of the year they are torpid during the day and predominantly active at night. They are very territorial in the breeding season.

The edible or fat dormouse (see Figure 14.11b) was introduced into Britain in Tring, Hertfordshire, in 1902. It is now established in the Chilterns and rarely seen elsewhere; it can be a pest in orchards and conifer plantations. Edible dormice are fairly sociable and largely arboreal. They can almost double their bodyweight before hibernation underground or in lofts during winter months.

European beaver

Characteristics and biological parameters of the European beaver (*Castor fiber*) are given in Figures 14.13 and 14.14.

This crepuscular species was once native to the British Isles, but the last recorded sighting in Scotland was near Loch Ness in 1527 (MacDonald, 1995). A formal trial reintroduction of beavers occurred in Scotland in 2009 and it has subsequently become apparent that an additional, large, free-living population is also present in eastern Scotland (Taylor, 1999). No reintroductions have presently occurred in England or Wales but beavers are present in several enclosed projects, with sightings of the odd free-living animal reported. There are also plans for their official trial release into Wales. Beavers of unknown origin are present in the wild in Devon, in the south-west of England (Withnall, 2013). Following Defra decision-making (Hansard, 2014), these animals have been screened for *Echinococcus multilocularis*, and re-released following negative results for this zoonotic disease. Such animals may be presented to the veterinary surgeon (veterinarian) as wildlife casualties, or for such testing (Gottstein *et al.*, 2014).

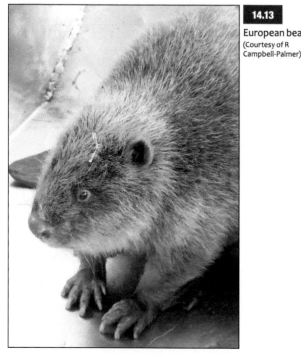

14.13

European beaver.
(Courtesy of R Campbell-Palmer)

Parameter	European beaver (*Castor fiber*)
Diet	Water plants, bark, roots, shoots and thistles
Distribution	Europe and Asia (see main text for current UK distribution) After loss of some populations, this species has been reintroduced through much of its former range in a number of separate projects. Currently occurs from Great Britain to China and Mongolia. Absent from Italy, Portugal and the southern Balkans.
Habitat	Riparian (rivers, streams and their banks and interfaces with woodland edges)
Bodyweight	12–30 kg
Size (head and body length)	850–1300 mm
Nipples	4 pairs
Dentition	$2 \times \left\{ I\frac{1}{1} \ C\frac{0}{0} \ P\frac{1}{1} \ M\frac{3}{3} \right\} = 20$
Breeding season	October–November
Oestrus	2-week oestrus cycle; receptive for 10–12h
Gestation	100–120 days
No. of litters per year	1
Litter size	2–4
Birthweight	230–630 g, born fully furred with open eyes
Development	Young not independent until 3 years of age; high juvenile survival rate
Age at weaning	3 months
Sexual maturity	2–2.5 years

14.14 Characteristics and biological parameters of European beaver.

Beavers are the second largest rodent species in the world (weights of up to 30 kg have been recorded for both the European and North American species (*Castor canadensis*), although 20–25 kg is the normal adult weight range) and have a large spatulate scaled tail, which is slapped on the water as an alarm signal and acts as a fat storage site. Scandinavian beavers are smaller and darker than the southern European subspecies. Beavers have webbed hind feet and smaller, more dextrous, non-webbed fore feet. Their adaptations to an aquatic environment include eyes that are covered by a nictitating membrane when swimming, ears and nostrils that can close when submerged and the ability to close off the throat with the base of the tongue, to enable them to carry sticks in their mouths underwater.

Beavers pair for life. Determining sex is complicated by the urogenital and anal orifices opening into a common cloaca and requires palpation or radiographic visualization of the os penis, present in adult males, or visualization of the nipples in pregnant or lactating females. The anal glands and large castor scent sacs (which are positioned inguinally) should not be confused with testes. Males have a more liquid yellowish brown anal gland secretion than females, which is of thicker consistency and greyish white.

There has been much recent discussion in the UK regarding the costs and benefits of the release of beavers into the UK. Scientific release trials should help to provide data to assist a formal decision on their official re-establishment in the wild. The main concerns regarding the effects of beavers on the ecology are interference with water courses and subsequent flooding and interference with fish migration. Generally speaking, any flooding in areas where it would interfere with human activities can be mitigated by fencing off areas or the placement of 'beaver deceivers' (outflow pipes used to mitigate damming effects). Fish migration (Atlantic salmon (*Salmo salar*) and sea trout (*Salmo trutta*)) may potentially be affected, but these species have coexisted naturally in Scandinavia for some time. Beavers cause minimal damage to coniferous trees due to their unpalatable sap. Their tree management around water courses is remarkably similar to human coppicing techniques and is generally beneficial to biodiversity.

Capture, handling and transportation

General handling techniques for these species are covered in greater detail in appropriate laboratory or domestic rodent texts (Fallon, 1996; Flecknell, 1998; Hrapkiewicz *et al.*, 1998; Lichtenberger and Hawkins, 2009; Campbell-Palmer and Rosell, 2013). However, wild rodents and insectivores are much more liable to bite than equivalent domestic species and are easily stressed, necessitating general anaesthesia for all but the most superficial examination (Fowler, 1995).

These animals should be handled or caught only when necessary. Indirect methods are less stressful – for example, catching/trapping in an appropriate net, box or tube and transporting them without direct handling.

Most small species are extremely fast and agile; some can jump and climb well and most immediately head for cover; all exits and hiding places should be blocked up in advance. Mice are most likely to jump away, and voles and shrews to run away. Nets can be useful for initially trapping or recapturing the animals (Gurnell and Flowerdew, 1994). The netting should be of solid material or very fine mesh, to avoid claws catching in the weave (Fowler, 1995), and the rims should be padded to avoid injury and escape.

Dim light should be used, to reduce activity levels and stress. Gloves increase the handler's confidence but severely reduce dexterity and control: the lightest gloves possible should be used. It is easy to grip smaller mammals too tightly and restrict breathing whilst wearing gloves (Fallon, 1996) and thick gloves only really have a place in the handling of the edible dormouse and the rat (A Hudson, personal communication). Even thick gloves are inadequate protection against adult beaver bites and encourage too tight a grip of the animal. They also make it difficult to obtain palpable early warning of the animal turning to bite. They may have a role in the handling of kits by inexperienced handlers only (R Campbell-Palmer, personal communication). Latex gloves should be used with the water shrew and beaver to protect from irritant sebaceous secretions and highly odiferous castor secretions. As zoonotic infections are potentially present in all the species described here (see 'Zoonoses and other risks to humans'), it would be prudent to wear latex gloves when handling all these species. Latex gloves may also be sufficient to prevent the bite of the smaller voles and shrews from breaking the skin.

Most species can be contained initially, and for medium-term accommodation, in small plastic pet boxes with securely fitting lids of the type sold for holding invertebrates, with a trapdoor opening in a removable top to allow the animal to be fed whilst minimizing the risk of escape (Stocker, 2005).

Moles

Moles can be held by the scruff of loose skin on the back of the neck and lifted very briefly by the tail, with the body supported (Bourne, 2002). It is important to avoid handling the sensitive nasal area.

Mice, rats, voles and shrews

These species can be caught in a net, then grasped by the head and neck and dropped into a suitable container (Bourne, 2002). They can be lifted briefly by the tail base only (to avoid sloughing); it is particularly important to avoid damaging the tail of harvest mice and common dormice (Poole, 1999). They can also be scruffed by the skin over the neck and back, with the tail held in the same hand (Bourne, 2002).

Dormice

To catch edible dormice, a net may be needed (Bourne, 2002), and robust housing and transport cages such as a cat basket are required (Stocker, 2005).

Common dormice are the only wild species described here that may routinely appear passive when they are handled (D Woods, personal communication). Such behaviour in any other small wild mammal is abnormal and denotes illness, shock or stress. Interfering with common dormice other than for veterinary treatment requires a licence (see 'Legal aspects').

Beavers

Whilst beavers may be fairly passive animals, they can be aggressive when being caught up, especially if cornered, and have the potential to cause severe bite wounds. They are also capable of causing severe, potentially fatal damage to conspecifics with whom they have not (yet) been socialized. Their main defence is to head for water if threatened. When capturing from a facility, pools should be drained where possible. In water they are very agile and difficult to catch. On land they are slow-moving and easily caught. Whilst strong and powerful, they are tractable and can be guided towards a box for capture and transport. Nets should be of sufficient size to enclose the animal, with frame joints reinforced to lift their weight. Injury to the animal with the frame must be avoided. Hessian sacks (Figure 14.15a) can be attached to a frame, as both a net and a carry sack after capture. Encompassing them and covering their eyes in this way greatly facilitates examination and short veterinary procedures, but experience is required to avoid being bitten. 'Bavarian' and other types of beaver traps are a useful alternative in wild settings, and may be baited with food or castoreum (exudate from the castor sacs) (Figure 14.15b). Beavers do not tend to readily bite or scratch, but any injuries are potentially serious given their powerful teeth and jaws, and strong claws (Campbell-Palmer and Rosell, 2013). Chemical immobilization to enable safe handling is a possibility, but should never be used with the animal free near open water due to the risk of drowning on induction or recovery.

It is not necessary to transport beavers in water or hose them down to keep them cool, but they should be offered food with high water content, such as apples, during transport. Adequate ventilation and shade from the sun should be provided during capture and transportation, as overheating in this species can easily occur. Wooden crates require a mesh lining to prevent escape.

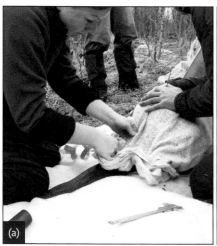 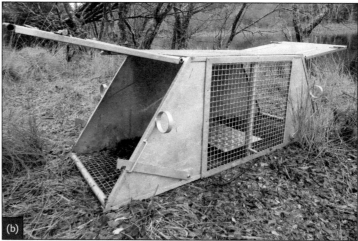

14.15
(a) A beaver being restrained using a hessian sac for examination and length measurements. (b) A Bavarian trap for catching beavers.
(Courtesy of R Campbell-Palmer)

Zoonoses and other risks to humans

Most of the species covered in this chapter can inflict bites of varying severity. In addition, the saliva of water shrews contains venom from the submaxillary glands, which is poisonous to vertebrate prey such as frogs and fish. Even if a bite does not break the skin, it will cause localized inflammation and pain in humans (Fowler, 1995). For these reasons latex gloves should be warn when handling these species and appropriate health and safety risk assessments carried out.

Wild rats in particular are extremely vicious and must be handled with great care. They should not be cornered and they should not be handled directly unless absolutely unavoidable, when thick gloves should be worn. To minimize the risks of leptospiral infection, it is advisable to wear goggles and masks as well as impermeable gloves. Medical advice should be sought in the event of a bite from a wild rat, or suspected ingestion or inhalation of leptospiral-infected material. Confirmation of leptospiral infection at post-mortem examination of the rat is advisable so that the need for human treatment can be assessed (A Hudson, personal communication).

Actual incidences of zoonotic or domestic animal infection appear of generally minimal significance, with the exception of leptospirosis. *Yersinia pseudotuberculosis* and *Campylobacter* spp. have been isolated from British rodents (Pocock *et al.*, 2001). *Cryptosporidium parvum* and *C. muris* have been isolated from house mice, wood mice and voles (Bull *et al.*, 1998) and constitute a risk to humans, especially in immunosuppressed individuals (Wells, 1937, cited in Rankin and McDiarmid, 1968), but the zoonotic potential of vole infection is unknown. *Encephalitizoon cuniculi* has been identified in wild rodents in the UK (Meredith *et al.*, 2015). *Mycobacterium bovis* was isolated from five rats and two moles in a study involving 5,700 wild mammals, including badgers, from 1971 to 1978 (Evans and Thompson, 1981), but was not found in 875 voles in another study (Kirkwood, 1991, citing a 1987 study by the then Ministry of Agriculture, Fisheries and Food). *M. tuberculosis* var. *muris* had an incidence of 1.4% in a study of 500 common shrews, but its zoonotic potential is unknown. Beard *et al.* (2001) found *M. avium* subsp. *paratuberculosis* (the causative organism of paratuberculosis) in rats and wood mice. There were 27 cases of human tuberculosis caused by *M. microti* reported in the literature over the past decade worldwide in one literature review (Panteix *et al.*, 2010).

Many zoonotic diseases are not currently present in the UK but could be introduced by the increasing numbers of people and animals moving around the world (Simpson, 1999). If introduced into the native rodent population, these infections (e.g. Omsk haemorrhagic fever, rabies, rat poxvirus, monkey poxvirus, Boutonneuse fever, Q fever and Rocky Mountain spotted fever) could conceivably achieve a foothold in the UK (Fraser *et al.*, 1991).

Seoul hantavirus has been detected in wild brown rats, and associated with human disease (Jameson *et al.*, 2013). A novel hantavirus, with zoonotic potential, has also been found in voles (Pounder *et al.*, 2013).

Examination and clinical assessment for rehabilitation

If possible, the exact location where the animal was found should be recorded, particularly in the case of the common dormouse, beaver and water vole. This is in order to help in planning an effective release strategy. If beavers are found, the organizations in the area responsible for their original release should be contacted (see 'Specialist organizations and useful contacts'), as release into the wild is illegal unless under licence. Beavers, and other species that are part of release programs, will have some form of identification. The standard implantation site for passive integrated transponders (PIT tag, microchip) is subcutaneously between the shoulder blades and dorsal neck. It is good practice to scan all wildlife admissions for microchips. Ear tags and telemetry devices may also have been applied to beavers (Campbell-Palmer and Rosell, 2013).

Examination

General anaesthesia is advisable for all but the most superficial examination (Fowler, 1995). Examination of the smaller mammals inside a transparent container (e.g. plastic box or glass jar) in dim light is more productive than attempting to examine the animal in the hand and permits better inspection of the head, underside and extremities as well as respiratory pattern, gait and locomotion.

Clinical assessment

Anything more than very minimal limb damage, especially in climbing species, is likely to lead to an increased risk of predation. Damage to the tail, especially in the common dormouse and harvest mouse (species that use their tails for climbing) and water shrew (which uses its tail for swimming), may be significant, depending on the extent. Damage to the forelimbs of moles is likely to have an effect on digging and therefore on feeding capabilities. Visual defects in moles and shrews do not necessarily preclude release.

Pest species

The treatment and release of 'pest' species is controversial, with the words 'vermin' and 'pest' being somewhat subjective and having no clear legal definition. The decision to euthanase or release such species is up to the individual veterinary surgeon, but the Wildlife and Countryside Act 1981 makes it an offence to release edible dormice and black rats (see 'Legal aspects' and Chapter 2). Consideration must be given to the release site, for example not releasing agricultural pest species, such as brown rats, into grain storage sites, or not releasing potential vectors of zoonotic diseases, into water bodies used by humans.

Euthanasia

Euthanasia is best performed by intravenous injection, or intracardiac injection following gaseous anaesthetic induction; intraperitoneal injection may also be used in an anaesthetized animal. Physical methods include cervical dislocation (carried out as described in laboratory animal texts (e.g. Redfern and Rowe, 1987) or skull crush (see Chapter 4).

First aid and short-term hospitalization

In many cases these animals require, and benefit from, only short periods of hospitalization. Their rapid metabolic rates, escape abilities, short lifespans and easily stressed nature make them generally poor candidates as longer term inpatients. Minor survivable injuries heal rapidly and more significant lesions are usually rapidly fatal. Small species can be housed short term in a plastic escape-proof container with newspaper or paper towelling on the floor and shredded paper to hide in.

Small mammals are prone to rapid heat loss and should be kept warm, but care should be taken to avoid overheating them, especially if they are debilitated and unable to move away from a source of heat. An ambient temperature of 25–28°C should be provided for smaller casualty species in particular, on initial presentation and if debilitated, after which ambient temperatures of 20–21°C are more appropriate.

These species generally require almost constant food intake. Suitable food (see 'Rehabilitation'), in particular the more palatable and easily digestible items, should be provided at once. Immediate fluid therapy should be considered, especially if the casualty does not eat readily. Hypoglycaemia should be addressed if it is a concern, or is diagnosed on blood glucose levels (see Chapter 5). Inappetant animals and those with higher energy requirements (especially those which are cold) should receive supplemental oral or parenteral glucose.

Fluid therapy

For a full discussion of oral dosing, injection sites and amounts that can be given, see Fallon (1996), Bauck and Bihun (1997), Hrapkiewicz et al. (1998) and Sayers and Smith (2010). Also see Chapter 5. All fluids must be given at the animal's normal body temperature, to avoid chilling the animal if too cold or causing local thermal damage if too hot (Saunders and Whitlock, 2012).

Administration of therapeutic agents
Intravenous injection and blood sampling

In small rodents the easiest venous access of choice is the cranial vena cava. General anaesthesia is required for sampling from this site and the animal is placed in dorsal recumbency. An area is clipped and swabbed with spirit just cranial to the manubrium on one side. A 25–27 G needle attached to a 1 ml syringe is inserted between the clavicle and first rib at a 45-degree angle, directed medially in line with the opposite hind leg. The vessel is just under the sternum, so the needle does not need to be advanced too deeply. Blood is seen in the hub of the needle and confirms correct placement. Maximum safe volumes for blood collection in small rodents are 0.6–0.7 ml per 100 g bodyweight at any one time.

Alternative sampling sites include the jugular and lateral tail veins in rats and larger species, under general anaesthesia. Warming the tail dilates the vessels. In mice, the use of these veins is limited to the removal of small volumes of blood and they are not suitable for injection purposes (Fallon, 1996).

In beavers, the ventral coccygeal vein is utilized (Figure 14.16). With the beaver in dorsal recumbency, the vein is located on the ventral aspect of the tail in the midline, and may be accessed in conscious or anaesthetized beavers. The medial saphenous vein, cephalic vein or jugular vein (following a cut-down) may be used for catheter placement, intravenous injections or smaller blood samples. Beaver blood clots rapidly, and may clot in heparinized containers. Ethylenediaminetetraacetic acid (EDTA) blood tubes should be used in preference to heparin (S Brown, personal communication) and should only be half filled and immediately gently rotated. Air-dried smears should be made immediately (Campbell-Palmer and Rosell, 2013).

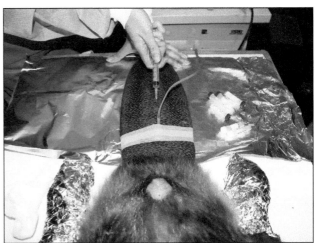

14.16 In beavers, the ventral coccygeal vein is utilized for blood sampling. With the beaver in dorsal recumbency, the vein is located on the ventral aspect of the tail in the midline. This animal is anaesthetized.
(Courtesy of R Campbell-Palmer)

Intramuscular injection

There is little difference in the rate of uptake from intramuscular and subcutaneous injections (McDiarmid, 1983). The intramuscular injection of irritant drugs or of excessive volumes can result in muscle necrosis and damage to adjacent nerves, in some cases resulting in self-mutilation (Hrapkiewicz *et al.*, 1998). Also, these species are easily stressed and fast-moving and subcutaneous routes are generally quicker and easier to use. If intramuscular injections are to be given, no more than 0.05 ml should be given in any one site to a mouse-sized rodent (Flecknell, 1996).

Intraosseous injection

This gives similar rates of uptake to that of intravenous injection but is useful if there is cardiovascular shock in these smaller species. The preferred sites are the proximal tibia or femur. Aseptic technique and general anaesthesia are required. Local anaesthetic should be injected at the site of insertion prior to placement (e.g. 0.01 ml of lidocaine 1%). Purpose-made intraosseous needles can be used. Alternatively, spinal or hypodermic needles of appropriate size can be used. The latter tend to become blocked with cortical bone unless the needle is attached to a syringe containing sterile saline (which is kept pressurized to maintain its patency) or a smaller needle or sterile stainless steel wire is used as a stylet.

Subcutaneous injection

Suggested volumes are up to 2 ml for a 30 g mouse and up to 5 ml for a 200 g rat (Flecknell, 1996). Sites include the nape of the neck and dorsolaterally over the ribs (Bourne, 2002). The addition of hyaluronidase at 1500 IU/l of fluids increases the rate of uptake of subcutaneous fluids. No more than 10 ml/kg should be given by this route at a time. Using multiple sites reduces the risk of local tissue damage (Saunders and Whitlock, 2012).

Oral dosing

Oral administration of drugs or fluids is likely to prove immensely stressful for many of these species. In many cases it will not be practicable, but in the case of debilitated individuals, or given as a free choice option, it may be a practical way of administering small quantities of fluids, especially if hypoglycaemia is a concern. Proprietary formulations, such as Vetark® Critical Care Formula, supplemented by either intravenous Vetark® formulations of glucose, oral glucose formulations (e.g. Glucogel®) or powdered dextrose may prove useful (see also Chapter 5).

Anaesthesia and analgesia

Light anaesthesia is advantageous as an aid to rapid, complete examination of these species. The current anaesthetics of choice are isoflurane (Fowler, 1993) or sevoflurane (Richardson and Flecknell, 2009), with induction taking place in a chamber at 4–5% for isoflurane and 5–8% for sevoflurane, and maintenance by mask at 1.5–3% and 3–5% respectively. Sevoflurane is preferable for induction as it causes less irritation to the mucus membranes. A purpose-designed concentric mask is preferable, as it permits more efficient scavenging of waste gases. A snugly fitting mask with a rubber or latex edge can provide a sufficient seal to aid in ventilating the animal if required.

Small mammals have a high ratio of surface area to bodyweight and therefore require good insulation and an external source of gentle warmth (e.g. Bair Hugger® or Hot Dog®) to avoid hypothermia whilst anaesthetized (Fowler, 1995; Flecknell, 1998). Conversely, it is important not to overheat them. Continuous real time temperature monitoring is the ideal.

Most species do not require preoperative starving to avoid vomiting. Due to their high metabolic rates, especially in the shrews, even short periods of starvation are likely to be fatal. Every effort to ensure a rapid return to consciousness and resumed food intake should be taken. The use of perioperative fluids should be employed (see 'Fluid therapy'). All fluids should be warmed to approximately 38°C before administration. Casualty wildlife patients can generally be assumed to be in state of dehydration and malnutrition, and this should be addressed prior to or during even a short anaesthetic.

If any invasive procedure is carried out, or the animal has presented with traumatic injuries, the use of analgesics is warranted, both for welfare reasons and to ensure a rapid return to normal feeding behaviour. Self-trauma of the affected part may be seen if inadequate analgesia is employed. Carprofen at 4 mg/kg by a single subcutaneous injection and meloxicam at 0.5–2 mg/kg by subcutaneous or oral administration have been widely used by this author in a number of these species. The high palatability of meloxicam makes oral administration practical. Buprenorphine (0.05–0.1 mg/kg s.c.), butorphanol (2 mg/kg s.c.) and morphine (2–5 mg/kg s.c.) can also be used as in small domestic rodents. For further more detailed discussion of anaesthesia and analgesia, see Richardson and Flecknell (2009).

Moles

Moles have a relatively high urine volume and they excrete bicarbonate in their urine. This may be an excretory mechanism to cope with a hypercapnic environment (Haim *et al.*, 1987). It may be advisable to provide parenteral fluids perioperatively in this species even more so than others, to assist this mechanism and avoid disturbances of acid–base balance. Intraperitoneal fluids may be given (M Brash, personal communication), but warmed subcutaneous fluids with added hyaluronidase will also be rapidly absorbed (E Keeble, personal communication).

Adaptation to a hypercapnic environment may also mean that the mole may not breathe spontaneously in a low carbon dioxide environment. Intermittent positive pressure ventilation (IPPV) or external chest compression during anaesthesia, and the use of carbon dioxide in inspired gases during the recovery period, might be required if apnoea occurs. However, no problems with recovery from isoflurane or sevoflurane have been noted (M Brash and E Keeble, personal communications).

Shrews

A combination of ketamine (20 mg/kg) and xylazine (1 mg/kg), given intramuscularly, has been reported to give 20–30 minutes of light anaesthesia in shrews (Fowler, 1993). Doses of 100 μg/kg medetomidine and 5 mg/kg ketamine, with reversal of the former with 300–500 μg/kg of atipamazole, are reported for laboratory insectivores (Fish *et al.*, 2011). Alternatively, gaseous agents may be used for induction and maintenance of anaesthesia (see above).

Voles

Alfaxalone has been used at 3 mg/kg i.m. in small Australian mammals (Dona, 2013). Pentobarbital has been used at a dose of 72 mg/kg intraperitoneal It was considered less safe in stressed voles and a further 24 mg/kg was required for excited voles (Poole, 1999). Overdose is very easy and such agents require very precise weighing of the animal beforehand and dose calculation. They also tend to result in prolonged recoveries with poor analgesia and so are not generally recommended by the author. Alternatively, gaseous agents may be used for induction and maintenance of anaesthesia and are safe and well tolerated (see above).

Beavers

The key concern regarding anaesthesia in beavers is whether post-anaesthetic recovery is to take place in a controlled environment (i.e. controlling access to water until it is considered safe) or field conditions (see Chapter 6). Regimes with long or variable recovery times should not be used in the latter situation, or the animals should be retained in captivity until they are safe to be released. Facemask induction with isoflurane was used by Wenger *et al.* (2010). Use of isoflurane as a sole induction and maintenance agent significantly reduces the risks of post-anaesthetic drowning (S Girling, personal communication). Injectable anaesthetic dose rates for beavers are given in Figure 14.17.

Drugs	Dosage	Comments
Ketamine (K) + medetomidine (M)	7.5 mg/kg (K) + 0.07 mg/kg (M) i.m.	After 20 minutes, reversal was carried out using atipamezole at 0.3 mg/kg i.m. No problems were associated with this regime (S Brown, personal communication)
Ketamine (K) + diazepam (D)	12.5 mg/kg (K) + 0.2 mg/kg (D) i.m.	Sedation generally occurred within 15–20 minutes, after which anaesthesia was induced using isoflurane delivered in 100% oxygen via a facemask (S Brown, personal communication)
Ketamine (K) + butorphanol (B) + medetomidine (M)	5 mg/kg (K) + 0.1 mg/kg (B) + 0.05 mg/kg (M)	Mean induction time was 8.4 ± 5.0 minutes (Ranheim *et al.*, 2004)
Ketamine (K) + butorphanol (B) + medetomidine (M) + midazolam (Mi)	5 mg/kg (K) 0.1 mg/kg (B) 0.05 mg/kg (M) 0.25 mg/kg (Mi)	Mean induction time was 7.8 ± 2.6 minutes (Ranheim *et al.*, 2004) NB better muscle relaxation was achieved with this regime compared with K+B+M alone

14.17 Injectable anaesthetic dose rates in beavers.

Mask induction and intramuscular injections may be performed with the beaver confined in a hessian sack (S Girling, personal communication; Campbell-Palmer and Rosell, 2013). Intubation is generally straightforward, although a laryngoscope or a blind technique is generally required. Tube sizes range from 2.5 for kits to 7.0 for large adults. For more detail on anaesthesia, the reader is referred to the captive management guidelines produced by the Royal Zoological Society of Scotland (Campbell-Palmer and Rosell, 2013).

Specific conditions

Injuries from predators can involve bites of varying degrees of severity, limb fractures (Figure 14.18), spinal damage or abdominal puncture and prolapsed intestines (Stocker, 2005). Even when only apparently minor injuries are noted, antibiotic therapy is warranted, as cat bites can commonly lead to *Pasteurella*-induced septicaemia, which may be rapidly fatal (Korbel, 1990; Korbel *et al.*, 1992). Euthanasia is likely to be the treatment of choice for any animal with significant internal injuries. Animals should be triaged under anaesthesia, including physical examination, with exploration of any wounds to see where they track, and radiography. Minor injuries unlikely to preclude release may be treated. Puncture wounds should not be sutured although lacerations may be cleaned and repaired if fresh. Fractures may heal with analgesia and cage rest. See also Chapter 30 for treatment of cat bite injuries.

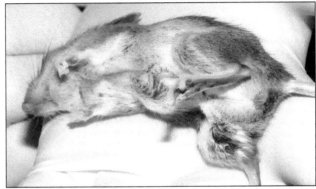

14.18 Wood mouse with a compound fracture of the tibia. Such fractures carry a poor prognosis and euthanasia at an early stage is the best course of action.
(Courtesy of G Cousquer)

Moles

Trauma

Bite wounds: Intraspecific fighting is common, as moles are territorial and aggressive outside the breeding season. Non-fatally injured moles with fight wounds may be seen but they frequently die in the 24 hours following admission (Small, 1994). This may be due to a number of reasons, not necessarily pathological.

Trapping injuries: Trapping is probably the main method of mole control used now in the UK, especially for smaller populations. In two studies, moles were shown not to have been instantaneously killed by traps. Atkinson *et al.* (1994) showed that whilst 22/22 moles were dead 24 hours after setting traps, some may have died from asphyxiation, starvation or hypothermia. Rudge (1963) found that 6/26 moles were caught by one or both forelimbs, and two of those moles were still alive when discovered. Mole traps do not require welfare approval, and their mechanical performance, and potentially their humaneness, vary widely (Baker *et al.*, 2012). Traumatic injuries as a result of non-fatal trapping may therefore be seen, especially if injuries to the limbs are sustained, non-lethal traps are not checked frequently enough, or if more than one mole is caught in a 'tube trap' and subsequently injure each other (Baker and Macdonald, 2012). Baker and Macdonald also note that there are potential welfare issues with capture/release or translocation of moles due to territoriality and lack of a suitable existing tunnel system (see also Natural England, 2011).

Poisoning

The use of strychnine to poison moles is now prohibited in the UK. In the absence of strychnine, other control options are being used such as traps and repellents. Other poisons have been trialled, but no other poison is currently approved for use in moles. European moles will only eat suitable baits (ideally worms) and will refuse unpalatably high levels of toxin. This limits the dose of poison that can be administered.

Alpha-chloralose was found to temporarily anaesthetize, but not kill, moles in one study. Whilst it is not approved for mole use, it may be considered as a differential if presented with a comatose or otherwise neurologically impaired mole (Universities Federation for Animal Welfare, 1983).

Phosphine gas produced from aluminium phosphide is an approved product for lethal fumigation of moles (e.g. Phostoxin® or Talunex®), but at suboptimal doses has resulted in prolonged deaths (up to 3–4 days) with incoordination, tachypnoea and convulsions (Quy and Poole, 2004).

Parasites

The host-specific fleas *Palaepsylla minor*, *P. kohauti* and *Ctenophthalmus bisoctodentatus* may be found (Lawson, 1999). The mites *Haemogamasus hirsutus*, *H. nidi* and *Eulaelaps stabularis* and an unnamed *Eimeria*-like coccidian, possibly *Elleipsisoma thomsoni*, have also been found on moles (Mohamed *et al.*, 1987). Their pathogenicity is unknown. Trematode species of the genus *Hyogonimus* have been found but again their pathogenicity is unknown (Corbet and Southern, 1977).

Juvenile animals

Juvenile moles spend more time above ground than adults when they first leave, increasing the risk of predation by birds of prey, foxes and cats. They may tunnel in unsuitable areas, leading to death by drowning. Non-fatally injured trapped moles may be seen.

Shrews
Parasites

Endoparasites such as *Porrocaecum talpae*, which is found coiled subcutaneously in the common shrew, and *Hymenolepis infirma* have been noted. These do not appear to have a significant effect on the host population, but the former is transmissible to owls (Small, 1994). A number of helminth parasites were detected in common and pygmy shrews in one study (Roots, 1992), which concluded that no serious pathogenic effects were noted as a result of infestation. Fleas, ticks and mites are commonly seen. Water shrews may have large endo- and ectoparasite burdens (The Mammal Society, 2001a).

Voles
Bacterial infections

Corynebacterium kutscheri infection has been reported in field voles. It may be more prevalent where there is a higher population density (Barrow, 1981).

Parasites

External parasites recorded for voles include fleas, lice, ticks and mites (Blackmore and Owen, 1968; Corbet and Southern, 1977; Healing and Nowell, 1985). Internal parasites are also well documented in the above references, but the significance of these parasitic infections on host health and population dynamics is largely unknown (Healing and Nowell, 1985).

Rats and mice
Viral infections

Kaplan *et al.* (1980) found a number of viral infections in experimentally immunosuppressed mice and voles, including pneumonia virus of mice (PVM), lymphocytic choriomeningitis virus, reovirus III, Theiler's mouse encephalomyelitis virus, ectromelia virus, mouse adenovirus, louping ill virus and encephalomyocarditis virus. Of these, only ectromelia and PVM were suspected of influencing population dynamics in wild mice and in general these diseases are of limited significance.

Parasites

Heligmosomoides polygyrus was found in 98% of wood mice in one study and this parasite does have a negative effect on the survival ability of the host (Gregory, 1991). In another study, nine helminth species were detected in wood mice, with 92% of the mice having at least one species present (Behnke *et al.*, 1999). Several species of *Eimeria* can infect wood mice, but their significance is uncertain (Nowell and Higgs, 1989).

Dormice
Parasites

The nematodes *Rictularia cristata* and *Syphacia obvelata* have been recorded in the common dormouse (Harris, cited by Sainsbury *et al.*, 1996). This paper also described orbital infestation with *Rhabditis orbitalis*, the incidence of which is unknown, but may be more of a problem at high population densities.

Diarrhoea of unknown origin, presumed to be related to sudden dietary changes and possible bacterial overgrowth, has been noted in dormice recently taken into captivity, and has responded to symptomatic treatment (H Ryan, personal communication).

Beavers
Trauma

Intraspecific fight wounds: These may develop into abscesses, often with thick pus similar to that found in rabbits. Tail and facial wounds from fighting are also very common and may provide sites for secondary bacterial infection. Species of *Pasteurella*, *Corynebacterium*, *Aeromonas*, *Pseudomonas* and *Staphylococcus* have all been isolated. This may lead to septicaemia and bacteraemia, and systemic bacterial disease and/or endocarditis may result, due to intracardiac turbulence from the combination of low blood pressure and an additional right atrial septum in this species. This may result in cardiovascular compromise, dramatic weight loss and may in some cases be fatal. Treatment is with appropriate antibiosis (e.g. systemic fluoroquinolones) and local treatment of infected wounds or abscesses (S Girling, personal communication). Echocardiography may be employed to detect endocarditis.

Parasites

A number of infectious diseases, including parasitic diseases, are reported in beavers. Some may be harboured in beavers, from other rodents. As these animals arise from stock imported from other countries, pre-release screening and vigilance for zoonotic species, or those with the potential to infect native wildlife, is important.

Ectoparasites: Beaver beetles (*Platypsyllus castoris*) are small wingless ectoparasites, which may be mistaken for fleas. However, they do not jump and are rusty orange/brown in coloration. Beavers do not appear to be bothered by these beetles feeding on skin secretions and epidermis, but heavy parasite burdens may indicate underlying health problems. They have been noted on Scottish beavers (Duff *et al.*, 2013).

Ear and skin mites (*Schizocarpus* spp.) may lead infected animals to shake, scratch or rub their ears and head, causing local trauma and secondary bacterial infection. There may be excessive ear wax production and a foul smell. Mites are usually spread through direct contact. Ticks have also been reported, and can indicate underlying health issues (R Campbell-Palmer, personal communication). Ticks may be manually removed, or direct treatment of the tick with surgical spirit may be applied (Stocker, 2005); fipronil or avermectins may also be used (S Girling, personal communication). Spot-on and spray treatments are not recommended as these are washed off in water. Systemic avermectins are used for endoparasites and appear safe in this species, and may be used in ectoparasite treatment also.

Endoparasites: Beaver nematode (*Travassosius rufus*) and beaver fluke (*Stichorchis subtriquetrus*) have been noted. These are species-specific organisms found in the stomach and caecum, respectively. The former has a direct life cycle, with eggs passed out in the faeces, and its infectious larval stage ingested by the beavers whilst feeding (Åhlén, 2001). The worms are seen on the stomach walls and within its contents. They are thin and pink/red in coloration. The latter has an aquatic snail as the intermediate host and beavers become infected when they ingest submerged plants. In one study, 100% of Swedish beavers (n=25) were found to be infected (Åhlén, 2001).

Cryptosporidium spp. is spread via the faeco–oral route. It can cause small intestinal disease, particularly in immunocompromised and/or immunologically naïve animals. It is difficult to eliminate the organism. It is widely present in wildlife and domestic animals; therefore, whilst released beavers should ideally be *Cryptosporidium*-free, they may become infected from native wildlife and domestic animals after release.

Beavers infected with *Giardia* spp. may show no evidence of disease, although clinical signs include diarrhoea and abdominal pain. Beavers have been implicated in human outbreaks, from faeco–oral transmission into human water sources. However, this organism is widely present in other species.

Echinococcus multilocularis is a pathogenic parasitic zoonotic disease present in central Europe. It could potentially be introduced to the UK via imported beavers acting as an intermediate host (Simpson and Hartley, 2011). Humans can be infected as an accidental intermediate host via faeco–oral transmission from the canid definitive hosts, which is potentially fatal, or can result in permanent organ, including brain, infection.

Infection can be determined through a combination of inspection of the beaver's liver at post-mortem examination or via minimally invasive exploratory laparoscopy in the live animal (Pizzi *et al.*, 2012), ultrasound examination of hepatic architecture, and blood tests (Gottstein *et al.*, 2014). Infection by this tapeworm was noted in a dead

Bavarian beaver from a captive population in England (Barlow *et al.*, 2011). Captive collections should ensure that any escaped animal originating from areas with this parasite are recaptured or accounted for, and ensure that any beaver carcasses are recovered and removed to prevent scavenging by other mammals, such as foxes, as soon as possible. Post-mortem examinations should include investigations for this parasite, particularly through examination of the liver for cysts (Barlow *et al.*, 2011), and rigorous standards of disease monitoring should be employed.

Tularaemia (*Francisella tularensis*) has not been reported in beavers in the UK, despite screening of imported animals. Beavers are susceptible to leptospirosis, and may acquire it from native rodents. (Campbell-Palmer and Rosell, 2013).

Other diseases

Dental disease: Abnormal incisor growth has been reported in wild beavers, which appear to survive, feed and breed despite these defects (Rosell and Kile, 1998). Fractures of the incisor teeth also appear to be common but rarely seem to cause long-term debility, owing to the rapid growth of these teeth. Birth defects or damage to teeth or jaw shortly after birth may lead to deformities (Rosell and Kile, 1998).

Therapeutics

Accurate weighing is important, for both drug administration and clinical assessment of these patients, and digital postal scales are particularly useful. However, even with reasonably accurate weighing, small body size and the relative uncertainty about dose rates suggest that drugs with a wide margin of safety should be used where possible. (For a more detailed discussion of rodent therapeutics, see de Matos, 2009.)

Dose rates

Using dose rates and frequencies established by pharmacological studies in domestic rodents will give the most accurate dose rates, which can be found in Fallon (1996), Flecknell (1996; 1998), Hrapkiewicz *et al.* (1998), Carpenter *et al.* (2001), de Matos (2009), Lennox and Bauck (2012) and Meredith (2015). In the absence of established dose rates and frequencies, doses calculated by allometric scaling (based on metabolic rate) rather than bodyweight are more accurate (see Chapter 7); the method is described by Flecknell (1998). Doses extrapolated from larger domestic mammals are likely to be much too low for these species in most cases.

It may also be necessary to dose more frequently in smaller species with high metabolic rates. Frequent medication of such animals, particularly orally, can be stressful and so the longest-acting preparation available should be used where possible. The addition of drugs to a highly palatable foodstuff may be useful (Flecknell, 1998). Sites of drug administration are noted in 'First aid'.

Parasiticides

Figure 14.19 gives dose rates for some parasiticides in rats and mice. Where dose rates are not available for relevant species allometric scaling can be used or doses extrapolated from similar species. It should be borne in mind, however, that use of products is unlicensed in these cases and potential toxic side effects are unknown.

Drug	Dose and application method	References	Notes
Flumethrin scab and tick dip	Animal totally immersed in dip for 10 seconds; repeated 2 weeks later	M Brash (personal communication)	Avoids direct handling Group of animals (e.g. rats) can be treated *en masse*
Fipronil spray	Used to wet cotton wool or gloved hand and then applied at lower end of dose range (i.e. 3 ml/kg)	Author's personal observation	Care must be taken to avoid chilling animal with solution, especially under anaesthetic, or allowing it to succumb to fumes of alcohol used as carrier
Praziquantel	No dose given; suggestions as follows: 5 mg/kg s.c. or 10 mg/kg orally 6–10 mg/kg orally	Wagner (1987) cited by Lipman and Foltz (1996) Carpenter *et al.* (2001) suggested for gerbils, mice and rats Orr (2002)	Treatment of *Hymenolepis* spp. Zoonotic
Niclosamide	100 mg/kg orally at 7-day intervals	Fraser (1991)	Treatment of *Hymenolepis* spp. Zoonotic
Ivermectin	0.2–0.4 mg/kg s.c., orally or topically q7–14d (NB Topically on the skin – applied between the shoulder blades at the back of the neck)	Fowler (1993) Carpenter *et al.* (2001) Orr (2002) Meredith (2015) Sayers and Smith (2010)	Effective against wide range of ecto- and endoparasites Appears to have wide margin of safety in these species; in view of their size, upper end of dose range should be used Percutaneous application may be absorbed via the skin or by grooming, and may be the method of choice in medicating animals which are difficult to handle See also Figure 13.13 for topical products and dose rates
Fenbendazole	20–50 mg/kg orally q24h for 5 consecutive days; the higher end of the range is suggested for giardiasis only	Meredith (2015)	Susceptible internal parasites (nematodes)

14.19 Parasiticides used in rats and mice and their dose rates.

Antibiotics

Some antibiotics can alter the normal gut flora of rodents and cause the development of fatal enterotoxaemias. Domestic rats and mice are rarely affected and wild ones are equally unlikely to have problems. Voles and dormice may be relatively more susceptible and it would be wise to avoid antibiotics that are particularly associated with such problems (e.g. penicillins, cephalosporins and especially lincosamides) unless there is a specific indication for their use. Parenteral antibiotics are generally safer in this regard than oral antibiotics. Fluoroquinolones and potentiated sulphonamides appear to be relatively safe to use both parenterally and orally in rodents and insectivores. Concurrent and subsequent dosing with probiotics may be of use in avoiding problems with bacterial overgrowth. In the event of an enterotoxaemia developing, cholestyramine resin may be of value in binding toxins within the gut (Flecknell, 1998). Figure 14.20 lists antibiotic doses for rats, mice and beavers. These species and the insectivores are less prone

Drug	Dose/comments
Amoxicillin	Mice, rats: 100–150 mg/kg i.m, s.c. q12h
Ampicillin (injection, 15% w/v; oral preparations)	Mice, rats: 25 mg/kg i.m., s.c. q12h[a] 50–200 mg/kg orally q12h[a]
Cephalosporins (cefalexin)	Mice: 30 mg/kg s.c. q24h Rats: 15 mg/kg s.c. q24h 60 mg/kg orally q12h
Chloramphenicol (injection; oral preparations)	Mice: 50 mg/kg i.m., orally q12h, 200 mg/kg orally q12h or 0.5 mg/ml drinking water[b] Rats and other rodents: 30–50 mg/kg i.v., i.m., s.c., orally q8–12h[b]
Amoxicillin/clavulanate (co-amoxiclav)	20 mg/kg orally q12h
Enrofloxacin	Mice, rats: 10 mg/kg s.c., orally q12h Beavers: standard formulation at 10 mg/kg q12–24h or long-acting formulation (Baytril Max) at 7.5–10 mg/kg every 2–4 days[c]
Marbofloxacin	10 mg/kg s.c. q24h[c] Other rodents and insectivores: 2–5 mg/kg i.m., s.c., orally q24h[b]
Neomycin (oral preparations)	Mice, rats: 25 mg/kg orally q12h[b] 2.6 mg/ml in drinking water[b]
Oxytetracycline (long-acting injection)	60 mg/kg i.m., s.c. q72h
Potentiated sulphonamides (e.g. trimethoprim/sulfadiazine)	50–100 mg/kg i.m., s.c., orally q24h 15–30mg/kg orally q12h
Sulfamerazine	0.02% in drinking water
Tetracycline (injectable; oral)	100 mg/kg s.c. (high dose used in respiratory disease) q72h 5 mg/kg in drinking water; 10–20 mg/kg orally q12h
Tylosin	10 mg/kg i.m., s.c., orally q24h

14.20 Antibacterial agents used in insectivores and rodents. Note that streptomycin and procaine penicillin are toxic to rats and mice.
([a] Ramsey, 2014; [b] Meredith, 2015; [c] Campbell-Palmer and Rosell, 2013)

to adverse gastrointestinal effects of antibiotics than hind-gut fermenting rodents. Where dose rates are not available for relevant species allometric scaling can be used or doses extrapolated from similar species. It should be borne in mind, however, that use of products is unlicensed in these cases and potential toxic side effects are unknown.

Antibiotic treatment of species with zoonotic bacterial infections is not recommended, due to the risk of the animal resuming shedding of bacteria after release and the effects on bacterial resistance. Euthanasia is recommended in such cases.

Management in captivity

Housing

Escape-proof housing is vitally important for these small fast-moving species. Housing requirements for different species are given in Figure 14.21. Some general guidelines are as follows:

- Secure plastic or glass vivaria or aquaria are best for smaller species, but may have poorer ventilation
- Ventilation must be good to avoid potential high humidity (relative humidity should not exceed 50–60%)
- The ceiling should consist of close-gauge mesh, with a small door opening in it (Stocker, 2005)
- Wood is warmer and cheaper than plastic, glass or wire, but difficult to clean and may be gnawed
- Wire cages are an option for species that gnaw

- Cages with walls at least partly of mesh rather than totally solid are another option but are less secure, more difficult to keep clean and will restrict normal nesting and burrowing behaviour
- Substrate options include sand, wood shavings, peat, hay, moss (Michalak, 1987), leaves and paper towels
- To reduce the stress of scent removal, avoid cleaning out too often (Poole, 1999) and leave some bedding in place after each clean
- Water for swimming should be provided for aquatic species, such as water shrews (Figure 14.22).

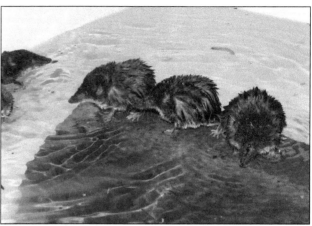

14.22 Hand-reared insectivores, such as this litter of water shrews, must be provided with a suitable environment during captivity in order that they can learn normal behaviour such as swimming. (Courtesy of G Cousquer)

Group	Structure	Nesting	Substrate	Humidity and water	Notes
Moles	Glass escape-proof vivarium No top required if container sufficiently tall (moles cannot climb)	Separate nesting boxes at each end	Layer of earth, peat and leaf litter deep enough to burrow into (Figure 14.23)	Regular watering of soil necessary: moles require moderately high humidity May result in nasal lesions if soil too dry (M Brash, personal communication)	'Collapse' the tunnels regularly to avoid stereotypy associated with lack of tunneling opportunities in longer-term accommodation
Shrews	Escape-proof plastic or glass vivarium with lid Hide tubes or boxes	Hay, moss, leaves	Not shredded paper (rustling noise can upset them) (Fowler, 1986; Dryden, 1975) Deep enough for burrowing	Can give water shrews some swimming water as part of enclosure but not essential (Henwood, 1985) (Figure 14.22)	Position food/water containers around edges of cage (shrews avoid exposed open centre of cage) (Dryden, 1975) If swimming water provided, water shrews also need a burrow in which to dry and groom themselves
Harvest mice	Cages at least 75 cm high	Dense vegetation (e.g. planting or by wedging entire tussock or bunches of oat/barley/wheat/ teasels tied together) (Henwood, 1985) for climbing and nest building		Humidity <50–60% Water in shallow containers at ground level	Fight if kept at high population densities
Rats and other mouse species	Escape-proof plastic or glass vivarium with lid Hide tubes or boxes	Hay, moss, leaves	Good depth of litter for burrowing	Humidity <50–60% Water in shallow containers at ground level	Hides are vital. Food should be placed in hidden or sheltered areas to allow them to feel secure when eating
Dormice	Robust housing to deter escape by gnawing Agile and jump well	Nest boxes with vegetation above ground level	Vegetation and branches	Nest needs to be moistened occasionally during hibernation to avoid dehydration	This housing information is applicable to the captive environment, and also to the provision of breeding nest boxes for wild dormice
Beavers	Robust fencing or walls. Beavers will escape by digging under, biting through, and even climbing over fences	Burrows into earth banks, and lodges constructed of branches	Wooded grassland, with access to water	Fresh, running water required for all but the most short-term captivity	Animals from different families should not be housed together, or fighting will ensue

14.21 Housing requirements for different species of insectivores and rodents in captivity.

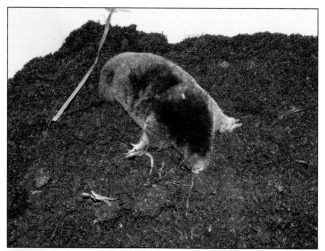

14.23 Moles require a deep substrate for digging in, and should ideally be fed live earthworms, rather than mealworms as illustrated here.
(© Richard Saunders)

For insectivores, further descriptions of husbandry can be found in Michalak (1987), Dryden (1975) and Rudge (1966). For rodents, accommodation requirements are well described in appropriate laboratory animal texts and by Michalak (1987) and Poole (1999). For common dormice, guidelines on long-term housing should be obtained from the Dormouse Captive Breeding Group (see 'Specialist organizations and useful contacts').

Wild species differ from laboratory animals in being more aggressive, more inclined to escape and more stressed by human contact. Therefore artefacts such as hide boxes, cardboard tubes, drainpipes and pots must be provided (especially for shrews), with adequate nesting material such as hay, leaves and moss. The substrate should be deep enough for burrowing but long-stranded material may entrap limbs and should be avoided (Bourne, 2002).

Beavers' requirements are more difficult to manage due to their size and aquatic requirements, as well as their potentially destructive nature. Short-term hospitalization has less exacting requirements, but they still need adequate space, and access to water. Access to water may be restricted if required in the short term (e.g. to allow wound closure), especially as beavers rapidly contaminate water with faeces. Veterinary surgeons treating beavers should contact the relevant authorities for husbandry guidelines or to make arrangements for the animal to return to such a facility (see 'Specialist organizations and useful contacts') (Campbell-Palmer and Rosell, 2013).

Feeding

The feeding requirements in captivity of insectivores and rodents are described below and in Figure 14.24.

Group	Suitable foods	Notes and special needs
Moles	Earthworms, slugs, insects, waxworms, mealworms, diets for insectivorous birds, dog food (preferably meat-in-jelly), chopped pinky mice	Place foods directly on substrate Water obtained mostly from food in wild but provide drinking water in shallow bowls in captivity (Small, 1994)
Shrews	Maggots, fly pupae, mealworms, fresh meat, egg, food for insectivorous birds, crushed dried cat food (Dryden, 1975) Ideal prey size 6–10 mm	Food must always be available (high metabolic rate) Often discard unpalatable parts and sometimes cache their food (Bourne, 2002) Refection of milky white fluid from anus is normal; contains fat globules and partially digested food
Water shrews	Minced mixture of beef offal, fish, chicken (or rabbit or guinea pig), egg, sprouted wheat grains, mealworms (Michelak, 1987)	As for other shrews Have been given milk instead of drinking water (Michelak, 1987)
Voles	Whole oats, meadow hay, chopped carrots, rodent pellets (Baker and Clarke, 1987) Chopped grasses, clover, garden flowers, seeds, dry oats, mouse food, crushed digestive biscuits, greens, leafy twigs with buds, hay	Field voles eat relatively more grass than other voles
Bank voles	Prefer seeds, fresh vegetables (e.g. carrot, apple, cabbage), fresh grasses, hedgerow fruits	High water requirement: drinking water must be available at all times
Rats and mice	Commercial diets available for pet rats and mice can be used	Additionally crushed oats, wheat, maize, fruit, vegetables and dog biscuits (broken or whole) can be fed
Wood mice	Prefer seeds, berries, rosehips, green plants, insects	Tend to avoid root vegetables
Harvest mice	Birdseed, blowfly pupae, millet, rape, linseed, growing grasses, hedgerow flowers and fruits, insects, small quantities of flaked fish food	Immune to toxins of berries that are poisonous to humans (e.g. black bryony (*Tamus communis*))
Common dormice	Sunflower seeds and peanuts (in moderation), hazelnuts, rich tea biscuits, ripe fruit (e.g. grape, apple, banana, strawberry, other berries), corn, tomato, clumps of hazel or sycamore branches, canary egg food, mynah bird food (D Woods, personal communication)	Also insectivorous in summer: moths, caterpillars On waking from hibernation, often eat pollen and nectar (D Woods, personal communication)
Edible dormice	As for common dormice plus dry puppy food, spinach, curly kale, pecan nuts (Stocker, 2005)	Will eat raw meat in captivity Drink large quantities
European Beavers	Green herbaceous vegetation, new woody growth, tree bark and aquatic plants. In captivity, small amounts of browse, supplemented with carrots, parsnip, beet, turnip, sweet potato, maize, pear, celery, cabbage, cucumber, broccoli and kale Grass hay may be used to at least partially provide fibre, although browse is preferred	High-sugar items such as fruits (e.g. apples and pears) should be excluded, or fed in very small amounts only (e.g. where tempting an ill animal to eat or in transit to provide dietary water) to avoid disrupting caecal bacteria populations

14.24 Feeding requirements of captive insectivores and rodents.

Drinking water

It should not be assumed that wild animals can operate a rodent drinker bottle, especially the smaller species. Water should also be offered in a bird drinker or bowl (which is not deep enough to permit drowning) or jam jar lid, and drinkers should be positioned very close to the ground.

Insectivores

Live food items for insectivores should be adequately nourished for at least 48 hours before they are consumed otherwise they will be of dubious nutritional value, have an empty gut and can be dehydrated when they are eaten. It is advisable to improve the nutritional status of invertebrates by feeding them with sliced fruit and vegetables, powdered dog biscuits, flaked fish food and proprietary or homemade insect foods or 'gut-loading' formulae, and to dust with proprietary nutritional supplementation.

Rodents

Commercial diets for a number of pet rodents exist and can be used as a basis for diets of wild rats and mice and as a supplementary diet for other wild small rodents. Additional ingredients for wild rodents include crushed oats, wheat, maize, fruit, vegetables and dog biscuits (broken or whole).

Beavers

Wild diets for beavers include green herbaceous vegetation, new woody growth, tree bark and aquatic plants. In captivity, small amounts of browse, supplemented with carrots, parsnip, beet, turnip, sweet potato, maize, pear, celery, cabbage, cucumber, broccoli and kale may be offered. High-sugar items such as fruits (e.g. apples and pears) should be excluded, or fed in very small amounts only (e.g. where tempting an ill animal to eat or in transit to provide dietary water) to avoid disrupting caecal bacteria populations. Grass hay may be used to at least partially provide fibre, although browse is preferred. Pelleted diets such as Mazuri® Leaf Eater Primate Pellet or Zoo Diet A and pelleted alfalfa cubes may be used as an addition to the diet; however, they should not form a significant proportion. Captive beavers have been known to develop hypervitaminosis D when fed on commercial primate pellets that contained vitamin D3 (Campbell-Palmer and Rosell, 2013). Beavers need access to fresh water of sufficient depth to submerge their mouths, including their lower jaw, as they cannot lick or lap water (Campbell-Palmer and Rosell, 2013).

Rearing of young

Orphaned rodents and insectivores are generally altricial, one exception being beavers. Rearing rodents and insectivores is extremely challenging and in many cases not possible unless they are sufficiently old (Spaulding and Spaulding, 1979). In some cases, euthanasia is likely to be the preferable course of action (Bourne, 2002). Age should be determined as accurately as possible at the outset (see Figures 14.3, 14.4, 14.6, 14.8, 14.10, 14.12 and 14.14). See also Chapter 8 for general information on rearing neonates.

Environmental temperature

These species exhibit poor thermoregulation and require well regulated temperatures of 35°C for a hairless infant and 32°C for one that is furred but has its eyes still closed. Once the eyes are open, the temperature can be dropped by 2.5°C weekly down to 20–21°C (Weber, 1978). A temperature gradient should be provided and soft comfortable disposable bedding is required.

Feeding

The special neonatal feeding requirements of different species are outlined in Figure 14.25. Given their comparatively low numbers in the wild, it is unlikely that orphaned beavers would be encountered. Anyone finding an abandoned neonatal beaver should contact the relevant specialist organizations for further information and advice (see 'Specialist organizations and useful contacts').

- The first feed should be of an oral rehydration solution followed by a gradual change to a milk substitute over several feeds.
- A syringe, catheter sleeve (Figure 14.26), paintbrush, Pasteur pipette or piece of string as a 'wick' can be used for smaller rodents; a kitten-feeder can be used for larger ones.

Group	Milk replacers	How often	Time for weaning	Weaning foods
Moles and shrews	Esbilac® or Zoologic® Milk Matrix 30/55® (mother's milk is concentrated and high-fat)	Hourly throughout day and night	As soon as possible	Live invertebrate food and finely chopped version of adult diet (Stocker, 2000)
Mice, rats and voles	Goat colostrum mixed 1:3 with milk replacer (e.g. Esbilac® or Zoologic® Milk Matrix 30/44®)	Every hour during daylight; every 2 hours overnight (a few drops per feed)	From 9 days of age	Mice: crumbled biscuits or rusks or cereal, soaked in milk replacer. Voles: chickweed, dandelion, clover (Stocker, 2000)
Dormice	Goat's milk or Lactol® made up 1:3 with water Vitamin drops (e.g. Abidec®) may be added	4 or 5 times daily, or every 2 hours from 6.30 am to 11.00 pm	2–3 weeks	Rusks (Stocker, 2000), dry puppy food, Milupa® baby food, wholemeal bread, apple, raspberries, cherries, rosehips, sycamore seeds, hazelnuts in shell, acorn, hazel twigs, honeysuckle (French, 1989)
Beavers	Esbilac® (beaver milk is higher in fat, protein and energy, but lower in sugar than that of most other mammals)	Every 2 hours until the kit starts to take food for itself	Solid food can be offered after the first week. Water (for drinking and swimming) should be made available from 3 days	Wild herbaceous plants and dark green leafy vegetables (Campbell-Palmer and Rosell, 2013); Weaning foods include sweet potato, sweetcorn (not including the outer fibrous sheath), apple, carrot, potato, willow (leaves and bark) and fresh vegetation (M O'Brien, personal communication)

14.25 Feeding requirements of orphan insectivores and rodents.

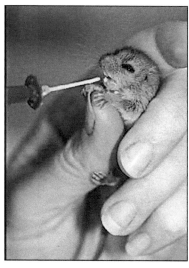

14.26 A juvenile common dormouse being syringe fed using a catheter sleeve as a dropper. Gloves should be worn when handling dormice.
(© Secret World Wildlife Rescue)

- Up to 35–40% of bodyweight can be fed daily, with no more than 25–50 ml/kg bodyweight given per feed.
- Toileting should be performed on admission and after each feed (Bourne, 2002) by gently rubbing the anogenital region with a damp wisp of cotton wool until urination and defecation take place.
- Records must be kept of weight, feeding amount, frequency, urination and defecation (Bourne, 2002).

Release

In most cases of individual release of adults, hard release (see Chapter 9) into suitable environments is preferred. For species bred or raised in captivity, soft release is preferred. For species with exacting habitat requirements (e.g. common dormice, water voles), liaison with experienced field workers is advised. Little research into the release or post-release success of other species has been carried out. The following release sites are recommended by Stocker (2005):

- Moles: deciduous woodland where there is no evidence of moles already present (to avoid territorial problems); they should be released in leaf litter and observed until underground
- Shrews, bank voles and field voles: hedgerows, gardens, verges and embankments
- Harvest mice: suitable fields of tall grasses or the hedgerows surrounding them
- Water voles: near small rivers and canals. The Mammal Society should be contacted before release, as there may be a release project in the area (The Mammal Society, 2001b).

Common dormice

A licence is required for any interventions with common dormice and can be obtained from Natural England. Immediate release *in situ* of uninjured adults is advised.

If a dormouse has been disturbed during hibernation, its nest should quickly be wrapped up again and covered over. If necessary, the nest and its occupant (with plenty of damp padding) may be transferred to a more secure ground location within 100 m of the original site, choosing a cool area out of direct sunlight. The nest can be covered with a flat stone to protect it from predators and to keep it

moist and cool. If the dormouse is partially active, release nearby at dusk may be preferable (Bright *et al.*, 1996).

The Dormouse Captive Breeding Group or Natural England should be contacted before release, which should be coordinated with release/reintroduction workers in the area. Any dormice not considered fit for release may be suitable for captive-breeding programmes. If maintained in permanent captivity the animal's 'five freedoms' (see Chapter 4) must be fulfilled and be able to be monitored for the rest of the animal's life.

Dormice are best released in pairs or small groups D Woods, personal communication) via a soft release (see Chapter 9) in early summer (French, 1989). A suitable environment without any existing dormice should be selected, as these animals live at much lower population densities than other rodents (Bright *et al.*, 1996).

Beavers

Beaver release should only be as part of a management programme, under licence, as they are technically a non-native species under the Wildlife and Countryside Act. The relevant authorities should be contacted (Campbell-Palmer and Rosell, 2013).

Legal aspects

Details of general legislation covering the species discussed in this chapter are given in Chapter 2 and the release of certain 'pest species' has previously been discussed in this chapter. The following points are specific:

- Schedule 6 of the Wildlife and Countryside Act (WCA) prohibits the taking and killing of shrews by certain methods
- Schedule 2 of the WCA covers the place of rest or shelter of voles
- Control of the brown rat is permitted by certain approved methods (e.g. spring traps and poisons)
- Release of the black rat or the edible dormouse is illegal under Schedule 9 of the WCA
- Under Schedule 6 of the WCA, neither species of dormouse may be taken or killed by certain methods. Common dormice are also afforded considerable protection under Schedule 5 of the WCA, which makes it an offence to interfere with them except under licence (Natural England should be contacted if a licence is required). Additional protection is given by the EU Conservation (Natural Habitats) Regulations, which covers habitats rather than the animals themselves
- The Eurasian beaver is protected under the Bern Convention and Annex IV of the EC Habitats directive, with disturbance only permitted under the latter under licence from the relevant statutory authority. However, this does not apply unless they have been formally reintroduced, and may also depend upon disease screening (Campbell-Palmer and Rosell, 2013).

Acknowledgements

The author would like to thank Matt Brash for information on the captive husbandry of moles and voles, Anne Hudson for her comments on wild rats and mice, Doug

Woods and Hazel Ryan for their comments on common dormice, Kate Long for her comments on water voles, Sandra Baker for her comments on moles, Adam Grogan for the admission figures for the species in this chapter, Derek Gow, Sarah Brown, Romain Pizzi, Roisin Campbell-Palmer and Simon Girling (RZSS) for their information on beavers, Tony Sainsbury for his comments on the dormice section, Debra Bourne and the Wildlife Information Network for information on a number of species covered here and Sian Saunders for her general comments.

References and further reading

Åhlén PA (2001) *The parasitic and commensal fauna of the European beaver (Castor fiber) in Sweden.* Honours thesis 2001: 3. Department of Animal Ecology, SLU, Umeå

Appleby BM, Anwar MA and Petty SJ (1999) Short-term and long-term effects of food supply on parasite burdens in tawny owls (*Strix aluco*). *Functional Ecology* **13**, 315–321

Atkinson R (2013) *Moles (The British Natural History Collection).* Whittet Books, Stansted

Atkinson RPD and Macdonald DW (1994) Can repellents function as a nonlethal means of controlling moles (*Talpa europaea*)? *Journal of Applied Ecology* **31**, 731–736

Atkinson RPD, Macdonald DW and Johnson PJ (1994) The status of the European mole *Talpa europaea* L. as an agricultural pest and its management. *Mammal Review* **24**, 73–90

Baker JP and Clark JR (1987) Voles. In: *UFAW Handbook on the Care and Management of Laboratory Animals, 6th edn*, ed. TB Poole. Longman, Harlow

Baker PJ, Bentley AJ, Ansell RJ and Harris S (2005) Impact of predation by domestic cats *Felis catus* in an urban area. *Mammal Review* **35(3–4)**, 302–312

Baker SE, Ellwood SA, Tagarielli VL and Macdonald DW (2012) Mechanical performance of rat, mouse and mole spring traps, and possible implications for welfare performance. *PLoS ONE* **7(6)**; e39334. doi.org/10.1371/journal.pone.0039334

Baker SE and Macdonald DW (2012) Not so humane mole tube traps. *Animal Welfare* **21(4)**, 613–615

Barlow AM, Gottstein B, and Mueller N (2011) *Echinococcus multilocularis* in an imported captive European beaver (*Castor fiber*) in Great Britain. *Veterinary Record* **169**, 339

Barrow PA (1981) *Corynebacterium kutscheri* infection in wild voles (*Microtus agrestis*). *British Veterinary Journal* **137**, 76–80

Beard PM, Daniels MJ, Henderson D *et al.* (2001) *Paratuberculosis* infection of nonruminant wildlife in Scotland. *Journal of Clinical Microbiology* **39**, 1517–1521

Behnke JM, Lewis JW, Zain SNM and Gilbert FS (1999) Helminth infections in *Apodemus sylvaticus* in southern England: interactive effects of host age, sex and year on the prevalence and abundance of infection. *Journal of Helminthology* **73**, 31–44

Blackmore DK and Owen DG (1968) Ectoparasites: their significance in British wild rodents. *Symposium of the Zoological Society of London* **24**, 197

Bourne D (2002) *UK Wildlife: First Aid and Care.* Wildlife Information Network, London (CD ROM)

Bright PW and Morris PA (1989) *A Practical Guide to Dormouse Conservation.* The Mammal Society, London

Bright PW and Morris PA (1990) Habitat requirements of dormice (*Muscardinus avellanarius*) in relation to woodland management in Southwest England. *Biological Conservation* **54**, 307–326

Bright PW and Morris PA (1992) Ranging and nesting behaviour of the dormouse (*Muscardinus avellanarius*) in coppice-with-standards woodland. *Journal of Zoology* **226**, 589–600

Bright PW and Morris PA (1993) Conservation of the dormouse. *British Wildlife* **4**, 154–162

Bright PW and Morris PA (1994) Animal translocation for conservation: performance of dormice in relation to release methods, origin and season. *Journal of Applied Ecology* **31**, 699–708

Bright PW and Morris PA (1996) Why are dormice rare? A case study in conservation biology. *Mammal Review* **26**, 157–187

Bright PW and Morris PA (2005) *The Dormouse.* The Mammal Society, London

Bright PW, Morris PA and Mitchell-Jones T (2006) *The Dormouse Conservation Handbook.* English Nature, Peterborough

Bull SA, Chalmers RM, Sturdee AP and Healing TD (1998) A survey of *Cryptosporidium* species in Skomer bank voles (*Clethrionomys glareolus skomerensis*). *Journal of Zoology* **244**, 119–122

Campbell-Palmer R, Girling S, Rosell F, Paulsen P and Goodman G (2012) *Echinococcus* risk from imported beavers. *Veterinary Record* **170**, 235

Campbell-Palmer R, Girling S, Pizzi R *et al.* (2013) *Stichorchis subtrequetrus* in a free-living beaver in Scotland. *Veterinary Record* **173(3)**, 72

Campbell-Palmer R and Rosell F (2013) *Captive management guidelines for Eurasian Beavers (Castor fiber).* Royal Zoological Society of Scotland, Edinburgh

Carpenter JW (2013) *Exotic Animal Formulary, 4th edn.* WB Saunders, Philadelphia

Carpenter JW, Mashima TY and Rupiper DJ (2001) *Exotic Animal Formulary, 2nd edn.* WB Saunders, Philadelphia

Chalmers RA, Sturdee AP, Bull SA, Miller A and Wright SE (1997) The prevalence of *Cryptosporidium parvum* and *C. muris* in *Mus domesticus, Apodemus sylvaticus* and *Clethrionomys glareolus* in an agricultural system. *Parasitology Research* **83**, 478–482

Churcher PB and Lawton JH (1987) Predation by domestic cats in an English village. *Journal of Zoology* **212(3)**, 439–455

Clark JD and Olfert ED (1986) Rodents. In: *Zoo and Wild Animal Medicine*, ed. ME Fowler. WB Saunders, Philadelphia

Corbet GB and Harris S (1991) *The Handbook of British Mammals, 3rd edn.* Blackwell Scientific, Oxford

Cosgrove GE (1986) Insectivores. In: *Zoo and Wild Animal Medicine: Current Therapy 2*, ed. ME Fowler. WB Saunders, Philadelphia

de Matos R (2009) Rodents: therapeutics. In: *BSAVA Manual of Rodents and Ferrets*, ed. E Keeble and A Meredith, pp. 52–62. BSAVA Publications, Gloucester

Dona M and Pyne M (2013) *Control and therapy series 270. Part 4: wildlife flashcard series – Mammals (small mammals).* Currumbin Sanctuary Wildlife Hospital. www.cve.edu.au

Dryden GL (1975) Establishment and maintenance of shrew colonies. *International Zoo Yearbook* **15**, 12

Duff AG, Campbell-Palmer R and Needham R (2013) The beaver beetle *Platypsyllus castoris* (Leiodidae: Platypsyllinae) apparently established on reintroduced beavers in Scotland, new to Britain. *The Coleopterist* **22**, 9–19

Edwards GR, Crawley MJ and Heard MS (1999) Factors influencing molehill distribution in grassland: implications for controlling the damage caused by molehills. *Journal of Applied Ecology* **36**, 434–443

Evans HTJ and Thompson HV (1981) Bovine tuberculosis in cattle in Great Britain. I. Eradication of the disease from cattle and the role of the badger (*Meles meles*) as a source of *Mycobacterium bovis* for cattle. *Animal Regulation Studies* **3**, 191–216

Fallon MT (1996) Rats and mice. In: *Handbook of Rodent and Rabbit Medicine*, ed. K Laber-Laird *et al.*, pp. 1–38. Elsevier Science, Oxford

Fish R, Danneman PJ, Brown M and Karas A (2011) *Anesthesia and Analgesia in Laboratory Animals*, p. 462. Academic Press, London

Flecknell P (1996) Anaesthesia and analgesia for rodents and rabbits. In: *Handbook of Rodent and Rabbit Medicine*, ed. K Laber-Laird *et al.*, pp. 219–238. Elsevier Science, Oxford

Flecknell P (1998) Developments in the veterinary care of rabbits and rodents. *In Practice* **20**, 6

Forder V (2006) *Captive Breeding and Reintroduction. The Hazel Dormouse (Muscardinus avellanarius).* Wildwood Trust. www.wildwoodtrust.org/files/dormice-captive-breeding.pdf

Fowler ME (1986) *Zoo and Wild Animal Medicine: Current Therapy 2.* WB Saunders, Philadelphia

Fowler ME (1993) *Zoo and Wild Animal Medicine: Current Therapy 3.* WB Saunders, London

Fowler ME (1995) *Restraint and Handling of Wild and Domestic Animals, 2nd edn.* Iowa State University Press, Ames

Fraser CM, Bergeron JA, Mays A and Aiello SE (1991) *Merck Veterinary Manual, 7th edn.* Merck and Co, Rahway, New Jersey

French HJ (1989) Hand rearing the common or hazel dormouse (*Muscardinus avellanarius*). *International Zoo Yearbook* **28**, 262

Gottstein B, Frey CF, Campbell-Palmer R *et al.* (2014) Immunoblotting for the serodiagnosis of alveolar *Echinococcus* in live and dead Eurasion beavers (*Castor fiber*). *Veterinary Parasitology* **205**, 113–118

Gregory RD (1991) Parasite epidemiology and host population growth: *Heligmosomoides polygyrus* (Nematoda) in enclosed wood mouse populations. *Journal of Animal Ecology* **60**, 805–821

Grogan A and Kelly A (2013) A review of RSPCA research into wildlife rehabilitation. *Veterinary Record* **172**, 211

Gurnell J and Flowerdew JR (1994) *Live Trapping Small Mammals – a Practical Guide, 3rd edn.* The Mammal Society, London

Haim A, van der Straelen E and Cooreman WM (1987) Urine analysis of European moles (*Talpa europea*) and white rats (*Rattus norvegicus*) kept on a carnivore's diet. *Comparative Biochemistry and Physiology, A: Comparative Physiology* **88**, 179–181

Hansard (2014) HC Deb, 26 June 2014, vol 583, c330W

Healing TD (1981) Infection with blood parasites in the small British rodents *Apodemus sylvaticus, Clethrionomys glareolus* and *Microtus agrestis*. *Parasitology* **83**, 179–189

Healing TD and Greenwood MH (1991) Frequency of isolation of *Campylobacter* spp., *Yersinia* spp. and *Salmonella* spp. from small mammals from two sites in southern Britain. International *Journal of Environmental Health Research* **1**, 54–62

Healing TD, Kaplan C and Prior A (1980) A note on some Enterobacteriaceae from the faeces of small wild British mammals. *Journal of Hygiene (London)* **85**, 343–345

Healing TD and Nowell F (1985) Diseases and parasites of woodland rodent populations. *Symposium of the Zoological Society of London* **55**, 193

Hellwing S (1973) Husbandry and breeding of white-toothed shrews (*Crocidurinae*) in the research zoo of the Tel-Aviv University. *International Zoo Yearbook* **13** 127–134

Henwood C (1985) *The Handbook of Rodents in Captivity*. Ian Henry Publications Ltd

Hrapkiewicz K, Medina L and Holmes DD (1998) *Clinical Medicine of Small Mammals and Primates – an Introduction, 2nd edn*. Manson Publishing, London

Jameson LJ, Logue CH, Atkinson B *et al.* (2013) The continued emergence of Hantaviruses: Isolation of a Seoul virus implicated in human disease, United Kingdom, October 2012. *Eurosurveillance* **18(1)**, 4–7

Kaplan C, Healing TD, Evans N, Healing L and Prior A (1980) Evidence of infection by viruses in small British field rodents. *Journal of Hygiene (London)* **84**, 285–294

Kirkwood JK (1991) Wild mammals. In: *BSAVA Manual of Exotic Pets, 3rd edn*, ed. PH Beynon and JE Cooper, pp. 122–149. BSAVA, Cheltenham

Korbel R (1990) Epizootiology, clinical aspects and therapy of *Pasteurella multocida* infection in bird patients after cat bites. *Tierarztliche Praxis* **18**, 365–376

Korbel R, Gerlach H, Bisgaard M and Hafez HM (1992) Further investigations on *Pasteurella multocida* infections in feral birds injured by cats. *Zentralblatt für Veterinarmedizin Reihe B* **39**, 10–18

Lennox AM and Bauck L (2012) Section 4: small rodents. Basic anatomy, physiology, husbandry and clinical techniques. In: *Ferrets, Rabbits and Rodents: Clinical Medicine and Surgery*, ed. EV Hillyer and KE Quesenberry, pp. 339–353. WB Saunders, Philadelphia

Lichtenberger M and Hawkins M (2009) Chapter 2. Rodents: physical examination and emergency care. In: *BSAVA Manual of Rodents and Ferrets*, ed. E Keeble and A Meredith, pp. 18–31. BSAVA Publications, Gloucester

Loss SR, Will T and Marra P (2013) The impact of free ranging domestic cats on wildlife of the US. *Nature Communications* **4**, 1396

MacDonald D (1995) *European Mammals: Evolution and Behaviour*. Collins, London

McDiarmid SC (1983) The absorption of drugs from subcutaneous and intramuscular injection sites. *Veterinary Bulletin* **53**, 9–23

Meehan TP (1993) Insectivora, medical problems of shrews. In: *Zoo and Wild Animal Medicine: Current Therapy 3*, ed. ME Fowler. WB Saunders, Philadelphia

Meredith A (2015) *BSAVA Small Animal Formulary, 9th edition – Part B: Exotic Pets*. BSAVA Publications, Gloucester

Meredith AL, Cleaveland SC, Brown J, Mahajan A and Shaw DJ (2015) Seroprevalence of *Encephalitozoon cuniculi* in wild rodents, foxes and domestic cats in three sites in the United Kingdom. *Transboundary and Emerging Diseases* **62**, 148–156

Michalak I (1987) Keeping and breeding the Eurasian water shrew (*Neomys fodiens*) under laboratory conditions. *International Zoo Yearbook* **26**, 223

Mohamed HA, Molyneux DH and Wallbanks KR (1987) A coccidian in haemogamasid mites; possible vectors of *Elleipsisoma thomsoni Franca, 1912*. *Annales de Parasitologie Humaine et Comparée* **62**, 107–116

Natural England (2011) *Moles; Options for Management and Control*. Technical Information Note TIN033. Natural England, Bristol http://publications.naturalengland.org.uk/publication/34015

Nelson M (2001) Mammal society maligns 'murdering' moggies. *Veterinary Times*, April, p. 10

Nowell F and Higgs S (1989) *Eimeria* species infecting woodmice (genus *Apodemus*) and the transfer of two species to *Mus musculus*. *Parasitology* **98**, 329–336

Panteix G, Gutierrez MC, Boschiroli ML *et al.* (2010) Pulmonary tuberculosis due to *Mycobacterium microti*: a study of six recent cases in France. *Journal of Medical Microbiology* **59(8)**, 984–989

Parker H, Rosell F and Holthe V (2000) A gross assessment of the suitability of selected Scottish riparian habitats for beaver. *Scottish Forestry* **54**, 25–31

Pizzi R, Cracknell J and Carter P (2012) *Echinococcus* risk from imported beavers. *Veterinary Record* **170**, 293–294

Pocock MJO, Searle JB, Betts WB and White PCL (2001) Patterns of infection by *Salmonella* and *Yersinia* spp. in commensal house mouse (*Mus musculus domesticus*) populations. *Journal of Applied Microbiology* **90**, 755–760

Poole T (1999) *The UFAW Handbook on the Care and Management of Laboratory Animals, 7th edn, Vol. 1*. Blackwell Scientific Publications, Oxford

Pounder KC, Begon M, Sironen T *et al.* (2013) Novel hantavirus in field vole, United Kingdom. *Emerging Infectious Diseases* **19(4)**, 673–675

Quy R and Poole D (2004) A review of methods used within the European Union to control the European Mole, *Talpa Europaea*: a report. Defra, London

Ramsey I (2014) *BSAVA Small Animal Formulary, 8th edn*. BSAVA Publications, Gloucester

Ranheim B, Rosell F, Haga HA and Arnemo JM (2004) Field anaesthetic and surgical techniques for implantation of intraperitoneal radio transmitters in Eurasian beavers (*Castor fiber*). *Wildlife Biology* **10**, 11–15

Rankin JD and McDiarmid A (1968) Mycobacterial infections in free living wild animals. *Symposium of the Zoological Society of London* **24**, 119

Redfern R and Rowe FP (1987) Wild rats and mice. In: *The UFAW Handbook on the Care and Management of Laboratory Mammals, 6th edn*, ed. TB Poole. Longman, Harlow

Richardson C and Flecknell P (2009) Rodents: anaesthesia and analgesia. In: *BSAVA Manual of Rodents and Ferrets*, ed. E Keeble and A Meredith, pp. 63–72. BSAVA Publications, Gloucester

Roots CD (1992) Morphological and ecological studies on helminth parasites of the British shrews. *Journal of Helminthology* **683**, 247–254

Rosell F and Kile NB (1998) Abnormal incisor growth in Eurasian beaver. *Acta Theriologica* **43**, 329–332

Rudge AJB (1963) A study of mole-trapping. *Proceedings of the Zoological Society of London* **149**, 330–334

Rudge AJB (1966) Catching and keeping live moles. *Journal of the Zoological Society of London* **149**, 42

Ruxton GD, Thomas S and Wright JW (2002) Bells reduce predation of wildlife by domestic cats (*Felis catus*). *Journal of Zoology (London)* **256**, 81–83

Sainsbury AW, Bright PW, Morris PA and Harris EA (1996) Ocular disease associated with *Rhabditis orbitalis* nematodes in a common dormouse (*Muscardinus avellanarius*). *Veterinary Record* **139**, 192–193

Saunders RA and Whitlock E (2012) Nursing hospitalized patients. In: *BSAVA Manual of Exotic Pet and Wildlife Nursing*, ed. M Varga, R Lumbis, and L Gott, pp. 129–166. BSAVA Publications, Gloucester

Sayers I and Smith S (2010) Mice, rats, hamsters and gerbils. In: *BSAVA Manual of Exotic Pets, 5th edn*, ed. A Meredith and C Johnson-Delaney, pp. 1–27. BSAVA Publications, Gloucester

Shore RF, Feber RE, Firbank LG *et al.*, (1997) The impacts of molluscicide pellets on spring and autumn populations of wood mice (*Apodemus sylvaticus*). *Agriculture, Ecosystems and Environment* **64**, 211–217

Simpson V (1999) Potential Wildlife Zoonoses in Britain. In: *Proceedings of the British Veterinary Association Congress, Bath*

Simpson V and Hartley M (2011) *Echinoccous* risk from imported beavers. *Veterinary Record* **169**, 689–690

Small M (1994) *Wildlife Welfare (Mammals)*. Intervet, Cambridge

Spaulding CE and Spaulding J (1979) *The Complete Care of Orphaned or Abandoned Baby Animals*. Rodale Press, Emmaus, Pennsylvania

Stocker L (2005) *Practical Wildlife Care, 2nd edn*. Blackwell Science, Oxford

Tabor R (2001) Cats are carnivores, not criminals. *The Cat*, May/June

Taylor K (1999) Scots eager for beavers. *BBC Wildlife*, January, p. 23

The Mammal Society (2001a) *Mammal Society Factsheets*. Mammal Society, London

The Mammal Society (2001b) *Mammal Society website*. www.mammal.org.uk

Universities Federation for Animal Welfare (1983) The use of alpha-chloralose for the control of moles. In: *UFAW Reports and Accounts*. www.ufaw.org.uk

US Fish and Wildlife Service (2008) *The Facts about Rats*. http://www.fws.gov/pacificislands/publications/ratsfactsheet.pdf

Weber WJ (1978) *Wild Orphan Babies, 2nd edn*. Holt, Rinehart and Wiston, New York

Wenger S, Gull J, Glaus T *et al.* (2010) Fallot's tetralogy in a European beaver. *Journal of Zoo and Wildlife Medicine* **41**, 359–362

Withnall A (2013) Wild beaver spotted in England for first time in 800 years. *The Independent*. www.independent.co.uk/news/uk/home-news/wild-beaver-spotted-in-england-for-first-time-in-800-years-8717543.html

Woods M, McDonald RA and Harris S (2003) Predation of wildlife by domestic cats (*Felis catus*) in Great Britain. *Mammal Review* **33(2)**, 174–188

Yalden DW and Dyckowski J (1998) An estimate of the impact of predators on the British field vole (*M. agrestis*) population. *Mammal Review* **28**, 165–184

Specialist organizations and useful contacts

See also Appendix 1

Beaver reintroductions:
England:
Department for Environment, Food and Rural Affairs (Defra)
www.gov.uk/government/organisations/department-for-environment-food-rural-affairs
Beaver Advisory Committee for England
www.beaversinengland.com

Scotland:
The Royal Zoological Society of Scotland, Edinburgh Zoo, 134 Corstorphine Road, Edinburgh EH12 6TS
www.rzss.org.uk/

Wales:
Wildlife Trusts Wales
www.wtwales.org
The Welsh Beaver project
www.welshbeaverproject.org/home/

Dormouse reintroductions:
Dormouse Captive Breeding groups (via Wildwood education centre 01227 712111 or www.wildwoodtrust.org)
or contact Natural England.

Small mammal information:
Mammal Research Unit
School of Biological Sciences, Bristol University, Bristol Life Sciences Building, 24 Tyndall Avenue, Bristol BS8 1TQ
www.bio.bris.ac.uk

Chapter 15

Bats

David Couper

Bats belong to the order Chiroptera (from the Greek for 'hand-wing'), which is traditionally divided into two sub-orders; the Megachiroptera (fruit bats) and Microchiroptera (insectivorous bats), although there has been much debate over this classification. There are over 1,100 species of bat in the world, accounting for around a fifth of all mammal species (Schipper *et al.*, 2008). In addition to being the only mammals to have developed powered flight, many aspects of their natural history are intriguing, including their use of echolocation, and low fecundity and marked longevity for mammals of their size.

Species seen in the UK

There are 18 species of the Microchiroptera native to the UK (Figure 15.1), belonging to two families, the vespertilionids (vesper bats) and the rhinolophids (horseshoe bats). Occasional vagrants from continental Europe are also reported. The majority of bats presented as wildlife casualties are common pipistrelle bats (*Pipistrellus pipistrellus*; Figure 15.2), soprano pipistrelle bats (*P. pygmaeus*) and brown long-eared bats (*Plecotus auritus*) (Bexton and Couper, 2010); these three species are synanthropic (roost in human habitations) and are widespread and common. The last 50 years has, however, seen dramatic declines in the British bat population (Stebbings, 1988; Harris *et al.*, 1995), with the result that some species are rare and endangered. Habitat loss and agricultural intensification are the likely major causes (Wickramasinghe *et al.*, 2003). All bats and their roosts are protected by legislation. The Bat Conservation Trust (BCT) provides extensive information about bats, and many of its members are licensed bat workers, who are of invaluable assistance in the re-habilitation of bat casualties (see 'Specialist organizations and useful contacts').

Species (common name)	Latin name	Bodyweight (g)[a]	Forearm length (mm)[a]	Distribution[b]	Population[b] (status[c])
Greater horseshoe bat	*Rhinolophus ferrumequinum*	18–24	53–62.4	South-west England and Wales	5,000 (Very rare and endangered)
Lesser horseshoe bat	*Rhinolophus hipposideros*	4–7	36.1–39.6	Wales, west England and Ireland	14,000 (Rare and endangered)
Greater mouse-eared bat	*Myotis myotis*	20–27	55–66.9	1 male found Sussex 2005	Extinct as a breeding population (Status unconfirmed)
Whiskered bat	*Myotis mystacinus*	4–7	32–36.5	Throughout UK; limited in Scotland	40,000 (Locally common)
Brandt's bat	*Myotis brandtii*	5–7	33–38.2	England and Wales	30,000 (Locally common)
Alcathoe bat	*Myotis alcathoe*	3.5–5.5	30.8–34.6	Yorkshire and Sussex but full distribution unknown	Status unconfirmed
Daubenton's bat	*Myotis daubentonii*	6–10	33.1–42	Widespread throughout UK	150,000 (Common)
Natterer's bat	*Myotis nattereri*	7–10	34.4–44	Throughout UK	100,000 (Widespread and common)
Bechstein's bat	*Myotis bechsteinii*	7–10	39–47.1	Southern England	1,500 (Very rare and endangered)
Common pipistrelle bat (see Figure 15.2)	*Pipistrellus pipistrellus*	3–7	28–34.5	Widespread throughout UK	2,000,000 (combined population of *P. pipistrellus* and *P. pygmaeus*; Widespread and common)
Soprano pipistrelle bat	*Pipistrellus pygmaeus*	4–7	27.7–32.3	Widespread throughout UK	2,000,000 (combined population of *P. pipistrellus* and *P. pygmaeus*; Widespread and common)
Nathusius' pipistrelle bat	*Pipistrellus nathusii*	6–10	32.2–37.1	Unknown	100 (Rare)
Noctule bat	*Nyctalus noctula*	21–30	47.3–58.9	England, Wales, southern Scotland	50,000 (Uncommon)

15.1 UK bat species. (continues) ▶
([a] Dietz *et al.*, 2009; [b] Harris *et al.*, 1995; [c] Bat Conservation Trust's (BCT) National Bat Monitoring Programme (NBMP))

Species (common name)	Latin name	Bodyweight (g)[a]	Forearm length (mm)[a]	Distribution[b]	Population[b] (status[c])
Leisler's bat	*Nyctalus leisleri*	13–18	38–47.1	Throughout England, Ireland. Occurs in Scotland	10,000 (Scarce)
Barbastelle bat	*Barbastella barbastellus*	7–10	36.5–43.5	South of the line from The Wash to Wales	5,000 (Rare)
Serotine bat	*Eptesicus serotinus*	18–25	48–58	Southern England and south-east Wales	Unknown (Uncommon and restricted)
Brown long-eared bat	*Plecotus auritus*	6–9	35.5–42.8	Widespread throughout UK	200,000 (Widespread and common)
Grey long-eared bat	*Plecotus austriacus*	6–10	36.5–43.5	Southern England	1,000 (Very rare)

15.1 (continued) UK bat species.
([a] Dietz *et al.*, 2009; [b] Harris *et al.*, 1995; [c] Bat Conservation Trust's (BCT) National Bat Monitoring Programme (NBMP))

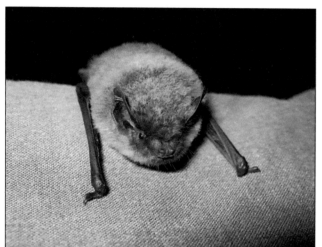

15.2 Common pipistrelle bat. Note rounded shape of a healthy bat.
(© RSPCA, David Couper)

Ecology and biology

Bats are nocturnal animals, emerging from their roosts at dusk or later to feed on insects and other invertebrates. By hunting at night using echolocation, they avoid diurnal avian predators and competition with avian insectivores.

A variety of hunting techniques and habitats are utilized by the different species; for instance, pipistrelle bats may be seen hunting in open spaces, catching insects in rapid flight (aerial hawking), the long-eared bats (*Plecotus* spp.) flutter slowly over vegetation, hovering to pick off any prey they hear (foliage gleaning), and Daubenton's bats (*Myotis daubentonii*) hunt over water courses, often picking insects off the water's surface with their feet (gaffing).

During the spring and summer, female bats congregate in maternity roosts to give birth and rear young. These roosts may be in roof spaces, whilst some species, for example noctule bats (*Nyctalus noctula*), will use natural cavities, such as holes in trees. The bats may change roost, with young attached, if the temperature or humidity becomes inclement. The generally singular young (pups), are born around June, begin to fly around July and August, and are fully independent by the end of the summer.

In most species, other than the long-eared bats and horseshoe bats, the males spend the summer individually or in male groups. In the autumn they attract females to their mating roosts, marked with odorous secretions from the buccal glands (see Figure 15.6b) and glands on the upper lips.

In the winter, as the abundance of their prey falls, insectivorous bats in temperate climates hibernate to avoid starvation, surviving on fat reserves built up during September and October. Many bats migrate to hibernacula, away from their normal hunting grounds. These are often underground in caves or mine shafts, and their conditions are cooler and more humid than those of the summer roosts, to minimize energy and moisture loss. The bats may become active during the winter if the temperature rises or, conversely, if there is a risk of freezing.

Although the common pipistrelle bat may live to 16 years of age in the wild, and brown long-eared bats to over 30, the average life expectancies in the wild of these species are only around 2 and 4 years, respectively (Dietz *et al.*, 2009). A free-living Brandt's bat (*Myotis brandtii*) has been reported at 41 years of age (Podlutsky *et al.*, 2005).

Anatomy and physiology

Apart from those with obvious identifying features, such as the eponymous large pinnae of the long-eared bats and the nose leaf of the horseshoe bats, many of the bat species in the UK appear very similar. Several excellent guides may be used to identify them (e.g. Dietz and von Helversen, 2004), utilizing features such as the presence or absence of the post-calcarial lobe, and the shape of the tragus (Figure 15.3), although certain *Myotis* species are so similar that they can only be differentiated by DNA analysis.

Sexing bats

The two sexes may be easily differentiated by the obvious penis of the male. The testes are intra-abdominal, although the swollen epididymae may be seen at the base of the penis in the autumn, when mating takes place. Following mating, sperm is stored in the uterus (in the receptaculum seminis) until ovulation occurs the following spring. The mammary glands are located in the axillary area, and are only obvious during lactation. Horseshoe bats have false nipples near the genital opening, to which the young attach in the roost.

Differentiating adult bats from juveniles

Differentiating adult bats from juvenile bats that have become independent is difficult on summary inspection, but scrutiny of the finger bones using transillumination will

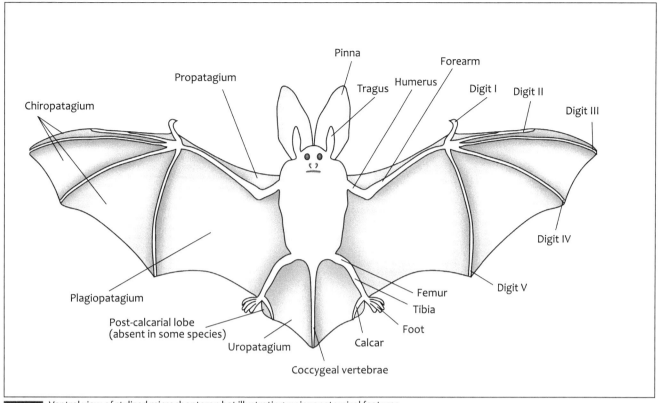

15.3 Ventral view of stylized microchopteran bat illustrating major anatomical features.
(Redrawn after Schober and Grimmberger, 1989)

reveal a terminal translucency of the phalanges in skeletally immature bats (Figure 15.4); those with such lucencies are in their first summer (Racey, 1999). Very young, dependent bats are easily identified by their relatively small size, underdeveloped wings and sparse pelage.

Adaptations for flight

The wing of a bat is formed from the elongated forelimb, which supports a thin membrane, or patagium, that also extends between the hindlimbs and tail. In addition to permitting flight, the patagium is used like a net to capture prey in some species. An obvious thumb is present on the wing, used for roosting, grooming and feeding. The uropatagium,

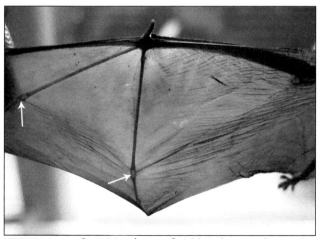

15.4 Lucent finger joints (arrowed) visible in the wing of a juvenile bat.
(© RSPCA, David Couper)

tail and calcar are important for flight in all species and integral to hunting in many (see Figure 15.3). The feet are also used for roosting and, in some species, for catching prey.

As adaptations to the high energy requirements of flight, the heart of a bat is relatively large, and the haemoglobin level, red blood cell count and haematocrit are relatively high when compared with those of small terrestrial mammals (Jürgens et al., 1981). An enormous relative lung size and respiratory surface area and a thin blood–gas barrier increase respiratory efficiency (Maina, 2000).

Heterothermic metabolism

The large surface area of bats relative to their body size results in the potential for the rapid loss of energy as heat. To conserve energy, bats have developed heterothermic metabolism. When active, they maintain their body temperature at around 37°C (heterothermic regulating). During periods of inactivity, they go into a state of torpor, actively dropping their body temperature in line with the environmental temperature (heterothermic conforming). This occurs during the daytime, and will also occur on a more protracted basis during periods of inclement weather if bats are unable to hunt. Female bats convert to homeothermy from mid-gestation, but during lactation they revert back to heterothermy and daily torpor (Altringham, 1996). Bats are able to arouse rapidly from daily torpor, and also if ambient temperatures fall to a critical level (usually freezing) during hibernation, to avoid fatal exposure to sub-zero temperatures.

Hibernation

Brown fat tissue, present over the dorsum, acts as the energy reserve for hibernation, over the course of which bats may lose more than one-third of their bodyweight. During hibernation, the heart rate of the greater mouse-eared bat (*Myotis myotis*) drops from 250–450 bpm (at rest) to 18–80 bpm, and the respiratory rate to one breath every 90 minutes (Kulzer, 2005, cited by Dietz *et al.*, 2009).

Capture, handling and transportation

The two main considerations during the capture and handling of bats are the fact that these animals are delicate and may be injured if excessive force is used, and their potential, albeit low in the UK, to carry European bat lyssavirus (EBLV, or bat rabies) (see 'Specific conditions').

Zoonotic risks

In the last two decades, the importance of chiropteran species worldwide as potential vectors of significant viral zoonoses has received growing attention (see 'Viral diseases'). However, EBLV is the only viral zoonosis carried by bats in Europe that is known to have resulted in human cases (Mühldorfer *et al.*, 2011a). Other zoonotic diseases that could potentially be contracted from bats in the UK include ringworm and salmonellosis (see 'Specific conditions').

A health and safety risk assessment should be in place in all veterinary practices and wildlife centres to cover the risks to staff and volunteers handling bats. Only trained, and rabies-vaccinated staff should be permitted to handle these animals and suitable gloves (see 'Handling') should be provided and worn at all times. If anyone is bitten or scratched by a bat, the wounds should be immediately irrigated and cleaned with soap and water or a suitable disinfectant, and medical advice urgently sought, regardless of vaccination status.

Capture and transportation

Capture of a confined flying bat is rarely necessary, and should only be performed by an experienced person with a soft-rimmed cloth net. In most cases opening a window or door will allow the animal to escape without the need for handling. In the field, free-flying bats may be caught in mist nets by licensed bat workers.

A bat found on the ground, especially during daylight, is always in need of attention. Its capture is best performed by an experienced bat handler; members of the public should be discouraged from handling bats wherever possible. Wearing suitable gloves, a small clean cloth can be placed over the bat, and the cloth and bat can then be transferred into an escape-proof container (towels should not be used, as bats can get their nails entangled in these). A shoebox, with a few small air holes made in the sides and the lid taped closed, will be adequate for transport. If available, the small plastic tanks with clip-on lids as sold for small pets are more substantial and secure. For a short journey to a veterinary surgeon (veterinarian) or rehabilitator, there is no need to provide food and water.

Handling

Gloves should always be worn when handling bats. Gardening gloves with an abrasion-resistant nitrile rubber palm (e.g. Showa® gloves) will provide protection against bites and scratches; these gloves are easily washed and latex gloves may be worn over them to prevent the spread of disease when handling multiple animals.

Bats are relatively easy to handle on account of their small size and generally passive behaviour. They should be handled gently, avoiding excessive pressure on the chest. With the wings held close to the body, they will tend to remain calm; a bat should never be restrained solely by holding the extended wings. Grasping bats by the scruff appears to cause them distress, and should also be avoided. A detailed description of how to handle bats can be found in Mullineaux and Brash (2009).

Throughout handling, capture and transport, attention should be paid to the prevention of escape. The small size and flat profile of bats enable them to escape from all but the most secure containers.

Examination and clinical assessment for rehabilitation

An accurate history and contact details should be taken from the finder (see Chapter 3). Taking note of the exact location where the bat was found will allow its release in familiar territory. Any evidence of illegal roost disturbance, cat predation, adverse weather or accidental indoor confinement should be noted.

The aim of the examination is to assess the suitability of the bat as a candidate for rehabilitation and release (see Chapter 4). The rehabilitation of bats often requires considerable expertise, time and facilities. This may be provided by local bat workers with experience of caring for injured bats, and knowledge of species identification and local bat populations. If at any point injuries are found that are not compatible with release, or the resources for successful rehabilitation are not available, euthanasia should be considered.

Clinical examination

Examination should be carried out in a secure room, with no gaps, such as air vents, through which the bat may escape, and should be deferred until after appropriate first aid has been administered; abnormalities of locomotion or behaviour cannot be assessed with the bat in a torpid state. Prior to handling the casualty, it should initially be observed on a flat, horizontal surface. Good lighting is essential, and a hand lens or magnifying loupes are advantageous. Placing white paper towel on the surface of the examination table will aid visualization of abnormalities, and will highlight tiny amounts of blood, urine, faeces or contaminant arising from the bat. A general appraisal should be made of body condition (a healthy bat has a rounded appearance (see Figure 15.2), whilst sunken flanks are seen with emaciation (Figure 15.5)), the state of hydration (the skin will tent and the wing membranes appear dull and more wrinkled in dehydrated individuals) and the presence or absence of ectoparasites. Whilst long bone fractures may result in obvious abnormalities of wing or leg carriage, less obvious lesions, such as injuries to the pectoral or pelvic girdles, may only become apparent as asymmetrical wing or leg movement when crawling. Occasionally bats with little or nothing wrong with them may fly at this point (for example, juvenile bats that have become trapped in a room when trying to find the roost) and an assessment of flight capability may be possible. See also 'Pre-release assessment'.

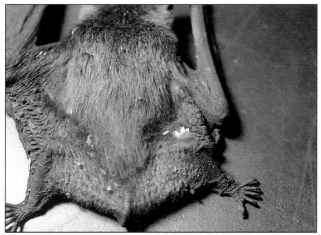

15.5 Thin juvenile bat with ectoparasites and blowfly eggs, showing 'tucked-in' abdomen.

Clinical examination in the hand should be systematic and ordered (see Figure 4.5); it is best facilitated by holding the bat dorsoventrally across the thorax, using the thumb and fingers in apposition (Figure 15.6).

The head and body should be examined, closely inspecting the eyes, ears and mouth, and any areas of wet or matted fur, which may signify the presence of wounds. Blowing the fur will allow visualization of the underlying skin, and may expose wounds, bruising or fly eggs. Whilst

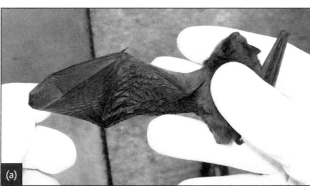

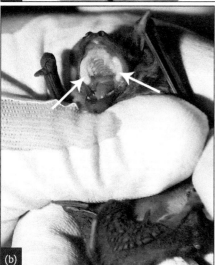

15.6 (a) For examination the bat is held dorsoventrally across the thorax using the thumb and fingers in apposition. Whilst supporting the body, each wing is extended and examined in turn. Note: photograph is of dead specimen. (b) Restraint of a noctule bat, one of the larger bat species in the UK. Note the large canines and location of the buccal glands (arrowed).
(a, © Steve Bexton; b, © Maggie and Bryan Brown)

the body is supported, each wing should be extended and examined in turn (Figure 15.6a). Transillumination of the wing will highlight bruising, and allow differentiation of adult and juvenile bats (see Figure 15.4). The integrity of each long bone should be assessed and the mobility of the joints gauged.

Comparison can be made with the contralateral wing. Any puncture or swelling or area of unexpected mobility should receive particular attention. The integrity of the wing membrane should be assessed and the size and situation of any holes or tears noted. The hindlimbs and the uropatagium should be examined in a similar manner and the animal can also be sexed at this stage (see 'Sexing bats').

Diagnostic techniques

Ancillary diagnostics are limited in bats due to their small size. Radiography can be useful to assess fractures, especially of the pectoral and pelvic girdles, which may not be obvious on clinical examination (Figure 15.7).

Kunz and Nagy (1988) described collection of blood into a 70 µl heparinized capillary tube from the veins in the uropatagium, or from the cardiac vein, which is prominent on the leading edge of the propatagium of the wing. Their technique was used on healthy bats weighing from 2 g to 15 g and therefore would be applicable to the species found in the UK. However, this is technically difficult, and the volumes obtained are insufficient for most tests. Consequently there is scant information available in the literature regarding normal haematology and biochemistry parameters in the different species. Wolk and Ruprecht (1988) detailed normal haematological values in the serotine bat (*Eptesicus serotinus*).

Ectoparasites can be examined by light microscopy, following removal with a fine slightly dampened paintbrush. Endoparasites such as coccidia may be detected by microscopic faecal examination, using wet smear and flotation techniques.

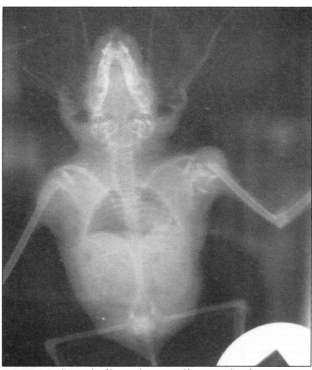

15.7 Radiograph of brown long-eared bat, revealing fractures around the left shoulder joint.
(© RSPCA, David Couper)

Euthanasia

Euthanasia of a bat should be seen as a positive welfare action rather than a negative veterinary action. Occasionally BCT bat workers will keep permanently disabled bats as educational tools. Veterinary treatment of a bat that will become permanently disabled, and therefore unreleasable, must be carried out with the bat's welfare as the paramount concern (see Chapter 4).

Pentobarbital sodium can be administered by intraperitoneal injection following induction of anaesthesia with an inhalational agent (see 'Anaesthesia and analgesia'), although if a post-mortem examination is to be performed, an overdose of inhalational agent is preferable. The small size of Microchiroptera species means that euthanasia by physical means is both feasible and humane (Routh, 1991; Racey, 1999) provided that the operator is both suitably trained and confident in performing the procedure. Techniques described are generally limited to the breaking of the neck (by placing a pencil across the cervical vertebrae with the bat held against a hard, flat surface and then pressure being applied to the pencil) or the application of a sharp blow to the cranium. The degree of trauma with these techniques can also reduce the value of the cadaver for post-mortem analysis (including rabies testing).

First aid and short-term hospitalization

The large surface area of bats relative to their body size results in the potential for the rapid loss of moisture and heat. As a consequence of this, and an inability to drink or hunt, grounded bats are frequently dehydrated and starved. The initial priorities when dealing with these animals are to provide warmth and fluid therapy. Warmth is best provided by placing the bat over a heat mat in an escape-proof container, such as the clip-top plastic tanks used for small pets. This will suffice as short-term accommodation (see 'Housing').

Fluid therapy

Once it has become active, oral electrolytes may be offered, with the bat restrained between thumb and fingers as for examination. Oral fluids may be provided using a fine artist's paintbrush, a small catheter or a pipette. They should be offered in small amounts, frequently, and the bat will often lap enthusiastically as its condition improves. Animals that show no interest in oral fluids, or improvement following them, may be given subcutaneous fluids in the form of 0.1 ml of sterile Hartmann's solution per 5 g bat (20 ml/kg), over the lower half of the dorsum. Once able to drink for itself, it should be left a small amount of water or oral electrolytes in a shallow dish.

Treatment of wounds

Care should be taken not to wet the fur excessively when performing wound lavage, to prevent cooling. Systemic antibiotic therapy and appropriate analgesia should be administered (see 'Therapeutics' and 'Anaesthesia and analgesia'); grooming will result in the ingestion of topical treatments, which should in general be avoided. Hydrocolloid gels, such as Intrasite®, may be applied.

Anaesthesia and analgesia

General anaesthesia

Anaesthesia is used mainly for carrying out ancillary diagnostic techniques such as radiography, and to allow surgical interventions. It should be deferred until after adequate patient stabilization and assessment, as complicating problems, such as dehydration, are common. Modern inhalational agents, such as isoflurane or sevoflurane, may be delivered in an induction chamber, followed by an improvised facemask, such as the connector for an endotracheal tube. Neither local anaesthetic agents nor injectable general anaesthetic agents can be advocated. Their narrow therapeutic ranges and long duration of action would be detrimental to the well being of the patient and may cause mortality. The monitoring of anaesthetic depth is complicated by the small size of the patient, and is largely restricted to the assessment of muscle tone in the wings, and observation of respiration. Bats should be kept warm throughout anaesthesia and during the recovery period. Subcutaneous fluids may be given during the procedure if necessary (see 'First aid').

Analgesia

Whilst acknowledging the need for analgesia to be a considered part of the therapeutic management plan for an injured bat, it is not easy in practice. The intention must be to achieve therapeutic levels without causing iatrogenic dose-related toxicity. It is difficult to advocate an analgesic agent that will safely accommodate both a bat's small size and its fluctuating metabolic pattern as there is a paucity of referenced information available in the literature.

The use of butorphanol by injection and buprenorphine sublingually (Lollar, 2010) has been described. Use of the non-steroidal anti-inflammatory drug meloxicam has also been described anecdotally in bats, to apparent good effect (Routh, 2003; Bexton and Couper, 2010) (see 'Therapeutics' and Figure 15.14).

Specific conditions

There have been limited investigations into the conditions of bats in the UK (e.g. Simpson, 1994; Daffner, 2001), apart from surveillance for EBLV and the fungus responsible for white-nose syndrome (Barlow et al., 2013). A post-mortem study of nearly 500 free-ranging bats (found dead, injured or moribund) belonging to 19 different species of European vespertilionids, many of which occur in the UK, has recently been carried out in Germany (Mühldorfer et al., 2011a; Mühldorfer et al., 2011b).

Trauma

Traumatic injuries have been described as a major cause of death in free-ranging European bat species, accounting for 65% of deaths in the study by Simpson (1994), and 40% in the study by Mühldorfer et al. (2011b). The large surface area and delicate structure of the wing render it very susceptible to damage (Bexton and Couper, 2010), and fractures and lacerations of the wings were the most common findings in traumatized individuals in the study by Mühldorfer et al. (2011b).

Cat attack

Injuries due to cat attacks account for around half of all trauma cases (Routh 1991; Simpson 1994; Mühldorfer *et al.*, 2011b), with those species roosting in human habitations being particularly susceptible. Some bats may have pre-existing illness leading to their predation, although cats have been observed waiting at roost entrances to catch healthy bats emerging at dusk. The injuries are frequently so severe as to warrant immediate euthanasia (Figure 15.8). Wound infection with *Pasteurella multocida* and subsequent septi-caemia are common sequelae (Simpson, 1994; Mühldorfer *et al.*, 2011b), and systemic antibiotic therapy and analgesia are indicated in any animals in which rehabilitation is attempted (see 'Therapeutics'). Subcutaneous emphysema can also develop as a sequel to cat attack. Deflation of the emphysema may lead to successful resolution if internal trauma is not too severe. However, serious occult injuries are not uncommon in victims of cat attack. See Chapter 30 for more information on systemic antibiotics for the treatment of cat bite injuries.

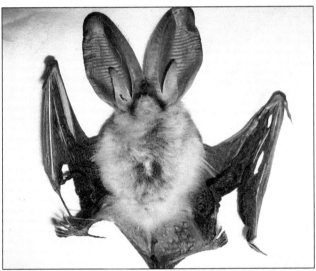

15.8 Brown long-eared bat showing massive trauma as a result of a cat attack: fracture of left forearm; holes in left wing membrane; phalanges exposed by large tear in right wing membrane; tear to uropatagium exposing right calcar. Note: photograph is of a dead specimen.
(© RSPCA, David Couper)

Fractures

Around 90% of bone fractures are seen in the humeri and forearms, and almost two-thirds of these are compound (Mühldorfer *et al.*, 2011b), with a correspondingly guarded prognosis. The repair of humeral and forearm fractures using splints or, in larger species, intramedullary pins (Lollar and Schmidt-French, 1998) or external fixators, has been described. However, all substantial fractures thus repaired carry a poor prognosis with respect to release; postoperative activity is reduced and subsequent movement in the wing is often restricted, thereby rendering the bat incapable of sustained flight. Such cases should therefore be euthanased.

Fractures of the metacarpals or phalanges may heal with rest, or with simple external coaptation, such as a 'Micropore™ sandwich' (an Altman splint, see Figure 5.18), although bone fragments are often devitalized, and splints can evoke self-trauma and deterioration of the patagium through impeded grooming. As the thumbs are important for roosting, grooming and feeding, fractures or injuries to these are likely to be significant. The debridement of

minor injuries to the wing tips and distal phalanges, and subsequent coaptation of the wound edges using an absorbable suture material with a swaged-on atraumatic needle, has been described (Routh, 2003). It should be considered that even apparently minor deficits in wing length or breadth may have significant effects on flight efficiency, and a critical pre-release flight assessment is necessary following the repair of any wing injury.

Fractures of the legs carry a guarded prognosis with respect to release. These, and other blunt trauma, including spinal injuries, rib fractures and pneumothorax, may be incurred when people attempt to catch a flying bat indoors (Bexton and Couper, 2010). As the legs are important for grooming and roosting, and catching prey in some species, perfect repair is required.

Fractures of the jaw are a possibility in an alert bat that steadfastly refuses to take solid food. These fractures cannot be repaired and carry a poor prognosis. A granulomatous glossitis as a consequence of penetration of the tongue by chitinous insect parts has been reported in a noctule bat (Mühldorfer *et al.*, 2011b), and this would be a differential diagnosis for oral trauma.

Patagial injuries

Many bats, on presentation, have discrete holes in the patagium (Figure 15.9a). These may be incidental findings, unrelated to the reason for admission. Bats in the wild incur minor injuries to the patagium and their flight can appear unimpeded by even relatively large holes. These holes, however, may be the relatively minor, visible manifestation of a cat attack, and systemic antibiotic therapy may be indicated. Small holes heal very quickly with no intervention necessary, and it is not necessary to wait for incidental holes to heal prior to release if the bat is flying well (Walsh and Stebbings, 1989).

Large holes and tears (i.e. holes that extend to and include the wing or tail margin) have a far more guarded prognosis, especially if these expose the finger bones or the calcar (Figure 15.9b). Attempts to repair tears using

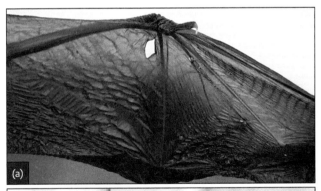

(a)

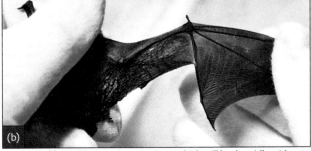

(b)

15.9 (a) Small hole in the patagium, which will heal rapidly without intervention. (b) Large tear in the patagium with a more guarded prognosis.
(a, © RSPCA, David Couper; b, © Maggie and Bryan Brown)

fine sutures, surgical glues and plastic membranes, 'sandwich fashion', have been described. Achieving apposition of the wound edges is difficult, as these naturally tend to curl inwards. Sutures often pull through and glue will prevent tissue–tissue union by coating the wound edges, unless applied at intervals rather than in a continuous line. The author has not found these techniques to offer any advantage over natural healing, during which new membrane forms to replace the deficit. Even extensive tears may heal naturally given time (several weeks), but the resultant scar tissue, by restricting full extension of the wing, often prevents functional flight.

Trapped and entangled bats

Inexperienced juvenile bats often end up trapped in houses, mistaking open windows for the entrance to their roost. If the bat is flying, the window can be left open and the bat observed to ensure it leaves. Bats may also come down chimneys, and can sustain burns and develop respiratory distress as a result of smoke inhalation. If bats are found grounded inside, they should be examined and treated, including rehydration, prior to release. Trauma as a result of attempted capture, inadvertent crushing under doors, or cat attack, is not uncommon.

Bats may become entangled in a variety of materials. Certain species are more prone to particular hazards, depending on their lifestyles. Species which glean, such as brown long-eared bats, may become stuck to flypapers or cockroach traps, or entangled in garden netting or vegetation. Daubenton's bats may become entangled in discarded fishing line whilst hunting over rivers, often becoming attached to the hook by the mouth, presumably having mistaken this for an insect. Synanthropic species such as pipistrelle bats may become covered with cobwebs and debris whilst entering or exiting their roosts (Figure 15.10). These cases may require euthanasia if the bat has been trapped for some time with resultant dehydration and starvation. Treatment of less severe cases involves the provision of appropriate first aid (see 'First aid'). Excess fly-paper should be cut away to prevent further entanglement; the removal of fly-paper adhesive is exhausting for the bat (see 'Contamination'). Fishing hooks may be removed under general anaesthesia, following removal of the barb. Injuries resulting from netting or fishing line should be carefully assessed with regard to their extent and any associated circulatory compromise, and disentangled bats should be monitored for the progression of pressure necrosis for a period of at least a week.

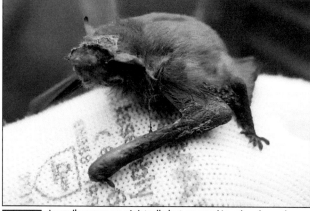

15.10 Juvenile common pipistrelle bat covered in cobwebs and debris.
(© RSPCA, David Couper)

Poisoning

The use of timber treatments in roof spaces represents a particular risk to bats that are using such areas to roost. Treatment of timbers and remedial building work are covered by wildlife legislation (see 'Legal aspects' and Chapter 2), thereby affording protection to bats and their roosts. In practical terms this gives the Statutory Nature Conservation Organizations (SNCOs) a role in advising how damage to bats and to their roosts can reasonably be avoided or minimized (Mitchell-Jones, 1999b). Older timber treatments, such as the organochlorine insecticide lindane, can remain toxic months after their application (Racey and Swift, 1986). Affected bats are likely to be found dead; they may be no more sensitive to these compounds than are other mammals, but stored liposoluble toxins may be released in fatal amounts when fat reserves are metabolized (Clark, 1988). Through enforcement of the law, increased public awareness, the use of newer, less toxic treatments, and the strict control of the antifungal pentachlorophenol (PCP), the number of future incidents should be minimized.

Toxic metals are readily transferred through insectivore food chains, resulting in their potential bioaccumulation in bats. Walker *et al.* (2007) analysed renal mercury, lead and cadmium concentrations in bats from south-west England. Residues were generally highest in whiskered bats (*Myotis mystacinus*). Overall renal levels were 6- to 10-fold below those associated with toxic effects, although 5% of *Pipistrellus* spp. had kidney lead residues diagnostic of acute lead poisoning.

Suspected poisoning from blue-green algal toxins has been recorded in the USA (Pybus *et al.*, 1986) and could potentially occur in the UK, especially in species such as the Daubenton's bat, which hunts over inland waters.

Agrochemicals, affecting both the bats and their insect prey, have contributed to the worldwide decline of bats (Stebbings, 1988).

Contamination

Contamination of the fur is a frequent presenting sign. Contaminants include oil, adhesives from fly-papers and cockroach traps, dust, paint, soot and cobwebs (see Figure 15.10). Chronically affected bats are often exhausted and emaciated, and euthanasia may be considered to prevent further suffering. As bats groom regularly, they are likely to have ingested some of the substance, possibly with toxic effects.

Cobwebs and dust can be removed with a soft brush. Water-soluble contaminants are most easily removed with a mild diluted household washing-up liquid (industrial degreasing agents are too severe), using warm water. Oils and adhesives may be removed by working butter, vegetable oil or margarine into the fur to loosen them. This can then be washed off with washing-up liquid, as before. The washed bat should be rinsed and dried thoroughly, to prevent cooling and loss of energy. Surplus water may be removed with a cloth, avoiding towels as thumbs and toenails can get caught in these. This process may need to be repeated several times to completely remove the contaminant, with rest and rehydration between washes. Oral kaolin and pectin gel act as an adsorbent to minimize effects from ingested oil (see 'Therapeutics' and Figure 15.14). Affected individuals should be monitored for a minimum of 2 weeks for adverse effects of ingestion or skin contact, such as skin sores or fur loss.

Infectious diseases

In the study by Mühldorfer *et al.* (2011b), one-third of mortalities were due to disease (principally respiratory disease), with fatal bacterial, viral and parasitic infections found in at least 12% of the bats investigated. Young bats and adult females were significantly more affected by disease, indicating that sex and age-related disease prevalence in bats are strongly correlated with the maternal season.

Viral diseases

European bat lyssavirus (bat rabies):
Incidence in the UK: Bats are the natural reservoir hosts for the European bat lyssaviruses, of which there are two strains. EBLV-1 is the most common strain in continental Europe, where it has been recorded over 850 times in several species (some of which occur in the UK), but most frequently in serotine bats. EBLV-2 is much less frequently isolated, only approximately 20 times to date, and appears to be limited to *Myotis* spp. bats (reviewed in Harris *et al.*, 2009).

In the UK, passive surveillance for EBLV in dead bats began in 1987 (see 'Specialist organizations and useful contacts' for more information). The findings suggest a low prevalence of EBLV-2 in Daubenton's bats, with virus isolated from approximately 4% of submitted specimens (Harris *et al.*, 2007). Serological testing of live Daubenton's bats has confirmed a low seroprevalence (less than 4%) (Scottish National Heritage, 2009; Harris *et al.*, 2009). To date, EBLV-1 has not been isolated from a bat in the UK, although antibodies to this strain have been recorded in two Natterer's bats (*Myotis nattereri*) (Scottish National Heritage, 2009) and one serotine bat (Harris *et al.*, 2009).

Clinical signs in bats: Infected bats may have non-specific signs, such as changes in behaviour or temperament, incoordination and tremors. However, virus may also be found in the saliva of seemingly healthy bats. It is still not fully understood why some bats exposed to the virus develop antibodies, whilst others develop fatal clinical disease.

Zoonotic potential: EBLV has been implicated in 'spill-over' infections in other animals, in which it causes clinical disease indistinguishable from classical rabies. There have been five human deaths associated with EBLV infection in Europe since 1977, including a Scottish bat worker in 2002 (Fooks *et al.*, 2003). Virus is transmitted in bat saliva, by a bite or scratch or through broken skin or mucous membranes. Should a bat be showing any behavioural or neurological signs leading one to suspect a case of rabies, it should be safely confined and the local Animal Health Office of Defra contacted for advice on how to proceed. All dead bats, not just those suspected of having rabies, should be submitted to the Animal and Plant Health Agency (APHA) for continued lyssavirus surveillance (see 'Specialist organizations and useful contacts'). Appropriate safe handling of bats has been described above (see 'Capture, handling and transportation').

Other viruses: Seven novel gammaherpesviruses and one novel betaherpesvirus have been discovered in seven European bat species (Wibbelt *et al.*, 2007). Each type of European bat herpesvirus appears to be primarily associated with a single bat species. A high prevalence of herpesvirus has been reported in bats in Germany (Mühldorfer *et al.*, 2011a). A 65% prevalence was observed for bat gammaherpesvirus 6 (BatGHV6) in common pipistrelle bats. The aetiological association of bat herpesvirus with pulmonary disease can presently not be excluded and remains to be elucidated (Wibbelt *et al.*, 2007).

A novel adenovirus has been reported in the intestines of common pipistrelle bats in Germany (Sonntag *et al.*, 2009), and was associated with mortality in the study by Mühldorfer *et al.* (2011a).

As stated earlier, bats worldwide are important as potential vectors of significant viral zoonoses, such as Hendra virus, Nipah virus, Ebola virus, severe acute respiratory syndrome (SARS) coronavirus and Middle East respiratory syndrome (MERS) coronavirus (Calisher *et al.*, 2006; Wong *et al.*, 2007: Lelli *et al.*, 2013). In Europe, SARS-like coronaviruses have been detected in *Rhinolophus* spp. bats, and MERS-like coronaviruses in vesper bats (mainly *Pipistrellus* spp.) (Lelli *et al.*, 2013).

Bacterial diseases

Bacterial infections in bats mainly involve invasive species and develop subsequent to traumatic injuries. *Pasteurella multocida* is most often isolated, frequently as a sequel to cat attack (Simpson, 1994; Mühldorfer *et al.*, 2011a). Given the frequency of cat attacks in bats (see 'Trauma'), the administration of systemic antibiotics is prudent where suggestive injuries of unknown origin are present (see 'Therapeutics' and Figure 15.14).

Other than invasive bacteria, the only bacteria recorded by Simpson (1994) were *Escherichia coli*, which were mostly associated with enteric disease. Culture of the intestines of 36 bats in the same study proved negative for *Salmonella* spp. Daffner (2001) isolated a *Salmonella* Group 4, 09, 12 sp. from a whiskered bat. *Salmonella enterica* serovar Typhimurium, *S. enterica* serovar Enteritidis and *Yersinia pseudotuberculosis* were identified as primary bacterial pathogens in bats in Germany (Mühldorfer *et al.*, 2011a).

Various other pathogenic bacteria have been reported in bats in the UK, including intra-erythrocytic *Bartonella* spp. (Concannon *et al.*, 2005) and *Sarcina*-like bacteria, recorded in the intestines of a brown long-eared bat (Barlow *et al.*, 2013). Evans *et al.* (2009) reported the discovery of a spirochaete causing fatal borreliosis in a *Pipistrellus* species bat in the UK, showing close relatedness to known causes of relapsing fever in Africa and Asia. An *Argas vespertilionis* tick was attached to the bat, and was presumed to be the source of the infection.

Fungal diseases

Ringworm: The survey by Simpson (1994) identified ringworm in bats, but did not specify the species found. Dermatophytes identified in bats in North America by Hill and Smith (1984, cited in Lollar and Schmidt-French, 1998) included *Trichophyton persicolor, T. mentagrophytes* and *Microsporum canis*. Lollar and Schmidt-French (1998) described ringworm as bald, circular patches within the fur or as pale iridescent areas where there is no hair. Scaly or yellowish crusting areas may also be seen. Given the frequency of hair loss in captive bats (see 'Conditions of the integument'), and the potential toxicity of antifungal medications, treatment should only be initiated following a definitive diagnosis (e.g. fungal culture). As ringworm is contagious and zoonotic, appropriate barrier nursing should be instituted.

White-nose syndrome: White-nose syndrome (WNS) is a cutaneous mycotic infection, caused by the psychrophilic (cold-loving) fungus *Pseudogymnoascus destructans* (Pd).

WNS was first discovered in the spring of 2006 in New York State, and since then has caused catastrophic declines amongst multiple cave-hibernating species of bats in North America (Figure 15.11). The fungus invades exposed membranes of the muzzles, ears and wings of hibernating bats. Affected bats present with white hyphae around the muzzle and a white tacky film on the wings. The low body temperature and suppressed cellular immune response of the hibernating bats favours the fungal growth (Meteyer *et al.*, 2011). Lorch *et al.* (2011) provided experimental evidence that the fungus is a primary pathogen, rather than an opportunist. WNS may lead to death due to premature depletion of stored fat during hibernation, likely as a result of altered hibernation patterns (Reeder *et al.*, 2012); affected bats spend significantly more time active during periodic arousal (Brownlee-Bouboulis and Reeder, 2013). Individuals surviving WNS often have notable wing damage (Meteyer *et al.*, 2011).

WNS has recently been confirmed by histopathology in bats in Europe, in association with sporadic deaths (Pikula *et al.*, 2012). Mass mortalities have not been recorded (Puechmaille *et al.*, 2011). Pd has been isolated from a white focus on the ear of a hibernating Daubenton's bat and from five hibernation sites in England, although mortality associated with WNS has not been reported in the UK to date (Barlow *et al.*, 2015).

Incidents involving abnormal winter behaviour, or unusual mortality involving bats with white fungus should be reported to the BCT.

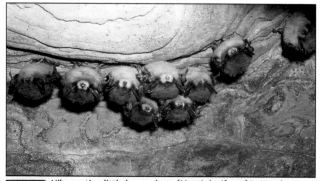

15.11 Hibernating little brown bats (*Myotis lucifugus*) in North America exhibiting white-nose syndrome.
(Courtesy of Nancy Heaslip, New York Department of Environmental Conservation)

Other fungal conditions: The APHA have been investigating cases of fungal infection in hibernating bats in Great Britain since January 2010. To date, they have reported a variety of saprophytic fungi on dead bats including *Rhizopus*, *Penicillium*, *Scopulariopsis*, *Mucor*, *Gliocoladium*, *Paecilomyces* and *Myceliophthora* spp. They also reported the presence of mycotic dermatitis in a live particoloured bat (*Vespertilio murinus*), an occasional vagrant species to Great Britain, on the Isle of Arran (Barlow *et al.*, 2011). Several small white lesions were present on the wing membranes. A *Cladosporium* sp. (probably *C. clado-sporioides*) and a *Rhodotorula* sp. were isolated. Both of these species are thought to be opportunistic pathogens.

Simpson *et al.* (2013) reported cutaneous mycosis in a barbastelle bat (*Barbastella barbastellus*), caused by *Hyphopichia burtonii*, presenting with grossly thickened skin over the face and muzzle, which in places was sloughing and ulcerated. Numerous nodules were present on the wings and pinnae. The bat was found alive, but emaciated, and it was felt that the muzzle lesions were likely to have contributed to the bat's condition by interference with feeding and grooming.

Cave sickness: *Histoplasma capsulatum* has been reported from more than 30 countries (Sanger, 1981, cited in Burek, 2001) and is recognized as a cause of disease of bats in the USA (Barnard, 1995; Lollar and Schmidt-French, 1998). Infection, known as 'cave sickness', may be contracted by people working in caves through their contact with bat guano (Burek, 2001). The organism requires moist conditions and large amounts of guano for multiplication. In the UK, even in large roosts, droppings usually remain dry and the disease is not currently identified as a risk for bat workers (Mitchell-Jones, 1999a).

Parasites

Ectoparasites: As in other animals, ectoparasites in bats are generally only present in significant numbers if the animal is otherwise debilitated and unable to groom. Several bat-specific parasites are found, presumed to be vectors of disease. Significant species differences in ectoparasite infestation exist, with those species primarily roosting in trees or nest boxes, like the noctule bat and Daubenton's bat, being more frequently infested (Mühldorfer *et al.*, 2011a).

Mites: There have been 64 species of mites reported in British and Irish bats and their roosts (Baker and Craven, 2003) including *Steatonyssus* spp., *Dermanyssus* spp. and larvae of *Neotrombicula autumnalis* (Simpson, 1994). Mites are found in their greatest numbers on debilitated juveniles, having been acquired in the maternity roost, and the numbers may be so large as to contribute to the debility. On adult bats, spinturnicid mites (Hutson and Racey, 1999) are often apparent on the wings, causing punctate damage to the patagium. *Psorergatoides nyctali* mites have been reported causing dermatitis and extensive depigmentation of the patagium of a noctule bat (Baker, 2005).

Other ectoparasites of bats: Bats in the UK are also hosts to the ticks *Argas vespertilionis* and *Ixodes vespertilionis* (Baker and Craven, 2003), ischnopsyllid fleas, cimicid bat bugs (Figure 15.12) and nycteribiid bat flies. All of these parasites feed on blood and are presumed to be disease vectors. If present, they are generally found in low numbers. The bat bugs and immature stages of other ectoparasites are often found in the roost. Debilitated bats may become the victims of flystrike (myiasis), which can be a feature of terminal decline.

Haemoprotozoal vectors: Ectoparasites are presumed to be vectors of the haemoprotozoa found in bats. *A. vespertilionis* is believed to transmit *Babesia vesperuginis* (Gardner and Molyneux, 1987). Infective forms of *Schizotrypanum* have been found in the gut of the bat bug *Cimex pipistrelli* (Gardner and Molyneux, 1988a), and the trypanosomes have been transmitted experimentally via *C. pipistrelli* (Gardner and Molyneux, 1988b). *Polychromophilus murinus* has been found in the bat fly *Nycteribia kolenatti* collected from a Daubenton's bat (Gardner and Molyneux, 1988c).

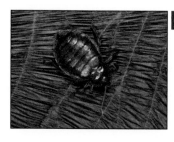

15.12 *Cimex* species bat bug.
(Courtesy of C Dietz)

Treatment: The safest method of treatment is often manual removal of the parasites, using a fine, slightly dampened artist's paintbrush. As the condition of the bat improves with rehydration and feeding, it will groom off parasites that are missed. Fly eggs are best removed by diligent grooming with a fine comb. Environmental parasitic stages will be removed with frequent (daily) changes of the substrate.

Various parasiticidal drugs have been used in bats, including permethrin flea powder (Bat Conservation trust, 2000), selamectin, amitraz (Brown and Brown, 2006) and oral ivermectin (Loller and Schmidt-French, 1998). The topical preparations should be applied sparingly between the shoulder blades where the bat cannot easily groom them off. Fipronil may be applied directly to ticks.

Endoparasites: In the study by Mühldorfer *et al.* (2011a), endoparasites were found in around 30% of bats, including protozoans (*Eimeriidae* and *Sarcocystidae* species) and helminths (nematodes, cestodes and trematodes). Helminths were predominantly found in the intestinal tracts, whilst in some animals granulomatous lesions in various organs were associated with larval migration of nematode species. The prevalence of endoparasitic infection increased significantly with increasing age. Larger species, like noctule and serotine bats, revealed higher endoparasite prevalence, compared to small- or medium-sized species.

Helminths: Barlow *et al.* (2013) reported *Molinostrongylus* species nematodes in the intestinal tract and free within the abdomen of a brown long-eared bat in the UK. They suggested that the large numbers were likely to have caused some degree of malabsorption or partial intestinal obstruction. The Natural History Museum's database lists three *Molinostrongylus* spp. (*M. alatus*, *M. ornatus* and *M. skrjabini*) reported in bats in the UK (Gibson *et al.*, 2005). Simpson (2013) reported finding many similar nematodes in 18 of 74 brown long-eared bats, which were identified as a *Seuratum* sp. (provisionally *S. mucronatum*). Multiple worms were present, some free within the abdominal and pleural cavities, in the absence of any significant pathology. Mühldorfer *et al.* (2011b) reported severe trematode (species not listed) infestation of the small intestine; gastritis, serositis and pancreatitis as a result of parasitic infection were present in 2% of bats in this study.

Haemoprotozoa: A number of studies of haemoprotozoa in British bats have been carried out, revealing trypanosomes (*Trypanosoma vespertilionis*, *T. dionisii* and *T. incertum*) in a range of species, malaria-like *Polychromophilus* species, and piroplasms assumed to be *Babesia vesperuginis* (summarized in Concannon *et al.*, 2005). *B. vesperuginis* has been found almost exclusively in *Pipistrellus* spp. in the UK, in association with splenomegaly, lowered haemoglobin and significantly raised white blood cell counts (Concannon *et al.*, 2005).

Coccidia: Renal coccidiosis has been reported sporadically in free-living bats in Europe (Gruber *et al.*, 1996; Mühldorfer *et al.* 2011b). White foci may be seen macroscopically on the external surface of the kidneys. The impact of renal coccidiosis remains unclear, but it seems likely that a progression of this disease might influence the health status of the infected host (Mühldorfer *et al.*, 2011b). Mild to severe intestinal coccidiosis was reported by Mühldorfer *et al.* (2011b) in a small number of bats.

Other protozoa: A suspected *Cryptosporidium* sp. was detected in heavy numbers in a faecal smear taken from a brown long-eared bat (Daffner, 2001). Cyst-forming *Sarcosporidia*-like protozoans have been reported in the myocardium and pharyngeal muscles of bats in Europe (Mühldorfer *et al.* 2011b).

Clinical signs attributable to endoparasitic infection are rarely, if ever, reported in bats in the UK, and routine treatment does not appear to be necessary in the author's experience.

Other conditions
Orphaned and abandoned juveniles

Young bats may be abandoned in the maternity roost if the temperature or humidity becomes unsuitable, or if insufficient prey is available for the adult bats to hunt. They may be found on the ground, having been driven by unfavourable conditions or hunger to leave the roost, and are often dehydrated, starved and covered in ectoparasites. For treatment see 'First aid'.

Occasionally, healthy juvenile bats may be found outside the roost, having fallen and been separated from their mothers. If, following a thorough examination, a juvenile bat appears healthy it should be kept warm and hydrated using an oral electrolyte solution, and returned to the roost at dusk in the hope that it will be picked up by its mother. This is best performed by a BCT licensed bat worker; the pup should be placed in a shallow container near the entrance to the roost, and observed to ensure it is safe from predators. This works in some cases and is the ideal conclusion. If release does not take place, either the bat will have to be taken into captivity for rearing (see 'Rearing of bat pups') or euthanasia will have to be carried out (Barnard, 1995).

Conditions of the integument

Bats spend a large amount of time grooming and keeping the various membranes that are essential for flight in good order. Care of the wing includes systematic licking of the patagium. Racey (1999) suggested that relative humidity is a key factor affecting health of the patagium; too dry an environment is deleterious, and too wet an atmosphere leads to fungal and bacterial skin infection. A relative humidity of 50–60% is generally adequate (Bat World Sanctuary, 2010).

Bat carers have noted the occurrence of various necrotic conditions of the wing, particularly in long-term captives. Conditions reported by Routh (2003) include areas of wing membrane loss through dry or ischaemic necrosis, approximating to tissues supplied by an end artery, and an advancing wet necrosis, occurring at the wing margin and causing progressive loss of the patagium. These differ in presentation from a moist, exudative lesion of the patagium causing areas of adhesion when the wing is folded in the natural resting position ('sticky wing'). Despite bacterial culture, fungal culture and histology, a definitive aetiology was not established in any of the cases listed above and all instances proved refractory to treatment.

Bats may also suffer from a condition analogous to wing tip oedema in raptors. Routh (2003) reported a noctule bat found grounded after a period of frost, which presented with fluid-filled blisters on both wings, distal to the carpus. The wing tips subsequently became oedematous, prior to the development of ischaemic changes, dry gangrene and sloughing. This sequence of events has been observed by other rehabilitators (Stocker, 2005).

Similar devitalizing changes to those seen in the patagium have also been observed in the pinna of a brown long-eared bat (Routh, 2003). The individual was, through amputation of a wing, a long-term captive and the changes were restricted to the ipsilateral pinna. This species roosts with the pinnae folded under the wings. The inability of this individual to do so with the affected pinna would affect its microenvironment, which could lead to the production of the lesions and, ultimately, to the loss of the pinna.

Fur loss occurs in some captive bats (Figure 15.13). Most frequently seen is a syndrome where the ventral head and neck are initially affected, but the alopecia may extend caudally to the ventral thorax and abdomen, with associated skin erythema. One speculated cause of this is that the fluid expressed from decapitated mealworms, as they are fed by hand to the debilitated bat, has a corrosive or irritant action on the skin. Barnard (1995) believed that quinones, excreted by the mealworms, may contribute to this condition. Affected individuals should not be released until the fur has grown back.

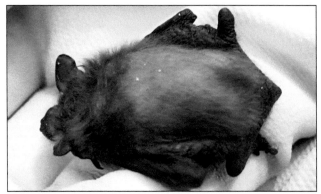

15.13 Common pipistrelle bat showing extensive fur loss. (© RSPCA, David Couper)

Joint conditions

Infected abrasions of the carpus through poor housing on harsh dirty surfaces are seen. Racey (1999) reported that horseshoe bats develop swollen carpal joints after even a few days in captivity. In an effort to avoid this, horseshoe bats should be provided with a perch or netting from which to hang by their feet.

Pneumonia

Pneumonia was the most common histopathological finding in the study by Mühldorfer et al. (2011b), with mild to severe interstitial pneumonia noted in almost 38% of specimens. Almost a quarter of these pulmonary lesions were clearly attributable to bacterial or parasitic infection. However, in most affected lungs, neither infectious agents nor viral inclusion bodies were detected during microscopic examination. The large respiratory surface area and thin blood–gas barrier may predispose bat lungs to injury from environmental toxicants and pathogenic microorganisms (Mühldorfer et al., 2011b).

Non-specific diarrhoea

Collapsed dehydrated bats may void mucoid or watery diarrhoea. This may be the primary cause of the debility or may be the manifestation of scant gut contents following starvation. Many respond to symptomatic treatment, including rehydration (see 'First aid') and judicious use of a kaolin and pectin gel (see Figure 15.14).

Therapeutics

There is no pharmacokinetic information available for any drugs used in bats; since bats are heterotherms, and thus do not conform to allometric principles, it is difficult to propose a logical course of action when considering the dosage regime of therapeutic agents. If one adheres to allometric principles, based on a metabolic weight, overdose would be likely in a bat that remained torpid. Conversely, allowance for torpor and appropriate reduction of drug dosage may mean that therapeutic levels are not achieved in the active bat. The author uses dosages extrapolated from those used in other small mammals, with the bat kept warm throughout treatment, to minimize the effects of torpor. Given the small size of bats, oral medication using a catheter or pipette is the safest method of administration, with injections being limited to those which can be given by the subcutaneous route, over the dorsum, via a 27–30 G needle (Bexton and Couper, 2010).

Bacterial culture and antibiotic sensitivity tests should be carried out prior to the use of antibiotics if at all possible. Antibiotics that appear to be well tolerated and that may, empirically, have a beneficial effect include the synthetic penicillins and augmented derivatives, the cephalosporins, enrofloxacin, clindamycin and lincomycin. Potentially ototoxic compounds (e.g. the aminoglycosides gentamicin and neomycin) should not be used and the use of tetracyclines and enrofloxacin would be contraindicated in growing individuals. The author has not observed gastrointestinal disturbances indicating adverse effects from the action of antibiotics on the gut flora, but some workers will supplement the diet of a bat undergoing antibiotic therapy with preparations containing lactobacilli (Barnard, 1995). Drugs used by the author are shown in Figure 15.14.

Drug	Formulation	Dose rate	Dilution	Volume of diluted product per 5 g bat	Comments
Antimicrobials					
Amoxicillin/ clavulanic acid (co-amoxiclav)	Dry powder containing 150 mg clavulanic acid plus 600 mg amoxicillin	30 mg/kg orally q12h	Reconstitute by adding 100 ml of water to dry powder Refrigerate after reconstitution and discard after 7 days	0.02 ml	Broad spectrum Duration of treatment according to response (minimum 5–7 days)
Enrofloxacin	2.5% oral solution	10 mg/kg orally q12h	Dilute 0.1 ml of solution with 0.9 ml of water	0.02 ml	Broad spectrum Duration of treatment according to response (minimum 5–7 days) Not to be used in growing animals Make up a fresh dilution daily

15.14 Medications used in bats. No products are licensed for use in bats; table is for guidance based on author's experience. (continues) ▶ (Adapted from Bexton and Couper, 2010)

Drug	Formulation	Dose rate	Dilution	Volume of diluted product per 5 g bat	Comments
Anti-inflammatories/analgesics					
Meloxicam	0.5 mg/ml oral suspension for cats	0.2 mg/kg orally q24h	Dilute 0.1 ml of suspension with 0.9 ml water	0.02 ml	NSAID for treatment of inflammation and mild to moderate pain Avoid use in dehydrated animals Avoid use in pregnant animals Make up a fresh dilution daily
Buprenorphine	0.3 mg/ml solution for injection	0.1 mg/kg s.c., orally q6–12h (Lollar, 2010)	Dilute 0.05 ml of solution with 0.95 ml of water	0.03 ml	For treatment of moderate pain
Miscellaneous					
Simethicone	40 mg/ml oral suspension	400 mg/kg orally q6h	Use undiluted	0.05 ml	For use in animals with bloat
Kaolin suspension	0.99 g Kaolin Light per 5 ml oral suspension	1 ml/kg as total daily dose Given as divided dose orally q6h	Dilute 0.05 ml of suspension with 0.95 ml of water Refrigerate after reconstitution and discard after 7 days	0.02 ml	For use in animals with non-specific diarrhoea

15.14 (continued) Medications used in bats. No products are licensed for use in bats; table is for guidance based on author's experience. (Adapted from Bexton and Couper, 2010)

Management in captivity

Housing

A hospitalized bat should have enough space to stretch its wings out fully and crawl around. Initially bats may be housed in the clip-top plastic tanks used for small pets. These are escape-proof, lightweight and easily disinfected. A cloth or paper towel hung over the edges of the container provides the bat with somewhere to hide, and should be replaced daily to maintain good hygiene (Figure 15.15). Care should be taken to avoid injury to the bat when removing and replacing the lid, as they will often rest inverted, with their feet at the lip of the container, and can quickly crawl up the side when returned to the tank. Wooden boxes are favoured by some bat workers on the grounds that they approximate more to the natural situation and are less acoustically harsh. These must be made from untreated timber. However, they are not so easily disinfected, and rough surfaces may harbour parasites and cause abrasions to the carpus. Horseshoe bats should be provided with plastic

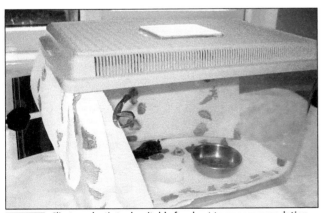

15.15 Clip-top plastic tank suitable for short-term accommodation. Paper towel hung over edges of container provides bat with somewhere to hide and hang from. Mealworms presented in a shallow, smooth-sided container, to allow easy access for bat, but to prevent mealworms from escaping. A heat mat is positioned behind the tank. (© RSPCA, David Couper)

netting from which they may hang freely by their feet from the 'roof' of the housing.

Heat should be provided at one end of the housing, thereby providing a temperature range of around 25–35°C. Water can be provided in a shallow dish, and should be available at all times. Ideally the relative humidity should be around 50–60%.

Socialization

Although social animals, there is no need to maintain bats in a group whilst they are hospitalized. Individual care is needed and there is the risk of transmission of undiagnosed disease between individuals. This can be reviewed for long-term captives, or when rehabilitating multiple animals from the same roost. In these cases, the collapsible mesh vivaria used by herpetologists provide more space.

Flight facilities

Whichever system is used to house the bat for the bulk of the day, it is essential that flight is permitted on a regular and frequent basis (see 'Pre-release assessment'). Initial flight may be poor, but it must be encouraged through persistence on the part of the rehabilitator. Failure of an apparently uninjured bat to fly within a few days indicates undiagnosed injuries; it carries a poor prognosis and warrants further investigation.

Bat researchers have learned that, in order to keep captive bats in good health, good flight facilities are a necessity. Post-release radiotelemetry studies have confirmed the importance of this, demonstrating that hand-reared bats exhibit improved survival if housed in a flight aviary prior to release (see 'Release') (Kelly et al., 2008). The greater space allows the bats to exercise and develop their echolocation and flight skills. Proprietary bat boxes can be provided, in which the bats can roost. Insects can be encouraged into the bat flight with the use of water, rotting vegetables, and moth lamps. Although free-living bats will only hunt if the density of their prey is above a certain threshold, hand-reared juvenile bats have, anecdotally, been observed to catch insects in bat flights (Brown and Brown, 2006). Kelly et al. (2012) recommended that obstacles approximating to 'entrance holes' be provided within the bat flight, to allow the young bats to develop the ability to navigate roost entrances. Close attention should be paid to disinfection, to avoid transmission of diseases and parasites between successive inhabitants.

Diet

The normal diet of bats in captivity is insects, bred primarily for use by aviculturalists and herpetologists. If these are not available, as an interim measure a commercial tinned cat food or convalescent diet (e.g. Hill's® Prescription Diet® a/d®), offered on a fine artist's paintbrush, is well accepted. The most common insect food offered is mealworms, the larvae of the beetle *Tenebrio molitor*. Whilst representing a good source of calories and being readily accepted, they are *per se* nutritionally deficient, in particular with reference to the calcium:phosphorus ratio. The deficiency is increased when the mealworms are feeding in bran, which is low in calcium and contains the calcium-binding compound phytate. Various methods of improving the nutritional value of mealworms have been described, including dusting them with proprietary vitamin and mineral supplements, and gut-loading with chick crumbs (feed for poultry), non-citrus fruit and milk replacer powder. Mealworms produce quinones which have been implicated in toxicities in captive bats, and are believed to be one of the factors responsible for fur loss. Some people appear to be sensitive to mealworms; in a few severe cases respiratory signs may be seen but, more commonly, there is local skin irritation. Wiping the face after handling mealworms may cause an acute conjunctivitis. Due caution is advised and the use of latex gloves is prudent.

Training bats to take mealworms

Bats can readily be trained to take mealworms. The bat is restrained gently in the cupped hand and the abdominal contents of a decapitated mealworm are extruded, toothpaste-like, into the bat's mouth (Figure 15.16). Once the bat starts chewing, the empty exoskeleton can be gently pushed into its mouth. When the bat has adapted to mealworms offered in this manner, it can be offered decapitated mealworms with tweezers and should ultimately progress to eating live mealworms offered in a shallow bowl. Horseshoe bats do not eat well when restrained, and prefer to be fed whilst hanging by their feet.

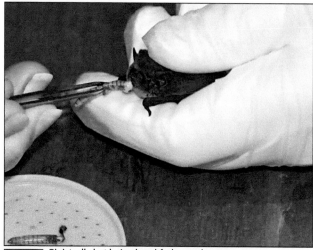

15.16 Pipistrelle bat being hand-fed a mealworm.
(© Maggie and Bryan Brown)

Continual assessment

Food intake, faecal quantity and quality, urination, bodyweight and condition should be monitored and recorded on a daily basis to gauge progress. As a rough guide, an adult pipistrelle species bat will eat around 40 'mini' mealworms per day (Bexton and Couper, 2010). Adjustment has to be made when the bat changes from the sedentary convalescing individual to the pre-release individual that is flying regularly. Failure of the bat to eat for itself after several days warrants further investigation and carries a guarded prognosis. Obesity has been recorded in captive bats (Daffner, 2001; Bexton and Couper, 2010). Simpson (1994) reported a white liver syndrome, in particular in hospitalized *Pipistrellus* spp. Due to its resemblance to a similar condition seen in lambs on low cobalt diets, he speculated that this could be dietary in origin.

Rearing of bat pups

The hand-rearing of bat pups through to flight, whilst being difficult and time-consuming, is achievable. Housing, feeding and weaning are all well documented (Barnard, 1995; Brown and Brown, 2006; Lollar, 2010). In summary, the young bats may be kept in incubators with a temperature range of around 25–35°C, at a relative humidity of around 50–60%, and fed a suitable milk replacer (Royal Canin® Babydog is recommended by the BCT at the time of writing) using a fine artist's paintbrush, a small catheter, or similar. Pipistrelle bat neonates will take as little as 0.1 ml per 2-hourly feed initially (see also Chapter 8). As with other young mammals, urination and defecation should be encouraged by stimulating the anogenital region at each feed. A few drops of water should be available in a shallow dish at all times. The young bats will start doing 'push-ups' with their wings when they are ready to begin flying. At this point weaning on to mealworms (see 'Diet') can commence.

Problems associated with hand-rearing

Metabolic bone disease is a common finding in hand-reared bats, manifesting as deformity of the bones, particularly the finger bones (Simpson, 1994), and folding fractures (Figure 15.17). Affected individuals may be reluctant to move and have poor or non-existent flight, and euthanasia is recommended. The condition is the result of dietary calcium:phosphorus imbalance, and would seem to be more common in individuals that are weaned on to mealworms too early.

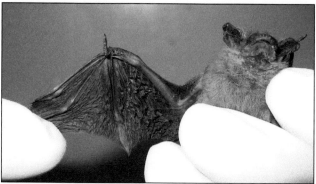

15.17 Metabolic bone disease in a juvenile common pipistrelle bat. The finger bones are deformed and there is a folding fracture of the forearm. Note: photograph is of a dead specimen.
(© RSPCA, David Couper)

Digestive upsets such as bloat and diarrhoea are also encountered. Predisposing factors include low body temperature, unsuitable milk composition or temperature, inconsistencies in the feeding regimen, and aerophagia. Pups should be rehydrated, and husbandry problems should be identified and corrected. Simethicone may be used to treat bloat (see Figure 15.14).

Aspiration pneumonia is also reported; to avoid this, the pup's head should be kept slightly below the body during feeding, and the feeding utensil introduced from below (Bexton and Couper, 2010). The pup should be fed slowly, to avoid covering the nostrils in milk.

Release

Pre-release assessment

Prior to release, the body condition and weight of the bat should be judged to be suitable for that species for the time of year. It is vital to ensure that a bat is capable of sustained flight and able to echolocate before its release is contemplated (see 'Flight facilities'). To assess flight a large escape-proof room is needed. The smaller species are more manoeuvrable and can be assessed adequately in a room of average size. The larger species, such as serotine bats and noctule bats, require more extensive facilities such as a large flight cage. It is best to carry out the assessment in the evening when the bat will be more metabolically active. The bat should be allowed to warm up thoroughly and become physically active before flight is attempted. This can be expedited by placing its container on a heat pad or similar. Once active, it should be encouraged to launch itself from a height of around 1.5 m. It should then, after an initial drop, climb to above head height and circle the room's airspace. Bats that are unfit either fail to gain height, or fly poorly before descending to the ground, or keep inverting themselves to brush against surfaces, using their hind feet to find a purchase on a wall or surface that will allow them to rest. Bats that are fit for release must fly vigorously for at least 10 minutes; those that show no signs of tiring (to the extent that one despairs of waiting for them to land) are ready for release.

A bat's ability to echolocate can be confirmed with a bat detector, used by conservationists and bat enthusiasts to observe bats and to study bat behaviour in the wild. These are tuned to pick up the ultrasound emissions through a microphone and then, in most versions, convert them down to 'real-time' sounds within the human auditory range. If possible, it should be tuned to the frequency that is characteristic of the species being flown. Ultrasound emissions should be detectable whilst the bat is flying and they coincide with the successful negotiation of objects.

Release of adults

Release should be undertaken only when the bat is deemed fit, as judged by the parameters outlined above. If the exact site where the bat was found is known, the bat should be returned to that site. Even if the social group has changed roost site in the interim, it is presumed that this lies within the bat's home range and therefore it should readily orientate itself within the release area. The release should take place at dusk and when weather conditions are favourable and conducive to flight. Heavy rain, wind, frost or snow, preclude release. The presence of conspecifics in the area would indicate conditions that are inherently suitable. Ideally a feed and warm-up flight should have been carried out that evening at the rehabilitation facility. The warmed-up and active bat should be held in a raised hand and allowed to launch itself.

Release of hand-reared juveniles

Prolonged pre-release flight training in a flight aviary is recommended prior to the release of hand-reared juveniles (Kelly *et al.*, 2012). Various soft-release techniques have been described, whereby bats are allowed to gradually acclimatize to new surroundings by provisioning post-release. This can be as simple as translocation of the bats in their bat boxes to an area used by wild conspecifics (Serangeli *et al.*, 2012). Kelly *et al.* (2012) recommended that hand-reared bats be allowed to self-release from a large flight cage situated in suitable bat habitat.

Post-release monitoring

Radiotelemetry has been used to demonstrate post-release survival of hand-reared pipistrelle bats in the UK, at least in the short-term (Kelly *et al.*, 2008). The length of time bats may be tracked is restricted by the small transmitter size, which in turn necessitates a small battery – the expected battery life of the transmitters in the study by Kelly *et al.* (2008) was 10–14 days. The survival of hand-reared Kuhl's pipistrelle bats (*P. Kuhlii*) has also been reported in Italy by Serangeli *et al.* (2012), who demonstrated that released bats were foraging and roosting in sites typically used by wild *P. Kuhlii* and were accepted in local conspecific colonies. Longer term survival was shown by Kelly *et al.* (2012) by the use of metal bat rings, with animals surviving hibernation (see also Chapter 9). Passive integrated transponder (PIT) tags have also been used successfully in bats in the UK (Rigby *et al.*, 2012), and could potentially be used to monitor the survival of rehabilitated bats post-release, by the placement of hoop PIT readers at roost entrances, as used in capture-recapture studies (Wimsatt *et al.*, 2005).

Legal aspects

The Wildlife and Countryside Act 1981 (WCA), the Conservation (Natural Habitats, &c.) Regulations 1994 (amended 2007), and the Countryside and Rights of Way Act (2000) (CRoW) afford protection to wild bats, their roosts and hibernation sites. It is an offence to capture, injure, kill or disturb a bat, or to destroy, damage, or block access to their roosts. Section 10(3)(a) of the WCA allows unlicensed persons to 'take' disabled bats, for the sole purpose of tending them, with the intention of releasing them when they are no longer disabled. Section 10(3)(b) permits the killing of bats that are so seriously disabled that no recovery is likely. It is an offence to possess, transport, sell or exchange any bat (alive or dead) or any part of a bat, including long-term captives. However, certain exceptions may be possible under licence from the Statutory Nature Conservation Organisation. See also Chapter 2 for more details.

The Abandonment of Animals Act (1960) would make it an offence to release any animal that is unlikely to survive in the wild, which would also include releasing bats into unsuitable habitat, or during unfavourable conditions.

Acknowledgements

The author is indebted to Andrew Routh for the bat chapter in the previous edition of this book, on which this chapter was founded, and to Maggie and Bryan Brown for advice and photographs.

References and further reading

Altringham JD (1996) *Bats: Biology and Behaviour.* Oxford University Press, Oxford

Arlettaz R, Christe P and Desfayes M (2002) 33 years, a new longevity record for a European bat. *Mammalia* **66**, 441–442

Baker AS (2005) *Psorergatoides nyctali* (Prostigmata: Psorergatidae), a new mite species parasitizing the bat *Nyctalus noctula* (Mammalia: Chiroptera) in the British Isles. *Systematic and Applied Acarology* **10**, 67–74

Baker AS and Craven JC (2003) Checklist of the mites (Arachnida: Acari) associated with bats (Mammalia: Chiroptera) in the British Isles. *Systemic and Applied Acarology Special Publications* **14**, 1–20

Barlow A, Jolliffe T and Tomlin M (2011) Mycotic dermatitis in a vagrant part-coloured bat (*Vespertilio murinus*) in Great Britain. *The Veterinary Record* **169**, 614

Barlow A, Wills D and Harris E (2013) Enteric nematodes and Sarcina-like bacteria in a brown long-eared bat. *Veterinary Record* **172**, 508

Barlow A, Worledge L, Miller H *et al.* (2015) The first confirmation of *Pseudogymnoascus destructans* in British Bats and hibernacula. *The Veterinary Record* **177(3)**, 73

Barnard SM (1995) *Bats in Captivity.* Wild Ones Animal Books, California

Bat Conservation Trust (2000) *Treatment of Bat Casualties for Veterinary Surgeons.* Professional Support Series. Bat Conservation Trust, London

Bat Conservation Trust (2008) *Bat care guidelines; a guide to bat care for rehabilitators.* Bat Conservation Trust, London

Bat Ward Sanctuary (2010) *Insectivorous bat care standards.* Bat World Sanctuary. www.batworld.org

Bexton S and Couper D (2010) Handling and veterinary care of British bats. *In Practice* **32**, 254–262

Brown M and Brown B (2006) *Bat Rescue Manual.* Otley, West Yorkshire Bat Hospital

Brownlee-Bouboulis SA and Reeder DM (2013) White-nose syndrome-affected little brown myotis (*Myotis lucifugis*) increase grooming and other active behaviours during arousals from hibernation. *Journal of Wildlife Diseases* **49**, 850–859

Burek K (2001) Mycotic diseases. In: *Infectious Diseases of Wild Mammals,* ed. ES Williams and IK Barker, pp. 514–531. Manson Publishing, London

Calisher CH, Childs JE, Field HE, Holmes KV and Schountz T (2006) Bats: important reservoir hosts of emerging viruses. *Clinical Microbiology Reviews* **19**, 531–545

Clark DR Jr (1988) How sensitive are bats to insecticides? *Wildlife Society Bulletin* **16**, 399–403

Concannon R, Wynn-Owen K, Simpson VR and Birtles RJ (2005) Molecular characterisation of haemoparasites infecting bats (*Microchiroptera*) in Cornwall, UK. *Parasitology* **131** 489–496

Constantine DG (1986) Insectivorous bats. In: *Zoo and Wild Animal Medicine,* ed. ME Fowler, pp. 650–655. WB Saunders, Philadelphia

Daffner B (2001) *Causes of morbidity and mortality in British bat species and prevalence of selected zoonotic pathogens.* Thesis for MSc in Wild Animal Health, Institute of Zoology and Royal Veterinary College, London

Dietz C and von Helversen O (2004) *Illustrated Identification Key to the Bats of Europe. Version 1.0,* released 15/12/2004 – electronic publication. Available from: http://biocenosi.dipbsf.uninsubria.it/didattica/bat_key1.pdf

Dietz C, von Helversen O and Dietmar N (2009) *Bats of Britain, Europe and Northwest Africa.* A & C Black Publishers Ltd, London

Done J (1998) (correspondence) *Veterinary Times* **28(7)**, 23

Duszynski DW and Upton SJ (2001) *Cyclospora, Eimeria, Isospora* and *Cryptosporidium* spp. In: *Parasitic Diseases of Wild Mammals,* ed. WM Samuel *et al.,* pp. 424–427. Manson Publishing, London

Evans NJ, Bown K, Tomifte D and Birtles RJ (2009) Fatal borreliosis in bat caused by relapsing fever spirochete, United Kingdom. *Emerging Infectious Diseases* **15**, 1331–1332

Findley JS (1993) *Bats: a Community Perspective.* Cambridge University Press, Cambridge

Fooks AR, Finnegan C, Johnson N *et al.* (2002) Human case of EBL type 2 following exposure to bats in Angus, Scotland. *Veterinary Record* **151**, 679

Fooks AR, McElhinney LM, Pounder DJ *et al.* (2003) Case report: isolation of a European lyssavirus type 2a from a fatal human case of rabies encephalitis. *Journal of Medical Virology* **71**, 281–289

Gardner RA and Molyneux DH (1987) *Babesia vesperuginis*: natural and experimental infections in British bats (*Microchiroptera*). *Parasitology* **95**, 461–469

Gardner RA and Molyneux DH (1988a) *Schizotrypanum* in British bats. *Parasitology* **97**, 43–50

Gardner RA and Molyneux DH (1988b) *Trypanosoma (Megatrypanum) incertum* from *Pipistrellus pipistrellus*: development and transmission by cimicid bugs. *Parasitology* **96**, 433–447

Gardner RA and Molyneux DH (1988c) *Polychromophilus murinus*: a malarial parasite of bats: life-history and ultrastructural studies. *Parasitology* **96**, 591–605

Gibson DI, Bray RA and Harris EA (2005) *Host-parasite database.* www.nhm.ac.uk/research-curation/scientific-resources/taxonomy-systematics/host-parasites/index.html.

Greenaway F and Hutson AM (1990) *A Field Guide to British Bats.* Bruce Coleman Books, Uxbridge

Gruber AD, Schulze CA, Brugmann M and Pohlenz J (1996) Renal coccidiosis with cystic tubular dilatation in four bats. *Veterinary Pathology* **33**, 442–445

Harris SL, Aegerter JN, Brookes SM *et al.* (2009) Targeted surveillance for European bat lyssaviruses in English bats (2003–06). *Journal of Wildlife Diseases* **45**, 1030–1041

Harris SL, Mansfield K, Marston DA *et al.* (2007) Isolation of European bat lyssavirus type 2 from a Daubenton's bat (*Myotis daubentonii*) in Shropshire. *Veterinary Record* **161**, 384–386

Harris S, Morris P, Wray S and Yaldon D (1995) *A review of British mammals: population estimates and conservation status of British mammals other than cetaceans.* Joint Nature Conservation Committee, Peterborough, UK

Hutson AM and Racey PA (1999) Examining bats. In: *Bat Workers' Manual,* ed. AJ Mitchell-Jones and AP McLeish, pp. 39–45. Joint Nature Conservancy Committee, Peterborough

Johnson N, Selden D, Parson SG and Fooks AR (2002) European bat lyssavirus type 2 in a bat found in Lancashire. *Veterinary Record* **151**, 455–456

Jones G, Duverge L and Ransome RD (1995) Conservation biology of an endangered species: field studies of greater horseshoe bats. *Symposia of the Zoological Society of London* **67**, 309–324

Jürgens JD, Bartels H and Bartels R (1981) Blood oxygen transport and organ weight of small bats and small non-flying mammals. *Respiratory physiology* **45**, 243–260

Kelly A, Goodwin S, Grogan A and Mathews F (2008) Post-release survival of hand-reared pipistrelle bats (*Pipistrellus* spp.). *Animal Welfare* **17**, 375–382

Kelly A, Goodwin S, Grogan A and Mathews F (2012) Further evidence for the post-release survival of hand-reared, orphaned bats based on radio-tracking and ring-return data. *Animal Welfare* **21**, 27–31

Kulzer E (2005) *Chiroptera, Vol. 3: Biologie – Handbuch der Zoologie VIII (Mammalia).* De Gruyter, Berlin

Kunz TH and Nagy KA (1988) Methods of energy budget analysis. In: *Ecological and Behavioral Methods for the Study of Bats,* ed. TH Kunz, pp. 277–302. Smithsonian Institution Press, Washington DC

Lelli D, Papetti A, Sabelli *et al.* (2013) Detection of Coronaviruses in bats of various species in Italy. *Viruses* **5**, 2679–2689

Lollar A (2010) *Standards and Medical Management for Captive Insectivorous Bats.* Bat World Publications, Mineral Wells, Texas

Lollar A and Schmidt-French B (1998) *Captive Care and Medical Reference for the Rehabilitation of Insectivorous Bats.* Bat World Publications, Texas

Lorch JM, Meteyer CU, Behr MJ *et al.* (2011) Experimental infection of bats with *Pseudogymnoascus destructans* causes white-nose syndrome. *Nature* **480**, 376–378

Maina JN (2000) What it takes to fly: The structural and functional refinements in birds and bats. *Journal of Experimental Biology* **203**, 3045–3064

Meteyer CU, Valent M, Kashmer J *et al.* (2011) Recovery of little brown bats (*Myotis lucifugus*) from natural infection with Geomyces destructans, white-nose syndrome. *Journal of Wildlife Diseases* **47**, 618–626

Mitchell-Jones AJ (1999a) Health and safety in bat work. In: *Bat Workers' Manual,* ed. AJ Mitchell-Jones and AP McLeish, p. 20. Joint Nature Conservancy Committee, Peterborough

Mitchell-Jones AJ (1999b) Timber treatment, pest control and building work. In: *Bat Workers' Manual,* ed. AJ Mitchell-Jones and AP McLeish, pp. 73–84. Joint Nature Conservancy Committee, Peterborough

Mitchell-Jones AJ and McLeish AP (1999) *Bat Workers' Manual.* Joint Nature Conservancy Committee, Peterborough

Mühldorfer K, Speck S, Kurth *et al.* (2011a) Diseases and causes of death in European bats: dynamics in disease susceptibility and infection rates. *PLoS ONE* **6**, 12

Mühldorfer K, Speck S and Wibbelt G (2011b) Diseases in free-ranging bats from Germany. *BMC Veterinary Research* **7**, 61

Mullineaux L and Brash M (2009) How to...handle bats. *Journal of Small Animal Practice* **50**, 8–11

Pikula J, Bandouchova H, Novotny L *et al.* (2012) Histopathology confirms white-nose syndrome in bats in Europe. *Journal of Wildlife Diseases* **48**, 207–211

Podlutsky AJ, Khritankov AM, Ovodov ND and Austad SN (2005) A new field record for bat longevity. *The Journals of Gerontology. Series A, Biological Sciences and Medical Sciences* **60**, 1366–1368

Puechmaille SJ, Wibbelt G, Korn V *et al.* (2011) Pan-European distribution of white-nose syndrome fungus (*Geomyces destructans*) not associated with mass mortality. *PLoS ONE* 6:e19167

Pybus MJ, Hobson DP and Onderka DK (1986) Mass mortality of bats due to probable blue-green algal toxicity. *Journal of Wildlife Diseases* **22**, 449–450

Racey PA (1999) Handling, releasing and keeping bats. In: *Bat Workers' Manual,* ed. AJ Mitchell-Jones and AP McLeish, pp. 51–56. Joint Nature Conservancy Committee, Peterborough

Racey PA and Swift SM (1985) Feeding ecology of *Pipistrellus pipistrellus* (Chiroptera: Vespertilionidae) during pregnancy and lactation. I. Foraging behaviour. *Journal of Animal Ecology* **54**, 205–215

Racey PA and Swift SM (1986) The residual effects of remedial timber treatment on bats. *Biological Conservation* **35**, 205

Ransome R (1990) *The Natural History of Hibernating Bats*. Christopher Helm, Bromley

Reeder DM, Frank CL, Turner GG *et al.* (2012) Frequent arousal from hibernation and low pre-hibernation body mass linked to severity of infection and mortality in bats with white-nose syndrome. *PLoS One* **7**:e38920

Richardson P (2000) *Guidelines on Bats in Captivity*. Bat Conservation Trust, London

Rigby EL, Aegerter J, Brash M and Altringham JD (2012) Impact of PIT tagging on recapture rates, body condition and reproductive success of wild Daubenton's bats (*Myotis daubentonii*). *Veterinary Record* **170**, 101

Routh A (1991) Bats in the surgery. *Veterinary Record* **128**, 316–318

Routh A (2003) Bats. In: *BSAVA Manual of Wildlife Casualties*, ed. E Mullineaux, RT Best and J Cooper, pp. 95–108. BSAVA Publications, Gloucester

Rupprecht CE, Stöhr K and Meredith C (2001) Rabies. In: *Infectious Diseases of Wild Mammals*, ed. ES Williams and IK Barker, pp. 3–36. Manson Publishing, London

Schipper J, Chanson JS, Chiozza F *et al.* (2008) The status of the world's land and marine mammals: diversity, threat and knowledge. *Science* **322**, 225–230

Schober W and Grimmberger E (1989) *A Guide to Bats of Britain and Europe*. Hamlyn, London

Scottish Natural Heritage (2009) *SNH releases latest bat lyssavirus monitoring results (03/07/2009)*. Scottish Natural Heritage

Serangeli MT, Cistrone L, Ancillotto L, Tomassini A and Russo D (2012) The post-release fate of hand-reared orphaned bats: survival and habitat selection. *Animal Welfare* **21**, 9–18

Simpson VR (1994) Pathological conditions in British bats. *Proceedings of Wildlife Diseases Association, First European Conference*, November 22–24, 1994, Paris, p. 47

Simpson VR (1999) Potential wildlife zoonoses in Britain. *Proceedings of BVA Seminar Day, Zoonotic Diseases of UK Wildlife, British Veterinary Association Congress*, September 23, 1999, Bath, pp. 1–8

Simpson VR, Borman AM, Fox RI and Mathews F (2013) Cutaneous mycosis in a Barbastelle bat (*Barbastella barbastellus*) caused by *Hyphopichia burtonii*. *Journal of Veterinary Diagnostic Investigation* **25**, 551–554

Sonntag M, Mühldorfer K, Speck S, Wibbelt G and Kurth A (2009) New adenovirus in bats, Germany. *Emerging Infectious Diseases* **16**, 2052–2055

Stallknecht DE and Howerth EW (2001) Pseudorabies (Aujeszky's disease). In: *Infectious Diseases of Wild Mammals*, ed. ES Williams and IK Barker, p. 166. Manson Publishing, London

Stebbings RE (1988) *Conservation of European Bats*. Christopher Helm, Bromley

Stocker L (2005) *Practical Wildlife Care, second edition*. Blackwell Science, Oxford

Walker LA, Simpson VR, Rockett L, Wienburg CL and Shore RF (2007) Heavy metal contamination in bats in Britain. *Environmental Pollution* **148**, 483–490

Walsh ST and Stebbings RE (1989) Care and rehabilitation of wild bats. In: *Proceedings of the Inaugural Symposium of the British Wildlife Rehabilitation Council*, ed. S Harris and T Thomas, pp. 64–72. British Wildlife Rehabilitation Council, c/o RSPCA, Horsham

Whitby JE, Heaton PR, Black EM *et al.* (2000) First isolation of a rabies-related virus from a Daubenton's bat in the United Kingdom. *Veterinary Record* **147**, 385–388

Wibbelt G, Kurth A, Yasmum N *et al.* (2007) Discovery of herpesviruses in bats. *Journal of General Virology* **88**, 2651–2655

Wickramasinghe LP, Harris S, Jones G and Vaughan N (2003) Bat activity and species richness on organic and conventional farms: impact of agricultural intensification. *Journal of Applied Ecology* **40**, 984–993

Wilson DE (1988) Maintaining bats for captive studies. In: *Ecological and Behavioral Methods for the Study of Bats*, ed. TH Kunz, pp. 247–264. Smithsonian Institution Press, Washington DC

Wimsatt J, O'Shea TJ, Ellison LE, Pearce RD and Price VR (2005) Anesthesia and blood sampling of wild big brown bats (*Eptesicus fuscus*) with an assessment of impacts on survival. *Journal of Wildlife Diseases* **41**, 87–95

Wolk E and Ruprecht AL (1988) Haematological values in the serotine bat *Eptesicus serotinus* (Schreber, 1774). *Acta Theriologica* **33**, 545–553

Wong S, Lau S, Woo P and Yuen KY (2007) Bats as a continuing source of emerging infections in humans. *Reviews in Medical Virology* **17**, 67–91

Yuill TM and Seymour C (2001) Arbovirus infections. In: *Infectious Diseases of Wild Mammals*, ed. ES Williams and IK Barker, pp. 98–118. Manson Publishing, London

Specialist organizations and useful contacts

See also Appendix 1

Bat Conservation Trust
15 Cloisters House, 8 Battersea Park Road, London SW8 4BG
0845 1300 228
enquiries@bats.org.uk
www.bats.org.uk

Carcasses for rabies analysis:
Bat carcasses are required for routine rabies screening. These do not need to be from suspected cases. They should be sent fresh, in a parcel that complies with current postal regulations, to:
Rabies Diagnostics Unit
Animal and Plant Health Agency, Woodham Lane, New Haw, Addlestone, Surrey KT15 3NB
www.gov.uk/rabies-in-bats

Current submission forms are available from the BCT (see above) or Defra

Chapter 16

Rabbits and hares

Jenna Richardson

Rabbits and hares are mammals from the order Lagomorpha and family Leporidae. Historically, lagomorphs were classified as rodents and it was not until 1912 that differentiation between the two was made. Lagomorphs display two pairs of upper incisors compared to the single pair of the rodent. Although there are similarities between rodents and lagomorphs, they are not closely related. It is through a parallel evolution that the two developed similarities in their dentition in correlation with a life of gnawing and chewing.

In the UK, there are three species of wild lagomorphs:

*   The European rabbit (*Oryctolagus cuniculus*) (Figure 16.1)
*   The brown hare (*Lepus europaeus*) (Figure 16.2)
*   The mountain hare (*Lepus timidus*) also known as the 'blue' or 'Irish' hare (Figure 16.3).

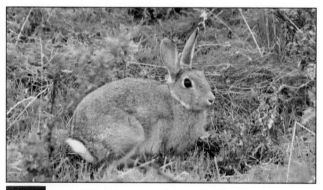

16.1 European rabbit.

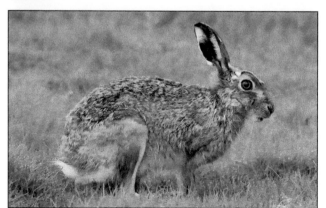

16.2 Brown hare.
(© Rob Barnett Photography)

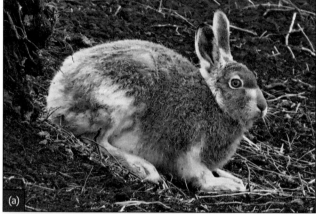

(a)

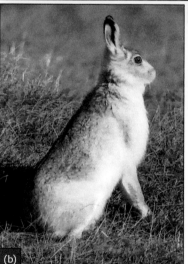

(b)

16.3 (a) Mountain hare with moulting of the winter coat in early springtime. (b) In late autumn the winter coat is almost complete, but provides poor camouflage on snow-free lowland ground.
(© Rob Barnett Photography)

Rabbits are one of the most common wild mammals found free-living in the British countryside and are widespread throughout mainland and island Britain. In correspondence with breeding seasons, population numbers peak during the spring and summer months.

Hares are markedly less common than rabbits in Britain. The brown hare is found well distributed throughout the UK, with the exception of northern Scotland. The mountain hare is seen in smaller numbers than the brown hare and is found in the Highlands of Scotland and parts of Ireland; there is also a small population in the Peak District.

Common reasons for presentation of lagomorph casualties are given in Figure 16.4.

BSAVA Manual of Wildlife Casualties, second edition. Edited by Elizabeth Mullineaux and Emma Keeble. ©BSAVA 2016

Category	Reason for presentation
Neonates	• Abandoned or apparently abandoned (leverets) by the dam • Found after disruption of the nest (rabbit kits) • Rescued from a predator (domestic cats and dogs are common culprits)
Juveniles	• Found in a debilitated state, often due to starvation and/or hypothermia • Rescued from a predator
Physical injury	• Road traffic accidents • Machinery incidents
Diseased	• Moribund or unable to evade capture; most common example is a rabbit with myxomatosis

16.4 Common reasons for the presentation of rabbit and hare casualties.

Ecology and biology

Habitat and diet

Rabbits can adapt to and live in a range of different environments, from farmlands and moorlands to woodlands and sand dunes. As part of their survival technique, their habitat requires areas of cover such as hedgerows and bushes to allow escape from predators. Rabbits spend most of the day underground in a communal warren. Warrens are composed of a series of underground chambers or burrows that are connected by numerous tunnels. Whilst some burrows are social areas, others are used as breeding chambers or 'stops'. It is common for a warren to have multiple entrances and exits. When above ground, if food is in plentiful supply, rabbits graze on grass and plants near to the warren. When food is scarce, for example during the winter months, a rabbit may have to travel further from the safety of the warren to forage. Winter diets are often composed of leaves, roots and bark.

The brown hare is mainly a lowland species, preferring flat countryside of open grass and farmland. They do not burrow, but instead use pre-existing cover to hide when threatened (e.g. hedgerows, woodland and uneven terrain). Brown hares dig shallow depressions known as 'forms' in open fields, in which they spend most of the day. When sitting in a form, only the top of the head and back is visible; this provides excellent camouflage from predators. Brown hares are deterred by livestock and are found in a greater abundance on arable farmland. The home range of an individual brown hare is large (20–40 hectares) and increases in accordance with food shortages.

Mountain hares, as the name might suggest, are found on higher ground. They live on heather moorlands and rocky upland ground. Although their preferred diet is grass, they can survive on heather, gorse, birch and older woody plants.

Social structure

Rabbits live in groups with a hierarchical social structure. Within the group there is a dominant buck and doe, along with subordinate and juveniles of both sexes. Group sizes can vary from two to ten adult animals. It is the role of the dominant male to defend the group's territory, whilst the adult females burrow to create and extend the warren. Juvenile bucks, after they have reached sexual maturity, will be driven from the group to either join another warren or live a solitary existence. If a younger stronger buck successfully challenges an older dominant male, the aged animal is driven from the warren. Females generally tend to stay within the group, even after they have become sexually mature.

Hares are less sociable than rabbits and during the day tend to live a solitary existence. They can congregate in the evenings to feed and this is particularly common if food is in abundant supply. When food is limited, the dominant hare will spend time defending the food source from both challenging and subordinate animals. Courtship behaviour involves 'boxing matches' as females try to ward off advances from unwelcome males. Fights between males attempting to achieve social dominance can be particularly violent and aggressive. The successful male does not bond to the females and mates with as many as possible in a short space of time.

Lifespan

Although wild rabbits could potentially live to similar ages seen in domestic rabbits (averaging 5 to 8 years of age); the reality is they have a far shorter lifespan. This is due to a number of factors including predation, disease, starvation and exposure to adverse weather conditions. In severe weather conditions, entire generations may be wiped out if a warren becomes flooded, drowning vulnerable kits still in the nest.

Hares in the wild can reach 4 to 5 years old, with records of up to 12 years of age being reported in captivity.

Role in the ecosystem

Lagomorphs, rabbits in particular, play a crucial role in many predator–prey food chains. Their intermediate size and population abundance makes them an easy target for numerous species of British wildlife predator. Rabbits supplement the diets of foxes, weasels, stoats, wildcats, larger species of gull and birds of prey.

Anatomy and physiology

Living under a constant threat of predation has forced lagomorphs to evolve skills and physiological variations to aid with both predator detection and escape.

Average adult weights of rabbits and hares are given in Figure 16.5. The lagomorph skeleton makes up less than 10% of the total bodyweight; by contrast the muscle mass contributes over 50% of bodyweight. This lightweight framework with strong powerful muscles aids with predator evasion. Rabbits and hares are light and agile, yet fast, due to powerful hindlimbs. Hares in particular are especially efficient runners. They can reach speeds of up to 75 km/hr for short bursts, which can allow them to escape from predators. In general the bones are quite brittle, so particular care should be taken when capturing and handling wild lagomorphs as fractures can readily

Species	Average adult bodyweight	
	Female	Male
European rabbit	1.5–2 kg	1.5–2 kg
Brown hare	3.4 kg	3.2 kg
Mountain hare	3 kg	2.7 kg

16.5 Average weights of adult rabbits and hares.

occur. The front feet have five digits, whilst the hind feet have four digits. The hind foot of a rabbit is approximately 8 cm long, compared to 14 cm for a mountain hare and 15 cm for a brown hare.

Rabbits have a heart rate range of 160–240 beats per minute, a respiratory rate of 30–60 breaths per minute and a body temperature of 38.5–40°C.

Digestive system

Rabbits and hares have 28 teeth with the following dental formula:

$$2 \times \left\{ I\, \frac{2}{1} \ \ C\, \frac{0}{0} \ \ P\, \frac{3}{2} \ \ M\, \frac{3}{3} \right\} = 28$$

The teeth are open-rooted and grow continuously. A natural diet high in fibre keeps the teeth worn to the correct length, preventing the overgrowths that are seen commonly in domestic rabbits.

Rabbits and hares are hindgut fermenters, with a digestive system designed to digest high-fibre diets (Figure 16.6). The abdominal cavity is proportionally very large, with the gastrointestinal tract accounting for between 10 and 20% of the total bodyweight. Gut transit time is fast to allow indigestible fibre to be rapidly eliminated from the gastrointestinal tract. This is advantageous in prey species as it allows overall bodyweight to remain low.

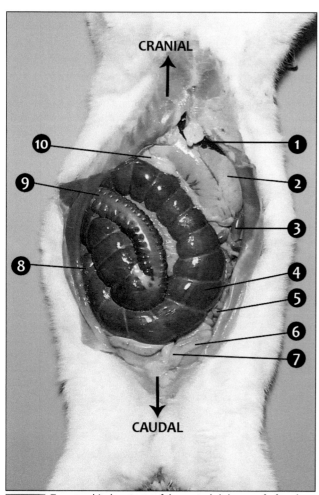

16.6 Topographical anatomy of the ventral abdomen of a female rabbit. Note the large ileocaecocolic complex that occupies most of the ventral abdomen. 1 = liver; 2 = stomach; 3 = small intestine; 4 = caecum; 5 = small intestine; 6 = uterus; 7 = bicornuate cervix; 8 = caecum; 9 = proximal colon; 10 = omentum.

Senses

As prey animals, rabbits and hares must be aware of both terrestrial and airborne predators and need to recognize even the most camouflaged of them. Their crepuscular activity also means that the ability to see in low light is essential. Group living (Figure 16.7) also ensures a 'herd effect' in predator detection.

The large eyes of rabbits and hares are located laterally near the top of the head (Figure 16.8). They are set wide apart and protrude beyond the orbital rim, which helps to provide an extensive vertical and horizontal (almost 360-degree) range of vision, but can also make the eyes more susceptible to injury and trauma.

Lagomorph eyes have a large corneal surface (occupying 30% of the globe), a spherical pupil and a heavily pigmented brown iris. The blood supply to the fundus at the posterior of the eye is quite unique when compared to other mammals. The fundus is merangiotic: it has blood vessels extending horizontally, along with myelinated nerve fibres, from the optic disc. This adaptation allows the presence of a 'visual streak', a long,

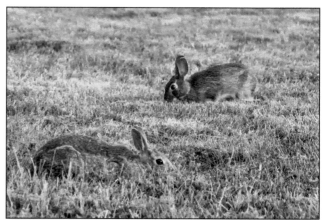

16.7 Two rabbits grazing together. When lagomorphs live in groups or congregate to graze, this provides the extra advantage of multiple fields of vision to detect predators.

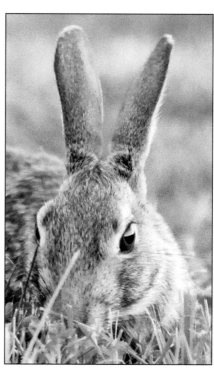

16.8 The lateral position of the eyes in rabbits and hares allows an extensive range of vision, with the horizontal visual streak promoting predator detection.

horizontal area with a very high density of photoreceptors located parallel to the retinal vessels (Williams, 2012). It is supplied completely through the choroidal vessel network. The horizontal positioning allows all points on the horizon to be monitored, therefore promoting predator detection. The predominant photoreceptors are rods, facilitating good low light vision. The intraocular pressure of a domestic rabbit is recorded at ranging from 5–23 mmHg.

The ears of both rabbits and hares are long, with a large surface area. Brown hares have the longest ears, with a black tip to the distal end. Lagomorph ears can move independently to one another to aid in pinpointing sound from different directions. The ears are well vascularized and are involved in thermoregulation.

Rabbits and hares have many scent glands: lacrimal, submandibular, Harderian, inguinal and anal. This scent is used to communicate between animals. 'Chinning' of a surface or object denotes territory and helps identify group members. Rabbits use scent-coated faecal pellets, creating latrines to mark the edges of territorial boundaries. Male rabbits may also spray urine scent on subordinate juveniles or as part of the courtship ritual with a female.

Reproduction
Rabbits
Female rabbits can reach full sexual maturity by 4 months of age, with bucks taking 1 to 2 months longer. It is therefore possible for offspring born at the beginning of the year to produce their own litters by the end of the breeding season, which can begin as early as February and continues through until September. Sexual behaviour is stimulated by lengthening photoperiod. Rabbits are induced ovulators and do not have a defined oestrous cycle. This very effective reproductive performance is one reason for rabbits' successful existence and widespread distribution in the British Isles.

The gestation period is short, at 30–32 days. Birthweights range from 40 to 100 g. Baby rabbits are known as kits (Figure 16.9a). A single female can produce between four and eight kits per litter and, in any one season, can produce up to five litters. Should a complication occur during pregnancy and the female aborts, foetuses are rarely expelled but instead are reabsorbed. Kits are born altricial (eyes closed and hairless) and are completely dependent on the nursing female for the first few weeks of life. Nursing females do not spend long periods of time tending to their offspring. In a 24-hour period, they can spend as little as 5 minutes with their young. This is likely due to the provision of high quality milk and a warm heat-retaining nest. A doe's milk has a high fat and protein composition and a low sugar content. Rabbits have four to five pairs of nipples and when the mother returns to the nest, there is a swarm of activity as the youngsters latch on to suck. As a prey species, returning to the nest infrequently greatly reduces the chance of highlighting the position to potential predators. If the mother is predated, kits will starve or freeze to death.

A doe plucks hair from her dewlap and ventrum to line the nest. When left unsupervised in the nest, kits are quiet and slowly rotate position with their littermates, each taking a turn in the warmest area in the centre. This constant movement allows heat to dissipate within the nest, keeping the litter warm. Due to the fur lining created by the mother, along with a large litter size, kits

can maintain a sufficient body temperature. For the first 7 days of life, they require a warm environmental temperature of 27–30°C.

Hares
Male hares generally reach full sexual maturity after only 6 months, with the females taking up to 8 months to fully develop. In the UK, the breeding season lasts from January to September and female hares can produce two to four litters per season. Research has shown that the breeding season is climate-dependent and in colder European countries, the breeding season may not begin until March. Equally, in populations of European hares introduced to the warmer climate of Australia, the breeding season can continue all year round.

The gestation period of hares is longer than that of the rabbit. In brown hares gestation can vary between 38 and 44 days, although 42 days is average. The average gestation period of the mountain hare is 50 days. A young hare is known as a leveret (Figure 16.9b). On average, brown hares produce four leverets per pregnancy, but numbers can vary from two to six. Mountain hares can produce as few as one to three young per litter. Young of all the hare species are precocious at birth, born fully furred, sighted and able to run within a few minutes of birth. Birthweights vary from 80 to 130 g.

Hares can also display superfoetation, whereby they have the ability to conceive and carry two concurrent pregnancies. This evolutionary adaptation allows maximum reproductive capacity to be reached within the breeding season. Studies have shown that, in brown hares, mating towards the end of pregnancy is able to induce a gonadotrophin surge and ovulation. Fertile matings are possible from day 34 of gestation with an increased frequency seen between day 38 and 40 (Caillol, 1991).

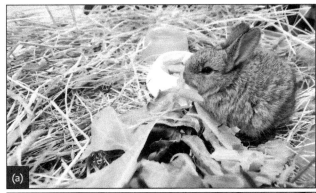
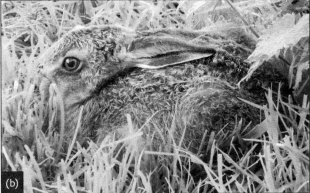

16.9 (a) Rabbit kit, approximately 2 weeks old. (b) Leveret in a 'form'.
(b, Courtesy of K Richardson)

Young leverets, like young rabbits, require feeding just once a day. The dam creates shallow depressions in the ground, known as forms, in which the young hares spend the day, lying low to avoid predators (see Figure 16.9b). A common misconception by members of the public is that these animals have been abandoned. As a result, healthy leverets may present for veterinary assessment under these circumstances. Public education is required to ensure such leverets are left alone, unless showing obvious signs of illness or injury or are at immediate risk of predation. The young congregate at dusk, when the mother returns to allow them to suck. Artificially rearing leverets adopts a similar approach to that described for rabbit kits.

Capture, handling and transportation

Capture and handling

Rabbits and hares consider humans as predators. It is therefore an extremely stressful event to be caught, handled and transported. Wild lagomorphs can panic to such an extent that spinal fractures can occur during a struggle. Acute stress when being handled has also been known to result in cardiac arrest. As lagomorphs have a thick coat, no sweat glands and an inability to open-mouth 'pant', overheating is also a concern if the transportation box is not suitably ventilated. Both rabbits and hares have extremely powerful back legs and can kick out and struggle in an attempt to avoid capture. It is unusual for a wild lagomorph to attempt to bite, but kicking and scratching can injure handlers. Care should therefore be taken to avoid injury to both handler and animal.

Capture should be planned in advance with all necessary tools and equipment readily available to significantly reduce the time spent interacting with the animal (see also Chapter 3). A long-handled net and towel are very useful for facilitating capture. The animal can initially be caught in the net before a towel is used to cover its head and restrain the body. If the animal is severely debilitated, a towel to aid capture will suffice.

Zoonoses

Wild lagomorphs have the potential to transmit a number of zoonotic conditions (Figure 16.10). As with all wildlife, strict hygiene should be maintained when handling, treating and emptying enclosures. Gloves should be worn and surfaces disinfected after contact with any animal (see also Chapter 7).

Transport

Once captured, the lagomorph can then be transferred into a solid box with non-slip floor and hay bedding. In order to help the patient to remain as calm as possible, it should be kept in darkness with minimum noise. Care should be taken to keep transportation times to a minimum. Rabbits and hares are at risk of hyperthermia when in transit, if the transport box is not well ventilated.

Potentially zoonotic infection	Transmission	Additional information
Brucellosis (*Brucella suis*, *B. bovis* or *B. melitensis*)	Direct contact with infected animals	• Hares appear more susceptible than rabbits
Encephalitozoon cuniculi	Oral ingestion of spores, most commonly shed in the urine of infected animals	• The condition is associated with domestic rabbits and is rare in wild lagomorphs • Immunocompromised humans at most risk of cross-infection
Escherichia coli	Oral ingestion following direct contact with infected animals, faeces or fomite	• A human outbreak was reported resulting from rabbits spreading *E. coli* O157 when grazing, travelling between a human picnic area and farmland housing cattle infected with *E. coli* (Scaife *et al.*, 2006)
Listeriosis (*Listeria monocytogenes*)	Direct contact, if agent is present in discharges from affected animals	• No confirmed links with human disease outbreaks and rabbits or hares
Leptospirosis (*Leptospira* spp.)	Infected urine	• No confirmed links with human disease outbreaks and rabbits or hares
Lyme disease (*Borrelia* spp.)	Tick (*Ixodes ricinus*) acting as a vector for the causal spirochaete	• Particular risk in areas with high tick burdens
Pseudotuberculosis (*Mycobacterium avium* subsp. *paratuberculosis*)	Infected faeces	• Zoonotic potential • Theories that rabbits may act as a vector in the transmission of bovine Johne's Disease (Greig *et al.*, 1999)
Salmonellosis (*Salmonella* spp.)	Infected faeces	• No confirmed links with human disease outbreaks and rabbits or hares
Toxoplasmosis (*Toxoplasma gondii*)	Infected cat faeces	• Toxoplasmosis due to *Toxoplasma gondii* infection is a rare condition seen in lagomorphs, resulting from contact with contaminated cat faeces • In experimentally infected individuals in captivity, clinical manifestations, including mortality, were much more pronounced in hares than in rabbits (Sedlák *et al.*, 2000) • Clinical signs can include central nervous signs (e.g. hindlimb paresis; haemorrhagic enteritis; enlarged mesenteric lymph nodes; pyrexia and death) • In brown hares and mountain hares it typically causes an acutely fatal disease
Tularaemia (*Francisella tularensis*)	Vector bite or by direct contact with an infected animal	• Zoonotic potential with a large reservoir for the disease in both wild and domestic animals.

16.10 Potentially zoonotic infections of rabbits and hares.

Examination and clinical assessment for rehabilitation

Restraint for examination

By following standard protocols, the risk of injury to both the handler and animal can be reduced. It is important to create the correct environment for examination of the compromised lagomorph. The room should be quiet and free from predator noises (e.g. barking dogs) and the light should be dimmed. In a compromised patient, examination is easier on the consulting room table. The table surface should be non-slip; if this is not the case, a towel can be placed on the table. If the patient is particularly lively, examination could occur at floor level. If the transportation box is top opening, the animal can stay in the box whilst a provisional examination is made. Movements around the patient should be calm, quiet and confident, with avoidance of sudden movements and loud noises.

The minimum restraint that is safely possible should be used to avoid stressing the rabbit or hare with excessive handling. Covering the eyes with a hand or a towel is often beneficial. At all times during lifting and carrying, the spine and hindlegs should be supported; having the patient wrapped in a towel is often safer and can prevent struggling. Although it is always important to be efficient when performing a lagomorph clinical examination, it is particularly important in the case of a wild animal. Once the examination is complete, the animal should immediately be placed back in the carry box or enclosure. Sometimes anaesthesia may be warranted to facilitate a more thorough clinical examination and reduce the negative effects seen with a panicking, struggling animal.

Clinical examination

A full standard clinical examination should be carried out, with consideration of all of the general factors required for a wild casualty animal to be suitable for rehabilitation and release (see Chapter 4).

Specific points of particular note in rabbits and hares include:

- Clinical signs associated with a respiratory tract infection, including discharge or crusting to the nares; as rabbits and hares are obligate nasal breathers, care should be taken when examining the nasal area to prevent accidently occluding the nostrils
- As dental disease is not a commonly encountered condition in wild lagomorphs, dental examination is not viewed with the same importance as it is in domestic rabbits
- The position of the eyes (see Figure 16.8) means that ocular injuries are not uncommon and may prevent release of the patient. The eyelids should be free of erythema and swelling; swelling of the eyelids and genital region can be indicative of myxomatosis, which would be grounds for euthanasia
- A pregnant uterus is palpable after the first trimester of gestation. Uterine neoplasia is not commonly seen in wild lagomorphs, unlike in domestic animals
- Unless debilitated, most wild lagomorphs will tense their abdomen when palpated; for thorough evaluation, the abdomen (see Figure 16.6) should be gently palpated with the animal sedated or anaesthetized. Small intestinal distension with ingesta or gas may be palpated together with any lesions or impactions.

Caecal impaction or gas accumulation can be readily palpated and are abnormal findings
- The skin and coat should be inspected, especially around the perineum and inguinal region as myiasis can affect this area in debilitated individuals.

Blood sampling

Blood collection techniques, volumes and sample types are described in Chapter 5. In conscious lagomorphs, blood can be taken from the marginal ear vein with minimal restraint. The use of EMLA® cream or similar is advised to desensitize the skin prior to venepuncture. In sedated or moribund individuals the lateral saphenous, cephalic or jugular vein are all viable options. The stress experienced by the animal should be considered before attempting to obtain conscious samples. The maximum volume removed should not exceed 10% of circulating blood volume, which is approximately 60 ml/kg.

Reference intervals for haematology and biochemistry values for rabbits and hares are given in Figure 16.11.

Euthanasia

It is advisable to sedate or anaesthetize wild lagomorphs prior to euthanasia in order to minimize unnecessary stress. Anaesthetizing the animal with inhalation anaesthetic alone prior to pentobarbital injection is not advised (see 'Anaesthesia'); poorly anaesthetized animals are likely to panic, struggle and vocalize. Once sedated or anaesthetized, the preferred method of euthanasia is intravenous, intracardiac, intrarenal or intrahepatic pentobarbital injection (see also Chapter 4).

Variable (units)	Reference interval	
	European rabbit (Oryctolagus cuniculus)	Brown hare (Lepus europaeus)
Haematology		
Red blood cell (RBC) count (x 10^{12}/l)	4–7	8.58–11.42
Haemoglobin (g/dl)	10–15	18.37–23.25
Packed cell volume (PCV) (l/l)	0.33–0.48	0.54–0.66
Mean corpuscular volume (MCV) (fl)	60–75	53.20–66.85
Mean corpuscular haemoglobin (MCH) ((pg) per cell)	19–23	18.68–22.49
Mean corpuscular haemoglobin concentration (MCHC) (g/l)	300–350	308–376.5
Platelet count (x 10^9/l)	250–600	105–618
Reticuloctyes (% RBC)	2–4	NDA
White blood cell (WBC) count (x 10^9/l)	5–12	0.59–6.06
Segmented neutrophils (x 10^9/l)	NDA	0–2.56
(%)	30–50	NDA
Lymphocytes (x 10^9/l)	NDA	0–4.11
(%)	30–60	NDA
Monocytes (x 10^9/l)	NDA	0–0.51
(%)	2–10	NDA
Eosinophils (x 10^9/l)	NDA	0–0.19
(%)	0–5	NDA
Basophils (x 10^9/l)	NDA	0–0.27
(%)	0–8	NDA

16.11 Haematology reference intervals in rabbits and hares. NDA = no data available (continues) ▶

(Harcourt-Brown, 2002; Marco et al., 2003; Carpenter, 2013; Wesche, 2014)

Variable (units)	Reference interval	
	European rabbit (Oryctolagus cuniculus)	Brown hare (Lepus europaeus)
Biochemistry		
Calcium (total) (mmol/l)	3.2–3.7	NDA
Calcium (ionized) (mmol/l)	1.6–1.82	NDA
Inorganic phosphate (mmol/l)	1.28–1.92	NDA
Sodium (mmol/l)	138–150	NDA
Potassium (mmol/l)	3.2–7	NDA
Creatinine (μmol/l)	44.2–229	87.4–140.6
Urea (mmol/l)	6.14–8.38	11.3–21.1
Bile acids (μmol/l)	<40	NDA
Bilirubin (μmol/l)	3.4–8.5	0.35–1.71
Glucose* (mmol/l)	4.2–7.8	3.5–18.8
Cholesterol (mmol/l)	0.3–3	0.33–0.77
Trigylcerides (mmol/l)	1.4–1.76	NDA
Alkaline phosphatase (ALP) (IU/l)	10–70	6–115
Alanine aminotransferase (ALT) (IU/l)	25–65	NDA
Aspartate aminotransferase (AST) (IU/l)	10–98	14–165
Gamma-glutamyl transferase (GGT) (IU/l)	0–7	NDA
Amylase (IU/l)	200–500	NDA
Total protein (g/l)	54–75	38.3–66.7
Globulin (g/l)	15–27	3.1–28
Albumin (g/l)	27–50	26.2–45.8

16.11 (continued) Biochemistry reference intervals in rabbits and hares. *Stress can cause a marked increase in glucose levels. NDA = no data available

(Harcourt-Brown, 2002; Marco et al., 2003; Carpenter, 2013; Wesche, 2014)

First aid and short-term hospitalization

Basic principles of first aid include ensuring the lagomorph remains at an optimum body temperature (see Chapter 5), is hydrated, has suitable analgesia (see 'Anaesthesia and analgesia') and has been provided with gastrointestinal stimulants.

Kits and leverets that appear to have been abandoned are commonly presented to veterinary surgeons (veterinarians) for assessment and treatment. The two most common conditions associated with very young animals are hypothermia and hypoglycaemia, both of which must be corrected appropriately (see Chapters 5 and 8).

Fluid therapy

Information on fluid therapy, including that suitable for rabbits and hares, has been described in Chapter 5. The placement of an intravenous catheter in the marginal ear vein is illustrated and described in Figure 16.12.

The author's preferred sites for placement of an intraosseous catheter are the trochanteric fossa of the proximal femur (medial to the greater trochanter and parallel to the long axis of the femur) or the proximal tibia (Figure 16.13). The proximal tibia is technically an easier site for placement; however, the needle enters the joint capsule of the stifle, which could result in complications. It is also possible to use the proximal humerus. General anaesthesia or sedation is required in animals that are not unconscious as the procedure is painful. Premedication with an opiate analgesic should be provided. A 1.5 inch (4 cm) spinal needle, intraosseous needle or 18–22 G 1 inch (2.5 cm) hypodermic needle with sterile surgical wire utilized as a stylet may be used.

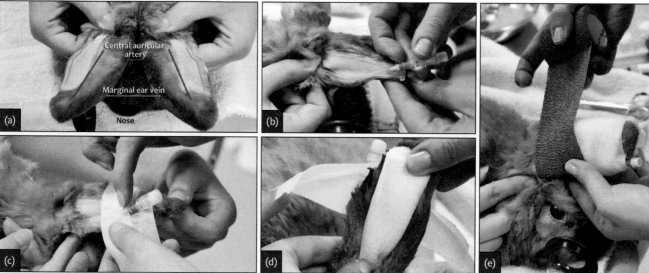

16.12 Intravenous catheterization using the marginal ear vein. Photographs of a domestic rabbit are used to illustrate this procedure. (a) The fur is clipped over the marginal ear veins of both ears and EMLA® cream applied and left for 15–20 minutes. Clipping both ears allows for a second attempt to be made at catheter placement should there be a complication with one vein. (b) The catheter is pre-flushed with heparinized saline to reduce the risk of blood clotting in it. The vein is raised by occluding the vessel at the base of the ear. The vein is very superficial and when the bevel of the catheter is through the skin, the angle of the catheter should be almost parallel to the ear. Once in the vein, the stylet and catheter are advanced approximately 0.3–0.5 cm before the catheter only is advanced further. Flashback of blood is not always seen due to the small vessel size. Holding a finger under the ear prevents the ear from bending whilst the catheter is advanced. (c) Once the catheter has been fully advanced into the vein, the stylet is removed and a bung fastened to the catheter. Tape is used to secure the catheter. (d) A rolled-up swab can be placed in the external ear canal to support the catheter and maintain the natural shape of the ear. The catheter is flushed to double-check correct positioning and patency. The fluid can often be seen running through the vessels of the ear or can be palpated entering the vessel at the level of the catheter. (e) If required, further bandaging material can then be added, but this is often less well tolerated in wild lagomorphs compared to domestic species.

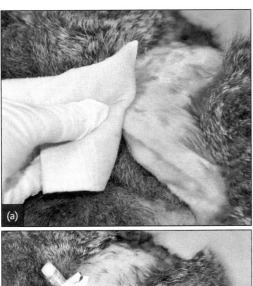
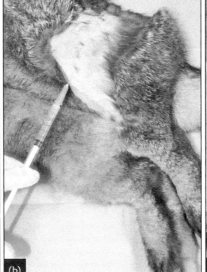
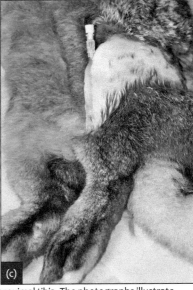

16.13 Intraosseous catheterization of the proximal tibia. The photographs illustrate intraosseous placement in the proximal tibia on a cadaver of a wild rabbit. (a) The site is clipped and surgically prepared. The procedure should be performed under sterile conditions. In a live rabbit, a sterile drape should be used. (b) Lidocaine 2% is infiltrated into the skin, muscle and the periosteum. A small incision can be made in the skin with a scalpel over the site of needle placement if needed. One hand should stabilize the target bone while the dominant hand inserts the needle along the long axis of the bone. Steady downward pressure is required, with a sudden release of pressure followed by a lack of resistance once the medullary cavity has been penetrated. The stylet is removed and the catheter flushed with heparinized saline. There should be no resistance to flushing and no swelling of surrounding soft tissues if the catheter is correctly placed. (c) A T-port or catheter bung should be attached and (d) butterfly tape can be applied to the hub and taped or sutured to the surrounding skin to secure the catheter.

Where there is doubt as to catheter placement, a radiograph can be taken to confirm positioning. Fluids or medication should be administered by a slow continuous infusion rather than a rapid bolus. The catheter should be flushed three times daily and after medication to prevent blockage.

Gastrointestinal stimulants

Capture and hospitalization are stressful events that can lead to gastrointestinal stasis in lagomorphs. Therefore, any hospitalized patient should receive gastrointestinal stimulants. Medications include ranitidine, metoclopramide and/or cisapride. The author's preferred first-line gastrointestinal stimulant is oral or injectable ranitidine, with oral cisapride added as required. Dose rates and administration routes and frequencies are described in Figure 16.24.

Short-term hospitalization

If wild lagomorphs need to be hospitalized they should be housed in a quiet dimly lit and escape-proof cage that is away from predator species. A cover can be placed over the enclosure to add further privacy and reduce visual stimulation. Newspaper lining, hay bedding and cardboard hide boxes should be provided (Figure 16.14). Grass, garden weeds and leafy greens should be scattered in one corner of the enclosure and water provided in a bowl.

Segregation and appropriate barrier nursing should be employed as necessary. This is especially important in wild lagomorphs where infectious diseases are confirmed or suspected (see 'Infectious diseases').

16.14 A typical hospital cage set-up for an injured lagomorph including the provision of a disposable hide box.

Anaesthesia and analgesia

The anaesthetic and analgesic doses and combinations used in domestic rabbits can be extrapolated and used in wild lagomorphs (Figures 16.15 and 16.16). Being prey animals, lagomorphs do not show overt signs of pain. It is crucial, therefore, to provide adequate analgesia if discomfort is at all suspected and not rely on the clinical signs shown by the patient.

It is not acceptable to anaesthetize a wild patient with inhalation anaesthetic agents alone as the animal is highly likely to panic and struggle. Breath-holding is also commonly seen and this greatly increases the risk of

Drug	Dosage	Drug type or indication	Comments
Acepromazine	0.1–0.5 mg/kg i.m., s.c.	Sedation	Does not provide analgesia
Alfaxalone	1–4 mg/kg i.v. 5 mg/kg i.m.	Induction agent	Give slowly to effect if using intravenous route, as can cause apnoea when administered too rapidly
Adrenaline	20 µg/kg i.v. or intratracheal	Cardiac arrest	0.1 ml/kg of 1 in 10,000 solution
Atipamezole	1 mg/kg i.v., i.m., s.c.	Reversal agent	Reverses medetomidine and dexmedetomidine
Buprenorphine	0.01–0.05 mg/kg i.v., i.m., s.c. q6–8h	Analgesic	Often used in combination for premedication
Bupivicaine 0.125%	1 mg/kg	Local anaesthetic	Slow onset of effect, duration of action 2–6 hours Can be used synergistically with lidocaine
Butorphanol	0.1–0.5 mg/kg i.v., i.m., s.c. q2–4h	Analgesic	Often used in combination for premedication
Carprofen	2–4 mg/kg i.v., i.m., s.c., orally q24h	Analgesic	Care using non-steroidal anti-inflammatory drugs (NSAIDs) in dehydrated patients
Dexmedetomidine	0.01–0.05 mg/kg i.v., i.m., s.c.	Sedation, anaesthesia	Some analgesic effects
Diazepam	1–2 mg/kg i.v., i.m.	Sedation	Anxiolytic and anticonvulsant
Fentanyl	0.005 mg/kg i.v.	Analgesic	May depress respiration and result in apnoea
Ketamine	10–20 mg/kg i.v., i.m., s.c.	Sedation, anaesthesia	Used in anaesthetic combinations
Ketoprofen	1–3 mg/kg i.v., i.m., s.c., orally	Analgesic	Care using NSAIDs in dehydrated patients
Lidocaine 2%	1 mg/kg	Local anaesthetic	Rapid onset of effect, duration of action 2–3 hours Can be used synergistically with bupivicaine
Medetomidine	0.1–0.3 mg/kg i.m., s.c.	Sedation, anaesthesia	Used in anaesthetic combinations Some analgesic effects
Midazolam	0.5–2 mg/kg i.v., i.m., s.c.	Premedication, tranquillizer	Give slowly i.v.
Meloxicam	0.2–0.6 mg/kg s.c., orally q12h	Analgesic	Care using NSAIDs in dehydrated patients
Morphine	2–5 mg/kg i.m., s.c. q2–4h	Analgesic	Potent analgesic therefore useful for example in orthopaedic-related pain
Propofol	2–3 mg/kg i.v.	Induction agent	Slow administration to reduce the risk of apnoea
Tramadol	11 mg/kg orally q24h	Analgesic	Available as an oral preparation, or can be made into an oral solution using soluble capsules

16.15 Anaesthetic and analgesic agents and their dose rates for use in rabbits and hares.
(Carpenter, 2013; Eatwell, 2014)

Suggested anaesthetic protocols	Drug	Dosage	Route	Comments
Combination 1	Dexmedetomidine (D) or medetomidine (M)	0.01–0.05 mg/kg (D) or 0.1–0.5 mg/kg (M)	i.m. or s.c.	Triple combinations are not recommended for sick or compromised patients Atipamezole (1 mg/kg) should be given to reverse the dexmedetomidine/medetomidine and hasten recovery The author commonly uses the lower to mid-range for the drug doses stated To reduce injections required, ketamine and dexmedetomidine/medetomidine can be mixed and administered in one syringe
	Ketamine	5–15 mg/kg		
	Buprenorphine (Bup) or butorphanol (But)	0.03–0.05 mg/kg (Bup) or 0.1–0.5 mg/kg (But)	s.c	
Combination 2	Buprenorphine	0.03 – 0.05 mg/kg	i.m. or s.c.	Onset of sedation can take 10–15 minutes
	Midazolam	1–2 mg/kg		

16.16 Anaesthetic drug combinations and their dose rates for use in rabbits and hares.
(Ivey, 2000; Orr, 2005; Marsh, 2009; Carpenter, 2013; Eatwell, 2014)

anaesthetic-associated deaths. Induction with injectable agents is preferable and intramuscular or intravenous routes can be used. Intubation in wild lagomorphs is recommended using the same method as in domestic rabbits. Successful intubation can be achieved using either the blind technique or via direct visualization of the epiglottis with the aid of an otoscope, laryngoscope or endoscope. Alternatively, a laryngeal mask can be used. Anaesthesia can be maintained with gaseous isoflurane or sevoflurane. There are also combinations of injectable anaesthetic drugs that can be used in lagomorphs (see Figure 16.16).

Specific conditions

Wild rabbits and hares can require veterinary treatment for a number of conditions; the most common presentations include predation with associated trauma, infectious conditions and 'orphaned' youngsters.

Trauma

A great variety of causes can lead to a traumatic injury in the wild lagomorph. These include gunshot wounds, traps, farm machinery, road traffic accidents, hare coursing and predation. Common injuries include fractured limbs (Figure 16.17) and soft tissue wounds. Any open wound is at risk of infection and myiasis (see 'Parasites'). Injuries involving the head can result in neurological clinical signs, jaw fracture and ocular damage, including corneal injury (Figure 16.18). Damage to the cornea can lead to impaired vision, with reduced ability to detect predators and find forage.

Whether to treat injuries in rabbits and hares is determined by the severity of the problem. The aim is for the patient to realize a full recovery without a prolonged treatment period so that it can be released back into the wild. If this is not possible the animal should be euthanased or permanent captivity carefully considered (see Chapter 4).

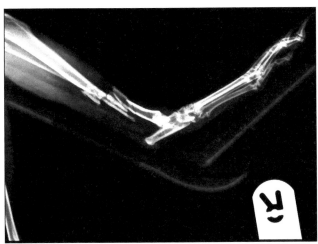

16.17 Lateral radiograph illustrating a comminuted fracture of the distal tibia and fibula (with a temporary supportive splinted bandage placed). This rabbit was euthanased based on radiographic findings.

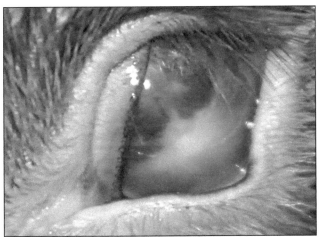

16.18 Corneal ulceration. This rabbit had an old healing ulcer with penetration of the corneal surface and purulent material visible in the anterior chamber. This animal would be unlikely to be suitable for rehabilitation and release.

Surgical considerations

There are some rabbit-specific surgical factors that must be considered if the decision is made to treat an injured animal.

Orthopaedic procedures are comparable to those in domestic rabbits, with the appreciation that rabbit bones are often small and brittle. During abdominal surgery, handling of the gastrointestinal system should be minimal to reduce the risk of adhesions and gastrointestinal stasis developing postoperatively. Catgut suture material should be avoided due to the increased risk of tissue reaction and postoperative adhesions developing. The author's preferred suture materials include poliglecaprone for ligating blood vessels and closing both subcutaneous and intradermal tissue layers, and polydioxanone for muscle layer closure. Lagomorphs are generally efficient at removing skin staples and sutures, therefore it is important to close the skin with a continuous intradermal technique. An Aberdeen knot can be used to bury the final knot.

Infectious diseases
Viral diseases
Myxomatosis:
Background: This fatal viral condition affects both wild and domestic rabbits. First introduced into Britain in 1953, myxomatosis is caused by a double-stranded DNA poxvirus. Other leporid genera, *Sylvilagus* and *Lepus*, encompass species with variable susceptibilities to myxomatosis virus, but these do not commonly develop the lethal form of the disease (Lemos de Matos *et al.*, 2014). The virus is naturally occurring in South America in wild 'jungle' rabbits (*Sylvilagus brasiliensis*). In these animals there are no systemic signs, but instead a cutaneous presentation is seen in the form of benign local fibroma. A recently confirmed case in a European brown hare in the UK demonstrated proliferative raised lesions around both ears. In this animal's case, the myxoma lesions appeared to be in a recovery phase and death was thought to have resulted from a secondary cutaneous *Staphylococcus aureus* infection causing systemic toxaemia or septicaemia (Barlow *et al.*, 2014). In the European rabbit, clinical signs are more severe and humans have utilized this fact over the past 70 years, using the virus as a method of biological control of wild rabbit populations.

Transmission: The rabbit flea *Spilopsyllus cuniculi* is the main vector of the myxomatosis virus in the UK, although sucking lice (Anoplura), fur mites (*Cheyletiella* spp.) and biting flies (e.g. midges) may also act as vectors. In warmer countries, the mosquitoes (Culicidae) are the main arthropod vectors. In the UK, the lifecycle of the insect plays a direct role in the prevalence of the disease and fleas are very effective reservoirs of the virus. They can overwinter on rabbits, allowing infection to resurface each year. The flea and doe lifecycle are synchronized, such that young susceptible kits can be exposed to heavy flea infestations. Rabbit-to-rabbit transmission of the disease is also possible with close contact.

Clinical signs: Clinical signs vary according to virulence of the pox strain and immune status of the rabbit population. In general, diseased animals follow a standard disease progression:

Day 1:	Exposure to infection
Day 4:	Blepharoconjunctivitis and thickening of the ears
Day 6:	Anogenital swelling: painful lesions can develop on the eyelids, ears, nares, lips, external genitalia and anus (Figure 16.19)
Day 8:	Mucopurulent nasal discharge
Day 10:	Secondary infections, e.g. pneumonia
Day 11–20:	Death

Death can occur more rapidly in young or diseased animals or where the strain of virus is highly virulent (Figure 16.19). Some individuals also appear to have a genetic resistance to infection, although most are susceptible.

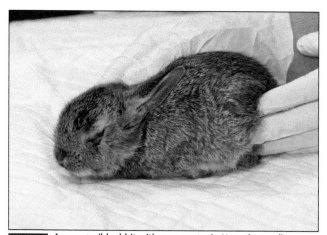

16.19 A young wild rabbit with myxomatosis. Note the swollen eyelids and subdued demeanour. Infected wild rabbits pose a serious risk to unvaccinated domestic pet rabbits.

Prognosis and treatment: Prognosis is very poor for affected individuals. Treatment with supportive care and systemic antibiosis for secondary infections is often unrewarding and euthanasia, on welfare grounds, is advisable.

Control and prevention: A new vaccine (Nobivac® Myxo-RHD) was launched in 2012 for domestic rabbits in the UK. The vaccine is composed of a rabbit haemorrhagic disease (RHD) capsid protein that has been inserted into the myxoma virus genome. This combination vaccine provides 12 months of immunity against myxomatosis and RHD. It is injected subcutaneously and can be given to rabbits as young as 5 weeks old. The decision to vaccinate adult rabbits prior to release should be based upon local risk factors and costs. Vaccination of hand-reared rabbits is carried out by most rescue centres, providing 1 year of immunity and therefore increasing the chance of survival immediately post-release.

In the face of an outbreak in a rehabilitation centre, vaccination is indicated in those animals not showing clinical signs of the disease. It should be remembered, however, that it takes 3 weeks for full immunity to be reached post-vaccination.

Vector control can also be promoted with the application of flea prevention (e.g. topical imidacloprid; see Figure 16.24) to rabbits. Biting flies can be discouraged by removing any areas of lying water which may attract them. Fly sheets and fly screens can also be installed.

Rabbit haemorrhagic disease:

Background: RHD (previously viral haemorrhagic disease), is a rapidly fatal disease caused by a host-specific calicivirus. The disease is endemic in wild rabbit populations in the UK, and can also affect domestic rabbits. The true number of losses in wild rabbits as result of the disease is unknown. It is thought many infected rabbits die underground in burrows, therefore the deaths go largely undetected by humans.

Recently a new genotype (RHDV2) has been identified in wild and pet rabbits in the UK causing fatalities (Westcott and Choudhury, 2014). This variant was found to be the predominant genotype in wild rabbit populations in France (Boucher *et al.*, 2015).

Wild hares can act as a reservoir host, carrying the virus without developing any clinical signs, further promoting spread of this highly infectious disease.

The virus is stable and resilient within the environment, remaining viable for 22–35 days at 22°C, and 3–7 days at a higher temperature of 37°C. It can also survive being frozen. The virus does not appear to affect rabbits under 4 weeks of age. When exposed, juveniles develop lifelong immunity, protecting them in future outbreaks. Adults are less fortunate, with mortality rates as high as 90–100%.

Transmission: Spread can occur via insect vectors (e.g. fleas, lice, flies and mosquitoes), as well as by direct contact between rabbits or with contaminated carcasses and fomites. The virus is excreted in urine and faeces and spreads via oral, nasal and parenteral transmission.

Infection is thought to have been introduced from mainland Europe to the UK via the movement of wild birds (Varga, 2014).

Clinical signs: The incubation period is 3–4 days. The disease causes a necrotizing hepatitis, with the virus replicating in the cytoplasm of hepatocytes. Disseminated intravascular coagulation (DIC) develops, producing numerous thrombi which can affect the heart, lungs and kidneys.

Death results either from hepatic failure or DIC. There are two presentations:

- Peracute – the rabbit is found dead
- Acute – the rabbit is found moribund; quiet, pale, pyrexic and tachypnoeic. Haematuria, haemorrhagic vaginal discharges or foamy exudate from the nostrils may be visible. Opisthotonus may be present in the agonal stage.

Prognosis and treatment: The prognosis is poor in adult rabbits. Treatment is ineffective and not advised in wild rabbits, those with clinical signs should be euthanased.

Control and prevention: There are three vaccines available in the UK against RHD (Cylap®; Lapinject VHD®; Nobivac® Myxo-RHD). All provide 12 months of immunity, with the Nobivac® combined vaccine providing 12 months of immunity against both myxomatosis and RHD (see 'Myxomatosis').

Cylap® and Lapinject VHD® can be administered from 10 weeks of age, and both are inactivated adjuvanted virus vaccines. All vaccinations are injected subcutaneously. Vaccines to protect against RHDV2 are available from other European countries and may be obtained using a Special Import Certificate (SIC).

Due to the highly infectious nature of the disease, strict hygiene should be adhered to, with protective clothing and gloves changed between handling animals. Enclosures used to house infected individuals should be thoroughly disinfected between patients. It should be remembered that infected grazing areas can also spread disease.

European Brown Hare Syndrome: European Brown Hare Syndrome (EBHS) was first recorded in Britain in the 1970s. Initially the aetiology was unknown and toxin ingestion was suspected. In 1989, researchers proposed a viral cause and this was confirmed in 1992 when a calicivirus was identified (Simpson, 2000). From historical frozen samples, it is now confirmed that the disease was present in hares in 1982. There is also some evidence of virus in suspected cases dating from 1976 (Duff *et al.*, 1994).

The virus is similar to, but distinct from, the calicivirus that causes RHD and EBHS does not appear to affect rabbits. Periodic die-offs of brown hares are attributed to EBHS. Affected animals suffer a severe and rapid hepatopathy and, due to the speed of disease progression, dead animals are often found in good body condition. Currently there is no treatment.

Bacterial diseases

Pasteurellosis: *Pasteurella multocida* is a Gram-negative bacterium found as a commensal in the respiratory tract of most rabbits. Respiratory infection with *Pasteurella* is uncommon as a primary disease in wild rabbits. If the animal is immunocompromised, however, the bacteria can multiply leading to secondary infection. It is common for rabbits with myxomatosis to have secondary *Pasteurella* infection. The physiological and immunological defences of the respiratory system cannot cope with the bacterial overgrowth and an upper respiratory tract infection can rapidly spread to cause a tracheitis, pneumonia, dacryocystitis, conjunctivitis or otitis media. Other bacterial overgrowths often develop and prompt antibiotic therapy (e.g. with enrofloxacin) is required for treatment.

Treponematosis: *Treponema cuniculi* is a highly contagious Gram-negative spirochaete bacterium that affects hares and, occasionally, wild rabbits. In common with other treponema infections, the disease is often referred to as 'syphilis'. The bacteria are long and slender with a characteristic spiral shape. They are propelled forward in a corkscrew-like motion by means of three flagella at either end.

Infection is spread by two routes:

- Venereal: the condition is seen in both sexes and is transmitted at coitus. Lesions around the genital area of one animal will spread disease to the breeding partner and infected males can readily spread disease to many females
- Direct contact: infection from the genital region is spread to the face due to direct contact when the lagomorph grooms itself. Offspring can also develop lesions if passing through an infected birth canal. Infected animals can spread disease to other group members when mutual grooming occurs, and vertical transmission is also possible.

Following exposure to infection there is a variable incubation period averaging 3 to 6 weeks before clinical signs appear. Infected animals develop painful crusty lesions around the nares, eyes, lips and genitals (Figure 16.20).

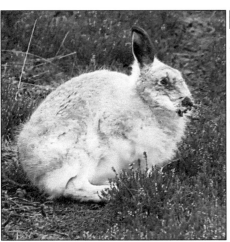

16.20 Mountain hare with clinical signs of *Treponema cuniculi* infection including crusting lesions around the eyes and mouth. (© Elizabeth Mullineaux)

Treponema has been recognized in brown hares in Europe for some years; however, it was not until 1992 that it was confirmed in brown and mountain hares in the UK (Figure 16.20). Histological examination of hares with 'orf-like' lesions revealed treponema-like spirochaetes in one brown and two mountain hares (Munro *et al*. 1995). The disease can be particularly serious in hares, increasing their risk of predation and the development of secondary amyloidosis.

Treatment, if appropriate, is by administration of procaine penicillin G, 42,000–84,000 IU/kg s.c., once weekly for 3 weeks.

Parasites

Ectoparasites:

Fleas: Rabbit fleas (*Spilopsyllus cuniculi*) often congregate around the head in rabbits and are particularly obvious around the edges of the pinnae. Flea infestations are irritating for the animal, with signs of pruritis including head-shaking and scratching. Diagnosis is made by the detection of flea dirt on the coat and by the presence of adult fleas, which are visible to the naked eye. Importantly, fleas can act as vectors for a number of fatal diseases including myxomatosis and RHD. Particularly in a veterinary practice or rehabilitation centre, treatment is warranted to prevent spread to other animals. Topical imidacloprid or selamectin are suitable treatments (see Figure 16.24).

Ticks: In some areas, tick infestations (*Ixodes ricinus*) (Figure 16.21) are a common problem, particularly in mountain hares who share grazing land with upland sheep. The rabbit tick is *Haemaphysalis leporispalustris*. Ticks attach mostly on the head and neck area and in large numbers can cause anaemia.

Lice: The sucking louse *Haemodipsus ventricosus* (Figure 16.22a) affects both rabbits and hares. It feeds on blood and can also act as a vector in the spread of a number of diseases including myxomatosis, RHD and tularaemia. They are visible with the naked eye at 1.5–2.5 mm in length and eggs can be visualized attached to individual hair fibres. Treatment is with imidacloprid or ivermectin (see Figure 16.24).

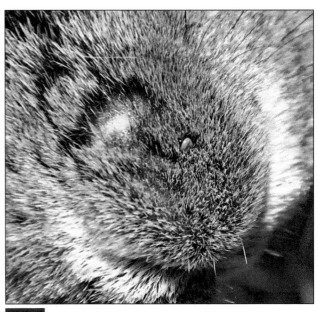

16.21 Tick (*Ixodes ricinus*) attached to the nose of a rabbit.

Mites: A variety of mites can be seen in wild lagomorphs (Figure 16.22). They are usually present in small numbers unless the animal is immunocompromised. It is unusual to see clinical signs associated with mite infestations.

Trombicula autumnalis, also known as the harvest mite, can often be found incidentally on wild lagomorphs during the summer and autumn months. They are often seen around the eyelids and ears as visible orange specks.

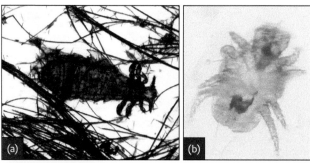
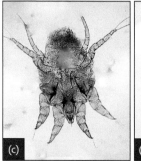
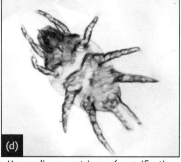

16.22 (a) The sucking louse, *Haemodipsus ventricosus* (magnification X40). (b) *Cheyletiella parasitovorax* (magnification X40). The body of the mite can be up to 0.4 mm in length. The legs are short and stubby and there are normally six long hairs present on the body. These create dandruff from disruption to the skin surface. (c) *Leporacarus gibbus* (magnification X40), previously known as *Listrophorus gibbus*, are fur mites. They are visible with the naked eye and have short legs, with a single rostral projection extending from the head over the mouthparts. (d) *Psoroptes cuniculi* (magnification X40). This oval shaped non-burrowing mite can have a body length of 0.75 mm. The legs have funnel-shaped suckers on the distal portion.

Myiasis: Myiasis (flystrike) can be seen in the warmer late spring and summer months. In wild lagomorphs this usually occurs secondary to another issue. Bluebottles (*Calliphora* spp.) and greenbottles (*Lucilia* spp.) are attracted to faecal contamination around the perineum or to open wounds. They then lay eggs, which hatch into L1 maggot larvae. The young maggots moult to L2 and L3 stages, during which they feed from the flesh of the infected lagomorph, causing invasive and painful tissue damage. Presenting animals should be treated promptly, or euthanased if the degree of damage is too great. Treatment should begin by clipping the fur around the affected area. Visible maggots and eggs should be removed from the wound and the area flushed with dilute antiseptic solution or saline. Insecticidal treatment can be administered to prevent any further larval development (e.g. ivermectin or cyromazine, see Figure 16.24). Supportive therapy should be given, including fluid therapy, analgesics and, where indicated, broad-spectrum antibiotics.

Endoparasites: The rabbit is the intermediate host for a number of tapeworms (e.g. *Echinococcus granulosus*, *Taenia pisiformis* and *Taenia serialis*) of which the dog or cat is the final host. Occasionally heavy burdens of

T. pisiformis can cause abdominal distension and discomfort in rabbits. Primary host cestodes are more common in hares, but are also seen in rabbits. *Oribatid* mites are the intermediate host, to allow completion of the parasite's lifecycle. It is believed that heavy infestations can cause clinical illness (Marcato and Rosmini, 1986).

Helminth parasites can be seen in different parts of the gastrointestinal system, including *Graphidium strigosum* in the stomach, *Trichostrongylus* spp. in the small intestine and the ascarid *Passalurus ambiguus* in the large bowel (Figure 16.23) (Allan *et al.*, 1999). In healthy individuals these are an incidental finding.

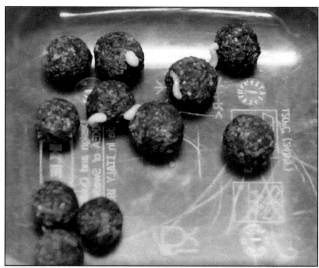

16.23 Pinworms (*Passalurus ambiguus*) clearly visible in faeces from an infested rabbit.

Protozoal parasites: Although *Encephalitozoon cuniculi* is a common disease seen in domestic rabbits, wild lagomorphs are rarely affected by this microsporidian parasite.

As with all mammals, infection with the protozoan *Toxoplasma gondii* is possible. This is particularly noteworthy as it is a zoonotic condition. Lagomorphs become infected by grazing on land contaminated with infected cat faeces. Clinical signs range from asymptomatic to neurological signs of hind limb paresis, pyrexia and death.

Coccidiosis: There are up to 14 *Eimeria* spp. that affect rabbits and hares. All except one (*E. steidae*), are found within the gastrointestinal tract, causing intestinal coccidiosis.

E. steidae is found in the epithelial cells of the bile ducts resulting in hepatic coccidiosis. The distended bile ducts, particularly on the gastric surface of the liver, resemble those seen in chronic liver fluke infection in ruminants. In chronic cases of hepatic coccidiosis, inspissated purulent material accumulates in the bile ducts. This condition causes high levels of mortality and is particularly common in young animals in rehabilitation centres, where emaciation and poor growth rates can be seen.

In young hares, infection with *E. leporis* is common. At times of hardship, either from sustained unfavourable weather, food shortages or concurrent disease, hares can become affected by clinical coccidiosis. In the UK, intestinal coccidiosis is the most common cause of mortality in young hares. Diagnosis is confirmed by the presence of oocysts in the faeces and post-mortem findings of lesions within the small intestines. Adult hares seem to have some immunity to the effects of coccidia. Treatment is using oral toltrazuril (Varga, 2014) or trimethoprim/sulfamethoxazole (see Figure 16.24).

In rehabilitation centres, burdens of oocysts can persist in the environment for many years. They are resistant to disinfectant, but do not survive in dry conditions. A blowtorch can be used to flame enclosures and kill oocysts. Strict hygiene should be adhered to when handling animals.

Miscellaneous conditions

Amyloidosis

This condition is seen in hares and occurs secondary to a chronic disease process, such as treponematosis. Whilst the inciting disease may not lead to death, the complication of amyloid deposition, particularly in the kidneys and liver, can lead to fatal renal or hepatic failure. Diagnosis is made at post-mortem examination.

Dental disease

Dental disease is very uncommon in wild lagomorph species, as their natural high-fibre diet helps wear down the elodont teeth. Cheek teeth erupt at approximately 3 mm per month, with incisors growing at 3 mm per week. Any misaligned teeth can rapidly lead to overgrowths with subsequent oral trauma and the potential for abscess formation within the oral cavity and sinuses. Dental disease can also occasionally occur in wild rabbits associated with trauma (particularly involving the incisors). In the majority of cases of dental disease, affected animals should be euthanased on welfare grounds.

Leporine dysautonomia

In the UK, leporine dysautonomia is the second most common cause of death in hares. There are many similarities between this condition and equine grass sickness. It was during fieldwork investigations of the equine disease that the condition in hares was incidentally found. The causal agent is still unknown.

Presenting signs include approachability, depression, muscle wasting, lethargy, large bowel impaction, gastric distension, inability to swallow, aspiration pneumonia and bladder distension. On post-mortem examination of hares, the autonomic ganglia lesions were indistinguishable from those seen in horses with grass sickness (Hahn, 2001).

If an animal is found alive, euthanasia should be carried out, to alleviate suffering.

Therapeutics

Therapeutic doses for domestic rabbits can be extrapolated for use in wild rabbits and hares (Figure 16.24).

Antibiotic-associated diarrhoea

Type and route of antibiotic administration are important to reduce the likelihood of drug-induced diarrhoea. Clindamycin, lincomycin and oral penicillins are all highly contraindicated and should not be administered in lagomorphs. Penicillin can be administered parenterally, whilst enrofloxacin, trimethoprim and tetracyclines can be given orally, with good safety margins.

Corticosteroids and non-steroidal anti-inflammatory drugs

Steroids are contraindicated in lagomorphs due to their immunosuppressive properties, which can lead to progression of latent infections resulting in clinical disease. Non-steroidal anti-inflammatory drugs (NSAIDs) provide anti-inflammatory and analgesic effects with good safety margins, although care should be taken in dehydrated individuals or where renal disease is suspected (see Figure 16.15).

Drug	Dosage/Application	Comments
Antibacterials		
Doxycycline	4 mg/kg orally q24h	Bacteriostatic agent Penetrates well in bronchial secretions
Enrofloxacin	5–10 mg/kg s.c., orally q12–24h	Antibiotic licensed for domestic rabbits Useful in pasteurellosis treatment Subcutaneous injections often associated with tissue necrosis
Fusidic acid (Isathal®)	Topically to eyes q12–24h	Licensed for domestic rabbits
Gentamicin (Tiacil®)	Topical eye ointment, 1–2 drops q8h for up to 7 days	Licensed for domestic rabbits for treatment of blepharitis, conjunctivitis, keratoconjunctivitis and anterior uveitis
Marbofloxacin	2 mg/kg i.v. q24h 5 mg/kg orally q24h	Broad-spectrum bactericidal antibiotic Particularly useful for soft tissue, urogenital and skin infections
Metronidazole	20 mg/kg orally q12h 40 mg/kg orally q24h	Antibacterial and antiprotozoal activity
Penicillin G (Procaine)	42,000–84,000 IU/kg s.c. q48h (Author's preferred dose 40–60 mg/kg s.c. q48h)	*Treponema cuniculi* treatment requires one injection weekly, for 3 weeks
Silver sulfadiazine cream (Silvadene®)	Topical q24h	Useful for supportive care of flystrike lesions
Trimethoprim/sulfamethoxazole	30 mg/kg orally q12h	Available as a paediatric suspension Antibacterial and anticoccidial

16.24 Drug formulary for rabbits and hares. Dosages are based on those used for domestic rabbits. NB Fipronil products are contraindicated in lagomorphs as they can cause neurological disease and death. (continues) ▶
(Carpenter 2013; NOAH, 2014)

Drug	Dosage/Application	Comments
Antiparasitic agents		
Cyromazine (Rearguard®)	Apply topically	Not effective on maggots, but does stop the development of blow-fly larvae
Fenbendazole (Lapizole®, Panacur®)	20 mg/kg orally q24h for 5–9 days	Treats endoparasites, including *Encephalitozoon cuniculi*
Imidacloprid (Advantage®)	10–16 mg/kg topically at base of neck. Can be repeated after 2 weeks	Designed for the treatment of fleas Licensed for use in domestic rabbits
Imidacloprid (I) 10% and moxidectin (M) 1% (Advocate®)	10 mg/kg (I) and 1 mg/kg (M) topically at base of neck once every 4 weeks, repeated three times (unlicensed in rabbits)	Fleas, lice and *Psoroptes cuniculi* treatment
Ivermectin (Xeno®, Panomec®)	0.1–0.2 mg/kg s.c. repeated every 14 days	Mites, fleas, lice and endoparasites
Permethrin (Xenex Ultra®)	See manufacturer's dose chart; see also Figure 13.13	For the prevention and control of infestations caused by flies (adult and immature stages), lice and surface mites NB Toxic to cats
Praziquantel (Droncit®)	5–10 mg/kg s.c., orally repeated every 10 days	Treats nematodes and cestodes
Selamectin	12 mg/kg topically at base of neck once	Used in treatment for fleas, ticks, lice and fur mites
Toltrazuril (Baycox®)	2.5–5 mg/kg orally, can be put in drinking water also. 2 day course repeatable after 5 days	Intestinal coccidiosis treatment
Prokinetics		
Cisapride	0.5 mg/kg orally q8–12h	Acts to promote gastrointestinal motility, with action on the large bowel
Domperidone	0.5 mg/kg orally q12h	Similar mode of action to metoclopramide
Metoclopramide	0.2–0.5 mg/kg s.c., orally q8–12h	Prokinetic, gastric protectant and anti-emetic effects.
Ranitidine	2 mg/kg i.v. q24h 4 mg/kg orally q12h	Author's preferred gastrointestinal stimulant
Miscellaneous		
Barium	10–14 ml/kg orally, one-off dose	Used for gastrointestinal contrast studies
Cholestyramine (Questran® Light)	2 g/animal/day orally	Toxin binder, useful in treatment of enterotoxaemia
Furosemide	1–3 mg/kg i.v., s.c., orally q8–12h	Loop diuretic
Miconazole (Mycozole®)	2 mg/kg applied topically q12h for up to 7 days	Anti-fungal

16.24 (continued) Drug formulary for rabbits and hares. Dosages are based on those used for domestic rabbits. NB Fipronil products are contraindicated in lagomorphs as they can cause neurological disease and death.
(Carpenter 2013; NOAH, 2014)

Management in captivity

Housing

For long-term management, a quiet, secluded and secure outdoor pen is required (Figure 16.25). The enclosure should be predator and weatherproof. As lagomorphs are skilled at digging and chewing, the enclosure should be designed with this in mind to prevent escape. Hide boxes and bolt-holes should be provided, as well as items to chew (e.g. fruit tree branches). Wild lagomorphs are likely to be very fearful of humans, and may injure themselves trying to evade capture; interactions with captive lagomorphs should be avoided.

Feeding

It is important to maintain a high-fibre diet with the provision of grass, good quality hay, herbs, weeds such as dandelion and plantain, and a small amount of fresh vegetable greens (e.g. spring greens, kale and cabbage). A small volume of commercial rabbit complete pellets can also be given.

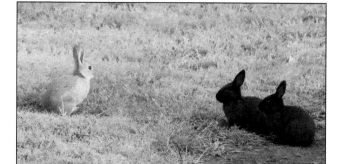

16.25 Orphaned litter of hybrid wild rabbits in a large outdoor enclosure. Individuals with a dark coat colour are more susceptible to predation and should not be released.

Rearing of kits and leverets

Kits and leverets can be hand-reared, but the mortality rate is often high, particularly associated with the time of weaning.

Feeding

The most common problems encountered when raising abandoned young include:

- Aspiration of milk at feeding time
- Development of fatal enterotoxaemia, bloat and diarrhoea.

Milk replacers are a nutritional compromise in comparison to lagomorph milk, therefore orphaned kits and leverets will require more frequent feedings than in the wild. Often up to six feeds are required daily in newborn animals, decreasing to two to three feeds as they get older. As a general rule, 10% of bodyweight should be fed in total every day (Figure 16.26). Commercial milk replacers for puppies and kittens can be used (e.g. Cimicat™ or Esbilac®). A suggested formulation for feeding rabbit kits is: 1 scoop Top Life Formula® Goats Milk for Puppies with 3 scoops of fresh goats milk. Young should be weighed twice daily using accurate scales. The frequency of feeding can be altered in accordance with weight gains observed.

Age and approx. bodyweight	Approximate volume of milk replacer (ml/feed)				Comments
	Kits	No. of feeds	Leverets	No. of feeds	
Newborn; 40 g	1–2	6	2–5	6	Unweaned
3 days; 50g	5–8	6	8–10	6	Unweaned
7 days; 80 g	12–14	4	15–20	4	Unweaned
10 days; 100 g	15–18	4	20–25	4	Offer solids (hay, parsley, grass)
14 days; 125 g	18–22	4	25–30	4	Junior rabbit pellets, dandelion and wild rocket
21 days; 160 g	23–28	4	30–40	4	Weaned by 28 days

16.26 Feeding volumes for kits and leverets. The actual amounts taken per feed will vary between individual animals.

Aspiration can occur if the rabbit is sucking incorrectly, or if fluids are fed too quickly by tube or syringe. When performed correctly, tube feeding is a reliable way to ensure youngsters obtain the correct volume of feed. It is also the most time efficient way of feeding a large litter. To prevent aspiration, care should be taken to ensure that the tube is correctly placed in the oesophagus and the milk should be administered slowly to prevent retrograde flow of liquid up the oesophagus.

The stomach and small intestines of suckling lagomorphs have very few microorganisms present. When fed an artificial milk substitute, the young are more susceptible to enteric bacterial infections, which can rapidly lead to the development of a fatal diarrhoea. Milk substitutes lack the protective substance 'milk oil', an antimicrobial fatty acid found as a natural component in the mother's milk. It is produced by an enzymatic reaction and provides protection against microbial overgrowths in the suckling animal's stomach (Mitchell and Tully, 2009). All feeding equipment should be thoroughly cleaned and sterilized between uses. Ideally, milk substitute solutions should be freshly reconstituted immediately before use. If storage is required until a later feed, the mixture should be refrigerated and kept for no longer than 24 hours; it must be warmed to body temperature before administration.

To stimulate urination and defecation, the perineal area should be wiped with a damp cloth to mimic the grooming behaviour of the mother. This can be done after feeding, before returning the youngster to the nest. Handling should be kept to a minimum.

Weaning

Young rabbits rely on a milk diet up until 10–15 days of age, at which point they will start supplementing their intake with small volumes of solid food. Weaning generally takes place at around 3–4 weeks of age. Leverets should be fully weaned after only 3 weeks of age. Good quality hay and grass should be offered. Where possible, caecotrophs from healthy lagomorphs can be fed to young to help populate the hindgut with healthy bacteria and protozoa. Transfaunation can occur through voluntary eating of caecotrophs or via syringe feeding of liquefied caecotrophs.

Weaning is a particularly high risk period for the development of gastrointestinal disease.

Instability in the caecal flora can lead to an imbalance of microbial activity after weaning (Gidenne et al., 2002). This can lead to non-specific enteropathies (i.e. without an identified pathogenic agent), giving rise to clinical signs such as bloat and diarrhoea. When pathogenic bacteria multiply, enterotoxaemia can develop. Involved pathogens can include Escherichia coli, Clostridium spiroforme, C. piliforme, Salmonella Typhimurium and S. Enteritidis.

Treatment is often unrewarding, but can include fluid therapy, analgesia, probiotics, transfaunation, nutritional support, antibiotics and toxin binders such as cholestyramine (see Figure 16.24), which helps prevent toxins reaching the systemic circulation. In many cases of enterotoxaemia, death occurs rapidly and euthanasia on welfare grounds may be necessary.

Prevention is better than cure in all cases and the importance of high-fibre diets cannot be overemphasized. Probiotic therapy (e.g. Bio-Lapis, Fibreplex™, Protexin® Pro-fibre or Vetark® Pro-C Probiotic) can be used around weaning time. Handling of animals should be kept to a minimum around this period to reduce any effects of stress on gastrointestinal motility. Strict hygiene is also crucial for limiting spread of pathogens between animals.

Housing

A suitable environment should be provided using blankets or towels as nesting material. The conditions should be warm, dry and clean. Heat pads, incubators or even an airing cupboard can all be used to keep young at a suitable body temperature (see also Chapter 8).

Release

Adults

Rabbits released in areas with low vegetation cover show higher mortality and dispersal distances than rabbits released in high cover areas (Letty et al., 2003). If an adult can be returned to the wild within a short timeframe, they can be released near to their original warren. If a prolonged amount of time has lapsed, a new environment should be selected that is rich in ground cover and vegetation.

Hares have a much larger home range. Again, if the original territory is known the animal can be released in this area. It should be remembered that hares prefer arable land and selection of a new release site would aim to be low in natural predators and provide enough food and ground shelter to sustain the hare.

Juvenile animals

If young animals are intended for release back into the wild, handling and other interactions should be kept to a minimum to avoid malprinting. The author recommends that any young rabbit being released back into the wild should be vaccinated to provide 1 year of immunity against myxomatosis and RHD.

Release sites for hand-reared juvenile animals should be carefully considered. In rabbits, release near to an already inhabited warren is not recommended. Rabbits are territorial and the newcomer is unlikely to be accepted into a pre-existing hierarchical system, with fighting likely to occur. Instead, release at a neutral site with good food supply and cover from predation is recommended.

With leverets, if a healthy youngster is brought in by a member of the public, it should be immediately returned to the location where it was found. For those kept in captivity for longer, a site with low predator numbers and a suitable habitat should be chosen.

Soft-release for juveniles is only possible if appropriate facilities are available at rehabilitation centres. The use of large escape-proof outdoor enclosures provides a safe environment for youngsters whilst allowing them to habituate to a more natural habitat, prior to full release.

Legal aspects

Rabbits are considered pests under the Pests Act 1954 due to the fact they can cause damage to crops on farmland. There is limited protective legislation and it is legal to kill them by lawful methods at any time of year.

Hares also have limited legal protection, with no closed season, and can be killed or taken by lawful means at any time of year. However, the Hare Preservation Act 1892 gives some protection by preventing the sale of adults or leverets during the main breeding season – between 1 March and 31 July.

The most commonly used method of wild lagomorph control is shooting. Although snares are also used, the use of self-locking snares is illegal. The Hunting Act 2004 (and Protection of Wild Mammals (Scotland) Act 2002) also banned hare coursing, making this activity illegal and therefore a prosecutable offence.

For further legal aspects relating to wild lagomorphs, see Chapter 2.

References and further reading

Allan JC, Craig PS, Sherington J et al. (1999) Helminth parasites of the wild rabbit Oryctolagus cuniculus near Malham Tarn, Yorskshire, UK. Journal of Helminthology 73, 289–294

Antoniou A, Kotoulas G, Magoulas A and Célio Alves P (2008) Evidence of autumn reproduction in female European hares (Lepus europaeus) from Southern Europe. European Journal of Wildlife Research 54(4), 581–587

Barlow A, Lawrence K, Everest D et al. (2014) Confirmation of myxomatosis in a European brown hare in Great Britain. Veterinary Record 175(3), 75–76

Beard PM, Daniels JM, Henderson D et al. (2001) Paratuberculosis infection of non-ruminant wildlife in Scotland. Journal of Clinical Microbiology 39(4), 1517–1521

Benson KG and Paul-Murphy J (1999) Clinical pathology of the domestic rabbit, acquisition and interpretation of samples. Veterinary Clinics of North America: Exotic Animal Practice 2(3), 539–551

Boag B, Lello J, Fenton A, Tompkins DM and Hudson PJ (2001) Patterns of parasite aggregation in the wild European rabbit (Oryctolagus cuniculus). International Journal for Parasitology 31(13), 1421–1428

Broderson JR and Gluckenstein FP (1994) Zoonotic and occupational health considerations. In: The Biology of the Laboratory Rabbit, 2nd edn. ed. PJ Manning et al. pp. 356–366. Academic Press, San Diego

Broekhuizen S and Maaskamp F (1981) Annual production of young in European hares (Lepus europaeus) in the Netherlands. Journal of Zoology 193, 499–516

Caillol M, Mondain-Monval M and Rossano B (1991) Gonadotrophins and sex steroids during pregnancy and natural superfoetation in captive brown hares (Lepus europaeus). Journal of Reproduction and Fertility 92, 299–306

Carpenter JW (2013) Exotic Animal Formulary, pp. 517–555. Elsevier Saunders, Philadelphia

Champan JA and Flux JEC (1991) Rabbits, Hares and Pikas – Status Survey and Conservation Action Plan. pp. 1–6. IUCN/SSC Lagomorph Specialist Group

Chasey D and Duff P (1990) European brown hare syndrome and associated virus particles in the UK. Veterinary Record 126, 623–624

Chasey D, Lucas M, Westcott D and Williams M (1992) European brown hare syndrome in the UK; a calicivirus related to but distinct from that of haemorrhagic disease of rabbits. Archives of Virology 124, 363–370

Daniels JD, Lees JD, Hutchings MR and Greig A (2003) The ranging behaviour and habitat use of rabbits on farmland and their potential role in the epidemiology of paratuberculosis. Veterinary Journal 165, 248–257

De Schaepdrijver L, Simoens P, Lauwers H and De Geest JP (1989) Retinal vascular patterns in domestic animals. Research in Veterinary Science 47, 34–42

Duff JP, Chasey D, Munro R and Wooldridge M (1994) European brown hare syndrome in England. Veterinary Record 134, 669–673

Eatwell K (2014) Analgesia, sedation and anaesthesia. In: BSAVA Manual of Rabbit Medicine, ed. A Meredith and B Lord, pp.138–159. BSAVA Publications, Gloucester

Fenner F and Fantini B (1999) Biological Control of Vertebrate Pests – The History of Myxomatosis – an Experiment in Evolution. CABI publishing, Oxford

Gidenne T, Jehl N, Segura B and Michalet-Doreau B (2002) Microbial activity in the caecum of the rabbit around weaning: impact of a dietary fibre deficiency and of intake level. Animal Feed Science and Technology 99(1–4,30), 107–118

Glass RL, Troolin HA and Jenness R (1967) Comparative biochemical studies of milks. IV. Constituent fatty acids of milk fats. Comparative Biochemistry and Physiology 22(2), 415–425

Graham JE (2014) Lagomorpha (Pikas, Rabbits and Hares). In: Zoo and Wild Animal Medicine, 8th edn, ed. ME Fowler and RE Miller, pp. 374–385. Elsevier Saunders, Philadelphia

Greig A, Stevenson K, Henderson D et al. (1999) Epidemiological study of paratuberculosis in wild rabbits in Scotland. Journal of Clinical Microbiology 37(6), 1746–1751

Greig A, Stevenson K, Perez V, Pirie A, Grant J and Sharp J (1997) Paratuberculosis in wild rabbits (Oryctolagus cuniculus). Veterinary Record 140, 141–143

Gustafsson K, Uggla A, Svensson T and Sjoland L (1988). Detection of Toxoplasma gondii in liver tissue sections from brown hare (Lepus europaeus) and mountain hare (L. timidus) using peroxidase anti-peroxidase (PAP) technique as a complement to conventional histo-pathology. Journal of Veterinary Medicine B35, 394–409

Hahn C, Mayhew IG and Whitwell KE (2001) Central nervous system pathology in cases of leporine dysautonomia. Veterinary Record. 149; 745–746

Harcourt-Brown FM (2002) Textbook of Rabbit Medicine and Surgery. Butterworth-Heinemann, Oxford

Harcourt-Brown FM and Chitty J (2014) BSAVA Manual of Rabbit Surgery, Dentistry and Imaging. BSAVA Publications, Gloucester

Ivey ES and Morrisey JK (2000) Therapeutics for rabbits. Veterinary Clinics of North America: Exotic Animal Practice 3,183–220

Judge J, Kyriazakis I, Greig A, Davidson RS and Hutchings MR (2006) Routes of intraspecies transmission of Mycobacterium avium subsp. paratuberculosis in rabbits (Oryctolagus cuniculus): a field study. Applied and Environmental Microbiology 72(1), 398–403

Le Gall-Reculé, Le Pendu J, Lemaitre E et al. (2015) Le nouveau virus de la maladie hémorragique virale du lapin (VHD): situation du RHDV2 en Europe et étude de la sensibilité des lapins à ce virus. 16èmes. Journées de le Recherche Cunicole, 21–22 Novembre 2015, Le Mans

Lemos de Matos A, McFadden G and Esteves PJ (2014) Evolution of viral sensing RIG-I-like receptor genes in Leporidae genera Oryctolagus, Sylvilagus, and Lepus. Immungenetics 66(1), 43–52

Letty J, Aubineau J, Marchandeau S and Clobert J (2003) Effect of translocation on survival in wild rabbit (Oryctolagus cuniculus). Mammalian Biology – Zeitschrift für Säugetierkunde 68(4), 250–255

Marcato PS and Rosmini R (1986) In: Pathology of the Rabbit and Hare. Societa Editrice Esculapio

Marco I, Cuenca R, Pastor J, Velarde R and Lavin S (2003) Haematology and serum chemistry values of the European brown hare. Veterinary Clinical Pathology 32(4), 195–198

Marsh MK, McLeod SR, Hansen A and Maloney SK (2009) Induction of anaesthesia in wild rabbits using a new alfaxalone formulation. Veterinary Record 164, 122–123

Meredith A and Lord B (2014) BSAVA Manual of Rabbit Medicine. BSAVA Publications, Gloucester

McBride A (1988) Rabbits and Hares. Whippet Books, London

Mitchell MA and Tully TN (2009) Manual of Exotic Pet Practice. Saunders Elsevier, Philadelphia

Motha MX and Kittelberger R (1998) Evaluation of three tests for the detection of rabbit haemorrhagic disease virus in wild rabbits. Veterinary Record 143(23), 627–629

Munro R, Wood A and Martin S (1995) Treponemal infection in wild hares. *Veterinary Record* **136**, 78–79

Natural England (2012) *Wild mammals: Management and Control Options*. www.gov.uk/wild-mammals-management-and-control-options

Orr HE, Roughan JV and Flecknell PA (2005) Assessment of ketamine and medetomidine anaesthesia in the domestic rabbit. *Veterinary Anaesthesia and Analgesia* **32**, 271–279

Paci G, Bagliacca M and Lavazza A (2006) Stress evaluation in hares (*Lepus europaeus Pallas*) captured for translocation. *Italian Journal of Animal Science* **5**, 175–181

Pehrson A and Lindlof B (1984) Impact of winter nutrition on reproduction in captive Mountain hares (*Lepus timidus*) (*Mammalia: Lagomorpha*). *Journal of Zoology* **204(2)**, 201–209

Quesenberry KE and Carpenter JW (2004) *Ferrets, Rabbits and Rodents: Clinical Medicine and Surgery, 2nd edn*. WB Saunders, St Louis

Ramsey I (2014) *BSAVA Small Animal Formulary, 8th edn*. BSAVA Publications, Gloucester

Rao SJ, Iason GR, Hulbert IAR, Daniels MJ and Racey PA (2003) Tree browsing by mountain hares (*Lepus timidus*) in young Scots pine (*Pinus sylvestris*) and birch (*Betula pendula*) woodland. *Forest Ecology and Management* **176(1–3)**, 459–471

Saunders R and Rees Davies R (2005) *Notes on Rabbit Internal Medicine*. Blackwell Publishing Limited, Oxford

Scaife HR, Cowan D, Finney J, Kinghorn-Perry SF and Crook B (2006) Wild rabbits (*Oryctolagus cuniculis*) as potential carriers of verocytotoxin-producing *Escherichia coli*. *Veterinary Record* **159**, 175–178

Sedlák K, Literák I, Faldyna M, Toman M and Benák J (2000) Fatal toxoplasmosis in brown hares (*Lepus europaeus*): possible reasons of their high susceptibility to the infection. *Veterinary Parasitology* **93(1)**, 13–28

Simpson VR (2000) Veterinary Advances in the Investigation of Wildlife Diseases in Britain. *Research in Veterinary Science* **69**, 11–16

Simpson VR (2002) Wild animals as reservoirs of infectious diseases in the UK. *The Veterinary Journal* **163**, 128–146

Small M (1994) *Wildlife Welfare (Mammals)*, pp. 13–14, 28–29. Intervet

Spibey N, McCabe VJ, Greenwood NM *et al.* (2012) Novel bivalent vectored vaccine for control of myxomatosis and rabbit haemorrhagic disease. *Veterinary Record* **170(12)**, 309

Stott P (2008) Comparisons of digestive function between the European hare (*Lepus europaeus*) and the European rabbit (*Oryctolagus cuniculus*): Mastication, gut passage, and digestibility. *Mammalian Biology – Zeitschrift für Säugetierkunde* **73(4)**, 27–286

Varga M (2014) *Textbook of Rabbit Medicine, 2nd edn*, pp. 88–90. Butterworth-Heinemann, Oxford

Walter N (2012) *Rabbit Myxomatosis: Where to Now?* Australasian Committee Association of Avian Veterinarians and Unusual and Exotic Pet Veterinarians (AVAC-UEP) Conference Proceedings

Wesche P (2014) Clinical pathology. In: *BSAVA Manual of Rabbit Medicine*, ed. A Meredith and B Lord, pp. 124–137. BSAVA Publications, Gloucester

Westcott DG and Choudhury B (2014) Rabbit haemorrhagic disease virus 2-like variant in Great Britain. *Veterinary Record* **176**, 74

Williams DL (2012) The Rabbit Eye. In: *Ophthalmology of Exotic Pets*, pp.15–52. Wiley-Blackwell, Chichester

Specialist organizations and useful contacts

See also Appendix 1

Hare Preservation Trust
www.hare-preservation-trust.co.uk

Rabbit Welfare Association and Fund
www.rabbitwelfare.co.uk

Chapter 17

Badgers

Elizabeth Mullineaux

The Eurasian badger (*Meles meles*) (Figure 17.1) is the largest of Britain's Mustelidae species. Eurasian badgers occur across the Palaearctic region in all states of Europe west of the border with the former Soviet Union, but are absent from arctic zones, high-altitude areas and some islands. In Great Britain and Ireland they are absent only in regions of altitudes over 500 m and most offshore islands. Population densities are greatest in the south-west of England, Wales and the east of Ireland, with estimates of over 1.2 animals per km². In some areas in the south of England populations have been estimated to be as high as 38 adults per km² (Macdonald and Newman, 2002).

The most common reasons for badgers requiring veterinary attention are road traffic accidents, injuries from baiting, snaring or poisoning, and intraspecific bite wounds (conspecific wounding). Orphaned badger cubs are commonly presented in some areas and require veterinary involvement in their rehabilitation. Local badger groups, usually branches of the Badger Trust, are available nationally to assist with the rehabilitation and release of casualties.

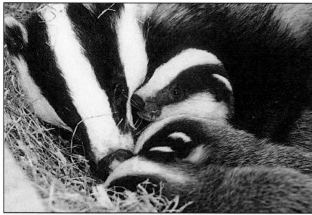

17.1 Badger and cubs.
(© Secret World Wildlife Rescue)

Ecology and biology

Setts and social groups

Badgers live in setts: networks of connecting underground tunnels and chambers with areas up to 1575 m². Setts typically have between three and ten large entrances, which can be differentiated from those of foxes (*Vulpes*

vulpes) or rabbits (*Oryctolagus cuniculus*) by their larger, more oval-shaped openings (30–60 cm across) and heaps of soil and discarded bedding material outside. No two setts are alike, their structure and size depending on the soil type, presence of tree roots and availability of food and bedding. As a general rule, badgers prefer well drained soil in deciduous and mixed woodland and copses where there is adequate food and bedding and an absence of human disturbance; they will, however, adapt to a variety of urban areas. Sett chambers are lined with bedding, which prevents heat loss, particularly for cubs. Bedding consists of hay, coarse grass, straw or other vegetation that the badger can carry to the sett bundled between its chest and front legs. Unsuitable bedding material such as plastic and baler-twine can result in entanglement of adults and deaths of cubs.

Each badger social group usually has one main sett within its territory, but may also have a variety of additional setts. There are well marked paths between the different sett areas, main feeding areas and latrines. Latrines are often on territory boundaries; underground latrines at the end of chambers and side tunnels are also seen. Territories vary from about 30 ha in high-density populations in optimal habitat to 300 ha in less ideal environments. Group and territory sizes are determined by the quality and distribution of food, respectively (Kruuk and Parish, 1982).

A typical social group consists of five animals, usually with a dominant male and a mixture of sexes and ages, but group size varies widely. Social groups of 2 to 35 animals and single-sex groups have been reported (Neal and Cheeseman, 1996). Communication between animals within social groups is mainly through scent marking, though vocalization and visual signs ('puffing up') are heard and seen, especially in cubs.

Population dynamics

In the wild it is unusual for badgers to reach more than 10 years of age, due to the high mortality rate in young animals. However, badgers of up to 15 years of age have been recorded in the wild and 19 years old in captivity (Neal and Cheeseman, 1996).

Starvation is thought to be a major cause of death in both cubs and adult badgers. Increases in group size are followed by increased mortality, reduced weight gain and reduced fertility within that group. Infectious disease is not thought to be a major factor in population dynamics (Cheeseman *et al.*, 1988; Rogers *et al.*, 1997).

Historically, the major cause of reduction in badger populations has been direct action by humans. In the 1960s and 1970s, digging, trapping, hunting and snaring kept badger numbers down. Legal protection from 1973 reduced these pursuits, though they still continue and can have a significant effect on numbers. Government operations to control tuberculosis in cattle by culling badgers can also have local and short-term effects. The greatest cause of identified badger deaths, even in tuberculosis-infected populations, is road accidents (Cheeseman *et al.*, 1988; Rogers *et al.*, 1997), which are estimated to number tens of thousands annually. It is thought unlikely that even these losses greatly influence overall population size (Neal and Cheeseman, 1996).

Activity

Badgers are crepuscular and nocturnal animals. Emergence from setts is usually at dusk in the spring and summer (May–August) and after dark at other times of the year. Urban badgers and those influenced by human activity tend always to emerge after dark. Activity is greatly reduced in the winter months (November–February), especially in northern areas of the UK. Food availability, environmental conditions and human activity affect the time of emergence. Cubs usually emerge before adults. Diurnal activity, usually related to foraging, is not uncommon during the summer.

Feeding

Badgers are opportunistic omnivores, eating a wide variety of plant and animal matter including earthworms (*Lumbricus terrestris*), fruit, insects, small mammals and birds. Earthworms are the single most important foodstuff in badger diets and provide a source of water, although badgers may also drink from other sources. The body-weight of badgers and weight gain during the summer and autumn is positively correlated to available permanent pasture and ley grassland (Delahay *et al.*, 2006). Badgers may take advantage of farm feeds made available in troughs and from open feed stores where they have a preference for cattle concentrates ('cake'). This feeding behaviour creates a possible risk of transmission of *Mycobacterium bovis* infection to cattle (see 'Tuberculosis').

When foraging, badgers usually amble along at a leisurely pace; they are, however, able to run fast, climb very well and swim if necessary.

Anatomy and physiology

Badgers are powerful mammals, well adapted for digging and life underground. They have short limbs with characteristics not dissimilar to those of chondrodystrophic breeds of dog. Hindlimbs and forelimbs are of a similar length, with five full digits with non-retractile claws that are often long, especially on the front feet. The back is relatively straight to support their weight and has less ability to arch than that of domestic carnivores. The skull has a prominent interparietal ridge that develops with age and is largest in adult male animals.

Dentition

The badger's skull supports well developed temporal muscles. Dentition reflects their omnivorous diet (temporary dentition in parentheses):

$$2 \times \left\{ I\ \frac{3\ (3)}{3\ (3)}\ C\ \frac{1\ (1)}{1\ (1)}\ P\ \frac{4\ (4)}{4\ (4)}\ M\ \frac{1\ (0)}{2\ (0)} \right\} = 38\ (32)$$

Incisors, canines and premolars are typical of a carnivore, whilst the last premolar and the molars are greatly modified for crushing and grinding, being broad and cusped like those of a herbivore. The first premolar is often vestigial or absent and supernumerary molars and premolars have also been described. Milk dentition erupts from the age of 4 to 6 weeks (canines, premolars, incisors – in that order) and permanent teeth from 10 to 16 weeks (incisors first) (Neal and Cheeseman, 1996). Tooth wear is a useful indicator of age in animals under 3 years old (see Figure 17.5).

Skin and coat

The skin is more mobile and tougher than that of dogs. There are long guard hairs and a dense undercoat. The melanin band in the guard hairs gives the badger a greyish look from a distance, apart from its distinctive black-and-white striped head. Melanistic, albino and erythristic pelage types are recognized (Figure 17.2), with intermediate varieties. There is no colour difference between the sexes. Badgers moult from the spring into the summer months, the undercoat shedding and regrowing first, followed by the guard hairs.

Size

Size and weight depend on age, sex, food availability and time of year. Population density has also been shown to have an influence on body condition and weight (Rogers *et al.*, 1997; Tuyttens *et al.*, 2000). Typical size and weight of adult male (boar) and female (sow) badgers is shown in Figure 17.3. Boars generally have broader heads than sows, but the sexes are virtually impossible to tell apart at any distance in the field. In a clinical environment boars are easily distinguished by their ventral prepuce, palpable os penis and visible scrotum (Figure 17.4a), whilst sows have a short anogenital distance (Figure 17.4b).

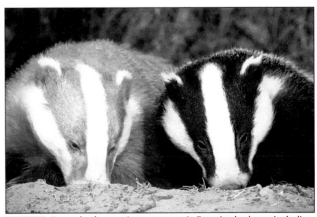

17.2 Several colour variants are seen in Eurasian badgers, including erythristic (left) and melanistic (right).
(© Secret World Wildlife Rescue)

Sex	Head and body length (mm)	Weight range (kg)
Male	686–803	9.1–16.7
Female	673–787	6.5–13.9

17.3 Body length and weight range for adult male and female badgers.
(Delahay *et al.*, 2008)

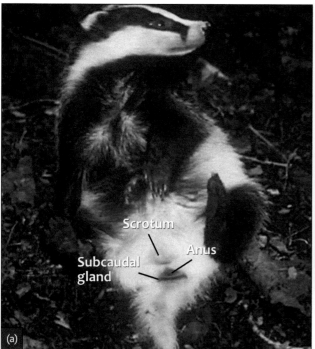

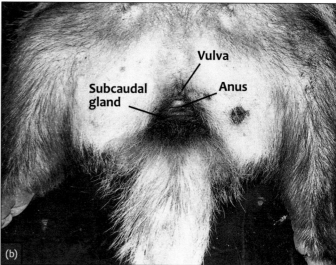

17.4 (a) Male badger showing position of subcaudal gland under the tail and dorsal to the anus. (b) Female badger showing short anogenital distance and subcaudal gland.
(a, Courtesy of C Seddon)

Normal physiological parameters

Body temperature is around 37°C (Bevanger and Brøseth, 1998) but can drop as low as 28°C in the winter months (Neal and Cheeseman, 1996). Resting heart and respiratory rates in individuals familiar with human contact appear to be not unlike those of domestic dogs of a similar size (heart rate 80–120 bpm, respiratory rate 10–30 bpm).

Special senses

The badger has a highly developed sense of smell, which is used in social communication. Scent is produced from several sources; subcaudal glands under the tail and above the anus (see Figure 17.4), anal glands similar to those of the dog, sweat and sebaceous glands and urine. Interdigital scent glands may also be present, though these have not been anatomically described in published literature.

Sense of hearing is good in badgers and the ears are protected by the small pinnae during digging. The eyes are adapted for night vision, with a predominance of retinal rods and a well developed tapetum; for this reason badgers are temporarily blinded by bright light. The eyes are not large for a nocturnal animal and cubs in particular are very short-sighted.

Reproduction

Male badgers become sexually mature at 12–15 months, whilst females usually ovulate for the first time in the spring of their second year, at 12–15 months old (Delahay *et al.*, 2008). Mating occurs year-round with a peak between February and March, when mature sows return to oestrus after cubbing and yearlings have their first oestrus. A second, smaller peak occurs during autumn in late-maturing animals and those sows that failed to conceive in the spring (Cresswell *et al.*, 1992). Implantation of embryos in the bicornuate uterus is usually delayed at the blastocyst stage following conception and does not take place until December. Implantation is affected by both photoperiod and body condition. True gestation lasts 6–7 weeks with the majority of cubs born in February (Neal and Cheeseman, 1996). Litter size is usually between one and five cubs although this may be reduced by the time the cubs are above ground. Deaths in cubs are thought to be due in part to infanticide by dominant sows. Growth rates are rapid between July and November, and cubs reach an average of 8 kg in the first year and 10 kg in the second (Figures 17.5 and 17.6).

Age of cub	Appearance	Eyes	Teeth	Size/weight	Notes
At birth (see Figure 17.6a)	Pink skin, sparse grey fur	Blind, eyes closed	No teeth	Body length 120 mm Tail length 30–40 mm Total length 150–160 mm 75–132 g	Below ground in sett
5 weeks (see Figure 17.6b)	Full black and white coat	Eyes open	Milk teeth erupt from 4–6 weeks	800 g	Below ground in sett
8 weeks	Full black and white coat	Eyes open	Milk teeth	1500 g	Seen above ground close to sett
12 weeks (see Figure 17.6c)	Full black and white coat	Eyes open	Permanent teeth erupt from 10–16 weeks	Approx. 3 kg	Weaning begins
15 weeks	Full black and white coat	Eyes open	Most permanent teeth erupted	Approx. 5 kg	Usually independent

17.5 Badger cub development.
(Neal and Cheeseman, 1996; Delahay *et al.*, 2008)

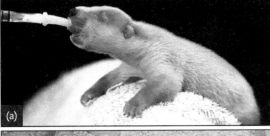
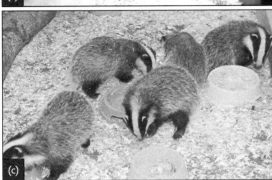
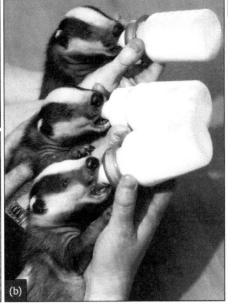

17.6 Badger cubs (a) syringe fed at around 1 week old, (b) bottle fed at around 5 weeks old, (c) weaned and within a newly formed social group at around 12 weeks old.
(© Secret World Wildlife Rescue)

Capture, handling and transportation

Badgers are powerful animals with a dangerous bite and should be treated with respect and suitable safety precautions taken at all times (see also Chapter 3). They should never be handled by untrained members of the public. If handled correctly, however, they are quite stoic and will rarely attack unless seriously provoked.

Capture and handling

In a field situation, a 'pig board' can be used to encourage injured badgers into a cage or other suitable container, such as a dustbin. Moribund animals can be gripped carefully, but firmly, by the scruff of the neck and a muzzle may be applied at this time (see 'Muzzles'). In less debilitated individuals, the scruff can be difficult to access and hold without danger to the handler and a more suitable option is to use a dog grasper. The hindquarters should be supported at all times if the animal is lifted by the scruff or with a grasper. Large heavy blankets (or a broom end) may assist with capture and handling and can be used to restrain the head once the animal is in a cage in order to allow injection of sedative drugs (see Figure 17.18). Heavy-duty gloves for handling tend to restrict grip and all but metal-enforced gauntlets offer little protection from bites. Disposable gloves (and ideally a facemask) should be worn to protect against zoonotic disease when handling badgers and cleaning up urine or faeces (see 'Tuberculosis' and Chapter 7).

Trapping cages

Trapping cages are available and organizations that frequently catch and transport badger casualties should use these or large crush cages. Cages should be of known weight, to allow easy calculation of bodyweight for sedation; they should also be free from blankets and bedding, to allow the crushing mechanism to work correctly. A blanket may be placed over the cage to darken it and reduce unnecessary stress.

Muzzles

Moribund animals must be treated carefully, as they can be unpredictable in their ability to move and bite, but may tolerate safe handling if muzzled. Baskerville™-type muzzles (Figure 17.7) are useful in allowing some normal jaw movement (e.g. in panting or vomiting); in their absence, a length of bandage material can be carefully tied around the muzzle and securely fastened.

Transportation

Badgers are best transported in metal trapping or crush cages, which should be covered with blankets to minimize noise and disturbance. Prolonged periods in inappropriate cages should be avoided, as nose and limb injuries may occur. Badgers should never be transported loose in cars or in insecure containers such as cardboard boxes, even if they appear comatose, as it is not uncommon for them to arouse whilst being transported, posing a significant risk to the handler.

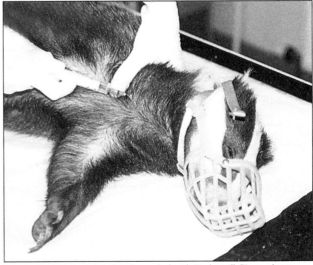

17.7 Badger sedated and muzzled with Baskerville™ muzzle to allow blood collection from the jugular vein.

Examination and clinical assessment for rehabilitation

History taking

A full history of the events leading to the presentation of a badger casualty, including its movement and behaviour during capture, should be obtained from the individuals involved. The exact location of where the animal was found must be recorded, since adult badgers must, as a general rule, be released back to the exact area where they were found (see 'Rehabilitation and release').

Restraint for examination

Whilst it may be necessary to administer immediate first aid to a casualty badger, care should be taken to ensure that this does not obscure the need for complete clinical assessment of the animal as soon as is practicable. Very young cubs and comatose or moribund adult animals will usually allow safe examination with minimal restraint, though a Baskerville™ muzzle (see Figure 17.7) is a useful precaution unless head injuries are severe. Most other casualties require some form of chemical restraint to facilitate a full clinical examination (see 'Anaesthesia and analgesia'); however, this may not be the most appropriate initial course of action until first aid has been provided (see 'First aid procedures').

Clinical examination

The clinical examination of a badger should, in principle, be no different from that for a dog or cat. Clinical examination gloves should always be worn and sensible hygiene precautions taken (see 'Tuberculosis'). Special attention should be paid to the animal's general condition (as evidence of chronic disease), mouth (tooth wear and jaw alignment), limbs and senses (especially vision). Full use should be made of available diagnostic facilities such as radiography, ultrasonography and laboratory tests (Figure 17.8). Due to the risk of tuberculosis, body cavities of badgers should not be drained or surgically entered until a reasonable assessment has been made, including auscultation, radiography or ultrasonography (see also 'Thoracic trauma').

Variable (units)	Reference interval
Haematology	
Red blood cell (RBC) count (x 10¹²/l)	6.93–12.99
Red cell distribution width (%)	19.11–24.14
Haemoglobin (g/dl)	10.73–19.12
Packed cell volume (PCV) (%)	30.09–53.23
Mean corpuscular volume (MCV) (fl)	38.05–45.71
Mean corpuscular haemoglobin (MCH) ((pg) per cell)	13.79–16.14
Mean corpuscular haemoglobin concentration (MCHC) (g/dl)	33.55–37.95
Platelet count (x 10⁹/l)	279.36–817.45
White blood cell (WBC) count (x 10⁹/l)	2.56–10.36
Neutrophils (x 10⁹/l) (%)	1.07–8.27 / 50.49–92.32
Lymphocytes (10⁹/l) (%)	0.09–2.66 / 2.96–41.04

17.8 Reference intervals for common blood parameters in captive badgers. (continues) ▶
(Courtesy of Dr S Lesellier, APHA)

Variable (units)	Reference interval
Haematology (continued)	
Monocytes (x 10⁹/l) (%)	0–0.63 / 0–9.66
Eosinophils (x 10⁹/l) (%)	0–0.33 / 0–5.11
Basophils (x 10⁹/l) (%)	0–0.15 / 0–2.23
Biochemistry	
Calcium (mmol/l)	2.01–2.54
Magnesium (mmol/l)	0.62–1.13
Creatinine (mmol/l)	68.39–121.12
Urea (mmol/l)	2.87–11.15
Bilirubin (µmol/l)	0.71–9.13
Cholesterol (mmol/l)	2.82–8.49
Alkaline phosphatase (ALP) (IU/l)	0–192.45
Alanine aminotransferase (ALT) (IU/l)	0–232.31
Gamma-glutamyl transferase (GGT) (IU/l)	1.02–4.32
Protein (g/l)	55.03–73.81
Globulin (g/l)	21.13–34.50
Albumin (g/l)	30.82–42.39
Cortisol (nmol/l)	0–264.20

17.8 (continued) Reference intervals for common blood parameters in captive badgers.
(Courtesy of Dr S Lesellier, APHA)

It should be remembered that sense organs (including vision) and the nervous system can only be assessed in the conscious animal and may require the assistance of someone with good knowledge of 'normal' badger behaviour or the use of remote monitoring devices.

Blood can easily be collected from the jugular vein of badgers (see Figure 17.7), or alternatively the cephalic or saphenous vein may be used. Reference intervals for healthy captive animals have been produced (Figure 17.8) and there are published values for wild populations (Winnacker *et al.*, 2008). Notably, urea levels in wild badgers are frequently elevated, related to their protein-rich diet containing earthworms.

Assessment for rehabilitation

The following questions should be asked before a treatment regime is decided (see also Chapter 4):

1. **Is the animal at the end of its natural lifespan?**
   - Old animals are easily identified by worn teeth, low bodyweight and poor body condition
   - Animals with chronic disease will be in poor body condition and may show specific signs of disease
   - Animals that have been displaced from setts because of age or disease may have 'territorial' bite wounds, often at several stages of healing.

   Animals should be euthanased where old age or chronic debilitating disease is suspected. It may be argued that removal of such animals may cause unnecessary disruption of social groups, but ethically it is difficult to justify the release of an animal that may shortly die and legally such release might be considered as 'abandonment'. ▶

2. **Would the healed injuries be expected to compromise the badger's life in the wild significantly?**
   This includes the ability to run, dig, feed, defend territory and reproduce.
3. **Are veterinary skills and finance available to treat the animal adequately?**
   If skills, time and finance are not available to treat the badger casualty to high standards, especially if orthopaedic surgery is required, the animal should either be referred quickly to a veterinary surgeon (veterinarian) with appropriate skills or be euthanased.
4. **Are suitable recovery and rehabilitation facilities available?**
   With the exception of a few minor casualties that can be released back to their site of capture within 24–48 hours, most casualties will need a period of recovery and suitable rehabilitation. Such a centre will have both the experience and facilities to deal with badgers. If a suitable centre is not available the casualty should be euthanased.
5. **Is a suitable release site available?**
   Adult badgers should be released at the exact spot where they were found. If this is not possible, euthanasia of these animals may be necessary (see 'Management in captivity and release'). Badger cubs need to be incorporated into release groups with other cubs and suitable new release sites found. This is a specialized process (see 'Rearing of badger cubs') and suitable facilities must be contacted as soon as the cub is admitted, to provide advice and ensure that rehabilitation facilities and release sites are available for that individual cub.

Euthanasia

Sedation or anaesthesia is usually required to examine badgers. Euthanasia, if indicated, is then most easily carried out using intravenous pentobarbital (150 mg/kg) into the cephalic, saphenous or jugular veins. If intravenous access is not possible, intracardiac or intraperitoneal injection may be used under general anaesthesia.

First aid and short-term hospitalization

First aid procedures

The principles of first aid treatment are broadly the same as in other species (see Chapter 5). Most of the injuries seen in badgers (road traffic accidents (RTA), bites, snares) require intravenous fluid therapy to treat dehydration and/or hypovolaemia. Intravenous access is easily achieved, usually via the cephalic vein, though saphenous and jugular veins are equally accessible. Fluid types and rates are as for domestic mammals and as described in Chapter 5. Mild sedation (diazepam, 0.25 mg/kg i.v. or i.m.) or the use of Baskerville™ muzzles prevents chewing of intravenous fluid administration lines, although most badgers requiring intravenous fluid therapy are indifferent to any intravenous line, as well as to dressings, bandages and splints.

Wounds should be dressed as necessary and limbs splinted as appropriate. Muzzles and Elizabethan collars may ensure that dressings remain in place in the short term, but are rarely tolerated for long.

Analgesics must be provided where indicated (see 'Anaesthesia and analgesia').

Warmth should be provided for all casualties. Badger cubs are most easily managed in incubators. Adults can be placed in heated kennels or under heat lamps, or provided with other forms of external heat, but pads and wires that can be chewed should be avoided for all except the most seriously ill or sedated individuals.

Short-term hospitalization
Accommodation

Kennels for short-term accommodation should be of stainless steel; badgers are able to bite and dig through other kennel materials and so escape would be possible. Suitable bedding material needs to be insulating and absorbent (e.g. shredded paper, straw, blankets) and should be used in amounts sufficient to allow the animal to bury itself. A large cardboard box on its side can also be used as a hide area.

Badgers are largely nocturnal and are disturbed by excessive light and by the noise and smell of other mammal species (e.g. dogs); they are also susceptible to disease from domestic animals. For these reasons they should be kept isolated where possible; cage doors should be covered and the animals should spend the minimum time necessary in a veterinary practice before being moved to a specially equipped facility. The long-term care of badgers in captivity requires specially constructed facilities, details of which are available from the Badger Trust or Secret World Wildlife Rescue (SWWR) (see 'Specialist organizations and useful contacts').

Feeding

The omnivorous nature of badgers means that they are able to eat a wide variety of foods. Suitable foods are given later (see 'Rearing of badger cubs' and Figure 17.20); in the short term, dog food (tinned or dried) can be offered. In reality many adult animals refuse to eat for several days in captivity, but go on to make uneventful recoveries. Fresh water should be provided in a heavy bowl.

Anaesthesia and analgesia

Figure 17.9 gives doses of commonly used anaesthetic and analgesic products in badgers.

Intramuscular combinations

General anaesthesia of badgers with ketamine alone has been used in field research. It is very safe, but produces poor muscle relaxation, making it unsuitable on its own for most veterinary procedures. The addition of acepromazine, an alpha-2 adrenoreceptor agonist or benzodiazepine improves the quality of surgical anaesthesia. The most common anaesthetic combinations now used for minor procedures in badgers by veterinary surgeons in practice and for sampling in research facilities are ketamine with medetomidine, or ketamine with medetomidine plus butorphanol (de Leeuw et al., 2004; McLaren et al., 2005; Figure 17.9).

Drug	Dosage
Ketamine (K) + medetomidine (M)	5–7.5 mg/kg (K) + 40 μg/kg (M) i.m.
Ketamine (K) + medetomidine (M) + butorphanol (B)	4 mg/kg (K) + 20 μg/kg (M) + 0.4 mg/kg (B) i.m.
Atipamezole	100–200 μg/kg i.m.
Diazepam	0.25–1 mg/kg i.v., i.m.
Propofol	4–6.5 mg/kg i.v. (dose depending on premedication)
Carprofen	4 mg/kg i.v., i.m., s.c. q24h 4 mg/kg orally q24h (or 2 mg/kg q12h)
Meloxicam	0.2 mg/kg s.c. single dose 0.1 mg/kg orally q24h, commencing 24 hours after injection
Buprenorphine	0.02 mg/kg i.m. q6h
Morphine	0.5 mg/kg i.m. q4h

17.9 Anaesthetic and analgesic drugs and dose rates commonly used in badgers.

The animal should be weighed prior to anaesthesia (pre-weighed cages assist with this procedure) and doses should be calculated accurately. Drugs are usually given by intramuscular injection into the quadriceps or lumbar muscles, through the bars of a crush cage (see Figure 17.18). As with all species, medetomidine causes respiratory and circulatory depression in the badger and this author prefers to supply oxygen (via mask or endotracheal tube) where possible to all badgers anaesthetized in this way and to monitor oxygen saturation levels and cardiac and respiratory functions throughout anaesthesia. Intravenous catheterization and appropriate fluid therapy should be administered as required (see 'First aid procedures'). Body temperature should be monitored and maintained at 37°C.

Medetomidine can be reversed with atipamezole given intramuscularly as soon as procedures have been completed. The addition of butorphanol to the combination reduces the amount of medetomidine required and provides additional analgesia but may render less effective other, more potent, opioids that may be more suitable for major procedures.

These anaesthetic combinations appear safe in badgers provided that good anaesthetic and post-anaesthetic monitoring is carried out. Both combinations can be supplemented with gaseous agents as required.

Intravenous agents

Propofol can be used, with the same safety considerations as in domestic animals. Most badgers will require some form of deep premedication (e.g. medetomidine sedation) to allow intravenous access, though it is possible to minimize this in small cubs or animals with intravenous catheters already placed. Intravenous propofol induction followed by intubation and gaseous maintenance anaesthesia would be the author's recommended protocol for major surgical procedures.

Gaseous anaesthesia

Both isoflurane and sevoflurane can be used safely in badgers for maintenance of general anaesthesia following intravenous induction and intubation in those animals in which intravenous access can be safely achieved. In other

cases mask induction following premedication with medetomidine or acepromazine may be preferred. The technique used will depend upon the clinical condition of the badger. Gaseous anaesthesia can be induced in cubs by mask, with gentle restraint and/or over a Baskerville™-type muzzle for safety. Intubation may be a little more difficult than in dogs due to more restricted jaw opening; a laryngoscope may help laryngeal visualization.

Analgesics

All injured badgers should receive appropriate analgesia, both for welfare reasons and to ensure most rapid return to normal feeding and behaviour patterns. Most of the non-steroidal anti-inflammatory drugs (NSAIDs) that are common in small animal practice have been used by the author without apparent problems in badgers. The author's preference is carprofen or meloxicam by injection for short-term use (e.g. before surgery) and meloxicam solution or carprofen palatable tablets in food for longer-term use (see Figure 17.9). This author's experience of using opioid analgesics such as buprenorphine and morphine in badgers has been unproblematic. Local anaesthetics may also be safely used (following the principles and doses applied in dogs) where appropriate.

Specific conditions

Trauma
'Territorial' wounds

Intraspecific (badger–badger) bite wounds, often referred to as 'territorial' wounds, are a normal part of badger social behaviour and are the most common reason for presentation of badgers to veterinary practices (Mullineaux and Kidner, 2011).

Fighting between badgers resulting in wounding has been described both at territorial boundaries and within sett areas. Bite wounds may be seen in both sexes at all times of year, but there are seasonal trends, being highest in male badgers in February to March, with a second, less distinct peak in September, and most common in females in April (Cresswell et al., 1992; Delahay et al., 2006). Veterinary admissions of badgers for bite wounds follow a similar seasonal pattern (Mullineaux and Kidner, 2011). Bite wounds occur more frequently in male than female animals (Mullineaux and Kidner, 2011) and may be of greater severity in male animals (Cresswell et al., 1992). There is an increased incidence of bite wounds in older badgers (Macdonald et al., 2004b), with cubs less affected (Delahay et al., 2006b).

Bite wounds are most commonly found on the rump, head, neck and shoulder areas, being more frequently located on the rump area (Figure 17.10) in adult male badgers and on the head in cubs and female badgers (Delahay et al., 2006).

Wounds vary from small tears and punctures to significant cutaneous defects (Figure 17.10). There is often secondary bacterial infection (beta-haemolytic *Streptococcus* spp., *Staphylococcus aureus* and coliforms) and, in the summer months, cutaneous myiasis. Bite wounds may be contaminated with *M. bovis* and biting represents a route of transmission of infection between badgers. Life-threatening bite wounds are, however, considered to be infrequent and wounds generally heal quickly in the wild.

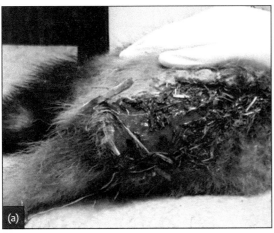 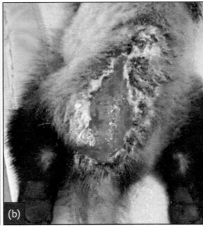

17.10 Large 'territorial' rump wound on an adult badger (a) before and (b) after cleaning. (© Elizabeth Mullineaux)

From a veterinary perspective, although the wounds appear large, with significant secondary infection and contamination, they are generally straightforward to treat and heal well with minimal or no intervention. Extensive wounds, however, may take several weeks to heal.

Assessment of territorial wounds: Animals with territorial wounds can be divided into two broad categories:

- *Young animals (both sexes) in good condition, with no concurrent injuries* – wounds in these badgers should be treated as described below and the animals released quickly where found or rehabilitated in the case of young cubs
- *Older animals (usually male), often with evidence of several episodes of wounding (wounds at various stages of healing), underweight and with worn or broken teeth* – these animals require careful assessment and all their clinical conditions must be treated if they are to be released. Euthanasia may be indicated in severe cases.

The latter category is the more common and old male badgers with serial wounds present the veterinary surgeon with an ethical dilemma regarding whether to treat or euthanase the animal. Territorial disputes are a normal part of badger social interaction, and rapid release with minimal intervention is probably the most ecologically sound approach in cases that are in good body condition and otherwise satisfy triage requirements (see 'Assessment for rehabilitation'). Tattooing of badger (under licence, see 'Legal aspects') with treated bite wounds prior to release, allowing post-release monitoring, is a useful aid to assessing the success of any intervention. The most severe cases, in poor body condition, however, would either require a protracted period in captivity or be likely to die on release. These animals should be euthanased on welfare grounds.

Treatment of territorial wounds:

1. The badger must be anaesthetized (see 'Anaesthesia and analgesia') for full examination and assessed as to its suitability for rehabilitation.
2. Clipping of excessive amounts of hair from around wounds should be avoided, as this prolongs the rehabilitation period while waiting for fur to regrow. Releasing an animal with excessive fur clipped leaves sensitive areas more vulnerable to further bite injuries, as the badger's thick hair coat provides some protection.
3. Wounds should be flushed and cleaned with sterile saline or diluted (1:40) 4% w/v chlorhexidine solution.

4. Wounds should not generally be sutured, as larger wounds require major debridement prior to suturing and generally heal much better by secondary intention. Flaps to areas such as the lips and ears may, however, require surgical apposition following adequate debridement.
5. Topical treatments such as hydrocolloid gel products (e.g. Intrasite®) and semi-permeable dressing sprays (e.g. Opsite®) should then be applied. Hydrocolloid dressings (Granuflex®) held in place with suture loops over the debrided area can be used as an alternative, but in the author's experience these are unnecessarily difficult to manage.
6. The short-term use of NSAIDs is advocated preemptively. A course of broad-spectrum antibacterials should be started where bacteraemia or cellulitis is suspected; amoxicillin/clavulanate (co-amoxiclav) (8.75 mg/kg i.m. q24h) is most suitable in the author's experience. Badgers often do not eat well in captivity and so injectable products rather than tableted medicine in food should be used. It should be noted that territorial bite wounds from other badgers, unlike bites from dogs, heal well with minimal intervention and rarely cause systemic signs; long-term medication is not normally required.
7. Daily topical cleaning and treatment should continue until wounds are healed. This is usually easily performed without sedation in the case of rump wounds: a thick blanket in the hands of an experienced carer is adequate to cover and restrain the animal's head (see Figure 17.18). A sterile plastic spatula is useful for the application of hydrocolloid gels. Head and neck wounds may require the animal to be sedated every few days for the wounds to be treated.

Digging and baiting injuries

Although badger baiting has been illegal since 1835, it was still legal to hunt, dig and kill badgers before the first Badgers Act of 1973. Despite being illegal (Protection of Badgers Act, 1992) and the focus of concern for animal welfare groups, badger digging and baiting continues throughout Britain.

Badgers subjected to baiting are generally dug from their setts, injured to prevent them from running away and then have dogs set upon them. Such badgers may present as dirty and muddy. There may be limb or skull injuries as a result of shooting or being hit with a spade. Hindlimb fractures and dislocations may result from being pulled down by larger dogs. Typical dogfight bites and tears to limbs and face will also be present, these are usually much more extensive than those associated with badger intraspecific wounding.

Treatment: Badgers with such injuries usually require emergency first aid, including aggressive intravenous fluid therapy (20 ml/kg initial i.v. bolus and then reassess), analgesics (see 'Anaesthesia and analgesia') and broad-spectrum antibacterials (amoxicillin/clavulanate, 8.75 mg/kg i.m. q24h) before being anaesthetized for more complete clinical and radiographic examination. Badgers with dog bite injuries require much more intensive treatment than those with bite wounds from other badgers. The decision to treat baiting injuries must be made on clinical assessment and consideration of the requirements for successful release.

Legal procedures: Badger baiting is illegal and any suspect badger cases should be reported to the police. Veterinary surgeons involved in suspect baiting cases must keep records of the badger's injuries (including dated photographs) and copies of radiographs in case prosecutions are possible. If dogs are presented that have been involved in baiting, they should be examined thoroughly and photographic and radiographic images taken as appropriate. Dogs usually have injuries to the face, especially the lower lips and jaw, and forelimbs, some of which may be old injuries from previous episodes of damage. Badger hairs found in a dog's mouth, faeces and vomit (induced as necessary) may be used as evidence in prosecution cases. Guidance in dealing with suspicious cases, with respect to client confidentiality, should be sought from the Royal College of Veterinary Surgeons. See Chapter 11 for further information on the investigation of wildlife crime.

Snares and trapping injuries

Although it is illegal in the UK to set snares intentionally to trap badgers, animals do get caught in snares set illegally or intended for other species (Figure 17.11a). The size and power of the badger in its attempts to release itself from the snare often result in considerable injury (Figure 17.11bc). Other traps and non-malicious materials such as netting may also prove hazardous to badgers. All such materials, traps and snares are best removed under general anaesthesia or sedation, preferably with the badger and trap brought to the veterinary surgery.

Careful examination of the whole badger for concurrent injuries must be carried out and radiography performed where necessary. It is common for the badger to have injuries to the jaw and limbs caused by the animal's attempts to escape.

Treatment: Intravenous fluid therapy, broad-spectrum antibiotics and analgesics are all usually required. It is not uncommon for there to be a delay in the development of tissue damage resulting from pressure necrosis around

and distal to the site of snare or trap injuries, and for this reason animals should be kept in captivity and monitored for at least a week prior to release.

Road traffic accidents

Road traffic accidents (RTAs) account for at least half the badger deaths in monitored populations and this is reflected in the frequency of their presentation to veterinary centres, accounting for over one third (37%) of all casualties (Mulineaux and Kidner, 2011). The range of injuries seen is not dissimilar to those encountered in dogs involved in RTAs. Badgers will be clinically shocked and require initial first aid treatment, as described earlier. Once stable, sedation or anaesthesia is usually required to allow a complete clinical examination.

Fractures: Bone damage following RTA typically includes fractures of the skull (Figure 17.12), pelvis and limbs. Simple jaw fractures (mandibular symphysis or ramus) and closed long bone fractures clear of joints can be successfully repaired using appropriate orthopaedic implants, with a reasonable prognosis. As in other wildlife species, fracture fixation planning should take into account the animal's tolerance of implants and the need to remove these prior to release (see Chapter 5). Young badgers appear to tolerate dressings and external skeletal fixators much better than adults. Badgers are robust animals and heal well, but their lifestyle requires near-perfect healing for normal function. Surgical skills and finances must be available to ensure the best possible outcome. If the best possible care is not available, the animal should be euthanased for welfare reasons.

In reality, few badgers will have orthopaedic injuries suitable for treatment. Compound fractures and those affecting joints carry an especially poor prognosis, as do fractures of the spine and pelvis. Euthanasia is a common necessary outcome and should be performed at an early stage.

Occasionally, badgers with healing or healed old fractures will be presented. These must be assessed on individual merit, considering the adequacy of healing and the normality of function. Female badgers with healed pelvic fractures that may result in dystocia should be euthanased.

Thoracic trauma: Because of the risk of *M. bovis* infection, haemothorax or pneumothorax following RTAs in badgers must be treated with caution and only following appropriate further diagnostic tests and clinical examination. Following radiographic and/or ultrasonographic assessment, simple closed drainage on a single occasion

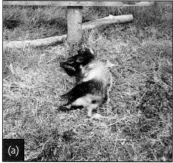
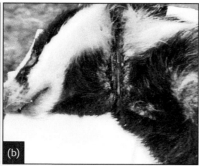
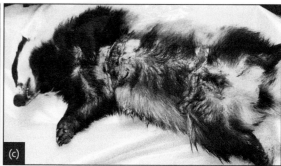

17.11 (a) Dead badger caught in a 'drag snare'. This type of snare is of dubious legality for any species, as the fact it can be dragged limits the ability to check it on a regular basis. In this case the snare has become trapped on a fence post. (b) Resulting wounds to the neck of the drag-snared badger. (c) Dead badger showing snare wounds around the chest and abdomen.
(Courtesy of M Brash)

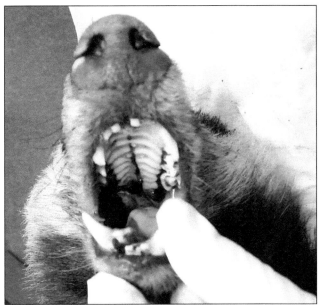

17.12 Road traffic accident injuries to an adult badger including fracture of the hard palate and fracture of the mandible. This casualty was euthanased following examination.
(© Elizabeth Mullineaux)

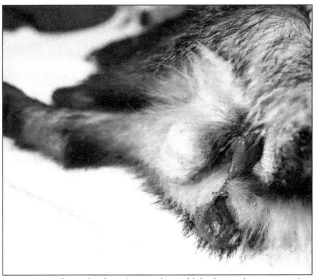

17.13 Badgers that have ingested metaldehyde may be presented with blue-green faeces.
(© Secret World Wildlife Rescue)

should be carried out, taking all relevant precautions, under appropriate sedation or local anaesthesia, to allow diagnosis and treatment of minor problems. Placing of chest drains and repeat drainage are unlikely to be well tolerated and are not recommended for reasons of human health and safety. Badgers requiring repeat chest drainage should be euthanased.

Ruptured diaphragms in badgers are generally straightforward to repair in the manner described in standard surgical texts for small animals. Badgers are easily intubated for positive pressure ventilation during surgery (see 'Gaseous anaesthesia'), and needle drainage of the chest at the end of surgery is usually adequate. Assuming good post-surgical recovery and lack of concurrent injury, release is possible 7–10 days later.

Abdominal trauma: Abdominal trauma in a badger following an RTA requires careful assessment to ensure that the animal is not released with long-term problems. To allow full assessment and treatment, general anaesthesia, appropriate diagnostic testing and subsequent exploratory laparotomy are usually required. With the exception of simple abdominal wall injuries (without intestinal prolapse) and splenectomy, most abdominal injuries carry guarded or unknown prognoses, and euthanasia may be the best course of action. Splenectomy is straightforward where indicated, but carries unknown risks of reduced immunity and should be considered carefully. Healed splenic and hepatic lesions from RTAs are incidental findings at post-mortem examination of free-living badgers (Gallagher and Nelson, 1979).

Poisoning

As well as malicious intent, the varied omnivorous diet of badgers makes them susceptible to accidental pesticide or rodenticide poisoning. Poisoning cases should be treated symptomatically, or specific antidotes given if the causal agent is known (see Chapter 5). Badgers that have ingested metaldehyde may present with blue-green faeces (Figure 17.13). Cases that do not respond quickly to treatment and general supportive care should be euthanased.

Infectious diseases
Viral diseases

Distemper: Canine distemper virus (CDV) has been described in badgers in mainland Europe, with clinical and pathological respiratory and central nervous system (CNS) signs, but not hyperkeratosis of the foot pads. The CNS signs may be confused with rabies in countries where that disease is endemic. A serological study in the south and south-west of England found no evidence of CDV in wild badgers (Delahay and Frölich, 2000).

Rabies: Badgers are not considered primary hosts for the rabies virus and only play a secondary role in the spread of disease throughout Europe. In the event of a rabies outbreak badger populations are severely affected. Contact between badgers and the main vectors of rabies, the red fox and the raccoon dog (*Nyctereutes procyonoides*), in Europe may increase the likelihood of badgers becoming vectors for rabies.

Viral enteropathogens (parvovirus and orthoreovirus): Mustelids are known to be susceptible to several strains of parvovirus, though there are no records of confirmed infection in free-living Eurasian badgers. Parvovirus infection has been suspected on histological findings as the cause of myocarditis in a wild badger (Burtscher and Url, 2007). Parvovirus in combination with an orthoreovirus has been described causing enteric pathology (Figure 17.14), associated with acute diarrhoea and death in badger cubs at a UK wildlife rescue centre. Sequencing of the parvovirus suggested it to be most closely related to feline panleukopaenia and related parvoviruses, such as mink enteritis virus. In these cases it was suggested that the orthoreovirus acted synergistically with the parvovirus, increasing the clinical severity of the cases (Barlow *et al.*, 2012).

Treatment of viral enteritis in badger cubs is the same as in dogs and cats; however, in the cases described above, treatment was unsuccessful.

The possible susceptibility of cubs in rehabilitation facilities to parvovirus suggests that suitable precautions should be taken to prevent infection. A live attenuated canine parvovirus vaccine (Nobivac® Parvo-C) has been

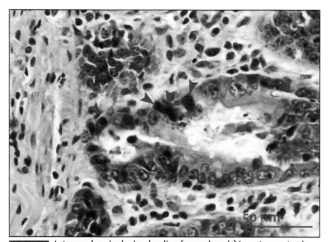

17.14 Intranuclear inclusion bodies (arrowheads) in enterocytes in the small intestine of a badger cub in which dual parvovirus and orthoreovirus infection were confirmed. Haematoxylin and eosin stain; bar = 50 μm.
(Courtesy of A Barlow, APHA Wildlife Group and WNDS)

used with apparent success and lack of complication by this author in badger cubs. Vaccination of wildlife is discussed in Chapter 7.

Bacterial diseases

Tuberculosis: *M. bovis* is a member of the *M. tuberculosis* complex, with a host range that includes many domestic and wildlife species as well as humans. *M. bovis* is considered to be a cattle disease (bovine tuberculosis, bTB) with zoonotic potential and its geographical range parallels distribution of livestock throughout the world. The disease has significant economic effects on communities as a result of effects in cattle, as well as public health, international trade and wildlife tourism. Infection of free-ranging wildlife is considered to be a spill-over effect from domestic animal populations, with very few species maintaining the infection within populations and acting as vectors of infection to other species. *M. bovis* infections have been identified in a broad range of UK wild mammals without evidence of the maintenance of infection. Several wildlife species are, however, able to maintain infection under the right circumstances and potentially pose a risk to cattle; these most notably include brushtail possum (*Trichosurus vulpecula*) in New Zealand, white-tailed deer (*Odocoileus virginianus*) in the Michigan area of the USA and badgers in Great Britain and Ireland.

Epidemiology in badgers: As is the case in tuberculosis in other species, aerosol infection of the respiratory tract is the main route for spread of *M. bovis* between badgers. Excretion of bacilli can occur in saliva, urine, faeces and pus from wounds and lymph node abscesses, although excretion appears to be intermittent. Most natural *M. bovis* infection occurs within the sett, but areas such as latrines act as foci of infection. Bite wounds (see 'Territorial wounds') are another possible method of horizontal infection via contaminated saliva and this may explain the higher infection rates found in male badgers compared to females. False vertical transfer of infection from mother to cubs is considered important in maintaining infection within social groups. In medium/high-density badger populations, a stable social structure appears to limit the spread of tuberculosis between groups of animals, conversely, disruption of social patterns (e.g. culling operation) increases disease transmission: 'perturbation effect' (Riordan *et al.*, 2011).

Tuberculosis in badgers: Most badgers infected with *M. bovis* do not have clinical tuberculosis and have no visible lesions when standard post-mortem examinations are carried out. Adult badgers infected with *M. bovis* may live and breed normally for many years despite infection (Corner, 2006).

The major clinical sign of tuberculosis in badgers is weight loss leading to emaciation. Auscultation of the chest and imaging (radiography or computed tomography) may suggest lung lesions or pleurisy consistent with the lung being the main focus of infection found at post-mortem examination. Lung lesions vary from miliary foci to caseous abscesses, frequently with involvement of the bronchiomediastinal lymph nodes. Lung lesions may be confused with adiaspiromycosis (see 'Fungal diseases').

The liver, spleen and kidney may become infected through haematogenous spread from the lungs or another primary lesion such as a bite wound. Clinical signs associated with organ damage may be evident. Superficial drainage lymph nodes associated with infected bite wounds may be palpably enlarged. Bone infection originating in growth plates (Figure 17.15) has been described, resulting in lameness.

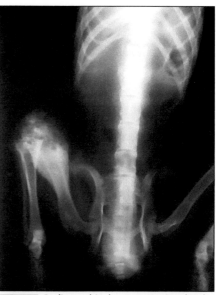

17.15 Radiographic changes associated with osteomyelitis of the right stifle joint, originating in the growth plates, in a young adult badger infected with *Mycobacterium bovis*.
(© Elizabeth Mullineaux)

Biochemical and haematological parameters associated with tuberculosis in badgers are non-specific and vary during the progression of the disease (Mahmood *et al.*, 1988; Chambers *et al.*, 2000). Abnormal organ-specific biochemical parameters may be linked to specific tuberculous lesions, but may equally be affected by other disease conditions.

RTA is considered to be the major cause of badger mortality, even in areas with endemic tuberculosis; however, tuberculosis is the predominant cause of natural deaths (Cheeseman *et al.*, 1988), although these are relatively uncommon (<10%) (Clifton-Hadley *et al.*, 1993).

Association between bTB in cattle and badgers: Badgers are considered the only wildlife maintenance host for *M. bovis* in the UK. Several properties of the infection in badgers make them good maintenance hosts and their social behaviour facilitates spread of infection. Epidemiologically, disease in badgers appears to lag behind that in cattle. There is limited scientific evidence for the direct spread of *M. bovis* between badgers and cattle, although transmission is likely to arise from shared use of pasture and farm resources (buildings, troughs and cattle feed).

Government reviews have concluded that badgers are a significant reservoir of *M. bovis* infection for cattle and several control policies involving the culling of badgers have been implemented in England in an attempt to control the disease in cattle (Figure 17.16). In recent years, the devolved governments of the UK have adopted differing policies for badger control; currently Scotland is OTF (officially tuberculosis free) and has no badger control, Wales has a policy of vaccinating badgers and Northern Ireland is implementing a TVR (test and vaccinate or remove) policy. This is an ever-developing subject and readers are directed to the websites of the national governments for the most current information.

1971	Badgers first implicated in spread of bTB to cattle (Muirhead *et al.*, 1974)
1973	The Badgers Act
1975	Gassing of badgers under licence
1980	Zuckerman review
1982–1985	'Clean ring strategy' – trapping, testing and culling of infected setts
1986	Dunnet review and 'Interim strategy' – badgers culled on farms where bTB had been confirmed in cattle
1992	Protection of Badgers Act
1997	Krebs report – recommended the establishment of the 'Randomised Badger Culling Trial' (RBCT) led by an Independent Scientific Group (ISG)
1998–2007	RBCT
2007	ISG final report on the RBCT finds that badger culling 'cannot meaningfully contribute to the future control of cattle TB in Britain' as a result of 'high costs and low benefits' and 'recommends that TB control methods focus on areas other than badger culling' (Bourne *et al.*, 2007). Findings considered contentious by others (King, 2007)
2010	BadgerBCG vaccine licensed
2011	Government policy document suggests badger culling in areas of 150 km² (plus a 2 km adjacent ring) using controlled shooting and cage trapping, to cull 70% of badgers, for at least 4 years
2012	Culling licences issued for areas in west Somerset and west Gloucestershire to carry out 'pilot culls' to test the humaneness, efficacy and safety of controlled shooting, assessed by an Independent Expert Panel (IEP). Culling is postponed until 2013
2013	Pilot badger culls begin in west Somerset and west Gloucestershire with a plan of culling annually for at least 4 years
2014	Defra produce *The strategy for achieving 'Officially Bovine Tuberculosis-free' status for England*, including 'zoning' of the country according to TB risk ('high-risk', 'edge', 'low-risk') with differing badger control methods in each area
2014	IEP report on badger pilot culls (Munro, 2014). Concerns raised regarding the effectiveness and humaneness of controlled shooting
2014	Pilot culls continue in west Somerset and west Gloucestershire
2015	Culls continue in west Somerset and Gloucestershire, and are extended to include areas of Dorset

17.16 Timeline of badger controls in the management of bovine tuberculosis in cattle and badgers in England. Note: This is an ever-developing area of government policy and the reader is directed to the Defra section of the Government website for the most current information.

Alternatives to badger culling to control bTB in cattle might include:

* Enhanced cattle testing and movement controls
* Improved farm biosecurity
* BCG vaccination of cattle together with use of a differential (DIVA) test
* BadgerBCG vaccination (see 'Vaccinating badgers')
* Reproductive control in badgers.

Zoonotic risk: M. bovis is classed by the OIE (World Organisation for Animal Health) as a Risk 3 (scale 1–4) pathogen for public health, although in most countries the risk is virtually negated through the pasteurization of milk. In the UK, only 0.5–1.5% of confirmed human tuberculosis cases annually are attributable to *M. bovis* and most of these are as a result of reactivation of long-standing latent infections acquired before widespread adoption of milk pasteurization, or *M. bovis* infections contracted abroad. Cases arising from an occupational risk in farm and veterinary situations have been described, but are very uncommon and the sources of such infections are poorly defined.

The potential zoonotic risks of *M. bovis* infection must, however, be addressed when treating badgers in veterinary practices and wildlife rehabilitation centres, and methods for controlling these risks are described below.

Diagnosis of M. bovis infection in badgers: The 'gold standard' for confirming *M. bovis* infection in all species is post-mortem examination combined with bacterial culture of tissue samples using selective media. The diagnosis of *M. bovis* infection in live animals relies upon the detection of cell-mediated immune responses (which may be protective), the detection of humoral responses (which are generally non-protective), or the culture of the causal organism from body secretions. Cell-mediated and humoral responses represent existing or historical (latent or resolved) infections, whilst organism culture confirms active infection.

Intradermal skin tests using purified protein derivatives (PPD) from mycobacterial cultures to generate a delayed type hypersensitivity (type IV) reaction, as used in cattle, are ineffective in badgers (Mahmood *et al.*, 1987) and should not be used. Interferon-gamma (IFN-γ) tests, involving the immunodiagnostic measurement of IFN-γ released by memory T-lymphocytes *in vitro* when re-exposed to antigens associated with the *M. tuberculosis* complex bacterium, are also used in cattle. A badger IFN-γ test has been developed (Dalley *et al.*, 2008) but is not currently commercially available. The need to complete such tests quickly after sampling might make them logistically difficult to use in practice. Culture of clinical samples from badgers (urine, faeces, lymph node aspirates, wound swabs) takes considerable time (6–12 weeks) at an approved laboratory. Collection of clinical samples is not without zoonotic risk.

Currently the only tests available for detecting *M. bovis* infection in live badgers in veterinary practice are antigen tests. These typically have low sensitivity (around 50%) but high specificity (around 90%) (Chambers *et al.*, 2002; 2008). Several serological assays are available to detect antibodies to *M. bovis* in badgers, although few have been fully validated. Some of the tests may be used 'badger side' in a field situation.

Most badger rehabilitators prefer to submit samples for bTB serological testing to the Animal and Plant Health Agency (APHA) (see 'Specialist organizations and useful contacts') which is able to carry out a commercially available validated test. A 1 ml serum sample is required, which can be collected most easily from the jugular vein in a sedated badger (see Figure 17.7).

The low sensitivity of antibody tests means that they are of limited use for detecting individual infected animals and, as a result of this, adult badgers for rehabilitation are not normally tested for bTB, but are instead isolated in captivity and released back to exactly where they were found to avoid any possible risk of spreading disease (Mullineaux and Kidner, 2011) (see 'Release – adults').

Where cub groups are reared and translocation is usually necessary, it is essential to ensure that animals released are disease-free. Multiple testing policies are therefore employed to improve the overall sensitivity of the test (Mullineaux and Kidner, 2011). Cubs testing positive on any occasion are euthanased and sent for post-mortem examination and culture for *M. bovis*. Multiple testing reduces the specificity of testing and it is not unusual for cubs that are serologically positive to be post-mortem and culture negative. In reality, few cubs test positive and the costs both financially and in terms of welfare are considered to be worthwhile to maintain land-owner confidence in the cub rehabilitation and release process. For more information on current testing policy for badger cubs, contact the Badger Trust, Royal Society for the Prevention of Cruelty to Animals (RSPCA) or SWWR (see 'Specialist organizations and useful contacts').

Vaccinating badgers: An injectable Bacille Calmette-Guérin (BCG) vaccine for badgers (BadgerBCG) has been commercially available in the UK since 2010. The vaccine reduces the severity and progression of tuberculosis in both experimental animals and free-living badgers and has been shown to have both direct and indirect effects in protecting individuals and in-contact cubs (Carter *et al.*, 2012). Vaccination of badgers aims to reduce transmission of bTB between badgers and from badgers to cattle by reducing the incidence of disease in badger populations. The vaccine was developed for field use, but has obvious applications to badger rehabilitation and release. Information for veterinary surgeons on using the vaccine has been published (Brown *et al.*, 2013).

Dealing with bTB in badgers in veterinary practice: Those dealing with badgers must be aware of the risk of bTB and must ensure that suitable risk assessments are put in place for staff and rehabilitators working with badgers (see Chapter 3). Suggested precautions include the following:

- Employers should be aware of the BCG vaccine status of staff dealing with badgers and advise discussion with their medical practitioner regarding vaccination
- Latex gloves must be worn when dealing with badgers and ideally masks should be worn, especially where there is a risk of aerosol spread from body fluids
- Care should be taken to avoid unnecessary direct contact with badger saliva, urine, faeces and bite wounds
- Surfaces coming into contact with badgers should be appropriately cleaned with a Defra-approved disinfectant of the correct strength and left for the recommended amount of contact time to kill mycobacteria
- Post-mortem examinations must not be carried out on badgers suspected of being infected with bTB. Some external laboratories are approved to carry out necropsies and appropriate *M. bovis* cultures; whole closed carcasses should be sent for this purpose
- Post-mortem examination of any badger is not recommended in a veterinary practice environment. If a post-mortem examination of a badger **not** suspected

of having tuberculosis is carried out, protective clothing (including masks) must be worn and the number of exposed staff kept to a minimum. Ideally, a closed area with extraction fans should be used
- Badgers suspected of having clinical bTB should be euthanased.

The following precautions should be taken to avoid the risk of spreading *M. bovis* infection when releasing badgers:

- Adult badgers must be isolated in captivity and released at the exact site at which they were found. For the reasons explained above, adult badgers are not normally blood tested for bTB
- If animals (usually cubs) are to be released in a different area, multiple blood tests should first be carried out (see 'Diagnosis of tuberculosis in badgers')
- Badgers found in areas with endemic bTB in cattle (Defra defined 'high-risk' or 'edge' zones, see Figure 17.16) should not be released into areas of a lower risk ('edge' or 'low-risk' zones, respectively)
- BadgerBCG vaccination should be considered for all badgers prior to release
- Badger cub groups should be BadgerBCG vaccinated prior to release.

Leptospires: Three strains of leptospires belonging to three serogroups have been isolated from badgers in England (*Leptospira australis*, *L. javanic* and *L. hebdomadis*), where infection was attributed to eating small rodents (Little *et al.*, 1987; Salt and Little, 1987); no clinical significance was attached to these infections.

Salmonellae: *Salmonella* spp. of a wide range of serovars are frequently cultured from badgers, with *S*. Agama being the principal isolate. Limited clinical significance has been attached to these bacteria, although they may occur concurrently with other infections that are clinically significant.

Other bacterial infections: Badgers are considered to be susceptible to anthrax, but there are no reports of incidence or clinical findings. Badgers have been used as serological sentinel species for monitoring of zoonotic *Yersinia pestis* in North America. They have been found to harbour *Mycobacterium avium* subsp. *paratuberculosis*, but no clinical significance has been attached to such isolation. *Borrelia burgdorferi sensu lato* has been isolated from badger skin, but there are no reports of clinical Lyme disease in badgers.

Fungal diseases

Dermatophytosis: Whilst there are no clinical reports of dermatophytosis in badgers, the dermatophyte *Arthroderma olidum* (part of the *Trichophyton terrestre* complex) has been isolated from a badger (Campbell *et al.*, 2006) and *Anthroderma melis* from a badger sett (Hancox, 1980).

Histoplasmosis: Lymphatic histoplasmosis (Hancox, 1980) and histoplasmosis caused by *Histoplasma capsulatum* var. *capsulatum* causing granulomatous skin lesions and lymph node lesions have been described in wild badgers (Bauder *et al.*, 2000).

Adiaspiromycosis: Adiaspiromycosis caused by *Emmonsia (Chrysosporium) crescens* is frequently found in the lungs of badgers at post-mortem examination, in common with findings in other digging mammals. In other Mustelidae such as otters (*Lutra lutra*) infection can prove fatal although there are no such reports in badgers. Adiaspiromycosis granulomas may be confused with tuberculosis lesions at post-mortem examination.

Parasites

Ectoparasites: The louse *Trichodectes melis* and flea *Paraceras melis melis* are the main badger ectoparasites, with especially high numbers found on debilitated individual badgers. Other flea species, *Pulex irritans* (human flea) and *Chaetopsylla trichosa*, have also been described in badgers (Hancox, 1980; Sleeman and Kelly, 1997). Fleas have been implicated in the transmission of *Trypanosoma pestanai* (see 'Protozoal infections').

Several tick species have been reported on badgers including *Ixodes canisuga*, *I. hexaganus* and occasionally *I. ricinus*. Ticks have been implicated as vectors of *Babesia missirolii* (Macdonald *et al*., 1999).

Cheyletiella parasitovorax infestation has been reported in badgers, especially cubs during the summer months (Newman *et al*., 2004). Mange caused by *Sarcoptes scabiei* has been reported in badgers in mainland Europe. *Trombicula autumnalis* has also been found in badgers.

Cutaneous myiasis (*Lucilia sericata*) has been reported in badgers and is often associated with territorial bite wounds.

Ectoparasites are rarely a clinical problem in badgers except in emaciated and debilitated individuals, where the number of lice in particular can become high. Ectoparasiticides, such as fipronil, should be used only where the burden is clinically significant or the animal requires a lot of human handling; this is especially the case in cubs.

Endoparasites: Parasites of all three helminth groups affect the digestive and respiratory tracts of badgers. *Capillaria erinacei* has been found in the stomach of badgers and *Uncinaria stenocephala* and *Molineus patens* in the intestines, with other helminth species less common and probably as a result of accidental infestation. No clinical significance has been attached to these infections.

Aelurostrongylus falciformis has been identified in the lungs of wild badgers at post-mortem and larvae have been identified in bronchoalveolar lavage fluid from captive badgers (McCarthy *et al*., 2009). Lungworm may result in verminous granulomas in the lungs, which may be confused with tuberculous lesions.

Both *Trichinella* spp. and *Echinococcus multilocularis* have been found in badgers in Italy (Di Cerbo *et al*., 2008); however, these have not been reported in the UK.

Protozoal infections:
Toxoplasmosis: Serological evidence of *Toxoplasma gondii* infection has been frequently found in badgers in southern England and elsewhere in Europe, but clinical signs of toxoplasmosis have not been reported.

Coccidiosis: Coccidiosis caused by *Eimeria melis* and *Isospora melis* has been reported occasionally in wild badgers, causing poor growth in cubs, with more severe infections resulting in deaths (Newman *et al*., 2000). Clinical disease (diarrhoea and dehydration) resulting in mortality has been described in captive badger cubs (Barlow *et al*., 2011). Animals have been successfully treated with toltrazuril at a dose of 30 mg/kg orally and repeated 10 days later as previously described in kittens and puppies (Lloyd and Smith, 2001).

Giardia: *Giardia duodenalis* assemblage E (Figure 17.17) has been found in badger cubs at a wildlife rehabilitation centre as a co-infection with *Emeria* spp. and *Salmonella* spp. (Barlow *et al*., 2011). In-contact badger cubs were successfully treated with fenbendazole at a dose of 50 mg/kg orally on 3 consecutive days.

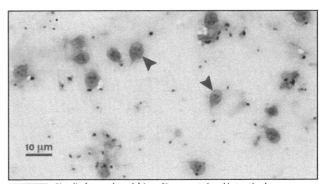

17.17 *Giardia* (arrowheads) in a Giemsa-stained intestinal scrape from a badger cub that died of giardiasis (bar = 10 μm).
(Courtesy of A Barlow, APHA Wildlife Group and WNDS)

Trypanosomiasis and babesiosis: *Babesia missirolii* and *Trypanosoma pestanai* have been reported with infection rates of 77% and 7.7%, respectively, in badgers in England (Peirce and Neal, 1974a; 1974b; MacDonald *et al*., 1999). Ticks, *Ixodes canisuga* and *I. hexaganus*, are suggested as potential vectors. In all cases, infections were asymptomatic.

Sarcocysts: Sarcocysts similar to *Sarcocystis gracilis* in roe deer (*Capreolus capreolus*) have been demonstrated in the tongue muscle of a badger in Germany (Odening *et al*., 1994), but there are no reports of this parasite in the UK.

Other diseases

A wide variety of diseases have been recorded post-mortem in individual badgers, usually in aged animals. These include arteriosclerosis, pulmonary ossification, polyarthritis, pyometritis, valvular endocarditis, liver haemangioma and cystic kidneys.

Neoplasia appears to be rare in badgers with few cases identified at necropsy and reported in the literature; these include lymphosarcoma, cutaneous papilloma, hepatic haemangiomas, mediastinal lymphoma and pelioid hepatocellular carcinoma.

Individual badgers with specific conditions should be treated on their own merit, following the principles of assessment outlined above.

Dental disease

Dental caries have been reported in healthy free-ranging badgers, especially older animals (Andrews and Murray, 1974). Tooth wear and caries may be the cause of emaciation in a small number of badgers. Fractured teeth may occur during road traffic accidents and have been associated with fatal osteomyelitis in untreated badgers.

Teeth must always be examined in badger casualties as an indicator of age and to assist in decision making for rehabilitation and release. As teeth are frequently fractured or have pulp cavities exposed by road traffic accidents, these cases must be especially carefully examined. An animal that is otherwise fit but has damaged teeth should have them treated or removed, as appropriate, before release. Animals with either severe dental disease or many teeth missing should be euthanased.

Therapeutics

Sites of injection

- Cephalic, saphenous and jugular veins are all accessible in badgers for the intravenous administration of fluids and medication.
- For intramuscular injections, the rump (gluteal muscle mass) is usually the most accessible area when a badger is in a crush cage and in most cases can be used safely in a kennel or pen with the badger's head simply covered and held with a heavy blanket. However, intramuscular injection into this area often produces a slow and unreliable response to sedative or anaesthetic drugs, presumably as a result of inadvertent injection into fat rather than muscle, and the quadriceps or lumbar muscles are preferred by the author if these alternative sites are presented upon restraint (Figure 17.18).
- Subcutaneous injections can easily be given into the scruff of an already restrained individual, or more caudally over the dorsum, with the head restrained and covered.

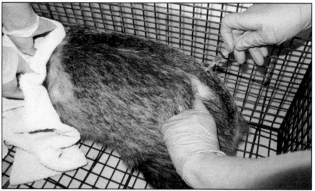

17.18 Intramuscular injection into the lumbar muscles of an adult badger restrained with a heavy blanket.
(Courtesy of M Gunn)

Dose rate

In the author's experience, the use of common veterinary drugs at the standard doses as for domestic dogs has been unproblematic, although it should be noted that there are no licensed products for use in badgers and in the UK the principles described under the cascade system for prescribing drugs should be followed. Suggested drugs have been given throughout this chapter for specific conditions as appropriate. Doses for anaesthetic and analgesic products are given in Figure 17.9.

Management in captivity

Adult badgers should generally be kept in isolation from other animals (including other badgers) during their captivity. Longer-term care of adults requires a specially constructed facility, details of which can be obtained from the Badger Trust, RSPCA or SWWR (see 'Specialist organizations and useful contacts').

Rearing of badger cubs

Most cubs brought into captivity are 8–10 weeks old, the age at which they first venture above ground. Younger cubs, from a few days old, may be presented as a result of

interference in setts by dogs, or because cubs have come above ground early in response to hunger after the death or injury of the sow. For guidance on ageing a cub, see Figures 17.5 and 17.6.

Feeding

The basic examination and assessment for rehabilitation of cubs are no different from those of adults. Badger cubs require the same care as other neonates (warmth, food and stimulation to pass faeces and urine) (see also Chapter 8), but will not wean until 8–10 weeks of age, which means that reasonably large cubs still require milk feeds (see Figure 17.6b). Most milk replacers suitable for puppies will be adequate for badger cubs; Esbilac® at half strength is preferred by many rehabilitators. Suggested frequencies and feeding volumes (approximately 0.5 ml/g/24h) are given in Figure 17.19, but these vary greatly between individual cubs.

When feeding, cubs tend to push out their subcaudal gland (see Figure 17.4). This is normal and should not be confused with straining for other reasons.

Cubs over 10 weeks of age (see Figure 17.6c) can begin to be weaned. Rehabilitators tend to use a wide variety of weaning foods (Figure 17.20) to mimic the badger's varied and omnivorous diet; tinned puppy food will usually be accepted in the short term.

Approximate age	Bodyweight	Total volume of milk (24 h)	No. of feeds (24 h)
1 week (see Figure 17.6a)	280 g	140 ml	9
4 weeks (see Figure 17.6b)	600 g	300 ml	5
8 weeks	1500 g	750 ml	4

17.19 Feeding volumes and frequencies for hand-rearing badger cubs.
(P Kidner, personal communication)

Stage of weaning	Age	Suitable weaning foods
Stage 1	8–10 weeks	Milupa® baby food, Weetabix®, scrambled eggs, yoghurt, porridge
Stage 2	10 weeks or more (see Figure 17.6c) and adults	Raw minced meat, raw minced tripe, puppy food, cooked sausages, cooked chicken, dead day-old chicks, peanut butter sandwiches, grapes, sunflower seeds, kitchen scraps

17.20 Food items suitable for weaning badger cubs.
(P Kidner, personal communication)

Pre-release management

In order to be released successfully, badger cubs need to be reared in social groups. Cubs kept as individuals tend to develop stereotypical behaviour and become unreleasable. People dealing with individual cubs should contact local or national Badger Trust groups at an early stage to ensure that suitable rearing and release facilities are available. Good record-keeping will help those involved in a cub's subsequent management.

Cubs should be identified by microchip as soon as possible and tattooed (both under licence, see 'Legal aspects') before release (Figure 17.21). Serological testing for tuberculosis should be carried out during rearing and BadgerBCG vaccine administered prior to release (see 'Tuberculosis'). For more information on cub rearing policy, contact the Badger Trust, RSPCA or SWWR.

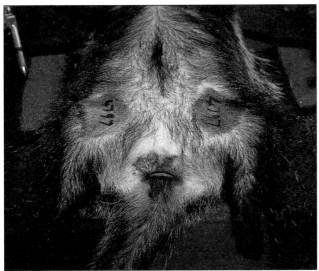

17.21 Bilateral medial thigh tattoos in a badger cub prior to release. This animal has been anaesthetized for this procedure. Tattooing of badgers requires an appropriate licence (see 'Legal aspects').
(Courtesy of C Seddon)

Release

Adults

Adult animals are not normally tested for tuberculosis prior to release, because of the limited sensitivity of a single serological test and the time and cost implications of multiple testing (see 'Tuberculosis'). The risk of potential disease transmission is minimized by isolating adult badgers in captivity and releasing them where they were found.

Because of that risk, and the territorial nature of badgers, adults should be released at the *exact* site where they were found. A good history is required for this to be possible. If there is no history of where the animal was found, the badger must either be euthanased or, if young, incorporated into a release group (see 'Rearing of badger cubs').

Badgers are best released from dusk onwards (Figure 17.22). To avoid further accidents where animals have been found at the roadside, it may be necessary to release them late at night when traffic is negligible.

There is some merit in tattooing adult animals (under licence) prior to release, at the time of pre-release veterinary examination, in order for post-release monitoring to be carried out (see Figure 17.21).

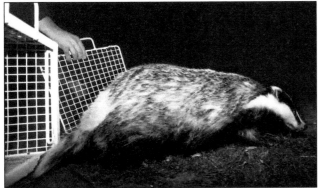

17.22 Adult badgers should be released at their place of origin at dusk.
(© Secret World Wildlife Rescue)

Cubs

Cubs are usually released via artificial setts at 6–8 months of age in groups of five to eight, with an appropriate sex ratio: there should be more females than males, and at least two males in the group (typically with four to six females). Cubs are routinely tattooed prior to release and radio frequency identification (RFID) microchips used for post-release monitoring (marking of badgers requires an appropriate licence, see 'Legal aspects'). More information is available from the Badger Trust, RSPCA and SWWR.

Legal aspects

Badgers are protected in England, Wales and Scotland under the Animal Welfare Act 2006/Animal Health and Welfare (Scotland) Act 2006 when captive, and under the Protection of Badgers Act 1992 in the wild. In Northern Ireland, they are protected under the Wildlife (Northern Ireland) Order 1985 as amended by the Wildlife and Natural Environment (Northern Ireland) Act 2011. General aspects of this legislation are discussed in Chapter 2.

Badgers have been given protection against digging and baiting under various legislation over the years. These were brought together under the Protection of Badgers Act 1992. This legislation is unusual in that it protects both the badger and its sett. The main features of this Act are as follows (Neal and Cheeseman, 1996):

- It is **illegal** to:
  - Kill, injure or take any badger or attempt to do so
  - Dig for a badger
  - Possess a dead badger, or any part of a dead badger, or an object derived from one if that badger was taken in contravention of the Act
  - Sell, have in possession or under control a live badger (see legal exceptions below)
  - Mark, ring or tag a badger (see licenced exceptions below)
  - Damage, destroy or prevent access to a badger sett
  - Cause a dog to enter a sett or disturb a badger in a sett.
- It is not an offence to kill a badger provided that it can be shown that it happened accidentally
- It is **legal** to:
  - Damage a sett unwittingly during lawful action
  - Euthanase an injured badger
  - Take and treat an injured badger or rear a cub, provided that the individual is released as soon as it is no longer incapacitated.

Licences are issued by the nature conservation agencies (Natural England, Scottish Natural Heritage, Natural Resouces Wales) to allow for the keeping of badgers in zoos, the translocation of badgers, the marking of badgers, and interference with setts for research, land development, archaeological investigation or the gathering of evidence about an offence.

Licences are issued by the relevant government bodies to allow badgers to be killed or setts interfered with for the prevention of spread of disease and to prevent damage to land, crops, poultry or property. They are also issued to allow interference with setts for agricultural and forestry work, or the maintenance or construction of watercourses, drainage or sea and tidal defences.

Acknowledgements

The author would like to thank Pauline Kidner (Secret World Wildlife Rescue), Richard Delahay (APHA), Matthew Brash, Chris Cheeseman and Phil Scott for their comments on earlier versions of this chapter.

References and further reading

Andrews AH and Murray RR (1974) Dental caries in the European badger (*Meles meles* L). *Veterinary Record* **95**, 163–165

Aznar I, Frankena K, More SJ *et al.* (2014) Optimising and evaluating the characteristics of a multiple antigen ELISA for detection of *Mycobacterium bovis* infection in a badger vaccine field trial. *PLoS ONE* **9(7)**, e100139. doi:10.1371/journal.pone.0100139

Barlow AM, Mullineaux E, Wood R, Tawenan W and Wastling JM (2011) Giardiosis in Eurasian badgers (*Meles meles*). *Veterinary Record* **167**, 1017

Barlow AM, Schock A, Bradshaw JM *et al.* (2012) Parvovirus enteritis in Eurasian badgers (*Meles meles*). *Veterinary Record* **170**, 416

Bauder B, Kübber-Heiss A, Steineck T, Kuttin ES and Kaufman L (2000) Granulomatous skin lesions due to histoplasmosis in a badger (*Meles meles*) in Austria. *Medical Mycology* **38**, 249–253

Bevanger K and Brøseth H (1998) Body temperature changes in wild-living badgers *Meles meles* through the winter. *Wildlife Biology* **4**, 97–101

Bourne FJ, Donnelly CA, Cox DR *et al.* (2007) *Bovine TB: The scientific evidence. A science base for a sustainable policy to control TB in cattle. An Epidemiological Investigation into Bovine Tuberculosis. Final Report of the Independent Scientific Group on Cattle TB.* Defra Publications, London

Brown E, Cooney R and Rogers F (2013) Veterinary guidance on the practical use of the Badger BCG tuberculosis vaccine. *In Practice* **35**, 143–146

Burtscher H and Url A (2007) Evidence of canine distemper and suggestion of preceding parvovirus-myocarditis in an Eurasian badger (*Meles meles*). *Journal of Zoo and Wildlife Medicine* **38**, 139–142

Campbell C, Borman A, Linton C, Bridge P and Johnson E (2006) *Arthroderma olidum*, sp. nov. A new addition to the *Trichophyton terrestre* complex. *Medical Mycology* **44**, 451–459

Carter SP, Chambers MA, Rushton SP *et al.* (2012) BCG vaccination reduces risk of tuberculosis infection in vaccinated badgers and unvaccinated badger cubs. *PLoS ONE* **7(12)**, e49833. doi:10.1371/journal.pone.0049833

Chambers MA, Crawshaw T, Waterhouse S *et al.* (2008) Validation of the BrockTB Stat-Pak Assay for detection of tuberculosis in Eurasian badgers (*Meles meles*) and influence of disease severity on diagnostic accuracy. *Journal of Clinical Microbiology* **46**, 1498–1500

Chambers MA, Gavier-Widen D, Stanley PA and Hewinson RG (2000) Biochemical and haematological parameters associated with tuberculosis in European badgers. *Veterinary Record* **146**, 734–735

Chambers MA, Pressling WA, Cheeseman CL, Clifton-Hadley RS and Hewinson RG (2002) Value of existing serological tests for identifying badgers that shed *Mycobacterium bovis*. *Veterinary Microbiology* **86**, 183–189

Cheeseman CL, Wilesmith JW, Stuart FH and Mallinson PJ (1988) Dynamics of tuberculosis in a naturally infected badger population. *Mammal Review* **18**, 61–72

Clifton-Hadley RS, Wilesmith JW and Stuart FA (1993) *Mycobacterium bovis* in the European badger (*Meles meles*): epidemiological findings in tuberculous badgers from a naturally infected population. *Epidemiology and Infection* **111**, 9–19

Corner LAL (2006) The role of wild animal populations in the epidemiology of tuberculosis in domestic animals: How to assess the risk. *Veterinary Microbiology* **112**, 303–312

Crawshaw TR, Griffiths IB and Clifton-Hadley RS (2008) Comparison of a standard and a detailed post-mortem protocol for detecting *Mycobacterium bovis* in badgers. *Veterinary Record* **163**, 473–477

Cresswell WJ, Harris S, Cheeseman CL and Mallinson PJ (1992) To breed or not to breed: an analysis of the social and density-dependent constraints on the fecundity of female badgers, *Meles meles*. *Philosophical Transactions of the Royal Society of London* **338**, 393–407

Dalley D, Davé D, Lesellier S *et al.* (2008) Development and evaluation of a gamma-interferon assay for tuberculosis in badgers (*Meles meles*). *Tuberculosis* **88**, 235–243

Davies PDO, Barnes PF and Gordon SB (2008) *Clinical Tuberculosis, 4th edn.* Hodder Arnold, London

Delahay RJ, Carter SP, Forrester GJ, Mitchell A and Cheeseman CL (2006) Habitat correlates of group size, bodyweight and reproductive performance in a high-density Eurasian badger (*Meles meles*) population. *Journal of Zoology* **270**, 437–447

Delahay RJ, de Leeuw ANS, Barlow AM, Clifton-Hadley RS and Cheeseman CL (2002) The status of *Mycobacterium bovis* infection in UK wild mammals: A review. *Veterinary Journal* **164**, 90–105

Delahay RJ and Frölich K (2000) Absence of antibodies against canine distemper virus in free-ranging populations of Eurasian badger in Great Britain. *Journal of Wildlife Diseases* **36(3)**, 576–579

Delahay R, Wilson G, Harris S and McDonald DW (2008) Family Mustelidae. In: *Mammals of the British Isles: Handbook, 4th edn*, ed. S Harris and DW Yalden, pp. 425–436. The Mammal Society, Southampton

de Leeuw ANS, Forrester GJ, Spyvee PD, Brash MGI and Delahay RJ (2004) Experimental comparison of ketamine with a combination of ketamine, butorphanol and medetomidine for general anaesthesia of the Eurasian badger (*Meles meles* L.). *Veterinary Journal* **167**, 186–193

Di Cerbo AR, Manfredi MT, Bregoli M, Milone NF and Cova M (2008) Wild carnivores as source of zoonotic helminths in north-eastern Italy. *Helminthologia* **45**, 13–19

Gallagher J and Nelson J (1979) Causes of ill health and natural death in badgers in Gloucestershire. *Veterinary Record* **105**, 546–551

Hancox M (1980) Parasites and infectious diseases of the Eurasian badger (*Meles meles* L.): a review. *Mammal Review* **10(4)**, 151–162

Jenkins HE, Morrison WI, Cox DR *et al.* (2008) The prevalence, distribution and severity of detectable pathological lesions in badgers naturally infected with *Mycobacterium bovis*. *Epidemiology and Infection* **136**, 1350–1361

King D (2007) Bovine tuberculosis in cattle and badgers. A report by the Chief Scientific Adviser, Sir David King. http://webarchive.nationalarchives.gov.uk/20130123162956/http://www.defra.gov.uk/animalh/tb/pdf/badgersreport-king.pdf

Kruuk H and Parish T (1982) Factors affecting population size, group size and territory size of the European badger (*Meles meles*). *Journal of Zoology (London)* **196**, 31–39

Little TW, Stevens AE and Hathaway SC (1987) Serological studies of British leptospiral isolates of the Sejroe serogroup. III. The distribution of leptospires of the Sejroe serogroup in the British Isles. *Epidemiology and Infection* **99**, 117–126

Lloyd S and Smith J (2001) Activity of toltrazuril and diclazuril against *Ispospora* species in kittens and puppies. *Veterinary Record* **148**, 509–511

Macdonald DW, Anwar M, Newman C, Woodroffe R and Johnson PJ (1999) Inter-annual differences in the age-related prevalences of *Babesia* and *Trypanosoma* parasites of European badgers (*Meles meles*). *Journal of Zoology* **247**, 65–70

Macdonald DW, Harmsen BJ, Johnson PJ and Newman C (2004) Increasing frequency of bite wounds with increasing population density in Eurasian badgers, *Meles meles*. *Animal Behaviour* **67**, 745–751

Macdonald DW and Newman C (2002) Population dynamics of badgers (*Meles meles*) in Oxfordshire UK: Numbers, density and cohort life histories, and a possible role of climate change in population growth. *Journal of Zoology* **256**, 121–138

Mahmood KH, Rook GA, Stanford JL, Stuart FA and Pritchard DG (1987) The immunological consequences of challenge with bovine tubercle bacilli in badgers (*Meles meles*). *Epidemiology and Infection* **98**, 155–163

Mahmood KH, Stanford JL, Machins S *et al.* (1988) The haematological values of European badgers (*Meles meles*) in health and in the course of tuberculosis infection. *Epidemiology and Infection* **101**, 231–237

McCarthy G, Shiel R, O'Rourke L *et al.* (2009) Bronchoalveolar lavage cytology from captive badgers. *Veterinary Clinical Pathology* **38**, 381–387

McLaren GW, Thornton PD, Newman C *et al.* (2005) The use and assessment of ketamine-medetomidine-butorphanol combinations for field anaesthesia in wild European badgers (*Meles meles*). *Veterinary Anaesthesia and Analgesia* **32**, 367–372

Muirhead RH, Gallagher J and Burn KJ (1974) Tuberculosis in wild badgers in Gloucestershire: epidemiology. *Veterinary Record* **95**, 552–555

Mullineaux E and Kidner P (2011) Managing public demand for badger rehabilitation in an area of England with endemic tuberculosis. *Veterinary Microbiology* **151**, 205–208

Munro R (2014) *Pilot badger culls in Somerset and Gloucestershire. Report by the Independent Expert Panel.* Defra Publications, London

Neal EG and Cheeseman C (1996) *Badgers.* T & AD Poyser Natural History, London

Newman C, Buesching CD and MacDonald DW (2004) First report of *Cheyletiella parasitovorax* infestation in the Eurasian badger (*Meles meles*). *Veterinary Record* **155**, 180–181

Newman C, MacDonald DW and Anwar MA (2000) Coccidiosis in the European badger, *Meles meles* in Wytham Woods: infection and consequences for growth and survival. *Parasitology* **123**, 133–142

Odening K, Stolte M, Walter G, Bockhardt I and Jakob W (1994) Sarcocysts (*Sarcocystis sp.*: Sporozoa) in the European badger, *Meles meles*. *Parasitology* **108**, 421–424

Peirce MA and Neal C (1974a) *Trypanosoma (megatryparum) pestania* in British badgers (*Meles meles*). *International Journal of Parasitology* **4**, 439–440

Peirce MA and Neal C (1974b) Piroplasmosis in British badgers (*Meles meles*). *Veterinary Record* **94**, 493–494

Riordan P, Delahay RJ, Cheeseman C, Johnson PJ and Macdonald DW (2011) Culling-induced changes in badger (*Meles meles*) behaviour, social organisation and the epidemiology of bovine tuberculosis. *PLoS ONE* **6(12)**, e28904. doi:10.1371/journal. pone.0028904

Rogers LM, Cheeseman CL, Mallinson PJ and Clifton-Hadley R (1997) The demography of a high-density badger (*Meles meles*) population in the west of England. *Journal of Zoology* **242**, 705–728

Roper T (2010) *Badger.* The New Naturalist Library, Harper Collins, London

Salt GFH and Little TWA (1977) Leptospires isolated from wild mammals caught in the south west of England. *Research in Veterinary Science* **22**, 126–127

Sleeman P and Kelly T (1997) Parasites and diseases of Irish badgers (*Meles meles*). *Small Carnivore Conservation* **17**, 20–21

Thoen CO, Steel JH and Gilsdorf MJ (eds) (2008) *Mycobacterium bovis infection in animals and humans, 2nd edn*. Blackwell Publishing, Ames, Iowa

Tuyttens FAM, Macdonald DW, Rogers LM, Cheeseman CL and Roddam AW (2000) Comparative study on the consequences of culling badgers (*Meles meles*) on biometrics, population dynamics and movement. *Journal of Animal Ecology* **69**, 567–580

Winnacker H, Walker NJ, Brash MGI, MacDonald JA and Delahay RJ (2008) Haematological and biochemical measurements in a population of wild Eurasian badgers (*Meles meles*). *Veterinary Record* **162**, 551–555

Specialist organizations and useful contacts

See also Appendix 1

APHA Starcross (for bTB blood testing)
Staplake Mount, Starcross, Exeter, Devon EX6 8PE, UK
Tel: 01626 891121; Fax: 01626 891766
Email: starcross@apha.gsi.gov.uk

Badger Trust (for general badger information)
P.O. Box 708, East Grinstead RH19 2WN, UK
Tel: 08458 287878
Email: enquiries@badgertrust.org.uk
www.badger.org.uk

Department for Environment, Food and Rural Affairs (approved disinfectants list)
http://disinfectants.defra.gov.uk/Default.aspx?Module=ApprovalsList_SI

Royal Society for the Prevention of Cruelty to Animals
www.rspca.org.uk

Secret World Wildlife Rescue
New Road, Highbridge, Somerset TA9 3PZ
Tel: 01278 783250 (daytime) or 07717 651515 (emergencies)
www.secretworld.org

Scottish Badgers
Email: info@scottishbadgers.org.uk
www.scottishbadgers.org.uk

Chapter 18

Otters

Vic Simpson and David Couper

Otters belong to the subfamily Lutrinae in the family Mustelidae. There are 13 species in the world but the Eurasian otter (*Lutra lutra*) is the only species native to the British Isles (Figure 18.1). Two other species, the Asian small-clawed otter (*Aonyx cinerea*) and the American river otter (*Lontra canadensis*), are commonly kept in captivity and, as they occasionally escape, they too may be presented to the veterinary surgeon (veterinarian) in the UK as a 'wild' animal.

In the late 1950s and early 1960s the otter hunts in England and Wales observed a sudden and dramatic crash in the population of otters. This led to almost immediate curtailment of hunting, followed by a ban in 1977, but there was no apparent improvement in numbers. Later studies provided circumstantial evidence that suggested that the crash was due to organochlorine pesticides or/and polychlorinated biphenyls (PCBs). These compounds were progressively banned or withdrawn and a study during the late 1980s and 1990s demonstrated a marked decline in pesticide and PCB residues in otter tissues (Simpson *et al.*, 2000). At the same time there was a strong population recovery, with otters spreading eastwards from their strongholds in south-west England and Wales, and otters are increasingly being submitted for veterinary attention.

Although the majority of otters submitted for post-mortem examination are the result of road traffic accidents (Simpson, 1997; Simpson *et al.*, 2011), in the authors' experience most of the otters submitted for veterinary treatment either have septic bite wounds or are abandoned or orphaned cubs suffering from exposure, dehydration and starvation. Occasionally the bite wounds are due to attack by domestic dogs, but the great majority are the result of intraspecific fighting (Simpson, 2006).

Ecology and biology

The Eurasian otter is essentially a solitary animal. An adult male (dog) may have a territory of up to 25 miles of waterway and within this area there may be two or three smaller territories occupied by breeding females (bitches) and their young (cubs). Otters mark their territory by depositing faeces (spraints) on features such as prominent stones and tree roots, and also by urine marking. The boundaries of the males' territories overlap and are continuously disputed. A post-mortem study of otters found dead in England and Wales between 1998 and 2003, however, showed that bite wounds from intraspecific aggression were equally common in both sexes (Simpson, 2006).

Otters are seldom seen, spending much of their time during the day resting up in a den (holt) or under bankside vegetation. Their tendency to be shy and nocturnal is probably a reflection of persecution by humans; in some areas (e.g. the Western Isles) they may be diurnal and relatively trusting. As the otter population expands, they are also being reported with increasing frequency in busy towns and cities in England.

The otter is essentially a fish eater (see Figure 18.1) and is therefore seldom found far from water. In England and Wales it is found mostly on freshwater systems, but in some areas, notably the west of Scotland, it inhabits the coast and feeds on marine species. Although otters do come into conflict with fishermen, particularly when they take salmonids or valuable carp (Cyprinidae), the preferred prey are eels (Anguilliformes) and, at certain times of the year, frogs (Anura). Otters occasionally eat birds and small mammals but they do not normally eat carrion.

Anatomy and physiology

The otter is a typical mustelid with short legs, an elongated head and a muscular neck of almost equal thickness that runs smoothly into the long body. There is little free skin over the neck and this makes the animal difficult to 'scruff'. These are important points to consider when trying to restrain otters, as they are powerful agile animals and can inflict severe bites. A mature dog will weigh around 7.5–10 kg, a bitch around 5–7 kg, with respective overall lengths of around 110–120 cm and 100–105 cm.

The eyes are set well forward in the skull and are small, possibly because otters do not rely as heavily on sight as

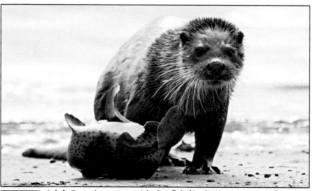

18.1 Adult Eurasian otter with dogfish (*Scyliorhinus canicula*).
(Courtesy of B Couper)

on some of their other senses. There are groups of long sensory bristles, called vibrissae, on the muzzle and cheek, above the eye and on the elbows; they form an almost complete circle around the anterior part of the body and are believed to be important as tactile organs where visibility is bad, particularly in the location of prey. The ear pinnae are small and rounded.

The feet are well adapted for swimming, with webs between all five toes. The front feet are larger and have longer toenails than those on the back. The coat is adapted for immersion, with a short outer coat and a dense undercoat that traps air. As with all mustelids, there are large scent glands either side of the anus. Otters are sexed as for domestic dogs except that in the male the penis does not protrude from the contour of the body. Only the tip of the prepuce is visible and, as a result, immature males with undeveloped scrotum and testes are sometimes mistaken for females. As in the domestic dog the penis has a baculum (or os penis). In the bitch there are usually four nipples but they tend to be very inconspicuous unless she is lactating; even then, it is often only the caudal pair that are active. The dentition is as follows (Harris, 1968) (with temporary dentition in parentheses):

$$2 \times \left\{ I\ \frac{3\ (3)}{3\ (3)}\ C\ \frac{1\ (1)}{1\ (1)}\ P\ \frac{4\ (1)}{3\ (2)}\ M\ \frac{1\ (1)}{2\ (0)} \right\} = 36\ (24)$$

The roots of the second lower incisors are set back, giving the impression of overcrowding, but this is normal (Figure 18.2). Eruption times are shown in Figure 18.3.

Much of the internal anatomy is typical of carnivores and has been summarized elsewhere (Simpson, 1997). The thyroid glands are unlike those in other mustelids. They are long, flat and tapering, usually with no isthmus, and are closely applied to the trachea. There is no cervical thymus but in healthy animals there is normally a bilobed cardiac thymus. The heart is unusually globular, with a thick-walled left ventricle and a much thinner right ventricle. Care should be taken not to interpret this as ventricular hypertrophy. The lungs resemble those of a

badger (*Meles meles*), with two lobes on the left, three on the right and an intermediate lobe that is also served by the right bronchus. The seven-lobed liver is similar to a dog's, but there are both common hepatic and cystic bile ducts, linked by a network of anastomoses, which join the duodenum adjacent to the pancreatic ducts. Unlike other British mustelids, the otter's kidneys are multilobular (see Figure 18.12) and more resemble those of a bovine or a cetacean.

Reproduction

Female otters do not breed until they are around 2 years of age and they produce no more than one litter a year, typically comprising two to three cubs. Cubs may be born during any month and it is thought that this is possible because, based on observations in captivity, otters appear to be continuously polyoestrous. However, studies on wild otters in Norway and also in south-west England suggest that they may be induced ovulators, or have periods of anoestrus. As far as is known, delayed implantation does not occur, although it does take place in the American river otter. Some data on reproduction and development are shown in Figure 18.3.

The cubs are born in a den, or holt, and are blind but with hair. They double their bodyweight every 10 days for the first 3 weeks and gain around 300 g every 10 days after that, weighing around 3 kg at 100 days (Reuther, 1999). They start to emerge from the holt at about 8–12 weeks, which coincides with weaning. An important feature, relevant to rehabilitation, is that the cubs then remain dependent on their mother until they are 10–12 months of age. It is believed that the dog plays no part in their rearing.

Stage/development indicator	Time
Oestrous cycle (captive)	45–50 days[a]
Oestrus duration	14 days[a]
Gestation period	61–63 days[bc]
Litter size	2–3 on average
Birthweight (captive)	100 g approx.[d]
Eyes open	30–35 days[e]
Permanent incisors erupt	13 weeks approx.[e]
Permanent canines erupt	15 weeks approx.[e]

18.3 Reproduction and development in the otter.
([a]Wayre, 1979; [b]Stephens, 1957; [c]Mason and Macdonald, 1986; [d]Reuther, 1999; [e]Heggberget, 1996)

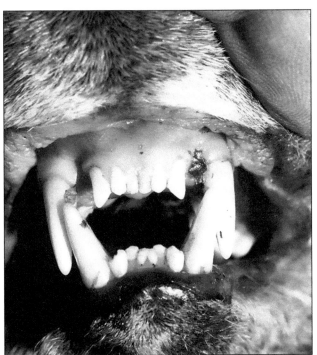

18.2 View showing staggered alignment of lower incisors. This is normal.
(© Vic Simpson)

Life expectancy

Although otters in the wild may live as long as 15 years, this is unusual and most die in the first few years. A study in the Shetlands showed that the life expectancy for a 1-year-old otter was 3.14 years and a similar study on specimens from mainland Scotland and England gave a figure of around 2.75 years (Kruuk, 1995). For otters in south-west England, the life expectancy may be even lower as a study between 1988 and 1994 gave a mean age at death of 2 years (Simpson, 1997). These figures should be interpreted with care as a high proportion of the otters examined in such studies are road traffic casualties and it is likely that immature animals are over-represented. There is little evidence of infectious disease in wild otters and the principal cause of natural mortality is intraspecific aggression (Simpson, 2006).

Capture, handling and transportation

Otters are difficult to handle safely on account of their muscular neck, lack of an obvious scruff and their powerful bite. During the capture of healthy otters, particular attention is paid to keeping the process brief, to avoid hyperthermia and to minimize trauma to the oral cavity (Spelman, 1999). Otter casualties are often very debilitated but due care should still be exercised during their capture and handling.

Otters can be manoeuvred into a pet carrier (ideally a pre-weighed crush cage) using pig boards, nets or dog-graspers. As the otter's head is the same width as its neck, it is necessary when using dog-graspers to involve one, or both, of the forelegs in the noose. Dog-graspers can, however, result in injuries to the teeth and their use should be avoided where possible.

Although otters in Britain do not normally carry any significant zoonotic infections, appropriate protective clothing should be worn during handling. Using gauntlets or a thick towel for protection, young cubs may be picked up with the thumb and fingers placed around the neck and chest, from the dorsal aspect (see Figure 18.6). This should not be attempted with adult otters unless they are totally collapsed. Transport in a pre-weighed crush cage will facilitate intramuscular injection of sedative prior to handling of these animals if necessary. A towel should be placed over the cage to minimize stress.

Examination and clinical assessment for rehabilitation

An accurate history taken from the finder, including details of the otter's behaviour and the exact location where it was found, will assist the examination and allow the animal to be returned to its territory if appropriate (see 'Release'). The aim of the examination is to assess the suitability of the otter for rehabilitation and release. To have allowed capture in the first place, adult otter casualties are generally severely debilitated and have a correspondingly guarded prognosis; a 79% mortality rate has been reported for injured adult animals at an otter rehabilitation centre in Scotland (Green and Green, 1998). Although the immediate prognosis for orphaned cubs is generally considerably more favourable, their rehabilitation is a long process, lasting a year or more, and requires specialized facilities. With these points in mind, euthanasia should be considered if successful rehabilitation is unlikely (see Chapter 4).

Otters are best examined in a quiet and escape-proof room. If the carrier has not been pre-weighed, the weight of the otter plus the carrier should be recorded, and the weight of the carrier subtracted from this after removal of the otter. Note should be taken of any discharges or abnormal faeces present in the carrier. Ideally, behaviour and locomotion are observed prior to examination in the hand, although in the confines of a veterinary practice this is generally only practical with cubs. In a confined area it is common for the animal to keep its body pressed flat to the floor whilst moving. Sedation or anaesthesia is often required to facilitate examination in adult animals, and an appraisal of the otter's general condition will determine what stabilization is appropriate beforehand.

The otter should be examined systematically, bearing in mind common findings that may be overlooked, such as bite wounds to the genitals. Particular attention should be paid to the teeth. Although the prognosis for those animals presenting with septicaemia subsequent to fractured teeth is poor, it may be advisable to extract the affected teeth; it may also be necessary to extract teeth damaged during the capture process. The significance of any injuries should be assessed by considering the consequences to the otter of loss of function of the affected area. Whilst these may be obvious, with severely traumatized limbs for example, other effects may be more subtle (see also Chapter 4). For instance, damage to the vibrissae may affect the otter's ability to hunt, as would significant damage to the tail. Bite wounds to the genital area resulting in castration would affect a dog otter's ability to defend its territory and fractures to the baculum could affect urine flow, whilst a fractured pelvis in a bitch may lead to subsequent dystocia. Euthanasia should be considered for all animals that are severely compromised.

Diagnostic techniques

Ancillary diagnostic tests may be performed in conscious cubs or very debilitated adults but generally require the use of sedation or anaesthesia. Blood samples for haematology and biochemistry are most readily taken from the jugular vein, with the animal placed in dorsal recumbency. Shaving or clipping of an otter's fur for venous access or any other reason should be kept to a minimum; if the guard hairs are significantly disrupted in such a way that the undercoat can become wet, hypothermia can develop (Spelman, 1999). Clipping is not necessary if liberal amounts of surgical spirit are applied. The haematological and biochemical characteristics of Eurasian otters collected from animals in a Scottish rehabilitation centre are listed in Figure 18.4. Similar results were obtained from 33 wild caught otters in Spain (Fernandez-Moran et al., 2001b). The other diagnostic modalities used in companion animals, such as

Variable (units)	Mean (SD)	Reference interval
Haematology		
Red blood cell (RBC) count (x 10^{12}/l)	7.01 (1)	4.8–9.11
Haemoglobin (g/dl)	15.7 (3.62)	7.6–20.5
Packed cell volume (PCV) (l/l)	0.53 (0.12)	0.28–0.74
Mean corpuscular volume (MCV) (fl)	75.8 (13.1)	46.7–96.6
Mean corpuscular haemoglobin (MCH) ((pg) per cell)	22.4 (4.2)	12.8–28
Mean corpuscular haemoglobin concentration (MCHC) (g/dl)	29.4 (2.27)	25.2–33.8
Platelet count (x 10^9/l)	676.8 9 (403)	43–1983
Reticulocytes (% RBC)	1.77 (2)	0.2–9.8
White blood cell (WBC) count (x 10^9/l)	6.44 (2.77)	3.03–13.9
Neutrophils (x 10^9/l)	3.99 (2.62)	1.62–12.1
Lymphocytes (x 10^9/l)	1.66 (0.84)	0.59–4.61
Monocytes (x 10^9/l)	0.2 (0.16)	0–0.62
Eosinophils (x 10^9/l)	0.57 (0.38)	0.07–1.73
Basophils (x 10^9/l)	0.016 (0.04)	0–0.2

18.4 Haematological and biochemical data from 41 and 47 otters, respectively, of both sexes and all ages. (continues) ▶
(Lewis et al., 1998)

Variable (units)	Mean (SD)	Reference interval
Biochemistry		
Calcium (mmol/l)	2.2 (0.13)	1.94–2.45
Inorganic phosphate (mmol/l)	2.51 (0.59)	1.58–4.5
Sodium (mmol/l)	150.2 (2.75)	145–159.3
Potassium (mmol/l)	4.77 (0.44)	3.68–5.77
Bicarbonate (mmol/l)	22.7 (3.93)	14.2–32
Creatinine (mol/l)	67.5 (23.5)	33–128
Urea (mmol/l)	11.4 (2.79)	7.42–22.6
Total bilirubin (mol/l)	1.13 (1.51)	0–4.5
Cholesterol (mmol/l)	2.38 (0.47)	1.26–3.57
Creatine kinase (IU/l)	434.7 (287.1)	183–1844
Alkaline phosphatase (ALP) (IU/l)	43.2 (24.3)	10–104
Alanine aminotransferase (ALT) (IU/l)	82.8 (46.6)	19–296
Aspartate aminotransferase (AST) (IU/l)	132.9 (75.5)	45–459
Gamma-glutamyl transferase (GGT) (IU/l)	20.5 (9.02)	4–45
Total protein (g/l)	63.2 (6.41)	48–77
Globulin (g/l)	30.3 (g/l)	19–44
Albumin (g/l)	32.5 (2.44)	27–38.2
Fibrinogen (g/l)	2.61 (1.21)	0–5.7

18.4 (continued) Haematological and biochemical data from 41 and 47 otters, respectively, of both sexes and all ages. (Lewis *et al.*, 1998)

radiography and ultrasonography, can also be used to investigate pathology in otters. Survey radiography is useful, and orthogonal views should be taken. Fur clipping for ultrasonography should be kept to a minimum. Faecal examination, by direct smear and flotation (see Chapter 10), may reveal the presence of parasites, and is easily performed as part of a health check.

Euthanasia

Euthanasia is best performed under anaesthesia. Pentobarbital (150 mg/kg) may be administered intravenously in the jugular or cephalic vein. Alternatively, the intracardiac or intrahepatic routes may be used (in an anaesthetized animal, although this will reduce the value of the carcass for post-mortem examination.

First aid and short-term hospitalization

The general principles applied to the first aid of companion animals should be adhered to, remembering that otter casualties may have been ill for some time prior to presentation and are often cold, dehydrated and in shock (see also Chapter 5).

First aid

Supplementary heat may be provided to hypothermic animals with a ceramic heat lamp, or cubs may be placed in an incubator. A warmed oral electrolyte solution may be given with a bottle and teat to mildly dehydrated cubs (at the rate of 5% bodyweight per feed) if they are sucking well (Myers, 2011), or they may be injected with sterile isotonic solutions subcutaneously between the shoulder blades. Intravenous fluid therapy is not easily administered in adult otters unless the animal is totally collapsed. However, an intravenous fluid bolus may be given during anaesthesia using the cephalic vein, and intraperitoneal and intraosseous injection routes may be used in more severely dehydrated or shocked individuals (see Chapter 5). The feeding by gavage of cubs, following rehydration, has been described (Myers, 2011) and has proved a useful technique in this author's hands (DC) for reviving individuals that are too weak to suckle. Wounds should be (minimally) clipped and lavaged, and appropriate analgesia should be provided where injuries are present (see 'Anaesthesia and analgesia'). Broad-spectrum antibiotic therapy (see Figure 18.14) should be started in otters with infected wounds and revised if necessary on receipt of culture and sensitivity results. Although bandages are not easy to manage in the conscious animal, Kollias (1999) reported that American river otters did not interfere significantly with bandages applied to the limbs.

Short-term hospitalization

In the first instance, otters may be housed in an escape-proof kennel. A walk-in kennel is most suitable, as it is not easy to handle or manage these animals in a confined space. They should be kept somewhere quiet away from domestic dogs, which are perceived as predators. Towels placed on the floor of the kennel allow them to rub and clean their fur. The animal should be provided with somewhere to hide, such as an upturned dog bed or cardboard box, and a towel should be placed over the door of the kennel to reduce visual stimuli and so minimize stress. Clean drinking water in a stable container should be available at all times.

Anaesthesia and analgesia

Anaesthesia is frequently required to facilitate the examination of otters and to carry out ancillary diagnostic tests and surgical interventions. As casualties are often seriously compromised, they present a particularly high anaesthetic risk and stabilization should be carried out beforehand wherever possible.

A variety of injectable agents have been used successfully in Eurasian otters, including ketamine in combination with benzodiazepines (Kuiken, 1988) or medetomidine (Fernandez-Moran *et al.*, 2001a) (Figure 18.5). The use of ketamine on its own has been associated with the development of hyperthermia (Reuther, 1983; Reuther and Brandes, 1984) and is no longer recommended. Intramuscular injections can be administered in the quadriceps or lumbar muscles, with the animal restrained in a crush cage if required.

Induction of anaesthesia with volatile inhalational agents has also been described (Spelman *et al.*, 1993); following appropriate premedication; isoflurane or sevoflurane in oxygen can be administered to debilitated adults via facemask, and cubs can be anaesthetized in an induction chamber. Whichever technique is used for induction, endotracheal intubation should be carried out (see Figure 18.9b) and the animal maintained on oxygen and an inhalational agent if required.

Drug	Dosage	Notes
Anaesthetic combinations		
Ketamine (K) + diazepam (D)[a]	18 mg/kg (K) + 0.5 mg/kg (D) i.m.	Good relaxation Risk of hyperthermia with ketamine
Ketamine (K) + midazolam (Mi)[b]	10–12 mg/kg (K) + 0.25–0.5 mg/kg (Mi) i.m.	Rapid induction 20–30 minutes anaesthesia Smooth recovery Risk of hyperthermia with ketamine
Ketamine (K) + medetomidine (M)[c]	5 mg/kg (K) + 50 µg/kg (M) i.m.	Rapid induction Good relaxation Can be reversed with atipamezole at dosage of 250 µg/kg i.m. Risk of hyperthermia with ketamine Risk of bradycardia and respiratory depression with medetomidine
Isoflurane/ sevoflurane in oxygen		Used for induction via face mask in cubs and debilitated adults following appropriate premedication Used for maintenance following intubation
Analgesics		
Meloxicam	0.2 mg/kg s.c., orally q24h (initial dose) 0.1 mg/kg s.c., orally q24h (maintenance dose)	Effective NSAID Oral preparation readily consumed in food
Carprofen	2–4 mg/kg i.v., s.c., orally q24h	Effective NSAID
Butorphanol	0.2–0.55 mg/kg i.v., i.m., s.c. q4h	Generally used as part of pre-anaesthetic medication
Buprenorphine	0.02 mg/kg i.v., i.m., s.c. q6h	Control of mild to moderate pain
Pethidine	2–10 mg/kg i.m., s.c. q1–2h	Control of mild to moderate pain
Morphine	0.5 mg/kg i.v., i.m. q2–4h	Control of moderate to severe pain

18.5 Anaesthetic and analgesic dose rates for use in otters. Note: the dose rates listed are those used in healthy animals.

([a] Kuiken, 1988; [b] Spelman, 1999; [c] Fernandez-Moran *et al.*, 2001a)

Respiratory depression can be expected in all anaesthetized otters, particularly during induction with injectable agents (Spelman, 1999). Kollias and Abou-Madi (2007) suggested that hypoventilation and subsequent hypoxaemia may be a primary cause of mortality in anaesthetized otters and recommended intermittent positive pressure ventilation. Monitoring of cardiac and respiratory function should be carried out throughout anaesthesia (see Chapter 6). Postoperatively, placing the animal in a quiet dark area will facilitate a smooth recovery, during which appropriate measures should be taken to maintain body temperature.

Analgesia should be considered in all animals with injuries, for welfare reasons and to ensure a rapid return to normal feeding and behaviour. Both non-steroidal anti-inflammatory drugs (NSAIDs) and opioids may be used at the dose rates used in domestic dogs (see Figure 18.5). Contraindications to the use of certain drugs, such as dehydration or pregnancy, should be borne in mind.

Specific conditions

Trauma

Bite wounds

Many otters submitted for veterinary attention are suffering from bite wounds, mostly to the face (Figures 18.6 and 18.7), the feet (where toes are often amputated), and around the anus and genitals (Simpson, 1997; Simpson, 2006). In most cases these are the result of fighting with other otters. Although some bite wounds are obvious, many are not and are easily overlooked, particularly those around the perineum (Figure 18.8). Their presence should be ascertained by close inspection and may be suggested by the presence of blood, pus or matted fur. However, in

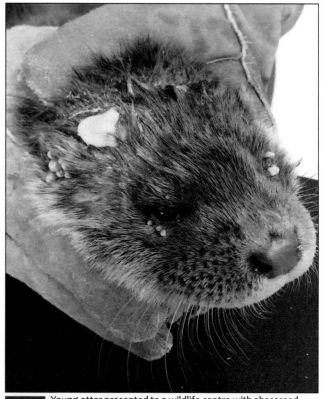

18.6 Young otter presented to a wildlife centre with abscessed wounds to the head, likely to be associated with intraspecific attack; there is also a heavy tick burden.

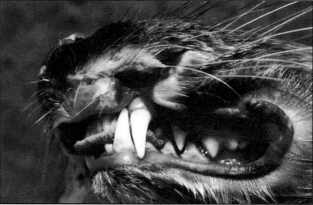

18.7 Healing bite wounds to the face of a young adult otter caused by intraspecific aggression. Note also the loss of lower incisors. The erosion of enamel on the anterior aspect of the lower canine is a common finding and of no clinical significance. This otter also had severe bite wounds around the perineum.
(© Vic Simpson)

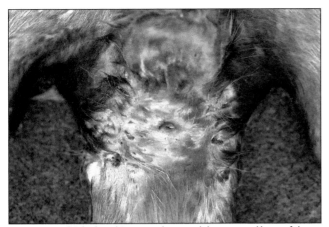

18.8 Multiple deep bite wounds around the anus and base of the tail caused by intraspecific aggression. In many cases the genital organs are also bitten.
(© Vic Simpson)

many cases bite wounds are only apparent after the fur has been wet with spirit or warm water and detergent. Bite wounds to the scrotum are common and in extreme cases the otter may have been castrated. Bites to the penis may result in fracture of the baculum and, in one study, 7.5% of 146 bacula examined showed evidence of a fracture (Simpson, 2006). Bite wounds are equally common in females and damage to the vulva can be severe. Apart from intraspecific attack, otters may be bitten by American mink (*Mustela vison*) and, less commonly, by domestic dogs. Dog bites are normally more extensive than otter bites and do not follow the typical pattern but have a random distribution. The skin may not be punctured but, especially where large dogs are involved, there may be internal haemorrhage associated with ruptured organs or fractured ribs (Simpson, 2006).

Secondary bacterial infection of bites is common and infection may track subcutaneously or between muscle layers well away from the puncture wounds. Impression smears from areas of cellulitis or necrosis around bite wounds usually show Gram-positive cocci and often Gram-negative coccobacilli. In addition there may be slender filamentous Gram-negative bacilli resembling *Fusobacterium* spp. (A Patterson and G Foster, personal communication; V Simpson, unpublished data). In a study of bite wounds in otters the predominant bacteria were Lancefield Group C *Streptococcus* sp., mostly *Streptococcus dysgalactiae* subsp. *equisimilis*, followed by Group L and Group G spp. Other commonly recovered bacteria were coliforms, *Staphylococcus* spp., *Aeromonas hydrophila* and *Corynebacterium ulcerans* (Simpson, 2006).

The signs exhibited by an otter with bite wounds may be associated with the location of the injuries. For instance, lameness may be seen if a leg or foot has been bitten, or dyspnoea if the otter has suffered thoracic trauma due to being bitten by a dog. However, these animals often present in a generally collapsed state. Radiography may be used to confirm the presence and extent of internal trauma, such as a fractured baculum as a result of intraspecific fighting, or fractured ribs and pneumothorax with dog bite wounds. Treatment, as a minimum, involves clipping and lavage, fluid therapy, analgesia and antibiotics. Although streptococcal isolates are normally sensitive to penicillin, most bite wounds have mixed bacterial infections and treatment with broad-spectrum antibiotics is therefore preferable (see Figure 18.14). The prognosis depends on the location and extent of injuries, and the degree of debilitation; it is typically

grave. A castrated otter is unlikely to be able to defend a territory in the wild and should be euthanased. A fracture of the baculum may heal, leaving it functional, if distorted. Provided urine flow is not obstructed throughout the healing process, euthanasia may not be necessary.

Missing and fractured incisors and canine teeth are common in otters and in many cases appear to be a result of fighting. Though less frequent, fractures of the cheek teeth occur, especially the carnassials (Figure 18.9a), and these may easily be missed on clinical examination. Fractured teeth, including cheek teeth, are common in road traffic casualties where they are often associated with fractures to the skull and significant lesions elsewhere: such cases carry a guarded prognosis (see Figure 18.9b). Dental radiography will assist with diagnosis, particularly where fractured roots are present. Fractures involving the root often lead to abscess formation, osteomyelitis and septicaemia. An upper carnassial root abscess in an otter is located almost directly below the eye, not anterior to it as in a domestic dog, and the sinus discharges laterally above the gum line into the facial tissues rather than through the skin and therefore the lesion may not be apparent. As with septic bite wounds, dental lesions such as these often prove fatal. A suitable antibiotic, such as clindamycin, should be administered. Fractured teeth or those with a root or gum infection should be removed. The removal of canine teeth does raise ethical concerns regarding the 'fitness' of the animal for release (see Chapter 4); otters with missing canines are, however, known to survive in the wild and, provided an otter is otherwise fit and in good body condition, the loss of a canine alone does not justify euthanasia.

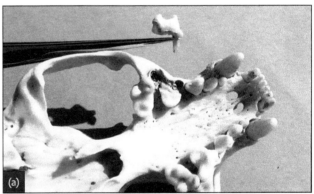

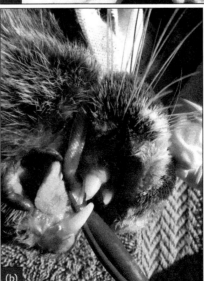

18.9

(a) Transverse fracture of an upper carnassial tooth (PM4) with resulting root abscess. Similar fractures of the lower carnassials (M1) occur but less frequently. (b) An intubated otter showing a shattered upper right canine tooth and loss of skin over the point of the lower jaw. These are highly typical injuries in road casualty otters and are often associated with serious traumatic lesions elsewhere in the body.
(a, © Vic Simpson)

Badly eroded footpads, particularly on the hind feet, are seen in animals that have been in prolonged conflict with another otter. These cases, mostly males, are usually in very poor physical condition and frequently have blackish, tarry material coming from the anus. This is quite distinct from normal spraints, which, although often soft, are formed (see 'Enteric disease'). The prognosis in such cases is poor, and euthanasia may be considered. Apart from bite wounds to the feet, severe cuts to the pads or webs are occasionally seen. Such cases normally require minimal treatment and heal well.

Snare injuries

Otters found caught in wire snares usually have such severe injuries that immediate euthanasia is indicated. In the event that the otter is not so severely injured, it should be taken into captivity and monitored for the development of pressure necrosis for at least a week. Treatment involves appropriate fluid therapy (considering the potential for reperfusion injury), clipping and lavage of the wound, analgesia and broad-spectrum antibiotics, pending the results of in vitro sensitivity tests. For additional information on snare injuries see Chapter 17.

Road traffic collisions

Otters involved in road traffic collisions are frequently killed outright or die shortly after. Those animals that survive should be thoroughly examined, as extensive internal trauma is common. Radiography can be used to confirm the presence of fractures and assess their suitability for repair. Treatment for shock and analgesia will be required and repair of injuries should only be attempted following adequate stabilization. Soft tissue repairs may be performed as in companion animals. Orthopaedic surgery should only be attempted if a full return to function is anticipated; compound fractures and those involving joints carry a grave prognosis. Any pins or plates involved in fracture repair must be removed prior to release. The likelihood of future dystocia in animals with a fractured pelvis, and (with all repairs) the stress involved with repeated interventions and prolonged confinement should be considered.

Infectious diseases
Viral diseases

Viral infections of otters appear to be rare, especially in free-ranging ones. A tentative diagnosis of Aleutian disease was made histologically on an otter from Norfolk (Wells et al., 1989). Canine distemper was diagnosed in two free-living otters in Austria (Loupal et al., 1998) and in captive otters in Germany (Geisel, 1979). Phocine distemper has been implicated in sea otter (Enhydra lutris) mortality in North America (Goldstein et al., 2009). There is a single record of rabies in a free-living otter in Germany (Wilhelm and Vogt, 1981). Feline infectious peritonitis has been suspected in a captive Asian small-clawed otter (Van de Grift, 1976) and canine adenovirus type 1 was shown to be the cause of fatal hepatitis in a captive Eurasian otter in Korea (Park et al., 2007). As these viral diseases are so rarely diagnosed, it is difficult to comment on their impact on wild populations. When diagnosed in otters in a rehabilitation centre the appropriate action in most cases would be euthanasia. Captive otters in zoological collections may be vaccinated against canine distemper and canine

adenovirus type 1. The authors do not consider that vaccination is appropriate for otters undergoing rehabilitation and release in the UK.

Bacterial diseases

There is little evidence of significant bacterial disease at population level in wild otters and most bacterial infections diagnosed in otters have arisen from post-mortem examinations. Mycobacterium avium subsp. avium was shown to be the cause of massive mesenteric lymph node lesions in an otter in Scotland (A Patterson, personal communication) and in 2009 the first confirmed case of Mycobacterium bovis in an otter was reported in Northern Ireland (Lee et al., 2009). The isolate was shown to be the same spoligotype (SB0140) as that affecting cattle in the area. However, no cases of tuberculosis were seen during a post-mortem study of 690 otters, mostly from south-west England where tuberculosis is common in badgers (Simpson, 2009). Tuberculosis could be suspected where an otter is presented in debilitated condition, especially if showing respiratory distress. Confirmation can be difficult but radiographic examination would be appropriate followed by microscopic examination of Ziehl–Neelsen-stained tracheal aspirates and/or cultural examination. Infected animals should be euthanased.

Other bacterial diseases occasionally recorded are pseudotuberculosis, salmonellosis and listeriosis. In most cases these would appear to be opportunistic infections in otters that were already in poor health. Keymer (1992) reported Yersinia pseudotuberculosis infection in an otter where the cause of death was uncertain. The organism has since been isolated from two otters, one with pleurisy and the other in debilitated condition (V Simpson, unpublished data). Salmonella Binza was recovered from the gut of an otter in Norfolk where Keymer (1992) considered that it could have derived from day-old poultry chicks: chicks were also thought to be the source of S. Enteritidis phage type 6 which caused fatal gastroenteritis in a captive Asian small-clawed otter (V Simpson, unpublished data). S. Enteritidis was also isolated from a free-living otter in Russia (Benkovskii et al., 1973). Other serotypes recorded include S. Dublin, a serotype typically associated with cattle, which caused a fatal septicaemia, S. Ajiobo and S. Typhimurium (DT56), which were isolated from the intestines of two wild otters that died in rehabilitation centres, and S. Ajiobo from one that was found dying on a trout farm (V Simpson, unpublished data). Listeria monocytogenes septicaemia was seen in a sick wild otter and the organism was also isolated in mixed culture from the lungs of a captive otter (V Simpson, unpublished data).

Aeromonas hydrophila was isolated from the heart and lungs of an otter that died from severe adiaspiromycosis (V Simpson and D Gavier-Widen, 2000) and also from the haemorrhagic lungs of an otter that had apparently died after eating toads (V Simpson and B Rule, unpublished data). However, the organism has been isolated from several other cases, mostly from lungs but also other internal organs and bite wounds (V Simpson, unpublished data). As A. hydrophila is ubiquitous in freshwater systems it is possible that in all these cases it was a terminal invader or inhaled contaminant rather than the primary pathogen.

A number of authors have suggested that otters may suffer from leptospirosis (Wayre, 1979; Chanin, 1985), with Keymer (1992) suggesting it may cause jaundice. However histological examination of a large numbers of livers and kidneys from south-west England showed no convincing evidence of leptospirosis (Simpson et al., 2011) and analysis of kidneys from 70 otters by polymerase chain reaction (PCR) assay showed leptospiral DNA in only three: one of these was sequenced and closely resembled *Leptospira interrogans* serogroup *canicola* (Jones, 2003). As yet, there does not appear to be any evidence that leptospirosis is significant in otters in the UK. *Brucella pinnipedialis* was isolated from an otter in Scotland in 1996. However, subsequent cultural and serological testing of more than 350 dead otters throughout the UK failed to isolate the organism and less than 5% were seropositive (Foster *et al.*, 2011). In view of this it appears that otters are rarely infected with *Brucella* spp. Tyzzer's disease, caused by *Clostridium piliforme*, was diagnosed in a cub that died in a rehabilitation centre in Scotland. It showed bilateral corneal oedema and had marked multifocal lesions of hepatic necrosis and petechial haemorrhage (Simpson *et al.*, 2008).

With the exception of salmonellosis, it is unlikely that any of these infections would be diagnosed in the live animal. The choice of antibiotic in a case of salmonellosis would depend on the results of *in vitro* sensitivity tests.

Fungal diseases

Small greyish granulomas, which, especially when mineralized, may resemble those of tuberculosis, are commonly seen in otters' lungs at post-mortem examination (Figure 18.10), and could possibly appear as multifocal radio-densities on thoracic radiography in the live animal. These are due to inhaled spores of the fungus *Emmonsia* sp. and the condition is referred to as adiaspiromycosis. Although severe infections may prove fatal (Simpson and Gavier-Widen, 2000), the condition is normally of little clinical significance and there is no accepted form of treatment.

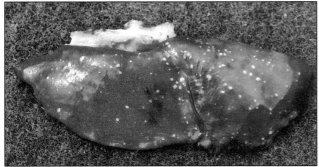

18.10 The left lung of an otter showing numerous lesions suggestive of tuberculosis. However, histopathological examination showed that they are partially mineralized granulomas due to adiaspiromycosis.
(© Vic Simpson)

Parasites

Small numbers of ixodid ticks are occasionally found on otters, mostly on debilitated animals (see Figure 18.6). There do not appear to be any confirmed reports of mange or significant lice infestation in otters.

Although various metazoan parasites have been recorded in otters, in most cases there is little evidence that they cause disease. The most significant is possibly the bile fluke, *Pseudamphistomum truncatum*. This was first described in the UK in otters and American mink in Somerset and Dorset (Simpson *et al.*, 2005); it was later found to be present in other areas, including East Anglia and South Wales (Sherrard-Smith *et al.*, 2009; Simpson *et al.*, 2009). Affected otters have shrunken, thickened gall bladders with liver pathology that ranges from mild bile duct hyperplasia and periportal fibrosis to severe

sclerosing cholangitis, hepatocyte necrosis and bile stasis. Some otters become jaundiced and may lose condition, but none have been shown to have died as a result of fluke infection (Simpson *et al.*, 2009). A second Opisthorchiid, *Metorchis albidus*, was described in 2009 causing similar gall bladder pathology (Sherrard-Smith *et al.*, 2009). Bile fluke infection due to either species could possibly be diagnosed by a zinc flotation test on faeces. Ultrasonography may be useful to assess gall bladder and liver pathology in the live animal. Attempted treatment would only be justified in an otter showing jaundice or raised serum gamma-glutamyl transferase (GGT) levels. Although there do not appear to be any records of attempted treatment in otters, praziquantel-based compounds are likely to be effective.

In North America, infection of the American river otter with the kidney worm *Dioctophyme renale* is not uncommon but, although the parasite has been recorded in Eurasian otters in Europe, the authors are not aware of any records of it in the UK. In a study in Denmark, larvae of the heartworm *Angiostrongylus vasorum* were seen in the lungs of a single otter (Madsen *et al.*, 1999), but this parasite has not been seen in otters in Britain, despite the fact that the infection is common in foxes (*Vulpes vulpes*) and domestic dogs (Simpson, 1996). Otters found dead in coastal areas of Scotland often had the nematode *Pseudoterranova decipiens* and the acanthophalan *Corynosoma strumosum* in their intestines, but there was no evidence that they were of pathogenic significance (Jefferies *et al.*, 1990).

There is little evidence of protozoal diseases. Although toxoplasmosis is a major cause of mortality in sea otters in North America and there is a high prevalence of antibody to *Toxoplasma gondii* in both Eurasian and American river otters (Tocidlowski *et al.*, 1997; Chadwick *et al.*, 2013), there is no evidence that the parasite causes disease in Eurasian otters. Histological examination of more than 140 otters, mostly from south-west England, showed no evidence of toxoplasmosis. One otter had *Sarcocystis* sp. in the external eye muscles, but there was no obvious pathology associated with the infection (Simpson, 1998; 2007).

Other conditions

Eye disease

Blindness was reported to be common in otters in England between 1957 and 1980. One or both eyes were affected, appearing white, but they were not examined by a pathologist and the precise nature of the lesion is uncertain (Williams, 1989). Lenticular cataracts were seen in a case of suspected Aleutian disease in Norfolk (Wells *et al.*, 1989). Unilateral corneal opacity is typically the result of trauma caused by fighting, as is puncture and collapse of the globe (Simpson, 2007). Investigations in south-west England showed histological lesions consistent with retinal dysplasia in approximately 12% of otters and suspected lesions in a further 25%. The cause was not established, but low vitamin A levels following exposure to organochlorine pesticides were suspected (Williams *et al.*, 1998; Simpson, 2007).

Respiratory disease

Otters that have septic bite wounds or a dental abscess are prone to developing a fibrinopurulent pleurisy and pericarditis. They are likely to present in a moribund dyspnoeic state. On post-mortem examination there is often a large amount of reddish-brown fluid in the thoracic cavity together with adhesions, pulmonary congestion, atelectasis, and in some cases, pneumonia. A range of bacteria can be isolated including *Pasteurella multocida*, *Streptococcus canis*, *S. equisimilis* and, less frequently, *Staphylococcus aureus* and *Moraxella* spp. Gram-negative bacilli resembling fusiforms may be seen in stained smears of pleuritic fluid. Treatment of such cases is futile. Dyspnoea due to pleurisy should be differentiated from that arising as a result of a road traffic collision; traffic casualties are likely to be in better body condition, unless suffering from concurrent problems. Radiography will help confirm the presence of internal injuries.

Inhalation pneumonia occurs in cubs that are being hand-reared, probably due to inhalation of milk, but also occurs in adults due to inhalation of plant material (V Simpson, A Philbey, unpublished data). Treatment of cubs may be attempted with appropriate broad-spectrum antibiotics (pending the results of *in vitro* sensitivity testing of a bronchoalveolar lavage) and supportive care.

Cardiac and vascular disease

An unusual lesion observed post-mortem in several otters was the formation of a large fibrinous plaque adherent to the endocardial surface of the right atrium. In some cases it extended back in to the caudal vena cava or through the tricuspid valve in to the right ventricle (V Simpson and A Tomlinson, unpublished data). The affected otters were all animals that had suffered severe septic bite wounds or dental abscesses and it is thought the lesions result from a bacterial, probably streptococcal, septicaemia. Arteriosclerosis involving the cranial mesenteric artery and adjacent abdominal aorta has been observed in a number of aged otters (Molenaar and Simpson, 2006; A Philbey, personal communication). The lumen of the mesenteric artery may be almost totally occluded by subintimal calcified deposits. In some cases other vessels, including the gastrosplenic artery, are affected and it would seem likely that the impaired blood flow to abdominal viscera would be of clinical significance.

Neurological disease

Incoordination: Wild otters in Ireland and England have been observed showing signs of incoordination or disorientation and possibly blindness (Wells *et al.*, 1989; Mason and O'Sullivan, 1992). However, histopathological examinations of brains were either not carried out or no lesions were seen and the aetiology remains obscure. Lesions of leucoencephalopathy affecting cerebrum, cerebellum and medulla were seen in a blind and ataxic otter in Cornwall. The otter had been submitted after being hit by a vehicle and it was thought the lesions could have resulted from a blow to the head (S Scholes, M King and V Simpson, unpublished data).

Hydrocephalus: Otters, especially cubs, showing signs of incoordination should be examined carefully for evidence of hydrocephalus, including radiographic examination (Green and Green, 1998). The cranium may be visibly rounded (Figure 18.11) and on post-mortem examination there is marked thinning of the cerebral hemispheres, flattening of the sulci and prolapse of the cerebellum through the foramen magnum. The prognosis in these cases is bad and euthanasia is recommended.

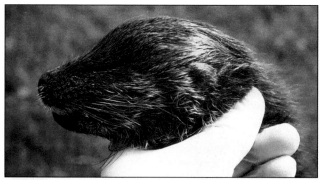

18.11 Otter cub suffering from hydrocephalus. Note the markedly domed cranium. The animal was showing signs of ataxia.
(© Vic Simpson)

Mercury poisoning: Chronic mercury poisoning may cause brain damage and has been suspected in otters in Shetland (Kruuk and Conroy, 1991). High tissue levels of mercury have also been recorded in otters in England (Mason *et al.*, 1986). Unfortunately, brains were not examined histologically in either case.

Renal disease

Urolithiasis is a well recognized condition of otters in zoological collections, especially in Asian small-clawed otters (Calle, 1988), but it also occurs in free-living populations, including the Eurasian otter (Keymer *et al.*, 1981; Weber, 2001, Simpson *et al.*, 2011). The prevalence varies greatly according to geographic region: for example, around 32% positive in Scotland, 16% in Denmark and 10% in south-west England (Weber, 2001; Simpson *et al.*, 2011).

In Eurasian otters the calculi are normally composed of ammonium urate (Keymer *et al.*, 1981; Weber 2001; Simpson *et al.*, 2011), whereas in Asian small-clawed otters they are typically calcium oxalate. The aetiology is unknown, but in the case of Eurasian otters it is thought that the otter's high purine, fish-based diet may predispose to the formation of calculi (Weber 2001; Ruff *et al.*, 2007). Keymer *et al.* (1981) suggested vitamin A deficiency as a possible cause, but Simpson (1998) found no evidence to support this hypothesis. A study of otters in south-west England (Simpson *et al.*, 2011) showed that otters with renal calculi frequently had enlarged adrenal glands. The results also suggested a possible link between an increased prevalence of renal calculi and an increase in intraspecific aggression in a rapidly expanding population.

Renal calculi may be observed during radiographic or post-mortem examination (Figure 18.12). They vary greatly in shape and size; larger calculi are 15 mm or more in length and occur mostly in the calyces, whilst the smallest ones are 1 mm or less and are seen mostly in the renal medulla. It would appear that the calculi have never been observed in ureters or the urethra and only once in a bladder (Simpson *et al.*, 2011). Kidneys containing large calculi often show cystic distension of one or more lobules and, in the most severe cases, hydronephrosis with multiple lobules reduced to fluid filled cysts that have no remaining parenchyma. In rare cases the cysts may rupture. However, despite the often striking lesions, there is little evidence that renal calculi are of clinical significance in free-living otters. The presence and extent of lesions may be confirmed by ultrasonography and intravenous urography and their effects on renal function assessed by performing biochemistry and measuring the urine protein to creatinine ratio, although there is no accepted form of treatment if renal function is compromised.

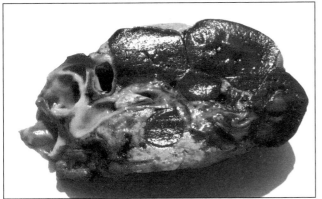

18.12 Sagittal section through a kidney affected by urolithiasis. One calculus has been left *in situ* in the grossly thickened calyx. Note the cystic degeneration of several lobules and the extensive replacement fibrosis.
(© Vic Simpson)

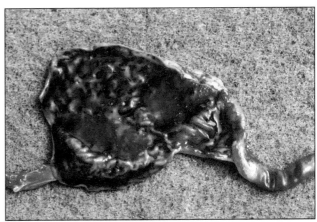

18.13 The opened stomach of an otter showing masses of blackish mucoid material, which also extended through much of the intestine. These changes are often seen in severely debilitated cases, especially those with severe bite wounds.
(© Vic Simpson)

Enteric disease

Intussusception and intestinal torsion are occasionally seen in cubs that are being hand-reared. The cause in some cases may be irregular feeding (V Simpson, unpublished data). Affected animals may present with abdominal pain, vomiting and scant diarrhoea. A tubular mass may be palpable in the abdomen in cases of intussusception, the presence and typical appearance of which may be confirmed by radiography and ultrasonography. Surgical correction may be attempted as per companion animals.

Fatal haemorrhagic gastroenteritis is not uncommon in otters in zoological collections, rehabilitation centres or during translocation (V Simpson, unpublished data; Kollias *et al.*, 1998). In some cases the otters are observed to be weak or lethargic, but most die unexpectedly. On post-mortem examination they are often in fat body condition, have areas of congestion and haemorrhage in lungs and other organs, straw-coloured fluid in body cavities, and marked distension of the stomach, and sometimes the intestines by reddish-black mucoid fluid. In most cases no significant pathogens are detected by aerobic culture, but anaerobic culture of gut contents reveals *Clostridium perfringens* Type A. Where treatment is possible Kollias *et al.* (1998) suggest metronidazole or parenteral trimethoprim-sulphonamide along with supportive care. The cause is uncertain, but may be due to a combination of stress, overeating or eating spoiled food (V Simpson, unpublished data; Kollias *et al.*, 1998) and consequently these should be avoided in rehabilitation situations.

Stress is also believed to be the prime reason for the gastric mucosal ulceration that is commonly seen in debilitated otters, especially those with extensive bite wounds. In these cases there is blackish haemorrhagic mucoid fluid in the stomach and intestine (Figure 18.13) and often blackish tarry material around the anus (Simpson, 1997; Simpson, 2007). Similar lesions of mucosal ulceration and gastric haemorrhage may be seen in abandoned cubs or ones which have died during attempted hand-rearing, especially by inexperienced people. Again it is believed that the lesions are the result of extreme stress (Simpson, 2007). If cubs are hand-reared appropriately (see 'Rearing of otter cubs'), the likelihood of these problems is considerably reduced. Cultural examination of gastric ulcers for *Helicobacter* spp. using specialist media and by PCR analysis has given negative results (Harris, 2004; Simpson, 2007). In the case of debilitated animals, the use of gastroprotectants may be considered, although the stress involved in repeated administration of medication, unless it can be successfully administered in food, may render this counterproductive and as a consequence this author (DC) does not use these routinely.

Oil pollution

Otters are vulnerable to oil spills and post-mortem examinations on 13 otters that died following an incident in Shetland showed that five were suffering from haemorrhagic gastroenteritis, believed to be due to ingestion of oil (Baker *et al.*, 1981). In Cornwall an otter that died after exposure to diesel oil had gastric ulceration and pulmonary inflammation and haemorrhage (V Simpson, unpublished data).

Following stabilization, the affected otter should be washed under light sedation using a suitable detergent and thoroughly rinsed and dried. Close attention should be paid to maintaining the body temperature within normal limits throughout. Activated charcoal may be administered in food to adsorb ingested toxins. Gastroprotectants and antibiotics may be used to treat haemorrhagic gastroenteritis. For general information on oil contamination in wildlife see Chapter 24.

Adrenal hyperplasia

The adrenal glands, especially that on the left, are often greatly enlarged and nodular in sick otters and also in bitches that are lactating or in late pregnancy. The reasons for this are not clear and although adrenal hyperplasia may result from prolonged stress, a positive correlation between adrenal size and the hepatic concentration of some PCB congeners has also been demonstrated (Simpson, 1998). Adrenal aplasia, together with renal aplasia, has been reported in *Lutra canadensis* in the USA and appears to be linked to levels of polyhalogenated hydrocarbons in the environment (Henny *et al.*, 1996).

Reproductive disorders

Evidence for reproductive disorders is uncommon although there was considerable concern during the 1980s that PCBs might be interfering with breeding, particularly in females. Heggberget (1988) described an otter in Norway with a cystic uterus and further cystic and convoluted uteri were reported in Denmark (Elmeros and Madsen, 1999).

Several, possibly similar, cases were recorded in south–west England between 1988 and 2003 (Simpson, 1997; Simpson, 2007). The aetiology and significance of these changes is uncertain, but is now thought that they could simply represent a normal stage of uterine development during early pregnancy. A single case of pyometra was seen in an otter from south-west England (Rivers, 1997).

Neoplastic disease

Neoplasia is rarely seen in Eurasian otters. Recorded conditions include hepatocellular adenoma (Bae *et al.*, 2007) malignant melanoma (Weber and Mecklenburg, 2000), and two cases of intestinal lymphoma (Bartlett *et al.*, 2010; V Simpson, unpublished data). In the latter case there was metastatic spread to the lungs. A uterine leiomyoma was seen in an otter from Norfolk (Keymer *et al.*, 1988) and in three from south-west England (V Simpson, unpublished data). It is notable that the otters in all these cases were judged by their dental wear to be aged animals.

Therapeutics

Many of the common medications used in domestic dogs can be used in otters, at similar dose rates (Figure 18.14). To minimize handling, palatable oral medications administered in food, should be used where possible. The administration of injections may be facilitated by the use of a crush cage. Subcutaneous injections may be given between the shoulder blades, and intramuscular injections may be given in the quadriceps or lumbar muscles. The administration of intravenous medications using the cephalic vein is generally only possible under anaesthesia or in very debilitated animals. Intraosseous injections may be given in the trochanteric fossa of the femur.

Management in captivity

Housing

The short-term housing requirements of otters have already been described (see 'First aid and short-term hospitalization'). Longer term, they require more specialized facilities, incorporating a large escape-proof outside run (Figure 18.15). Otters will easily scale fencing, and an over-hang should be provided if a roof is not present, or electric fencing used. They will also dig under fencing, which should be buried to a depth of at least 0.75 m. Clean water must be available for the otter to swim in, allowing it to develop fitness and to keep its fur in good condition. A suitable artificial holt should be provided; this is often a wooden box, in which the otter can also be transported for release. Natural materials such as branches and logs will allow the otter to develop agility and find resting sites. Closed circuit television (CCTV) cameras may be employed to allow remote monitoring of the animal's health, helping to keep stress to a minimum.

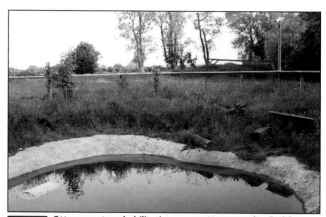

18.15 Otter pen at a rehabilitation centre. Note wooden 'holt', provision of water for swimming and observation using CCTV camera. The high secure fences are electrified when the pen is in use.
(© Secret World Wildlife Rescue)

Drug	Dosage	Comments
Antimicrobial drugs		
Amoxicillin/clavulanate (co-amoxiclav)	8.75 mg/kg i.m., s.c. q24h 12.5–25 mg/kg orally q12h	Broad-spectrum Useful for treatment of bite wounds Duration according to response (minimum of 5–7 days)
Enrofloxacin	5 mg/kg s.c., orally q24h	Reserved for infection when first-line antimicrobials would not be effective Duration according to response (minimum of 5–7 days) Not to be used in growing animals
Marbofloxacin	2 mg/kg s.c., orally q24h	Reserved for infection when first-line antimicrobials would not be effective Duration according to response (minimum of 5–7 days) Not to be used in growing animals
Clindamycin	5.5 mg/kg orally q12h 11 mg/kg orally q24h	For treatment of bite wounds, and oral infection Duration according to response (minimum of 5–7 days)
Antiparasitic drugs		
Ivermectin	200 µg/kg s.c., orally	Rarely indicated
Selamectin	15 mg/ up to 2.5 kg topically 30 mg/2.6–5 kg topically 60 mg/5.1–10kg topically	Rarely indicated
Fipronil 0.25% w/v spray	3–6 ml/kg topically	Rarely indicated For the treatment of ticks
Fenbendazole	50 mg/kg orally q24h for 3 days	For the treatment of nematodes and cestodes
Praziquantel	5 mg/kg orally	For the treatment of trematodes

18.14 Therapeutics commonly used in otters. None of these drugs are licensed for use in otters and doses are extrapolated from those used in domestic dogs.

Diet

Otters can be fed a variety of fish but, for the purposes of short-term rehabilitation, trout is suitable and readily available (Figure 18.16). Thiamine depletion in frozen fish should be corrected for with appropriate vitamin supplementation (e.g. Mazuri® Fish Eater tablets). Fish can be fed whole to adults, but should be skinned, filleted and flaked for young cubs or weaker individuals. As a rough guide, an adult otter will eat around 1.5–2 kg of fish per day but this should be adjusted with respect to appetite, weight gain and activity levels. Otters will also eat day-old chicks and other types of meat; these are provided for a more balanced diet to longer term captives.

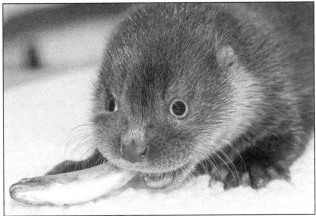

18.16 Otter cub at a rehabilitation centre, eating a small trout. The fish should be skinned, filleted and flaked for very young cubs or weaker individuals.
(© Secret World Wildlife Rescue)

Rearing of otter cubs

Otter cubs are often presented at 2–4 months of age, around the time when they would naturally start emerging from the holt. Although they can be born at any time of year, those cubs born in winter are at greater risk of being separated from the bitch during stormy weather, or when rivers are in spate (Green and Green, 1998). They should all receive a thorough examination, as they are often cold and dehydrated, and injuries and behavioural abnormalities (e.g. as a result of hydrocephalus) are occasionally encountered.

At this age, cubs would naturally be starting to eat solid food (see Figure 18.16). However, many will require bottle feeding initially to encourage intake and younger cubs will require anogenital stimulation of defecation and urination. Otter's milk is high in fat (24%) and protein (11%), and low in lactose (1%) (Shaul, 1962), and supplementation of proprietary milk replacers for puppies and kittens has been recommended by some rehabilitators. The Royal Society for the Prevention of Cruelty to Animals (RSPCA) wildlife centres and the New Forest Wildlife Park use Esbilac® with no apparent problems, although younger cubs that are bottle fed for longer periods may be weaned on to a 'fish soup' (blended trout and Esbilac® and multivitamins) before introduction to solid food, such as finely flaked trout (minus the skin and bones) and chopped up day-old chicks. Very young cubs (less than 2 weeks old) will require hand-feeding at 2-hourly intervals initially, gradually increasing this to 4-hourly. They should be provided with supplementary heat using a heat lamp with a ceramic bulb, from which they can move away if they become too hot. The hand-rearing process is best performed by one person, in a quiet stress-free environment, to minimize the likelihood of gastric ulceration. Less severe digestive upset (manifesting as diarrhoea, bloat and inappetence) is occasionally reported in hand-reared otter neonates; it may be associated with several factors, including inappropriate milk formula, feeding frequency, overfilling of the stomach and rapid changes in the diet (Myers, 2011). Upper respiratory infections are also occasionally encountered (see 'Respiratory disease'), and should be treated promptly with appropriate broad-spectrum antibiotics (see Figure 18.14). To reduce stress and the likelihood of malprinting and habituation developing, and to improve social and physical development, cubs should be kept in pairs, and human contact kept to a minimum. This is particularly important as otter cubs are normally kept in captivity until they are around a year old, at which age they would become independent in the wild. A brief period of quarantine (3–4 days) prior to mixing will enable accurate monitoring of individual food intake of cubs that are self-feeding.

Release

Only animals with a chance of survival comparable to that of their wild conspecifics should be released. Adult otters should be returned to where they were found, in order that they have a chance to reoccupy their territory. They should be kept cool during transport to the release site and given ample ventilation to avoid hyperthermia. Their release should be carried out at dusk, when the dangers posed by traffic, humans and domestic dogs are minimal. Otter cubs are soft-released in suitable habitat, following a period of site acclimation in an escape-proof release pen (see also Chapter 9). The animals are held in the pen for a period of 2 weeks, and food is provided post-release for as long as it is taken. The choice of site is very important, bearing in mind that it must be suitable habitat, and yet, ideally, in an area of low otter density to reduce the likelihood of intraspecific fighting. Every effort should be made to reduce the introduction of novel pathogens to an area, by barrier nursing within the rehabilitation facility, treatment of identified parasites prior to release, and the release of healthy animals into their original territory where possible.

Passive post-release monitoring may be achieved with microchips, implanted subcutaneously between the shoulder blades, although these depend on the animal being recaptured or found dead. Radiofrequency identification (RFID) microchips may be used to assess whether animals are making use of back-up feeding in the release pen (see also Chapter 9).

Legal aspects

Otters are protected principally under the Conservation of Habitats and Species Regulations (2010), with additional protection under the Wildlife and Countryside Act (1981), as amended. It is an offence to deliberately capture, injure or kill otters, or to damage, destroy or obstruct their breeding or resting places, or to disturb otters in their breeding or resting places. There is provision within the legislation to kill, take, disturb or possess otters under licence, in certain defined circumstances, if the issue cannot be resolved by any alternative means. It is not an offence to capture an otter for the purpose of rehabilitation and release, and euthanasia on welfare grounds is permitted. Under Section 1 of the Abandonment of Animals Act (1960), an offence may be committed if a released rehabilitated animal does not have a reasonable chance of survival (i.e. a chance similar to that of its wild conspecifics).

References and further reading

Bae IH, Pakhrin B, Jee H, Shin NS and Kim DY (2007) Hepatocellular adenoma in a Eurasian otter (*Lutra lutra*). *Journal of Veterinary Science* **8**, 103–105

Baker JR, Jones AM, Jones TP and Watson HC (1981) Otter *Lutra lutra* mortality and marine oil pollution. *Biological Conservation* **20**, 311–321

Bartlett SL, Imai DM, Trupkiewicz JG et al. (2010) Intestinal lymphoma of granular lymphocytes in a fisher (*Martes pennanti*) and a Eurasian otter (*Lutra lutra*). *Journal of Zoo and Wildlife Medicine* **41**, 309–315

Benkovskii LM, Golovina TI and Scherbina RD (1973) Studying the diseases and parasites of the otter from Sakhalin Island. *Vestnik Zoologie* **7**, 21–24

Ben Shaul DM (1962) The composition of milk of wild animals. *International Zoo Yearbook* **4**, 333–342

Calle PP (1988) Asian small-clawed otter (*Aonyx cinerea*) urolithiasis prevalence in North America. *Zoo Biology* **7**, 233–242

Chadwick EA, Cable J, Chinchen A et al. (2013) Seroprevalence of *Toxoplasma gondii* in the Eurasian otter (*Lutra lutra*) in England and Wales. *Parasites and Vectors* **6**, 75

Chanin P (1985) *The Natural History of Otters*. Croom Helm, London

Elmeros M and Madsen AB (1999) On the reproductive biology of otters (*Lutra lutra*) from Denmark. *Zeitschrift fur Saugetierkunde* **64**, 193–200

Fernandez-Moran J, Molina L, Flamme G, Saavedra, D and Manteca-Vilanova X (2001b) Hematological and biochemical reference intervals for wild caught Eurasian otter from Spain. *Journal of Wildlife Diseases* **37**, 159–163

Fernandez-Moran J, Perez E, Sanmartin M, Saavedra D and Manteca-Vilanova X (2001a) Reversible immobilization of European otters with a combination of Ketamine and medetomidine. *Journal of Wildlife Diseases* **37**, 561–565

Foster G, Davison N, Simpson V et al. (2011) Brucella serology of otters (*Lutra lutra*) in the UK. Brucellosis 2011, International Research Conference Including the 64th Brucellosis Research Conference Buenos Aires, Argentina, September 21st to 23rd, 2011

Geisel O (1979) Staupe bei Fischottern (*Lutra lutra*). *Berliner und Munchener Tierarztliche Wochenschrift* **92**, 304

Goldstein T, Mazet JAK, Gill VA et al. (2009) Phocine distemper virus in northern sea otters in the Pacific Ocean, Alaska, USA. *Emerging Infectious Diseases* **15**, 925–927

Green R and Green J (1998) Disease and Health Problems in British Otters (*Lutra lutra*) at a Rehabilitation Centre. *Proceedings of the VIIth International Otter Colloquium, Trabon, Czech Republic, March 14–19, 1998*

Harris CJ (1968) *Otters: A study of the recent Lutrinae*. Weidenfeld and Nicholson, London

Harris R (2004) *Furthering the search for Helicobacter mustelae in British mustelids*. Thesis (BSc Veterinary Conservation Medicine), Liverpool University

Heggberget TM (1988) Reproduction in the female European otter in central and northern Norway. *Journal of Mammalogy* **69**, 164–167

Heggberget TM (1996) Age determination of Eurasian otter (*Lutra lutra* L.) cubs. *Fauna norvegica Serie A* **17**, 30–32

Henny CJ, Grove RA and Hedstrom OR (1996) *A field evaluation of mink and river otter on the Lower Columbia River and the influence of environmental contaminants*. Final report to The Lower Columbia River Bi-State Water Quality Program, USA, February 12, 1996

Jefferies DJ, Hanson HM and Harris EA (1990) The prevalence of *Pseudoterranova decipiens* (Nematoda) and *Corynosoma strumosum* (Acanthocephala) in otters *Lutra lutra* from coastal sites in Britain. *Journal of the Zoological Society of London* **221**, 316–321

Jones G (2003) *The prevalence of leptospirosis in British wildlife*. Submitted in partial fulfilment of the requirements of the BSc in Veterinary Conservation Medicine, Liverpool University

Keymer I (1992) Diseases of the otter (*Lutra lutra*). *Proceedings of the National Otter Conference, Cambridge, September 1992* pp. 30–33

Keymer I, Lewis G and Don P (1981) Urolithiasis in otters (Family Mustelidae, Subfamily Lutrinae) and other species. *Sonderdruck aus Verhandlungsbericht des XXII Internationalen Symposiums uber die Erkrankungen der Zootier, Halle/Saale*, pp.391–401

Keymer I, Wells G, Mason C and Macdonald S (1988) Pathological changes and organochlorine residues in tissues of wild otters (*Lutra lutra*). *Veterinary Record* **122**, 153–155

Kollias GV (1999) Health assessment, medical management, and prerelease conditioning of translocated North American river otters. In: *Zoo and Wild Animal Medicine, Current Therapy 4*, ed. ME Fowler and RE Miller. WB Saunders, Philadelphia

Kollias GV and Abou-Madi N (2007) Procyonids and mustelids. In: *Zoo Animal and Wildlife Immobilization and Anaesthesia*, ed. G West, D Heard, and N Caulkett. Blackwell Publishing, Oxford

Kollias GV, McDonough P, Valentine B et al. (1998) *Clostridium perfringens* enterotoxicosis in recently captured North American river otters (*Lontra canadensis*). Annual Conference of the American Association of Zoo Veterinarians, Omaha, Nebraska, October 1998

Kruuk H (1995) *Wild Otters: Predations and Populations*. Oxford University Press, Oxford

Kruuk H and Conroy J (1991) Mortality of otters (*Lutra lutra*) in Shetland. *Journal of Applied Ecology* **28**, 83–94

Kuiken T (1988) Anaesthesia in the European otter. *Veterinary Record* **123**, 59

Lee J, Hanna R, Hill R, McCormick CM and Skuce RA (2009) Bovine tuberculosis in an Eurasian otter. *Veterinary Record* **164**, 727–728

Lewis JCM, Pagan L, Hart M and Green R (1998) Normal haematological and serum biochemical values of Eurasian otters (*Lutra lutra*) from a Scottish rehabilitation centre. *Veterinary Record* **143**, 676–679

Loupal G, Weissenbock H, Bodner M and Stotter C (1998) Distemper in free-living European otters in Austria. *Proceedings VIIth International Otter Colloquium – March 14–19, 1998, Trebon*, pp.211–213

Madsen AB, Dietz HH, Henriksen P and Clausen B (1999) Survey of free-living otters (*Lutra lutra*) – a consecutive collection and necropsy of dead bodies. *IUCN Otter Specialist Group Bulletin* **16(2)**, 65–75

Mason C, Last N and Macdonald S (1986) Mercury, cadmium and lead in British otters. *Bulletin of Environmental Contamination and Toxicology* **37**, 844–849

Mason CF and O'Sullivan WM (1992) Organochlorine pesticide residues and PCBs in otters (*Lutra lutra*) from Ireland. *Bulletin of Environmental Contamination and Toxicology* **48**, 387–393

Molenaar F and Simpson V (2006) Arteriosclerosis in a wild Eurasian otter (*Lutra lutra*). *British Veterinary Zoological Society Proceedings November 11–12th, 2006, Bristol*

Myers G (2011) *Summary of Veterinary Care Guidelines for Otters in Zoos, Aquariums, Rehabilitation and Wildlife Centres*. IUCN/SSC Otter Specialists Groups Otters in Zoos, Aquaria, Rehabilitation and Wildlife Sanctuaries Task Force (OZ)

Park NY, Lee MC, Kurkure NV and Cho HS (2007) Canine adenovirus type 1 infection of a Eurasian river otter (*Lutra lutra*) *Veterinary Pathology* **44**, 536–539

Reuther C (1983) Immobilization of European otter with ketamine hydrochloride. *Berliner-und-Munchener Tierarztliche Wochenschrift* **96**, 401–405

Reuther C (1999) Development of weight and length of Eurasian otter (*Lutra lutra*) cubs. *IUCN Otter Specialist Group Bulletin* **16**, 11–25

Reuther C and Brandes B (1984) Occurrence of hyperthermia during immobilization of European otter (*Lutra lutra*) with ketamine hydrochloride. *Deutsche Tierarztliche Wochenschrift* **91**, 66–68

Rivers SA (1997) *Histology of the ovaries and uterine horns of the European otter (Lutra lutra)*. Project report, MSc in Veterinary Pathology, University of London

Ruff K, Kruger HH, Sewell AC et al. (2007) Dietary risk factors for urate urolithiasis in Eurasian otters (*Lutra lutra*). In: *Nutritional and energetic studies on captive Eurasian otters (Lutra lutra)*. Dissertation for degree of Doctor of Natural Sciences, University of Hannover.

Sherrard-Smith E, Cable J and Chadwick EA (2009) Distribution of Eurasian otter biliary parasites, *Pseudamphistomum truncatum* and *Metorchis albidus* (Family Opisthorchiidae) in England and Wales. *Parasitology* **136(9)**, 1015–1022

Simpson VR (1996) Angiostrongylus vasorum infection in foxes (*Vulpes vulpes*) in Cornwall. *Veterinary Record* **139**, 443–445

Simpson VR (1997) Health status of otters (*Lutra lutra*) in south-west England based on postmortem findings. *Veterinary Record* **141**, 191–197

Simpson VR (1998) *A post-mortem study of otters (Lutra lutra) found dead in south west England*. R&D Technical Report W148, Environment Agency, Bristol

Simpson VR (2006) Patterns and significance of bite wounds in Eurasian otters (*Lutra lutra*) in southern and south west England. *Veterinary Record* **158**, 113–119

Simpson VR (2007) *Health status of otters in southern and south west England 1996–2004*. Science Report SCO10064/SR1 Environment Agency, Bristol

Simpson VR (2009) Bovine tuberculosis in Eurasian otters. *Veterinary Record* **164**, 790

Simpson VR, Bain M, Brown R, Brown B, and Lacey R (2000) A long-term study of vitamin A and polychlorinated hydrocarbon levels in otters (*Lutra lutra*) in south west England. *Environmental Pollution* **110**, 267–275

Simpson VR and Gavier-Widen D (2000) Fatal adiaspiromycosis in a wild European otter (*Lutra lutra*). *Veterinary Record* **147**, 239–241

Simpson VR, Gibbons LM, Khalil LF and Williams JLR (2005) Cholecystitis in otters (*Lutra lutra*) and mink (*Mustela vison*) caused by the fluke *Pseudamphistomum truncatum*. *Veterinary Record* **157**, 49–52

Simpson VR, Hargreaves J, Birtles RJ, Marsden H and Williams DL (2008) Tyzzer's disease in a Eurasian otter (*Lutra lutra*) in Scotland. *Veterinary Record* **163**, 539–543

Simpson VR, Tomlinson AJ and Molenaar FM (2009) Prevalence, distribution and pathological significance of the bile fluke *Pseudamphistomum truncatum* in Eurasian otters (*Lutra lutra*) in Great Britain. *Veterinary Record* **164**, 397–401

Simpson VR, Tomlinson AJ, Molenaar FM, Lawson B and Rogers KD (2011) Renal calculi in wild Eurasian otters (*Lutra lutra*) in England. *Veterinary Record* **169**, 49

Spelman LH (1999) Otter anaesthesia. In: *Zoo and Wild Animal Medicine, Current Therapy 4*, ed. ME Fowler and RE Miller. WB Saunders, Philadelphia

Spelman LH, Sumner PW, Levine JF and Stoskopf MK (1993) Field anesthesia in the North American river otter (*Lutra canadensis*). *Journal of Zoo and Wildlife Medicine* **24**, 19–27

Spelman LH, Sumner PW, Levine JF and Stoskopf MK (1994) Anesthesia of North American river otters (*Lutra canadensis*) with medetomidine-ketamine and reversal by atipamezole. *Journal of Zoo and Wildlife Medicine* **25**, 214–223

Tocidlowski ME, Lappin MR, Sumner PW and Stoskopf MK (1997) Serologic survey for toxoplasmosis in river otters. *Journal of Wildlife Diseases* **33**, 649–652

Van de Grift ER (1976) Possible feline infectious peritonitis in short clawed otters, *A. cinerea. Journal of Zoo Animal Medicine* **7**, 18

Wayre P (1979) *The Private Life of the Otter.* Book Club Associates, London

Weber H (2001) *Untersuchungen zur Urolithiasis beim Eurasischen Fischotter, Lutra lutra.* Inaugural Dissertation, Institut fur Zoologie der Tierarztlichen Hochschule, Hannover

Weber H and Mecklenburg L (2000) Malignant melanoma in a Eurasian otter (*Lutra lutra*). *Journal of Zoo and Wildlife Medecine* **31**, 87–90

Wells G, Keymer I and Barnett K (1989) Suspected Aleutian disease in a wild otter (*Lutra lutra*). *Veterinary Record* **125**, 232–235

Wilhelm A and Vogt D (1981) Rabies in an otter, *Lutra lutra. Monatshefte fur veterinarmedizin* **36**, 361

Williams DW, Flindall A and Simpson VR (1998) Retinal dysplasia in wild otters: a pathological survey. In *Abstracts of the 3rd European Wildlife Disease Association Conference, Edinburgh, 1998*

Williams J (1989) Blindness in otters. *IUCN Otter Specialist Group Bulletin* **4**, 29–30

Specialist organizations and useful contacts

See also Appendix 1

International Otter Survival Fund (IOSF)
Website provides useful general otter information.
Broadford, Isle of Skye, Scotland IV49 9AQ
Tel: 01471 822 487 Fax: 01471 822 975
www.otter.org

IUCN/SCC Otter Specialist Group
This group is a valuable source of information, with otter specialists located Worldwide. They can be contacted at: www.otterspecialistgroup.org.

Chapter 19

Other mustelids

Debra Bourne

There are several small mustelids from what has been commonly known as the subfamily Mustelinae in the UK (classification of these species is presently in flux and the *Martes* spp. may be separated into a different subfamily, the Martinae). There are both native and introduced species and whilst they are not often presented for veterinary attention, this does happen occasionally. All of these species are closely related to the domestic ferret (*Mustela putorius furo*), therefore many aspects of their medical care can be extrapolated from that of the ferret.

The weasel (*Mustela nivalis*) (Figure 19.1), the smallest species, is found throughout England, Wales and Scotland, but is absent from Ireland and Northern Ireland. It is sandy-brown dorsally and creamy ventrally. The junction between the brown and creamy areas is irregular and the ventral pattern can be used to identify individuals; they do not change colour in winter.

Stoats (*Mustela erminea*) (Figure 19.2) are found throughout the British Isles. Like weasels they also have a sandy-brown head and upper parts and creamy-white underparts, but the division between the pigmentation areas is usually straight (less so in many stoats in Ireland). In winter in northern England and Scotland they may develop a completely white coat, whilst further south in England and Wales, they may become mottled. The tail is longer than in the weasel and has a black tip.

The polecat (*Mustela putorius*) (Figure 19.3) is the probable ancestor of the domestic ferret. Polecats are widely distributed across Europe, but presently have a limited distribution in the UK, found primarily in Wales and the

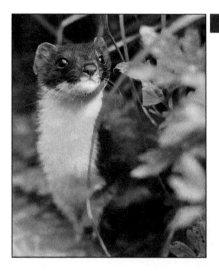
19.2 Stoat.
(© British Wildlife Centre, Surrey)

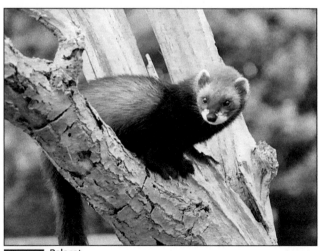
19.3 Polecat.
(© British Wildlife Centre, Surrey)

English Midlands, extending eastwards to the Peak District and the Home Counties; there are also re-established populations in Argyll, Perthshire, Cumbria, the Chilterns and central southern England following reintroductions. They are absent from Ireland. They have a dark brown or purplish black coat with a creamy undercoat, and have a distinct facial mask, dark around the eyes, with an outer pale ring and white on the muzzle and ear margins. It is important to distinguish polecats from 'polecat ferrets':

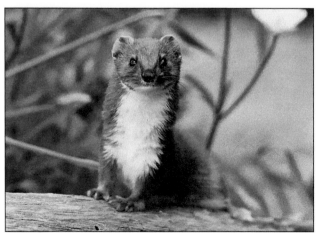
19.1 Weasel.
(© British Wildlife Centre, Surrey)

domestic ferrets with polecat-type coloration, but usually less distinct markings. Escaped ferrets may be presented as 'wildlife' casualties. Note that ferrets can hybridize with polecats and should not be released into the wild.

The pine marten (*Martes martes*) (Figure 19.4) is the largest of these mustelids. In the British Isles its distribution is now limited mainly to western counties of Northern Ireland/Ireland (with some strongholds further east) and the Scottish Highlands, with expansion to other parts of Scotland, plus a few remnant populations scattered in England and Wales. Pine martens are basically brown except for a cream-to-yellow or orange throat patch, which extends from the underside of the chin down to the chest; dark spots of brown in this area can be used for identification of individuals.

The introduced American mink (*Mustela (Neovison) vison*) (Figure 19.5) is widespread throughout the British Isles, due to both escapes and misguided large-scale releases from fur farms by activists. They have unfortunately, to the detriment of many small native species, survived and thrived. These are similar in size to polecats, are dark chocolate brown, usually have a white chin patch and often have white spots on the chest, abdomen and groin area.

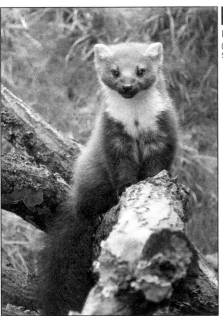

19.4

Pine marten.
(© British Wildlife Centre, Surrey)

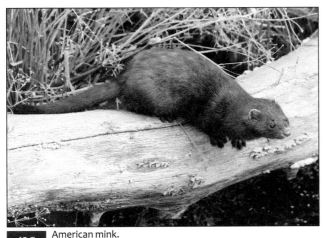

19.5 American mink.
(© British Wildlife Centre, Surrey)

Ecology and biology

These small carnivores – weasels are the smallest of the Carnivora – are fast and agile. All of the mustelids are found in a variety of habitats, but they have distinct preferences. Weasels are found in the widest range of habitats including lowland pasture and woodland. They rapidly make use of new habitats even in urban areas, so long as cover and their favoured prey, small mammals (mice and voles – *Microtus*, *Apodemus* and *Myodes* spp.), are available. Stoats are found in broadly similar habitats to weasels, but also use moorland and higher altitudes. With their larger body size, they can catch a wider range of prey than weasels, taking mammals up to the size of rabbits. In the British Isles and in New Zealand (where they are considered pest species) they are found in forests, but they are generally absent from forests in mainland Europe, Asia and North America.

Polecats are primarily woodland animals within Europe; their remaining strongholds in the UK are mainly river valleys holding prey of all types (mammals, birds, reptiles and amphibians), although this may be a reporting bias. They are also found in habitats such as sand dunes, farmland and sea cliffs. About 75–90% of their diet comprises mammals, with rabbits forming an important part, but birds, amphibians, reptiles and occasionally fish and invertebrates may be eaten.

Pine martens are more arboreal and are generally found in mature woodland, although they are also found in moorland, rocky hills and even seashore areas. They are opportunistic generalists, eating small mammals such as mice, voles and shrews, birds (particularly passerines), carrion (deer), amphibians, berries, honey and invertebrates.

American mink are semi-aquatic and are often found in riverine habitats. They are opportunistic in their diet, preying on a wide variety of mammals, birds, fish and invertebrates.

Generally, territories of males of each of these species overlap with territories of one or more females, but not with the territories of other males. Territories of females are separate from one another. The presence of secure dens is important. Multiple dens are used, for resting and for breeding; these are commonly nests and burrows of prey (weasels never make their own dens).

Anatomy and physiology

Basic anatomical and physiological data for the British small mustelids are given in Figure 19.6.

The small mustelids all have a long thin body, a small head and short legs; the tail is shortest (as a percentage of body length) in the weasel and longest and bushiest in the pine marten. There are five toes on each foot.

The dental formula of the *Mustela* spp. is:

$$2 \times \left\{ I\ \frac{3}{3}\ C\ \frac{1}{1}\ P\ \frac{3}{3}\ M\ \frac{1}{2} \right\} = 34$$

and that of the pine marten is:

$$2 \times \left\{ I\ \frac{3}{3}\ C\ \frac{1}{1}\ P\ \frac{4}{4}\ M\ \frac{1}{2} \right\} = 38$$

The teeth are specialized for a carnivorous diet, the upper carnassials being long and narrow and the upper molars elongated transversely. These carnivorous species have a short gut and rapid gut transit time (about 2.5–4.5 hours). All the species have multiple scent glands including anal glands, which they can express resulting in a strong scent.

Species	Head–body length (mm)	Tail length (mm)	Weight (g)	Longevity (years)	Heart rate (beats per minute)	Respiratory rate (breaths per minute)	Body temperature (°C)
Weasel (*Mustela nivalis*)	195–248 (m) 175–194 (f)	32–62 (m) 35–46 (f)	81–195 (m) 48–107 (f)	2–3; longer in captivity	451 (range 420–480) (m) 468 (range 420–510) (f)	96–104 (even higher in younger animals)	39–40 (36.6 when at rest, 39.5 when active)
Stoat (*Mustela erminea*)	260–318 (m) 244–278 (f)	67–119 (m) 69–100 (f)	252–471 (m) 180–303 (f)	6–8, although this age is rarely reached in the wild	402 (range 360–480) (m) 421 (range 360–510) (f)	86–100	38–40
Polecat (*Mustela putorius*)	330–450 (m) 318–388 (f)	125–190 (m) 125–169 (f)	800–1913 (m) 500–1123 (f)	Up to 14 in captivity In wild probably 4–5	150 (5 minutes after induction with ketamine/ medetomidine)	Approx. 85 (5 minutes post-injection with ketamine/ medetomidine)	38–39 (5 minutes post-injection with ketamine/ medetomidine)
Pine marten (*Martes martes*)	480–520 (m) 410–460 (f)	225–270 (m) 220–240 (f)	1500–1850 (m) 1100–1450 (f)	Up to 18 reported in the wild in Lithuania (but only 26% over 3 years old)	116–129 (15 mins post-injection with ketamine/ medetomidine) (In *Martes pennanti*, 120 at rest, up to 389 when running)	57–71 (15 minutes post-injection with ketamine/ medetomidine)	37.9–40.1 (15 minutes post-injection with ketamine/ medetomidine)
American mink (*Mustela (Neovison) vison*)	330–450 (m) 320–370 (f)	150–220 (m) 135–190 (f)	840–1805 (m) 450–810 (f)	Up to 6 in wild	Approx. 254; lower when diving 90–210	40–70	39.5–40.1

19.6 Basic anatomical and physiological data for the British small mustelids. (f = female; m = male).
(Corbet and Harris, 1991; Dunstone, 1993; Arnemo *et al.*, 1994; Sheffield and King, 1994; Fournier-Chambrillon *et al.*, 2003; Harjunpää and Rouvinen-Watt, 2004; Harris and Yalden, 2008)

Species	Number of nipples	Age at sexual maturity	Litter size	Litters per year	Gestation
Weasel (*Mustela nivalis*)	3–4 pairs, visible only in adult female	3–4 months: females may breed in their first year, males usually unsuccessful in birth year	4–8	2	34–37 days total Implant at 10–12 days after development to blastocysts; no delayed implantation
Stoat (*Mustela erminae*)	4–5 pairs, visible only in adult female	10–11 months in males; 2–3 months in females	<12	1	Initial 2–3 weeks development of blastocyst then delayed implantation of 9–10 months Active gestation 4 weeks Births April–May
Polecat (*Mustela putorius*)	Up to 10 active Visible in lactating females	1 year	2–12; usually 5–10	1, but a second litter is possible if first litter lost	40–43 days No delayed implantation Births May–June
Pine marten (*Martes martes*)	Two pairs, larger in adult females	>2 years	2–6; average 3	1	Mating takes place June–August Delayed implantation 5.5–6.5 months Active gestation 30–35 days Births March–April
American mink (*Mustela (Neovison) vison*)	1–8 palpable during lactation	1 year	2–8; average 4, but more in captivity	1	39–76 days Approx. 28 days active gestation after implantation

19.7 Small mustelid reproductive parameters.
(Larivière, 1999; Harris and Yalden, 2008)

The anogenital distance is notably larger in males than in females, and usually the os penis is palpable in males on the ventral midline. During the breeding season the testes in their furred scrotum may be evident; in winter these are smaller and in first-year individuals barely visible. The vulva is swollen when females are in oestrus. The uterus is simple and bicornuate. Reproductive parameters are described in Figure 19.7.

Most species breed just once a year. Weasels are the exception and breed twice a year. Pole cats may have a second litter if the first is lost. Delayed implantation is a feature of most species, but does not occur in weasels

or pole cats. In all species the kits are born altricial (blind, deaf and with no fur). Weaning age varies between species, but most kits are able to hunt for themselves by 8 weeks old.

Young kits (the young of all species) are unable to keep themselves warm in cold conditions. For example, stoat kits are unable to maintain body temperature under 5–7 weeks of age and if subjected to temperatures below 10–12°C they enter reversible cold rigor (characterized by reduced cardiac and respiratory functions and reduced sensitivity). Landmarks in neonatal development are described in Figure 19.8.

Species	Birth weight (g)	Pelage	Eyes/ears	Dentition	Lactation/feeding	Hunting/dispersal
Weasel (Mustela nivalis)	1.5–4.5	Birth: naked 4 days: white downy fur 10 days: darker fur visible dorsally	Neonates blind and deaf Eyes open at 4 weeks	Deciduous teeth erupt at 2–3 weeks Canine teeth emerge at 5 weeks	Weaned at 3–4 weeks (lactation may last 12 weeks)	Able to kill efficiently by 8 weeks Family disperses at 9–12 weeks
Stoat (Mustela erminae)	3–4	Birth: white down 3 weeks: prominent temporary mane 6–7 weeks: tail tip black 8 weeks: fully furred	Eyes open at 5–6 weeks	Deciduous teeth erupt at 3 weeks	Take solid food at four weeks Weaned at 7–12 weeks	Innate killing behaviour by 10–12 weeks Dispersal at 12 weeks or older
Polecat (Mustela putorius)	9–10	By 1 week: silky white hair 3–4 weeks: brownish woolly coat By 50 days: adult markings	Neonates blind and deaf	Eruption of permanent dentition starts at 7–8 weeks, finished by 11–13 weeks	Weaning starts at 3 weeks	Young are independent at 2–3 months
Pine marten (Martes martes)	30	Birth: whitish fur By 3 weeks: soft brown fur	Neonates blind and deaf Eyes open 32–38 days	Permanent dentition erupts at 4 months, carnassials last	Start eating solid food at 34–38 days Weaned at 6–7 weeks	First emerge from den at 7–8 weeks, very active by 3 months Independent at about 6 months of age
American mink (Mustela (Neovison) vison)	Approx. 6	Birth: short, fine white fur	Eyes open 25 days	Deciduous teeth erupt at 16–49 days Permanent teeth erupt at 44–71 days	Weaning starts 5–6 weeks	Juveniles hunt from 8 weeks

19.8 Landmarks in neonatal development of small mustelids.
(Sleeman, 1989; Larivière 1999; Harris and Yalden, 2008)

Capture, handling and transportation

Conscious small mustelids must be handled with caution: these animals will bite and either hold on, or release but bite again repeatedly (this may vary with species and individual). Where rabies is absent, as in the British Isles, there are no major zoonotic risks from bites, but all these animals have very strong jaws and the larger species can bite fingers through to bone. At all times, hands must be kept away from the animal's face/mouth. Whilst stout leather gloves or padded motorcycling gloves can be worn for protection, dexterity is greatly reduced by the use of these; a combination of latex or nitrile examination gloves, plus thin leather gloves may provide the best compromise between protection and loss of dexterity. Whilst a recently arrived juvenile or frightened and injured adult may freeze, enabling initial restraint on one occasion, the animal is less likely to be cooperative on future occasions. Manual restraint of these agile, flexible and fast-moving species is difficult and should be avoided whenever possible; general anaesthesia is recommended for examination and treatment. See also Chapters 3 and 6.

Handling

A dog-grasper can be used to briefly pick up the larger species (pine marten, polecat and American mink). This should be placed just behind the forelegs of the animal, tightened and used to lift the mustelid quickly into a suitable transport container. Nets can also be used for restraint, and the larger species can be restrained using a crush cage to enable intramuscular injections (e.g. for induction of anaesthesia). If restraint by hand is necessary, one gloved hand grasps the back of the neck and the forequarters whilst the other extends the hind legs and tail.

If a stoat or weasel is to be caught and restrained by hand, one method that can be used is to cover the animal with a towel, then (noting which way the head is pointing) firmly grasp the skin at the back of the neck with one hand whilst supporting the rest of the body with the other hand. Do **not** pick up any of these species by the tail.

Transportation

For brief transportation, for example between two cages, a tube can be offered with one end blocked; once the mustelid enters the tube to inspect it, the other end is blocked off using a solid object (e.g. a wooden spoon to block the end of a kitchen roll tube for weasels) and the tube then moved to a new enclosure. Alternatively, and for longer periods of transport, offer a tube leading to a box, and close off the entrance once the mustelid enters the box, after which the animal can be transported within the box, or the box placed into a transport cage. Transport within an escape-proof carrier, not by hand, is highly recommended when transferring mustelids between rooms and on the way to release. A metal mesh cage with small-aperture mesh and a tight-fitting lid would be appropriate, or a standard metal cage for the larger species. A towel is suitable for bedding. Plastic containers may be used for brief transportation of weasels and stoats.

Examination and clinical assessment for rehabilitation

Initial assessment may be carried out visually (observation without restraint), but anaesthesia is likely to be needed for a full, hands-on assessment of a wild mustelid that is not already unconscious (see 'Capture, handling and transportation'). As part of the initial examination, the species and age of the animal should be determined, to ensure that correct handling, housing and feeding are used.

If the clinical examination reveals severe injuries that are likely to prevent the mustelid from living a normal life in the wild, then euthanasia or, very rarely, permanent captivity is indicated (see Chapter 4). Such injuries would include loss of a limb (or loss of use of a limb), loss of an eye and tooth loss or jaw injury such that the animal would be unable to kill prey effectively. In females, pelvic injury likely to obstruct parturition would also come under this category. For most severely injured individuals, considering the likely stresses of prolonged treatment for severe injuries, euthanasia will be the most humane option. Occasionally, if housing that can fulfil the 'five freedoms' and provide an appropriate environment and a high standard of care is available, permanent captivity may be considered for some casualty animals, for example after hand-rearing if the animal is not considered suitable for release (see also Chapter 4). Pine martens and polecats may in some instances be appropriately passed to a captive breeding programme following treatment. The welfare of the individual animal must be the primary consideration, recognizing that not all individuals will adapt to a captive situation.

American mink, an introduced species, should be euthanased unless an appropriate licensed centre or individual can be found that can take the animal, as a licence is required to either keep or release this species (see 'Legal aspects' and Chapter 2).

Incoming mustelids should be kept quarantined from each other and from other carnivores for the first 10 days to reduce the risk of transfer of infectious diseases (particularly canine distemper). After this initial quarantine period adults should continue to be maintained individually, whilst juveniles of the same species may be mixed.

Euthanasia

Euthanasia normally should be carried out in the anaesthetized or unconscious animal to minimize stress and pain. The mustelid may be anaesthetized using an inhalation anaesthetic; injection of pentobarbital can then proceed via the intravenous, intracardiac or intraperitoneal routes (McClure and Anderson, 2006; Sikarskie and Hollamby, 2006; AZA Small Carnivore Taxon Advisory Group, 2010). Alternatively, stunning/killing with a blow to the back of the head, followed by exsanguination, can be used (HSA/UFAW, 1993). For animals in a trap, use of a high-velocity 0.22 air rifle, aiming to penetrate the brain, may be appropriate (not for mink) (HAS/UFAW, 1993). General principles of euthanasia and information on acceptable euthanasia methods have been compiled (AVMA, 2013).

Diagnostic techniques

Blood samples can be collected from the jugular vein, cranial vena cava, cephalic vein or saphenous vein in an anaesthetized mustelid (the latter two veins being used for small samples only and not in the smaller species). Haematological and biochemical data are given in Figures 19.9 and 19.10; where data are not available for a species, the information given here, and for other mustelid species, and/or published data for ferrets, should be used as guidelines.

Note that male mustelids have dark urine, which may give a false positive reading for ketones when tested using a urine dipstick. A degree of proteinuria is normal in mustelids.

Imaging techniques as described for domestic ferrets may be used in these species. Direct microscopy of wet faecal smears for endoparasites should be performed as routine (see Chapter 10).

Variable (units)	Stoat (Mustela erminae)		Polecat (Mustela putorius)	Mink (Mustela (Neovison) vison)	
	Mean (range) (data 3 days after capture)	Mean (range) (data 12+ weeks after capture)	Mean ± SD	Mean ± SD (data for males)	Mean ± SD (data for females)
Red blood cell (RBC) count (x 10^{12}/l)	9.87 (6.6–11.8)	12.28 (10.1–14.9)	8.39 ± 1.86	8.07 ± 0.67	7.44 ± 0.51
Packed cell volume (PCV) (l/l)	0.42 (0.31–0.47)	0.47 (0.39–0.54)	0.436 ± 0.087	0.459 ± 0.031	0.473 ± 0.03
Haemoglobin (g/l)	140.8 (99–159)	166.9 (139–190)	143 ± 27	156 ± 11	155 ± 9
Mean corpuscular volume (MCV) (fl)	43.0 (39–47)	39.1 (34–43)	52.1 ± 407	56.9 ± 1.9	61.2 ± 2.2
Mean corpuscular haemoglobin (MCH) ((pg) per cell)	14.3 (13.2–15.2)	13.8 (12.1–14.9)	17.3 ± 1.1	NDA	NDA
Mean corpuscular haemoglobin concentration (MCHC) (g/l)	332 (315–344)	353 (340–365)	332 ± 19	340 ± 5.2	327 ± 10
Platelets (x 10^9/l)	NDA	NDA	303 ± 1.33	729.58 ± 125.4	840.70 ± 259.36
White blood cell (WBC) count (x 10^9/l)	1.60 (0.3–2.9)	2.15 (0.3–6.2)	6.20 ± 2.36	6.49 ± 2.02	5.28 ± 1.68
Neutrophils (x 10^9/l)	1.23 (0.15–2.67)	1.10 (0.15–2.42)	2.88 ± 1.63 (bands 0.09 ± 0.05)	2.64 ± 1.27 (bands 0.008 ± 0.020)	2.32 ± 1 (bands 0.003 ± 0.012)
Lymphocytes (x 10^9/l)	0.215 (0.004–0.99)	0.778 (0.04–3.35)	2.98 ± 1.73	3.12 ± 1.05	2.37 ± 0.82
Monocytes (x 10^9/l)	0.122 (0.05–0.16)	0.127 (0.02–0.33)	0.15 ± 0.11	0.19 ± 0.13	0.18 ± 0.11
Eosinophils (x 10^9/l)	NDA	NDA	0.24 ± 0.19	0.47 ± 0.44	0.38 ± 0.47
Basophils (x 10^9/l)	NDA	NDA	0.10 ± 0.07	0.05 ± 0.54	0.03 ± 0.031

19.9 Haematological data in small mustelids. NDA = no data available.
(Weiss et al., 1994; Fernandez-Moran, 2003; O'Connor et al., 2006)

Variable (units)	Mean ± SD			
	Polecat (Mustela putorius)	Pine marten[a] (Martes martes)	Mink (Mustela (Neovison) vison)	
			Males	Females
Calcium (mmol/l)	2.28 ± 0.23	2.2 ± 0.1, 2.3 ± 0.4	2.39 ± 0.98	2.37 ± 0.1
Phosphorus (mmol/l)	2 ± 0.55	0.9 ± 0.3, 1.6 ± 0.3	1.71 ± 0.26	1.68 ± 0.35
Sodium (mmol/l)	152 ± 6	155 ± 3, 165 ± 3	153.7 ± 1.3	153.4 ± 1.3
Potassium (mmol/l)	4.7 ± 0.6	3.8 ± 0.4, 4 ± 0.2	4.34 ± 0.23	4.51 ± 0.52
Chloride (mmol/l)	116 ± 8	120 ± 3, 126 ± 1	114.5 ± 1.7	114.6 ± 1.6
Blood urea nitrogen (BUN) (mmol/l)	12.5 ± 3.99	8.2 ± 4, 12.1 ± 4.9	15.2 ± 5.6	16.2 ± 6.7
Creatinine (μmol/l)	43.3 ± 17.7	60 ± 5, 70 ± 16	62.8 ± 7.1	55.6 ± 6.2
Glucose (mmol/l)	5.93 ± 1.6	11.6 ± 0.8, 17.2 ± 3.9	7 ± 1.04	6.88 ± 1.08
Cholesterol (mmol/l)	191.9 ± 52.6	4.6 ± 0.6, 5 ± 0.5	NDA	NDA
Creatine kinase (IU/l)	379 ± 384	237 ± 251, 599 ± 616	NDA	NDA
Lactate dehydrogenase (LDH) (IU/l)	474 ± 403	1103 ± 129, 1875 ± 520	NDA	NDA
Alkaline phosphatase (ALP) (IU/l)	64 ± 79	77 ± 29, 115 ± 35	NDA	NDA
Alanine aminotransferase (ALT) (IU/l)	102 ± 56	1723 ± 120, 222 ± 106	71.6 ± 56.9	80 ± 68.7
Aspartate aminotransferase (AST) (IU/l)	74 ± 28	113 ± 20, 159 ± 18	67 ± 13.7	76.3 ± 37.4
Gamma-glutamyl transferase GGT (IU/l)	10 ± 8	17 ± 12, 25 ± 19	NDA	NDA
Total protein (g/l)	57.7 ± 80	60 ± 4, 62 ± 12	59.4 ± 3.1	60.9 ± 3.1
Albumin (g/l)	33 ± 4	30 ± 4, 37 ± 2	29.8 ± 1.4	30 ± 1.7
Globulin (g/l)	24 ± 7	23 ± 2, 31 ± 4	NDA	NDA

19.10 Serum biochemistry data in small mustelids. [a]Lowest and highest mean values from three sets of results (same animals tested three times over a period of 6 months).

(Arnemo et al., 1994; Weiss et al., 1994; Fernandez-Moran, 2003)

First aid and short-term hospitalization

First aid

Immediate first aid for these species should follow standard principles (see Chapter 5): control bleeding, control seizures, provide fluids, provide supplemental oxygen if there are breathing difficulties, provide appropriate analgesia (see below). Considering the high metabolic rate, particularly in the weasel and stoat, blood glucose measurements should be made where possible and fluids given should include dextrose. It may be more practical to give fluids by the subcutaneous, intraosseous or peritoneal routes than intravenously, particularly in the smaller animals (see Chapter 5). Wounds should be cleaned and dressed, although dressings may be poorly tolerated.

Short-term hospitalization

For hospitalization, small cages are acceptable. The cage must be escape-proof; the ability of these species to squeeze though small spaces must be taken into account. For initial/emergency accommodation a wire mesh box with a close-fitting lid can be used; a hide box and a towel for bedding should be provided.

Weak, inappetant mustelids may be fed semi-liquid diets by syringe into the mouth. Convalescent diets specifically designed for carnivores are available, such as Oxbow Carnivore Care® and Emeraid® Carnivore; calculated energy requirements and feeding guides for small carnivores are provided with these products. Other products that have been used include vanilla-flavoured Ensure® (a human enteral product) and convalescent food designed for cats and dogs (Hills® Prescription Diet® a/d) mixed with electrolyte solution. If necessary, similar foods can be given by stomach tube. Further principles of initial management of wildlife casualties are given in Chapter 7. (See also 'Rearing of mustelid kits'.)

Anaesthesia and analgesia

Anaesthesia

Isoflurane and sevoflurane are suitable anaesthetic agents and may be used for induction and maintenance of general anaesthesia in all of these species; sevoflurane, being less irritant to the mucous membranes, is preferable for induction. Note that the American mink (being semi-aquatic) may breath-hold, leading to an increased induction time. The least stressful method of anaesthesia is the use of an induction chamber into which the mustelid, within a small travel cage, can be placed. Once the mustelid becomes recumbent it can be removed from the container and anaesthesia maintained using a small facemask over the nose. Alternatively, the mustelid can be restrained and anaesthesia induced with isoflurane or sevoflurane administered via facemask, if this can be carried out without causing excessive stress to the animal and risk to the handler. If the animal can be persuaded to enter a narrow tube in which it cannot turn around, then the head is available for mask induction and the hind end for injection.

Injectable agents which may be used for induction of anaesthesia are ketamine or, preferably, ketamine combined with a benzodiazepine or alpha-2 agonist (Figure 19.11). Once the mustelid is anaesthetized it should be

Drug(s)	Dosage	Comments
Ketamine	5–10 mg/kg i.m. [a]	For restraint of mink
	20–30 mg/kg i.m. [b]	For stoats and weasels
Ketamine (K) + diazepam (D)	25 mg/kg (K) i.m. + 25 mg/kg (D) i.m. [b]	For stoats and weasels
	25–35 mg/kg (K) + 2–3 mg/kg (D) i.m. [c]	For ferrets. Moderate anaesthesia with poor analgesia
Ketamine (K) + medetomidine (M)	10 mg/kg (K) + 0.2 mg/kg (M) i.m. [d]	For polecats
	5 mg/kg (K) + 0.1 mg/kg (M) i.m. [e]	For stoats
	10 mg/kg (K) + 0.2 mg/kg (M) i.m. [f]	For pine martens
	5–8 mg/kg (K) + 0.08–0.1 mg/kg (M) i.m. [c]	For ferrets
Ketamine (K) + midazolam (Mi)	0.25 mg/kg (Mi) i.m. followed 10 minutes later by 5–10 mg/kg (K) i.m. [c]	In ferrets, for heavy sedation/induction; then use inhalation anaesthesia
Meloxicam	0.2 mg/kg i.m., s.c., orally q24h [c]	Use with a histamine (H2) receptor antagonist (see Figure 19.12)
Carprofen	1 mg/kg orally q12–24h [c]	Use with a histamine (H2) receptor antagonist (see Figure 19.12)
Ketoprofen	0.5–1 mg/kg i.m., s.c., orally q24h [c]	Use with a histamine (H2) receptor antagonist and for less than 5 days (see Figure 19.12)
Buprenorphine	0.01–0.05 mg/kg i.v., i.m., s.c. q8–12h [g]	Can be used in addition to NSAID
Atipamezole	1.0 mg/kg i.m. (five times the dose of medetomidine)	For the reversal of medetomidine given at 0.2 mg/kg (e.g. for polecats [d] and pine martens [f] given medetomidine at 0.2 mg/kg)
	0.5 mg/kg (half i.v., half i.m.) [e]	For stoats given medetomidine at 0.1 mg/kg i.m. [e]

19.11 Anaesthetics and analgesics used in small mustelids. None of these drugs are licensed for use in these species and some are extrapolated from commonly used doses in domestic ferrets.
([a] Fowler, 1995; [b] Hall et al., 2001; [c] Johnson-Delaney, 2009; [d] Fournier-Chambrillon et al., 2003; [e] Kreeger, 1997; [f] Arnemo et al., 1994; [g] Carpenter, 2005)

intubated (which is relatively simple in these species) and anaesthesia maintained using isoflurane or sevoflurane.

Mustelids, particularly the smaller animals, rapidly lose heat and develop hypothermia. Always provide protection from heat loss, and supplemental warmth, whilst the animal is anaesthetized and during recovery (see Chapters 5 and 6). Their high metabolic rates also mean that they quickly become hypoglycaemic and food should be reintroduced shortly after recovery from anaesthesia. For this reason food should also not be withheld for more than an hour before elective surgery.

Analgesia

As analgesic dose rates specific for these mustelid species have not been calculated, analgesia should be provided based on ferret dosages (see Figure 19.11). Use of a histamine (H2) receptor antagonist is recommended when non-steroidal anti-inflammatory drugs (NSAIDs) are used in ferrets to reduce the risk of gastrointestinal ulceration; it would be prudent to maintain this practice with these species also. Buprenorphine can be used in addition to a NSAID.

Specific conditions

Trauma

Probably the most common reason for presentation of small mustelids is trauma. Bite wounds from cats or dogs are relatively common and juvenile stoats and weasels in particular may suffer from cat bite wounds. Snaring or trapping injuries are also seen, plus injuries (including fractures and internal injuries) following falls. The possibility of internal injuries should always be considered when an individual is presented with even apparently minor bite wounds. The

subsequent formation of abscesses, especially around the head and neck, may be fatal.

Puncture wounds or abscesses (e.g. from a cat bite) should be flushed twice daily with an appropriate antiseptic solution, such as dilute chlorhexidine solution, and the surface kept open to ensure that healing occurs from the base of the wound. Broad-spectrum systemic antibiotics should be administered (see Figure 19.12).

Broken teeth are especially common in polecats and may be a reason for euthanasia (see 'Examination and clinical assessment for rehabilitation').

Burn wounds may result from an individual getting caught in a fire (e.g. a bonfire in which it has denned, or a forest, heath or grass fire). Electrocution may occur occasionally if the mustelid climbs an electric fence, particularly with a wet coat (Cooper, 2003). These cases should be treated as for burns in any species, or euthanased if their injuries are too severe.

Mustelids may be presented with hypothermia and associated hypoglycaemia and exhaustion after becoming trapped in a water container; hypothermia could also occur if a mustelid, particularly of the smaller species, was exposed to cold wet conditions whilst caught inside a live trap. Hyperthermia may occur occasionally, for example if the animal becomes trapped in a metal container exposed to the sun. All of these conditions should be treated by standard methods.

Poisoning

Secondary poisoning with anticoagulant rodenticides is recognized in weasels, thought to be common in polecats and stoats, and has been confirmed in pine martens. The possibility of such poisoning should be considered in wildlife casualties, both as a possible primary reason for presentation and as a potential complicating factor following trauma. Deliberate poisoning should also be considered; deliberate (illegal) poisoning of weasels with an organophosphate (mevinphos) has been reported (see also Chapters 5 and 11).

Mustelids are also susceptible to botulism, particularly to type C toxin, causing paralysis, dyspnoea and death.

Infectious diseases
Viral infections

Mustelids are susceptible to canine distemper virus, although there are few reports of the disease in free-living individuals. Clinical and fatal disease has been seen in stoats, weasels and in at least one free-living polecat (Trebbien *et al.*, 2014), as well as in domestic ferrets; vaccination against this disease should be considered in orphans and long-term captive animals. In stoats and weasels, reduced activity, photophobia, bilateral watery ocular discharge, reddening of foot pads, crusting of the nose/upper lip and, less commonly, recurrent fits/muscular spasms and diarrhoea were seen; fatal infection occurred in both species (Keymer and Epps, 1969). Mucopurulent oculonasal discharge, respiratory signs, diarrhoea, hyperkeratosis of the foot pads and a rash both under the chin and in the inguinal area have also been seen in affected mustelids. Some affected individuals have survived infection, but euthanasia may be the least stressful option for wild casualties.

Mustelids are considered susceptible to feline pan-leucopaenia virus and rabies, and may be susceptible to infectious canine hepatitis and Aujezsky's disease. Mink and domestic ferrets are known to be susceptible to Aleutian disease and quarantine animals should be anti-body tested for this before being added to any captive collection of mustelids.

Bacterial diseases

Mycobacterium avium subsp. *paratuberculosis* has been isolated from stoats and weasels on farms in Scotland with a known Johne's disease problem. In some of the mustelids, histopathological lesions consistent with infec-tion with a slow-growing mycobacterial species were found, but there is no information regarding whether infection is clinically significant (Beard *et al.*, 2001). Isolations of *Mycobacterium bovis* have been made occa-sionally from stoat, polecat and mink in the UK (Delahay *et al.*, 2002; Delahay *et al.*, 2007). Antibodies against *Leptospira sejroe* were detected in one of eight weasels in one study (Michna and Campbell, 1970). Mustelids are susceptible to salmonellosis.

Parasites

A variety of parasites can be found on and in the small mustelids, including ticks, mites, lice, fleas (picked up from other species), nematodes, trematodes and cestodes. Ticks are most likely to be found around the ears and on the shoulders. The possibility of *Sarcoptes* or *Demodex* infection should be remembered as these have been found in ferrets (McDonald and Larivière, 2001), and signs of mange have been found in stoats. Standard antiparasitic agents can be used, such as fenbendazole and ivermectin (see Figure 19.12).

Angiostrongylus vasorum (lungworm) has been detected in stoats and weasels in south-west England (Simpson, 2010; 2014).

The nematode *Skrjabingylus nasicola* may be found in stoats, weasels, polecats and pine martens. The adult worms are found in the nasal sinuses and frontal sinuses and, if present in large numbers, can result in distortion and perforation of the frontal bones, with resultant pressure on the brain; infestation may be associated with spasms and fits. On the European mainland, cranial bone lesions have also been described associated with *Troglotrema acutum* flukes in pine martens (Kierdorf *et al.*, 2006). Sarcocystosis has been reported in the weasel and mink. There are no reported treatments for these infections.

Further information on diseases and parasites is available in Petrini, 1992; McDonald and Larivière, 2001; McDonald *et al.*, 2001; and Harris and Yalden, 2008.

Therapeutics

Drug doses extrapolated from those suggested for domestic ferrets can be used in these species. None of these drugs are licensed for use in these species. Dose rates for commonly used products are given in Figure 19.12. Where possible drugs should be administered in food to avoid the stress of handling.

Drug	Dosage	Comments
Amoxicillin/clavulanate (co-amoxiclav)	12.5–25 mg/kg orally q8–12h[a]	General broad-spectrum antibacterial use
Enrofloxacin	10–20 mg/kg i.m., s.c., orally q12–24h[a]	Injectable form can cause inflammation and necrosis
Fenbendazole	20 mg/kg orally once daily for 3 days[a]	For the treatment of nematode infestation
Ivermectin	0.2–0.4 mg/kg s.c. or orally Repeat after 14 days[a]	For the treatment of nematode and mite infestations
Ranitidine	3.5 mg/kg orally q12h[bc]	Histamine (H2) receptor antagonist For the prevention/treatment of gastric ulceration
Sucralfate	25–125 mg/kg orally q8–12h[b]	For the treatment of gastric ulcers Give before meals (requires acidic pH)

19.12 Dose rates for commonly used therapeutic products in small mustelids. None of these drugs are licensed for use in these species and are extrapolated from commonly used domestic ferret doses.
([a] Morrisey, 2009; [b] Carpenter, 2005; [c] Johnson-Delaney, 2009)

Management in captivity
Housing

Mustelids have been successfully kept in a variety of cages and enclosures. For medium-term hospitalization, a glass vivarium with a tight-fitting wire lid can be used for weasels and a small-mesh (10 mm aperture) wire cage is suitable for both weasels and stoats, whilst for the other species a strong metal cage is suggested; adequate ventilation must be present in all cases. Newspaper or sawdust can be used on the floor. A hide box should be provided, with a towel as bedding. Make sure that the cage can be cleaned without having to catch the animal or risk it escaping; this is most easily achieved by providing a nest chamber that can be locked shut. For weasels and stoats a small plastic vivarium with a hinged lid is useful. For the larger species it is preferable to use a dividable cage, with the mustelid shut into one side whilst the other side is cleaned.

For longer term captivity outside enclosures should be used. These should have metal walls buried to 0.75 m to prevent the inhabitants from digging out, or be wired under the whole ground surface, and either be covered overhead with wire mesh or have an inwards-facing smooth metal overhang to prevent the animals from climbing out.

Enrichment

In all enclosures, environmental enrichment should be provided. Initially this may only be a box for hiding in and a towel for bedding. Even in a hospital environment simple enrichment can be provided, for instance cardboard tubes from kitchen rolls (for stoats and weasels) or appropriate-diameter pieces of plastic piping for the animal to hunt through, table-tennis balls for weasels and stoats to bat around, whole dead prey items and whole raw eggs for mustelids to 'hunt' and eat and scent trails of herbs, etc.

In long-term housing there should be soil for digging and burrowing, water for swimming, vegetation, rocks, leaves, pine cones and logs and branches for climbing (particularly lots of branches for pine martens) and always one or more den boxes.

Diet

All of these species eat several small meals per day, rather than one or two large meals. Weasels in particular require frequent meals (2–4 g, 5–10 times daily); they cannot survive without food for more than approximately 24 hours. Guideline food quantities are provided in Figure 19.13.

Diets should be chosen with consideration of the normal carnivorous diet of these species; a familiar form to the diet is preferable, for example mice, rats, day-old chicks, rabbit, strips of meat and occasional raw eggs for stoats, weasels and polecats. White fish may be added for American mink. Pine martens have been kept long-term on day-old chicks, raw lean meat (beef, rabbit, chicken), locusts, fish and fruit (apple, banana, seasonal berries), with a vitamin and mineral supplement. Dry cat food can also be offered; some stoats will eat this in preference to meat from large rodents. Weak individuals may be unable to digest fur, feathers or bones; therefore, meat should be provided without these (perhaps with a small piece of appropriate skin attached to make the offered food more likely to be accepted). A varied diet should always be provided, as once habituated to a single type of food, captive small mustelids may then refuse to change to a different diet.

Since mustelids commonly cache food, it is important to regularly remove excess cached food from the nest box (or other cache site) and clean this as required. A balance is needed, however, because cleaning the cage invades the mustelid's territory and may cause stress. Overfeeding should also be avoided to reduce development of obesity.

Rearing of mustelid kits

Landmarks in the development of small mustelids are given in Figure 19.8 and these can be used to estimate the age of neonates. Hand-rearing of young kits is difficult and should not be attempted lightly. Handling and general exposure to humans should be minimized if release is to be possible. If a lactating female ferret is available it might be possible to foster kits on to her.

Hand-rearing requires feeding the kits every 2 hours initially. As with other species, feeding rehydration solution first, then changing to full-strength milk formula over the following three feeds is suggested. An appropriate feeder would be a plastic pipette, or a Catac teat or a catheter attached to a small syringe (1 ml syringe initially for weasels and stoats, 2.5 ml for larger species). The kits are fed in sternal recumbency. At each feed, the kit should be fed until it is satisfied. KMR® Kitten Milk Replacer, Esbilac® puppy milk replacer or goat milk have been used; enrichment of the percentage fat to 20% by combining three parts Esbilac® with one part whipping cream has been suggested for ferrets (McKimmey, 2002).

Weaning

From about 3–4 weeks for stoats, formula can be supplemented with small pieces of dry kitten food (soaked), cat food and pinkie mice or other appropriate dead prey items chopped up into small pieces, preferably from a dish. Once the eyes are open (5 weeks in stoats), kits should be

Species	Food requirement	Recommended amount and frequency
Weasel (*Mustela nivalis*)	Approx. 33% of bodyweight daily; slightly more for females and about 80–100% extra during lactation	2–4 g, 5–10 times daily (this amounts to about one 30 g vole per day – or two during lactation) Note: require frequent meals; cannot survive without food more than about 24 hours Avoid preoperative starvation
Stoat (*Mustela erminae*)	Approx. 23% of bodyweight in food per day More variable in females Lactating females need 200–300% of normal intake	At least 70 g per day for males At least 50 g per day for non-lactating females Approx. 100–150 g per day for lactating females
Polecat (*Mustela putorius*) (based on data for ferrets)	Approx. 125 g/kg (wet weight) bodyweight, 42 g/kg (dry weight) for males Approx. 145 g/kg (wet weight) bodyweight, 49 g/kg (dry weight) for females	Approx. 225–245 g wet weight (80 g dry weight) per day for males Approx. 105–125 g wet weight (40 g dry weight) per day for females
Pine marten (*Martes martes*)	Approx. 10% of bodyweight per night	140–160 g per night
Mink (*Mustela (Neovison) vison*)	Approx. 40 g/kg (dry matter) per day for males Approx. 53 g/kg (dry matter) per day for females Or about 152 calories digestible energy per kg per day Requirements may triple during lactation	207–227 g wet weight (73 g dry weight) per day for males 125–145 g wet weight (46 g dry weight) per day for females

19.13 Daily food requirements of small mustelids.
(Bleavins and Aulerich, 1981; Partridge, 1995; Larivière, 1999; Bourne et al., 2001; McDonald and Larivière, 2002; Harris and Yalden, 2008)

fully weaned from milk formula on to small dead prey items and good quality kitten food (wet, dry and dry food which has been soaked), and finally on to dead prey items and hard food only.

Housing juveniles

Appropriate housing for newborn kits would be a high-sided basket or bowl with soft bedding, kept inside an incubator. The kits should then (at 2–5 weeks of age for stoats) be moved to a vivarium with a heated pad under half of the floor surface and a box for denning, along with a stuffed toy if a single kit is being reared. At 5–7 weeks of age kits need a larger pen (e.g. a Petmate® Vari-Kennel with small-gauge wire on the door) with supplemental heat as required, then by 7–8 weeks (for a stoat) they should be moved to an outdoor pen with a den box, soil for digging in and multiple logs for climbing.

Release

It is important to ensure that the small mustelid is capable of surviving in the wild after release. Prior to release, the mustelid must be acclimatized to outdoor temperatures, be fully sighted, have all four limbs functional, have its scent glands intact (important for social signalling) and be able to efficiently catch and kill live prey. It should be noted that a true full testing of this last aspect would require provision of live prey of the appropriate species, which is illegal under most circumstances in the UK. Consider vaccinating against canine distemper (using a vaccine licenced for use in ferrets), feline panleucopaenia and perhaps leptospirosis in juveniles in high risk situations before release (see Chapter 7 for general considerations in relation to prophylaxis).

Whilst adult casualties which have been in care for only a short length of time should be fully capable of survival once returned to health, release of hand-reared animals, which may not know how to hunt, is more problematic. Typical prey-killing behaviour is innate, not learned, but juveniles that have not observed their mother hunting may be less efficient at killing and may not know how to search for prey. Juveniles should have reached the normal age of dispersal from their mother and should have shown that they have appropriate climbing, digging and preferably hunting skills. Preferably a soft-release should be used, with initial provision of a den box and supplementary food. Care must be taken to select release sites that provide suitable habitat and prey but are free from persecution.

Animals which have become habituated to humans and/or to domestic animals, such as cats or dogs, cannot be released (see Chapter 9) and every effort should be made to avoid such habituation. If animals have become too tame, euthanasia is required unless an appropriate long-term facility for their care is available as described previously (see 'Examination and clinical assessment for rehabilitation').

Release should not take place in severe weather, which would make it harder for the animal to hunt. If an individual is only fit for release in late autumn or winter, consider whether it should be maintained in an appropriate enclosure over winter and released in spring once plenty of prey is available. The correct release location is important. Individuals which were independent from their mother when brought into captivity (i.e. able to hunt) should be released as close as possible to where they were found, unless this is dangerous (e.g. on a road), or if they were brought to a human by a cat or dog, in which case they should be released into appropriate habitat near to where they were found.

Legal aspects

Mink cannot be released, nor kept in captivity under the Destructive Imported Animals Act 1932 and the Mink Keeping (Prohibition) (England) Order 2004, except under licence. There are some centres in the UK with appropriate licences to allow keeping these species for exhibition purposes; in the absence of space at such centres mink would need to be euthanased.

Pine martens and polecats are protected under the Wildlife and Countryside Act 1981 and all the species are protected under the Wild Mammals (Protection) Act 1996. See Chapter 2 for more information. Since there have been a number of releases of polecats from breeding programmes, all polecats presented, whether or not surviving to release, should be scanned for a microchip. If a microchipped animal is found, details of its identity together with when and where it was found should be passed on to The Mammal Society (see Appendix 1) and/or the Vincent Wildlife Trust (see 'Specialist organizations and useful contacts'). Both organizations would also be very interested to hear about the location at which any polecat (microchipped or otherwise) or pine marten was found, to assist in studies on the re-expansion of areas in which these species are present.

References and further reading

American Veterinary Medical Association (2013) *AVMA Guidelines for the Euthanasia of Animals: 2013 edition.* www.avma.org/KB/Policies/Documents/euthanasia.pdf

Arnemo JM, Moe RO and Søli NE (1994) Immobilization of captive pine martens (*Martes martes*) with medetomidine-ketamine and reversal with atipamezole. *Journal of Zoo and Wildlife Medicine* **25**, 548–554

Association of Zoos and Aquariums (AZA) Small Carnivore Taxon Advisory Group (TAG) (2010) *Mustelid (Mustelidae) Care Manual.* Association of Zoos and Aquariums, Silver Spring, Maryland

Beard PM, Daniels MJ, Henderson D et al. (2001) Paratuberculosis infection of nonruminant wildlife in Scotland. *Journal of Clinical Microbiology* **39**, 1517–1521

Bleavins MR and Aulerich RJ (1981) Feed consumption and food passage time in mink (*Mustela vison*) and European ferrets (*Mustela putorius furo*). *Laboratory Animal Science* **31**, 268–269

Bourne DC, Lawson B and Boardman S (2001) *Wildpro UK Wildlife: First Aid and Care.* http://wildpro.twycrosszoo.org/List_Vols/Wildpro_Gen_Cont.htm

Carpenter JW (2005) *Exotic Animal Formulary, 3rd edn.* Elsevier, St Louis, Missouri

Cooper JE (2003) Other mustelids. In: *BSAVA Manual of Wildlife Casualties, 1st edn*, ed. E Mullineaux, D Best and JE Cooper, pp. 147–151. BSAVA Publications, Gloucester

Corbet GB and Harris S (1991) *The Handbook of British Mammals 3rd edn.* Blackwell Scientific Publications, Oxford

Delahay RJ, De Leeuw AN, Barlow AM, Clifton-Hadley RS and Cheeseman CL (2002) The status of *Mycobacterium bovis* in UK wild mammals: a review. *The Veterinary Journal* **164**, 90–105

Delahay RJ, Smith GC, Barlow AM et al. (2007) Bovine tuberculosis infection in wild mammals in the south-west region of England: a survey of prevalence and a semi-quantitative assessment of the relative risks to cattle. *The Veterinary Journal* **173**, 287–301

Dunstone N (1993) *The Mink.* T and AD Poyser, London

Elmeros M, Christensen TK and Lassen P (2011) Concentrations of anticoagulant rodenticides in stoats (*Mustela erminea*) and weasels (*Mustela nivalis*) from Denmark. *The Science of the Total Environment* **409**, 2373–2378

Fernandez-Moran J (2003) Mustelidae. In: *Zoo and Wild Animal Medicine 5th edn*, ed. ME Fowler and EM Miller, pp. 501–516. Saunders, St. Louis, Missouri

Fournier-Chambrillon C, Chusseau JP, Dupuch J et al. (2003) Immobilization of free-ranging European mink (*Mustela lutreola*) and polecat (*Mustela putorius*) with medetomidine-ketamine and reversal by atipamezole. *Journal of Wildlife Diseases* **29**, 393–399

Fowler ME (1995) *Restraint and Handling of Wild and Domestic Animals, 2nd edn.* Iowa State University Press, Ames, Iowa

Hall LW, Clarke KW and Trim CM (2001) *Veterinary Anaesthesia, 10th edn.* WB Saunders, London

Harjunpääa S and Rouvinen-Watta K (2004) The development of homeothermy in mink. *Comparative Biochemistry and Physiology Part A: Molecular and Integrative Physiology* **137**, 339–348

Harris S and Yalden DW (2008) *Mammals of the British Isles: Handbook, 4th edn.* The Mammal Society, Southampton

Hines C (2003) Environmental enrichment in wildlife rehabilitation. *Wildlife Rehabilitation* **21**, 137–145

Hines C (2005) Natural history and rehabilitation of weasels (*Mustela* spp.). *Wildlife Rehabilitation* **23**, 63–69

HSA/UFAW (1993) *Humane Killing of Animals.* Humane Slaughter Association and Universities Federation for Animal Welfare, Wheathampstead

Iacarusco TL (1999) Rehabilitation of least weasels (*Mustela nivalis*). *Wildlife Rehabilitation* **17**, 113–116

Johnson-Delaney CA (2009) Ferrets: anaesthesia and analgesia. In: *BSAVA Manual of Rodents and Ferrets*, ed. E Keeble and A Meredith, pp. 245–253. BSAVA Publications, Gloucester

Keymer IF and Epps HBG (1969) Canine distemper in the family Mustelidae. *Veterinary Record* **85**, 204–205

Kierdorf U, Kierdorf H, Konjević D *et al.* (2006) Remarks on cranial lesions in the European polecat (*Mustela putorius*) caused by helminth parasites. *Veterinarski arhiv* **76**, S101-S109

King CM (1983) *Mustela erminea. Mammalian Species* **195**, 1–8

Kreeger TJ (1997) *Handbook of Wildlife Chemical Immobilization.* Wildlife Pharmaceuticals, Inc. Fort Collins, Colorado

Larivière S (1999) *Mustela vison. Mammalian Species* **608**, 1–9

Lloyd M (2002) Veterinary care of ferrets 1. Clinical examination and routine procedures. *In Practice* **24**, 90–95

McClure D and Anderson N (2006) Rodents and small mammals. In: *Guidelines for Euthanasia of Nondomestic Animals*, pp. 61–65. American Association of Zoo Veterinarians, Yulee

McDonald RA, Day MJ and Birtles RJ (2001) Histological evidence of disease in wild stoats (*Mustela erminea*) in England. *Veterinary Record* **149**, 671–675

McDonald RA, Harris S, Turnbull G *et al.* (1998) Anticoagulant rodenticides in stoats (*Mustela erminea*) and weasels (*Mustela nivalis*) in England. *Environmental Pollution* **103**, 17–23

McDonald RA and Larivière S (2001) Diseases and pathogens of *Mustela* spp., with special reference to the biological control of introduced stoat (*Mustela erminea*) populations in New Zealand. *Journal of the Royal Society of New Zealand* **31**, 721–744

McDonald RA and Larivière S (2002) Captive husbandry of stoats (*Mustela erminea*). *New Zealand Journal of Zoology* **29**, 177–186

McKimmey V (2002) Ferret kits. In: *Hand-rearing Wild and Domestic Mammals*, ed. LJ Gage, pp. 203–206. Iowa State Press, Ames, Iowa

Michna SW and Campbell RSF (1970) Leptospirosis in wild animals. *Journal of Comparative Pathology* **80**, 101–106

Morrisey J (2009) Ferrets: therapeutics. In: *BSAVA Manual of Rodents and Ferrets*, ed. E Keeble and A Meredith, pp. 237–244. BSAVA Publications, Gloucester

O'Connor C, Turner J, Scobie S *et al.* (2006) *Stoat reproductive biology.* Science for Conservation 268. Department of Conservation, Wellington, New Zealand

Partridge J (1995) *Husbandry Handbook for Mustelids.* Association of British Wild Animal Keepers, Bristol

Petrini K (1992) The medical management and diseases of mustelids. *Proceedings of the Joint Meeting of the American Association of Zoo Veterinarians and the American Association of Wildlife Veterinarians. Oakland, California, 15–19 November 1992*

Sheffield SR and King CM (1994) *Mustela nivalis. Mammalian Species* **454**, 1–10

Sikarskie JG and Hollamby SR (2006) Carnivores. In: *Guidelines for Euthanasia of Nondomestic Animals*, pp. 78–81. American Association of Zoo Veterinarians, Yulee

Simpson V (2010) *Angiostrongylus vasorum* infection in a stoat. *Veterinary Record* **166**, 182

Simpson V (2014) *Angiostrongylus vasorum* infection in Cornwall. *Veterinary Record* **175**, 178–179

Sleeman P (1989) *Stoats and Weasels, Polecats and Martens.* Whittet Books, London

Stocker L (2005) *Practical Wildlife Care 2nd edn.* Blackwell Publishing, Oxford

Trebbien R, Chriel M, Struve T *et al.* (2014) Wildlife reservoirs of canine distemper virus resulted in a major outbreak in Danish farmed mink (*Neovison vison*). *PLoS One* **9**, e85598

Weiss DJ, Wustemberg W, Bucci TJ *et al.* (1994) Hematologic and serum chemistry reference values for adult brown mink. *Journal of Wildlife Diseases* **30**, 599–602

Specialist organizations and useful contacts

See also Appendix 1

National Ferret Welfare Society
For general ferret information including information specifically for vets
www.nfws.net

The Vincent Wildlife Trust
For notification of pine marten sightings and useful information on pine marten, polecat and stoat
3 and 4 Bronsil Courtyard, Eastnor, Ledbury, Herefordshire HR8 1EP
Tel: 01531 636441
www.vwt.org.uk

Chapter 20

Wildcats

Anna Meredith

The Scottish wildcat (*Felis silvestris grampia;* Figure 20.1) is the only remaining indigenous member of the cat family in Britain. It was once found across the British mainland but is now confined to the Scottish Highlands and is sometimes considered a distinct subspecies of the European wildcat (*Felis silvestris silvestris*), although further research is required to determine this (Miller, 1907). Scottish terms for the wildcat are 'will cat' or 'wullcat' and, in Gaelic, 'cat fiadhaich'. In addition to habitat loss and historical persecution, a major threat to the Scottish wildcat population is introgressive hybridization with the domestic cat (*Felis silvestris catus*), which has probably been occurring for hundreds, if not thousands, of years (Kitchener *et al.*, 2005).

The current status of the Scottish wildcat is unclear and there are only two population density estimates available for Scotland. These are Glen Tanar, Deeside, with 30 wildcats per 100 km² and Ardnamurchan with an estimated eight wildcats per 100 km² (Davis and Gray, 2010). A 1995 study resulted in an estimate of 3500 pre-breeding animals of independent age (over 5 months old) across Scotland (Harris *et al.*, 1995). However, there may be as few as 400 cats considered to be uninfluenced by introgression, and it is possible that very few genetically pure wildcats remain (Macdonald *et al.*, 2004). If so, this population would be classified as critically endangered (Kitchener *et al.*, 2005).

The Scottish wildcat has been identified in Scotland's Species Action Framework as one of 22 key Scottish species 'requiring targeted management action to improve prospects for its future survival as a distinct native species'. In 2013 the Scottish Wildcat Conservation Action Plan (SWCAP) was launched by Scottish Natural Heritage (SNH), a collaborative multi-organizational plan of conservation actions aimed at halting the decline of wildcats over a 6-year period (SNH, 2013).

Ecology, biology and behaviour

Habitat

Wildcat habitat typically consists of woodlands and woodland margins, and areas of dense gorse or juniper thickets. Young forestry plantations are an important habitat as they support a high population density of small mammal prey. Wildcats require open patches, such as pasture or riparian areas, for hunting but for movement they prefer to avoid open areas, using woodland, scrub, forest clear-fell, hedge lines and stream edges for cover. They are also strong climbers.

There are regional differences in habitat, depending largely on prey type and prey abundance; in the east of Scotland, wildcats prefer the moorland, pastureland and woodland margins, whereas in the west, where rabbit population densities are low, they prefer uplands with rough grazing and moorlands. Scottish wildcats will live up to an altitude of around 800 m, but are not generally found higher than 650 m.

Diet in the wild

The preferred prey of the Scottish wildcat is the European rabbit (*Oryctolagus cuniculus*), which can form up to 70% of the diet in eastern Scotland, but they also eat small mammals, mainly voles (*Microtus agrestis* and *Myodes glareolus*) and wood mice (*Apodemus sylvaticus*), which form the majority of their diet in other areas where rabbit population densities are lower. They will also take birds, reptiles and invertebrates where these are easily available.

Home range and marking

Wildcats are generally considered to be nocturnal or crepuscular and are solitary, except during mating or when females are raising young. The home range of a male overlaps with the ranges of one or more females. Home ranges overlap to a greater or lesser extent depending

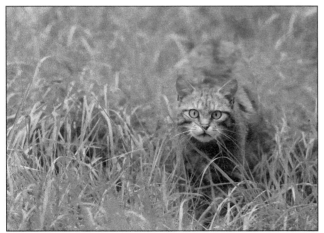

20.1 Scottish wildcat.
(© Jean Manson)

on prey abundance. In areas of high rabbit abundance (e.g. Cairngorms National Park) the home range is between 0.3 and 6 km², but in the west of Scotland where prey population density is lower, home ranges can vary from 8 to 18 km². Wildcats use faeces (scats) deposited in prominent places, such as on rocks or in the middle of paths, and urine sprayed on trees or bushes to mark their home range. They also scent mark by scratching and rubbing their cheek glands against trees and other objects to communicate.

Breeding

Dens are created in rock piles, large logging piles, brush piles or among tree roots. Wildcats will also use empty rabbit warrens, fox dens and badger setts as dens. Females are reflex ovulators and can breed from December to August, but the main mating season is in late winter (January to March). Gestation is 63–68 days and usually one litter of up to eight kittens (average three or four) is produced in the spring (April to May). In some cases, a second litter may be produced later in the year, for example if the first litter dies. Kittens begin to hunt with their mother from 10–12 weeks old and are fully weaned by 10–14 weeks old. They reach independence between 5 and 6 months of age, when they will disperse to seek new potential home ranges. Males reach sexual maturity at 9–10 months old, and females at 12 months. Male kittens normally leave the maternal home range before their first winter, and can travel large distances (up to 55 km) on dispersal. Female kittens can stay within their natal range during the first winter before dispersing. Dispersal is associated with a high risk of mortality due to road traffic accidents or predation by other species such as foxes (*Vulpes vulpes*) and eagles (Accipitridae).

Longevity

Although wildcats have been known to live 15–16 years in captivity, it has been shown in Scotland that only 7% of wildcats live longer than 6 years in the wild, with females living up to 10 years and males up to 8 years. The main causes of mortality in wild populations are believed to be human-related; prior to legal protection in 1988 it is estimated that approximately 92% of wildcat deaths in Scotland were due to hunting. The Game Conservancy's National Game Bag Census for 1984–85 recorded the death of 274 wildcats on 40 shooting estates in Scotland, an annual mortality of nearly 10% of the estimated wildcat population, although some may have been hybrids (Kilshaw, 2011). Illegal persecution may still be a significant threat, and wildcats are also at risk of mortality due to road traffic accidents.

Anatomy and physiology

In general, the Scottish wildcat is larger than the domestic cat and has longer legs, a larger more robust head and skull and a more muscular appearance. The intestinal length of the wildcat is shorter than that of the domestic cat. Males are 82.3–98.1 cm long including the tail, with bodyweights of 3.77–7.26 kg. Females are smaller, being 73–89.5 cm long and weighing 2.35–4.68 kg. There are genetic differences between wildcats and domestic cats (Driscoll *et al.*, 2007). The ability to robustly identify true wildcats from hybrids is the overriding conservation issue affecting Scottish wildcat survival (Pierpaoli *et al.*, 2003; Oliveira *et al.*, 2008). Seven key pelage markings have been identified that show consistent differences in appearance between wildcats and domestic tabby cats (Figure 20.2) (Kitchener *et al.*, 2005).

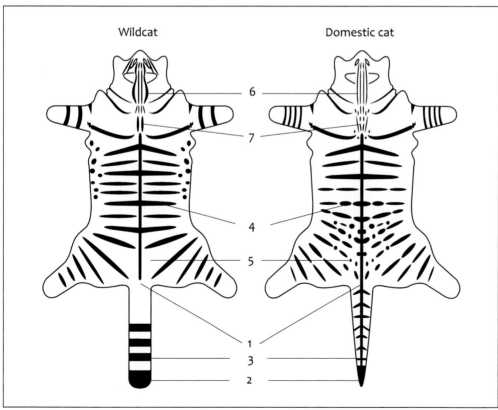

20.2 Seven key pelage markings can be used to distinguish between wildcats and domestic tabby cats. In wildcats:

1. Dorsal stripe on the lower back always stops at the root of the tail.
2. Tip of tail blunt and black.
3. Distinct aligned tail bands.
4. Unbroken flank stripes.
5. No spots on rump; stripes may be broken, but distinct.
6. Four nape stripes: broad, wavy and unfused.
7. Two shoulder stripes.

(© The Zoological Society of London, reproduced from Kitchener *et al.*, 2005, with permission)

These provide a useful way to visually distinguish the species and are used as a field definition, but how this phenotypical assessment relates or corresponds to genetic purity is still a subject of research. Current findings indicate that there is a continuum between wild and domestic cat genetic types in the wild/feral cat population, and the population is a hybrid swarm. Hybrids are of variable appearance but are generally larger than domestic cats, with a tabby coat that can be confused with wildcats. Domestic tabby cats and hybrids can have patches of white in their coat (e.g. white paws or white patches on their back or sides), but the Scottish wildcat has no such markings. A major problem for conservation is the difficulty in using morphology solely to determine the hybridization status of an individual wildcat (Beaumont *et al.*, 2001; Lecis *et al.*, 2006) and genetic markers to differentiate pure wildcats from hybrids have recently been identified (Driscoll *et al.*, 2011; Nussberger *et al.*, 2013). Currently, as a precautionary approach for gamekeepers, landowners and those involved in feral cat control, striped tabby cats in Scotland that are living wild, with a thick ringed and blunt-tipped tail with no stripe down the middle, and no white paws, are considered a potential wildcat, even though this might include some hybrids.

Anatomically, apart from the differences mentioned above, wildcats are very similar to domestic cats. Gender determination is by the greater anogenital distance, round preputial opening and presence of testicles in the male (>6–10 weeks). In females the vulva lies directly beneath the anus and is slit-like.

Capture, handling and transportation

Wildcats are very aggressive and dangerous animals and can elicit severe bite and claw injuries. General principles of capture, handling and transportation are given in Chapter 3. Any wildcat that can be caught easily will be severely debilitated or injured. Targeted capture can be achieved using a pre-baited trap (Figure 20.3) and the wildcat can then be transferred to a crush cage for sedation. Alternatively, a dog-grasper or large net can be used. Unless very debilitated or comatose the animal should then be sedated or anaesthetized, to minimize stress and facilitate handling and examination (Figure 20.4). Scruffing

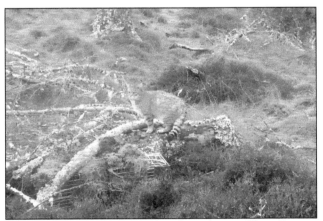

20.3 Pre-baited traps are used to effectively trap wildcats. For efficiency traps should be placed where prior use of camera traps has identified the presence of a suspected wildcat. (Courtesy of R Campbell)

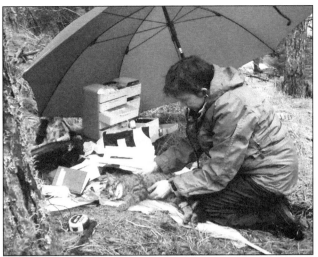

20.4 Scottish wildcat being examined under anaesthesia by the author in the field.

of fully conscious adult cats should not be attempted as they are very strong and can still inflict serious injuries with teeth and claws, and escape. Transportation can be carried out with the cat still in the trap or crush cage, or within a suitable robust domestic cat carrier (not cardboard), which should be covered with a cloth or towel to reduce stress. Wildcat kittens can be handled with care using the scruff.

Puncture-type bite injuries from wildcats during handling, as with domestic cats, frequently lead to infections in the handler, including non-purulent wounds with cellulitis and lymphangitis and purulent wounds without abscess formation, due to injection of mixed aerobic and anaerobic bacteria, predominantly *Pasteurella* and *Fusobacterium* spp. (Abrahamian and Goldstein, 2011). *Bartonella henselae*, the causative agent of cat-scratch disease, has also been detected in wildcats (Gerrikagoitia *et al.*, 2012).

Examination and clinical assessment for rehabilitation

Examination and assessment of a sedated or anaesthetized wildcat uses the same techniques as those for domestic cats (see Figure 20.4). Euthanasia will also be achieved in the same manner as for domestic cats (i.e. by overdose of barbiturates by the intravenous or intra-organ route), in a sedated or anaesthetized animal (see Chapter 4).

Diagnostic techniques

There is only one published study of normal haematological and serum biochemical values from 20 captive animals from Spain (Marco *et al.*, 2000), which showed that results for most parameters fall within the reference range for domestic cats (Figure 20.5). However, mean values for alanine aminotransferase (ALT), aspartate aminotransferase (AST), creatine kinase (CK), lactate dehydrogenase (LDH), blood urea nitrate (BUN), glucose and sodium were higher than the upper limit of the domestic cat reference range in the wildcats sampled. The author has analysed blood samples from 15 clinically healthy Scottish wildcats and the results are also presented in Figure 20.5.

Variable (units)	European wildcats[a]			Scottish wildcats[b]		
	n	Mean	Reference interval	n	Mean	Reference interval
Haematology						
Red blood cell (RBC) count (x 10^{12}/l)	20	9.4	7.9–11.4	15	9.3	6.7–11.8
Haemoglobin (g/dl)	20	12.1	9.6–14.9	15	12.6	8.9–16.4
Packed cell volume (PCV) (%)	20	37.7	31–46	15	39	27–51
Mean corpuscular volume (MCV) (fl)	20	40.4	34.7–47.7	15	42.2	39.4–44.9
Mean corpuscular haemoglobin (MCH) ((pg) per cell)	20	13	10.8–14.6	NDA	NDA	NDA
Mean corpuscular haemoglobin concentration (MCHC) (g/dl)	20	32.2	30–34.9	15	32.4	30–34.9
White blood cell (WBC) count (x 10^9/l)	20	14.7	9.2–26.1	15	14.4	3.3–25.6
Neutrophils (x 10^9/l)	20	8.7	3.7–14.9	15	7.8	1.5–27.4[c]
Lymphocytes (x 10^9/l)	20	4.1	1.8–7.4	15	4.5	0.8–8.2
Monocytes (x 10^9/l)	20	0.4	0.1–1	15	0.8	0.09–4.3[c]
Eosinophils (x 10^9/l)	20	1.5	0.3–3.7	15	1.3	0.17–5.3[c]
Basophils (x 10^9/l)	20	0	0	15	0	0
Neutrophil band (x 10^9/l)	20	0.1	0–0.5	NDA	NDA	NDA
Biochemistry						
Sodium (mmol/l)	14	166.7	156–172	15	152.9	150.7–155.1
Potassium (mmol/l)	14	5.2	4.7–5.6	15	4.94	3.8–6.1
Chloride (mmol/l)	9	123.6	118.8–130.2	15	112.1	108.2–116
Blood urea nitrate (BUN) (mmol/l)	18	13.6	5.5–21.2	NDA	NDA	NDA
Creatinine (µmol/l)	18	114.9	68.0–152.1	15	118.5	76.2–160.8
Urea (mmol/l)	NDA	NDA	NDA	15	11.2	3.5–18.9
Total bilirubin (µmol/l)	18	1.54	0–0.4	NDA	NDA	NDA
Glucose (mmol/l)	9	9.3	5.6–17.5	NDA	NDA	NDA
Cholesterol (mmol/l)	18	2.9	1.1–5	NDA	NDA	NDA
Triglycerides (mg/dl)	18	46.4	14.3–106	NDA	NDA	NDA
Creatine kinase (CK) (IU/l)	18	304.4	58–623	NDA	NDA	NDA
Lactate dehydrogenase (LDH) (IU/l)	18	452.8	20.4–1,236	NDA	NDA	NDA
Alkaline phosphatase (ALP) (IU/l)	NDA	NDA	NDA	15	36.8	13.1–82.7[c]
Alanine aminotransferase (ALT) (IU/l)	18	55.8	22.0–94.2	NDA	NDA	NDA
Aspartate aminotransferase (AST) (IU/l)	18	46.2	23–74	NDA	NDA	NDA
Gamma-glutamyl transferase (GGT) (IU/l)	18	2	0.5–5	NDA	NDA	NDA
Total protein (g/l)	20	77.4	70–88	15	67.9	61.6–74.3
Albumin (g/l)	18	34.9	21.2–42.7	15	33.7	29.1–38.4
Alpha-1 globulins (g/l)	18	3.5	2–6.2	NDA	NDA	NDA
Alpha-2 globulins (g/l)	18	8.2	4–11.3	NDA	NDA	NDA
Beta-1 globulins (g/l)	18	3.2	1.6–6.1	NDA	NDA	NDA
Beta-2 globulins (g/l)	18	5.1	3.4–10.8	NDA	NDA	NDA
Gamma globulins (g/l)	18	22	10.1–37.7	NDA	NDA	NDA
Albumin:globulin	18	0.9	0.4–1.5	NDA	NDA	NDA

20.5 Haematological and serum biochemical values for captive European wildcats and Scottish wildcats. NDA = no data available.

([a] Adapted from Marco et al., 2000. [b] Meredith, unpublished data from 15 Scottish wildcats. [c] Data have undergone log transformation)

First aid and short-term hospitalization

Wildcats are extremely powerful animals and a strong metal caging should be used to house them. A divider, or internal cage that can be closed securely, will be necessary to enable cleaning without handling. Apart from the issues associated with dealing with a potentially aggressive and dangerous wild animal, the principles of immediate first aid and hospitalization will be the same as for a feral or domestic cat (see Chapters 5 and 7).

Anaesthesia and analgesia

Administration of anaesthetic drugs by the intramuscular route can be achieved by hand injection using a crush cage, or if necessary via blowpipe or dart gun in a captive situation. However, the risk of trauma using the latter route may be high. A combination of medetomidine (40–80 µg/kg) and ketamine (5 mg/kg) i.m. is used by the author in field situations for trapped wildcats, but doses may need to be reduced in debilitated or injured animals. Reversal of the effects of medetomidine can be achieved with atipamezole at 2.5–5 times the dose of medetomidine used (the author uses five times the dose in field situations). Butorphanol at 0.4 mg/kg can be added to this combination ('triple combination') if desired (e.g. for surgical procedures). Alternatively, in debilitated individuals ketamine at 5 mg/kg plus midazolam at 0.25 mg/kg can be used in combination by intramuscular injection, although this gives deep sedation/light anaesthesia only and the animal should still be handled with care. Intubation is advisable and anaesthesia can be prolonged or deepened using gaseous agents such as isoflurane.

Other anaesthetic and analgesic agents can be used at the same doses as for domestic cats.

Specific conditions

Trauma

Many wildcat casualties are presented with traumatic injuries as a result of road traffic accidents, shooting or trapping for example. Dental trauma is also common. Techniques for assessing and treating injuries are the same as for domestic cats, although treatment decisions and outcomes must be made with the aim of rapid return to the wild, unless specific licensed permission has been given to retain the cat in captivity (e.g. to enter a captive breeding programme).

Infectious diseases

Viral diseases

There are very limited data available on the health and diseases of Scottish wildcats. Scottish studies report evidence of feline leukaemia virus (FeLV) infection in two out of 23 live trapped animals, but no evidence of infection with feline coronavirus (FCoV) or feline immunodeficiency virus (FIV) (McOrist et al., 1991; McOrist, 1992). Antibodies to Toxoplasma gondii were found in all samples, and three cats had clinical signs associated with upper respiratory tract infection ('cat flu'). A subsequent Scottish study (Daniels et al., 1999) surveyed 50 trapped wildcats and confirmed that they are commonly infected with the major viruses of the domestic cat (FeLV, feline calicivirus (FCV), feline herpesvirus (FHV), FCoV, as well as feline foamy virus (FeFV)), with the exception of FIV. Other information for free-living wildcats comes from studies on European wildcats also demonstrating exposure to many common feline pathogens including feline parvovirus (FPV, feline panleukopaenia, feline infectious enteritis) and canine distemper virus (Leutenegger et al., 1999; Millán and Rodriguez, 2009; Duarte et al., 2012). A captive wildcat from Spain was found to have gross and histological post-mortem findings consistent with FPV infection, confirmed by immunohistochemistry and polymerase chain reaction (PCR) (Wasieri et al., 2009).

Bacterial diseases

Corynebacterium felinum was isolated from the mouth of a Scottish wildcat that had died of feline influenza (FHV), along with Escherichia coli, a Streptococcus sp. and a Pseudomonas sp. (Collins et al., 2001). Antibodies to Chlamydia sp. were found in 27% of 25 wildcat serum samples in Spain (Millán and Rodriguez, 2009), and Candidatus Mycoplasma turicensis has been detected by PCR in European wildcats (Willi et al., 2007).

Preliminary findings from Scottish wildcats/hybrids trapped and sampled in 2013/2014 have detected FeLV, FPV, Mycoplasma haemominutum, M. felis, Chlamydia felis and Clostridium perfringens (A Meredith, unpublished data). Thus there is strong evidence that pathogen transmission between domestic cats and wildcats and their hybrids is occurring, and diseases caused by these pathogens could have a major impact on the health and survival of the remaining wildcat population.

Parasites

A variety of parasites have been reported in wildcats. Ectoparasites include the cat flea (Ctenocephalides felis), rabbit flea (Spillopsyllus cuniculi), rodent flea (Hystrichopsylla talpae), ticks (Ixodes ricinus) and lice (Filicola subrostratus) (Corbett, 1979). The author has also noted ear mites (Otodectes spp.) causing mild otitis in free-living and captive wildcats. These, and endoparasites (e.g. Toxocara spp. and Taenia spp.), can be treated as for domestic cats if deemed necessary (see Chapters 1 and 7).

Therapeutics

Standard drug doses as used for domestic cats can be used in wildcats. Injectable agents can be given to a conscious animal using a crush cage; oral medication can be offered in the food if the animal is eating, but this may be rejected unless it is finely crushed or in liquid form, well mixed and a palatable formulation. The use of long-acting injectable products should be considered to minimize the requirement for restraint.

Management in captivity

Housing and feeding

Strong metal cat or dog kennels can be used for short-term housing but should be away from domestic cats and dogs. This is essential for biosecurity, both to prevent any indirect or direct contact with potential feline pathogens whilst in captivity, and also to prevent any possible introduction of previously unencountered feline pathogens back into wild populations after release. Provision of a hide box and visual security is vital. Feeding should mimic the wild diet and include fresh, or frozen and thawed, rabbits, quail, day-old chicks and small rodents. Commercial wet domestic cat food or raw chicken can be used in the short term if whole prey is unavailable.

Longer term housing and accommodation for soft-release requires a more specialist large outdoor high-roofed pen with plenty of cover and branches or platforms.

Rearing of wildcat kittens

Wildcat kittens can be reared in a similar manner to domestic kittens, ideally in conspecific groups and with minimal human exposure (see Chapter 8 for general guidelines on hand-rearing mammals).

Release

Phenotypic identification, and preferably genetic identification (by blood sample), of wildcats to distinguish them from domestic cats or hybrids must be carried out prior to release. If presented with a tabby feral cat (e.g. for neutering and release as part of a trap-neuter-return (TNR) programme) or a suspected hybrid, advice on identification and protocols for testing and release should be sought from SNH in line with the SWCAP. It is important to note that in Scotland the legal situation is that unowned (feral) cats are considered non-native invasive species (Wildlife and Natural Environment (Scotland) Act 2011), and cannot be released after capture (e.g. for neutering) without specific licence authority from SNH.

In general, true wildcats that have only been in captivity for a short time should be released at the site where they were found but advice from SNH should be sought as this may vary depending on area, presence or absence of feral cats, and current conservation advice in line with the SWCAP. Wildcats that have been in captivity for longer periods or reared from orphans are likely to need more specialist soft-release procedures and expert advice and assistance from experienced rehabilitators will be required.

Wildcats should be screened for feline pathogens prior to release wherever possible in order to avoid the potential of introducing disease to wild populations, particularly if translocation is being considered.

Vaccination has been shown to elicit an excellent immune response after administration of one dose of standard modified-live or inactivated feline vaccine against FPV, FCV and FHV at the time of neutering in feral cats in TNR programmes (Fischer *et al.*, 2007), and thus it is advisable to vaccinate wildcats prior to release due to the risk of contact with unvaccinated feral or domestic cats. Individual identification with a microchip, and also detailed photographic records of pelage markings, are also strongly advised.

Legal aspects

The wildcat (*Felis silvestris*) is listed as of 'Least Concern' in the International Union for Conservation of Nature (IUCN) Red List of Threatened Species. However, the European wildcat (*Felis silvestris silvestris*) is classed as threatened at the national level in many range states. It is a European protected species (EPS) and receives protection through inclusion on Schedule 2 of the Conservation (Natural Habitats, etc.) Regulations 1994 that transpose the EU Habitats Directive into UK law. In the UK it was formerly listed on Schedule 5 for protection under the Wildlife and Countryside Act 1981, but was removed from this domestic legislation through an amendment to the Conservation (Natural Habitats etc.) Regulations in Scotland in 2007.

In captivity wildcats are covered by the Dangerous Wild Animals Act 1976, and the Animal Health and Welfare (Scotland) Act 2006.

As mentioned above (see 'Release'), in Scotland unowned (feral) cats are considered non-native invasive species (Wildlife and Natural Environment (Scotland) Act 2011), and cannot be released after capture (e.g. for neutering) without specific licence authority from SNH.

References and further reading

Abrahamian FM and Goldstein EJC (2011) Microbiology of animal bite wound infections. *Clinical Microbiological Review* **24(2)**, 231–246

Beaumont M, Barratt EM, Gottelli D *et al.* (2001) Genetic diversity and introgression in the Scottish wildcat. *Molecular Ecology* **10(2)**, 319–336

Collins MD, Hoyles L, Hutson RA, Foster G and Falsen E (2001) *Corynebacterium testudinoris* sp. nov., from a tortoise, and *Corynebacterium felinum* sp. nov., from a Scottish wild cat. *International Journal of Systematic Evolutionary Microbiology* **51**, 1349–1352

Corbett LK (1979) *Feeding ecology and social behaviour of wildcats (Felis silvestris) and domestic cats (Felis catus) in Scotland.* PhD Thesis, University of Aberdeen

Daniels MJ, Golder MC, Jarrett O and MacDonald DW (1999) Feline viruses in wildcats from Scotland. *Journal of Wildlife Diseases* **35(1)**, 121–124

Davis AR and Gray D (2010) *The distribution of Scottish wildcats (Felis silvestris) in Scotland (2006–2008).* Scottish Natural Heritage Commissioned Report No. 360. Inverness, Scottish National Heritage

Driscoll CA, Menotti-Raymond M, Roca AL *et al.* (2007) The Near Eastern origin of cat domestication. *Science* **317(5837)**, 519–523

Driscoll CA, Yamaguchi N, O'Brien SJ and Macdonald DW (2011) A suite of genetic markers useful in assessing wildcat (*Felis silvestris* ssp.) domestic cat (*Felis silvestris catus*) admixture. *Journal of Heredity* **102 Supplement 1**, S87–S90

Duarte A, Fernandes M, Santos N and Tavares L (2012) Virological survey in free-ranging wildcats (*Felis silvestris*) and feral domestic cats in Portugal. *Veterinary Microbiology* **158**, 400–404

Fischer SM, Quest CM, Dubovi EJ *et al.* (2007) Response of feral cats to vaccination at the time of neutering. *Journal of the American Veterinary Medical Association* **230(1)**, 52–58

Gerrikagoitia X, Gil H, García-Esteban C *et al.* (2012) Presence of *Bartonella* species in wild carnivores of northern Spain. *Applied Environmental Microbiology* **78(3)**, 885–888

Harris S, Morris P, Wray S and Yalden D (1995) *A review of British Mammals; population estimates and conservation status of British mammals other than cetaceans.* JNCC, Peterborough

Kilshaw K (2011) *Scottish wildcats: Naturally Scottish.* www.snh.org.uk/pdfs/publications/naturallyscottish/wildcats.pdf

Kitchener AC, Yamaguchi N, Ward JM and Macdonald DW (2005) A diagnosis for the Scottish wildcat: a tool for conservation action for a critically-endangered felid. *Animal Conservation* **8**, 223–237

Lecis R, Pierpaoli M, Birò ZS *et al.* (2006) Bayesian analyses of admixture in wild and domestic cats (*Felis silvestris*) using linked microsatellite loci. *Molecular Ecology* **15**, 119–131

Leutenegger CM, Hofmann-Lehmann R, Riols C *et al.* (1999) Viral infections in free-living populations of the European wildcat. *Journal of Wildlife Diseases* **35(4)**, 678–686

Macdonald DW, Daniels MJ, Driscoll CA, Kitchener AC and Yamaguchi N (2004) *The Scottish Wildcat: analyses for conservation and an action plan.* The Wildlife Conservation Research Unit, Oxford

Marco I, Martinez F, Pastor J and Lavin S (2000) Hematologic and serum chemistry values of the captive European wildcat. *Journal of Wildlife Diseases* **36(3)**, 445–449

McOrist S (1992) Diseases of the European wildcat (*Felis silvestris* Schreber, 1777) in Great Britain. *Revue scientifique et technique (International Office of Epizootics)* **11(4)**, 1143–1149

McOrist S, Boid R, Jones TW *et al.* (1991) Some viral and protozool diseases in the European wildcat. *Journal of Wildlife Diseases* **27(4)**, 693–696

Millán J and Rodriguez A (2009) A serological survey of common feline pathogens in free-living European wildcats (*Felis silvestris*) in central Spain. *European Journal of Wildlife Research* **55(3)**, 285–291

Miller GS (1907) Some new European Insectivora and Carnivora. *The Annals and Magazine of Natural History, 7th Series* **20**, 389–398

Nussberger B, Greminger MP, Grossen C, Keller LF and Wandeler P (2013) Development of SNP markers identifying European wildcats, domestic cats, and their admixed progeny. *Molecular Ecology Resources* **13(3)**, 447–460

Oliveira R, Godinho R, Randi E, and Alves PC (2008). Hybridization *versus* conservation: are domestic cats threatening the genetic integrity of wildcats (*Felis silvestris silvestris*) in Iberian Peninsula? Philosophical Transactions of the Royal Society of London. *Series B Biological Sciences* **363(1505)**, 2953–2961

Pierpaoli M, Biro ZS, Herrmann M *et al.* (2003) Genetic distinction of wildcat (*Felis silvestris*) populations in Europe, and hybridization with domestic cats in Hungary. *Molecular Ecology* **12(10)**, 2585–2598

Scottish National Heritage (2013) *Scottish Wildcat Conservation Action Plan.* Inverness, Scottish National Heritage

Wasieri J, Schmiedeknecht G, Förster C, König M and Reinacher M (2009) Parvovirus infection in a Eurasian lynx (*Lynx lynx*) and in a European wildcat (*Felis silvestris silvestris*). *Journal of Comparative Pathology* **140(2–3)**, 203–207

Willi B, Filoni C, Catão-Dias JL *et al.* (2007) Worldwide occurrence of feline hemoplasma infections in wild felid species. *Journal of Clinical Microbiology* **45(4)**, 1159–1166

Specialist organizations and useful contacts

See also Appendix 1

National Museum of Scotland,
Chambers Street, Edinburgh EH1 1JF, UK
Tel: 0300 123 6789 (for wildcat identification and deposition of wildcat carcasses)

Scottish National Heritage,
Great Glen House, Leachkin Road, Inverness IV3 8NW, UK
Tel: 01463 725000
www.snh.gov.uk

Scottish Wildcat Action
www.scottishwildcataction.org

Chapter 21

Foxes

David Couper

There are 23 species of fox in the world. Red foxes (*Vulpes vulpes*) (Figure 21.1) have the largest distribution and are found throughout most of the northern hemisphere, as well as being an introduced species in Australia. In the UK they are almost ubiquitous, although they are absent from the Scilly Isles, the Channel Islands and most of the Scottish islands (Baker and Harris, 2008). Their resourceful behaviour and opportunistic diet have allowed them to establish a large urban population in the UK and elsewhere in Europe. Like many urban-adapted species, red foxes occur at much higher densities in urban environments than in less disturbed areas, supported by abundant resources that are not prone to seasonal fluctuation (Bradley and Altizer, 2007). These high population densities can elevate contact rates within and among wildlife species and favour the transmission of parasites (Deplazes, 2004). Red foxes are frequently studied as they are a wildlife reservoir of several important diseases of humans and domestic animals, including rabies virus, and the fox tapeworm (*Echinococcus multilocularis*) in continental Europe.

Common reasons for the presentation of foxes as wildlife casualties include orphaned and abandoned cubs, trauma and sarcoptic mange. Whilst medically and surgically foxes can generally be treated like domestic dogs, various vulpine peculiarities must be taken into account for successful rehabilitation.

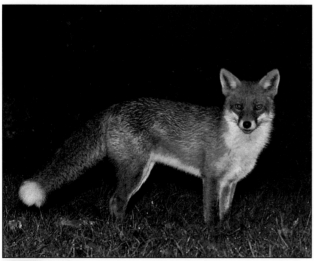

21.1 Red fox.
© Paul Cecil

Ecology and biology

Red foxes are highly adaptable and occupy a wide variety of rural and urban habitats; in cities, low-density residential areas with large gardens are favoured. They are mainly nocturnal and during the day will often lie-up above ground, under dense cover. In the spring they give birth in dens, or earths, which may be former badger setts, abandoned rabbit holes or under garden sheds. Foxes live in family groups, composed of a dominant pair (the male (dog) and female (vixen)), their cubs, and often young from previous years which may help to rear the cubs of the dominant pair. The cubs start to come above ground at around 4 weeks of age, and the vixen often leaves them for long periods. From September onwards, some cubs will disperse and can travel large distances in search of territories. Red foxes are omnivores; their natural diet consists mainly of small mammals, although they also eat birds, beetles and a wide variety of invertebrates, caught using their keen senses of hearing and smell. In addition to hunting, they will eat carrion, fallen fruits and discarded human food. The life expectancy for free-living foxes is up to 9 years (Harris and Smith, 1987), although on average most foxes in urban areas will only live until around 12 months of age, largely as a result of road traffic collisions (Harris, 1981).

Anatomy and physiology

Red foxes are readily identified by their typical canid form; the coat is red with black ears and socks, a slender red and white muzzle, a white bib and often a white tail tip (see Figure 21.1). Occasionally, colour variants of the coat are seen, for instance melanistic (referred to as 'silver') foxes. The irises are amber and the pupils are oval and vertically orientated. Dog foxes weigh 5.5–9 kg and vixens 3.5–7.5 kg. The two sexes can be differentiated by their typical canine reproductive anatomy, although this may not be readily visible unless the fox is restrained. From the age of 10 months, the head of the dog fox appears larger than that of the vixen, on account of a more prominent interparietal ridge (saggital crest). The thick tail, or brush, is used to keep the fox warm and for behavioural posturing, such as expressing submission and dominance. It is held horizontally when running. The feet are heavily furred between the digits, with five digits on the forefeet, and four on the hind. Moult occurs twice yearly, in the spring and autumn; only the spring moult is clearly visible with loss of the thick winter coat.

The dental formula (with temporary dentition in parentheses) of red foxes is as follows:

$$2 \times \left\{ I \; \frac{3 \, (3)}{3 \, (3)} \; C \; \frac{1 \, (1)}{1 \, (1)} \; P \; \frac{4 \, (3)}{4 \, (3)} \; M \; \frac{2 \, (0)}{3 \, (0)} \right\} = 42 \; (28)$$

The eruption patterns of the temporary and permanent dentition are described in Figure 21.2. The canine teeth are more slender and the premolars less tightly packed than those of domestic dogs (Figure 21.3). Foxes may be roughly aged by the condition of their teeth, with wear being apparent on the teeth of older animals, although this is also affected by factors other than age, such as diet. Age determination may be performed more accurately by a variety of techniques on post-mortem examination (reviewed in Harris, 1978a), for example by counting the incremental lines in the cementum.

Reproduction

Foxes are monoestrous spontaneous ovulators. The breeding season, or rut, occurs between December and February (in the northern hemisphere), and the oestrous period lasts for 3 weeks. The scrotum of the dog fox is enlarged during the rut. Vixens can breed from the age of 10 months, although breeding is most common between 2 and 4 years of age. Subordinate females may breed, but often fail to produce viable cubs due to social stress. The gestation period lasts for 53 days, with most cubs born in March. Whilst the mean litter size is four or five, litters of up to ten have been reported. Peak lactation lasts, on average, for 7 weeks, and during this time the fur around the mammary glands assumes a reddish hue. Female foxes generally have eight nipples, although up to ten is not uncommon (Baker and Harris, 2008). Cub development is described in Figure 21.2.

Age	Description	Comments	Image
Birth–2 weeks	80–120 g at birth 250–350 g by 2 weeks Short chocolate-black fur Eyes and ears open 11–14 days	Unable to thermoregulate for first 2–3 weeks – vixen stays with cubs	
3 weeks	350–500 g Black eye streak appears Irises slate-blue	Temporary incisors erupt at approx. 18 days Temporary canines erupt at approx. 21 days	
4 weeks	500–800 g White muzzle and red patches on face are apparent Ears erect, muzzle starts to elongate Irises change to amber	Progressively weaned on to solids Begin to emerge above ground	
5–6 weeks	800–1200 g By 6 weeks, the fur colour is similar to that of the adult but appears woolly	Already eating a wide variety of solid items Catching insects and earthworms by themselves	
7 weeks–12 months	Coat loses woolly appearance by 9–12 weeks and cubs appear like small adults From 10 months, heads of male cubs appear larger than those of females	Permanent incisors erupt at approx. 15 weeks Permanent canines erupt at approx. 18 weeks Full complement of permanent dentition by 6 months Become progressively more independent until July or August, at which point they may disperse, or stay on in the range Young males may disperse large distances	

21.2 Red fox cub development.
(Baker and Harris, 2008; dentition eruption patterns from Linhart, 1968)

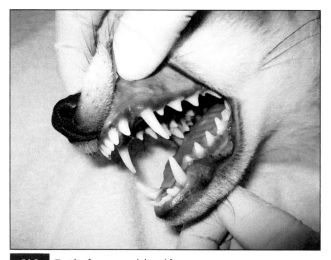

21.3 Teeth of a young adult red fox.

Normal parameters

The average heart rate of a red fox is around 125 beats per minute (bpm) at rest, and can increase to 320 bpm whilst running (Kreeger *et al.*, 1989). The respiratory rate at rest is around 10–30 breaths per minute. The normal rectal temperature is 39–40°C (Kreeger *et al.*, 1989).

Capture, handling and transportation

Suitable personal protective equipment should be worn when handling foxes, considering the potential for physical injury and zoonotic infection. Leather gauntlets may be worn but these reduce the dexterity of the handler. Red foxes are reservoirs of a wide variety of zoonoses (see Chapter 7 and 'Specific conditions'); latex gloves and long sleeves should always be worn to reduce the likelihood of transmission of infections such as sarcoptic mange and leptospirosis.

Capture

Capture may be attempted with a baited trapping cage, although foxes are often wary about entering these. A strong net with a padded rim is useful to catch loose foxes, whilst metal dog graspers may be necessary when removing foxes from narrow spaces. However, the use of dog graspers can result in fractured teeth as the animal tries to bite its way free, and should be avoided where possible. In the confines of a rehabilitation centre, a large towel placed over the fox is often adequate for capture (see 'Handling').

Transportation

Adult foxes are best transported in a top-opening wire pet carrier or crush cage; it is more difficult to extract them safely from front-opening pet carriers. Cardboard pet carriers are sufficient for young cubs up to 4–5 weeks old, but are unsuitable for larger cubs and adult foxes, as they will easily escape from these. Pre-weighing of the carrier aids the calculation of sedative drug doses. A towel should be placed over the carrier to minimize stress during transport, and young cubs and shocked animals should be kept warm.

Handling

The fox should be removed from the cage in a quiet escape-proof room. Although apt to try to bite, foxes are generally easier to handle than a fractious domestic dog, particularly when debilitated. The fox will usually be lying pressed to the floor of a top-opening carrier (Figure 21.4a). A thick towel can be placed over the fox, and the neck area restrained through the towel (Figure 21.4b). A hand can then be placed under the towel to grasp the scruff, as far cranially as possible. The body of the fox is supported with the other hand when lifting. A standard dog muzzle may be applied, which should be thoroughly cleaned after use to prevent the spread of infectious diseases such as sarcoptic mange. Cubs are not difficult to restrain; very young ones are generally quiet when scruffed, whilst older cubs can bite and should initially be restrained as for adults.

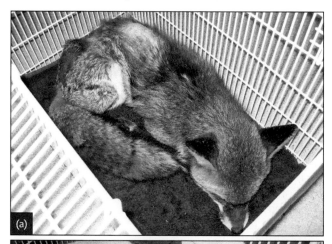

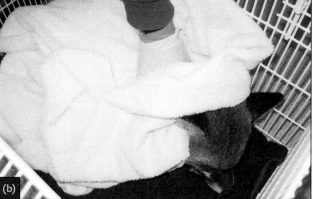

21.4 Restraint of a red fox. (a) The fox will usually be lying pressed to the floor of a top-opening carrier. (b) A thick towel can be placed over the fox, and the neck area restrained through the towel. (Note: Lesions of sarcoptic mange are evident in this fox.)

Examination and clinical assessment for rehabilitation

History

A thorough history should be taken from the finder. This will help determine what has happened to the fox and will allow the animal to be returned to familiar territory following rehabilitation. Allegedly abandoned or orphaned cubs are frequently presented, and the circumstances surrounding this should be noted; whilst they may genuinely be abandoned, they will start venturing from the den at around 4 weeks of age, and it is normal practice for the vixen to leave them for extended periods. With adult foxes particularly, it is advisable to ascertain if the finder observed the animal's behaviour and locomotion prior to its capture, as it is difficult to assess this in the confines of a consulting room. Members of the public finding foxes should be discouraged from handling them (see Chapter 3); if the finder has already been bitten, they should be advised to seek immediate medical attention.

Examination

The aim of the examination is to assess the suitability of the fox as a candidate for rehabilitation and release (see also Chapter 4). If its condition is such that it is unlikely to survive the rehabilitation process, or that its chances of survival post-release are not comparable with its conspecifics, then euthanasia should be considered. Likewise, if suitable rehabilitation facilities are not available to rear cubs (see 'Rearing of orphans'), together with suitable available release sites, then euthanasia may need to be performed on welfare grounds.

Ideally, the fox should be observed loose in a quiet area prior to handling. However, livelier older cubs and adult foxes will tend to leap up the walls and can be awkward to catch in a consulting room. The author examines these animals in an escape-proof corridor, giving them space to exhibit a normal gait, vision and behaviour. Behavioural abnormalities are not uncommon in foxes (e.g. aimless wandering as a result of encephalitis and tameness as a result of hand-rearing in isolation). If in any doubt about the behaviour, the advice of an experienced rehabilitator should be sought.

For the physical examination of very lively animals, sedation may be necessary (see 'Anaesthesia and analgesia'). A fox should be examined systematically and thoroughly (see Chapter 4), as for a domestic dog. Weighing the animal on initial removal from its carrier, or by calculation using a pre-weighed carrier, will aid with the assessment of body condition, and give a baseline from which to proceed. The body condition can be judged by feeling the ribs, spine and pelvis, which should be palpable but not overly prominent. This will give an idea as to the chronicity of any longer-term problems, being aware that body condition varies with the time of year; for example, a vixen may be very lean when rearing cubs.

Certain conditions must not be overlooked in foxes during the clinical examination. For instance, septicaemia and jaundice secondary to wound infection may be present in an animal admitted with another more obvious condition, such as sarcoptic mange. The subtle lesions of early onset mange may be missed on the hocks and elbows of young cubs. A thorough examination of allegedly orphaned and abandoned cubs should be carried out, considering their age, and assessing their body condition and behaviour for any abnormalities that may suggest they are actually orphaned or abandoned, such as dehydration, emaciation and myiasis. If it has not been possible to observe the animal's locomotion, the presence of lameness may be suggested by muscle wastage, reduced flexibility of joints and long claws on the affected limb. When considering the significance of any abnormalities found during the examination, it should be borne in mind that for an adult fox to allow itself to be easily captured, unless it has been entangled or trapped, it is likely to be seriously debilitated. For example, a fox presenting with a fractured leg following a road traffic collision is likely to be suffering from more serious conditions, such as concussion, hypovolaemic shock or pelvic trauma.

Diagnostic techniques

Blood samples for haematology, biochemistry and serology can be taken from cephalic, jugular and saphenous veins, either with the animal conscious if it is well re-strained, or under sedation. The author's favoured vein is the cephalic, as it is familiar in terms of restraint and access, and requires minimal clipping, while the jugular vein is more suitable if larger samples are required. Ethylenediaminetetraacetic acid (EDTA) and lithium heparin are suitable anticoagulants for most diagnostic blood tests (see Chapter 5). Haematology and biochemistry data for red foxes are shown in Figure 21.5.

Variable (units)	Mean	SD	Reference range	Sample size[a]	Animals[b]
Haematology					
Red blood cell count (RBC) (x 10^{12}/l)	12.14	15	6.6–92.8	31	23
Haemoglobin (g/l)	158	17	110–189	34	25
Packed cell volume (PCV) (l/l)	0.44	0.095	0.23–0.59	48	31
Mean corpuscular volume (MCV) (fl)	48.3	8.9	5.3–55.7	31	23
Mean corpuscular haemoglobin (MCH) ((pg) per cell)	16.2	2.9	1.7–55.7	29	21
Mean corpuscular haemoglobin concentration (MCHC) (g/l)	337	29	294–452	34	25
Platelet count (x 10^{12}/l)	0.39	0.14	0.24–0.66	13	9
Nucleated RBC per 100 WBC	0	0	0–1	7	7
Reticulocytes (% RBC)	15.3	30.5	0–61	4	3
White blood cell (WBC) count (x 10^9/l)	5.78	2.07	2.5–11.2	45	29
Segmented neutrophils (x 10^9/l)	3.17	1.41	0.55–7.31	39	25
Lymphocytes (x 10^9/l)	1.77	1.16	0.16–4.29	43	27
Monocytes (x 10^9/l)	0.21	0.15	0.00–0.62	37	23
Eosinophils (x 10^9/l)	0.61	0.65	0.001–3	42	27
Basophils (x 10^9/l)	0.11	0.14	0–0.27	3	3
Neutrophilic bands (x 10^9/l)	0.35	0.49	0.078–1.69	10	8

21.5 Reference ranges for haematological and biochemical parameters in red foxes. (Adapted from International Species Information System reference ranges. [a] Number of samples used to calculate the reference range; [b] Number of different individuals contributing to the reference values). (continues) ▶

Variable (units)	Mean	SD	Reference range	Sample size[a]	Animals[b]
Biochemistry					
Calcium (mmol/l)	2.38	0.25	1.7–2.8	45	31
Phosphorus (mmol/l)	1.42	0.65	0.52–2.94	40	27
Sodium (mmol/l)	146	7	129–156	35	23
Potassium (mmol/l)	4.3	0.4	3.5–5	35	23
Chloride (mmol/l)	114	3	109–119	31	19
Bicarbonate (mmol/l)	17.2	2.3	15–21	6	1
Carbon dioxide (mmol/l)	19.6	4.6	11–29	23	15
Iron (µmol/l)	27.21	10.56	13.78–46.18	13	6
Magnesium (mmol/l)	0.7	0.12	0.58–1	10	4
Blood urea nitrogen (mmol/l)	8.21	3.21	3.57–21.78	48	32
Creatinine (µmol/l)	80	27	35–194	41	28
Uric acid (mmol/l)	0.018	0.006	0.006–0.03	15	10
Total bilirubin (µmol/l)	15	5	7–26	37	24
Direct bilirubin (µmol/l)	5	2	3–7	13	7
Indirect bilirubin (µmol/l)	14	3	5–19	13	7
Glucose (mmol/l)	7.10	2.05	3.72–13.32	48	32
Cholesterol (mmol/l)	4.95	1.94	2.23–12.64	40	27
Triglyceride (mmol/l)	0.49	0.31	0.14–1.09	17	11
Creatine kinase (CK) (IU/l)	225	199	37–891	28	18
Lactate dehydrogenase (LDH) (IU/l)	299	261	50–1206	22	17
Alkaline phosphatase (ALP) (IU/l)	61	54	19–249	40	27
Alanine aminotransferase (ALT) (IU/l)	127	123	39–607	41	27
Aspartate aminotransferase (AST) (IU/l)	56	31	9–160	34	21
Gamma-glutamyl transferase (GGT) (IU/l)	5	5	0–20	15	9
Amylase (IU/l)	100.3	69.38	0–191.1	14	9
Lipase (IU/l)	61.72	0	NDA	1	1
Total protein (colorimetry) (g/l)	58	8	35–76	43	28
Globulin (colorimetry) (g/l)	27	6	18–40	31	20
Albumin (colorimetry) (g/l)	34	5	23–44	33	22
Cortisol (nmol/l)	246	105	171–320	2	2

21.5 (continued) Reference ranges for haematological and biochemical parameters in red foxes. (Adapted from International Species Information System reference ranges. [a] Number of samples used to calculate the reference range; [b] Number of different individuals contributing to the reference values). NDA = no data available.

Radiography is generally performed to confirm fractures (e.g. of the limbs and pelvis) and assess their suitability for repair. As for companion animals, orthogonal views are advisable. Survey radiography is useful, and may reveal incidental findings such as healed fractures and air gun pellets. Other diagnostic imaging techniques such as ultrasound, endoscopy and computed tomography (CT) can be employed although the cost involved may be prohibitive; the equipment should be cleaned thoroughly after use if it is also used for companion animals.

Other simple tests may be performed to confirm conditions such as sarcoptic mange and lungworm infections (see 'Specific conditions').

Euthanasia

Euthanasia is performed by chemical means, using intravenous injection of pentobarbital (150 mg/kg) generally into the cephalic vein, although the jugular and saphenous veins can also be used. The use of sedation or anaesthesia (see 'Anaesthesia and analgesia') will reduce stress on the part of the fox and the handler, and will allow intrahepatic or intracardiac injection if venous access is not possible.

First aid and short-term hospitalization

First aid should be provided according to the same principles applied in domestic dogs, remembering that fox casualties, unlike most dogs, have often been compromised for some time prior to presentation and are more likely to be suffering from confounding factors such as dehydration, hypothermia and starvation (see Chapter 5). Warmth should be provided for shocked animals and young cubs. This can be achieved with heat lamps or mats, although no cables should be accessible for the fox to chew. Young cubs may be placed in an incubator. Dehydration can be treated by various means depending on the condition of the fox. Access to water or an electrolyte solution may be sufficient in animals that are bright enough to drink voluntarily. Young cubs (less than 2–3 weeks) may be given electrolytes via a bottle and teat. Subcutaneous fluids can be administered in the loose skin of the scruff and may be considered for mildly dehydrated individuals. Intravenous fluids may be administered via a catheter in the cephalic vein for the treatment of more severe dehydration and shock. A bolus can be given if the animal is under sedation, but a conscious fox is unlikely to tolerate a drip unless it is very weak and will chew it out unless it is has an Elizabethan collar in place. The intraosseous route may be used where intravenous access is not possible. Wounds should be (minimally) clipped and lavaged, and may require antibiotic therapy (see Figure 21.12); dressings and splints can also be protected from chewing by the use of an Elizabethan or inflatable collar. Analgesia can be provided using the drugs listed in Figure 21.6 and should be considered for all animals with injuries.

Short-term hospitalization

Foxes should be housed somewhere quiet, away from humans and domestic dogs. An easily sterilized walk-in kennel will suffice for adults and older cubs in the short term, with a towel placed over the door and somewhere for the fox to hide. Young cubs may be housed in a pet carrier or a standard dog kennel, as they are easier to handle in a confined space. Suitable quarantine measures should be in place. Human interaction with cubs must be kept to a minimum to prevent the development of malprinting and habituation (see Chapter 9). A proprietary dog food may be offered, tinned food being more appetizing, and a convalescent diet being more appropriate for starved individuals. Dead day-old chicks, if available, are often more readily consumed. Young cubs may need to be fed promptly with a proprietary milk replacer (see 'Rearing of fox cubs'). Drinking water should be provided at all times.

Anaesthesia and analgesia

The efficacy of various injectable anaesthetic combinations has been assessed in the field, including medetomidine in combination with ketamine or midazolam (Shilo et al., 2010). A medetomidine, ketamine and butorphanol combination is easily administered intramuscularly in the quadriceps or lumbar muscles, and is favoured by the author for anaesthetizing livelier individuals for examination, or facilitating euthanasia. Oxygen may then be supplied by facemask or following intubation, which is performed as for domestic dogs. However, as fox casualties are likely to present a higher anaesthetic risk than a healthy domestic dog undergoing an elective procedure, drugs should be chosen and dosed accordingly; for example, use of suitable premedication and an intravenous induction agent followed by maintenance of anaesthesia with an inhalational anaesthetic, such as isoflurane, may be more appropriate for the fox than using an alpha-2 adrenoreceptor agonist/ketamine combination, but requires increased competency on the part of the handler. As foxes are often a lot lighter than dogs of comparative size, it is imperative to weigh the animal prior to the administration of anaesthetic drugs. Monitoring of cardiac and respiratory function, including oxygen saturation levels, should be carried out throughout anaesthesia. Body temperature should be monitored and maintained at 39°C.

Analgesia may be achieved with the same non-steroidal anti-inflammatory drugs or opioids used in domestic dogs, which should be chosen appropriately considering the likely severity of pain (Figure 21.6). Beware of early (and hence not clinically obvious) pregnancy in vixens, considering the time of year, when using drugs that are not licensed for use during pregnancy.

Drug	Dosage	Notes
Sedatives and anaesthetics		
Medetomidine (Me) + midazolam (Mi)	0.07 mg/kg (Me) + 0.8 mg/kg (Mi) i.m.[a]	Allows physical examination for a period of at least 20–25 minutes. Medetomidine can be reversed with atipamezole at 0.35 mg/kg
Medetomidine (Me) + ketamine (K)	0.07 mg/kg (Me) + 2 mg/kg (K) i.m.[a]	Allows physical examination for a period of at least 20–25 minutes. Supplementation of oxygen, and close monitoring of body temperature is paramount with this combination. Medetomidine can be reversed with atipamezole at 0.35 mg/kg
Medetomidine (Me) + ketamine (K) + butorphanol (B)	0.02 mg/kg (Me) + 4 mg/kg (K) + 0.4 mg/kg (B) i.m.[b]	Useful immobilization achieved for 30 minutes. Medetomidine can be reversed with atipamezole at 0.1 mg/kg
Acepromazine (ACP) + buprenorphine (Bup)	0.05 mg/kg (ACP) + 0.02 mg/kg (Bup) i.m.	Premedication
Alfaxalone	2 mg/kg i.v.	Induction. Useful in animals with i.v. line already placed
Propofol	4 mg/kg i.v.	Induction. Useful in animals with i.v. line already placed
Isoflurane/sevoflurane in oxygen		Can be used for induction via facemask in cubs and debilitated adults, following appropriate premedication. Used for maintenance of anaesthesia following intubation
Analgesics		
Meloxicam	0.2 mg/kg s.c., orally (initial dose) 0.1 mg/kg s.c., orally q24h (maintenance dose)	Oral formulation readily consumed in food
Carprofen	2–4 mg/kg s.c., orally q24h	Palatable oral formula readily consumed in food
Buprenorphine	0.02 mg/kg i.m., s.c. q6–8h	Mild to moderate pain
Morphine	0.5 mg/kg i.v., i.m. q2–4h	Moderate to severe pain
Methadone	0.1–0.5 mg/kg i.m. q3–4h	Moderate to severe pain

21.6 Anaesthetic and analgesic drugs and their dose rates which can be used in red foxes. Note that the doses stated are for use in healthy foxes and should be lowered appropriately in debilitated animals. None of these drugs are licensed for use in foxes. Doses are those commonly used in domestic dogs.
([a] Shilo et al., 2010; [b] Brash, 2003)

Specific conditions

Trauma

Trauma, for example as a result of road traffic collisions and bite wounds, is a relatively common reason for admission. The signs exhibited by the fox will obviously depend on the injuries sustained and any secondary complications, such as septicaemia. Fractured limbs are common in urban areas; in a post-mortem study in London, 32.4% of foxes older than 6 months of age had one or more fractures (Harris, 1978b). Loss of part or all of the tail is also frequently reported. Historic trauma, such as healed fractures or shooting injuries, may be seen as an incidental finding on radiography, and its significance must be considered in relation to the reason for admission.

Fracture repair

Fracture repair may be performed using similar principles to those in domestic dogs but only when a near-perfect result is anticipated. The prognosis for compound fractures and fractures involving joints is much more guarded. Casts and bandages will be chewed and, likewise, external fixators may result in self-trauma, and will likely be chewed by cagemates. Intramedullary pins or bone plates may be used, and should be removed before release. Repairs involving frequent interventions or prolonged confinement are stressful for adult foxes and may result in malprinting and habituation in young cubs. However, cubs heal relatively quickly and may be kept in a pair to avoid malprinting and habituation where the repair permits. Strict cage rest of an adult fox (e.g. for a fractured pelvis) is difficult to achieve, as they cannot be managed easily in a confined space, and a very nervous fox may not settle in a larger pen. The likelihood of future dystocia in a vixen with a fractured pelvis, where the pelvic canal will be narrowed, should be considered and compromised animals should be euthanased.

Bite wounds

Bite wounds inflicted by conspecifics may result in abscesses, cellulitis and septicaemia, frequently involving *Streptococcus* spp. (see 'Bacterial infections'). Foxes may also be attacked by domestic dogs, and this is a common cause of mortality in cubs in urban areas (Harris, 1981). The signs exhibited by the fox may be associated with the location of the bite; for instance lameness may be seen if a leg is involved, and the author has seen vestibular disease as a sequel to a bite wound to the base of the pinna. However, often animals are septicaemic when captured, and are presented in a collapsed state as a consequence. Bite wounds may be treated according to the same principles as in other species for infected puncture wounds, including (minimal) clipping, lavage, broad-spectrum antibacterials, fluid therapy and analgesia as appropriate; however, septicaemic animals generally require euthanasia.

Entanglement

Foxes present fairly frequently as a result of becoming entangled, commonly by their hind legs in wire fences (Figure 21.7). The circulation to the distal limb is often badly compromised, with serious injuries and infection, and euthanasia may be required. With less severe or unapparent damage, the fox should be taken into captivity

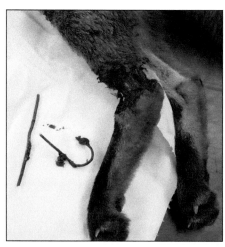

21.7 Hindlimb of red fox damaged by fencing (removed and shown to left). The animal was euthanased on account of this injury. (© Steve Bexton)

and monitored for a week, given the risk of subsequent wound breakdown due to ischaemic necrosis. The teeth and mouth should be examined for damage resulting from the fox's attempts to bite its way free. Treatment following entanglement may involve fluid therapy (considering the possibility of reperfusion injury), clipping, wound lavage, broad-spectrum antibacterial cover and analgesia. The above also applies to foxes caught in snares; the use of illegal snares should be reported to the police (Wildlife Crime Officer), the Royal Society for the Prevention of Cruelty to Animals (RSPCA) or the Scottish Society for the Prevention of Cruelty to Animals (Scottish SPCA) (see Chapters 2 and 11).

Poisoning

Blackmore (1964) reported that poisoning with organochlorine insecticides was the most common cause of mortality in his study of red foxes in the UK, and the fox is still a very common victim of accidental and deliberate poisoning with pesticides, biocides and rodenticides (Shore *et al.*, 2003). The Wildlife Incident Investigation Scheme (WIIS) (Health and Safety Executive) produces a list of incidents of poisoning in foxes and other wildlife species annually, and suspected cases should be reported to them (see Appendix 1). The signs exhibited by a poisoned fox will depend on the poison ingested; for instance neurological signs may be seen with organophosphate toxicity. More 'novel' poisonings may also be encountered, for example the author has been presented with an apparently anaesthetized fox that had dug up and ingested a domestic cat which had been euthanased with pentobarbital. Treatment is supportive and symptomatic, but poisoned foxes are generally found dead, and diagnosis is made on post-mortem examination (see also Chapters 5 and 11).

Contamination

Contamination of the fur with harmful substances such as diesel may result from misadventure, particularly in urban areas. There may be skin irritation, and possibly internal effects due to ingestion of toxins on grooming. The fur should be washed with a suitable agent (e.g. a washing up detergent for oil-based substances) and thoroughly rinsed and dried, under sedation. Activated charcoal can be given in food to adsorb toxins, and antibiotics may be required to treat secondary infection of inflamed skin. Haematology and biochemistry should be performed to assess any internal effects, such as liver and kidney damage. Diesel and other contaminants can result in the fur falling out 1 or 2 weeks after the initial incident and the fox should not be released until sufficient re-growth has occurred, especially during winter.

Infectious diseases

Viral diseases

Infectious canine hepatitis: Infectious canine hepatitis (ICH) is caused by canine adenovirus (CAV) type 1. It was first reported in farmed silver foxes in North America, and was referred to as fox distemper or epizootic fox encephalitis (Green, 1925, cited by Woods, 2001). Spontaneous ICH occurs sporadically in red foxes in the UK although its epidemiology is uncertain (Thompson *et al.*, 2010). In a recent study, CAV type 1 antibodies were detected in 19% of fox carcasses from England and Scotland (Thompson *et al.*, 2010). Spread between foxes occurs via urine, nasal and conjunctival secretions, and in faeces. Clinical signs appear after an incubation period of 2–6 days, and include anorexia, rhinitis, haemorrhagic diarrhoea, jaundice, hyperexcitability, seizures, paralysis, coma and death (Woods, 2001). Death may occur after a brief clinical course, or suddenly without clinical signs. Uveitis and keratitis (blue eye) have been reported in non-fatal cases of ICH in silver foxes (Woods, 2001). On gross post-mortem examination, congestion of the liver with mild accentuation of the hepatic lobular pattern is seen, and mesenteric and hepatic lymph nodes are enlarged and congested. On histopathology, generalized necrosis and dissociation of hepatocytes is present with typical intranuclear inclusion bodies visible within the hepatocytes (Woods, 2001). Diagnosis in the live animal is based on clinical signs, and may be confirmed with serological testing, virus isolation, immunofluorescent evaluation and polymerase chain reaction (PCR). Treatment would be supportive and symptomatic, but the prognosis for animals with ICH is guarded, and recovering individuals go on to excrete virus in urine for at least 6 to 9 months following infection. The vaccination of foxes against ICH is discussed later in the chapter (see 'Therapeutics').

Canine distemper virus: Epidemics of canine distemper virus (CDV) are reported in continental Europe (Nouvellet *et al.*, 2013) and CDV antigen has recently been detected in tissues from foxes in the UK (S Bexton, unpublished data). Transmission of the virus is primarily by aerosol or contact with oral, respiratory and ocular fluids and exudates containing the virus. The clinical signs are similar to those in domestic dogs, and include mucopurulent oculonasal discharge, coughing, fever, depression, anorexia, vomiting and diarrhoea. Central nervous signs may be concurrent or follow systemic disease, usually within 5 weeks post-infection, and include aimless wandering, diurnal behaviour in this nocturnal species and inappropriate interactions with humans. If the animal recovers from infection it may shed virus for 2–3 months. On post-mortem examination, an important diagnostic feature of CDV is the presence of intracytoplasmic and intranuclear inclusion bodies in epithelia, neurons and astroglia. Secondary bacterial or protozoal infections due to the immunosuppressive effect of CDV may complicate microscopic evaluation (Williams, 2001). Diagnosis in the live animal is based on clinical signs, and can be confirmed by various tests. Smears of conjunctiva or buffy coats may be examined for inclusion bodies or by fluorescent antibody

staining for CDV antigen. Serology may be performed, although animals dying of the disease often do not have antibodies against CDV. RT-PCR on urine samples is highly sensitive in domestic dogs. Given the poor prognosis and the potential for spread within groups of cubs, euthanasia of affected animals is recommended. The vaccination of foxes against CDV is discussed later in the chapter (see 'Therapeutics').

Canine parvovirus: Although red foxes seroconvert to canine parvovirus (CPV) following experimental infection, they do not develop clinical signs of disease (Barker and Parrish, 2001). A new parvovirus (tentatively named 'fox parvovirus') has recently been demonstrated by PCR in red fox faeces in continental Europe – further work is required to discover whether this virus is pathogenic for foxes (Bodewes *et al.*, 2013).

Rabies virus: The UK is free from classical rabies virus at the time of publication. Red foxes are the most important wildlife reservoir of this disease in continental Europe, where it has largely been controlled by oral vaccination within bait, although outbreaks continue to occur (e.g. Nouvellet *et al.*, 2013). The disease is spread in saliva, generally through biting, and is characterized by acute behavioural alterations. At the end of the incubation period (which may last from a few days to several months), a short non-specific prodromal phase is followed by encephalopathy and death within a few days. Neurological signs include hyperaesthesia to auditory, visual or tactile stimuli, and sudden unprovoked agitation and aggressive behaviour (furious rabies). A paralytic phase (dumb rabies) may follow the furious phase, or immediately follow the prodromal phase (Rupprecht *et al.*, 2001). If rabies is suspected the animal should be contained if this is possible without risk, and the Animal and Plant Health Agency (APHA) should be notified (see Appendix 1). Diagnosis is confirmed on post-mortem examination by fluorescent antibody testing (FAT) on brain tissue. Contingency plans for dealing with the disease in foxes are in place in the event that the virus enters the UK, involving vaccination and poisoning – for more information on the current UK rabies strategy, consult the Defra website (see Appendix 1).

Other viral infections: Many other viruses have recently been demonstrated by PCR in red fox faeces in continental Europe, including a bocavirus, adeno-associated virus, hepevirus, astroviruses and picobirnaviruses (Bodewes *et al.*, 2013). These viruses were discovered during a study investigating possible zoonoses in red foxes. CAV-2 has been reported in the faeces of a red fox in Italy (Balboni *et al.*, 2013). In Belgium, foxes have been shown to carry the rodent-borne *Puumala Hantavirus*, a causative agent of haemorrhagic fever with renal syndrome in humans (Escutenaire *et al.*, 2000). The low seroprevalence and virus titres found in positive animals suggest that foxes are probably a dead-end host. Further work is required to show whether any of the viruses listed above are pathogenic for red foxes.

Foxes exhibiting reduced fear of humans and aimless wandering are occasionally presented for rehabilitation in the UK. Post-mortem examination of these animals frequently reveals non-suppurative encephalitis of presumed viral origin, although the histopathology is inconsistent with that reported for ICH in foxes and research is ongoing as to the aetiology (S Bexton, unpublished data).

Bacterial diseases

Leptospirosis: Leptospirosis occurs sporadically in red foxes in the UK, and *Leptospira interrogans* serovars Copenhageni and Icterohaemorrhagiae have been detected in fatal cases (Duff, 2002). Many other serovars have been reported from serological studies in red foxes in Europe (reviewed in Philbey and Thompson, 2009). The specific characteristics of the red fox life cycle, namely the high reproductive potential, migration of young individuals and opportunistic food habits, identify the red fox as an epizootiologically important species in the chain of leptospirosis transmission (Slavica *et al.*, 2011). Affected individuals are usually found dead or moribund and exhibit marked jaundice (Figure 21.8). Given the poor condition of affected animals on presentation, euthanasia is strongly advised. On histopathological examination, there are varying degrees of hepatic necrosis and hepatocyte dissociation, along with necrotizing, haemorrhagic or non-suppurative interstitial nephritis (Philbey and Thompson, 2009). Differential diagnoses would include other causes of jaundice, such as ICH and streptococcal septicaemia, all of which have a poor prognosis. The vaccination of foxes against leptospirosis is discussed later in the chapter (see 'Therapeutics').

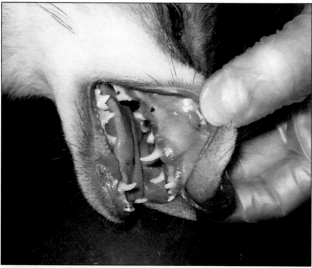

21.8 Jaundice in a red fox evident on examination of the oral mucosa.

Streptococcal infection: Streptococcal infection is a common cause of natural mortality in wild foxes in the UK and may be the result of bite wounds or other penetrating injuries (Blackmore, 1964). Beta-haemolytic streptococcal infections result in septicaemia and jaundice, with suppurative cellulitis being found at the primary focal lesion (Barrat *et al.*, 1985). On post-mortem examination, abscesses may be seen in the spleen, liver, lungs and kidneys, and pericarditis and septic arthritis may be apparent (Blackmore 1964; Barrat *et al.*, 1985). *Streptococcus* spp. can be isolated in pure culture from the blood of sick or dead foxes. In a study by Barrat and colleagues (1985), the extremely brief course of the disease (24–48 hours) precluded specific antibiotic therapy, although the bacteria were usually susceptible *in vitro* to penicillin and erythromycin at standard canine doses.

Other bacterial infections: Various other bacterial infections have been reported in foxes in the UK. These often involve invasive species, such as *Proteus vulgaris*,

subsequent to snare wounds, shooting injuries and other penetrative lesions. Septicaemia and jaundice would appear to be common sequels (Blackmore, 1964). Blackmore (1964) also reported pyometra in a vixen, from which he cultured haemolytic *Escherichia coli*. The significance of many bacterial infections in foxes, however, is related to their potential threat to human and companion animal health.

Salmonella spp. have been reported in red foxes in Cornwall (Euden, 1990); with their opportunistic diet, foxes are a useful indicator species for *Salmonella* serovars in the environment. A study in Norway revealed that red foxes were frequently infected with *Salmonella* Typhimurium during the winter months, and suggested that this was a result of the ingestion of small passerines dying of salmonellosis (Handeland *et al.*, 2008).

Foxes in the UK have been shown to have a high (41.2%) seroprevalence to *Coxiella burnetii*, the aetiological agent of Q fever in humans and other animals, providing evidence that predator species could act as indicators for the presence of *C. burnetii* in rodents (Meredith *et al.*, 2015b).

Reports of mycobacterial infection in free-living canid species are rare. There is, however, evidence of enzootic natural *Mycobacterium avium* subsp. *paratuberculosis* infection of foxes in Scotland; 85% of foxes examined in a study showed evidence of this infection (Beard *et al.*, 2001). It was conjectured that the foxes were infected by eating infected rabbits. The significance of the fox as a vector has yet to be established. *Mycobacterium bovis* was cultured from the tissues of 1.15% of 954 foxes examined in the UK (Krebs, 1997). A more recent study produced similar findings, with 12 of 993 foxes being positive on culture (Delahay *et al.*, 2001). Foxes have not been implicated as maintenance hosts for *M. bovis* infection and (like domestic cats) are likely to be spill-over hosts following exposure to infected prey species or environmental contamination of wounds.

Anaplasma phagocytophilum (the aetiological agent of granulocytic ehrlichiosis of animals and humans) was discovered in 16.6% of red foxes by PCR in a study in central Italy (Ebani *et al.*, 2011). The pathogen is transmitted by *Ixodes* spp. ticks. Foxes seem not to suffer from the infection, yet the high prevalence of infection suggests they may play a role in the epidemiology of the disease, especially in wild animals, and act as a potential reservoir. *A. phagocytophilum* has not been recorded in foxes in the UK to the author's knowledge, but a prevalence of 0.7% in ticks infesting domestic dogs has been reported (Smith *et al.*, 2013).

Lyme disease spirochaetes have been reported in a red fox found dead in Japan (Isogai *et al.*, 1994). On histopathology, spirochaetes were found in the skin, brain, heart, kidney and liver. Red foxes have also been shown to carry *Ixodes canisuga* ticks infected with *Borrelia valaisiana* in the UK (Couper *et al.*, 2010).

Fungal diseases

Dermatophytes: Ringworm occurs occasionally in red foxes. Both *Microsporum* and *Trichophyton* spp. (Knudtson *et al.*, 1980; Brash, 2003) have been recorded. Diagnosis is made by culture on an appropriate medium, and although treatment may theoretically be carried out with azole drugs, the necessary prolonged isolation of affected individuals means that this is rarely practical. Underlying immunosuppression and concurrent diseases should be considered and addressed.

Parasites

Ectoparasites:

Sarcoptic mange: Infection with *Sarcoptes scabiei* is the most significant ectoparasitic mite infection of red foxes, and results in a chronic, debilitating disease. Although, untreated, the condition normally results in the death of the animal, low-grade or sub-clinical infections, and even natural recoveries, are possible (Davidson *et al.*, 2008). A severe crusting form of sarcoptic mange has been present in England since the early 1990s, causing heavy mortality in foxes in some areas. The disease has apparently been responsible for numerous secondary cases in dogs and humans; presumed spill-over infection in badgers, as a result of sharing a sett with foxes, has also been reported (Collins *et al.*, 2010).

Infection is most obvious initially at the hind end (Figure 21.9), with marked fur loss and crusting extending cranially to include the whole body and head in advanced cases. Chronically infected foxes are generally very thin on presentation. Early onset infection is occasionally seen in young cubs, with subtle scaly lesions on the hocks and elbows, and at the tail head. Diagnosis is based on clinical signs (which should be differentiated from the patchy fur loss seen during the moult), and skin scrapes. Deep scraping as performed in dogs is rarely necessary in advanced cases, and sarcoptes mites are often easily identified by light microscopy in a sample of the thick crust present on the hindquarters, using potassium hydroxide to aid visualization.

Treatment for sarcoptic mange consists of repeated administration of an avermectin (see Figure 21.12) and suitable antibiotics to treat secondary bacterial infection of the skin. However, advanced cases are often emaciated as a result of the debilitating nature of the disease and concurrent problems such as bite wounds, and may require euthanasia. Occasionally, physical removal of crusts, with the aid of an emollient, may be indicated in advanced cases to alleviate signs (e.g. to permit eyelids to function normally). This is best performed under sedation, with appropriate analgesia being provided. The fox should not be released until the fur has grown back, particularly during the winter. However, prior to treatment, consideration should be given to both the immune competence of the fox and the ethics of keeping a wild animal in captivity for a prolonged period that may get reinfected upon release.

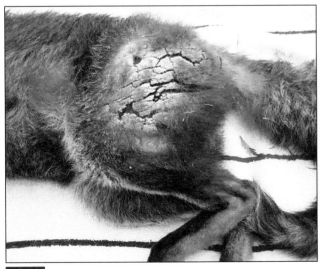

21.9 Severe crusting sarcoptic mange on the hindlimb of a red fox.

Other ectoparasites: Various other ectoparasites have been reported in red foxes (reviewed in Baker and Harris, 2008); they are generally present in low numbers and are of little consequence to the animal.

There is no host-specific flea of red foxes in the UK; some species (e.g. *Spilopsyllus cuniculi*) are probably acquired from prey, whilst others, such as *Archaeopsylla erinacei*, may be acquired from the environment. *Pulex irritans*, *Ctenocephalides canis* and *Paraceras melis* are all believed to feed on foxes.

Mites described include: *Otodectes cyanotis*, which is frequently found in the ear canal; skin mites, such as *Demodex folliculorum* and *Notoedres* spp.; and the penta-stomid mite *Linguatula serrata*, found in the nasal passages.

Ticks, such as *Ixodes ricinus* and *I. hexagonus*, are common, particularly on nursing vixens and juveniles, and *I. canisuga* has also been reported.

Myiasis may be seen in debilitated animals, generally in young cubs. Removal of fly eggs and maggots must be accompanied by aggressive treatment of the underlying condition. However, in these cases the prognosis is poor as the animals are usually already severely compromised.

Treatment of low-grade ectoparasitic infection may not be necessary for adult animals, but can be carried out with products licensed for use in domestic dogs to prevent transmission within groups of cubs (see Figure 21.12).

Endoparasites: Studies across Europe have found at least 58 helminths capable of infecting foxes, the majority of which were found in the intestines. However, only a narrow range of species appear to affect any one population of foxes (Wolfe *et al.*, 2001, citing various references).

Parasites of the gastrointestinal system: The most common parasites in foxes in the UK are *Toxocara canis* (prevalence 61.6%), and the fox hookworm *Uncinaria stenocephala* (prevalence 41.3%) (Smith *et al.*, 2003). Although these parasites are of little clinical significance to adult foxes, they may cause symptomatic infections in young cubs, with poor body condition and distended abdomens being seen (Blackmore, 1964; Brash, 2003). A low prevalence of *Toxascaris leonina* was reported by Smith *et al.* (2003). Foxes may act as a reservoir of endoparasites for domestic dogs (Epe *et al.*, 1999).

Cestodes reported in red foxes in the UK include *Dipylidium caninum*, *Taenia serialis*, *T. pisiformis*, *T. taeniaeformis*, *T. ovis* and *T. hydatigena*. None of these parasites cause clinically apparent infections in foxes (Brash, 2003). *Echinococcus granulosus* was suspected in only six of 588 animals in a study of zoonotic parasitic infections of foxes by Smith *et al.* (2003), suggesting that *E. granulosus* may not be widespread in the UK fox population.

Echinococcus multilocularis, the fox tapeworm, involves rodents as its intermediate host. Human infection, referred to as alveolar echinococcosis, is acquired from food contaminated by fox faeces, and is considered to be one of the most lethal helminthic zoonoses. Over the last 20 years, the parasite's distribution in continental Europe has been increasing, and several countries have reported it in foxes for the first time (Davidson *et al.*, 2012). *E. multilocularis* does not occur in the UK at the time of publication, although it has been reported in an imported beaver (*Castor fiber*) (Barlow *et al.*, 2011). Risk assessments have been performed assessing the likelihood and consequences of importation of the parasite to the UK (Torgerson and Craig, 2009; Kosmider *et al.*, 2013): there are a number of suitable intermediate hosts for *E. multilocularis* in the UK, including the field vole

(*Microtus agrestis*) (Kosmider *et al.*, 2013), which constitutes a significant proportion of the diet of foxes. These studies have suggested that the long-term consequences would be a prevalence of 40% in red foxes in the UK, with high levels in urban foxes. Diagnosis depends on demonstration of the adult worms in the intestine, or the eggs in faecal samples; these cannot be distinguished morphologically from the eggs of other taeniid worms, but may be identified by coproantigen enzyme-linked immunosorbent assays (cELISAs) or PCR (Al-Sabi *et al.*, 2007). Given the zoonotic potential of the parasite, it is recommended that carnivore faeces and intestines are frozen for at least 3 days at -80°C prior to processing in endemic regions (Eckert *et al.*, 2001).

Trematodes, such as *Brachylaima recurva*, *Cryptocotyle lingua* and *Alaria alata* are occasionally reported (Richards *et al.*, 1995; Wolfe *et al.*, 2001). *A. alata* has been reported in foxes in Wales and is zoonotic, causing respiratory and ophthalmic problems in humans following ingestion of the intermediate or paratenic hosts (reviewed in Wolfe *et al.*, 2001). A low prevalence of the acanthocephalans *Plagiorhynchus* (*Prosthorhynchus*) *transversus* and *Macracanthorhynchus catulinus* has been reported in foxes in southern England (Richards *et al.*, 1995).

Treatment of gastrointestinal parasites may be necessary, generally in symptomatic cubs, and can be carried out with the anthelmintics used in domestic dogs (see Figure 21.12). Treatment during the quarantine period (see 'Rearing of fox cubs') will prevent the transmission of parasites when cubs are mixed in groups.

Parasites of the respiratory system: Nematodes were found in the respiratory tract of 44% of foxes in the UK in a post-mortem study by Morgan *et al.* (2008). *Eucoleus aerophilus* (syn. *Capillaria aerophila*) is common in foxes in all parts of Great Britain. *Crenosoma vulpis* was infrequently recovered. Clinical signs associated with these parasites have not been reported in infected foxes, to the author's knowledge.

Angiostrongylus vasorum, French heartworm, is a metastrongyle parasite, which typically inhabits the right ventricle and pulmonary artery of members of the family Canidae, although it has also been reported in Mustelidae (Simpson, 2010). It has become an increasing problem in domestic dogs in the UK in recent years. Animals become infected by ingesting snails and slugs containing infective third-stage larvae. *A. vasorum* was reported in red foxes in the UK by Simpson (1996) in Cornwall (south-west England) and since then, the parasite has been found in foxes as far north as Scotland (Philbey and Delgado, 2013). A prevalence of 32% in foxes in Cornwall since 2002 has been observed (V Simpson, personal communication), and Morgan *et al.* (2008) reported a national prevalence of around 7%. Research in Denmark has suggested there is a good degree of adaptation between the parasite and its fox host, although Simpson (1996) reported foxes with significant *A. vasorum* burdens and associated pathology, possibly as a result of immunosuppression due to concurrent sarcoptic mange infection. On post-mortem examination, the adult worms may be identified in the right ventricle and pulmonary artery, with associated changes in the lungs, including ventral consolidation, multiple haemorrhagic foci and a brownish discoloration due to haemoglobin from phagocytosed red blood cells (Figure 21.10). Right ventricular hypertrophy has also been reported in infected foxes (Morgan *et al.*, 2008). Diagnosis in the live animal may be performed by identification of the L1

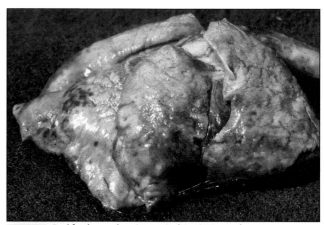

21.10 Red fox lungs showing typical *Angiostrongylus vasorum* pathology.
(© Vic Simpson)

larvae, with a characteristic kink in their tails, on microscopic examination of faeces (using the Baermann test or faecal smears, see Chapter 10) or on bronchoalveolar lavage. The finding of large numbers of larvae in tracheal mucus post-mortem suggests that a tracheal wash could also be a useful diagnostic technique in foxes (V Simpson, personal communication). Affected foxes can be treated with anthelmintics used for *A. vasorum* infection in domestic dogs (see Figure 21.12).

Protozoal infections:

Toxoplasmosis: Toxoplasma gondii is an apicomplexan intracellular protozoan that infects a large number of animals and humans as intermediate hosts (Verin *et al.*, 2013), with cats as definitive hosts. In European red foxes, antibody prevalence has been measured in several countries, using an indirect fluorescent antibody test, ranging from 20% in the UK (Hamilton *et al.*, 2005) to 98% in Belgium (Buxton *et al.*, 1997). *T. gondii* infections are generally subclinical in red foxes, although acute toxoplasmosis has been reported on multiple occasions in association with concurrent CDV infection (reviewed by Dubey *et al.*, 1990). In one case, acute disseminated toxoplasmosis was reported in a red fox in North America without CDV, that was exhibiting signs of incoordination and lack of awareness of its surroundings (Dubey *et al.*, 1990). On post-mortem examination, central nervous system (CNS) lesions are characterized by multifocal to coalescing foci of mild non-suppurative encephalitis with mononuclear infiltration and areas of gliosis. Given the increasing urbanization of foxes and their opportunistic eating habits, they can be considered sentinels of *Toxoplasma* infection in wildlife (De Craeye *et al.*, 2011; Verin *et al.*, 2013).

Neosporosis: Neospora caninum is a protozoan parasite with the domestic dog as its definitive host. However, there is still interest as to whether wild canids can also serve as definitive hosts (Hamilton *et al.*, 2005). Coyotes (*Canis latrans*) have been shown to excrete oocysts following experimental infection (Gondim *et al.*, 2004). Antibodies have been found in the serum of wild red foxes in the UK, indicating they are at least an intermediate host of the parasite. Hamilton *et al.* (2005) reported a seroprevalence of 0.9% in foxes in the UK. In a more recent study, Bartley *et al.* (2013) detected *N. caninum* by PCR in 4.8% of foxes, and demonstrated that other wild carnivores in the UK, such as badgers (*Meles meles*) and European polecats (*Mustela putorius*), could also act as intermediate hosts.

Other protozoal infections: Cryptosporidium parvum was isolated from the faeces of 9% of foxes in a study by Sturdee *et al.* (1999). *Sarcocystis* species and *Isospora* species are reported infrequently (Farmer *et al.*, 1978; Wolfe *et al.*, 2001). A recent UK study of *Encephalitozoon cuniculi* (the causal agent of encephalitozoonosis in humans and animals) revealed a seroprevalence of around 50% in foxes, providing some evidence that foxes could act as sentinels for the presence of *E. cuniculi* in rodents, and may be a significant reservoir of infection (Meredith *et al.*, 2015a).

Other conditions

Hydrocephalus

Hydrocephalus is seen relatively frequently in fox cubs; a domed skull may be obvious, with the ears wide-set (Figure 21.11), although the skull deformity can be more subtle. Affected cubs are dull and unresponsive, and may exhibit aimless wandering (Blackmore, 1964; author's personal experience). It is possible that they are abandoned by the vixen due to abnormal behaviour at the time when they would start becoming more mobile and emerging from the den (from 4 weeks), as they are generally admitted around this age. The condition is progressive, with seizures developing, and euthanasia is the only option. Ljungan virus, a member of the *Parechovirus* genus in the family *Picornaviridae*, has been suspected as a possible cause of hydrocephalus in fox cubs. Ljungan virus was first isolated from bank voles (*Myodes glareolus*) in Sweden in 1998. It has been linked, speculatively, to malformations in human foetuses, including hydrocephaly and anencephaly (reviewed in Koenen *et al.*, 2013).

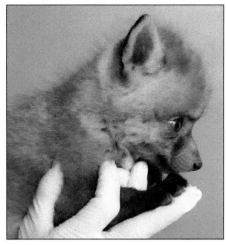

21.11 Hydrocephalus in a red fox cub.

Therapeutics

In general, foxes may be treated with the same drugs licensed for use in domestic dogs, at the same dose rates, being aware of the contraindications and side effects (Figure 21.12). Intramuscular injections can be given in the quadriceps or lumbar muscles, and subcutaneous injections in the scruff of the neck. To avoid excessive handling, oral medications administered in food are preferable. Dead day-old chicks are useful for delivering oral medications, which may be inserted through the open beak into the crop of the chick. When using antibiotics, where possible the choice of drug should be based on the results of culture and sensitivity testing.

Drug	Dosage	Comments
Antimicrobial drugs		
Amoxicillin	15 mg/kg s.c. q48h	For treatment of mild infection when minimal handling is required
Amoxicillin/clavulanate (co-amoxiclav)	8.75 mg/kg i.m., s.c. q24h 12.5–25 mg/kg orally q12h	Broad-spectrum Useful for treatment of bite wounds Duration according to response (minimum of 5–7 days)
Cefalexin	10–25 mg/kg i.m., s.c. q24h 10–25 mg/kg orally q12h	Useful for treatment of bacterial infection of skin secondary to sarcoptic mange
Enrofloxacin	5 mg/kg s.c., orally q24h	Reserved for infection when first-line antimicrobials have been shown to be ineffective on culture and sensitivity Duration according to response (minimum of 5–7 days) Not to be used in growing animals
Marbofloxacin	2 mg/kg s.c., orally q24h	Reserved for infection when first-line antimicrobials have been shown to be ineffective on culture and sensitivity Duration according to response (minimum of 5–7 days) Not to be used in growing animals
Clindamycin	5.5 mg/kg orally q12h 11 mg/kg orally q24h	For treatment of bite wounds and oral infections Duration according to response (minimum of 5–7 days)
Anti-parasitic drugs		
Ivermectin	200–400 µg/kg s.c., orally	For treatment of sarcoptic mange – administer at 2-week intervals a minimum of three times (until negative skin scrape)
Selamectin	15 mg/up to 2.5 kg topically 30 mg/2.6–5 kg topically 60 mg/5.1–10kg topically	For treatment of sarcoptic mange – apply at monthly intervals a minimum of twice (until negative skin scrape) Also treats fleas, ear mites and roundworms
Fipronil 0.25% w/v spray	3–6 ml/kg topically	For the treatment of fleas
Fenbendazole	50 mg/kg orally q24h	For the treatment of roundworms and tapeworms during the quarantine period, treat for 3 days For the treatment of *Angiostrongylus vasorum*, treat for 7–21 days

21.12 Therapeutic drugs and doses that are commonly used in red foxes. None of these drugs are licensed for use in foxes; the suggested doses are those commonly used in domestic dogs.

Vaccination

Vaccination of red foxes using multivalent domestic dog vaccines is performed in some rehabilitation centres in the UK, generally to provide protection against ICH and leptospirosis. The age at which the primary course may be completed renders them of limited use as a means of preventing disease spread within groups of cubs in a rehabilitation facility, given that cubs are usually mixed much in advance of this. The practice of vaccination to prevent infection post-release raises ethical questions, as this may give the rehabilitated animals an advantage relative to their wild conspecifics (see also Chapter 7).

Management in captivity

Housing

Adult foxes should be housed in isolation in a pen which is easily sterilized and will not harbour mites. The accommodation must be secure and have a roof; foxes are expert escape artists and will easily leap in excess of 1.8 m up a fence. Electrical cables, on which the fox can chew or become entangled, must be avoided. Towels and sheets can be used as a short-term substrate, whilst shavings are indicated longer term, as they require less intensive management. Foxes should be provided with somewhere to hide, such as an upturned plastic dog bed. The size of the pen may need to be restricted to a small indoor area initially, for example to provide heat to a debilitated animal or to encourage fracture healing. Thereafter, access to an outside run will give the fox space to improve fitness. Some adult foxes will spend a lot of time trying to escape, which will negate the benefits of cage rest and can result in serious injuries, such as broken teeth and spinal trauma. This may only be apparent with remote monitoring of the fox's behaviour, as it often occurs at night. Foxes will make use of food puzzles, and these can be provided to alleviate boredom. Euthanasia of particularly stressed individuals that are likely to be in captivity for some time may have to be considered on welfare grounds.

Diet

Adult foxes and weaned cubs can be fed a proprietary tinned dog food, with amounts as per a similarly sized domestic dog, remembering the increased requirements of a debilitated animal. Dead day-old chicks and quail can be added for environmental enrichment and to encourage the consumption of oral medications. Water should be available at all times, in a stable container.

Rearing of fox cubs

Housing

Young cubs may be kept in a pet carrier initially. Heat should be provided as, like puppies, they are unable to thermoregulate for the first few weeks of life. Ideally, quarantine would be carried out for 10 days to prevent the spread of diseases such as ICH. However, young cubs (approx. 0–4 weeks of age) kept on their own for this length of time run the risk of becoming malprinted and habituated and being unreleasable. The author isolates such cubs for only 3–4 days, during which period they are

treated for endoparasites (and ectoparasites, if necessary) and monitored closely for signs of disease, such as purulent nasal or ocular discharge. They are then mixed into small groups of 2–3 animals for another week before being mixed into larger groups. Older, wilder cubs can generally be kept in isolation for longer.

Cubs can be kept in groups of up to six, and only cubs of a similar age should be mixed together to avoid unfair competition for food and potentially serious fighting. Housing of much larger numbers of cubs together, or of multiple groups in the vicinity of one another, results in social stress, manifesting as reduced weight gain (Robertson and Harris, 1995). Implantation of microchips allows identification of cubs in a group, enabling their condition to be monitored throughout the rehabilitation process, and potentially following release. Access to an outside run from the age of 6 weeks provides the cubs with more space to exercise and explore, and exposes them to the elements prior to release. At the age of 12–16 weeks, they can be moved to a soft-release pen. Environmental enrichment may be provided in the form of cage furniture such as logs and branches. This will help cubs develop agility, fitness and the ability to find dens. Food items such as dead quail can be provided for the cubs to squabble over (developing social skills) and practise caching food.

Feeding

Unweaned cubs (see Figure 21.2 for aging of cubs) can be given a puppy milk replacer (such as Welpi™), and should be hand-reared as per a puppy, with feeding intervals and toileting practices being the same (see Chapter 8). They should be encouraged to feed independently as quickly as possible: a proprietary puppy food and chopped up day-old chick should be introduced from 4 weeks of age. The cubs can be weaned at 6 weeks. Ideally a range of foods should be provided to prepare cubs for the wild. However, a study by Robertson and Harris (1995) showed that pre-release training is not necessary for rehabilitated red fox cubs to develop hunting skills, which are either innate or learned quickly, large unfamiliar prey being caught almost immediately after release.

The main problems encountered when rearing cubs are nutritional and behavioural. Cubs may get diarrhoea following the introduction of food, or as a result of overfeeding. This is generally self-resolving. Of more concern when rearing young cubs, is the development of malprinting or habituation, manifested by the cub wagging its tail frantically and seeking human contact, which may render it unreleasable (see 'Release'). Handling should be limited in young cubs to avoid this, and every attempt should be made to limit any association of feeding with humans. Ideally, the health of the cubs should be monitored remotely, for example with closed circuit television (see Chapter 9). The author performs a health check at fortnightly intervals, at which point the animals are weighed and their body condition is assessed.

Release

Adults

Adult foxes should be released where they were found at the earliest possible juncture, in order that they have a chance to reoccupy their territory. Although rehabilitated foxes may lose their territory within a number of days, they have already developed the skills necessary to establish a new one if required (S Harris, personal communication). Release should be performed on a calm night, when the fox would be naturally active and hazards such as dogs, people and traffic are minimal. A suitable alternative spot in the vicinity should be chosen if they were found beside a busy road.

Cubs

As stated, cubs may be picked up under the false assumption that they have been orphaned or abandoned, whilst the vixen is away from the den. If the cub appears in good health and circumstances permit, it may be returned to the same location in the evening, within 24–48 hours of being found, and monitored. Harris and MacDonald (1987) suggest that in the majority of cases, such cubs will be found and reared by their parents. Orphaned cubs that are already weaned can be provisioned with food near their den until fully independent (Harris and Macdonald, 1987).

Hand-reared cubs are kept until they are able to survive independently, which means that they are usually released around August to September, when natural dispersal would occur in the wild. Subsequent to a study by Robertson and Harris (1995) showing poor survival of rehabilitated fox cubs, a soft-release approach is used, whereby a period of site acclimatization in a release pen is carried out. They are kept in this pen for 2 weeks, and provisioned with food for at least another 2 weeks post-release. Those cubs that are presented after weaning, from 8–10 weeks of age onwards, can often be released where they were found, although post-release provisioning of food may be required.

The post-release monitoring of fox cubs has historically been hindered by the fact that they are not skeletally mature at the time of release, and hence the fitting of radiotelemetry/global positioning system (GPS) collars is problematic. The implantation of subcutaneous/intra-abdominal transmitters, although feasible, must be performed surgically under Home Office Licence. Recent advances in technology allow the remote drop-off of collars and, at the time of publication, the RSPCA is undertaking a post-release survival study involving global system for mobile communication (GSM) technology (RSPCA, unpublished information). More passive monitoring may be achieved using ear tags and radiofrequency identification (RFID) technology.

Legal aspects

Foxes are not protected by the Wildlife and Countryside Act 1981 (see Chapter 2). It is legal to kill them with a shotgun or a rifle, and free-running snares. It is not legal to poison them (the legislation regarding poisoning is complex; the use of pesticides for poisoning foxes is illegal under the Food and Environment Protection Act (FEPA) 2005 and the Control of Pesticide Regulations (COPR) 2006). Red foxes may be kept as pets. When in captivity, they are protected by the Animal Welfare Act (2006), and thus must be provided with appropriate care, including veterinary attention. Rehabilitated foxes must be released in a responsible manner, i.e. not when this would be considered an offence under the Abandonment of Animals Act 1960; they must have a chance of survival post-release equal to that of their non-rehabilitated peers.

References and further reading

Al-Sabi MNS, Kapel CMO, Deplazes P and Mathis A (2007) Comparative copro-diagnosis of *Echinococcus multilocularis* in experimentally infected foxes. *Parasitology Research* **101**, 731–736

Baker PA and Harris S (2008) Foxes. In: *Mammals of the British Isles: Handbook, 4th edn*, ed. S Harris and DW Yalden, pp. 407–423. The Mammal Society, Southampton

Balboni A, Verin R, Morandi F et al. (2013) Molecular epidemiology of canine adenovirus type 1 and type 2 in free-ranging red foxes (*Vulpes vulpes*) in Italy. *Veterinary Microbiology* **162**, 551–557

Barker IK and Parrish CR (2001) Parvovirus infections. In: *Infectious Diseases of Wild Mammals, 3rd edn*, ed. ES Williams and IK Barker, pp. 131–146. Iowa State University Press, Iowa

Barlow A, Gottstein B and Mueller N (2011) *Echinococcus multilocularis* in an imported captive European beaver (*Castor fiber*) in Great Britain. *The Veterinary Record* **169**, 339

Barrat J, Blancou J, Demantke C and Gerard Y (1985) Beta haemolytic streptococcal infection in red foxes (*Vulpes vulpes* L.) in France: the natural disease and experimental studies. *Journal of Wildlife Diseases* **21**, 141–3

Bartley PM, Wright SE, Zimmer IA et al. (2013) Detection of *Neospora caninum* in wild carnivorans in Great Britain. *Veterinary Parasitology* **192**, 279–283

Beard PM, Daniels MJ, Henderson D et al. (2001) Paratuberculosis infection of non-ruminant wildlife in Scotland. *Journal of Clinical Microbiology* **39**, 1517–1521

Blackmore DK (1964) A survey of disease in British wild foxes. *The Veterinary Record* **76**, 527–533

Bodewes R, van der Giessen J, Haagmans BL, Osterhaus ADME and Smits SL (2013) Identification of multiple novel viruses, including a parvovirus and a hepevirus, in feces of red foxes. *Journal of Virology* **87**, 7758–7764

Bradley CA and Altizer S (2007) Urbanization and the ecology of wildlife diseases. *Trends in Ecology and Evolution* **22**, 95–102

Brash MGI (2003) Foxes. In: *BSAVA Manual of Wildlife Casualties*, ed. E Mullineaux, D Best and JE Cooper, pp. 154–165. BSAVA Publications, Gloucester

Buxton D, Maley SW, Pastoret P-P, Brochier B and Innes EA (1997) Examination of red foxes (*Vulpes vulpes*) from Belgium for antibody to *Neospora caninum* and *Toxoplasma gondii*. *The Veterinary Record* **141**, 308–309

Collins R, Wessels ME, Wood R, Couper D and Swift A (2010) Sarcoptic mange in badgers in the UK. *The Veterinary Record* **167**, 668

Couper D, Margos G, Kurtenbach K and Turton S (2010) Prevalence of *Borrelia* infection in ticks from wildlife in south-west England. *The Veterinary Record* **167**, 1012–1014

Davidson RK, Bornstein S and Handeland K (2008) Long-term study of *Sarcoptes scabiei* in Norwegian red foxes (*Vulpes vulpes*) indicating host/parasite adaptation. *Veterinary Parasitology* **156**, 277-283

Davidson RK, Romig T, Jenkins E, Tryland M and Robertson LJ (2012) The impact of globalisation on the distribution of *Echinococcus multilocularis*. *Trends in Parasitology* **28**, 239–247

De Craeye S, Speybroeck N, Ajzenberg D et al. (2011) *Toxoplasma gondii* and *Neospora caninum* in wildlife: common parasites in Belgian foxes and cervidae? *Veterinary Parasitology* **178**, 64–69

Delahay RJ, Cheeseman CL and Clifton-Hadley RS (2001) Wildlife disease reservoirs: the epidemiology of *Mycobacterium bovis* infection in the European badger (*Meles meles*) and other British mammals. *Tuberculosis* **81**, 43–49

Deplazes P, Hegglin D, Gloor S and Romig T (2004) Wilderness in the city: the urbanization of *Echinococcus multilocularis*. *Trends in Parasitology* **20**, 77–84

Dubey JP, Hamir AN, and Rupprecht CE (1990) Acute disseminated toxoplasmosis in a red fox (*Vulpes vulpes*). *Journal of Wildlife Diseases* **26**, 286–290

Duff JP (2002) *Wildlife Diseases in the UK 2002. Report to the Department of Environment, Food and Rural Affairs (DEFRA) and the Office International des Epizooties (OIE)*. Veterinary Laboratories Agency

Ebani VV, Verin R, Fratini F, Poli A and Cerri D (2011) Molecular survey of *Anaplasma phagocytophilum* and *Ehrlichia canis* in red foxes (*Vulpes vulpes*) from central Italy. *Journal of Wildlife Diseases* **47**, 669–703

Eckert J, Gemmell MA, Meslin FX and Pawlowski ZS (2001) *WHO/OIE Manual of echinococcosis in humans and animals: a public health problem of global concern*. World Health Organization and World Organization for Animal Health, Paris

Epe C, Meuwissen M, Stoye M and Schnieder T (1999) Transmission trials, ITS2-PCR and RAPD-PCR show identity of *Toxocara canis* isolates from red fox and dog. *Veterinary Parasitology* **84**, 101–112

Escutenaire S, Pastoret P-P, Brus Sjolander K et al. (2000) Evidence of *Puumala Hantavirus* in red foxes (*Vulpes vulpes*) in Belgium. *The Veterinary Record* **147**, 365–366

Euden PR (1990) *Salmonella* isolates from wild animals in Cornwall. *British Veterinary Journal* **146**, 228–232

Farmer JN, Herbert IV, Partridge M and Edwards GT (1978) The prevalence of *Sarcocystis* species in dogs and red foxes. *Veterinary Record* **102**, 78–80

Gondim LFP, McAllister MM, Pitt WC and Zemlicka DE (2004) Coyotes (*Canis latrans*) are definitive hosts of *Neospora caninum*. *International Journal for Parasitology* **34**, 159–161

Hamilton CM, Gray, R, Wright SE et al. (2005) Prevalence of antibodies to *Toxoplasma gondii* and *Neospora caninum* in red foxes (*Vulpes vulpes*) from around the UK. *Veterinary Parasitology* **130**, 169–173

Handeland K, Nesse LL, Lillehaug A *et al.* (2008) Natural and experimental *Salmonella* Typhimurium infections in foxes (*Vulpes vulpes*). *Veterinary Microbiology* **132**, 129–134

Harris S (1978a) Age determination in the red fox (*Vulpes vulpes*) – an evaluation of technique efficiency as applied to a sample of suburban foxes. *Journal of Zoology* **91**, 91–117

Harris S (1978b) Injuries to foxes (*Vulpes vulpes*) living in suburban London. *Journal of Zoology* **186**, 567–572

Harris S (1981) An estimation of the number of foxes (*Vulpes vulpes*) in the city of Bristol, and some possible factors affecting their distribution. *Journal of Applied Ecology* **18**, 455–465

Harris S and Macdonald D (1987) Orphaned foxes – Guidelines on the Rescue and Rehabilitation of Fox Cubs. Royal Society for the Prevention of Cruelty to Animals (RSPCA), Horsham, UK

Harris S and Smith GC (1987) Demography of two urban fox (*Vulpes vulpes*) populations. *Journal of Applied Ecology* **24**, 75–86

Isogai E, Isogai H, Kawabata H *et al.* (1994) Lyme disease spirochaetes in a wild fox (*Vulpes vulpes schrencki*). *Journal of Wildlife Diseases* **30**, 439–444

Knudtson WU, Gates CE and Ruth GR (1980) *Trichophyton mentagrophytes* dermatophytosis in wild fox. *Journal of Wildlife Diseases* **16**, 465–468

Koenen F, Gibbs, EPJ Ruiz-Fons F and Barlow AM (2012) Picornavirus Infections. In: *Infectious Diseases of Wild Mammals and Birds in Europe, 1st edn*, ed. D Gavier-Widen, JP Duff and A Meredith, pp. 168–180. Blackwell Publishing Ltd, Oxford

Kosmider R, Paterson A, Voas A and Roberts H (2013) *Echinococcus multilocularis* introduction and establishment in wildlife via imported beavers. *The Veterinary Record* **172**, 606

Krebs JR (1997) *Bovine tuberculosis* in cattle and badgers. Ministry of Agriculture, London

Kreeger TJ, Monson D, Kuechle VB, Seal US and Tester JR (1989) Monitoring heart rate and body temperature in red foxes (*Vulpes vulpes*). *Canadian Journal of Zoology* **67**, 2455–2458

Linhart SB (1968) Dentition and pelage in the juvenile red fox (*Vulpes vulpes*). *Journal of Mammalogy* **49**, 526–528

Meredith AL, Cleaveland SC, Brown J, Mahajan A and Shaw DJ (2015a) Seroprevalence of *Encephalitozoon cuniculi* in wild rodents, foxes and domestic cats in three sites in the United Kingdom. *Transboundary and Emerging Diseases* **62(2)**, 148–156

Meredith AL, Cleaveland SC, Denwood MJ, Brown JK and Shaw DJ (2015b) *Coxiella burnetii* (Q-fever) seroprevalence in prey and predators in the United Kingdom: evaluation of infection in wild rodents, foxes and domestic cats using a modified ELISA. *Transboundary and Emerging Diseases* **62(6)**, 639–649

Morgan ER, Tomlinson A, Hunter S *et al.* (2008) *Angiostrongylus vasorum* and *Eucoleus aerophilus* in foxes (*Vulpes vulpes*) in Great Britain. *Veterinary Parasitology* **154**, 48–57

Nouvellet P, Donnelly CA, De Nardi M *et al.* (2013) Rabies and canine distemper virus epidemics in the red fox population of northern Italy (2006–2010). *PLoS ONE* **8**, e61588

Philbey AW and Delgado D (2013) Detection of *Angiostrongylus vasorum* in red foxes in Scotland. *The Veterinary Record* **173**, 148

Philbey AW and Thompson H (2009) Leptospirosis and infectious canine hepatitis in foxes (*Vulpes vulpes*). *Proceedings of the British Veterinary Zoological Society*, Spring Meeting 2009, pp. 39–40

Richards DT, Harris S and Lewis JW (1995) Epidemiological studies on intestinal parasites of rural and urban red foxes (*Vulpes vulpes*) in the United Kingdom. *Veterinary Parasitology* **59**, 39–51

Robertson CPG and Harris S (1995) The behaviour after release of captive-reared fox cubs. *Animal Welfare* **4(4)**, 295–306

Rupprecht CE, Stohr K and Meredith C (2001) Rabies. In: *Infectious Diseases of Wild Mammals, 3rd edn*, ed. ES Williams and IK Barker, pp. 3–36. Iowa State University Press, Iowa

Shilo Y, Lapid R, King R, Bdolah-Abram T and Epstein A (2010) Immobilization of red fox (*Vulpes vulpes*) with medetomidine-ketamine or medetomidine-midazolam and antagonism with atipamezole. *Journal of Zoo and Wildlife Medicine* **41**, 28–34

Shore RF, Fletcher MR, Walker LA (2003) Agricultural pesticides and mammals in Britain. In: *Conservation and conflict – mammals and farming in Britain*, ed. F Tattersall and W Manly, pp. 37–50. Linnean Society Occasional Publication No. 4, London

Simpson VR (1996) *Angiostrongylus vasorum* infection in foxes (*Vulpes vulpes*) in Cornwall. *The Veterinary Record* **139**, 443–445

Simpson VR (2000) Wildlife on a knife edge – a veterinary perspective. *Biologist* **47**, 131–135

Simpson VR (2010) *Angiostrongylus vasorum* infection in a stoat. *The Veterinary Record* **166**, 182

Slavica A, Dezdek D, Konjevic D *et al.* (2011) Prevalence of leptospiral antibodies in the red fox (*Vulpes vulpes*) population of Croatia. *Veterinarni Medicina* **56**, 209–213

Smith FD, Ellse E and Wall R (2013) Prevalence of *Babesia* and *Anaplasma* in ticks infesting dogs in Great Britain. *Veterinary Parasitology* **198**, 18–23

Smith GC, Gangadharan B, Taylor Z *et al.* (2003) Prevalence of zoonotic important parasites in the red fox (*Vulpes vulpes*) in Great Britain. *Veterinary Parasitology* **118**, 133–142

Sturdee AP, Chalmers RM and Bull SA (1999) Detection of *Cryptosporidium oocysts* in wild mammals of mainland Britain. *Veterinary Parasitology* **80**, 273–280

Thompson H, O'Keeffe AM, Lewis JCM *et al.* (2010) Infectious canine hepatitis in red foxes (*Vulpes vulpes*) in the United Kingdom. *The Veterinary Record* **166**, 111–114

Torgerson PR and Craig PS (2009) Risk assessment of importation of dogs infected with *Echinococcus multilocularis*. *The Veterinary Record* **165**, 366–368

Verin R, Mugnaini L, Nardoni S *et al.* (2013) Serologic, molecular and pathologic survey of *Toxoplasma gondii* infection in free-ranging red foxes (*Vulpes vulpes*) in Central Italy. *Journal of Wildlife Diseases* **49**, 545–551

Williams ES (2001) Morbilliviral diseases. In: *Infectious Diseases of Wild Mammals. 3rd edn*, ed. ES Williams and IK Barker, pp. 37–76. Iowa State University Press, Iowa

Wolfe A, Hogan S, Maguire D *et al.* (2001) Red foxes (*Vulpes vulpes*) in Ireland as hosts for parasites of potential zoonotic and veterinary significance. *The Veterinary Record* **149**, 759–763

Woods LW (2001) Adenoviral diseases. In: *Infectious Diseases of Wild Mammals, 3rd edn*, eds. ES Williams and IK Barker, pp 202–212. Iowa State University Press, Iowa

Specialist organizations and useful contacts

See also Appendix 1

The Fox Project
Southern Wildlife Ambulance Network website with useful fox information.
www.foxproject.org.uk

The Fox Website
Contains useful information on foxes including aspects of ecology, behaviour, management and human conflict, run by the Mammal Group, University of Bristol.
www.thefoxwebsite.net

Chapter 22

Deer

Molly Varga

There are six species of deer found in the UK. Only red deer (*Cervus elaphus*) (see Figure 22.6) and roe deer (*Capreolus capreolus*) (Figure 22.1a) are indigenous. Fallow deer (*Dama dama*) (Figure 22.1b) are considered 'naturalized': they existed in the UK in prehistoric times, but their distribution was significantly altered during periods of climate change, meaning that they were absent from the UK for millennia, before being reintroduced by the Romans. Sika deer (*Cervus nippon*) (Figure 22.1c), Chinese water deer (*Hydropotes inermis*) (Figure 22.1d) and muntjac deer (*Muntiacus reevesi*) (Figure 22.1e) are all introduced species.

Over the past decade the number of wild deer in the UK has doubled to an estimated 2 million individuals, meaning that the numbers are higher now than at any time in the last thousand years. Consequently, deer casualties, as well as the incidence of infectious diseases, are increasing. Common reasons for presentation to a veterinary surgeon (veterinarian) include road traffic accidents, apparently abandoned young and animals caught in fencing.

Red deer are the UK's largest free-living mammals. All deer species are potentially dangerous and should be treated with caution, especially in an emergency situation. Ideally, injured deer should be referred to a wildlife hospital or rehabilitation centre with suitable facilities for treating and housing the animal, either directly, or as soon as possible after triage (see Chapter 4).

Ecology and biology

As a general rule most species of deer are found in woodland habitats, often close to arable land, but usually close to cover (Figure 22.2). Because they are adaptable they may also be found in semi-urban environments and some species are comfortable on open heath or moorland. There are distinct species and seasonal differences in habitat preference and usage. Red deer are active primarily at

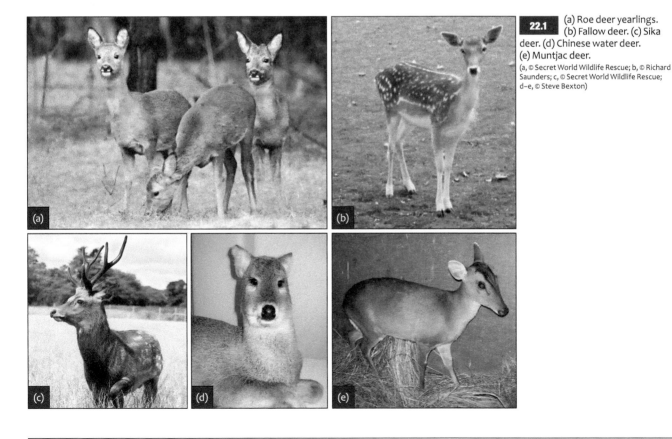

22.1 (a) Roe deer yearlings. (b) Fallow deer. (c) Sika deer. (d) Chinese water deer. (e) Muntjac deer.
(a, © Secret World Wildlife Rescue; b, © Richard Saunders; c, © Secret World Wildlife Rescue; d–e, © Steve Bexton)

dawn and dusk are usually found in mature woodland and on moorland; roe deer are found in woodland, but will venture towards field edges; and fallow deer prefer open parkland or open areas within woodland. Chinese water deer have a preference for areas adjacent to water courses, sika like dense woodland but can be found in deer parks and muntjac can be found in various habitats from dense woodland to farmland. Deer play an important role in woodland ecosystems; however, they may pose a threat to biodiversity in situations where over-browsing occurs.

Deer most commonly occur as herd animals, although solitary animals (often males) are also seen. Solitary individuals tend to be territorial, whilst herd groups have areas of preference (core areas) which can vary seasonally, with the groups being noted frequently in these core areas but not on adjacent land. Where herds of different species occupy the same area, there may be competition for resources. Whilst this is often passive, aggressive encounters can occur.

Deer both graze and browse, meaning that they will eat grass and cover plants as well as the leaves and bark of trees and shrubs. The pattern of feeding (particularly the height to which trees are browsed) is characteristic of the species. Typically fallow deer will both browse and graze, feeding from standing crops, woodland trees and the undergrowth layer. Red deer tend to be more selective grazers; however, when they browse in woodland they can reach a height of up to 1.6 m. Sika are also primarily grazers, with a maximum browse reach of 1.6 m. Muntjac are typically browsers, reaching up to around 90 cm in height; they will also rear up on their hind legs to access higher browse or to knock plants over in order to eat. Chinese water deer and roe deer tend to be less destructive to woodland and crops. In some circumstances where there is sufficient deer population, lack of food resource can force deer out of woodland and on to arable land or into peri-urban environments. This brings deer into conflict with farmers due to crop damage, as well as increasing the likelihood of road traffic accidents. Factors such as these, as well as rapid population increase, have led to the decision to cull deer in some areas. Where there is a chronic high deer population in an area, significant and permanent changes to the flora of that area can occur, leading to the suggestion that deer can adversely affect biodiversity within an ecosystem. With a lack of large wild carnivores in the UK, deer have no natural predators except humans.

Biological and ecological data for British deer species can be found in Figures 22.2 and 22.3.

Species	Description	Field observations	Distribution (shaded)	Other characteristics
Red deer (Cervus elaphus) (see Figure 22.6)	Red to dark brown coat; spots only in juveniles	Live in mature woodland, grazing on the edges and in adjacent grassland May also be seen on moorland and scrub Active primarily at dawn and dusk		Will travel considerable distances in their herds Herds consist of females and young led by a matriarch Males are usually solitary except during the rut
Roe deer (Capreolus capreolus) (see Figure 22.1a)	Small and fine-boned Red in summer becoming greyer during the winter Muzzle is black, chin is white, and caudal patch is white or cream	Found in woodland and field edges Rest in dense scrub during daylight		Non-herding and usually seen as individuals or small family groups Males are solitary except during the rut This species is very strongly territorial
Fallow deer (Dama dama) (see Figure 22.1b)	Spotted, including young (see Figure 22.5a) Colour can vary from dark brown/black (melanistic) through sandy brown with white spots (menil) to albino (whitish cream) Black stripes down the caudal thigh are common	Found in parkland and prefers open woodland, but also found in mature and coniferous woodland as well as open areas		More likely to be found in semi-urban/urban areas than other deer Active at dawn and dusk, but active diurnally if not disturbed Non-territorial: herds of females with young and separate male herds are found, mixing only during the rut
Sika deer (Cervus nippon) (see Figure 22.1c)	Red to reddish brown with a prominent paler patch over the rump, perineum and caudal thighs Often retain juvenile white spots as adults	Found in deer parks, dense woodland and mixed fields		Will interbreed with red deer leading to hybridization

22.2 UK deer species and some of their ecological characteristics. (continues) ▶

Species	Description	Field observations	Distribution (shaded)	Other characteristics
Chinese water deer (*Hydropotes inermis*) (see Figure 22.1d)	Woolly coat type, greyish to sandy brown	Found in wet woodland and reed beds adjacent to fields		Solitary
Muntjac deer (Reeves muntjac: *Muntiacus reevesi*) (see Figure 22.1e)	Reddish in summer becoming more brown in the winter	Habitat is variable: dense woodland and scrub to farmland		Almost pig-like in appearance with a roached (hunched) back Active throughout the day and night They are shy and solitary, but can be seen in pairs

22.2 (continued) UK deer species and some of their ecological characteristics.

Species	Size	Ageing and lifespan	Gender determination	Antlers (see Figure 22.4)
Red deer (*Cervus elaphus*) (see Figure 22.6)	Up to 250 kg in males, females are smaller Head to rump length 165–260 cm; height at shoulder 114–122 cm	Young are spotted at birth but the spots are lost at first moult at approximately 2 months of age (see Figure 22.5a) Animals get broader across back as they age Adult dentition at 29–30 months (deciduous premolar 3 lost at 27–28 months), last cusp of 3rd molar may not come into wear until 36 months Lifespan 14 years	Males are larger and have a mane and thicker neck in the autumn Adult males usually have antlers	Usually only males Tines and beam have an oval cross-section; several tines extend from the beam Cast in winter Antler tine numbers increase with age, but size and pedicle length reduce with increasing age
Roe deer (*Capreolus capreolus*) (see Figure 22.1a)	Up to 25 kg in both sexes Head to rump length 95–135 cm; height at shoulder 63–67 cm	Young are spotted (see Figure 22.5a) Broader across back with age Adult size reached at 1 year Adult dentition present at 12–13 months Lifespan 8 years	Females may have a prominent anal tuft of hair Adult males usually have antlers	Usually only males Usually fairly simple, with one forward and one backward pointing tine on each antler Cast between October and January Antlers are not a good indicator of age
Fallow deer (*Dama dama*) (see Figure 22.1b)	Up to 100 kg in both sexes Head to rump length 130–170 cm; shoulder height 85–110 cm	Get stockier and broader with age Deciduous 3rd premolar lost at 19–22 months Adult dentition present at 26–30 months Last cusp of 3rd molar in wear by 36 months Lifespan is 12 years	Males have a thicker neck with no mane, and may have a tuft of preputial hair Females have a shorter coat, with a longer neck Adult males usually have antlers	Usually only males Males have distinctive flattened or 'palmate' antlers Cast in April–May Increase in complexity with age, but size and pedicle length reduce
Sika deer (*Cervus nippon*) (see Figure 22.1c)	Up to 60 kg in both sexes Shoulder height up to 85 cm	Older animals are stockier and broader across the back Deciduous premolar 3 is lost at 18–20 months and adult dentition is present at 24–26 months Last cusp of 3rd molar comes into wear at 36 months Lifespan is 12 years	Adult males are larger and darker than the females, and may have a mane in the winter Adult males usually have antlers	Usually only males Round or oval cross section, with several tines extending from each beam; shorter and more upright than red deer Antlers increase in complexity with age, but size and pedicle length reduce

22.3 Biological characteristics of common UK deer species. (continues) ▶

Species	Size	Ageing and lifespan	Gender determination	Antlers (see Figure 22.4)
Chinese water deer (*Hydropotes inermis*) (see Figure 22.1d)	Up to 18 kg; legs are proportionally longer compared to other species Up to 60 cm at the shoulder	Difficult to age Adult weight achieved at 1 year Individuals become stockier with age Upper canines reach full length at 18–24 months, but the length is not a good indicator of age Lifespan is 8 years	Can be difficult to distinguish even in adults The upper canines (tusks) may be visible in mature males	None present
Muntjac deer (Reeves muntjac: *Muntiacus reevesi*) (see Figure 22.1e)	Up to 20 kg, distinctive due to the heavier muscling and short thin legs Head to rump length 90–100 cm; shoulder height 45–52 cm	Fawns have spots until 2 months of age (see Figure 22.5b) Adult weight is reached at 1 year Individuals become stockier with age Lifespan is 10 years	Males are larger and darker than females, with a more yellowy forehead Tusks, antlers and pedicles may be visible in males	Usually only males Simple short spikes, may have a small brow tine at base Antlers cast from May to July Antlers are not a good indicator of age

22.3 (continued) Biological characteristics of common UK deer species.

Anatomy and physiology

The physical characteristics of the UK deer species are described in Figures 22.2 and 22.3. A glossary of terms used to describe deer, including the names of males, females and young of each species, is given in Figure 22.4.

Term	Definition
Male; female; neonate	
Stag	Male red or sika deer
Hind	Female red or sika deer
Calf	Juvenile red or sika deer
Buck	Male fallow, roe, Chinese water or muntjac deer
Doe	Female fallow, roe, Chinese water or muntjac deer
Fawn	Juvenile fallow, roe, Chinese water or muntjac deer
Kid	The juveniles of the smaller species (roe, muntjac and Chinese water deer) are also sometimes termed kids
Behaviour	
Rut	Deer breeding season
Hefting	Territorial/behavioural ties of certain species/sexes of deer to a specific geographical area
Antlers	
Pedicle	The base of the antler, the portion which attaches to the skull
Velvet	The living skin that covers antlers whilst they are growing
Beam	The central stalk of the antler
Tines	Points off the main antler branches
Bey	The second anterior tine
Trey	The third anterior tine
Perruque	Abnormal uncontrolled antler growth which occurs with interruption or removal of testosterone production (serious illness or castration) May have the appearance of a tumour and become secondarily infected

22.4 Glossary of terms used to describe deer.

Coat

All British deer are spotted as juveniles (Figure 22.5), but the spots are lost in most species at the time of the first moult at around 2 months of age (see Figure 22.3). Deer hair is hollow, brittle and easily epilated. The hair coat changes twice a year, with the winter coat typically being darker and thicker. Summer coats can be very thin. Late coat changes may be an indication of poor health (through illness or injury). Deer possess pre-orbital and limb scent glands, the number and location of which varies with

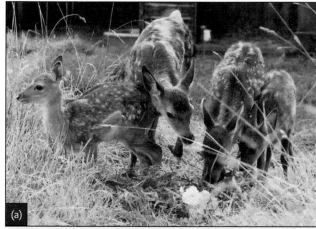
(a)

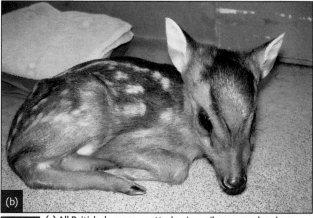
(b)

22.5 (a) All British deer are spotted as juveniles: examples shown here from left to right are fallow, red, red, roe. (b) Muntjac kid.
(a, © Secret World Wildlife Rescue; b, © Steve Bexton)

species; for example, all species found in the UK (except roe deer) have pre-orbital glands, whilst only roe deer have interdigital glands. These are used for marking territory as well as recognition of individuals, status and young.

Senses

Deer have several adaptations that are characteristic of prey animals, including the ability to feed in short intense bursts and then to ruminate once safety is reached. They have good eyesight with very laterally placed eyes, giving a wide field of view; they are also much better at seeing moving objects and may miss stationary ones. Deer possess a very acute sense of smell, and can identify individual deer or human scent over a distance of hundreds of metres. They also have very sensitive hearing; each ear is able to move independently giving a 360-degree range.

Antlers

Antlers are unique to deer and are usually only present on males (Figure 22.6), except in caribou (*Rangifer tarandus*) where they are also present on females. Occasionally older females will have small continuously growing antlers (particularly roe deer). This condition appears to be rare, and is associated with levels of testosterone that are high relative to oestrogen levels within an individual. Antlers form on top of pedicles (permanent bony outgrowths situated on top of the skull). Each year, under the hormonal influence of testosterone and increasing day length, new antlers grow under a layer of skin (velvet) that contains blood vessels and nerves. Antler growth takes between 3 and 4 months, after which the velvet dies and is shed, exposing the hard bone of the fully grown antler. Handling live animals in velvet should be avoided because damage to the velvet will cause pain and haemorrhage. Equally the

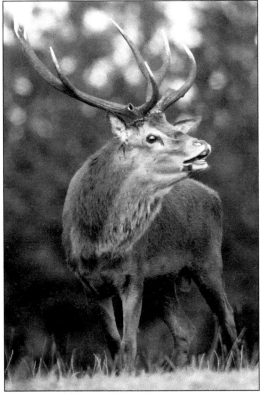

22.6 Red deer stag with antlers.
(© Secret World Wildlife Rescue)

cutting of velvet antlers from live animals in the UK is illegal except for defined welfare reasons. The fully grown antler is retained for a period and then cast (different species cast at different times of year). The oldest animals in best condition will usually lose their antlers first. Because antler production is under hormonal control, factors that affect hormone production (e.g. illness or injury) will affect antler growth. If testosterone production is reduced or stopped then antlers will fail to harden and the velvet will not be shed. This leads to a condition of abnormally grown soft velvet antlers known as 'perruque' head (see Figure 22.4). These antlers are at risk of infection and flystrike. Damage or illness during growth can cause abnormalities, but as long as the pedicle is not damaged then usually the next set of antlers will be normal. As an individual animal ages, the antlers produced often reduce in size, a process known as 'going back'. Both genetic and environmental factors can affect antler quality and shape.

Digestive system

Most deer species have the following dental formula:

$$2 \times \left\{ I \frac{0}{3} \ C \frac{1}{1} \ P \frac{3}{3} \ M \frac{3}{3} \right\} = 34$$

Roe and fallow deer do not have upper canines. Deer lack upper incisors and instead there is a hard pad on the upper jaw for the lower incisors to butt against. Dentition can be used as a means of ageing (see Figure 22.3) and in some species (e.g. muntjac) the growth of the upper canines (tusks) can be an aid to sex determination.

Deer are ruminants, similar to cattle and sheep. In common with other ruminant species they are adapted to eating a fibrous poorly-digestible diet, although the strategies adopted are not always exactly the same. Different species of deer have adapted to a greater or lesser extent to the type of diet they normally eat. For example, roe and muntjac deer are often regarded as less evolved and 'older' forms of deer with slightly simpler digestive tracts than other ruminant species. The rumen functions as a large fermentation vat containing microorganisms that initiate the breakdown of plant material. The rumen microbial population is sensitive both to extremes of temperature and rapid changes in diet. Failure of the microbial digestion can prove fatal. Once food is prehended and chewed, it is swallowed and stored in the rumen until the animal reaches a place of safety in which to ruminate. The food is then regurgitated and chewed for a second time before being swallowed and passing from the rumen to the reticulum, the omasum and then to the abomasum (the equivalent of the true stomach). Digestion then follows a similar path to monogastric species, with food passing to the small and then large intestines, with digestion and absorption continuing as it travels along the gut. In contrast to most other ruminant species, deer do not have a gall bladder.

Reproduction

Reproductive strategies vary between deer species (Figure 22.7). Most deer species are polyoestrous; however, roe deer are monoestrous with delayed implantation of the embryo, meaning young are produced in the summer when food resources are abundant. Most species are seasonal breeders, with the exception of the muntjac, which breeds all year round. High pregnancy rates in all species allow deer to maintain population levels. The short period of parental dependency further facilitates this.

Species	Oestrus cycle	Rut	Pregnancy rate	Gestation	Birthing season	Number of young	Lactation
Red deer (*Cervus elaphus*)	Polyoestrous	September/ October	90%	7 months	May/June	1 (occasionally 2)	5–6 months
Roe deer (*Capreolus capreolus*)	Monoestrous, but 5 months delayed implantation	July/August	Up to 100%	5 months	May/June	1–2	5–6 months
Fallow deer (*Dama dama*)	Polyoestrous	October/ November	90%	8 months	June/July	1 (occasionally 2)	5–6 months
Sika deer (*Cervus nippon*)	Polyoestrous	September/ November	90%	9 months	June/July	1	5–6 months
Muntjac deer (*Muntiacus reevesi*)	Polyoestrous	No defined season: breed year round	Up to 100%	7 months	Year round	1	2 months
Chinese water deer (*Hydropotes inermis*)	Polyoestrous	November/ December	No data available	6 months	May/June	2 (4–5 possible)	3–4 months

22.7 Reproductive data for common UK deer species.

Capture, handling and transportation

Adults of all deer species are potentially dangerous and should only be handled by trained and experienced personnel. Members of the public should never be advised to approach an injured deer, and any wild deer that allows a human to approach is likely to have significant injury or illness that is life-threatening. Deer have various means of defence: antlers, hooves, size and the ability to run away. They also have the instinct to avoid contact and handling, such that deer attempting to escape human contact will act in an apparently irrational manner to avoid capture. Deer may also carry a variety of potentially zoonotic infections (Figure 22.8).

Capture

By its nature all wildlife work is unpredictable and often does not allow for choosing the time and place of capture and handling. There are several factors to consider that will maximize the success and minimize the risk (to both humans and patients) when planning a deer handling intervention.

- **Why?** Consideration should be given to whether the benefits of capture and evaluation outweigh the (significant) risks, particularly in cases where an injured animal appears otherwise well, active and able to feed (on distant observation). In all circumstances the welfare of the individual must be paramount; however, many wild deer survive apparently serious injuries such as antler damage and long bone fracture. A short 'field' intervention with the provision of first aid and pain relief may be preferable to confinement in a hospital facility. This approach is particularly applicable, for example, in cases where an animal is trapped in fencing. It may also be appropriate when juveniles are brought in by well meaning individuals thinking, erroneously, that they have been abandoned.
- **Where?** Away from traffic and members of the public, avoiding obvious hazards like river banks or steep hillsides/cliffs, attempting to drive a wild animal into an area where it can be safely manually restrained or darted. This ideal may not be achievable, but thought must be given particularly to protection of the public from potential harm. The police and/or appropriate local wildlife charities (e.g. Royal Society for the Prevention of Cruelty to Animals (RSPCA) or Scottish Society for the Prevention of Cruelty to Animals (Scottish SPCA)) should be contacted where an animal may escape on to a public highway.
- **When?** Avoiding both very hot (see 'Capture myopathy') and very cold/icy conditions (potential injury due to slipping/falling) – early in the morning is often the ideal time. If it is not possible to avoid an intervention during adverse conditions, then provision should be made to mitigate the problems that this can cause.
- **How?** Using a familiar and appropriate method of restraint for both the species and the situation. Always approach recumbent deer with caution as they are prone to jumping up suddenly and may charge through/past an approaching human even if apparently injured.
- **What equipment?** Something to cover the head/eyes as a blindfold (e.g. a towel, blanket or sacking), sturdy ropes, netting (e.g. freight netting: this must be strong and with a suitable size of mesh to avoid causing additional injury), thick blankets/rugs, equipment for sedation (appropriately licensed syringe pole/dart gun; see Chapters 2 and 6), sedative drugs (see 'Anaesthesia and analgesia') and equipment for euthanasia (see 'Euthanasia'). Some method for transportation (see 'Transportation') will also need to be considered.

Handling

Small or juvenile deer can be safely restrained manually. The animal should be approached quietly from behind and a blanket (or net) thrown over the head and body. The animal can then be blindfolded and rope hobbles applied. The response to blindfolding varies between species: roe, and juvenile red, sika and fallow deer will remain calm, whilst muntjac will often vocalize persistently and panic if they cannot see. Rope hobbles are used to restrict the

Disease	Route of infection	Clinical signs in deer	Clinical signs in humans
Bacterial infections			
Actinomycosis (*Trueperella pyogenes*)	Contact (both direct and indirect)	Mastitis/mammary abscessation, bronchopneumonia/pulmonary abscesses, metritis and septicaemia	Nodular skin lesions, granulomas, abscesses, chronic pneumonia, chronic abdominal masses
Anthrax (*Bacillus anthracis*)	Contact (both direct and indirect)	Fever, depression, lethargy, staggering. Often acute death. Bloody discharge from nose/mouth may be seen	Ulcerative skin lesions, pneumonia, septicaemia
Borreliosis (Lyme disease) (*Borrelia burgdorferi*)	Tick bites	May be asymptomatic. Lameness and fever possible	'Target lesions', arthritis, sepsis, pyrexia, headaches and myalgia
Brucellosis (*Brucella* spp.)	Ingestion, mucous membrane contact	May be asymptomatic. Signs typical of other ruminants such as abortion and epididymitis are reported leading to reduced fertility. Septic arthritis may also be noted	Undulant fever, septicaemia
Campylobacteriosis (*Campylobacter* spp.)	Ingestion of contaminated faeces	May be asymptomatic carriers. Placentitis and abortion reported in deer. Enteritis may also be noted	Usually enteritis, possibly arthritis/septicaemia
Clostridiosis (*Clostridium* spp.)	Contact (both direct and indirect), ingestion	Signs dependent on species of clostridium involved. Enterotoxaemia, malignant oedema/blackleg and tetanus are all possibilities. See also 'Infectious diseases'	Enteritis, gangrene, septicaemia
Colibacillosis (*Escherichia coli*)	Contact, ingestion of contaminated faeces	Depend on age of deer and strain of bacterium. Vary from mild diarrhoea to haemorrhagic diarrhoea, CNS signs and collapse or death from endotoxic shock	Enteritis, haemolytic uraemic syndrome
Dermatophilosis (*Dermatophilus congolensis*)	Direct contact	Exudative dermatitis, scabby skin with patchy hairloss. Underlying skin can be red and inflamed. Ranges from superficial to deep skin infection. Often around feet, but can be seen on any area of the body	Pustular desquamative dermatitis
Erysipeloid (*Erysipelothrix rhusiopathiae*)	Contact (both direct and indirect)	Mild skin lesions. Potentially vegetative endocarditis	Cellulitis, septicaemia
Leptospirosis (*Leptospira* spp.)	Exposure or ingestion of contaminated urine	Asymptomatic. See also 'Infectious diseases'	Fever, rash, other significant systemic effects including liver/kidney failure
Mycobacteriosis (*Mycobacteria* spp. avium-intracellulare complex and non-tuberculous forms)	Environmental contact	A variety of signs may be noted. Because deer are very susceptible to some forms of mycobacteriosis it is advised that any form of abscess (does not need to be caseated or calcified) found on a deer should be treated as a potential case unless proven otherwise	Variety of granulomatous infections depending on route of entry
Nocardiosis (*Nocardia asteroides*)	Environmental exposure, wound contamination	Pulmonary abscessation	Pneumonia, skin lesions, abscesses, disseminated disease in immunocompromised individuals
Salmonellosis (*Salmonella* spp.)	Ingestion of contaminated faeces	Enteritis, septic arthritis, CNS signs and septicaemia	Variety of conditions ranging from enteritis to sepsis
Tetanus (*Clostridium tetani*)	Wound infection, penetrating wound	Stiff legged gait proceeding to generalised muscle stiffness and hyper reaction to stimulation, possibly seizures. Eventual death	Muscle spasm, seizures, potentially fatal
Yersiniosis (*Yersinia pseudotuberculosis*)	Ingestion of contaminated material	Watery to bloody diarrhoea. May cause death without premonitory signs. See also 'Infectious diseases'	Enteritis, possibly mesenteric adenitis or arthritis and septicaemia
Rickettsial infections			
Anaplasmosis (*Anaplasma phagocytophilum*; human granulocytic anaplasmosis)	Tick bites	N/A	Asymptomatic to non-specific febrile illness, immunocompromised individuals may have more severe disseminated disease
Q fever (*Coxiella burnetii*)	Airborne, exposure to infected excretions/secretions	Serologically detected but no clinical signs	Fever, pneumonia, endocarditis, hepatitis
Fungal infections			
Blastomycosis (*Blastomyces dermatitidis*)	Environmental	Pyogranulomatous lesions often in skin, but can occur in various tissues	Pneumonia, skin or bony lesions
Cryptococcosis (*Cryptococcus neoformans*)	Environmental	Upper respiratory disease progressing to lower respiratory granuloma formation	Self-limiting pulmonary granulomas, can disseminate in immunocompromised individuals

22.8 Diseases of deer with zoonotic potential, where handling or close contact with deer carrying these infections can result in human infection. (continues) ▶

Disease	Route of infection	Clinical signs in deer	Clinical signs in humans
Fungal infections continued			
Dermatophytosis (*Trichophyton and Microsporum* spp.)	Direct contact, arthropod vectors	Discrete scaley alopecic skin lesions. May be asymptomatic	Typical skin lesions
Sporotrichosis (*Sporothrix schenckii*)	Direct contact	Cutaneous, lymphocutaneous and disseminated forms reported. Small firm subcutaneous nodules found near to previous skin wound. These can track into the lymphatic system causing secondary swellings. Lymph and/or haematogenous spread leads to disseminated disease	Ulcerative skin lesions, may affect draining lymphatics
Parasitic infections			
Babesiosis (*Babesia microti*)	Tick bites	Deer remain asymptomatic	Fever and haemolytic anaemia
Cryptosporidiosis (*Cryptosporidium* spp.)	Faecal–oral ingestion	Diarrhoea, particularly in hand-reared orphans	Enteritis possibly cholecystitis
Giardiasis (*Giardia* spp.)	Faecal–oral ingestion	Diarrhoea, may be asymptomatic	Enteritis, possibly persistent
Coenuriasis (*Taenia multiceps*)	Ingestion of tapeworm cysts from meat or during surgery/post mortem (human infection); ingestion of eggs from the environment (passed from an infected carnivore)	Dependent on where cysts are located, however may be asymptomatic, or demonstrate signs of abdominal discomfort or hepatic dysfunction. Deer are not the definitive host, therefore the risk to humans is primarily from exposure to cyst contents	Skin swellings, occasionally neurological or ocular involvement
Echinococcosis (*Echinococcus granulosus*, *E. multilocularis*)	Ingestion of tapeworm cyst contents	Dependent on where the cysts are located, i.e. organ dysfunction if located within organ parenchyma. May be asymptomatic	Cause space-occupying lesions, clinical signs depend on the organ affected
Acariasis (Mange: various types)	Direct or indirect contact	Typical scaley skin lesions that are often pruritic	Typical, often pruritic, skin lesions
Tick paralysis	Due to envenomation of ticks (*Dermacentor, Ixodes, Rhipicephalus* and *Haemaphysalis* spp.)	Presence of ticks, enteritis followed by progressive lower motor neurone (LMN) paralysis	Gastroenteritis followed by LMN paralysis
Viral diseases			
California encephalitis virus (Bunya virus)	Mosquito bites	Prevalent serologically (dependent on geographical location) but clinical signs not reported	Fever, encephalitis, neurological signs
Contagious ecthyma (Orf) (Parapox virus)	Contact (both direct and indirect)	Scabby lesions around face, lips, udder and above hooves	Ulcerative lesions, often on the hands can be disabling
Foot-and-mouth disease (Aphthovirus, family picornaviridae)	Contact (both direct and indirect)	May not show obvious outward signs seen in cattle and sheep (i.e. lameness/drooling) Blisters seen in mouth/around hooves. Will appear lethargic and unwell. See also 'Infectious diseases'	Humans can get a mild form of the illness, and become carriers without becoming ill
Hepatitis E (Hepeviridae)	Faecal–oral spread, contact with infected tissues	Deer remain unaffected, the disease is detected serologically	Fever, gastrointestinal signs, jaundice
Louping ill (Flaviviridae)	Tick bites, wound contamination	Neurological signs and death, serologically positive animals may remain asymptomatic. See also 'Infectious diseases'	Undulating illness with encephalitis a feature subsequent to initial mild malaise

22.8 (continued) Diseases of deer with zoonotic potential, where handling or close contact with deer carrying these infections can result in human infection.

kicking movements of the legs and are applied at the level of the metacarpus/metatarsus, tying all legs together. These measures are suitable for short restraint (a few minutes for initial assessment/first-aid); however, if longer restraint or transport is indicated then the animal should be covered and secured into a large blanket or net.

Larger adult deer present more of a challenge and are undoubtedly severely injured or ill if they can be easily approached. Care must be taken because even injured deer can suddenly jump up and cause injury.

Transportation

Most deer cannot be transported safely without physical or chemical restraint. Smaller animals can be blindfolded and hobbled or trussed in a blanket; large crush cages, wooden crates (see Figure 22.24), or a dog-sized Vari-Kennel® may also be used. Larger animals may need to be sedated and transported in a crate or horsebox. The safety of the driver and other road users is paramount and the veterinary surgeon must ensure that transportation can be safely undertaken.

Examination and clinical assessment for rehabilitation

Initial assessment

Deer should always be observed from a distance prior to approach. The veterinary surgeon should look for evidence of normal vision, alertness, haemorrhage, fractures, obvious lameness and traumatic wounds. This allows approach, handling methods and clinical assessment to be planned.

Assessment should categorize those animals that are suitable for first-aid treatment and immediate release in the field, those that require transportation to a suitable facility for treatment/rehabilitation and release, and those that require immediate euthanasia. For general triage information see Chapter 4; some key points for consideration when triaging deer are as follows:

- Animals with superficial injury, or trapped in a fence, or similar, should be carefully assessed, treated on site (see 'First aid') and then released
- Animals with very severe or chronic wounds, or more than one fractured leg, or with damage to teeth, or females with pelvic damage should be immediately euthanased
- Animals that are recumbent with no obvious external injury, or have suspected capture myopathy, may be transported for assessment and treatment.
  Alternatively, these animals should be euthanased, if there are concerns regarding their welfare
- Be cautious about attempting treatment and/or rehabilitation where treatment will last more than a few days
- If no suitable facilities are available euthanasia is necessary
- Be very cautious about attempting to treat or release male deer of any species, and hand-reared males in particular, due to the danger they pose to humans when released. Seek specialist rehabilitator assistance and choose release sites with care (see 'Release'). Euthanasia should be considered in cases where there is a significant risk to human safety
- Sika/muntjac cannot be released without a license (see 'Legal aspects').

Reference ranges for rectal temperature and heart rate in deer (white-tailed deer (*Odocoileus virginianus*)) have been suggested as 38.6–39.3°C (Demaris *et al.*, 1986) and 50–75 bpm (Turbill *et al.*, 2011), respectively. Stress of handling will cause significantly elevated respiratory and heart rates as well as elevated core temperature. In addition basic parameters may show seasonal variations. These are therefore not reliable indicators of the animal's true condition, although they do provide useful information on trends within an individual animal.

The limitations of field assessment are obvious; however, the attending veterinary surgeon should try to avoid transporting animals that are likely to be suitable for minimal/no treatment and should be immediately released where they are found, for example juveniles or neonates in good condition or animals with minimal injuries trapped in fencing. With juveniles and neonates it is worth bearing in mind that the animal may be orphaned and a period of post-release observation, to ensure parental care, is sensible.

Clinical evaluation

Full clinical evaluation is most easily accomplished with a sedated animal (see 'Anaesthesia and analgesia');

however, accurate neurological assessment, particularly of vision, is not possible in a sedated animal.

Examination should progress in a logical manner, typically in a cranial to caudal direction (see Chapter 4), noting any conditions that will affect the animal's ability to feed, be mobile or breed. Orthopaedic and ophthalmic examinations (Figure 22.9, see 'Post-capture blindness') are essential in deer. Any injuries/illnesses that are likely to require prolonged hospitalization should be a cause for concern and euthanasia should be considered in these cases. This is particularly the case in adult deer (males especially), which can be aggressive in captivity, and will certainly suffer from significant stress.

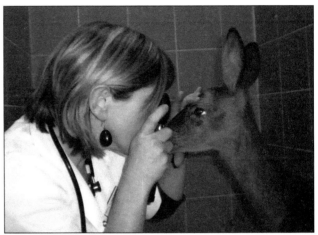

22.9 Ophthalmic examination is essential in deer casualties. This adult roe deer was exhibiting reduced mentation following a road traffic accident, enabling a complete ophthalmological examination in a conscious animal.
(© Emma Keeble)

Diagnostic techniques

Blood samples may be taken from the jugular, cephalic or saphenous vein (Figure 22.10), if the patient is adequately restrained and it is safe to do so. The ventral coccygeal vein may also be used, although some species have very short tails, which makes sampling at this site more difficult. Reference intervals for haematological and biochemical parameters are given in Figures 22.11 and 22.12, respectively.

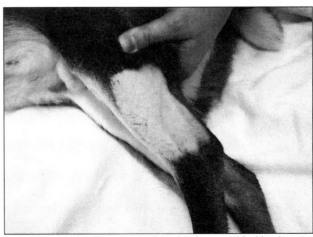

22.10 Lateral saphenous vein clipped and prepared for blood sample collection in a roe deer.
(© Steve Bexton)

Variable (units)	Red deer (Cervus elaphus)	Roe deer (Capreolus capreolus)	Fallow deer (Dama dama)	Sika deer (Cervus nippon)	Muntjac deer (Muntiacus reevesi)	Chinese water deer (Hydropotes inermis)
Haemoglobin (g/l)	113–206	166–171	112–19.6	53–207	76–220	124–206
Red blood cell (RBC) count (x 10¹²/l)	6.8–11.1	9.10–11.72	6.7–13.2	4.78–15.7	3.1–27.9	7.9–14.5
Packed cell volume (%)	31–55	45.0–53	30–54	17.5–60	21.3–71.6	34–55
Mean corpuscular volume (MCV) (fl)	36.4–59.4	35.94–36.85	35.4–48.7	24.2–89.8	16.7–143.3	32.5–47.4
Mean corpuscular haemoglobin (MCH) ((pg) per cell)	13.6–22	13.45–13.66	13.1–17.9	4.8–29	6.2–43.6	12.3–17.4
Mean corpuscular haemoglobin concentration (MCHC) (g/l)	342–401	292–460	343–394	161–423	190–648	350–393
Platelets (x 10⁹/l)	85–405	NDA	119–587	25–82.4	57–497	16.85–541
Reticulocytes (x 10⁹/l)	0	NDA	0–13.1	0.0–214	0–14	0–41.3
White blood cell (WBC) count (x 10⁹/l)	1.49–6.72	1.22–2.96	0.4–4.18	1.2–9.1	1.2–17.8	0.06–4.14
Neutrophils (x 10⁹/l)	0.21–3.58	0.65–4.11	0–2.55	0.13–6.79	0.192–13	0–2.6
Lymphocytes (x 10⁹/l)	0.01–3.73	1.79–2.12	0–2.08	0.016–2.91	0.088–12	0.21–1.9
Eosinophils (x 10⁹/l)	0–1.31	0–1.43	0–0.81	0–0.67	0–1.27	0–0.23
Monocytes (x 10⁹/l)	0–0.19	0.06–0.1	0–0.15	0–0.8	0–1.74	0–0.58
Basophils (x 10⁹/l)	0–0.41	0–1.73	0–0.13	0–0.073	0–0.24	0–0.08
Fibrinogen (g/l)	1.17–4.59	NDA	0.41–4.09	0–8	0–6	0.65–4.34

22.11 Reference intervals for haematological variables of certain deer species. NDA = no data available.
(ISIS database; Ursache et al., 1980; Montané et al., 2002; Flach, 2003)

Variable (units)	Red deer (Cervus elaphus)	Roe deer (Capreolus capreolus)	Fallow deer (Dama dama)	Sika deer (Cervus nippon)	Muntjac deer (Muntiacus reevesi)	Chinese water deer (Hydropotes inermis)
Calcium (mmol/l)	2.38–2.55	2.35–2.61	1.9–2.53	1.78–3.13	1.73–3.5	2.21–2.85
Phosphorus (mmol/l)	1.49–2.24	0.96–1.97	1.2–3.07	1–4.75	1.42–6.3	1.96–3.79
Sodium (mmol/l)	135.4–156.4	145.3–150.7	135.6–148.8	136–156	132–174	143–160.7
Potassium (mmol/l)	2.51–10.1	6.02–6.52	3.95–5.88	3.1–7.6	3–10.1	5.29–9.59
Chloride (mmol/l)	106–160	103–116	104–207	92–113	96–131	78–138
Creatinine (μmol/l)	93.70–141.44	115–127	91.94–182.99	62–345	0–212	68.95–121.99
Urea nitrogen (mmol/l)	5.57–16.92	8.65–11.85	2.95–12.1	3.57–16.07	0–21.42	7.39–15.49
Glucose (mmol/l)	2–19.24	9.08–10.98	2.44–21.98	2.054–21.09	1.832–23.53	4.107–18.48
Cholesterol (mmol/l)	0.36–2.9	NDA	1.38–2.52	0.518–6.061	1.399–6.786	1.166–5.232
Creatine kinase (IU/l)	89–595	NDA	56–320	83–1067	97–9888	80–230
Lactate dehydrogenase (LDH) (IU/l)	550–1463	1198–2152	86–5721	225–1057	336–6070	118–2805
Alanine phosphatase (ALP) (IU/l)	72–303	53–85	54–301	3–3220	18–2205	46–90
Aspartate aminotransferase (AST) (IU/l)	32–80	285–2291	51–394	30–198	24–757	86–411
Gamma-glutamyl transferase (GGT) (IU/l)	27–58	NDA	18–354	17–595	6–1058	64–362
Total protein (g/l)	62.4–76.6	70.6–75.5	55.7–70.3	48–88	41–94	53.9–66
Globulin (g/l)	17.9–35.8	23.45–34.4	20.7–34	15–56	13–62	16.7–32.4
Albumin (g/l)	32.8–53.5	30.6–37.7	28.9–42.4	22–62	17–60	30.1–40.6

22.12 Reference intervals for biochemical variables of certain deer species. NDA = no data available.
(ISIS database; Ursache et al., 1980; Montané et al., 2002; Flach, 2003)

Ultrasonography can be used to demonstrate evidence of internal bleeding and/or organ damage. In a recumbent animal with no obvious external injury this can be very useful. Ultrasound guided abdominocentesis can be used to demonstrate haemorrhage, peritonitis and intestinal perforation/rupture.

Any recumbent animal should have a comprehensive radiographic orthopaedic survey performed. This means that, subsequent to clinical examination, any areas considered potentially abnormal should be radiographed to determine whether the injuries are treatable, with a view to release of the animal. From a practical perspective, mobile equine radiographic units may be the most useful option, although for smaller individuals standard small animal machines may be used. Damage to joints, the pelvis (particularly of significance in females) (Figure 22.13), the spine (Figure 22.14), the skull, jaws or teeth, or more than one limb should bring the possibility of release into question and euthanasia is the preferred option at this stage.

Cytology may be a useful and rapid technique where there are lesions or fluid accumulations that need to be evaluated during the decision-making process. Basic categorization of lesions as infected or non-infected, inflammatory or neoplastic, and of bacterial or fungal causes can often be made in the clinical setting (see Chapter 10).

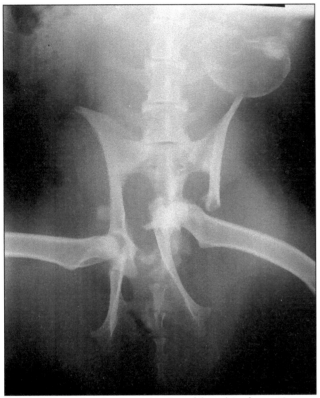

22.13 Ventrodorsal radiographic view of the pelvis of a muntjac deer, showing pelvic fractures following a road traffic collision; note fetal skull on the right of the figure.
(© Steve Bexton)

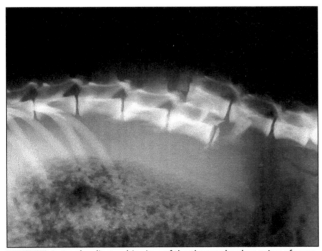

22.14 Lateral radiographic view of the thoracolumbar spine of a roe deer showing dislocation at L4/L5 with a fractured spine following a road traffic collision.
(© Steve Bexton)

Euthanasia

Euthanasia of injured deer is often necessary. The likelihood is that it may need to take place in public view (e.g. at the scene of a road traffic accident) and public safety as well as public perception of the actions undertaken must be borne in mind.

Deer can be euthanased by either chemical or mechanical means. Intravenous barbiturates (pentobarbital 0.7 ml/kg i.v.; secobarbital plus cinchocaine 1 ml/10 kg i.v.) can be used, but this obviously means that the carcass poses a risk to carrion-eating wildlife so it must be moved and disposed of safely. This method also relies on being able to safely achieve intravenous access. Sedation administered intramuscularly (see 'Anaesthesia and analgesia') to allow placement of an intravenous catheter is the practical method, as large volumes of intravenous drugs may be required. Screens or windbreaks may be advisable to avoid the public viewing the euthanasia procedure.

Mechanical options for euthanasia include shooting with a pistol, rifle or captive bolt gun. These methods allow for use of the carcass afterwards to feed other captive wildlife; however, not every veterinary surgeon attending an injured deer will have a firearms license and a suitable licensed firearm (see Chapter 2), or have access to someone who has. There are also legal issues relating to shooting of deer (see Chapter 2 and 'Legal aspects'); however, animal welfare (euthanasia) is an exception to most legal restrictions. Small animal practitioners in particular may not have access to firearms, so they must ensure that they have suitable contacts with reliable huntsmen or gamekeepers, or the local RSPCA/Scottish SPCA, in the event of being called out to a deer that requires euthanasia.

To achieve instant loss of consciousness the deer must be shot in the head, with the aim of destroying the brainstem. Should the deer not be under restraint (i.e. if it is being shot from a distance) then the side of the head, aiming at the base of the ear, should be the target; rifles of a calibre greater than .240 must be used (Deer Act, 1991). Chest shots should be avoided as they do not cause immediate death, and during the ensuing throes the animal can cause itself further damage and potentially put human bystanders at risk. If the deer is amenable to restraint then a pistol (.32 horse-slaughtering pistol) or captive bolt gun (.22) may be used. The deer should be held securely and the gun placed on the back of the head, low down between the ears aiming towards the nose. This orientation should produce rapid loss of consciousness with minimal reflex movement. The law in Scotland is defined by the Deer (Firearms, etc.) (Scotland) Order 1985, which lays out the method in which shotguns, rifles and slaughtering instruments may be used and the types of bullet to be employed.

First aid and short-term hospitalization

Basic principles of first aid are described in Chapter 5 and apply to deer. These include the early provision of analgesia (see 'Anaesthesia and analgesia'), fluid therapy, appropriate wound care and fracture management (see 'Specific conditions'). Post-capture blindness is not uncommon in deer and is discussed under 'Specific conditions' below.

Fluid therapy

In cases where an animal is in shock or suffering from capture myopathy (in reality this is every casualty deer) then intravenous fluids are essential. A catheter can be secured into the jugular, cephalic or saphenous vein (see Figure 22.10) and lactated Ringer's (Hartmann's) solution infused at shock rates (90 ml/kg/hour). As the animal improves and starts to move around it may be useful to consider the use of a coiled equine infusion line that allows for extension without displacing the catheter. Some animals may benefit from the addition of diazepam (0.5–2 mg/kg i.v.) to keep them calm in order to tolerate intravenous fluids for longer periods. Crystalloid preparations are very useful for treatment of dehydration and volume deficits; however, the use of colloids or plasma expanders (volumes equal to 25% of the estimated blood loss infused over the first 24 hours) should be considered when there are significant perfusion problems, for example when internal haemorrhage is suspected (see also Chapter 5).

Short-term hospitalization

Short-term hospitalization of deer within a veterinary practice should be avoided. The stress experienced by wild deer in captivity is significant, and a conscious deer will react adversely to human contact. Self-trauma is common and may delay or prevent eventual release. If hospitalization is unavoidable then deer must be hospitalized in an area separate from cats and dogs and away from human noise or passing human traffic. For larger deer, a quiet stable or outbuilding with straw bedding is suitable, whilst smaller animals can be housed in a quiet isolation area, cage, or Vari-Kennel®. Keeping the areas where deer are hospitalized quiet, covering any windows and padding the interior (e.g. with hay bales) can all be helpful.

The use of anxiolytics (long-acting neuroleptics) to calm animals whilst in hospital should be considered, such as zuclopenthixol acetate at a dose of 1 mg/kg i.m. (Diverios *et al.*, 1996) (see also Chapter 6). Transfer to suitable housing for rehabilitation should be made at the earliest opportunity.

Deer may be fed in the short term on vegetables such as carrots and cabbage and leafy branches of deciduous trees that have not been treated with pesticides (e.g. hawthorn, blackthorn, wild rose, hazel). Water should always be provided, even though deer will often not eat or drink for the first 24 hours of captivity. Whilst hay and commercial ruminant pellets should be offered, they will often be ignored (see 'Management in captivity').

Anaesthesia and analgesia

Anaesthesia and sedation

Most deer, unless moribund, will require some form of chemical restraint to allow complete examination and veterinary treatment. Specific considerations when anaesthetizing deer include:

- Capture myopathy
- Hyperthermia
- Self-trauma during induction
- Passive regurgitation and aspiration of ruminal contents
- Ruminal tympany
- Hypoxia.

Peri-anaesthetic considerations

There is some debate as to whether starving ruminant animals, including wild deer, prior to anaesthesia is desirable. The consequences of not fasting include regurgitation of ruminal contents, with aspiration into the lungs leading to potentially fatal aspiration pneumonia, and ruminal tympany, which can exacerbate hypoxia. The consequences of fasting can include ruminal impaction and electrolyte derangements. Withholding water and concentrate feed for 6 hours before and after an elective anaesthetic procedure is an acceptable compromise.

Any elective procedures should be planned for the coolest time of day, and prolonged chases avoided. The consequence of capture during the hotter parts of the day is an increased risk of hyperthermia and capture myopathy developing. Prolonged stalking and chasing will also significantly increase the risk of capture myopathy (Spraker, 1993; Bateson and Bradshaw, 1997).

The location chosen for a field anaesthetic procedure should be one where there is no risk to members of the public, should the animal attempt to escape after being injected or darted. If a dart is used, the empty dart must be found and members of the public prevented from entering any area where a dart is missing. Measures should be taken to make the area as safe as possible for the animal, reducing the likelihood of the deer running on to adjacent roads, into rivers, or into cover where they cannot be located.

Once anaesthetized the animal should be maintained in sternal recumbency with the head and neck extended and elevated, with the mouth lower than the poll to encourage drainage of ruminal contents and prevent aspiration. Positioning in lateral or dorsal recumbency can contribute to hypoxia and make ruminal tympany more likely.

Deer are prone to both hyperthermia and hypoxia during anaesthesia, so rectal temperature and oxygen saturation should be monitored throughout any procedure. A rectal temperature rising towards 40°C is cause for concern and a temperature consistently at or above 41°C should be viewed as an emergency. In this situation the anaesthetic procedure should be terminated if it is safe to do so, and cooling procedures initiated (e.g. intravenous fluid therapy if not already being given, use of fans, wetting the extremities/ears, cold water enemas) whilst the temperature is monitored regularly.

The risk of hypoxia is dependent both on the drugs used and the animal's position whilst it is anaesthetized. Endotracheal intubation (Figure 22.15), with the patient in sternal recumbency is the ideal. This can be difficult to

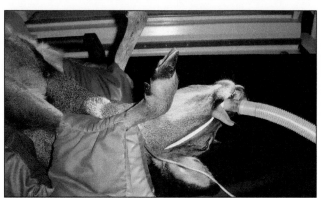

22.15 Roe deer intubated and positioned for ventrodorsal radiography of the spine and pelvis following a road traffic collision. NB positioning in lateral or dorsal recumbency can contribute to hypoxia and make ruminal tympany more likely and where possible sternal recumbency is preferred.
(© Emma Keeble)

achieve in deer, but is essential in order to maintain oxygenation. A laryngoscope with a long blade is helpful, and should be placed on the dorsal aspect of the epiglottis, pushing this ventrally. This allows the operator to see the glottis. An endotracheal tube can then be inserted into the trachea. A standard pulse oximeter can be used on the tongue to monitor blood oxygen saturation levels.

As many deer will be suffering from shock, capture myopathy, malnutrition and/or dehydration, perioperative fluid therapy should be provided. This can be administered during the anaesthetic procedure via a sutured jugular or taped cephalic catheter, and discontinued once the animal is fully recovered. Where necessary fluids should be continued for a longer period.

Anaesthetic drugs

For most wild deer, sedation alone will not be sufficient for full clinical examination, and a combination of drugs is required to achieve general anaesthesia. Drug dosage requirements are higher for wild deer than for captive individuals of a similar size. When wild deer are sedated it must be noted that, if released back into the wild, there is the potential for them to enter the human food chain (through stalking and culling) so drugs that are not licensed in food-producing animals should be avoided (Fletcher, 2005).

Anaesthetic and sedative drugs commonly used for deer are described in Figure 22.16 and in Chapter 6. The alpha-2 adrenoreceptor agonists xylazine and medetomidine are often used in deer sedation; xylazine can be used alone (this is often not reliable in wild deer, or does not produce sufficient sedative effect) or in combination with ketamine or tiletamine/zolazepam. The combination of tiletamine and zolazepam is particularly useful for wild deer as it can be used intramuscularly and will give 45–60

minutes of anaesthesia. The proprietary combinations (e.g. Zoletil® and Telazol®) are available only via a special import license in the UK. Xylazine, administered intranasally at 1.5–2 mg/kg, has produced reliable sedation and stress reduction in North American elk (*Cervus canadensis*) (Cattet *et al.*, 2004) and it would be worth considering its use in this manner in wild British species of deer.

Medetomidine is usually used in combination with ketamine; the 10 mg/ml formulation is very useful for large deer. The advantage of medetomidine over xylazine is that it significantly reduces the required ketamine dose. From a practical perspective, this means that the medetomidine can be reversed sooner (using atipamezole), with less risk of ketamine producing side effects such as convulsions or muscle rigidity. For most emergency cases medetomidine and ketamine is a good first choice general anaesthetic combination.

Potent narcotics such as etorphine, carfentanil and fentanyl have been used for the immobilization of several species of deer. They are in general used in combination with other agents, for example with acepromazine maleate (etorphine plus acepromazine combination, e.g. Large Animal Immobilon®) or with xylazine. These drugs require great care when handling them and when injecting/darting (see Chapter 6). They can be antagonized using naltrexone or diprenorphine. These drugs are unlikely to be available to the general practitioner. Large Animal Immobilon® is no longer authorized for use in food-producing animals in the UK and so should not be used in wild deer.

Gaseous anaesthesia is required for prolonged or invasive procedures. Isoflurane or sevoflurane may be used. Sevoflurane is especially useful alone for induction and maintenance of anaesthesia in fawns. Because passive regurgitation can occur during induction and maintenance of anaesthesia, an endotracheal tube should be inserted as soon as possible (see Figure 22.15).

Drug	Dosage	Comments
Sedatives and anaesthetics		
Diazepam	0.5–2 mg/kg i.v., orally 1 mg/kg i.m.	Mild sedation to reduce stress during handling Contraindicated in shock Can be reversed using flumazenil
Etorphine (E) + acepromazine (ACP)	0.02–0.05 mg/kg (E) + 0.08–0.2 mg/kg (ACP) i.m.	Large Animal Immobilon® No longer licensed for food-producing animals
Medetomidine (M) + ketamine (K)	0.05–0.1 mg/kg (M) + 0.8–3.2 mg/kg (K) i.m.	The combination of choice at time of publication due to ease of availability Medetomidine reversed with atipamazole (see below)
Tiletamine/zolazepam	2.9–20 mg/kg i.m.	Most species of deer will not require a high dose (highest dose is for fallow deer, when used without an alpha-2 adrenoreceptor agonist) Zolazepam may be reversed with flumazenil (see below)
Tiletamine/zolazepam (T/Z) + medetomidine (M)	0.7–1.3 mg/kg (T/Z) + 0.08–0.12 mg/kg (M) i.m.	Medetomidine should be reversed with atipamazole at the end of the procedure
Xylazine	0.5–2 mg/kg i.m. 1.5–2 mg/kg intranasally	Xylazine is associated with more significant side effects than other alpha-2 adrenoreceptor agonists
Xylazine (X) + ketamine (K)	0.5–2 mg/kg (X) + 2.7–18.7 mg/kg (K) i.m	Dose of ketamine required is much higher when used in combination with xylazine, compared to medetomidine
Butorphanol (B) + azaperone (A) + medetomidine (M)	0.41–0.62 mg/kg (B) + 0.14–0.21 mg/kg (A) + 0.9–0.25 mg/kg (M) i.m.	This combination provides a smooth induction with the deer rapidly becoming recumbent, and a quick recovery Butorphanol and medetomidine can be reversed using naltrexone and atipamezole respectively 'BAM' (a mixture of butorphanol, azaperone and medetomidine) is marketed by Wildlife Pharmaceuticals Inc. USA Has been used extensively in fallow and white-tailed deer

22.16 Drugs used for chemical immobilization and provision of analgesia in wild deer. (continues) ▶
(Haskell and Anttila, 2001; Miller *et al.*, 2004; Miller *et al.*, 2007; Tranquilli *et al.*, 2007; West *et al.*, 2007; Clarke and Trim, 2013; Scala *et al.*, 2015)

Drug	Dosage	Comments
Reversal agents		
Atipamezole	0.5 mg/kg i.v, i.m.	Medetomidine antagonist Atipamezole is not authorized for reversal of xylazine; however, a limited amount of data (NOAH Compendium) has suggested it may be useful
Yohimbine	0.3 mg/kg i.v., i.m.	No authorized product available in UK
Tolazoline	2 mg/kg i.v.	Mixed alpha-1 and alpha-2 antagonist developed for reversal of xylazine. No UK product available. Seizures have been reported in Asian deer
Flumazenil	5 mg/deer i.v., i.m.	Used to reverse benzodiazepines Half-life is short, so repeated dosing may be required Can be difficult to source in the UK
Diprenorphine	Same volume as the volume of etorphine/acepromazine administered i.m.	Structurally similar to etorphine; therefore is used to reverse its action Same volume (of a 3 mg/ml solution; Large Animal Revivon®) as the volume of etorphine and acepromazine (2.25 mg/ml and 7.38 mg/ml; Large Animal Immobilon®) administered i.v. or i.m. As it is a partial agonist, overdosage can produce side effects
Naltrexone	0.25 mg/kg i.v. or 0.75 mg/kg s.c.	Reversal of opioid sedation
Analgesics		
Methadone	0.5 mg/kg i.v., i.m.	Half-life is approximately 8 hours No adverse effects were noted at this dose
Fentanyl	0.3–0.66 mg/kg i.v., i.m.	Can also be used in combination with xylazine for sedation
Buprenorphine	10–20 µg/kg i.v., i.m.	Short acting potent analgesia
Butorphanol	0.2 mg/kg i.v., i.m.	Can be used in combination with azaperone and medetomidine for sedation
Carprofen	1 mg/kg i.v., s.c. q48h	Analgesic and anti-inflammatory
Ketoprofen	3 mg/kg s.c. q24h for 3 days	Analgesic and anti-inflammatory
Flunixin	2 mg/kg i.v., s.c. q24h	Analgesic and anti-inflammatory
Meloxicam	0.5 mg/kg i.v., s.c. once only	Analgesic and anti-inflammatory

22.16 (continued) Drugs used for chemical immobilization and provision of analgesia in wild deer.
(Haskell and Anttila, 2001; Miller et al., 2004; Miller et al., 2007; Tranquilli et al., 2007; West et al., 2007; Clarke and Trim, 2013; Scala et al., 2015)

Recovery from anaesthesia

Following field anaesthesia, the animal should be kept quiet and confined until fully recovered (with normal mentation and able to walk without ataxia). If definitive treatment has been undertaken then the animal can be released directly; otherwise transfer to a suitable short-term rehabilitation centre can be undertaken.

When anaesthetized in the veterinary practice or rehabilitation centre then consideration must be made for the period of recovery where the animal is ataxic and disorientated. It is advisable to let the endotracheal tube remain in position for as long as possible to reduce the risk of aspiration. Intranasal oxygen could be considered to reduce the risk of hypoxaemia. The recovery area should be quiet, dark and padded (e.g. with hay bales) to reduce the risk of self-trauma.

Analgesia

Any deer with a wound or condition that is likely to cause pain should receive some form of pain relief on welfare grounds. In animals that are being immediately released this would obviously only be of short-term (36 hours) benefit. Analgesic drugs suitable for deer are described in Figure 22.16.

Non-steroidal anti-inflammatory drugs (NSAIDs) such as meloxicam, ketoprofen or carprofen are suitable for those animals being immediately released. Opioid agonists such as fentanyl and methadone are the drugs of choice for conditions resulting in severe pain, but may cause sedation/mental alteration so should not be employed in animals prior to immediate release. It is worth noting that in wild deer species, drug side effects such as central nervous system (CNS) stimulation and arousal, hypo- or hyperthermia, cardiac and respiratory depression and gastrointestinal motility suppression may prove clinically significant. Opioid partial agonists or agonist/antagonists such as butorphanol, buprenorphine or pentazocine have varying affinities for opioid receptors, and whilst they do not produce the profound analgesia that full agonists do, they are associated with fewer side effects. The utility of some of these drugs (butorphanol is a good example) is limited by their short half-lives and the need for repeated injections. Corticosteroids are advocated by some clinicians for the treatment of capture myopathy (see 'Specific conditions'), but carry general and specific risks in wildlife species (see Chapter 5) and should certainly not be used at the same time as NSAID drugs.

For information on the use of drugs in deer see 'Therapeutics'.

Specific conditions

Trauma

Road traffic accidents

Collisions of deer with motor vehicles are increasingly common, with between 31,000 and 45,000 estimated to have occurred in England and Wales annually between 2003 and 2005 (Langbein et al., 2007). It is the most common reason for presentation of deer to a veterinary surgeon. In some instances the collision will have been witnessed, or alternatively the animal will just be found recumbent at the side of the road.

A good clinical assessment (see 'Examination and clinic assessment for rehabilitation') in these cases is important. Signs that a deer has been hit by a car can include bruising around the head, eyes and/or lips (Figure 22.17), scuffing damage to the hooves, scratches and scrapes to the skin, reduced mentation and central blindness (see 'Miscellaneous conditions'). These deer commonly have life-threatening injuries such as internal haemorrhage and intracranial bleeding or oedema. Haemorrhage will present as signs of distributive shock and can be confirmed ultrasonographically (see 'Diagnostic techniques'). Use of appropriate fluid therapy (see 'Fluid therapy') can be life-saving in this instance. Signs of intra-cranial bleeding or oedema can include reduced mentation or unconsciousness as well as anisocoria (in the case of bleeding in a discrete area). Mannitol is indicated in the case of cerebral oedema (but contraindicated if there is a suggestion of intracranial bleeding or pulmonary oedema), at a dose of 0.25 g/kg i.v. over 30–60 minutes.

Wounds

Wounds should be treated in a similar way to other species, with the primary aim of rapid resolution and subsequent release. Lavage and treatment to allow healing by primary or secondary intention are both suitable strategies, depending on the type and location of the wound (see Chapter 5). Any suture material placed should be absorbable.

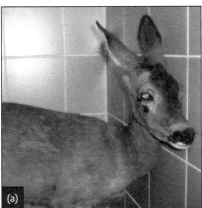

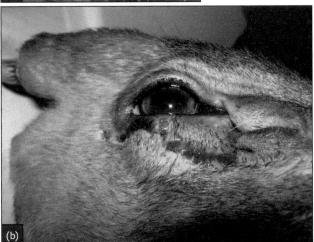

22.17 Facial trauma in (a) a roe deer and (b) a muntjac deer following road traffic collisions.
(a, © Emma Keeble; b, © Steve Bexton)

Fencing or snare wounds usually affect the distal limbs and are often linear in appearance (Figure 22.18). Degloving injuries may also be seen and may result in loss of the portion of the limb distal to the vascular injury (Green, 2003). Proximal limb injuries (e.g. hip luxations) may be associated with these distal wounds, as a result of the deer struggling to free itself from entrapment. These injuries should be ruled out prior to any treatment of the distal wound as they will significantly affect the prognosis for release. Although amputation of the distal part of the limb has been described (Green, 2003) the prognosis for such cases is in doubt and euthanasia is usually the recommended course of action.

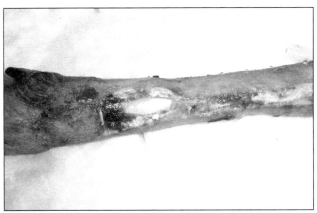

22.18 Distal limb injury in an adult roe deer following entrapment of the animal in fencing. Note the linear shape of the wound. The distal area had bone exposed with significant soft tissue damage and this animal was euthanased.
(© Emma Keeble)

Wounds may be sutured in the same manner as in other species; however, closure is often complicated by a lack of free skin with which to close the wound in this area and wound contamination. The most important factors affecting successful treatment are the degree of compromise of the vascular supply to the distal limb and the extent of any damage to tendons and ligaments. In all cases a long-acting broad-spectrum systemic antibiotic (e.g. enrofloxacin 5 mg/kg s.c. q24h; long-acting oxytetracycline 20 mg/kg i.m.; see also Figure 22.21) should be used. During the summer months wounds are at risk of fly-strike and proprietary ectoparasiticides should be used (see 'Ectoparasites').

Dog bite wounds are more commonly seen in juvenile animals, on the neck or hindquarters. They are typically puncture wounds and, as with any bite wound, need to be thoroughly assessed for deep tracts and secondary infection. These wounds should be treated as for bite wounds in other species. Suturing should be avoided, wounds should be copiously lavaged with sterile saline and indwelling drainage considered. The animal should also be monitored for signs of capture myopathy, which can ensue after being chased by dogs. Broad-spectrum systemic antibiosis is indicated (see above and Figure 22.21) as is analgesia (see Figure 22.16). The animal can often be released after 3–4 days.

Gunshot wounds (e.g. Figure 11.6) should be treated in a similar way to other puncture wounds. It is not necessary to remove the bullets/pellets. Deer are often shot face-on by stalkers, therefore eye damage can occur. If the deer has compromised eyesight it is at greater risk of predation. Blind or partially sighted deer should be euthanased (however, see also 'Post-capture blindness').

Fractures

Proximal limb fractures: Although grossly visible and significantly able to affect mobility, particularly in the acute phase post-injury, fractures of this type have been reported to resolve without intervention, such that the animal is weight-bearing by 4–5 weeks post-injury (Green, 2003). In view of this, proximal long bone fractures may be best left untreated as long as the animal is in good bodily condition and in an area with little prospect of human interference, whilst at the same time allowing for continued remote observation. Prolonged captivity is stressful for the animal and release immediately after surgical fixation is liable to cause implant failure and impede healing. Non-intervention however, brings its own legal and ethical concerns particularly where injuries are obviously painful and the animal is considered to be suffering. This may lead to the animal being reported repeatedly to local wildlife agencies (this is particularly true when the animal is in an area with lots of human interaction) and may well constitute 'unnecessary suffering' and abandonment. If the animal is not in good body condition or has other concurrent problems then euthanasia on humane grounds is indicated.

Distal limb fractures: As discussed above (see 'Wounds') distal fractures may result in ischaemic necrosis of the distal limb and the best option for treatment is euthanasia on humane grounds.

Pelvic fractures: Pelvic fractures (see Figure 22.13) occur often as a consequence of road traffic accidents and, depending on where the pelvis is damaged, can result in uni- or bilateral lameness. These animals may often still be able to stand, and crepitus can be felt over the pelvis on clinical examination. Animals with unilateral lameness may be released without surgical intervention, with the caveat that the animal is a good weight and in a relatively safe area with little human interference as described above). Initial monitoring in captivity for return to function of the limb, urination and defecation allows the clinician to be certain that release is likely to be successful, as well as allowing for short-term analgesia to be provided. In females where the pelvic canal diameter may be affected resulting in future dystocia (see Figure 22.13), euthanasia is the best course of action. The pelvis can be palpated for both symmetry and alignment during the clinical examination, and injuries likely to reduce the diameter of the pelvic canal can be confirmed radiographically. Deer with bilateral lameness have a poor prognosis, as there is often concurrent neurological damage resulting in urinary and faecal incontinence (cauda equina), and these animals should be euthanased.

Spinal fractures: As in other species, radiographic evaluation of spinal trauma (see Figure 22.14) may not always reflect the neurological damage that has occurred. Full neurological assessment is therefore vital in these cases. Hemiplegia or paraplegia are both grounds for immediate euthanasia.

Antler damage

Treatment of antler injuries is dependent on the time of year when the injuries occur. Growing antlers are covered in 'velvet', a delicate skin that is well supplied with both blood vessels and nerves (see Figure 22.4). Damage therefore causes pain and haemorrhage. The underlying bone is spongy and not fully ossified and therefore is easily damaged. Damaged or unstable antlers may be removed. This will require anaesthesia if the antler is still in velvet and haemostasis will also be necessary. Most individuals will at least require sedation prior to antler removal, and a local anaesthetic ring block around the antler base should be administered. This ring block is designed to anaesthetize the branches of the trigeminal nerve that innervate the antler and, in the absence of specific landmarks established for all species, is likely to prove the most effective method of local anaesthesia. Avoid damaging the 'pedicle' in the course of amputation, so that subsequent antler growth is not affected, by removing the antler 2 to 3 cm above the coronet. A tourniquet placed around the base of the antler provides haemostasis.

Infectious diseases

Deer may be infected with a range of infectious diseases, some of which are notifiable. See the Department for Environment Food and Rural Affairs (Defra) website for current information.

Viral diseases

Foot-and-mouth disease: Foot-and-mouth disease (FMD) is caused by a picornavirus. FMD is a highly contagious notifiable disease that causes significant economic impact. All species of deer found in the UK may be affected to varying degrees (roe and muntjac exhibit severe disease, whilst signs may go unnoticed in other species) and can potentially be vectors for infection in farm animals; however, they were not considered important in FMD transmission in previous outbreaks in livestock in the UK, such as in 2001 (Weaver *et al.,* 2013). Transmission is by direct contact, via ingestion or inhalation of infected respiratory excretions. Clinically, vesicles may be seen in the mouth and around the coronary band and interdigital space. Secondary infection may ensue. Mortality may be high in the smaller deer species (roe and muntjac). If FMD is suspected in deer then Defra should be informed (see Appendix 1) and the animal and premises immediately quarantined.

Equine encephalomyelitis viruses: Eastern, Western, Californian and Venezuelan equine encephalomyelitis viruses (arboviruses) are reported occasionally in wild deer and are potentially zoonotic. The diseases are notifiable in horses and should be reported to Defra if suspected in deer. At the time of publication these diseases are not present in the UK; however, clinical disease has been reported in white-tailed deer in the USA. Clinical signs are related to CNS dysfunction and include ataxia, depressed mentation and somnolence.

Louping ill: Louping ill is a tick-transmitted viral (flavivirus) disease that affects the CNS of ruminants. It may be seen in wild deer where *Ixodes ricinus* ticks are present. Affected deer become febrile and then, when the virus reaches the CNS, develop clinical signs such as muscle tremors, ataxia, weakness, collapse, seizures and death. Louping ill is a potential zoonosis.

Malignant catarrhal fever: Malignant catarrhal fever (MCF) is a gamma-herpesvirus that affects many species of artiodactylids, including deer. MCF is typically fatal although some animals may have subclinical infection or recover. It may present as chronic hair loss and weight loss, but typically causes pyrexia, marked lymphadenopathy, ocular and nasal discharge, corneal oedema/opacity, oral lesions and diarrhoea. It is an important concern in farmed deer. It is also relevant because of the potential of disease transmission to cattle. Sheep may be asymptomatic carriers of the disease. Biocontainment measures such as the use of dedicated or disposable clothing when dealing with infected individuals, gloves, aprons, foot covers and footbaths as well as enhanced general hygiene should also be implemented.

Bluetongue: Bluetongue is an arthropod-borne orbivirus transmitted by biting flies and midges. Bluetongue is almost exclusively a disease of sheep and cattle; however, some species of deer can develop severe clinical signs, which include severe pulmonary oedema and dyspnoea. On examination oral ulcers and cyanosis ('bluetongue') may be noted as well as difficulty walking due to inflammation of hoof coronets. During an outbreak, vaccination of at-risk livestock can be considered (as long as the DIVA principle – differentiating infected from vaccinated animals – can be applied). Control of vectors using pour-on pyrethroids has not proved useful in cattle and sheep. Bluetongue was recognized in the UK in 2008 but the UK is, at the time of publication, free from infection.

Schmallenberg virus: Initially recognized in 2011 as a cause of reduced milk yield, inappetence and poor body condition in cattle and sheep in Europe, Schmallenberg virus (SBV), an orthobunyavirus, was reported in cattle in the UK in 2012. It has also been recognized serologically in the UK deer population. Currently no clinical disease or neonatal malformations have been recognized in UK deer, they may however act as a reservoir for disease in farm animals (Barlow *et al.*, 2013). SBV is notifiable to Defra.

Prion diseases

Chronic wasting disease: Chronic wasting disease (CWD) is seen in mule deer (*Odocoileus hemionus*), white-tailed deer and elk in North America. This disease is not currently present in the UK. CWD is a transmissible spongiform encephalopathy that was first identified in Colorado in the 1960s. It causes a progressive fatal central nervous disease in adult animals. As a prion disease it is similar to scrapie and bovine spongiform encephalopathy (BSE). Animals with CWD are always older than 16 months, and may display a spectrum of signs ranging from subtle behavioural changes and weight loss to loss of wariness, hyperexcitability on handling, somnolence and ataxia. Death occurs more commonly in CWD-affected deer than normal animals following routine chemical immobilization where aspiration pneumonia is a frequent post-mortem finding. If this disease is suspected, then Defra must be informed, and appropriate samples (brain, tonsils, lymph nodes) obtained and sent to the Animal and Plant Health Agency (APHA) (see Appendix 1). Europe-wide surveillance for this disease is ongoing.

Bacterial diseases

Tuberculosis: Deer (particularly red and fallow) may be seriously affected by both *Mycobacterium bovis* and *M. avium* infection. These organisms are frequently isolated from wild deer, and notification (to Defra, see Appendix 1) of suspected infection is mandatory. Deer do not appear to be as resistant to *M. avium* infection as other ruminant species, and infection with this organism may be indistinguishable from *M. bovis* infection. Clinically, affected animals may have abscessed lymph nodes (especially in the head) and abscesses in lungs and liver. Deer may just be presented as 'emaciated'. Any deer with an internal abscesses should be regarded as a possible tuberculosis case, and samples submitted to the APHA. Suitable

precautions to prevent zoonotic infection must also be taken (e.g. the use of masks, gloves and protective clothing). Euthanasia of animals where tuberculosis is a real possibility should be considered on welfare grounds as well as to mitigate the risks posed. In the UK, deer are not a maintenance host of *M. bovis* infection. This is different from the situation in certain parts of the USA where white-tailed deer are considered to be maintenance hosts. See also Chapter 17.

Johne's Disease: Deer (primarily red, fallow, and occasionally roe) are susceptible to infection with *M. avium paratuberculosis* resulting in Johne's disease, which is characterized by diarrhoea, weight loss and emaciation. The clinical course in deer is much more rapid (several weeks) than that in cattle (several months). Thickening of the gut wall can be found in the jejunum, ileum and ileo-caecal junction; however, in some cases only enlargement of the mesenteric lymph nodes is noted. Diagnosis should be based upon identification of the causal organism (see Chapter 10), rather than clinical signs alone. There is no effective treatment and affected animals should be euthanased. Wild ruminants are considered a maintenance reservoir for disease in domestic ruminants.

Yersiniosis: *Yersinia enterocolitica* is occasionally seen as a cause of systemic disease or enteritis in wild deer (roe and fallow). Faeco–oral transmission in a heavily contaminated environment leads to haemorrhagic diarrhoea, dehydration, collapse and death. Enlarged oedematous lymph nodes and septic arthritis (Figure 22.19) may also be seen associated with this infection. Diagnosis can be

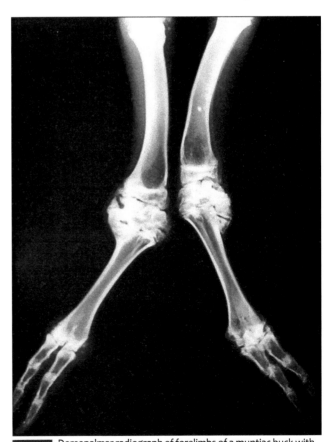

22.19 Dorsopalmar radiograph of forelimbs of a muntjac buck with severe carpal and metacarpophalangeal valgus secondary to septic arthropathy. Note the extensive proliferative carpal arthropathy, with destruction of the joint structure and production of new bone. *Yersinia* sp. was cultured from these joints. This animal was euthanased. (Courtesy of P Green)

confirmed by culturing the organism from faeces, lymph node aspirates or peritoneal fluid; serology can be performed (there is an enzyme-linked immunosorbant assay (ELISA) commercially available) or the organism detected using polymerase chain reaction (PCR) technology. *Y. enterocolitica* is carried by wild animals and birds and survives in a wet cold environment (temperate areas and during the cooler parts of the year). Treatment can be attempted with intravenous fluids, antibiosis and reduction of stress, however yersiniosis is zoonotic and may be contracted by direct contact or faecal–oral transmission. The decision to treat confirmed or suspected cases must be carefully considered, and appropriate measures taken to protect human health; euthanasia of the deer may be a sensible alternative.

Leptospirosis: Serological evidence of infection (not necessarily disease) has been noted in red, fallow and roe deer in the UK. Whilst specific serovars do not appear to infect deer, in areas where rats are the maintenance hosts, the same serovar tends to be found in other mammals, possibly as incidental hosts (Birtles, 2011). There are no current reports of *Leptospira*-induced pathology in European deer.

Clostridial disease: *Clostridium perfringens* type D is an uncommon cause of enterotoxaemia in deer (Sato and Matsuura, 1998).

Lyme disease: Borreliosis (Lyme disease) is spread by *Ixodes ricinus*. Deer are unlikely to be clinically affected; however, they may act as a reservoir of infection and this impacts on humans having close contact with wild deer, as Lyme disease is zoonotic (see Figure 22.8). Any persons handling wild deer regularly should look for and remove, or treat, ticks found either on themselves or the animals they care for. Because ticks feed only once a year, the risk comes from ticks allowed to remain in the environment and potentially bite humans in the following season rather than from ticks that have fed on deer that year.

Other bacterial diseases: Salmonellosis, campylobacteriosis, nocardiosis, erysipeloid and colibacillosis have all been found with varying frequency in deer in the UK and are important as potential causes of infection within the host as well as sources of zoonotic disease (see Figure 22.8). Infections with these organisms generally follow similar courses to those in domestic ruminant species.

Septic arthritis: Septic arthritis is a common finding in casualty deer. Implicated organisms include *Escherichia coli*, *Staphylococcus aureus*, *Chlamydia psittaci*, *Mycoplasma* spp. and *Erysipelothrix rhusiopathiae*. Both haematogenous spread as well as extension from other lesions have been implicated. Several joints may be affected, and periarticular exostosis and partial joint ankylosis may occur in chronic surviving cases. In some cases angular limb deformities may result. Any animal with swollen joints should be radiographed. Due to the potential for subsequent deformities and severe pain and lameness, affected animals should be euthanased rather than treated.

Fungal disease

Deer can be affected by various types of fungal infection including; blastomycosis, cryptococcosis, dermatophytosis and sporotrichosis. These are however, rarely diagnosed in casualty animals pre-mortem and are only of note because they are potentially zoonotic (see Figure 22.8).

Parasites

Ectoparasites: Deer can be infested with a range of external parasites that can have implications for their welfare through the discomfort caused, as well as vectors for disease. Commonly seen species include ticks (*Ixodes* spp., *Dermacentor* spp., *Haemaphysalis* spp.), lice (*Damalinia* spp., *Trichodectes* spp.), and keds (*Lipoptena cervi*). Parasite burdens also provide indirect information on the general health of the individual whereby sick or debilitated individuals can have very high burdens indeed. In general terms ectoparasites do not require treatment in individuals that are going to be released immediately (see Chapter 7). In heavy infestations, a single dose of a commercially available pour-on (e.g. doramectin or moxidectin) may be employed. Where myiasis is a risk in open wounds, individuals benefit from large animal fly-repellents (e.g. cypermethrin).

Endoparasites: Parasitic infestations of importance include babesiosis, cryptosporidiosis, giardiasis, coenurosis, cysticercosis, echinococcosis and taeniasis. Deer also host many species of internal parasites in common with livestock (*Dictyocaulus viviparus*, *Ostertagia ostertagii*, *Elaphostrongylus cervi*, *Chabertia ovina*, *Trichostrongylus* spp.). Some parasites can be a zoonotic risk as well as contributing to reduction in wellness in captive individuals. Deer may be wormed in a similar manner to cattle or sheep, but for animals that are being released immediately this is unnecessary.

Lungworm (*Dictyocaulus* spp.; *D. eckerti* in red deer, *D. capreolus* in roe; *D. vivaparus* can cause issues but is less well adapted to deer) can be a significant cause of mortality in juvenile deer and may result in problems in hand-reared individuals and groups in wildlife rescue centres as well animals in the wild. Clinical signs include coughing, evidence of pneumonia, weight loss, tachycardia, tachypnoea and fever. Diagnosis is using a modified Baermann method (see Figure 10.9). Avermectins, levamisole (dose-dependent) and benzimidazoles groups are effective against migrating larval stages and adult parasites. Consideration should also be given to the use of 'clean' grazing following worming where this is available. In the later stages of disease the damage to the lung is significant and antibacterials and anti-inflammatories may be required. See 'Therapeutics' and Figure 22.21.

Other conditions
Dental disease

Deer teeth are closed-rooted permanent teeth that erupt at differing times during maturation (see Figure 22.3). Any traumatic damage to teeth preventing prehension or mastication of food will affect an individual's ability to survive in the wild. Animals with dental arcades that do not occlude (e.g. following a road traffic accident) should be euthanased. Aged individuals may have very worn teeth with periodontal disease and missing teeth. These animals are usually extremely old and in poor body condition. Deer with evidence of dental disease compromising their welfare should be euthanased.

Capture myopathy

Capture myopathy is a common metabolic condition of deer that can lead to significant mortality. It is associated with pursuit, capture, restraint and transportation of wild deer (or indeed any prey species). It shares many similarities with exertional rhabdomyolysis in horses. Characteristically, it is associated with metabolic acidosis, muscle necrosis and myoglobinuria.

Capture myopathy affects both skeletal and cardiac muscle and is seen in response to extreme stress and muscular exertion. Whilst some authors (Spraker, 1993) believe this condition is seen in natural circumstances (after stalking and capture by a predator) others argue that it is iatrogenic associated with unnatural degrees of stress and physical exertion experienced during hunting or capture (Harthoorn, 1980; Bateson and Bradshaw, 1997). Regardless of aetiology this condition impacts the success of deer casualty treatment and release. The aetiology of the condition, together with possible management and medical intervention, is illustrated in Figure 22.20.

Clinical signs include muscle pain and/or stiffness, ataxia, weakness, torticollis, collapse and paralysis. Animals become anorexic, obtunded and unresponsive within minutes or hours of capture, although problems can occur days to weeks after the capture event. Animals may die suddenly after pursuit, or may develop myoglobinuria and ataxia or ruptured muscle syndrome over a longer period.

Clinicopathological changes that support a diagnosis of capture myopathy include: myoglobinaemia, myoglobinuria, elevated creatine kinase levels (levels of ≥ 10,000 IU/l indicate myopathy in horses (Volfinger et al., 1994)), hyperkalaemia and coagulopathy. Differential diagnoses include white muscle disease, plant toxicoses, malignant hyperthermia, tetanus, botulism, hypocalcaemia and myositis.

There are various strategies that can be employed to minimize the risk of causing capture myopathy:

- Avoiding planned captures during the warmer parts of the day and when it is very humid
- Avoiding prolonged pursuit, particularly at high speed
- Minimizing the time spent in restraint, particularly if the animal is struggling
- Minimizing repeated restraint interventions
- Minimizing the time spent in transport.

Treatment and prevention of capture myopathy should include fluid therapy (this should be viewed as the core therapy for this condition and for all casualty deer), analgesia (see Figure 22.16), benzodiazepines (e.g. diazepam 0.5–1 mg/kg i.v. or midazolam at 0.03 mg/kg i.v.) for muscle spasm, water-soluble vitamins B and C, and sodium bicarbonate (5–10 mmol/kg slowly i.v.; the 8.4% injectable solution is equal to 1 mmol/ml) to counteract acidosis. Corticosteroids may help preserve lysosomal membrane and capillary integrity, but are now controversial in the treatment of capture myopathy.

Post-capture blindness

Many deer that are found recumbent and approachable by the roadside are blind. These cases are thought to occur subsequent to head trauma and the blindness is central rather than peripheral in origin. These animals will have no menace response, but pupillary light reflexes are normal as is ophthalmological examination (see Figure 22.9). Several cases examined by ophthalmologists indicated cortical blindness, which in humans can be associated with ischaemia, hypoxia and head trauma. Blind deer with a previous history of head trauma without obvious ocular damage should not be euthanased (unless for other specific clinical reasons), as their sight may slowly return over a period of days to weeks (S Bexton, personal communication). If suitable facilities are available and cases are otherwise treatable, these deer can often be rehabilitated back to the wild once their sight returns.

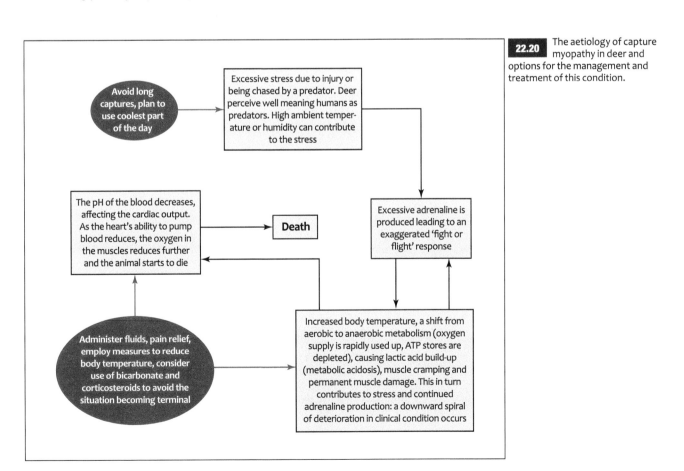

22.20 The aetiology of capture myopathy in deer and options for the management and treatment of this condition.

Therapeutics

Deer are farmed extensively in the UK, but at the time of publication there are no drugs specifically licensed for these species available in the UK. Any veterinary surgeon attending an injured deer should consider the prescribing cascade when treating these animals. Doses for some commonly used drugs in deer are given in Figure 22.21. Anaesthetic and analgesic drug doses are given in Figure 22.16. Specific precautions when prescribing for deer include:

- Absorption from the gastrointestinal tract is affected by the volume and pH of the ruminal contents and whether the drug is metabolized by the ruminal microflora
- There is some evidence that drugs given orally to deer need to be given at higher doses (compared with cattle/sheep) due to relatively greater gastrointestinal motility
- Oral antibiotics affect the ruminal microflora and therefore digestion, so should generally be avoided

Drug	Dosage	Comments
Oxytetracycline	20 mg/kg i.m. every 2 days	Broad-spectrum systemic antibiotic
Enrofloxacin	5 mg/kg s.c. q24h	Broad-spectrum systemic antibiotic Do not administer orally Fluoroquinolones should not be used in growing animals
Trimethoprim/ sulfamethoxazole	20 mg/kg i.m. q24h	Broad-spectrum systemic antibiotic
Dexamethasone	5 mg/kg i.v. usually once	For capture myopathy Can be used at lower doses (0.8 mg/kg i.v., i.m.) for its anti-inflammatory properties in severe cases of lungworm
Fenbendazole	10 mg/kg in feed for 3 days	Activity against mature, immature and egg stages of roundworms including Ostertagia and lungworm. Short-acting, therefore no persistence; metabolized in 24 hours
Albendazole	7.5–10 mg/kg orally once	Lower end of dose range used for roundworms and tapeworm, whilst the upper range is used for fluke infestation
Levamisole	7.5 mg/kg s.c. or orally 10 mg/kg pour-on	Active against gastrointestinal worms but not effective against lungworm in deer
Ivermectin	400 µg/kg s.c. every 14 days	Has a shorter persistence than other avermectins
Moxidectin	500 µg/kg pour-on (efficacy lasts approximately 28 days)	Has a longer persistence than ivermectin for the treatment and prevention of reinfestation of lungworm
Doramectin	299 µg/kg i.m. or s.c.	Intermediate persistence compared with other avermectins

22.21 Dose rates of commonly used therapeutic drugs for deer casualties.
(Haskell et al., 2001; Fowler, 2003; Mackintosh, 2013)

- The rate of parenteral drug absorption can vary with location of intramuscular injection, and in summer/ autumn there may be thick layers of fat subcutaneously. Suitable injection locations include the neck and the shoulder area; the rump should be avoided in summer when there is fat deposition
- Anthelmintics are thought to be more rapidly metabolized in deer, and therefore it is recommended to give these at twice the cattle dose (Fletcher, 2005).

Routine antiparasitic treatments are not usually required for wildlife casualties (see Chapter 7), however those with significant ectoparasite infestation require treatment (see 'Parasitic infections') and de-worming may also be considered for animals in poor general condition where faecal analysis is not possible. Ideally, such treatments should be based upon identification of both the parasites involved (e.g. using faecal analysis) and the level of infection (see Chapter 10).

Any animal that is treated and immediately released is potentially introducing the drugs it has received into the wildlife food chain. Even though there are no large carnivores to prey on deer in the UK, should the animal die, carrion eaters could be affected. There is also the potential for drugs to enter the human food chain through stalking and culling of deer. This is not to say an animal that has received drugs should not be released, more that veterinary surgeons and wildlife rehabilitators should be aware of the potential consequences and legal implications when prescribing drugs in game species. When there is a real risk of treated deer entering the food chain (e.g. in areas of known stalking and shooting), veterinary surgeons must only prescribe a medicinal product whose active ingredient appears in Table 1 of the EU Commission Regulation 37/2010; drugs in Table 2 of EU 37/2010 must not be used. Alternatively a 'no eat' ear tag can be applied to the deer prior to release.

Management in captivity

Housing

Deer should be housed away from areas with lots of noise and human traffic. A low stable bedded with hay or straw is suitable. Juveniles or small deer can be housed in sheds 1.5 m x 1.8 m x 1.8 m high at most (they are less stressed in smaller spaces) and larger individuals in sheds of up to 3 m x 2 m x 1.8 m high. Deer, being prey species, appear to prefer sheds without windows; however, ventilation must be provided and vents at ceiling level are ideal. Since deer are very good at jumping and escaping, the shed needs to have a full door, although practically for observation purposes, a split stable door is more useful. Ideally the top portion of this door should be fairly shallow so that the gap left when it is open is small relative to the whole depth of the door. Deer may jump towards the light when the shed door is opened, so care must be taken when attempting to enter. Double doors on enclosures are ideal.

Outdoor accommodation should be secure with fences that are high enough to prevent escape (2 m high for smaller species, 3 m for the larger species, with an in-facing overhang also being beneficial) (Figure 22.22). The fencing used should be made of material that will not harm the inhabitants (e.g. tensile deer-fence mesh) so that should a deer attempt to rush the fence it will not

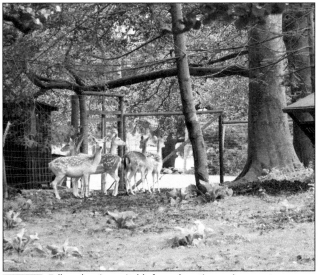

22.22 Fallow deer in a suitably fenced captive environment.
(© Emma Keeble)

inflict self-trauma. Areas of cover should also be provided to allow the animal to hide and so reduce stress. Planting is ideal for this purpose; however, shelters made of straw bales or even small sheds are also suitable. Whilst any outdoor space is desirable, small deer should ideally have an area of 100 m^2 and large deer, 400 m^2.

Feeding

Deer are ruminant herbivores but unlike cattle they are more reliant on succulent food than grass and hay. Some species (fallow and red deer) will make use of grazing if provided; however, most deer prefer items such as cabbages, feed potatoes or turnips, which should be of a suitable size to avoid choking. The smaller deer in particular rely on browse (leaves, branches and shoots) and this should be provided fresh daily. Items should not have been sprayed with pesticides. Brambles, other fruit bushes, ivy (this is not poisonous to deer) and leaves of trees such as hawthorn, wild rose, willow, sweet chestnut and horse chestnut can be offered. Small amounts of seasonal fruits may also be eaten. Deer maintained in captivity for any length of time may learn to eat commercial ruminant (goat) pellets; however, succulent food should always be available. Deer in the wild are observed using natural 'salt-licks' and often appreciate provision of soil to lick when in captivity; this is particularly true of fawns. Fresh water should be provided daily in a heavy bowl.

Rearing of young deer

Young deer (called kids, calves or fawns, depending on species; see Figure 22.4) are frequently admitted to veterinary surgeries and wildlife rehabilitation centres having been picked up by members of the public who believe they have been abandoned. Ideally, uninjured juveniles should be returned to where they were found and observed at a distance for evidence of the doe/hind returning to feed them.

Hand-rearing of deer is both time- and labour-intensive. Professional wildlife rehabilitation centres, however, have good success with hand-rearing and release programmes. A suitable centre should be sourced at admission to the veterinary surgery and well before weaning. This means that once initial veterinary treatment is complete, the animal is placed in the hands of an experienced rehabilitator to continue the rearing process. Malprinting and habituation are common in deer unless appropriate measures are taken to avoid these (see Chapters 8 and 9). This can be a particular problem in male animals that become unafraid of humans; they may seek out human contact and in some cases be aggressive towards people.

Diet

Where a fawn or calf has been abandoned, it is sensible to make the first couple of feeds an oral rehydration solution. Ideally all neonates should receive colostrum. Goat, cow or ewe colostrum are all suitable; however, artificial colostrum can be used if nothing else is available. Deer milk is 2 times higher in protein and 2–4 times higher in fat than cow milk, so rearing on cow milk alone affects growth rate and may lead to diarrhoea. Several 'recipes' for feeding deer neonates have been suggested, based on cow, goat or sheep milk. These include:

- Ewe milk replacer can be used on its own, or with the addition of one beaten egg, 5 ml of oil (vegetable or rapeseed) and 1 teaspoon of glucose (glucose BP powder) per litre
- Goats milk can also be used on its own, or with the addition of one beaten egg, 5 ml of oil and 1 teaspoon of glucose per litre
- Full cream cows milk with the addition of one beaten egg, 5 ml of oil and 1 teaspoon of glucose per litre has also been used successfully.

A feeding schedule is given in Figure 22.23 and additional information on rearing neonates is provided in Chapter 8.

Age	Red deer (*Cervus elaphus*)	Fallow deer (*Dama dama*)	Roe (*Capreolus capreolus*), sika (*Cervus nippon*), muntjac (*Muntiacus reevesi*), Chinese water deer (*Hydropotes inermis*)	Frequency
	Volume per feed			
0–1 week	30–100 ml, increasing to 300 ml by the end of the week	15–40 ml, increasing to 120 ml by end of first week	7–25 ml, increasing to 75 ml by end of first week	Every 2–3 hours, with longer breaks during the night
2–5 weeks	300–500 ml increasing to 1000 ml by the end of this the fifth week	120–200 ml, increasing to 400 ml by the end of the fifth week	75–125 ml increasing to 250 ml by the end of the fifth week	Every 3–4 hours, with the times in between feeding increasing slowly Suitable browse should be provided from 4–5 weeks old
5 weeks onwards	Minimum of 1000 ml per feed, dependent on size	Minimum of 400 ml per feed	Minimum of 250 ml per feed	Every 6 hours, with frequency reducing as individual starts to eat solid food Suitable browse should be provided from 4–5 weeks old

22.23 Feeding schedule for hand-rearing deer. Note: individual and species variation may require an increase or decrease in volume, dependent on weight gain.

The young of larger species can be fed using a lamb feeding bottle, whilst smaller species will do better with a human infant feeding bottle. Stomach (orogastric) tubing of deer neonates can be a quick and easy alternative to bottle feeding if the animal will not suck.

Very young animals will require perineal stimulation in order to stimulate toileting. Perineal stimulation can be accomplished by wiping the area around the anus with a wet cloth or wet cotton wool to mimic maternal licking. Burping or winding is sometimes required when fawns are bottle fed, this is achieved by keeping the animal's head up (the animal can be held vertically close to the handler's body if small enough) and gently rubbing the ventral abdomen in small circles to dislodge pockets of gas.

Release

As discussed in Chapter 2 and below ('Legal aspects'), the legal implications of releasing deer must be considered before releases are made, especially where muntjac and sika deer are involved.

Adults

In most cases hard release is appropriate for adult deer (see Chapter 9). Release should take place near to where the animal was found (as long as this is a safe area). Releases should take place at dawn or dusk and close to suitable 'cover' (Figure 22.24).

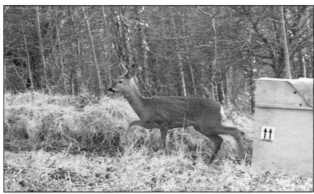

22.24 Roe deer release. Adult deer releases should be made at dawn or dusk, close to where the deer was found and close to suitable cover.
(© Secret World Wildlife Rescue)

Young deer

Where fawns or calves have been released after hand-rearing a 'soft-release' approach is used (see Chapter 9). Large outdoor enclosures are built in suitable areas where animals of the same species range (Figure 22.25). Nutritional support is provided for some time until the enclosure is eventually opened up to allow dispersal, with consideration taken to avoid malprinting and habituation (see 'Rearing of young deer' and Chapter 9).

Legal aspects

Deer Acts

Deer are protected by most of the wildlife and animal welfare legislation described in Chapter 2. In addition they are also protected by the Deer Act 1991 and the Deer (Scotland) Act 1996 (and its amendment). These Acts protect the welfare of deer generally and specifically the 'taking/killing of deer in close season and the taking/killing of deer at night'. There are exemptions to the Acts for 'prevention of suffering of an injured or diseased' deer. In these cases the 'setting in position or using any traps or net' and the humane killing of deer are permitted. The method of killing with a firearm is defined. In England and Wales the Deer Act defines this as a 'smooth-bore gun which is of not less gauge than 12 bore; has a barrel less than 24 inches (609.6 mm) in length; and is loaded with a cartridge purporting to contain shot none of which is less than .203 inches (5.16 mm) in diameter (that is to say, size AAA or any larger size)'. In Scotland the regulations are defined by the Deer (Firearms etc.) (Scotland) Order 1985.

The Regulatory Reform (Deer) (England and Wales) Order 2007 amended the Deer Act in an attempt to improve deer management and welfare. These changes included:

- The use of 0.22 calibre fire rifles for shooting smaller species of deer (namely muntjac and Chinese water deer)
- Allowing any reasonable means of humanely dispatching deer that are suffering due to illness or disease
- Allowing dependent deer to be taken or killed if they have been, or are about to be, deprived of their mother, at any time of the year

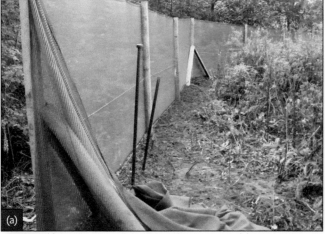
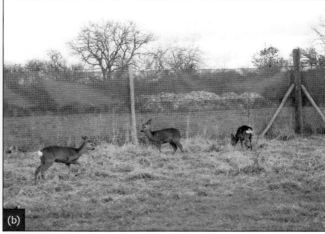

22.25 (a) Construction of roe deer soft-release pen. (b) Roe deer in soft-release pen.
(© Secret World Wildlife Rescue)

- Enabling licensed killing or taking of deer during the close season to prevent deterioration of the natural heritage or to preserve public health and safety
- Enabling licensed killing or taking of deer at night to prevent deterioration of the natural heritage, to preserve public health and safety or to prevent serious damage to property
- Shortening the close season for all female deer to allow better control of population numbers by moving the commencement date to 1st April
- Introducing close seasons for Chinese water deer from 1st April to 31st October inclusive and for red/sika hybrids the same as the parent species. To maintain protection for female Chinese water deer the close season will also apply to males as it is difficult to distinguish between the two sexes
- Amending the meaning of mechanically propelled vehicle in the Deer Act to permit discharging of firearms or projecting missiles from a mechanically propelled vehicle that is stationary and the engine is not running.

In recent years there has been much discussion of the risk of deer populations to environments and habitats and to people as a result of road traffic accidents. Various codes of practice have been written in relation to deer management. Guidance and the current position on controls are available from the relevant government bodies (Appendix 1) and non-governmental organizations (see 'Specialist organizations and useful contacts').

Release of non-indigenous species

As muntjac and sika deer are not indigenous the Wildlife and Countryside Act 1981 (and its amendments) makes it an offence to: 'Release or allow to escape into the wild' 'Sika (Cervus nippon) and Muntjac (Muntiacus reevesi)' deer and 'any hybrid one of whose parents or lineal ancestors was a species of 'cervus' deer'. Under certain circumstances, in some parts of England where the species are already established, they may be released under licence (from Natural England) within 1 km of where they were found. Release in Wales, Scotland and Northern Ireland is currently not permitted.

References and further reading

Barlow A, Green P, Bonham T and Healy N (2013) Serological confirmation of SBV infection in wild British deer. Veterinary Record 172(16), 429

Bateson P and Bradshaw EL (1997) Physiological effects of hunting red deer (Cervus elaphus). Proceedings of the Royal Society of London Series B 264, 1707–1714

Benato L and Bexton S (2011) Management of an injured roe deer (Capreolus capreolus) with a metacarpal fracture and cortical blindness resulting from a vehicle collision. Journal of Wildlife Rehabilitation 31(1), 15–20

Birtles R (2012) Leptospiral infection. In: Infectious Diseases of Wild Mammals and Birds in Europe, ed. D Gavier-Widen, JP Duff and A Meredith. Wiley-Blackwell, Oxford

Carreno RA, Diez-Baños N, Rosaro Hidalgo-Argüello M and Nadler SA (2009) Characterization of Dictyocaulus species (Nematoda: Trichostrongyloidea) from the three species of wild ruminants in northwestern Spain. Journal of Parasitology 95(4), 966–970

Cattet MRL, Caulkett NA, Wilson C, Vandenbrink T and Brook RK (2004) Intranasal administration of xylazine to reduce stress in elk captured by net gun. Journal of Wildlife Diseases 40(3), 562–565

Clarke KW and Trim CM (2013) Veterinary Anaesthesia, 11th edn. Elsevier, Oxford

Demarais S, Fuquay JW and Jacobson HA (1986) Rectal temperatures of white-tailed deer in Mississippi. The Journal of Wildlife Management 50, 702–705

Diverios S, Goddard PJ, Gordon IJ (1996) Physiological responses of farmed red deer to management practices and their modulations by long acting neuroleptics. Journal of Agricultural Science 126(2), 211–220

Flach E (2003) Cervidae and tragulidae. In: Zoo and Wild Animal Medicine 5th edn, ed. ME Fowler and RE Miller. Elsevier Science, St Louis, Missouri

Fletcher J (1987) Veterinary aspects of deer management 2: Disease. In Practice 9(3), 94–97

Fletcher J (1995) Handling farmed deer. In Practice 17(1), 30–37

Fletcher TJ (2005) Prescribing for deer. In: The Veterinary Formulary 6th edn, ed. YM Bishop, p.40. British Veterinary Association Pharmaceutical Press, London

Fowler ME (1996) Horns and antlers. In: Zoo and Wild Animal Medicine Current Therapy 3. WB Saunders, Philadelphia

Green P (2003) Deer In: BSAVA Manual of Wildlife Casualties, ed. E Mullineaux, D Best and J Cooper. BSAVA Publications, Gloucester

Harthoorn AM (1980) Exertional myoglobinuria in black wildebeest, and the effect of graduated exercise. Journal of the South African Veterinary Medical Association 47, 219–222

Haskell SRR and Anttila TA (2001) Small Ruminant Diagnosis and Therapy. University of Minnesota, Minnesota

Hofman RR (1989) Evolutionary steps of ecophysial adaptation and diversification of ruminants: a comparative view of their digestive system. Oecologia 78, 443–457

Kusak J, Špicić S, Süjepčević V et al. (2012) Health status of red deer and roe deer in Gorski Kotar, Croatia. Veterinarski Arhiv 82(1), 59–73

Langbein J (2007) National deer–vehicle collisions project – England (2003–2005), pp. 1–96. The Deer Initiative Ltd., Wrexham

Lewis J (1994) Spinal fractures in deer. Veterinary Record 135(17), 415

Linden A (2012) Paratuberculosis or Johnes Disease. In: Infectious Diseases of Wild Mammals and Birds in Europe, ed. D Gavier-Widen, JP Duff and A Meredith. Wiley-Blackwell, Oxford

Miller BF, Miller LI, Doherty T et al. (2004) Effectiveness of antagonists for tiletamine/zolazepam/xylazine immobilization in female white-tailed deer. Journal of Wildlife Diseases 40(30), 533–537

Miller LI, Osborn DA, Ramsey EC et al. (2007) Use of xylazine/ketamine or medetomidine combined with either ketamine, ketamine/butorphanol or ketamine/telazol for immobilization of white-tailed deer (Odocoileus virginianus). Journal of Animal and Veterinary Advances 6(3), 435–440

Montané J, Marco I, López-Olvera J et al. (2003) Effects of acepromazine on capture stress in roe deer (Capreolus capreolus). Journal of Wildlife Diseases 39(2), 375–386

Montané J, Marco I, Manteca JX, López J and Lavín S (2002) Delayed acute capture myopathy in three roe deer (Capreolus capreolus). Journal of Veterinary Medicine Series A 49, 93–98

Nadjenski H and Speck S (2012) Yersinia infections. In: Infectious Diseases of Wild Mammals and Birds in Europe, ed. D Gavier-Widen, JP Duff, and A Meredith. Wiley-Blackwell, Oxford

Sato Y and Matsuura S (1998) Gastric mucormycosis in sika deer (Cervus nippon) associated with proliferation of Clostridium perfringens. Journal of Veterinary Medical Science 60(8), 981–983

Scala C, Marsot A, Limoges MJ et al. (2015) Population pharmacokinetics of methadone hydrochloride after a single intramuscular administration in adult Japanese Sika deer (Cervus nippon nippon). Veterinary Anaesthesia and Analgesia 42(2), 165–172

Spraker TR (1993) Stress and capture myopothy in artiodactylids. In: Zoo and Wild Animal Medicine: Current Therapy. ed. ME Fowler, pp. 481–488. WB Saunders, Philadelphia

Tranquilli WJ, Thurman JC and Grimm KA (2007) Lumb and Jones' Veterinary Anaesthesia and Analgesia, 4th edn. Wiley-Blackwell, Oxford

Turbill C, Ruf T, Mang T, and Arnold W (2011) Regulation of heart rate and rumen temperature in red deer: effects of season and food intake. Journal of Experimental Biology 214, 963–970

Ursache O, Chevrier L, Blancou JM and Jaouen M (1980) Biochemical and haematological values in roe deer (Capreolus capreolus). Reevue de Medecine Veterinaire 131(7), 547–552

Volfinger L, Lassourd V, Michaux JM et al. (1994) Kinetic evaluation of muscle damage during exercise by the calculation of amount of creatinine kinase released. American Journal of Physiology. Regulatory, Integrative and Comparative Physiology 226, 434–441

Weaver GV, Domenech J et al (2013) Foot and mouth disease: a look from the wild side. Journal of Wildlife Diseases 49(4), 759–785

West G, Heard D and Caulkett N (2007) Zoo Animal and Wildlife Immobilization and Anaesthesia. Blackwell Publishing, Iowa

Specialist organizations and useful contacts

See also Appendix 1

Best Practice Guides
Website contains useful information on deer ecology, health, management and slaughter
Tel: 01463 725000
www.bestpracticeguides.org.uk

National Deer–Vehicle Collisions Project
Administered by The Deer Initiative, this website provides information on how to report on deer vehicle collisions and advice on what to do should you be involved.

Greenleas, Chestnut Avenue, Chapel Cleeve,
Minehead, Somerset TA24 6HY, UK
Tel: 01984 641366
www.deercollisions.co.uk

The British Deer Farms and Parks Association
A deer farming website
PO Box 7522, Matlock DE4 9BR, UK
Tel: 08456 344758
www.bdfpa.org

The British Deer Society
Information about native and alien deer species found in the UK, as well as
information on farming
The Walled Garden, Burgate Manor,
Fordingbridge, Hampshire SP6 1EF, UK
Tel: 01425 655434
www.bds.org.uk

The Deer Initiative
A partnership for the management of the wild deer population in England and
Wales. Provides useful information on deer species and biology, as well as
administering the National Deer–Vehicle Collisions Project
The Deer Initiative, The Carriage House, Brynkinalt Business Centre,
Chirk, Wrexham LL14 5NS, UK
Tel: 01691 770888
www.thedeerinitiative.co.uk

The Deer Study and Wildlife Centre
Trentham Gardens, Stoke-on-Trent ST4 8AX, UK
www.deerstudy.com

The Veterinary Deer Society
General information, including help on finding deer vets, aimed primarily at
farmed deer.
Moredun, Pentlands Science Park, Bush Loan, Edinburgh EH26 OPZ, UK
Tel: 0131 445 5111
www.vetdeersociety.com

Chapter 23

Marine mammals

James Barnett and Steve Bexton

British marine mammals primarily belong to two groups: cetaceans and pinnipeds. Cetaceans, in particular, are rarely seen by most veterinary surgeons (veterinarians) in general practice and specialist advice should be sought at an early stage of involvement with them.

The order Cetacea can be divided into two suborders: the Mysticeti (baleen whales) and the Odontoceti (toothed whales, dolphins and porpoises). The identification and distribution of those species found around British coasts is considered in Figure 23.1.

The taxonomic group Pinnipedia ('flipper-footed') contains three closely-related families within the order Carnivora: the Phocidae (true seals), Otariidae (sea lions and fur seals) and Odobenidae (walrus). The two resident

Species	Group	Size	Appearance	Distribution	Group size
Harbour porpoise (*Phocoena phocoena*) (Figure 23.2)	Coastal odontocete	Up to 1.8 m (0.67–0.9 m at birth, 0.9–0.95 m at weaning)	Dark grey dorsally, paler on flanks; no 'beak'; small rounded pectoral flippers, small central triangular dorsal fin	Widely distributed and resident	Solitary or small pods
Bottlenose dolphin (*Tursiops truncatus*)	Coastal and pelagic odontocete	Up to 4 m (0.98–1.3 m at birth, approx. 1.75 m at weaning)	Dark grey or brown dorsally, light grey flanks, white ventrally; short 'beak'; centrally placed fairly tall usually sickle-shaped dorsal fin	Resident locally (Moray Firth, Cardigan Bay, south-west England)	Usually small pods <25
Common dolphin (*Delphinus delphis*) (Figure 23.3)	Pelagic odontocete	Up to 2.6 m (0.8–0.85 m at birth, nearly 1.5 m at weaning)	Dark grey dorsally, 'hour glass' pattern of yellow/tan/grey on sides; long 'beak'; centrally placed sickle-shaped or erect dorsal fin	Seen off Atlantic and Irish Sea coasts	Forms large pods, sometimes of hundreds
Striped dolphin (*Stenella coeruleoalba*)	Pelagic odontocete	Up to 2.4 m (1 m at birth)	Black dorsally, white ventrally, black lines from eye to anus and eye to pectoral fins, white blazes from eye to dorsal fin and eye to tail; mid-length 'beak'; centrally placed, sickle-shaped or erect dorsal fin	Seen off Atlantic and Irish Sea coasts	Forms large pods, sometimes of hundreds
Atlantic white-sided dolphin (*Lagenorhynchus acutus*)	Pelagic odontocete	Up to 2.8 m (1.08–1.12 m at birth)	Black dorsally, elongated yellow-ochre band on flanks extending back from upper edge of long white oval blaze; short thick 'beak'; large often erect sickle-shaped centrally placed dorsal fin	Prefers colder northern waters: seen northern Scotland to Shetland and Atlantic coasts	Forms large pods, of tens to low hundreds
White-beaked dolphin (*Lagenorhynchus albirostris*)	Pelagic odontocete	Up to 3.1 m (1.2–1.6 m at birth)	Black dorsally around base of dorsal fin, pale grey/white areas on upper flanks cranial to fin and caudally over back and tail stock; short thick often white 'beak'; large often erect sickle-shaped centrally placed dorsal fin	Prefers colder northern waters, seen northern Scotland to Shetland, north and central North Sea and Atlantic coasts	Often in pods of up to 30, sometimes in larger groups
Risso's dolphin (*Grampus griseus*)	Pelagic odontocete	Up to 3.8 m (1.2–1.5 m at birth)	Dark grey dorsally and on flanks, lightening with age to light grey, particularly on head; multiple scratches and scars; no 'beak'; tall sickle-shaped centrally placed dorsal fin	Seen off northern Scotland, Irish Sea and Atlantic coasts	Normally in pods of 5 to 50+

23.1 Ecological and biological data for cetacean species found around British coasts. (continues)
(Evans, 1995; Shirihai and Jarrett, 2006; Barnett *et al.*, 2013b; www.seawatchfoundation.org.uk) ▶

Species	Group	Size	Appearance	Distribution	Group size
Long-finned pilot whale (*Globicephala melas*)	Pelagic odontocete	Up to 6.3 m (1.75–1.78 m at birth, 2.3–2.5 m at weaning)	Grey-black dorsally, grey/white patch on chin; square, bulbous head; no 'beak'; low sickle/flag-shaped dorsal fin set well forward	Seen off Atlantic and northern coasts	Can form large pods
Northern bottlenose whale (*Hyperoodon ampullatus*)	Pelagic odontocete	Up to 9.8 m (3.6 m at birth)	Brown/green-brown dorsally, lighter on flanks; bulbous forehead; short beak; erect hooked dorsal fin two-thirds along back	Uncommon off Atlantic and northern coasts	Small pods of 3–10
Minke whale (*Balaenoptera acutorostrata*)	Pelagic mysticete	Up to 8.5 m (2.6 m at birth, 4.5 m at weaning)	Dark grey to black dorsally, pale grey/white ventrally, white band on dorsal surface of pectoral flippers; tall sickle-shaped dorsal fin set two-thirds along back	Seen off northern Scotland, north North Sea and Atlantic coasts	Solitary or small pods < 5

23.1 (continued) Ecological and biological data for cetacean species found around British coasts.
(Evans, 1995; Shirihai and Jarrett, 2006; Barnett *et al.*, 2013b; www.seawatchfoundation.org.uk)

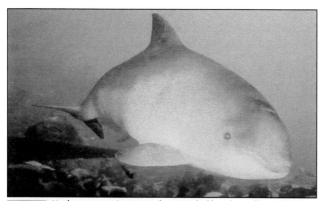

23.2 Harbour porpoise. Note the rounded head, small rounded pectorals and triangular dorsal fin.
(Courtesy of Florian Grana, International Fund for Animal Welfare)

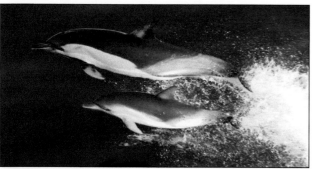

23.3 Common dolphin and calf. Note long beak, hour glass pattern on sides and centrally placed dorsal fin.
(Courtesy of Stephen Marsh, British Divers Marine Life Rescue)

species of seal found in British coastal waters are phocids: the grey seal (*Halichoerus grypus*) (see Figure 23.7) and the common or harbour seal (*Phoca vitulina*) (see Figure 23.8). Occasionally, Arctic ice-breeding vagrants are encountered, including the ringed seal (*P. hispida*), harp seal (*P. groenlandica*), hooded seal (*Cystophara cristata*), bearded seal (*Erignathus barbatus*) and walrus (*Odobenus rosmarus*). There are no sea lions or fur seals in European waters.

Common seal numbers have been in sharp decline in some parts of the UK, especially the Northern Isles and east coast of Scotland (Thompson *et al.*, 2010). In contrast, grey seal numbers are generally stable or increasing over most of their range (Special Committee on Seals, 2012).

Ecology and biology

Cetaceans

Cetaceans are usually considered to be coastal or pelagic (oceanic) in range (see Figure 23.1). Mysticetes feed on plankton, krill or small fish; they take large quantities of water into their mouths, expelling it through the hairy plates of keratinous baleen that have replaced their teeth, and retain any prey. Odontocetes hunt fish and squid, primarily using echolocation (see 'Anatomy and physiology').

Seals

Basic ecological and biological data for the two resident seal species found in the UK is outlined in Figure 23.4.

Species	Adult size	Lifespan	Appearance	Distribution	Diet
Grey seal (*Halichoerus grypus*) (see Figures 23.6 and 23.7)	Males can be over 300 kg and 2.5 m long Females 150–200 kg and 1.8 m long	Males up to 25 years Females up to 40 years	Long broad muzzle with straight or convex nose (most pronounced in males); nostrils almost parallel; coat colour variable although generally darker in males	Over 80% of UK population is in Scotland, especially exposed coasts of Outer Hebrides and Northern Isles; smaller colonies exist on mainland North Sea coast, south-west England and Wales	Generalist feeders on a range of fish, particularly sand eels (Ammodytidae), gadoids (Gadidae) and flatfish (Pleuronectiformes), with geographical and seasonal variations
Common or harbour seal (*Phoca vitulina*) (see Figure 23.8)	Males up to 120 kg and 1.8 m long Females up to 100 kg and 1.7 m long	Males around 20 years Females 20–30 years	Small dog-like head with concave forehead/muzzle; v-shaped nostrils; coats generally paler than grey seals and patterned with spots or rings	80% of UK population is found in Scotland, especially west coast, Hebrides and Northern Isles; along eastern coasts, populations are concentrated around estuaries including The Wash	Feed on a wide variety of prey including sand eels, herring and sprats (Clupeidae), gadoids, flatfish, octopus and squid (cephalopods), crustaceans and molluscs with seasonal and geographical differences

23.4 Ecological and biological data for resident pinniped species of the British Isles.

Grey seals range further out to sea and may undertake feeding trips lasting several days, before returning to rest socially on communal haul-out sites. Common seals generally remain closer to shore, preferring to feed in sheltered coastal waters, and haul out in the same area throughout the year. It is not unusual to see mixed groups of both species hauled out on land.

Anatomy and physiology

Cetaceans and seals have no intra-abdominal or intra-muscular fat. Instead, all their fat is stored in a thick subcutaneous layer: the blubber. This not only stores energy, but also provides insulation and aids streamlining. Countercurrent heat-exchange systems in the flippers, flukes and fins control heat loss to the periphery.

Cetaceans achieve laminar flow over their smooth skin, lubricated by the continual shedding of epithelial cells and oil droplets. They propel themselves by vertical movement of the broad flat fibrous tail fluke. Seals swim by flexing the caudal spine and hind flippers laterally, spreading their webbed digits. The pectoral fins of cetaceans and fore flippers of seals are used for steering and balance.

The nares ('blowholes') of cetaceans are on top of the head; they are single in odontocetes and paired in mysticetes. Cetaceans inhale before diving and exhale explosively on resurfacing, before immediately inhaling. Seals exhale on diving. In both groups of animals, the alveoli collapse at depth and air is diverted into larger airways where there is no gas exchange. This prevents the absorption of nitrogen, thereby eliminating the risk of decompression sickness, which occurs when nitrogen absorbed into the circulation at depth comes out of solution on resurfacing, forming harmful gas bubbles in blood vessels and tissues (Elsner, 1999). Marine mammals have a large oxygen storage capacity, with a relatively large blood volume, large red blood cells with high haemoglobin content and a high concentration of muscle myoglobin. During long dives, deoxygenated blood is pooled in large venous sinuses and there is pronounced bradycardia. The remaining oxygenated blood is diverted solely to nervous tissue and heart, whilst the muscles respire anaerobically (Elsner, 1999).

Marine mammals obtain water from food, as both free and metabolic water, and through the oxidation of fat in fasting animals. Water conservation and salt balance are ensured by the production of concentrated urine and by restricted ingestion of seawater.

The eyes of marine mammals are adapted to low light intensities. The elastic lens of cetacean eyes allows effective focusing in water and air. The less elastic spherical lens of seals allows effective focusing underwater, but they suffer from astigmatism above water. Pupillary constriction corrects this in bright sunlight, but vision is blurred in dim light. The cornea of marine mammals is heavily keratinized. A continually-produced tear film also provides protection; it is particularly viscous in cetaceans. There are no functional nasolacrimal ducts and so tears continually overflow.

Marine mammals have well developed directional hearing underwater. Odontocetes also use 'echolocation': high-frequency clicks, emitted from the upper nasal passages, are focused by the 'melon' (fat pad in front of the skull) and, on being reflected, are received by the mandible and transmitted via 'acoustic fat' within the mandible to the inner ear. Seals use their sensitive vibrissae to detect vibrations and 'feel' their way along the seabed and detect prey. They have a sigmoid flexure in the neck and can hunt in water of zero visibility by swimming with the neck flexed and suddenly extending it when prey motion is detected.

Reproduction
Cetaceans

In cetaceans, single births are normal and maternal care is highly developed. Lactation periods range from 4 months in the minke whale (*Balaenoptera acutorostrata*) to 22 months in the pilot whale (*Globicephala melas*). The learning of life skills during prolonged lactation is considered critical for survival, throwing doubt on the wisdom of attempting to rehabilitate unweaned orphans. Harbour porpoises (*Phocoena phocoena*) (see Figure 23.2) strand more frequently as dependent calves than other species: the calves are born mainly in June and July and are suckled for 7–10 months.

Seals

Reproductive data for British seal species are found in Figure 23.5.

Adult males (bulls) of both seal species are aggressive and fight over females and territory at breeding sites. Dominant males are polygynous and mate with several females. In general, females return to the same breeding site each year, which is also often the same site where they were born (natal philopatry). Females generally produce a single pup, which is suckled for a comparatively short period on high fat milk and then abruptly weaned. Females then moult and mate and return to sea. Delayed implantation ensures a 12-month pupping interval. After weaning, pups starve initially and must learn to forage for themselves; their survival potential is highly dependent on their blubber reserves at weaning.

Female grey seals give birth in the autumn/winter. The pupping season varies according to geographical location; colonies in the south-west of England pup earliest,

Species	Peak pupping season	Birthweight and length	Lactation period	Sexual maturity
Grey seal (*Halichoerus grypus*) (see Figures 23.6 and 23.7)	South-west England and Wales Aug–Oct North-west Scotland Sep–Nov North-east Scotland Oct–Nov Eastern England Nov–Dec (NB grey seal births have been recorded throughout the year)	Birthweight 13–14 kg, length 0.9–1.1 m	16–23 days Weight at weaning 45–55 kg	Males about 6 years but rarely breed before 10 years of age Females about 5 years
Common or harbour seal (*Phoca vitulina*) (see Figure 23.8)	Jun–Jul	Birthweight 10–12 kg, length 0.7–1.0 m	3–4 weeks Weight at weaning 20–30 kg	Males 4–5 years Females 3–4 years

23.5 Reproductive data for resident pinniped species of the British Isles.

with peak pup production becoming progressively later around the coast in a clockwise direction, with the last pups being born in eastern England (see Figure 23.5). Grey seal pups are born with a long coat of creamy white hair ('lanugo') and are known as 'white coats' (Figure 23.6). Although able to swim, they do not regularly take to the water and remain mostly on land until after weaning, except in south-west England and south Wales where pups are born in caves and coves often flooded at high tide. Traditionally, their breeding sites have been areas of coast protected from disturbance, such as uninhabited islands, inaccessible coves, sea caves and secluded beaches. They are suckled for 16–23 days and are then abandoned abruptly by their mother and moult into their adult-like pelage (Figure 23.7). They then remain at the breeding site and undergo a period of starvation before taking to the sea; they may lose more than 25% of their bodyweight whilst they learn to forage.

Common seals (Figure 23.8) are adapted to life in the intertidal zone. The pups are born in summer, having shed their white coat *in utero* unless born prematurely (see Figure 23.33). They are able to swim and dive shortly after birth and so can be born on sand bars, estuaries and beaches below the high-tide line. Common seal pups accompany their mothers into the sea and suckle for 3–4 weeks.

Juvenile seals can be sexed by the anogenital distance; the vulva is adjacent to the anus, the preputial opening is located further cranially on the ventral abdomen.

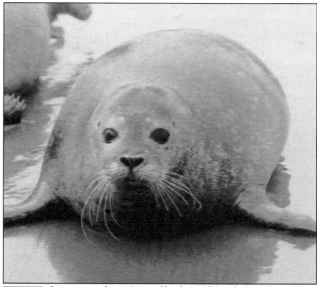

23.8 Common seal pup, in good body condition, being released into The Wash.
(Courtesy of Anglian Newspapers Ltd)

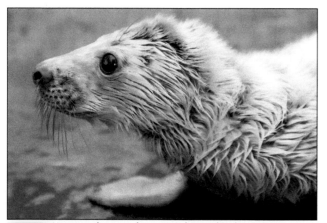

23.6 Unweaned grey seal pup. Note long, white lanugo coat.
(Courtesy of A Fowles)

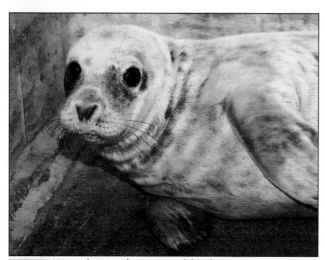

23.7 Weaned grey seal pup. Note adult pelage.
(Courtesy of A Fowles)

Capture, handling and transportation

Health and safety aspects of handling

A wide range of potentially zoonotic pathogens may be carried by marine mammals (see also Chapter 7) and even young seal pups are capable of delivering a nasty bite. Adult seals, particularly greys, have the potential to be very dangerous. Examples of zoonotic infections include:

- Marine mammal *Brucella* spp.: reported infections in humans have included headaches, lassitude and severe sinusitis (Brew *et al.*, 1999), intracerebral granuloma (Sohn *et al.*, 2003) and spinal osteomyelitis (McDonald *et al.*, 2006). Interestingly, in none of these cases was there evidence of direct contact with marine mammals. To date, two species have been characterized: *B. ceti* from cetaceans and *B. pinnipedialis* from seals (Foster *et al.*, 2007)
- Seal pox: a parapoxvirus isolated from seals; rarely may cause skin nodules in humans from handling infected seals (Hicks and Worthy, 1987; Clark *et al.*, 2005; Roess *et al.*, 2011)
- *Mycoplasma* spp.: a number of different species have been isolated from seals – one species, *M. phocacerebrale* has been associated with infected bite wounds in humans ('seal finger'); infection is unresponsive to most commonly-prescribed antibiotics and tetracyclines are the treatment of choice (Baker *et al.*, 1998). Infection can also gain entry through broken skin during seal handling without the handler actually being bitten
- *Mycobacterium* spp.: the primary species in pinnipeds is *M. pinnipedii* and internationally there are a small number of reports of zoonotic infections with this pathogen. However, following a recent case of *M. bovis* infection in a grey seal pup (Barnett *et al.*, 2013a), this known zoonosis also needs to be considered when handling pinnipeds. Transmission of mycobacterial infections to humans may occur through inhalation or contamination of wounds

- Leptospiral infection has been recorded in pinnipeds (Cameron *et al.*, 2008) and could potentially be zoonotic to handlers
- Influenza viruses have been isolated from seals and pose a potential risk of human infection; conjunctivitis in humans following contact with influenza-infected seals has been reported (Webster *et al.*, 1981)
- Opportunistic bacteria: isolated from cetaceans and seals; may infect humans via inhalation or contamination of wounds. With both seals and cetaceans, it is advisable to wear masks particularly where there is evidence of respiratory infection.

For further information, Waltzek *et al.* (2012) provide a useful review of marine mammal zoonoses.

Capture and handling methods

Cetaceans

Cetaceans on the beach can thrash about when stressed, particularly during handling for moving or stomach tubing. It is important to take great care around the tail as this has the potential to inflict serious injury, especially with larger species. Appropriate clothing includes dry suits or (less preferable) wet suits and the use of disposable gloves when handling the animal out of the water and neoprene dive gloves (with no plastic ribbing) when handling the animal in the water.

- To reduce lung compression, the animal should be supported in sternal recumbency. The animal is righted on to its sternum by gently rolling the animal with the flats of the hands after folding the uppermost pectoral fin ventrocaudally to prevent it being bent back when the fin contacts the substrate.
- Smaller animals, if necessary, can be moved in a tarpaulin, with the pectoral fins folded ventrocaudally against the body, or in a stretcher specifically designed for dolphins with padded holes for the pectoral fins.
- Support on uncomfortable substrates can be provided with an air mattress (Figure 23.9) or foam padding
- Lifting by the dorsal fin, fins or tail should be avoided.
- Animals too large to move should be made comfortable, with shade and support, until the tide comes in; if available, a pontoon can be used for support (Figure 23.10).

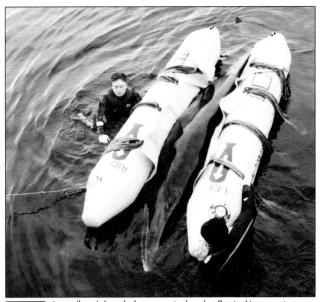

23.10 Juvenile minke whale supported and refloated in a pontoon. (Courtesy of British Divers Marine Life Rescue)

Seals

- Seals can be aggressive and unpredictable, and suitable training in their capture and restraint is recommended. Protective clothing (e.g. gloves, waterproof bib overalls and boots) should be worn when handling seals. Juvenile seals weighing up to 50 kg (less if the handler is inexperienced) can be caught by approaching from behind, covering their head with a towel and dropping on to the knees whilst grasping the neck with both hands, just behind the head (seals can markedly extend their necks). Once restrained, the pup is then positioned in sternal recumbency and straddled without putting any weight on it (Figure 23.11). The fore flippers can be tucked underneath its body to help with restraint and prevent injury from kneeling on them. It is not recommended to attempt capture of seals in water. The major risk when handling seals is from being bitten and it is important to keep control of the head at all times. Seal bites can become infected (typically 3–5 days later) and result in 'seal finger' (see 'Health and safety aspects of handling'), which causes swelling,

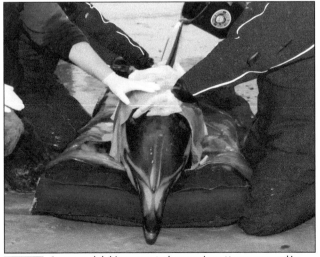

23.9 Common dolphin supported on an air mattress, covered in damp sheets and doused with seawater.
(Courtesy of British Divers Marine Life Rescue)

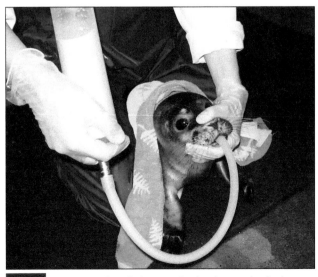

23.11 Common seal pup being restrained and stomach tubed.

stiffness and often joint involvement. If bitten, the wounds should be immediately lavaged and medical attention sought according to an established practice protocol.
- Larger seals can be restrained against a solid barrier with a herding board (e.g. large pig board) for minor examination, injections and sedation. Sedation is needed for more detailed or painful procedures.

Transport requirements

Legal requirements should be borne in mind before transporting a marine mammal (see Chapter 2).

Cetaceans

- Transport is stressful and should only be carried out if absolutely necessary (e.g. to move an animal to a more suitable location for reflotation).
- Journey times should be minimized and certainly should not exceed 2 hours.
- The animal should be supported on an air mattress (see Figure 23.9) or foam padding.
- Adequate temperature control (see 'First aid procedures') and ventilation are essential.
- Poor transport can induce muscle damage and predispose to respiratory infections.

Seals

- Adult seals require purpose-built crates or cages, but loose transport in a horsebox is feasible.
- Transit hyperthermia is a common problem especially in larger seals transported in vehicles with inadequate ventilation during warm weather. This can be rapidly fatal, and susceptible animals should be closely monitored during the journey and periodically sprayed with water and/or bedded on damp towels to reduce the risk of overheating.
- Good ventilation is important. Ideally, seals should be given oral fluids prior to departure (see 'Fluid therapy') and monitored regularly during the journey (including demeanour, hydration and temperature). They should never be transported in water.
- Pups should be transported in cages, sky kennels, seal stretchers or another suitable escape-proof container. They generally travel well and do not seem particularly stressed by the experience; in spite of this, journey times should always be kept as short as possible.
- Neonates and emaciated pups are prone to chilling as they lack sufficient blubber reserves for insulation. They should be kept on dry towels, and monitored regularly during transportation for signs of hypothermia and hypoglycaemia.

Examination and clinical assessment for rehabilitation

Cetaceans

Rehabilitation has not proved to be a viable option for stranded cetaceans in the UK. Unlike countries such as the USA and the Netherlands, the UK at present has no dedicated facilities built to accommodate the rehabilitation of cetaceans and there are few pools capable of suitably accommodating a stranded cetacean, even for a few weeks. Survival rates historically have been poor and the option has not been used in the UK since the mid-1990s.

Stranded cetaceans, therefore, fall into one of two categories:

- **Candidates for reflotation** (i.e. release after a short period of treatment on the beach of origin or close by) include any weaned individual in moderate to good body condition (Figure 23.12), with no evidence of significant clinical disease or trauma, or with dehydration that is considered rapidly reversible. With prompt action, reflotation is a viable option primarily for pelagic species, which often strand in a healthy state through navigational error. However, it should be remembered that such animals might become severely compromised by the stranding event itself. Reflotation of some large cetaceans, though complicated by size and weight, has been achieved, but there is no information on their medium- to long-term survival post-release. Sperm (*Physeter macrocephalus*), beaked and bottlenose whales are unlikely to remain viable once fully beached
- **Candidates for euthanasia** are those individuals with any disease, trauma or condition loss likely to compromise their welfare and survival after reflotation. Dependent calves should also be euthanased, the only possible exception being if there is evidence of conspecifics in the immediate vicinity of the stranding.

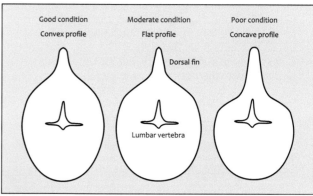

| 23.12 | Lumbar muscle profile as an indicator of body condition in cetaceans. |

(Courtesy of M Barnett; reproduced with kind permission of *In Practice*)

Adoption of a two-option strategy in the UK does not appear to have hindered decision-making on the beach. A clinical triage to aid veterinary surgeons with this and the assessment of stranded cetaceans was first produced by veterinary surgeons of the Marine Animal Rescue Coalition (Baker *et al.*, 2000) and has been updated regularly with increasing knowledge of the most appropriate means of assessing stranded cetaceans in the UK (Barnett *et al.*, 2013b). The most recent version of the triage is reproduced in Figure 23.13. Mass strandings raise additional considerations for triage (see 'Specific conditions').

Methods of euthanasia

Euthanasia can be considered using either chemical or physical methods. Whatever the method utilized, selection must consider humane destruction, operator safety, appropriate and practical delivery method, the availability of effective volumes in the case of chemical methods and

Step 1: determine whether the animal is alive or dead.	
Small- and medium-sized cetaceans	Look for opening and closing of the blowhole
Big whales	May hold breath for up to 20 minutes, so (carefully) assess corneal and other reflexes (see Step 9)

Step 2: determine whether any abnormal behaviour was observed before stranding.	
Abnormal behaviour	Twitching, muscle tremors, pronounced and sustained lateral or ventral flexion, listing, lack of responsiveness and movement
May take several hours to correct. If it does not cease, the animal should be euthanased	

Step 3: determine how long the animal has been stranded for.	
Porpoises, pelagic dolphins	If <4 m long, may remain viable on the beach more than 12 hours after stranding
Toothed whales	If >4 m long, may not be viable if stranded more than 6 hours If <4 m long, may not be viable if stranded more than 12 hours
Baleen whales	If >6 m long, may not be viable if stranded more than 6 hours If <6 m long, may not be viable if stranded more than 12 hours
Sperm, beaked and bottlenose whales	In all but the most exceptional circumstances, these animals are not likely to be viable once stranded
Animals that are not deemed viable should be euthanased. If animals have not been stranded for the guide times given above but cannot be refloated within these times, they may also need to be euthanased	

Step 4: determine whether the animal is likely to be maternally dependent.	
Neonates	Umbilicus present; vibrissae may be present on maxilla
Older unweaned calves	With some species, dependent calves can be identified from length and season (see 'Ecology and biology' and Figure 23.1). May see lingual papillae
In the majority of cases, dependent calves will need to be euthanased, although, very occasionally, the mother may still be offshore	

Step 5: assess the animal's body condition (see Figure 23.12).	
Poor condition	Lumbar muscles below dorsal fin concave. A visible neck may be present
Moderate condition	Lumbar muscles below dorsal fin flat
Good condition	Lumbar muscles below dorsal fin rounded
Animals in poor condition should be euthanased. Interpretation is complicated by a number of factors: blubber thickness is often season- and age-dependent and may be maintained despite atrophy of the underlying muscles. The shape of the animal may be distorted when beached and animals in good body condition may, of course, be suffering from acute illness	

Step 6: assess the extent of any injuries.	
Superficial trauma	Often occurs on stranding and is generally not clinically significant, despite often heavy bleeding
Significant injuries	Deeper wounds penetrating the muscle layer, extensive abscesses or haematomas, fractures and dislocations
Animals with significant injury should be euthanased. Some significant injuries may be difficult to detect and the stress and trauma of stranding can cause significant muscle damage, which may not be clinically apparent	

Step 7: assess degree of deterioration in skin condition due to being out of the water.	
Signs of early skin deterioration	Wrinkling
Signs of more severe skin deterioration	Peeling, cracking and blistering
Animals with excessive skin loss should be euthanased, due to fluid loss and increased risk of secondary infection. Wind and high temperatures exacerbate rate of deterioration	

Step 8: assess hydration.	
Hydrated	Firm tone, no sponginess when hands placed against flanks
Dehydrated	Loss of tone, sponginess when hands placed against flanks (PCV >58% also likely to be indicative of dehydration (see Step 15))
Animals that cannot be easily rehydrated should be euthanased	

Step 9: assess muscle tone and reflexes.	
Parameters to assess	Jaw and tongue tone, blowhole, flipper and palpebral reflexes
Poor reflexes and muscle tone	May be associated with shock and a decreased level of consciousness
Improvement in reflexes and muscle tone	May be seen with supportive treatment (oral fluids, NSAIDs, etc.) and moving the animal into the water
If no reflexes or evidence of jaw and tongue tone are seen over the course of an hour, the animal should be euthanased.	

Step 10: check for deep bleeding from anus, blowhole and mouth.	
If these are seen, the animal should be euthanased	

Step 11: check for evidence of respiratory disease.	
Signs of respiratory disease	Shallow respirations, strong-smelling exhalations, mucopurulent blowhole discharge, occasionally coughing and sneezing, adventitious lung sounds (usually only detectable in animals under 3 m in length)
Animals with respiratory disease should be euthanased	

23.13 Clinical triage for stranded cetaceans. (continues)
(Baker *et al.*, 2000, Barnett *et al.*, 2013b) ▶

Step 12: determine the respiratory rate	
Small cetaceans (e.g. harbour porpoise (*Phocoena phocoena*), common dolphin (*Delphinus delphis*))	2–5 breaths per minute: normal >6 breaths per minute: mild stress, hyperthermia or respiratory compromise >10 breaths per minute: severe stress, hyperthermia or respiratory compromise
Pilot whale (*Globicephala melas*)	1 breath per minute: normal
Sperm whale (*Physeter macrocephalus*)	As low as 1 breath per 20 minutes: normal when stranded
If increased rate is due to stress, then removal of stressors should bring rate down in a few minutes. If due to hyperthermia, rate should come down quickly after extensive cooling. If no significant reduction is seen with time and moving the animal into the water, the animal should be euthanased	

Step 13: determine gap between expiration and inspiration	
Expiration–inspiration gap >4 seconds	May be seen with respiratory disease, or with onset of shock
If due to shock, improvement may be seen with supportive treatment and moving the animal into the water. If no improvement is seen, the animal should be euthanased	

Step 14: if possible, take a rectal temperature	
36–37.5°C	Normal temperature
40–42°C	Critical. If no positive response to cooling, the animal should be euthanased
Above 42°C	Likely to be terminal: the animal should be euthanased
Temperatures can be taken with a thermistor probe. In animals <50 kg, it should be inserted at least 20 cm into the rectum; in larger animals, it should be inserted at least 30 cm. A sealed digital thermometer securely attached to a length of stomach tubing may be a suitable alternative. A positive response to cooling in hyperthermic animals is a good prognostic sign	

Step 15: if possible, take a blood sample (see Figure 23.14)	
Check PCV, creatinine, muscle enzymes	As a rough guide: PCV should be between 40 and 58% Creatinine should be below 200 µmol/l Aspartate aminotransferase (AST) should be below 500 U/l Creatine kinase (CK) should be below 1000 U/l
Blood sampling site of choice: central tail veins, running near the midline of the ventral and dorsal surfaces of each tail fluke. Exceptions: can use caudal peduncle vein in very small animals (e.g. juvenile harbour porpoises) and, for safety in larger animals (pilot whales and upwards), use the central arteriovenous complex in the midline of the dorsal fin (see Figure 23.14). NB Some risk of necrosis distal to sampling sites. Needle sizes: see 'Therapeutics'. Limited reference ranges are available, such as for the harbour porpoise (Koopman et al., 1995; 1999) and there is considerable individual and between species variation in levels for the above parameters. Improvements in some parameters may be seen with support and fluid therapy. Therefore, levels should be evaluated alongside clinical assessment and only elevations significantly in excess of the levels above should be used as poor prognostic indicators. Serial bleeding during prolonged refloats may help indicate stability of condition. As speed of response is important, delaying refloat for results is not advisable. Animals with marked azotaemia should be euthanased. Where there is marked elevation in muscle enzymes, the levels should be reassessed after the animal has been moved into the water and refloating initiated. Any decrease may take several hours to occur, but if levels remain persistently markedly elevated, the animal should be euthanased	

Step 16: assess behaviour during reflotation	
Abnormal behaviour	See Step 2, plus inability to lift head to breathe, no closure of blowhole on immersion, no coordinated, forceful efforts to swim
Some signs of abnormal behaviour are not necessarily associated with a poor prognosis, as they may take several hours to correct during the reflotation procedure. However, if they do not correct, the animal should be euthanased	

23.13 (continued) Clinical triage for stranded cetaceans.
(Baker et al., 2000, Barnett et al., 2013b)

the logistical considerations of the environment including geography, scavenger exposure to residues and the impact that the method may have on members of the public, in terms of safety and also perception of what is often a highly emotive subject (J Cracknell, personal communication). As with euthanasia of any animal in public view, an appropriate briefing of observers is advisable to warn them of the potential adverse responses the animal may exhibit to different methods of euthanasia. Where possible, animals should be screened from public view using, for example, beach windbreaks.

Chemical:
Etorphine: This opioid is now extremely difficult to obtain in the UK, but it has been used effectively for the euthanasia of cetaceans. It is currently available only on import from South Africa as M99.

Large Animal Immobilon® (containing 2.45 mg/ml etorphine and 10 mg/ml acepromazine) was previously used but stock has been discontinued. It is the only validated and effective method of cetacean euthanasia using opioids and is included here for completeness and in the (perhaps unlikely) event of it becoming available again. Etorphine/acepromazine is injected intramuscularly at the following doses (RSPCA, 1997):

- Dolphins and porpoises: 0.5 ml per 1.5 m length
- Whales: 4.0 ml per 1.5 m length.

M99 (9.8 mg/ml etorphine) can be imported from South Africa. It is four times the concentration of Large Animal Immobilon® and so one quarter of the volume should be used (the effective dose being the same):

- Dolphins and porpoises: 0.125 ml per 1.5 m length
- Whales: 1 ml per 1.5 m length.

A sedative can be administered prior to euthanasia with etorphine.

Ideally, injections should be given through the blubber into the lumbar muscles (Figure 23.14). 18–21 G needles are indicated depending on the size of the animal. 5 cm needles can be used in dolphins and porpoises up to 2 m in length, 6.25 cm needles from 2 to up to 3 m in length and 8.75 cm needles from 3 m long dolphins to 8.5 m long

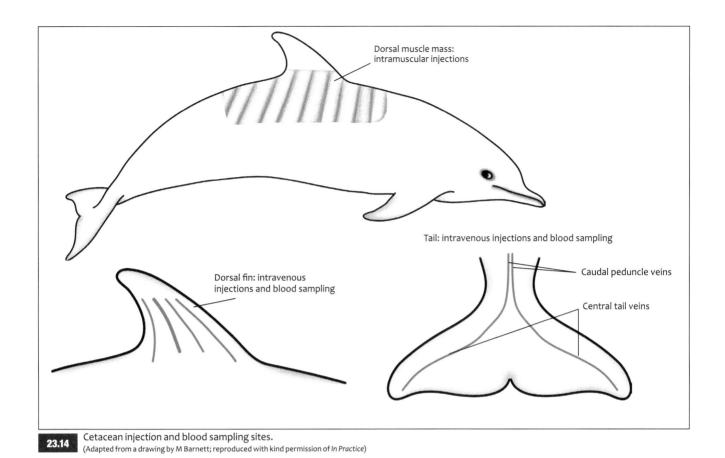

Dorsal muscle mass: intramuscular injections

Tail: intravenous injections and blood sampling

Caudal peduncle veins

Central tail veins

Dorsal fin: intravenous injections and blood sampling

23.14 Cetacean injection and blood sampling sites.
(Adapted from a drawing by M Barnett; reproduced with kind permission of *In Practice*)

small whales; needles of up to 25 cm may be needed for large whales. Injections with shorter needles should still prove effective, as the blubber layer is vascular. Blubber is fibrous, it is difficult to force in the liquid and care should be taken. It is advisable to use Luer-Lock syringes and the injection should be given over several different sites.

In addition to considerations of public safety and carcass disposal associated with its use, animals euthanased with etorphine may take several minutes to die, particularly if the injection was given into the blubber layer. A marked excitatory phase also may be seen prior to death, which can be distressing to onlookers; this is even more likely with M99 due to its lack of combination with a sedative. Prior administration of a sedative combination, such as diazepam (0.11 mg/kg) and ketamine (1.1 mg/kg) intramuscularly or ketamine (1.75 mg/kg) and medetomidine (0.04 mg/kg) intramuscularly (used in small cetaceans) or midazolam (0.025 mg/kg) and butorphanol (0.15 mg/kg) intramuscularly (used in a pilot whale), may help reduce the risk of excitation but also may reduce cardiac output and slow the time to effective euthanasia.

Barbiturates: Barbiturates can be used intravenously (via blood sampling sites) or intraperitoneally in animals as large as pilot whales. Pentobarbital doses of 60–200 mg/kg are recommended (Greer and Rowles, 2000). When large volumes have to be administered, pre-loading the syringes and having these handed in turn to the operator is advisable. Alternatively flutter valves can be employed. Volumes to be administered can also be reduced by using large animal barbiturate combination preparations (e.g. secobarbital sodium and cinchocaine hydrochloride (Somulose®; 40 mg/kg and 2.5 mg/kg, respectively)). Again, prior administration of a sedative combination is advisable before infusing large volumes in larger species.

Potassium chloride: Large cetaceans have proved difficult to euthanase so, historically, these have tended to be left to die naturally. Outside the UK, intravenous or intracardiac potassium chloride has been used successfully in a number of cases (Daoust and Ortenburger, 2001; Harms *et al.*, 2014). Harms *et al.* (2014) use 1 kg of potassium chloride dissolved in 3 litres of water to provide a 330 g/l solution. This is administered as a minimum dose of 75 mg/kg, or more if possible, using an intracardiac approach and always following deep sedation and analgesia. The delivery system is a commercial garden sprayer, clear-plastic tubing and a custom-made, metre-long needle. This method has the advantage of being low risk to scavengers if the carcass is to remain on the beach (depending on the sedative agents used) and a number of these delivery systems have been produced for use in the UK.

Neuromuscular blocking agents: The use of neuromuscular blocking agents, such as succinylcholine, is contraindicated in the conscious cetacean. Whilst they may be effective, the welfare of the individual is severely compromised as the animal will still experience pain and fear prior to death. The only possible exception is as a last resort in cases of large stranded cetaceans that remain alive for prolonged periods of time, where previous euthanasia attempts have failed and when more suitable euthanasia agents are not available. Here it may be considered that the animal's welfare may be more compromised if such an agent is not administered.

Physical:
Shooting: Small cetaceans can be shot from close range through the blowhole, with a rifle of at least .30 calibre using a solid bullet of at least 140 grains, aiming towards an

imaginary line midway between the pectoral fins (RSPCA, 1997). In New Zealand, whales up to 6 m in length are shot successfully using .303, .306 or .308 rifles using 180 grain, soft or solid, round nosed projectiles (Donoghue *et al.*, 2003). Present guidance in the UK is that shooting is only appropriate for animals under 3 m in length, only solid bullets should be used due to concerns over rapid loss of penetration by hollow or soft-nosed bullets and the use of shotguns is contraindicated (RSPCA, 1992). Before using a firearm, the police should be notified and requested to attend to ensure public safety and the firearm should be discharged only with the agreement of the attending police officer. Legislation governing the use of firearms must be adhered to at all times (see Chapter 2).

Explosive charge: Controlled explosions have been used outside the UK to euthanase large cetaceans successfully (Coughran *et al.*, 2012). Practical and legal difficulties associated with using this method in the UK may prove difficult to overcome.

Seals

The majority of seals brought into care are pups; generally either pre-weaned animals that have become separated from their mother ('orphans'), or post-weaned animals suffering from starvation and parasitism. Seals breed seasonally in, or close to, colonies and so local knowledge of breeding sites and timing of pup production is useful to aid decision-making. When there is doubt, the animal should be observed *in situ* without disturbance before the decision is made to rescue it. Dependent pups may be left ashore whilst the mother is foraging at sea, so isolated pups that appear to be healthy should be observed from a distance for return of the mother before intervention. Solitary white coat pups (see Figure 23.6) that are found away from

established breeding sites have probably been swept away and warrant further investigation.

Recently weaned grey seal pups naturally lounge on the shore and can appear lethargic and apathetic, but should become more alert and vocal when approached. Naïve weaned juveniles also occasionally haul-out in unsuitable locations (such as public beaches) and may need moving or taking into care to prevent harm. Assessment of the body condition of these animals is the most useful guide in determining whether intervention is needed.

When faced with a stranded seal, three options are available:

- Immediate release may be appropriate if the seal is weaned, healthy and well nourished, after allowing recovery from handling and transport
- Malnourished, sick or injured seals should be transported to the nearest suitable rehabilitation facility (see 'Specialist organizations and useful contacts')
- Animals in terminal condition should be euthanased.

Figure 23.15 contains a protocol for the triage of seal pups that are presented to the veterinary surgeon. A full clinical examination of the seal should be carried out with the animal restrained on the floor by an assistant (see 'Capture, handling and transportation'). The head and neck must be controlled at all times as seals can snap and bite very quickly. Generally, the head is covered with a towel, although some animals seem more relaxed if the head is uncovered. Older seals can be assessed using the same guidelines, but animals that weigh over 50 kg may need sedation or anaesthesia to allow a full examination; adult male grey seals can weigh in excess of 200 kg. Most adult seals that present as wildlife casualties will be suffering from severe disease, injury or old age and most require immediate euthanasia.

Step 1: identify species: identifying the species is helpful for decisions about when intervention is needed.	
Grey seal (*Halichoerus grypus*) (see Figures 23.6 and 23.7)	Elongated broad snout, parallel nostrils, flat or convex 'Roman' nose (especially adult males)
Common seal (*Phoca vitulina*) (see Figure 23.8)	Dog-like head, concave forehead/muzzle, v-shaped nostrils, short nose
Arctic species	Rare but occasional individuals are reported (e.g. harp seal (*Pagophilus groenlandicus*), ringed seal (*Pusa hispida*) and hooded seal (*Cystophora cristata*) – refer to appropriate text for identification)
Step 2: determine age: especially important to differentiate between weaned and dependent pups.	
Neonate (or premature)	Newborn pups of both species, less than 1 week old, still have an umbilical cord or fresh umbilical remnant. Neonatal **grey seals** have a pale fluffy coat that may be stained yellow due to amniotic fluid. Premature **common seal** pups are occasionally found (usually in May or early June) but are rare. They are easily identifiable as they still have the white lanugo coat that is naturally shed before birth (see Figure 23.33)
Unweaned pup	Dependent **grey seal** pups have fluffy white fur (which is moulted around weaning time) and are known as 'white coats' (see Figure 23.6). Precise age determination is more difficult in **common seal** pups, but most pups found abandoned in June and July will be unweaned
Recently weaned pup	**Grey seal** pups moult at 16–21 days, so a pup that is moulting or recently moulted (with a few white tufts remaining) is freshly weaned. Knowledge of the timing of the local breeding season can also help with age determination in grey seals (see Figure 23.5). It can be difficult to differentiate weaned from unweaned **common seal** pups. Most are born in June/July and weaned after about 4 weeks, so the time of year can be a useful guide to age. NB Weight at weaning influences likelihood of future survival
Older juvenile	Fully moulted **grey seal** pups (see Figure 23.7) are independent. After weaning they naturally remain on land for many days before venturing into the sea. They are vulnerable to parasitism and starvation, especially if they had insufficient fat reserves at weaning. Most **common seals** found between August and April are independent juveniles (less than a year old)
Adult or subadult	Adults are large with typical body lengths of 1.5–2.5 m in **grey seals** and 1.3–2 m in **common seals**

23.15 Clinical triage for stranded seals. (continues) ▶

Step 3: assess body condition.	
Good body condition	Visibly rounded with no obvious bony protuberances and smooth tight skin (see Figure 23.8)
Underweight	Body contours visible, particularly pelvis, and there is a distinct neck
Emaciated	Bones visible especially hips, pelvis and ribs. Skin may appear loose (see Figure 23.18). Risk of hypoglycaemia
NB Pups are born with very little blubber and therefore even healthy neonates can appear thin (check for umbilicus). Otherwise, all individuals in poor body condition that strand and tolerate human proximity need further assessment	
Step 4: determine hydration status: seals have no nasolacrimal ducts so hydration can be assessed by presence of tears around the eyes.	
Hydrated	Tear film visible around eyes (see Figure 23.28) (assuming rest of head is dry)
Dehydrated	Eyes appear dry and sunken and eyelids may be crusty
NB Assessing the skin turgor (skin tent or pinch test) is unreliable in seals as their skin is taut and firmly attached to underlying tissues	
Step 5: assess demeanour and alertness: best observed from a distance with minimal disturbance.	
Bright	Animals are alert and responsive to stimuli, lying on side or with elevated head and tail ('banana' posture)
Dull	Quiet and reduced responsiveness, head down and arched back ('hump-backed' posture)
Moribund	Unresponsive, unable to lift head, fore flippers spread out laterally ('aeroplane' posture)
Healthy seals generally have a large flight zone and will not tolerate human approach within a certain distance. NB Neonatal pups often appear to be quiet and unresponsive and are also thin (check for umbilicus); monitor for maternal presence. Occasionally older pups are observed asleep (especially weaned grey seal pups which are sometimes naturally lethargic and apathetic)	
Step 6: assess the extent of any injuries: see 'Specific conditions'.	
Superficial wounds and abrasions	Clinically insignificant – heal rapidly and usually require no intervention
Deep or infected wounds	Bite wounds are very common, sometimes penetrating into deeper tissues including bones and joints. Localized infection, abscessation, cellulitis, arthritis and osteomyelitis are possible sequels
Traumatic injuries	Fractures to jaw, face and limbs are not uncommon
Eye lesions	Very common. Bilateral ocular disease carries a grave prognosis
Blood around face	Very common, usually indicative of lungworm (occasionally due to traumatic injury, see Figure 23.27)
Step 7: rectal temperature: it is best to base decisions on multiple thermometer readings due to body temperature fluctuations.	
Less than 35.5°C	Hypothermia (common in young and thin seals). NB In large seals subnormal temperatures may be due to the rectal thermometer not being inserted far enough
36–38.5°C	Normal range (taking into account minor increases associated with physical activity, capture and restraint)
39–41°C	Elevated temperature, usually pyrexia (possibly hyperthermia if recent transportation)
Above 41°C	Most likely hyperthermia ('heatstroke') (natural fevers rarely exceed 41°C), usually recent transportation, or prolonged exposure to direct sun. Temperatures exceeding 42°C can result in brain damage or reflect existing brain damage
Based on the initial findings decide whether to leave, relocate, euthanase or remove for rehabilitation	
Step 8: further examinations.	
Respiratory system	• Observe breathing pattern for signs of hyperpnoea or dyspnoea and coughing • The respiratory rate can be very variable and is affected by stress, fear and breath-holding ('normal' respiratory rate 5–15 breaths/min) • Note any oculonasal discharge (mucopurulent discharge is indicative of bacterial/viral infection) • Haemorrhage visible around the nose/mouth is usually the result of haemoptysis due to lungworm (see Figure 23.27) • Auscultation and percussion of the respiratory system is essential
Cardiovascular system	• Examine mucous membrane colour and capillary refill time (should be less than 2 seconds) to assess peripheral perfusion and for evidence of anaemia, toxaemia, icterus, etc. • Auscultation often reveals tachycardia (usually related to handling stress) ('normal' heart rate in pups 80–120 bpm) • Sinus dysrhythmia is not unusual but is usually of little clinical significance • Murmurs are usually haemic associated with dehydration, but persistent murmurs can be due to congenital cardiac defects (especially patent ductus arteriosus)
Buccal cavity	• It can be difficult to open the mouth in some individuals • Gingivitis and gingival erosion are relatively common • Tooth laxity, fracture, attrition and discolouration are relatively common • Check for palatal ulceration especially in weaned common seal pups (see Figure 23.26)
Ophthalmic examination	• Can be difficult because seals retract the globe when the palpebrae are touched • Fundoscopy is hampered by miosis under natural light conditions • Phthisis bulbi is a common finding • Corneal oedema, ulceration (see Figure 23.28) and keratitis are very common • Cataracts are occasionally seen
Faecal examination	• Diarrhoea is common and usually due to diet change and stress of captivity; usually resolves spontaneously • Persistent diarrhoea can be due to helminthiasis, coccidiosis or infectious enteritis • Melaena often accompanies severe parasitic pneumonia due to swallowing of coughed-up blood

23.15 (continued) Clinical triage for stranded seals.

Methods of euthanasia

Chemical: The method of choice for the euthanasia of seals is the intravenous administration of a barbiturate into the extradural intravertebral vein (see 'Blood collection' and Figure 23.16). Prior sedation is occasionally required (see Figure 23.23). The intraperitoneal injection of barbiturates is generally unsatisfactory as the effects are unpredictable and the onset of unconsciousness is usually delayed; this route should therefore only be used as a last resort. Canine doses are applicable and needles of up to 9 cm may be required for large animals.

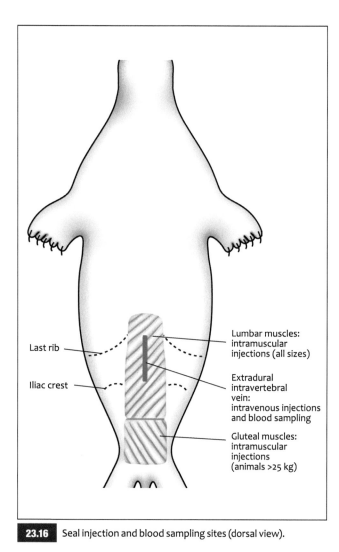

Last rib

Iliac crest

Lumbar muscles: intramuscular injections (all sizes)

Extradural intravertebral vein: intravenous injections and blood sampling

Gluteal muscles: intramuscular injections (animals >25 kg)

23.16 Seal injection and blood sampling sites (dorsal view).

Physical: Seals *in extremis* on the beach can be euthanased by a headshot from point-blank range with a free-bullet humane killer. If the seal cannot be approached, it can be shot from distance with a rifle by a competent licensed marksman. A powerful rifle is necessary to ensure a humane death; details of the legal requirements for suitable firearms can be found in the Conservation of Seals Act 1970 and the Marine (Scotland) Act 2010 (although strictly speaking, the dispatch of injured and disabled seals is exempt). Shotguns are not generally effective unless firing a single slug. In Scotland only, it is a requirement to notify Marine Scotland (see 'Specialist organizations and useful contacts') when a seal is euthanased (Marine Scotland, 2010).

First aid and short-term hospitalization

Cetaceans

In addition to the handling procedures already described above, trenches can be dug under the pectoral fins to reduce cramping and overheating. Hyperthermia (see Step 14, Figure 23.13) can be corrected by applying cool water (see Figure 23.9); the tail stock appears to be an important site of heat dumping. Very cold water or ice on the flukes and fins, however, may cause peripheral vasoconstriction (T Williams, personal communication). If the animal is in direct sunlight, shade can be erected over the animal or, if possible, the animal can be moved into the shade. The skin can be kept moist with damp sheets and obstetrical jelly or zinc oxide cream. Hypothermic individuals should be sheltered from the wind and covered with sheets soaked in mineral oil. The animal's eyes can be flushed with saline and ocular lubricants; topical ocular antibiotics may also be beneficial. Noise and disturbance should be minimized, although there are anecdotal reports that individual human contact and quiet talking may help to calm nervous animals (NB such actions tend to increase rather than decrease stress in many other wildlife species).

Dehydration, a common finding in stranded animals, can be corrected with oral fluids. Proprietary farm animal oral rehydration solutions, Ringer's and Hartmann's solutions have been used. Stomach tubing can be carried out in the water, with adequate support, or out of the water on, for example, an air mattress. Many small cetaceans open their mouths when a lubricated equine stomach tube is introduced, but towels can also be used to pull the jaws apart gently. After negotiating the central dorsally pointing larynx, the tube is passed to a point between the pectoral and dorsal fins to enter the first stomach. Before fluids are passed, the animal is allowed to take a breath to ensure that the larynx has not been dislodged.

Due to the small size of the cetacean first stomach, fluids should be given at a maximum of 1% v/w, up to 1 litre for small cetaceans and, to minimize stress, no more frequently than every 6 hours. Oral rehydration of animals over 4 m in length is unlikely to be practicable. Intraperitoneal fluids have also been used (Sweeney, 1989).

As rehabilitation is not used in the management of stranded cetaceans in the UK at present, the remainder of this section for cetaceans will focus on the option of reflotation.

Reflotation

At the earliest opportunity, small cetaceans suitable for refloating should be carried into waist-deep water; larger animals can be refloated on the tide in a pontoon (see Figure 23.10). The animal is supported with its blowhole above water, until control of breathing is regained, and rocked gently to alleviate any muscle stiffness or circulatory impairment and to help to restore equilibrium. Careful attention should be paid to the animal's behaviour and response to being in the water (see Step 16, Figure 23.13). Handlers supporting cetaceans in the water are at risk from hypothermia and should keep clear of thrashing tails.

When the animal appears to be able to support itself and is making an effort to swim, it should be moved into deeper water to see whether it can swim unaided. If it can, it should be guided quietly seawards. Boats (and pontoons) can be used to take an animal further out to sea before final release, for example if the animal has stranded in a relatively enclosed body of water. A successful refloat may take several hours to complete.

In mass strandings, ensuring adequate assessment and care for all individuals requires a high level of organization. Early detection, assessment, triage and euthanasia of those unsuitable for refloating is required. Refloating involves amassing suitable candidates in sheltered shallow water and releasing them together when tidal and weather conditions are suitable (Needham, 1993) (Figure 23.17).

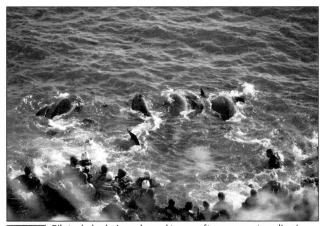

23.17 Pilot whales being released to sea after a mass stranding in Scotland.
(Courtesy of British Divers Marine Life Rescue)

Seals

Fluid therapy

Seal pups, particularly if malnourished, are usually dehydrated and fluid therapy is given as a routine. With the pup restrained in sternal recumbency, (warmed) proprietary oral rehydration solutions are given via a lubricated stomach tube (such as portex silicone tubing) with approximately 1 cm external diameter at initial volumes of 150–300 ml for common seal pups and 250–350 ml for grey seal pups (depending on their size). This can be supplemented with additional glucose (1–2 g/kg/day oral glucose solution) where there is increased risk of hypoglycaemia (see 'Nutritional diseases'), especially in emaciated individuals, and stomach tubing should be carried out every 3–4 hours. Severely debilitated pups can be given intravenous fluids at standard mammalian flow rates and volumes using blood sampling sites (see 'Blood collection' and Figures 23.16 and 23.18). The tight application of the skin to the blubber layer makes it difficult to give adequate volumes of fluids subcutaneously. The intraperitoneal route is possible, but sterility is always in question as the skin of the abdomen is in constant contact with contaminated surfaces.

Oral rehydration of adult seals will be possible only in weaker animals. More lively adults can be encouraged to drink from a freshwater pool or hose, or fed fish injected with fluids. Intravenous fluids can be given to moribund adult individuals, or to animals sedated for examination.

Correction of hypothermia

Hypothermia (<35.5°C) (often combined with hypoglycaemia) is common in very young and very thin pups (see Step 7, Figure 23.15 and 23.18). Treatment involves drying the skin with towels and covering the body with a blanket, space blanket or bubble wrap. Supplementary

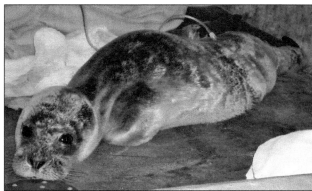

23.18 Intravenous fluid administration in a common seal pup via the extradural intravertebral vein. This pup is very thin, with loose skin evident.
(Courtesy of K Price)

heat sources, especially heat lamps, can be used in severe cases and warmed fluids with additional glucose (see 'Fluid therapy') should be given orally and/or intravenously. The rectal temperature should be monitored every 15 minutes and the heating/insulating materials removed once it reaches 37°C to avoid overheating.

Correction of hyperthermia

When faced with a seal with elevated body temperature, it is important to differentiate between pyrexia and hyperthermia (heatstroke). Hyperthermia (>40°C) is caused by environmental heat such as transportation in a poorly ventilated vehicle, being wrapped in a blanket, or simply hot weather and exposure to direct sun. The risk is greatest in seals with good blubber layers. It is an emergency and affected seals must be cooled immediately due to the risk of brain damage. Wet towels are usually used but they must be replenished every few minutes and desktop fans are also useful. It is also essential to administer fluids. The rectal temperature should be checked regularly to monitor the response and avoid overcooling. The prognosis depends on the degree and duration of overheating.

Diagnostic techniques

Cetaceans

Clinical pathology

Blood collection is covered in Step 15 of Figure 23.13 and collection sites illustrated in Figure 23.14. Other samples, such as blowhole discharge and faeces samples for bacteriology and parasitology are generally only of retrospective interest as results are unlikely to be available for, or are unlikely to affect, the decision-making process (see Chapter 4).

Seals

Clinical pathology

Blood collection: Blood samples can be obtained from the extradural intravertebral vein, with the pup held in sternal recumbency. This vein is accessed via the L3/L4 intervertebral space, halfway between the last rib and the iliac crests (see Figure 23.16). In pups under 25 kg, the space can be palpated and a 2.5–5 cm, 21 or 20 G needle can be used. In larger seals, the space is found by 'walking' a 6–9 cm, 18–20 G spinal needle over the vertebrae. Adults may need to be sedated for blood sampling if no suitable physical restraint (e.g. a crush cage) is available. Fasting for several hours before blood collection is necessary to prevent lipaemia, which reduces the usefulness of the blood sample; however, fasting is not recommended in debilitated animals prior to stabilization.

Blood samples clot rapidly and should be placed immediately in tubes containing standard anticoagulants (see Chapter 5). Samples can also be collected for retrospective serology. Hypoglycaemia in severely malnourished pups can be assessed quickly with blood glucose test strips and/or a glucometer. Haematology and biochemistry results can be compared with reference intervals (Greig *et al.*, 2010) (Figure 23.19).

Other samples: Deep nasal and pharyngeal swabs may help to isolate underlying pathogens in bacterial pneumonia. Bacterial isolates from traumatic lesions may be clinically significant, but faecal contaminants are a problem. Infected lesions such as abscesses, septic arthritis and corneal ulcers can be swabbed for culture and sensitivity testing; antimicrobial resistance is common in seal pathogens. Faeces can be screened for helminth ova and larvae (see 'Lungworm' and Figure 23.20) and subjected to bacterial culture. Baermann technique larval counts (see Chapter 10) can be helpful to assess patent lungworm burdens and to monitor response to anthelmintic therapy.

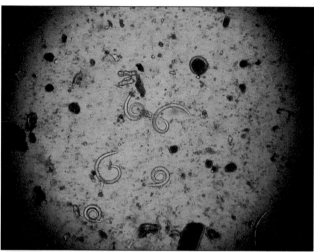

23.20 *Otostrongylus* larvae and an ascarid ovum in a seal faecal sample (direct microscopy, magnification X100).

Other diagnostic aids

Radiography is useful, particularly in the assessment of injuries involving bone (Figure 23.21). Sedation or anaesthesia will often be required. Thoracic radiographs can be useful in cases of respiratory disease. Suspected megaoesophagus and diaphragmatic herniation (Figure 23.22) can be investigated radiographically with contrast techniques, particularly barium swallows, if necessary.

Variable (units)	Common seal (*Phoca vitulina*)	Grey seal (*Halichoerus grypus*)
	Reference interval (No. of samples)	
Haematology		
Red blood cell (RBC) count (x 10¹²/l)	4–7 (134)	4–7 (78)
Haemoglobin (g/dl)	15–26 (144)	17–24 (79)
Packed cell volume (PCV) (l/l)	0.45–0.7 (136)	0.45–0.7 (78)
Mean corpuscular volume (MCV) (fl)	90–125 (134)	90–130 (78)
Mean corpuscular haemoglobin (MCH) ((pg) per cell)	30–45 (134)	30–50 (78)
Mean corpuscular haemoglobin concentration (MCHC) (g/dl)	30–40 (136)	30–40 (78)
Platelet count (x 10⁹/l)	80–740 (116)	180–780 (68)
Reticulocytes (% RBC)[a]	0–8 (134)	0–4 (78)
Heinz bodies (% RBC)[a]	0–1 (130)	0–3 (79)
White blood cell (WBC) count (x 10⁹/l)	3–17 (142)	5–19 (79)
Segmented neutrophils (x 10⁹/l)	2–11 (137)	2–12 (79)
Lymphocytes (x 10⁹/l)	0–5 (137)	0–6 (79)
Monocytes (x 10⁹/l)[a]	0–4 (137)	0–3 (79)
Eosinophils (x 10⁹/l)[a]	0–3 (139)	0–2 (79)
Basophils (x 10⁹/l)[a]	0–1 (139)	0–1 (79)
Fibrinogen (g/l)	2–6 (109)	1–5 (66)
Biochemistry		
Phosphate (mmol/l)	0.7–3 (41)	1.3–2.7 (24)
Sodium (mmol/l)	145–160 (38)	145–155 (25)
Potassium (mmol/l)	3.5–5.5 (38)	3.8–5.5 (25)
Creatinine (μmol/l)	0–100 (41)	0–100 (25)
Urea (mmol/l)	7–23 (41)	7–22 (25)
Bilirubin (μmol/l)	0–10 (39)	0–10 (25)
Cholesterol (mmol/l)	4–8 (40)	4–10 (25)
Alkaline phosphatase (ALP) (IU/l)	0–200 (41)	0–600 (25)
Alanine aminotransferase (ALT) (IU/l)	0–200 (41)	0–100 (25)
Aspartate aminotransferase (AST) (IU/l)	0–500 (39)	0–200 (24)
Gamma-glutamyl transferase (GGT) (IU/l)	0–80 (39)	0–100 (25)
Total protein (g/dl)	50–90 (41)	50–90 (25)
Albumin (g/dl)	29–50 (41)	29–50 (25)

23.19 Haematology and biochemistry reference intervals for common and grey seals, originally calculated as mean ± 2SD.
[a] Observed range.
(Haematology values adapted from Bennett *et al.*, 1991; biochemistry values adapted from unpublished data, RSPCA Norfolk Wildlife Hospital)

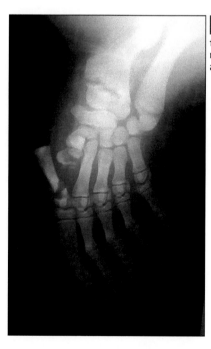

23.21 Dorsopalmar radiograph of a fractured metacarpal and radius in a seal with associated osteomyelitis.

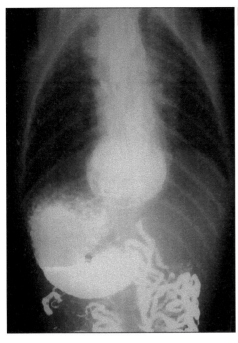

23.22
Dorsoventral radiograph with barium contrast illustrating a hiatus hernia in a seal pup.

Abdominal radiographs are less useful because seals lack abdominal adipose tissue and contrast is therefore poor. Radiography is particularly useful in adult seals because of the relatively high incidence of shooting, foreign bodies, end-stage lung disease and skeletal abnormalities, all of which are best diagnosed radiographically. Ultrasonography has been used to assess suspected cardiac problems. Flexible endoscopy can also be useful to investigate upper alimentary tract disorders.

Anaesthesia and analgesia

Cetaceans

Anaesthesia is not an option in the management of stranded cetaceans except as premedication as part of the euthanasia techniques outlined above.

Intramuscular diazepam and midazolam (Figure 23.23) have been used to sedate cetaceans before transport to rehabilitation facilities in Europe and the USA, but their use prior to refloating is not advisable. Most sedatives are contraindicated in animals to be refloated, due to their effects on respiration and thermoregulation (Sweeney and Ridgway, 1975). However, their use should be considered prior to euthanasia.

Non-steroidal anti-inflammatory drugs (NSAIDs) should be considered if indicated (Figure 23.23). These drugs have been used at doses similar to those used in dogs; however, due to the considerable variation in size of cetaceans encountered, allometric scaling of doses should be considered in larger animals (Kirkwood, 1983). If NSAIDs are used, the animal should be fully assessed and confirmed viable for reflotation before they are administered to prevent masking of clinical signs that may lead to a decision to euthanase. There is also a potential for renal injury if NSAIDs are used in an animal not fully rehydrated prior to reflotation. Most of these drugs are licensed in domestic animals for use by the subcutaneous and/or intravenous routes, which are not the most suitable routes in cetaceans. Subcutaneous injections, particularly in animals in moderate to good body condition, are difficult to administer without drugs entering the blubber layer, with subsequent delayed absorption and increased risk of abscess formation. Intravenous injections can be given into vessels used for blood sampling (see Figures 23.13 and 23.14) and

Drug	Dosage in seals	Dosage in cetaceans	Indications, side effects and comments
Analgesics/anti-inflammatories			
Carprofen	4 mg/kg i.m., orally q24h	4 mg/kg i.v. single dose	Musculoskeletal disorders and postoperative analgesia
Meloxicam	0.1 mg/kg orally q24h	0.2 mg/kg i.v., i.m. single dose	Musculoskeletal disorders and postoperative analgesia
Ketoprofen	1 mg/kg i.m., orally q24h (max. 5 days i.m.)	Not used	Musculoskeletal disorders, pulmonary inflammation
Flunixin	1 mg/kg i.m., i.v. q24h	1 mg/kg i.v. single dose	Musculoskeletal disorders and severe pulmonary inflammation Maximum 3 days' use due to risk of gastric ulceration
Butorphanol	0.2 mg/kg i.m.	Not used	Postoperative analgesia, repeat as needed; duration of activity unknown
Buprenorphine	0.01–0.02 mg/kg i.m.	Not used	Postoperative analgesia, repeat as needed; duration of activity unknown
Sedatives			
Medetomidine	0.05–0.1 mg/kg i.m.	Not used	Light to heavy sedation in grey seal pups, lasting up to 1 hour; reverse with atipamezole (5x medetomidine dose rate in mg, i.m.)
Medetomidine (M) + butorphanol (B)	0.02 mg/kg i.m. (M) + 0.08 mg/kg i.m. (B)	Not used	Sedation of grey seal pups for radiography and ocular examination; reverse medetomidine with atipamezole (5x medetomidine dose rate in mg, i.m.)
Midazolam	0.5 mg/kg i.v., i.m.	0.1 mg/kg i.m.; for transport – not advisable to use in animals to be refloated within 4 hours of transport	Light to moderate, 10–15 min sedation of adult seals and pups for minor procedures; premedication before induction of general anaesthesia with propofol or isoflurane
Diazepam	0.1 mg/kg i.v. (not i.m.)	0.15–0.2 mg/kg i.m.; for transport – not advisable to use in animals to be refloated within 8 hours of transport	Light to moderate sedation of adult seals and pups for minor procedures; premedication Can also be used at low doses orally as an anxiolytic and appetite stimulant to encourage fractious seals to eat

23.23 Analgesics, sedatives and anaesthetics and their dose rates used in seals and cetaceans. (continues)
(Sweeney, 1989; Kastelein et al., 1997; Barnett et al., 2013b) ▶

Drug	Dosage in seals	Dosage in cetaceans	Indications, side effects and comments
Anaesthetics			
Medetomidine (M) + ketamine (K)	0.06 mg/kg i.m. (M) + 2.0 mg/kg i.m. (K)	Not used	Grey seal pups; up to 1 hour of anaesthesia
Medetomidine (M) + butorphanol (B) + ketamine (K)	0.025 mg/kg i.m. (M) + 0.1g/kg i.m. (B) + 2.0–2.5 mg/kg i.m. (K), 15 min after M+B	Not used	Grey seal pups; up to 1 hour of anaesthesia
Ketamine + midazolam	6 mg/kg i.m. (K) + 0.15 mg/kg i.m. (M)	Not used	Common and grey seals; induction agent or short periods of anaesthesia
Tiletamine and zolazepam	Up to 1 mg/kg combined dose i.m.	Not used	Field use primarily; sedation and light anaesthesia; not licensed for use in UK and not easily available to UK practitioners
Propofol	5–6 mg/kg i.v.	Not used	Induction agent; short periods of anaesthesia
Isoflurane, sevoflurane	To effect; mask induction	Not used	Use with or without initial sedation in seals of any size, but handling can be a problem for larger animals

23.23 (continued) Analgesics, sedatives and anaesthetics and their dose rates used in seals and cetaceans. (Sweeney, 1989; Kastelein et al., 1997; Barnett et al., 2013b)

the same risks of ischaemic necrosis apply (see Step 15 in Figure 23.13). However, meloxicam is licensed for intramuscular use in certain domestic species (e.g. pigs), suggesting there is scope for using NSAIDs by this route.

Seals

Figure 23.23 lists analgesics, sedatives and anaesthetic drugs that have been used in seals. Anaesthesia in seals has inherent risks due to their dive physiology and should not be undertaken lightly. Elective procedures should be delayed until patients are in optimum condition, especially with regards to their respiratory function. Breath-holding during induction and apnoea and bradycardia during maintenance are very common. Premedication with atropine sulphate (20 µg/kg i.m.) is advisable (Huuskonen et al., 2011). Induction agents with the least potential for cardiopulmonary depression are generally preferred. Alpha-2 agonists have been associated with bradycardia, reduced cardiac output, prolonged recovery periods and mortality (Lynch and Bodley, 2007). Endotracheal intubation and intermittent positive pressure ventilation (IPPV) are strongly advised (even when spontaneous breathing is present) to prevent hypoxia and hypercapnia. The tongue is relatively short and inflexible and intubation can be facilitated by using a tongue grasper. The anaesthetic circuit and flow rate must be suitable for IPPV (e.g. Bain). As a minimum, an oesophageal stethoscope and respiratory monitor are required for monitoring during anaesthesia and recovery. Pulse oximetry and capnography can also be valuable. Core body temperature monitoring is advisable as thermoregulation is often affected, probably due to the dive reflex. Intravenous access is discussed under 'Blood collection' and may be useful for administration of emergency drugs and fluid therapy during anaesthesia. Recovery can be prolonged, depending on the pre-anaesthetic condition, duration of anaesthesia and anaesthetic agents used. Adequate provision should be made for a long recovery period before starting the procedure. Doxapram can be useful to stimulate respiration and recovery at a dose of 2 mg/kg intravenously or sublingually.

NSAIDs are particularly useful for analgesia in seals, but should be used with caution when renal perfusion is reduced, for example in hypovolaemia, dehydration and anaesthesia (Barnett, 1998). Opioid analgesics (see Figure 23.23) appear to have prolonged effects in seals (Huuskonen et al., 2011), which may contribute to protracted recoveries from general anaesthesia.

Specific conditions in cetaceans

As cetacean rehabilitation is not an option in the UK at present, prognosis is made on the basis of clinical signs in the stranded animal, rather than the diagnosis of specific conditions. Discussion of specific conditions will therefore be largely limited to seals.

Deaville et al. (2010) summarized the findings from the post-mortem examination of 933 live individual and mass stranded cetaceans in the UK between 1990 and 2008. Of these, infectious disease (n=149), poor nutritional condition (n=110) and trauma or non-infectious disease (n=53) were significant conditions likely to have caused individuals to live-strand in extremis. 318 animals were found to be in apparent good health and nutritional status with no significant pathologies that might explain the stranding. A number of factors have been suggested to explain why such animals may strand, including following prey inshore, adverse weather conditions, geomagnetic disturbances or errors in navigation whilst following geomagnetic contours, disturbance of echolocation in shallow water and anthropogenic noise (Deaville et al., 2010). Examples of infectious diseases encountered in live stranded cetaceans include Brucella-associated meningoencephalitis, parasitic and bacterial pneumonia, and septicaemia.

Mass strandings

These involve pelagic species with highly evolved social structures. Here, animals may strand with no evidence of significant infectious disease or trauma prior to the event (Jepson et al., 2013), or only one key animal is compromised (Rogan et al., 1997). In other mass strandings, most animals involved have not been healthy at the time of intervention (Walsh et al., 2001).

Both reflotation (see Figure 23.17) and euthanasia may need to be carried out in any mass stranding event. Assessment and treatment is essentially the same as for single strandings, but ensuring adequate care for all stranded individuals requires a high level of organization. Early detection and euthanasia of those unlikely to survive is required: this often includes the animal that initiated the stranding and those suffering from significant trauma and other complications associated with stranding. The technique for refloating involves amassing all those suitable in the shallows and releasing them together when the conditions are appropriate.

There have been a number of notable mass strandings in the UK in recent years, including around 70 pilot whales in the Kyle of Durness, north-west Scotland in 2011 (see Figure 23.17), of which 44 were returned to the sea, and the UK's largest mass stranding of common dolphins (*Delphinus delphis*) in Falmouth Bay, Cornwall in 2008, when at least 26 dolphins died and a similar number were refloated or herded back to sea (Jepson *et al.*, 2013).

Specific conditions in seals

Trauma

Bite wounds

Abandoned pups can get bitten by other seals, especially in crowded breeding sites. Weak seals that strand on shores with public access are also vulnerable to attack by dogs. Bite wounds can penetrate deeper tissues such as bones and joints. Suturing is generally contraindicated as wounds are usually contaminated and/or infected. Wounds should be bathed and flushed with dilute chlorhexidine, and analgesia and parenteral broad-spectrum antibacterial therapy (see 'Therapeutics') are indicated. Ideally the choice of antimicrobial agent should be based on culture and sensitivity results, although wounds are often secondarily contaminated. Infection can progress to abscessation, cellulitis, septic arthritis and osteomyelitis, and surgical debridement is occasionally necessary. Once strong enough, the seal should be allowed access to regular swimming in clean saltwater, which helps promote healing. See also 'Infected wounds'.

Netting entanglement

Seals can become entangled in discarded fishing nets ('ghost nets'), rope and synthetic line, which often becomes entangled around the neck (Stewart and Yochem, 1987). Many seals cope initially and can be impossible to catch, and some individuals manage to free themselves. However, in many cases, the drag of the net impairs the ability to dive and hunt, and the seal becomes progressively weaker. In addition, the netting can tighten resulting in deep 'cheese-wire' lacerations with infection and pressure necrosis (Figure 23.24). By the time they are captured, many animals have secondary problems such as pneumonia and malnutrition. Even when the wounds are deep, the prognosis is generally favourable providing there is no permanent damage (e.g. to bone or eyes). Animals must be stabilized

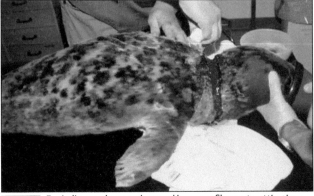

23.24 Encircling neck wound caused by monofilament netting in a grey seal pup.
(Courtesy of A Charles, RSPCA Norfolk Wildlife Hospital)

and rehydrated before tight material is removed as this can be associated with the sudden liberation of toxins and inflammatory mediators into the circulation, with potentially fatal results. Sedation or anaesthesia may be necessary for the removal of deeply embedded line and treatment of long-standing lesions. Seals with these injuries need to be observed closely for 7–10 days for evidence of reperfusion injury and delayed ischaemic necrosis.

Other injuries and fractures

Traumatic injuries such as wounds and fractures (especially to the jaw, digits and ribs) can be caused by rough seas, when animals may be thrown against rocks, or by falling or crawling along rocky terrain. Swelling and bruising can be difficult to detect, especially in well nourished seals, due to their thick blubber layer and tight skin. Radiography is useful to demonstrate fractures, dislocations, osteomyelitis and bone sequestra (see Figure 23.21). Simple fractures can heal, but compound fractures carry a grave prognosis. Phalangeal injuries are particularly common, and may result from bites or other trauma. There is a risk of osteomyelitis and sequestrum formation; bacterial culture and antibacterial sensitivity testing are useful, especially in refractory cases. Surgical intervention is often necessary and infected, exposed or fractured phalanges can be removed and digits amputated, using tension-relieving sutures to minimize the risk of dehiscence (Lucas *et al.*, 1999). Seals with single amputated digits appear able to swim and dive normally (J Barnett, personal observation), but amputation or permanent disability of an entire limb is likely to significantly reduce their long-term survival prospects and such animals should be euthanased.

Boat collision

Traumatic injuries can be sustained during collisions with marine vessels, particularly fast-moving vessels such as powerboats and jet skis. Propeller strike typically produces sequential parallel chop wounds that can be very deep (although they generally heal well with time).

Foreign body ingestion

Ingestion of fishing hooks and tackle is rare, but should be considered when an older seal is admitted without an obvious reason. Sea fishing hooks and wire booms have been identified in the stomachs of seals. Gastroliths (pebbles and sand) are also occasionally visible on radiographs, particularly in ice-breeding seals; their exact function is unknown, but they are probably ingested deliberately to assist with digestion or buoyancy (Nordoy, 1995).

Shooting

The Grey Seals Protection Act (1914) and the Grey Seals Protection Act (1932) limited hunting of grey seals to outside the breeding season, which allowed their numbers to recover from the effects of hunting in the 1800s. Commercial hunting of common seal pups in the UK began in the 1950s and became such a serious threat to many populations that a new law (Conservation of Seals Act 1970) was introduced that protected both species of seals in Great Britain during their breeding seasons. However, the law does not prevent fishermen from shooting seals outside the breeding season or even during the breeding season if they can claim that a seal was near their nets. The 1970 law also provides for government-sanctioned culls to be carried out with the view of protecting fisheries by reducing the seal population. Major culls of grey seals were carried out in the 1970s until these were stopped in 1981. The Marine (Scotland) Act 2010 Part 6 replaced the Conservation of Seals Act 1970 in Scotland. Part 6 seeks to balance seal conservation with sustainable fisheries and aquaculture and its introduction means it is an offence to kill or injure a seal except under licence or for welfare reasons, outlawing unregulated seal shooting that was permitted under previous legislation (Barnett *et al.*, 2013b) (see also Chapter 2). Non-fatal shooting injuries are occasionally seen in adult seals. Affected animals usually have head and eye injuries; radiography is required to confirm the diagnosis and the prognosis is usually poor.

Idiopathic alopecia

Occasionally seals are admitted with patches of bald skin, especially around the head, neck and trunk, as an incidental finding. In most cases, no specific cause is identified and microscopic examination of the hairs reveals broken shafts, consistent with abrasion on rough surfaces. Lesions are usually chronic but non-progressive and probably resolve during annual moulting.

Pollutants and toxins

The effects of contaminants on seal health are poorly understood, but high levels of persistent organic pollutants may adversely affect immunity and reproduction (Reijinders, 1986; Hall *et al.*, 1992; Swart *et al.*, 1994). Algal blooms in the marine environment are capable of producing neurotoxins such as domoic acid and brevetoxin, which can affect seals (McHuron *et al.*, 2013). Contamination of seals with oil is usually superficial, with systemic effects unlikely. The oil can be removed by washing in detergent and thorough rinsing. See also Chapter 24 for further details.

Infectious diseases

Viral diseases

Morbillivirus: Phocine distemper virus (PDV) is a morbillivirus, closely related to canine distemper (CDV, which can also occasionally cause disease in seals). This disease principally affects common seals, although grey seals can have subclinical infections. PDV is capable of causing epidemics associated with high morbidity and mortality and can affect seals of different ages. The population of common seals in The Wash was dramatically reduced by two PDV epidemics, with a 52% decline in 1988 and a 22% decline in 2002 (Thompson *et al.*, 2005; Lonergan *et al.*, 2010). It has been suggested that PDV is endemic in some ice-breeding seal species and disease may be introduced to common seal colonies by vagrant animals from the Arctic (possibly via grey seals) (Härkönen *et al.*, 2006). Infected animals typically have acute pneumonia that can be accompanied by pulmonary and subcutaneous emphysema. They are dull and lethargic and may have a fluctuating rectal temperature. PDV infection also causes immunosuppression and secondary bacterial and viral infections are common. Some individuals develop seizures due to central nervous system (CNS) involvement. The diagnosis can be confirmed in live animals by virus isolation and polymerase chain reaction (PCR) on nasal and pharyngeal swabs. Serology can also be useful and commercial canine serum neutralizing

antibody tests (for CDV) are sensitive enough to be useful for the antigenically similar PDV. Treatment is largely supportive, but the survival rates for confirmed cases are low. Once recovered, however, strong immunity lasts for several years. Broad-spectrum antibacterials, bronchodilators and mucolytics may provide helpful supportive treatment in some cases.

Herpesvirus: Phocine herpesvirus-1 (PhHV-1) is an alphaherpesvirus, antigenically similar to canine and feline herpesviruses. PhHV-1 is endemic in free-living European common seals and disease can occur in the wild (Gulland *et al.*, 1997), although outbreaks of disease are mostly seen in pups undergoing rehabilitation (Goldstein *et al.*, 2004). Clinical signs include nasal discharge, coughing, vomiting, diarrhoea, pyrexia, anorexia and lethargy. Diagnosis can be challenging because the clinical signs are non-specific. Virus isolation can be attempted from oronasal discharge and measurement of serum neutralizing antibody titres can be useful (Harder *et al.*, 1997). The morbidity and mortality rates can be high, especially in very young seals, and in many cases the diagnosis is only confirmed at necropsy. Therapy includes antibiotics to control secondary pathogens, fluid/nutritional support and symptomatic treatment for respiratory signs (Borst *et al.*, 1986; Robinson, 1995).

Poxvirus: Seal pox can infect several species of pinniped and disease has been reported in free-living animals, but is most common in rehabilitation centres. Common seals can be infected (Muller *et al.*, 2003), but lesions are more often seen in grey seal pups (Simpson *et al.*, 1994). Stress, malnutrition and concurrent disease may predispose animals to infection. Clinical disease is usually caused by a parapoxvirus, but an orthopoxvirus is capable of causing similar lesions and mixed infections involving both viruses have been reported. The lesions consist of firm pale cutaneous nodules, principally on the head, ventrum and flippers (Figure 23.25). The gross lesion appearance is pathognomonic, but histopathology or electron microscopy can be used to confirm the diagnosis (Hicks and Worthy, 1987). Affected seals usually develop one or two discrete lesions, but occasionally there can be multiple widespread coalescing lesions. Most infections are self-limiting and produce no other signs. No specific treatment is needed and lesions regress after 6–8 weeks. In severe cases there can be lethargy, discomfort, inappetance and secondary pyoderma,

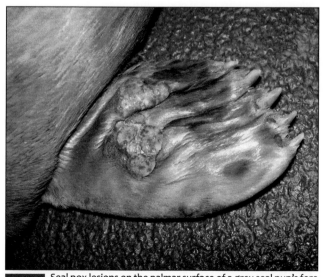

23.25 Seal pox lesions on the palmar surface of a grey seal pup's fore flipper.

and symptomatic treatment is occasionally needed with analgesia and broad-spectrum antibacterials. Allowing animals to bathe in (warm) saltwater or Epsom salts can help alleviate discomfort. The antiviral drug cidofovir has been shown to have good *in vitro* activity against parapoxvirus and may have potential therapeutic uses (Nollens, 2005). Pox is very contagious so attempts to reduce virus spread are advisable. Seal pox has zoonotic potential, occasionally causing nodules on the fingers of handlers (Hicks and Worthy, 1987).

Influenza viruses: Influenza A and B viruses have been isolated from seals with respiratory disease and are often fatal (Lang *et al.*, 1981; Osterhaus *et al.*, 2000). During 2014 in Northern Europe an outbreak of avian influenza A virus (H10N7) was associated with a mass mortality event of common seals. The virus was detected using RT-PCR and it is likely that seals were infected through exposure to infected wild birds or their droppings (Zohari *et al.*, 2014). Influenza viruses also pose a risk of human infection (Webster *et al.*, 1981).

Flaviviruses: Recently, West Nile Virus, a mosquito-borne flavivirus, has been recognized as an emerging pathogen in phocids in North America and the virus is present in continental Europe. The virus has not to date been detected in the UK, however this situation could change. Clinical infection in seals manifests as progressive neurological dysfunction with head tremors, weakness and clonic spasms (Del Piero *et al.*, 2006). Seals are dead-end hosts, similar to equids and humans.

Bacterial diseases

Infected wounds: Bites and traumatic wounds are prone to contamination and infection, often with mixed aerobic and anaerobic bacteria. Infections are often suppurative and may progress to cellulitis, abscessation, arthritis and osteomyelitis. Acute cellulitis (especially of the muzzle or flipper) frequently develops suddenly and pyothorax and peritonitis are also not uncommon in juvenile seals. There is a risk of rapid progression to sepsis, with high mortality rates especially in debilitated animals. Immediate antibacterial therapy (with intravenous administration in severe cases) is essential.

Common organisms from infected wounds include *Streptococcus* spp. (especially *S. phocae*), *Pseudomonas* spp. (especially *P. aeruginosa*), *Pasteurella haemolytica*, *Arcanobacterium phocae* and *Mycoplasma* spp. Antimicrobial therapy should ideally be based on culture and sensitivity results; however, contamination of wounds by environmental organisms often results in a mixed bacterial growth (S Bexton, personal observation).

In young seal pups, the umbilicus should be checked for infection. In neonates, the umbilical cord should be treated prophylactically with iodine tincture or a similar strong antiseptic solution.

Bacterial pneumonia: Primary bacterial pneumonia can occur, especially in younger animals, but most cases are secondary to parasitic bronchopneumonia or concurrent disease (e.g. PDV). Typical signs include coughing, hyperpnoea and a mucopurulent nasal discharge. Lung fields are harsh on auscultation, often with adventitious sounds. Thoracic radiography can be used to confirm the diagnosis. Various treatments have been used including systemic antibacterials, NSAIDs, mucolytics, bronchodilators, steam inhalation and nebulization. In secondary pneumonia,

treatment of the underlying cause (usually lungworm, see 'Parasites') is also necessary. Affected animals should not be allowed access to water due to the risk of drowning, but recovering cases may benefit from swimming exercise later on to assist with lung clearance.

Septicaemia: Most rescued juvenile seals are suffering from malnutrition and are often immunodeficient and particularly vulnerable to septicaemia as a result of traumatic injuries or pneumonia (Barnett, 1998). Most cases are acute and can result in death within 48 hours. Clinical signs can include dullness, anorexia, pyrexia, hyperpnoea and oedema or cellulitis. Many are caused by opportunistic pathogens acquired from the natural environment or from within the seal rescue centre (e.g. *Pseudomonas aeruginosa*, *Pasteurella haemolytica*, *Escherichia coli* and *Klebsiella pneumoniae*). The warm moist environment of seal rehabilitation units is ideal for the survival of potentially pathogenic bacteria. Regular antibacterial use within these facilities can also encourage the development of antimicrobial resistance. Strict hygiene, disinfection, steam cleaning, barrier nursing and isolation procedures can help reduce environmental contamination but it can be difficult to completely eliminate the problem due to the persistence of organisms in inaccessible places such as drains and pipework. Viral infections (e.g. herpesvirus, poxvirus) and coccidiosis can also spread rapidly within facilities in spite of rigorous biosecurity measures.

Pyorrhoea: Gingivitis, stomatitis and palatal ulceration (Figure 23.26) are relatively common, especially in weaned common seal pups. Suitable treatments include chlorhexidine sprays, broad-spectrum antibiotics (see Figure 23.31) and NSAIDs (see Figure 23.23). Superficial lesions heal well but severe gum erosion, osteomyelitis, tooth loss and development of large oronasal fistulae carry a grave prognosis.

Bacterial enteritis: Diarrhoea is common in the early stages of rehabilitation and is usually secondary to dietary change and stress. More persistent or severe diarrhoea (especially with blood) can indicate bacterial enteritis or dysbiosis of the gut flora. Faecal culture and sensitivity may be useful and microscopic examination for parasites

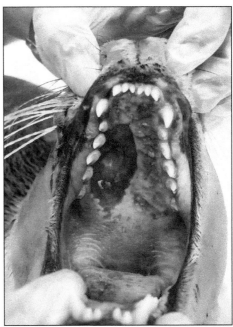

23.26

Palatal ulceration in a common seal pup.

should be considered. *Salmonella* spp. (e.g. *S.* Bovis-morbificans), *E. coli* and *Proteus* spp. are occasionally isolated. Antibacterial therapy (e.g. enrofloxacin) can be combined with symptomatic antidiarrhoeal treatment (e.g. kaolin), and possibly probiotics. Melaena is relatively common in weaned seals with lungworm and is usually due to ingestion of blood coughed up from the lungs. Occasional cases of melaena are due to gastric ulceration and gastroenteritis and these animals should be treated with oral fluids and appropriate gastrointestinal therapy (see Figure 23.31).

Otitis externa: Purulent aural discharge is sometimes noticed in seals during rehabilitation. The ear canal is relatively short and most cases resolve spontaneously without treatment. Providing access to clean water for swimming is beneficial, with the addition of salt to the water if practical. Antibiotics can be used but are rarely effective or necessary.

Parasites

Lungworm: Parasitic bronchopneumonia is extremely common in seals and is the major reason for the rescue and admission of weaned juveniles. Any compromise to the respiratory system affects the seal's ability to dive and feed. Significant disease may be more likely in animals that are already struggling with pre-existing problems such as malnutrition. Two species of lungworm, *Parafilaroides gymnurus* and *Otostrongylus circumlitus*, infest seals. Both have intermediate hosts and therefore only weaned animals tend to be infested. *P. gymnurus* infests the lung parenchyma and alveoli, causing oedema, inflammation, excessive mucus production and, occasionally, pulmonary and pleural haemorrhage; *O. circumlitus* infests the bronchial tree causing obstruction (and can also sometimes be found in the right ventricle and pulmonary artery). Clinical signs include malaise, lethargy, hyperpnoea or dyspnoea, coughing, haemoptysis and epistaxis (Figure 23.27). Larvae can be found in the sputum and faeces (see Figure 23.20), and adult worms may be coughed up. Baermann technique larval counts (see Chapter 10) can be useful to identify the species of lungworm involved (both species can occur together) and give

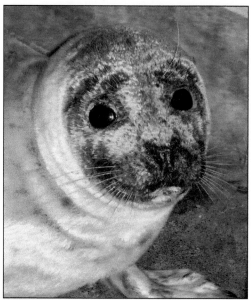

23.27 Haemoptysis and epistaxis in a common seal pup with lungworm.

an indication of severity. Pre-patent infestations are also seen with severe clinical signs due to mass larval migration through the pulmonary vasculature. Fatal haemorrhage and anaemia can occasionally result.

The timing of anthelmintic treatment is crucial and in many animals it is advisable to delay anthelmintic treatment until lung function and in particular clearance mechanisms have improved; otherwise, there is a significant risk of fatal airway obstruction caused by dead lungworms and bronchial exudates. Most cases have secondary bacterial pneumonia, which should be controlled with broad-spectrum antibacterials (e.g. amoxicillin/clavulanate). Potent NSAIDs (e.g. flunixin) or corticosteroids (in severe cases) and bronchodilators are beneficial in the early stages to reduce lung inflammation, exudation and bronchospasm and facilitate clearance of the airways. Mucolytics and steam inhalation also help to loosen bronchial secretions and oral fluids are given routinely. Oxygen therapy and nebulization of therapeutic agents may also be beneficial. Ivermectin is very effective against lungworm and therefore carries the greatest risk of airway occlusion or anaphylaxis from sudden lungworm die-off. Some veterinary surgeons prefer to use less effective (but safer) anthelmintics (such as fenbendazole) initially to reduce lungworm burden, followed by ivermectin at a later date (authors' personal experience).

Gastrointestinal helminthiasis: Most gastrointestinal worms of seals are of low pathogenicity and are generally well tolerated. Their significance increases, however, in individuals already debilitated by other diseases, and gastric mucosal erosion can be caused by large ascarid burdens (*Anisakis* spp. and *Contracaecum* spp.) with perforation and peritonitis possible. Cestodes and acanthocephalans are occasionally seen as an incidental finding. Concurrent lungworm infestation is likely and routine anthelmintics used for lungworm are equally effective against gastrointestinal nematodes.

Coccidiosis: *Eimeria phocae* can cause fatal dysentery in seal pups that are undergoing rehabilitation. Diagnosis is confirmed by observing coccidial oocysts in the faeces of clinically affected animals. Clinical signs include malaise, anorexia and watery diarrhoea. Prompt treatment with potentiated sulphonamides (see Figure 23.31) and supportive therapy, including rehydration, is essential. Outbreaks can be controlled by pen cleaning and water changes at least every 48 hours, i.e. under the likely sporulation time of the parasite (Munro and Synge, 1991). Overcrowding and poor water quality increases the risk of disease outbreaks. Oocysts are less likely to survive in pools and pipework if saltwater or chlorinated water is used.

Ectoparasites: Seal lice, *Echinophthirius horridus*, are of little clinical significance but are possible intermediate hosts for the heartworm *Dipetalonema spirocauda* (Geraci *et al.*, 1981). Nasal mites (*Halarachne halichoeri*) are often found on post-mortem examination and heavy infestations may be associated with nasal mucosal inflammation.

Other conditions
Ocular conditions

Eye disease is relatively common and it is not unusual to see one-eyed seals in the wild seemingly coping with their disability. Their eyes are relatively large which makes them vulnerable to injury. Dehydrated seals may be more prone to corneal irritation due to reduced production of protective tears. Ocular conditions include: corneal oedema; corneal ulceration (Figure 23.28) (including melting ulcers with *Pseudomonas aeruginosa* infection, which can rapidly progress to globe rupture); anterior uveitis; hypopyon; conjunctivitis; conjunctival or bulbar abscesses; and bilateral persistent pupillary membranes. Cataracts are occasionally seen in old animals.

Treatment is usually topical, with antibiotic eye drops for corneal ulcers and NSAID eye drops for painful conditions. Eye preparations containing gentamicin or fluoroquinolone have been the most effective in the authors' experience. Seals have to be kept dry whilst on treatment, which can be stressful. As an alternative, milder cases can be managed with saltwater floats, which can be combined with concentrated salt water sprays for corneal oedema. Subconjunctival injections of antibiotics, administered under sedation, can be used in intractable cases. Non-responsive corneal ulcers have been managed with corneal debridement and conjunctival pedicle grafts, protected by third-eyelid flaps. Severely traumatized and infected eyes or those where glaucoma has developed, can be enucleated.

Loss of sight in one eye does not rule out release, as many such seals have been observed surviving well in the wild. The decision to release such animals should be made on an individual case basis and following close observation of the animal's behaviour and feeding habits prior to release. Such animals should ideally be monitored post-release (see 'Release').

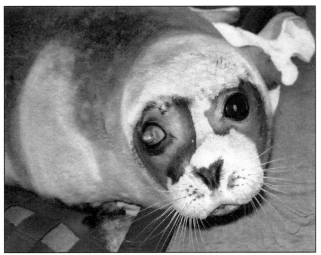

23.28 Corneal ulceration with descemetocele in a common seal pup. The left eye is 'normal'. This animal is well hydrated with an obvious tear film around both eyes.

Nutritional diseases

Starvation: Seal pups suckle for a relatively short time and are entirely dependent on their mother for food, therefore, unweaned seal pups that have become separated rapidly lose condition and are in need of rescue. They can be abandoned if the pup–dam bond is weak or can become separated by severe weather during the pupping season or following disturbance by people and dogs. Once in care, they need rehydration and the gradual introduction of nutritional support, with vitamin and mineral supplementation (see 'Rearing of seal pups').

Older (weaned) pups are also at risk of starvation especially if they were underweight at weaning and/or struggle to adapt to independent life. Research into juvenile grey seals suggested that a minimum weight at weaning of

25 kg for females and 35 kg for males was necessary for survival (Hall *et al.*, 2001), and 18 kg has been suggested as the equivalent minimum for common seals. Animals less than these weights lack the necessary blubber reserves to survive the period of post-weaning fasting and transition to independent feeding. Weaned pups in poor body condition are commonly rescued and taken into care; many have concurrent problems, in particular lungworm.

Hypoglycaemia: Hypoglycaemia is a significant risk in premature, neonatal and emaciated seal pups, with clinical disease most commonly observed within the first few days after rescue. They lack sufficient insulating fat and, under cold and wet conditions, their limited energy reserves can be rapidly depleted. Clinical signs of hypoglycaemia include muscle twitching, unresponsiveness and stiff vibrissae. The diagnosis can be quickly confirmed by measuring a blood glucose of less than 2 mmol/l. In an emergency, the immediate administration of glucose (1–5 ml of 50% glucose solution i.v. diluted with equal part saline or water for injection) is followed by rapid short-term improvement and can be life-saving, but relapses are common and susceptible animals require close monitoring of both blood glucose and rectal temperature. They often have poor thermoregulation and should be kept warm and dry. High-energy feeds should be given at regular intervals (including through the night if possible). Intravenous fluid infusions (see Figure 23.18) with additional glucose are often helpful in the short term. To prevent recurrence of this condition the underlying cause must also be addressed.

Thiamine deficiency: During rehabilitation, there is a risk of dietary thiamine deficiency due to the seal's fish-based diet. The risk of thiaminase activity is greatest in poor quality fish, especially if it has been incorrectly defrosted or stored. As a precaution, it may be necessary to provide thiamine supplementation (see Figure 23.31).

Iron-deficiency anaemia: This can be a problem following blood loss, especially with chronic or intermittent bleeds. Affected animals are pale and often weak. The diagnosis can be confirmed on haematology and by the response to treatment with injectable iron dextran (see Figure 23.31).

Congenital defects

Patent ductus arteriosus (PDA) is occasionally diagnosed in unweaned seal pups. Affected animals fail to thrive, although can still put on weight if sedentary. There is usually exercise intolerance, hyperpnoea and a pansystolic cardiac murmur. Mucous membrane colour and capillary refill time can be surprisingly normal at rest, but usually deteriorate with exercise. The ductus arteriosus can naturally take up to 6 weeks postpartum to close (Dennison *et al.*, 2011), so suspected cases should be allowed sufficient time to resolve, before making the decision to euthanase. Lesions can be confirmed at post-mortem examination. Coexisting patent foramen ovale has also been reported (Dennison *et al.*, 2011).

Megaoesophagus can be a problem in seal pups and usually presents as chronic intermittent regurgitation, failure to thrive and sometimes dysphagia. Affected animals are also prone to aspiration pneumonia. The diagnosis can be confirmed radiographically using barium contrast techniques, but care is needed with radiographic interpretation as the oesophagus of normal seals is comparatively wide. Once a diagnosis is confirmed the animal should be euthanased.

Hiatal hernia and paraoesophageal herniation have also been seen in seal pups. Clinical signs are similar to megaoesophagus with regurgitation, vomiting and ill thrift. Lesions can often be seen on radiographs (see Figure 23.22), although repeat procedures may be necessary. (It should be noted that the pylorus of seals is normally tight and easily mistaken for pyloric stenosis on radiographs).

Umbilical herniation also occurs in seal pups, and these cases should be treated as in other mammals.

Albinism is a rare disorder that is occasionally seen in common seals. Most individuals have poor vision, with photophobia or total blindness, and therefore have poor survival prospects. Melanistic grey seals are also occasionally seen. Seals are occasionally reported with red-tinged pelage; this is thought to be due to high levels of iron oxide in the local environment.

Therapeutics

Cetaceans

Drugs and their dose rates used in the treatment of stranded cetaceans are listed in Figure 23.29. Many drugs used in animals taken into rehabilitation facilities are of limited use or, in some cases, contraindicated for animals to be refloated (e.g. anthelmintics). Due to considerable variation in the weight of animals encountered, allometric scaling of doses may be appropriate for larger animals (Kirkwood, 1983). Some species-related (e.g. Stoskopf et al., 2001) and weight-related (e.g. Sweeney, 1989) doses are given in the literature. Length–weight data for a number of cetacean species is provided in Figure 23.30.

Intravenous injections can be given into vessels used for blood sampling and the same risks of ischaemic necrosis apply. Needles of 2.5–9 cm, 18–21 G, will be required, depending on patient size. Intramuscular injections are

Drug	Dosage	Indications and comments
Antibiotics		
Amoxicillin	15 mg/kg i.m. long-acting preparation as single injection	May be beneficial to reduce risk of secondary infection of wounds sustained upon stranding
Oxytetracycline	20 mg/kg i.m. long-acting preparation as single injection	May be beneficial to reduce risk of secondary infection of wounds sustained upon stranding
Topical eye treatments		
Ocular lubricant	As required (monitor for desiccation)	To minimize ocular desiccation, irritation, trauma
Chloramphenicol	q4–8h	To minimize ocular desiccation, irritation, trauma and prevent secondary bacterial infection (Gram-positive, Gram-negative and anaerobic activity, useful in the treatment of bacterial conjunctivitis)
Gentamicin	q4–6h	To minimize ocular desiccation, irritation, trauma and prevent secondary bacterial infection (often Gram-negative bacteria isolated)

23.29 Drugs and their dose rates used in the treatment of cetaceans undergoing reflotation in the UK.
(Unpublished data from UK stranding records; RSPCA, 1997; Barnett, 1998; Barnett et al., 2013b)

Species	Length (metres)	Maximum likely weight (kg)
Harbour porpoise (*Phocoena phocoena*)	0.7	6.5
	1	25
	1.5	70
	1.8	80
Common dolphin (*Delphinus delphis*) and striped dolphin (*Stenella coeruleoalba*)	1	20
	1.5	60
	2	125
	2.5	150
Atlantic white-sided dolphin (*Lagenorhynchus acutus*)	1.2	40
	1.5	60
	2	140
	2.5	190
	2.7	200
White-beaked dolphin (*Lagenorhynchus albirostris*)	1.2	40
	1.5	75
	2	150
	2.5	260
	2.8	300
Risso's dolphin (*Grampus griseus*) and bottlenose dolphin (*Tursiops truncatus*)	1.5	65
	2	150
	2.5	260
	3	370
	3.5	480
	4	600
Pilot whales (*Globicephala macrorhynchus*)	1.75	75
	2	150
	4	2000
	6	3500
Minke whales (*Balaenoptera acutorostrata*)	2	150
	2.5	350
	7	5000
	8.5	7000

23.30 Length–weight data for various cetacean species.
(UK Cetacean Strandings Investigation Programme (Barnett et al., 2013b))

administered into the lumbar muscles (see Figure 23.14); see 'Methods of euthanasia' for suitable needle lengths. Asepsis is important to minimize the risk of infection, for example with clostridial species, which has been reported after intramuscular injections in marine mammals. Subcutaneous injections should be avoided (see 'Anaesthesia and analgesia').

Wound care

Superficial wounds can be cleaned and flushed, but topical preparations usually wash off on immersion, except possibly Orabase®. Suturing of wounds is not advisable, as dehiscence is likely.

Seals

Drugs and their dose rates used in the treatment of seals are included in Figure 23.31. Canine doses are generally applicable in seal pups, though allometric principles should be borne in mind with large adult seals (up to 300 kg). It is

Drug	Dosage	Indications and comments
Antibiotics		
Amoxicillin	7 mg/kg i.m. q24h 10 mg/kg orally q12h	First line broad-spectrum
Amoxicillin/clavulanate (co-amoxiclav)	12.5 mg/kg orally q12h (double dose in refractory cases) 8.75 mg/kg i.m. q24h	First line broad-spectrum
Clindamycin	11 mg/kg orally q12h	Abscesses, osteomyelitis, gum disease
Enrofloxacin	5 mg/kg i.m., orally q24h	Septicaemia
Gentamicin	5 mg/kg i.m. q12h on first day, q24h thereafter	*Pseudomonas* infections
Cefalexin	10–15 mg/kg orally q12h	Use based on sensitivity results
Ceftazidime	25 mg/kg i.v., i.m. q12h	Use based on sensitivity results: restrict use for multiple antibiotic resistance (e.g. *Pseudomonas* infections)
Trimethoprim/sulfadiazine	30 mg/kg i.m., orally q24h	Use based on sensitivity results; also effective against *Eimeria phocae*
Oxytetracycline	50 mg/kg initial dose then 25 mg/kg thereafter orally q12h; 10 mg/kg i.m. q24h	Use based on sensitivity results
Mucolytics and bronchodilators		
Bromhexine	2 mg/kg orally q12h 0.5 mg/kg i.m. q24h	Mucolytic
Dembrexine	0.3 mg/kg orally q12h	Mucolytic
Carbocisteine	75–125 mg orally q6h	Mucolytic
Clenbuterol	0.8–5 µg/kg i.m., i.v., orally q12h	Reduces bronchospasm and aids mucociliary clearance
Anthelmintics		
Fenbendazole	10 mg/kg orally q24h for 3 days	Respiratory and gastrointestinal nematodes (repeat treatments usually necessary, based on faecal parasitology results)
Ivermectin	0.2–0.3 mg/kg i.m.	Respiratory and gastrointestinal nematodes (recommended 3 injections at 10–14 day intervals for lungworm treatment, but risk of resultant airway obstruction in severe infestations)
Drugs acting on the gastrointestinal tract		
Butylscopolamine and metamizole	0.4 mg/kg and 50 mg/kg respectively i.m., i.v.	Gut sedation
Cimetidine	5–10 mg/kg i.m., orally q6h	Gastric ulceration
Ranitidine	2–3 mg/kg orally q12h initially, then q24h	Gastric ulceration
Kaolin	1 ml/kg/day orally in divided doses	Diarrhoea
Liquid paraffin	1 ml/kg/day orally in divided doses	Constipation
Ispaghula husk	5–15 ml orally q24h	Constipation
Attapulgite and bone charcoal	2.5–5 g/feed	Diarrhoea
Sucralfate	0.25–1 g orally q8h	Gastric ulceration
Topical eye treatments		
Chloramphenicol	2 drops q4–8h	Use based on sensitivity results
Gentamicin	1–2 drops q4–6h	Use based on sensitivity results; treatment of choice for melting corneal ulcers caused by *P. aeruginosa*; improved response often seen if enriched with injectable gentamicin
Fusidic acid	1–2 drops q4–8h	Use based on sensitivity results
Cloxacillin	Applied q4–8h	Use based on sensitivity results
Ofloxacin	1–2 drops q4–6h	Use based on sensitivity results; also used for melting corneal ulcers caused by *P. aeruginosa*
Ciprofloxacin	2–3 drops q4–6h	Use based on sensitivity results; often treatment of choice for persistent corneal ulcers
Dexamethasone, hypromellose, neomycin and polymyxin B	3–4 drops q4–8h	To reduce scarring

23.31 Drugs and their dose rates used in the treatment of seals. (continues) ▶
(Unpublished data from UK seal rehabilitation records; Robinson,1995; Barnett, 1998)

Drug	Dosage	Indications and comments
Vitamin and mineral supplementation		
Injectable multivitamin/vitamin B complexes	2–10 ml i.m. depending on product and size of animal	May be given when pup is first admitted
Oral multivitamin preparations for fish-eaters (e.g. International Zoo Veterinary Group, Aquavits)	1 tablet q12h	Alternatively use human oral multivitamin preparations at twice recommended dose rate, ensuring 50 mg thiamine per kg feed and 100 mg vitamin E per kg feed
Ferrous sulphate	200 mg orally q12h	Dose can be increased in non-regenerative anaemias

23.31 (continued) Drugs and their dose rates used in the treatment of seals. (continues)
(Unpublished data from UK seal rehabilitation records; Robinson,1995; Barnett, 1998)

advisable to use precautionary antibiotics in all casualty seals due to the high incidence of secondary infections (e.g. pneumonia, infected wounds) and subclinical infections, and the risk of nosocomial bacterial infections whilst in captivity. Most pups will be suffering from some degree of immunosuppression due to malnutrition, immaturity and/or reduced passive immunity.

Intravenous injections are given via the extradural intravertebral vein. Intramuscular injections are into the lumbar muscles, or the gluteal muscles in larger animals (see Figure 23.16). Needles of up to 9 cm, 18 G, may be required in adults. Oral drugs may not be appropriate during stabilization due to poor gastrointestinal absorption but later in rehabilitation these can be added to liquidized tube feeds, or tablets/capsules can be inserted into fish gills once individuals are eating whole fish.

Management in captivity

Cetaceans

As stated earlier, rehabilitation has not proved to be a viable option for stranded cetaceans in the UK and is not available at present. Rehabilitation of cetaceans requires more expensive facilities than those required for seals, with a need for larger, deeper pools, saltwater systems and more sophisticated filtration where closed water systems are used. The details of requirements for USA facilities can be found in Gage and Whaley (2009). Rehabilitation in suboptimal facilities cannot be condoned.

Seals

Housing of adults

Adult seals, particularly greys, are potentially very dangerous and require specialist accommodation, which is unlikely to be available in the ordinary veterinary practice or most rehabilitation centres. Immediately after initial assessment and treatment, these animals should be moved to a facility that is able to house them appropriately. (See 'Specialist organizations and useful contacts'.)

Housing of seal pups

Seal pups can be temporarily housed indoors in a suitably sized enclosure (minimum 1.5 x 2 m) before being transferred to a suitable rehabilitation facility (see 'Specialist organizations and useful contacts'). They should be isolated from other animals initially, to minimize stress and reduce the potential for disease spread. Supplementary heat and some floor insulation (e.g. rubber matting, towels) may be necessary, especially in the early stages. Unlike

cetaceans, seals have no physiological requirement to be immersed in water; in fact, in the initial stages of rehabilitation, access to swimming water may be contraindicated due to the risk of hypothermia and drowning. Once stronger and healthier, regular exercise in water improves fitness and well being and seals are also more likely to self-feed in water. Access to water is gradually increased in line with clinical and physical progress and seals are grouped with others for socialization and competition for food resources to mimic a more natural environment.

Feeding

After initial assessment and treatment, seal pups are given rehydration fluids by stomach tube at intervals of 3–4 hours throughout the first 24 hours (see 'First aid'). After 24 hours a liquid diet (see Figure 23.11) is gradually mixed with the rehydration fluid in increasing proportions until the pup is on full-strength diet (see 'Rearing of seal pups'). The speed of transfer to liquid diet depends on the progress of the individual but on average takes 3–4 days. Volumes of feeds are initially small (see 'First aid') and build up to a maximum of 350 ml for common seals and 500 ml for grey seals over a period of 3–5 days.

The feeding of older seals, including adults, is similar, but general handling is more difficult. Most adults begin eating for themselves within a few days, especially if fish is provided whilst the seal is in water of sufficient depth. Mackerel and herring are most commonly fed, as they are widely available, though smaller fish such as sprats and whitebait may be used in the first instance to help stimulate self-feeding.

Rearing of seal pups

Although initial management of seal pups in captivity can be carried out in a veterinary practice or wildlife centre isolation facility, it is advisable to move seals at an early stage to an appropriately equipped rehabilitation centre. The full rehabilitation process cannot be attempted without access to adequate facilities, including suitable pools (Figure 23.32).

Feeding

Seals have evolved a short lactation period with high-fat milk (40–50%) and, as a result, pups rapidly lay down blubber and put on weight (up to 2 kg per day in grey seals). These fat reserves enable them to survive a period of natural starvation in the immediate post-weaning period. During rehabilitation, seal pups are under less pressure to accumulate blubber reserves rapidly and it is more

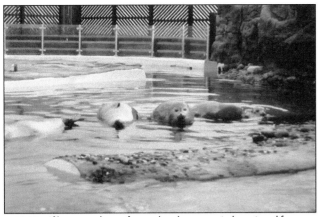

23.32 If large numbers of reared seal pups are to be catered for, large outdoor pools, such as this one at Scarborough Sea Life Sanctuary, need to be provided.

important that they learn how to feed themselves on fish. Therefore, it is not necessary to feed such a high-fat diet and attempts to replicate the high fat content of seal milk can even result in digestive disturbances such as regurgitation, vomiting, colic and steatorrhoea. Some seal rescue centres feed modified milk replacement formula; others feed liquidized fish and encourage pups to take fish as soon as possible (and often before they would have done naturally in the wild). Suitable diets easily available include the following:

- **Fish soup**. Ingredients: 500 ml rehydration fluid, three (500 g) medium-sized mackerel or herring (heads and tails removed, but not gutted), vitamin/mineral supplement (see Figure 23.31). Liquidize until of a consistency that will pass down a stomach tube. The fat content of the final mix is variable, as the fat content of the fish varies with the season in which they are caught. However, it is simple and readily available. It is the first choice for older pups that have been weaned for some time and will rapidly progress to a diet of whole fish and is also widely used for unweaned pups instead of artificial milk
- **Lactose-free milk replacer**. Zoologic® 30/55, mixed at maximum recommended concentration with water (1:1 by weight) provides a good milk substitute for unweaned pups, but the fat content of the reconstituted milk is only about 15%
- **Oil-enriched mixtures**. By adding fish oil to the milk replacer, a higher fat content can be achieved. Up to one-third salmon oil by volume can be added. Lecithin, readily available from health food shops, can be added as an emulsifier. A vitamin/mineral supplement is also added. The fat content of the final diet is about 40%. Cream can be used as an alternative fat source, but as seals are intolerant of lactose, the enzyme lactase must be added to the mixture before it is fed; thus such diets are best avoided unless in experienced hands.

All diets should be freshly made up each day and kept refrigerated.

Weaning

When pups start to thrive and gain weight, they begin to show swallowing movements as the tube is passed. The next step is for the seal to learn to feed on fish for itself and from this time on, a fish is always left with the seal in its

enclosure. Some individuals will eat fish as soon as it is offered (especially those that had already been eating for themselves in the wild); other seals take longer to learn and may progress through several stages. Herring or mackerel is commonly used as a fish feed for the high oil content and tube and fish feeds can be combined during the transition period. The fish are initially 'force-fed' by restraining the pup in sternal recumbency, introducing a fish into the corner of its mouth and then gently pushing the fish over its tongue until swallowing is stimulated. The use of gags or heavy gloves to force open the mouth is discouraged, as it tends to increase aggressive resistance, causes discomfort and can increase the time until self-feeding is established. The next stage is hand-feeding, where the seal is not held and will take fish from the handler, but still requires the fish to be pushed over its tongue to stimulate swallowing. Afterwards, many seals start chomping fish in water; this is a natural step towards eating fish whole. Each seal progresses at its own pace and this process can depend on the skill and experience of the handler.

Once self-feeding is established, feed quantity is increased according to appetite to a maximum of 4.5 kg/day divided into three feeds. Seals should be weighed weekly to assess progress.

Seals are able to obtain water from the fish in their diet and it is not necessary to provide drinking water; even where water is provided (in a bowl), not all seals will take it.

As soon as possible, seals are paired up for company and once eating well they are moved into larger groups for competition and to stimulate natural interactions (see Figure 23.32).

Premature pups

Premature common seal pups (Figure 23.33) are difficult to rear successfully. Initially, they require tube feeding every 2–3 hours with 100 ml of a suitable liquid diet (see 'Feeding'), including through the night. The volume can be gradually increased according to response up to a maximum of 200 ml. They often have poor thermoregulation and immunity and have a high risk of developing hypothermia, hypoglycaemia and septicaemia.

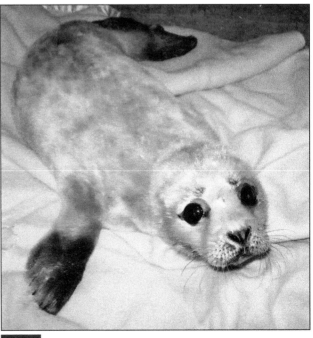

23.33 Premature common seal pup with pale lanugo coat.

Release

Cetaceans

Survival rates

Records collated by the charity carrying out the majority of strandings response in the UK, British Divers Marine Life Rescue (BDMLR), indicated that a little over half (71 of 123) of live animals attended in mass strandings between 1995 and 2012 were refloated and not found restranded. Of the live single strandings attended, less than a quarter (27 of 128 animals) were refloated and not found restranded (Barnett *et al.*, 2013b).

Assessing survival in the days immediately post-release can be aided by photo identification, by tying biodegradable ribbon around the tail stock, by writing an identifier on the dorsal fin with, for example, a raddle stick marker, or by microchipping the animal at the base of the dorsal fin. However, these techniques are only likely to provide information on short-term survival, due to their limited lifespan, or because they rely on the animal being resighted at sea or restranding. To monitor medium- to long-term success requires satellite telemetry (see Chapter 9). There are legal, logistical and, certainly in the past, welfare considerations associated with its use, including the need to attach tags to the dorsal fin with bolts and potential effects on hydrodynamics, health and behaviour. However, with tags becoming smaller and lighter, and casings more hydrodynamic, drag effects and energy costs associated with dorsal fin mounted satellite tags have been reduced considerably and some tags can now be attached with a single pin. Satellite tags have been successfully deployed on refloated cetaceans in the USA and are soon to be deployed in the UK.

Seals

Seals are released when they are clinically and behaviourally normal and in good body condition. They must be able to dive and self-feed and compete with others for food. Allowance should be made for some post-release weight loss as animals acclimatize to the natural environment and locate food sources. Therefore, as a guideline, pups should be released at their average expected weaning weight, although they will be considerably older when this weight is achieved. The authors recommend release weights of 40–45 kg for grey seals and 30–35 kg for common seals. Generally, seals are released back to sea as close as possible to where they were initially discovered. Shore release or boat release are equally suitable. In the UK, there are distinct populations on the east and west coasts and, even though they can travel great distances, they should be released back to the appropriate coastline.

On average the rehabilitation process can take from 3 to 6 months. A short-term rehabilitation option has been advocated for very young common seal pups (Wilson, 1999).

Survival rates

Survival rates of over 80% (grey seal pups) and 70% (common seal pups) can be expected during rehabilitation. Post-release studies from satellite telemetry (Figure 23.34) suggest that rehabilitated animals behave normally and have similar survival expectations to their wild counterparts (Lander *et al.*, 2002; Vincent *et al.*, 2002; Morrison *et al.*, 2012). Sightings based on plastic livestock ear tags that are routinely attached to hind flippers before release indicate that rehabilitated seals can survive well and may go on to breed successfully (A Charles, personal communication).

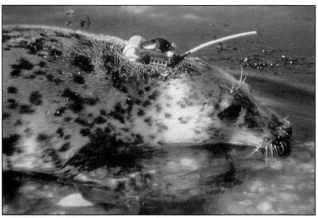

23.34 Satellite tag on a grey seal pup.
(Courtesy of C Vincent, University of La Rochelle)

Legal aspects

General aspects of the law relating to wildlife rehabilitation which are pertinent to marine mammals are covered in Chapter 2.

Legislation specific to cetaceans includes the Statute Prerogative Regis, 17 Edward II (AD 1324), which states that cetaceans are classified as 'Royal Fish' and belong to the Crown. The exceptions to this are animals that strand within the limits of a Manor, where title passes to the Lord of the Manor. In Scotland, pilot whales, northern bottlenose whales and cetaceans less than 7.5 m in length are not classed as 'Royal Fish' (see www.gov.uk and www.gov.scot and Figure 23.35 for more information).

In practical terms, current law requires that stranded cetaceans be reported to the Receiver of Wrecks in England and Wales and the Marine Directorate in Scotland. Strandings should also be reported to the relevant Cetacean Strandings Investigation Programme (CSIP) national co-ordinators for England, Scotland and Wales, which work under contract to Defra and the respective Devolved Governments (see www.ukstrandings.org for more information on reporting both live and dead stranding incidents). Strandings in Northern Ireland should also be reported to the Department of the Environment Northern Ireland (DOENI) (see also Figure 23.35). Disposal of carcasses is usually the responsibility of the Local Authority (where it occurs on public beaches) or private landowner (on privately owned land). Cetaceans are listed in the EU Habitats Directive (see www.gov.uk).

Relevant authority	Web reference
Maritime and Coastguard Agency, Receiver of Wrecks (England and Wales)	www.gov.uk/government/ publications/protected-marine-species
Marine Scotland Directorate (Scotland)	www.gov.scot/Topics/marine/ Licensing/marine/Applications/ royalfish
Cetacean Strandings Investigation Programme (CSIP) (England, Scotland and Wales strandings)	www.ukstrandings.org/CSIP_ leaflet.pdf
Department of the Environment Northern Ireland (DOENI) (Northern Ireland strandings)	www.doeni.gov.uk

23.35 Useful websites for more information about legal aspects associated with marine mammals.

Legislation specific to seals includes the Conservation of Seals Act 1970 in England and Wales, which makes it an offence to capture, injure or kill seals. This protection lasts all year round in east and south-east England (Conservation of Seals (England) Order 1999), and during the close season elsewhere (1 September to 31 December for grey seals and 1 June to 31 August for common seals). There are exceptions to this to allow the taking or killing of seals that are sick or injured. A further exception is the 'netsman's defence' that permits the killing of an individual seal in the vicinity of nets and tackle if it is causing damage. A licence is not necessary in this situation, but an approved firearm must be used. In Scotland, the Marine Scotland Act 2010 makes it an offence to kill seals except under licence and grey seals are legally protected during their breeding season (1 September to 31 December). In Northern Ireland, the Wildlife (Northern Ireland) Order 1985 provides protection for seals and prohibits killing (except under licence) and disturbance. Additionally, both native seal species are listed in Annex II of the EU Habitats Directive implemented by the Conservation (Natural Habitats, &c.) Regulations 2010 in England and Wales and the Conservation (Natural Habitats, &c.) Regulations 1994 as amended in Scotland.

Acknowledgements

The authors would like to thank: Alison Charles, Ian Robinson, Jon Cracknell, Sean Langton, Andrew Greenwood, Paul Jepson, Rob Deaville, Richard Lucas, Paul Riley and Terrie Williams for their technical input into this chapter; the Zoological Society of London for use of data from the Lynx programme; and *In Practice* for the use of illustrations previously published in an article by James Barnett in 1998. They would also like to thank the staff of the RSPCA East Winch Wildlife Centre and the Cornish Seal Sanctuary, the directors and other volunteers of British Divers Marine Life Rescue and their families for their support and patience over the years.

References and further reading

Baker AS, Ruoff KL and Madoff S (1998) Isolation of *Mycoplasma* species from a patient with seal finger. *Clinical Infectious Diseases* 27, 1168–1170

Baker J, Barnett J, Cooke M et al. (2000) Assessment of stranded cetaceans. *Veterinary Record* 147, 340

Barnett J (1998) Treatment of sick and injured marine mammals. *In Practice* 20, 200–211

Barnett J, Booth P, Brewer JI et al. (2013a) *Mycobacterium bovis* infection in a grey seal pup (*Halichoerus grypus*) *Veterinary Record* 173, 168

Barnett J, Knight A and Stevens M (2013b) *Marine Mammal Medic Handbook*, 7th edn. British Divers Marine Life Rescue, Uckfield, East Sussex

Barnett J, Woodley AJ, Hill TJ et al. (2000) Conditions in grey seal pups (*Halichoerus grypus*) presented for rehabilitation. *Veterinary Record* 147, 98–104

Bennett PM, Gascoyne SC, Hart MG et al. (1991) Development of Lynx: a computer application for disease diagnosis and health monitoring in wild mammals, birds and reptiles. *Veterinary Record* 128, 496–499

Borst GHA, Walvoort HC, Reijnders PJH et al. (1986) An outbreak of a herpesvirus infection in harbor seals (*Phoca vitulina*). *Journal of Wildlife Diseases* 22, 1–6

Brew SD, Perrett LL, Stack JA et al. (1999) Human exposure to *Brucella* recovered from a sea mammal. *Veterinary Record* 144, 483

Cameron CE, Zuerner RL, Raverty S et al. (2008) Detection of pathogenic *Leptospira* bacteria in pinniped populations via PCR and identification of a source of transmission for zoonotic leptospirosis in the marine environment. *Journal of Clinical Microbiology* 46, 1728–1733

Clark C, McIntyre PG, Evans A et al. (2005) Human sealpox resulting from a seal bite: confirmation that sealpox virus is zoonotic. *British Journal of Dermatology* 152, 791–793

Coughran D K, Stiles I and Mawson PR (2012) Euthanasia of beached humpback whales using explosives. *Journal of Cetacean Research and Management* 12, 137–144

Daoust PY and Ortenburger AI (2001) Successful euthanasia of a juvenile fin whale. *Canadian Veterinary Journal* 42, 127–129

Deaville R, Baker J, Brownlow A et al. (2010) A review of live stranded cetaceans in the UK between 1990 and 2008. *24th Conference of the European Cetacean Society, 22nd–24th March, Stralsund, Germany*

Del Piero, F, Stremme DW, Habecker PL and Cantile C (2006) West Nile Flavivirus Polioencephalomyelitis in a harbor seal (*Phoca vitulina*). *Veterinary Pathology* 43(1), 58–61

Dennison SE, Boor M, Fauquier D et al. (2011) Foramen ovale and ductus arteriosus patency in neonatal harbour seal (*Phoca vitulina*) pups in rehabilitation. *Aquatic Mammals* 37, 161–166

Dierauf LA and Gulland FMD (2001) *CRC Handbook of Marine Mammal Medicine: Health, Disease and Rehabilitation, 2nd edn.* CRC Press, Boca Raton, Florida

Donoghue M, Bamber C and Suisted R (2003) *Euthanasia of stranded cetaceans in New Zealand.* Submitted by New Zealand to the IWC Workshop on Whale Killing Methods

Elsner R (1999) Living in water: solutions to physiological problems. In: *Biology of Marine Mammals*, ed. JE Reynolds and SA Rommel, pp. 73–117. Smithsonian Institution Press, Washington

Evans PGH (1995) *Guide to the Identification of Whales, Dolphins and Porpoises in European Seas.* Sea Watch Foundation, Oxford

Foster G, Osterman BS, Godfroid J et al. (2007) *Brucella ceti* sp. nov. and *Brucella pinnipedialis* sp. nov. for *Brucella* strains with cetaceans and seals as their preferred hosts. *International Journal of Systematic and Evolutionary Microbiology* 57, 2688–2693

Gage L and Whaley JE (2009) *Policies and best practices for marine mammal strandings response, rehabilitation and release. Standards for rehabilitation facilities.* NOAA Fisheries, Office of Protected Resources. http://www.nmfs.noaa.gov/pr/pdfs/health/rehab_standards.pdf

Geraci JR, Fortin JF, St. Aubin DJ et al. (1981) The seal louse, *Echinophthirius horridus*: an intermediate host of the seal heartworm, *Dipetalonema spirocauda* (Nematoda). *Canadian Journal of Zoology* 59, 1457–1459

Geraci JR and Lounsbury VJ (2005) *Marine Mammals Ashore. A Field Guide for Strandings, 2nd edn.* National Aquarium in Baltimore, Baltimore, Maryland

Goldstein T, Mazet JAK, Gulland FMD et al. (2004) The transmission of phocine herpesvirus-1 in rehabilitating and free-ranging Pacific harbour seals (*Phoca vitulina*) in California. *Veterinary Microbiology* 103, 131–141

Greer L and Rowles T (2000) Humane euthanasia of stranded marine mammals. *Proceedings AAZV and IAAAM conference, New Orleans*, pp. 374–375

Greig DJ, Gulland FMD, Rios CA et al. (2010) Haematology and serum chemistry in stranded and wild-caught harbour seals in central California: reference intervals, predictors of survival, and parameters affecting blood variables. *Journal of Wildlife Diseases* 46, 1172–1184

Gulland FMD, Lowenstine LJ, Lapointe JM et al. (1997) Herpesvirus infection in stranded Pacific harbour seals of coastal California. *Journal of Wildlife Diseases* 33, 450–458

Hall AJ, Law RJ, Wells DE et al. (1992) Organochlorine levels in common seals (*Phoca vitulina*) which were victims and survivors of the 1988 phocine distemper epizootic. *Science of the Total Environment* 115, 145–162

Hall AJ, McConnell BJ and Barker RJ (2001) Factors affecting first year survival in grey seals and their implications for life history strategy. *Journal of Animal Ecology* 70, 138–149

Harder TC, Vos H, de Swart RL et al. (1997) Age-related disease in recurrent outbreaks of phocid herpesvirus type-1 infections in a seal rehabilitation centre: evaluation of diagnostic methods. *Veterinary Record* 140, 500–503

Härkönen T, Dietz R, Reijnders P et al. (2006) A review of the 1988 and 2002 phocine distemper virus epidemics in European harbour seals. *Diseases of Aquatic Organisms* 68, 115–130

Harms CA, McLellan WA, Moore MJ et al. (2014) Low-residue euthanasia of stranded mysticetes. *Journal of Wildlife Diseases* 50, 63–73

Hicks BD and Worthy GAJ (1987) Sealpox in captive grey seals (*Halichoerus grypus*) and their handlers. *Journal of Wildlife Diseases* 23, 1–6

Huuskonen V, Hughes L and Bennett R (2011) Anaesthesia of three young grey seals (*Halichoerus grypus*) for fracture repair. *Irish Veterinary Journal* 64, 1–6

Jepson PD, Deaville R, Acevedo-Whitehouse K et al. (2013) What caused the UK's largest common dolphin (*Delphinus delphis*) mass stranding event? PLoS ONE 8: e60953. doi:10.1371/journal.pone.0060953

Kastelein RA, Bakker MJ and Staal C (1997) The rehabilitation and release of stranded harbour porpoises (*Phocoena phocoena*). In: *The Biology of the Harbour Porpoise*, ed. AJ Read et al., pp. 9–61. De Spil Publishers, Woerden, The Netherlands

King JE (1983) *Seals of the World.* Oxford University Press, Oxford

Kirkwood JK (1983) Influence of body size on animals in health and disease. *Veterinary Record* 113, 287–290

Koopman HN, Westgate AJ and Read AJ (1999) Haematology values of wild harbour porpoises (*Phocoena phocoena*) from the Bay of Fundy, Canada. *Marine Mammal Science* 15, 52–64

Koopman HN, Westgate AJ, Read AJ et al. (1995) Blood chemistry of wild harbour porpoises (*Phocoena phocoena*) (L.). *Marine Mammal Science* 11, 123–135

Lander ME, Harvey JT, Hanni KD *et al.* (2002) Behaviour, movements, and apparent survival of rehabilitated and free-ranging harbour seal pups. *The Journal of Wildlife Management* **66**, 19–28

Lang G, Gagnon A and Geraci JR (1981) Isolation of an influenza A virus from seals. *Archives of Virology* **68**, 189–195

Lonergan M, Hall A, Thompson H *et al.* (2010) Comparison of the 1988 and 2002 phocine distemper epizootics in British harbour seal (*Phoca vitulina*) populations. *Diseases of Aquatic Organisms* **88**, 183–188

Lucas RJ, Barnett J and Riley P (1999) Treatment of lesions of osteomyelitis in the hind flippers of six grey seals (*Halichoerus grypus*). *Veterinary Record* **145**, 547–550

Lynch M and Bodley K (2007) Phocid seals In: *Zoo Animal and Wildlife Immobilization and Anaesthesia*, ed. G West, D Heard and N Caulkett, pp. 459–468. Blackwell Publishing, Iowa

Marine Scotland (2010) *Killing of a seal to alleviate suffering*. Topic Sheet No. 79 v1. www.scotland.gov.uk/Resource/Doc/295194/0104462.pdf

McDonald WL, Jamaludin R, Mackereth G *et al.* (2006) Characterisation of a *Brucella* sp. strain as a marine-mammal type despite isolation from a patient with spinal osteomyelitis in New Zealand. *Journal of Clinical Microbiology* **44**, 4363–4370

McHuron EA, Greig DJ, Colegrove KM *et al.* (2013) Domoic acid exposure and associated clinical signs and histopathology in Pacific harbour seals (*Phoca vitulina richardsii*). *Harmful Algae* **23**, 28–33

Morrison C, Sparling C, Sadler L *et al.* (2012) Post-release dive ability in rehabilitated harbour seals. *Marine Mammal Science* **28**, 110–123

Muller G, Groters S, Siebert U *et al.* (2003) Parapoxvirus infection in harbour seals (*Phoca vitulina*) from the German North Sea. *Veterinary Pathology* **40**, 445–454

Munro R and Synge B (1991) Coccidiosis in seals. *Veterinary Record* **129**, 179–180

Needham DJ (1993) Cetacean strandings. In: *Zoo and Wild Animal Medicine*. Current Therapy 3, ed. ME Fowler, pp. 415–425. WB Saunders, Philadelphia

Nollens H (2005) *Poxvirus infections in North American pinnipeds*. PhD thesis, University of Florida

Nordoy ES (1995) Gastroliths in the harp seal *Phoca groenlandica*. *Polar Research* **14**, 335–338

Osterhaus ADME, Rimmelzwaan GF, Martina BEE *et al.* (2000) Influenza B virus in seals. *Science* **288**, 1051–1053

Reijinders PJH (1986) Reproductive failure in common seals feeding on fish from polluted coastal waters. *Nature* **324**, 456–457

Robinson I (1995) The rehabilitation of seals at the RSPCA Norfolk Wildlife Hospital. *Journal of the British Veterinary Zoological Society* **1**, 13–17

Roess AA, Levine RS, Barth L *et al.* (2011) Sealpox virus in marine mammal rehabilitation facilities, North America, 2007–2009. *Emerging Infectious Diseases* **17**, 2203–2208

Rogan E, Baker JR, Jepson PD *et al.* (1997) A mass stranding of white-sided dolphins (*Lagenorhynchus acutus*) in Ireland: biological and pathological studies. *Journal of the Zoological Society of London* **242**, 217–227

RSPCA (1992) *Stranded Whales, Dolphins and Porpoises. A First Aid Guide*. Royal Society for the Prevention of Cruelty to Animals, Horsham

RSPCA (1997) *Stranded Cetaceans: Guidelines for Veterinary Surgeons*. Royal Society for the Prevention of Cruelty to Animals, Horsham

Simpson VR, Stuart NC, Stack MJ *et al.* (1994) Parapox infection in grey seals (*Halichoerus grypus*) in Cornwall. *Veterinary Record* **134**, 292–296

Sohn AH, Probert WS, Glaser CA *et al.* (2003) Human neurobrucellosis with intracerebral granuloma caused by a marine mammal *Brucella* sp. *Emerging Infectious Diseases* **9**, 485–488

Special Committee on Seals (SCOS) (2012) *Scientific advice on matters related to the management of seal populations: 2012*. www.smru.st-andrews.ac.uk

Stewart BS and Yochem PK (1987) Entanglement of pinnipeds in synthetic debris and fishing net and line fragments at San Nicolas and San Miguel Islands, California, 1978–1986. *Marine Pollution Bulletin* **18**, 336–339

Stoskopf MK, Wilson S and McBain JF (2001) Pharmaceuticals and formularies. In: *CRC Handbook of Marine Mammal Medicine: Health, Disease and Rehabilitation, 2nd edn*, ed. LA Dierauf and FMD Gulland pp. 703–727. CRC Press, Boca Raton, Florida

Swart RL de, Ross PS, Vedder L *et al.* (1994) Impairment of immune function in harbour seals (*Phoca vitulina*) feeding on fish from polluted waters. *Ambio* **23**, 155–159

Sweeney JC (1989) What practitioners should know about whale strandings. In: *Small Animal Practice, 10th edn*, ed. R Kirk, pp. 721–727. WB Saunders, Philadelphia

Sweeney JC and Ridgway SH (1975) Procedures for the clinical management of small cetaceans. *Journal of the American Veterinary Medical Association* **167**, 540–545

Thompson D, Duck CD and Lonergan ME (2010) The status of harbour seals (*Phoca vitulina*) in the United Kingdom. *NAMMCO Scientific Publication* **8**, 117–128

Thompson D, Lonergan M and Duck C (2005) Population dynamics of harbour seals (*Phoca vitulina*) in England: monitoring population growth and catastrophic declines. *Journal of Applied Ecology* **42**, 638–648

Vincent C, Ridoux V, Fedak MA *et al.* (2002) Mark-recapture and satellite tracking of rehabilitated juvenile grey seals (*Halichoerus grypus*): dispersal and potential effect on wild populations. *Aquatic Mammals* **28**, 121–130

Walsh MT, Ewing RY, Odell DK *et al.* (2001) Mass strandings of cetaceans In: *CRC Handbook of Marine Mammal Medicine: Health, Disease and Rehabilitation, 2nd edn*. ed. LA Dierauf and FMD Gulland pp. 83–96. CRC Press, Boca Raton, Florida

Waltzek TB, Cortés-Hinojosa G, Wellehan JFX Jr *et al.* (2012) Marine Mammal Zoonoses: A Review of Disease Manifestations. *Zoonoses and Public Health* **59**, 521–535

Webster RG, Geraci J, Petursson G *et al.* (1981) Conjunctivitis in human beings caused by influenza A virus of seals. *The New England Journal of Medicine* **304**, 911

Wells RS, Fauquier DA, Gulland FMD *et al.* (2013) Evaluating post intervention survival of free-ranging odontocete cetaceans. *Marine Mammal Science* **29**, E463–E483

Wilson S (1999) Radiotelemetry study of two rehabilitated harbour seal pups released close to the natural time of weaning in the wild. *Journal of Wildlife Rehabilitation* **22**, 5–11

Zohari S, Neimanis A, Harkonen T, Moraeus C and Valarcher JF (2014) Avian influenza A (H10N7) virus involvement in mass mortality of harbour seals (*Phoca vitulina*) in Sweden, March through October 2014. *Eurosurveillance* **19(46)**, 1–6

Specialist organizations and useful contacts

Marine mammal rescue organizations

British Divers Marine Life Rescue
Tel: 01825 765546 (during office hours)
Out of hours mobile: 07787 433412

Royal Society for the Prevention of Cruelty to Animals (RSPCA)
Tel: 0300 1234 999

Scottish Society for the Prevention of Cruelty to Animals (SSPCA)
Tel: 03000 999 999

Major seal rehabilitation facilities in the UK

(This list is not exhaustive)

Cornish Seal Sanctuary
Gweek, Cornwall, UK
Tel: 01326 221361

Exploris NIE Seal Sanctuary
Portaferry, Co. Down, UK
Tel: 028 427 28062

Hunstanton Sea Life Sanctuary
Norfolk, UK
Tel: 01485 533576

Mablethorpe Seal Sanctuary and Wildlife Centre
Mablethorpe, Lincolnshire, UK
Tel: 01507 473346

Orkney Seal Rescue
South Ronaldsay, Orkney, UK
Tel: 01856 831463

RSPCA East Winch Wildlife Centre
See Appendix 1

Scarborough Sea Life Sanctuary
North Yorkshire
Tel: 01723 373414

Scottish Sea Life Sanctuary
Oban, Argyll
Tel: 01631 720386

Skegness Natureland Seal Sanctuary
Skegness, Lincolnshire
Tel: 01754 764345

Scottish SPCA National Wildlife Rescue Centre
See Appendix 1

Welsh Mountain Zoo
Colwyn Bay, Conwy
Tel: 01492 532938

National strandings coordinators

(To whom live and dead marine mammal strandings should be reported.)

England and Wales
Institute of Zoology, Cetacean Strandings Investigation Programme (CSIP)
Tel: 0800 652 0333

Scotland
Scottish Marine Animal Stranding Scheme, Inverness
Tel: 01463 243030

In Scotland, seals euthanased to alleviate suffering should be reported to Marine Scotland, Marine Planning and Policy, Area 1-A South, Victoria Quay, Edinburgh EH6 6QQ

Northern Ireland
Department of the Environment Northern Ireland (DOENI)
Tel: 028 7082 3600

Chapter 24

Seabirds

Emma Keeble

Seabirds are defined as birds whose normal habitat and food source is the sea. Seabirds encountered in veterinary practice belong to three main orders (Figure 24.1): Procellariiformes ('tube-noses' such as albatrosses, fulmars, shearwaters, petrels and storm petrels); Pelecaniformes (gannets, pelicans, cormorants and shags); and Charadriiformes (waders, skuas, gulls, terns, and auks such as razorbills, guillemots and puffins). A fourth order (Sphenisciformes – comprising the penguins) is commonly included with seabirds; however, these species are not seen in the wild in the United Kingdom. This chapter will consider only the common species of seabirds that may be presented in the UK. For wading birds and divers, see Chapters 25 and 26, respectively.

The coastlines of Britain and Ireland provide the most important breeding sites for seabirds in the northeast Atlantic Ocean and 25 species breed here regularly. There are great variations in adaptive anatomical features and in nutritional and captivity requirements for the different species; therefore, species identification is of great importance (Figures 24.1 and 24.2).

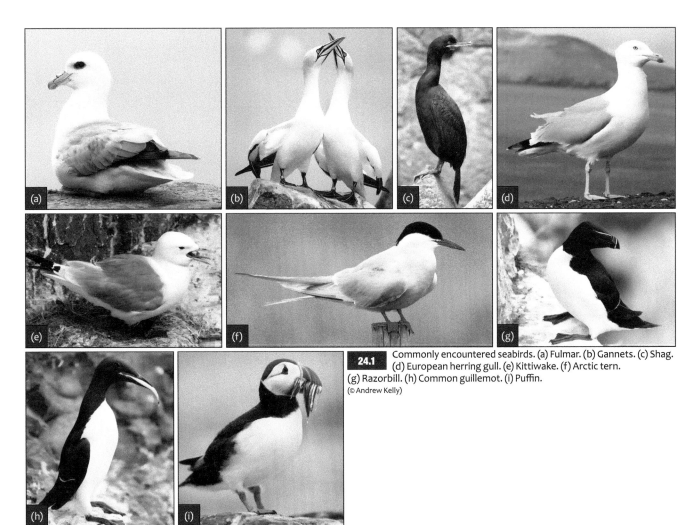

24.1 Commonly encountered seabirds. (a) Fulmar. (b) Gannets. (c) Shag. (d) European herring gull. (e) Kittiwake. (f) Arctic tern. (g) Razorbill. (h) Common guillemot. (i) Puffin.
(© Andrew Kelly)

	Commonly encountered species	Bodyweight range[a]	Natural diet
Order Procellariiformes			
Procellariidae	Fulmar (*Fulmarus glacialis*) (see Figure 24.1a)	650–1000 g	Zooplankton, live fish
	Manx shearwater (*Puffinus puffinus*)	350–545 g	Pilchards, herrings, sprats
Hydrobatidae	European storm petrel (*Hydrobates pelagicus*)	20–38 g	Small fish, zooplankton, crustaceans and small cephalopods
Order Pelecaniformes			
Sulidae	Northern gannet (*Morus bassanus*) (see Figure 24.1b)	2.1–3 kg	Herring, mackerel, sprats, whiting
Phalacrocoracidae	Cormorant (*Phalacrocorax carbo*)	2.1–3.6 kg	Trout, eels, flatfish, perch
	Shag (*Phalacrocorax aristotelis*) (see Figure 24.1c)	1.8–2.2 kg	
Order Charadriiformes			
Laridae	European herring gull (*Larus argentatus*) (see Figure 24.1d)	720–1500 g	Omnivorous: crustaceans, echinoderms, molluscs, earthworms, bird eggs and their young, scavenged refuse from landfill sites Kittiwake diet: small fish, marine invertebrates and plankton
	Black-headed gull (*Chroicocephalus ridibundus*)	200–400 g	
	Lesser black-backed gull (*Larus fuscus*)	650–1000 g	
	Kittiwake (*Rissa tridactyla*) (see Figure 24.1e)	305–525 g	
Sternidae	Sandwich tern (*Sterna sandvicensis*)	180–300 g	Whiting, herring, squid, sand eels, crustaceans
	Common tern (*Sterna hirundo*)	110–141 g	
	Arctic tern (*Sterna paradisaea*) (see Figure 24.1f)	86–127 g	
Alcidae	Razorbill (*Alca torda*) (see Figure 24.1g)	372–645 g	Sand eels, small sprats, crustaceans, molluscs
	Common guillemot (*Uria aalge*) (see Figure 24.1h)	618–870 g	
	Puffin (*Fratercula arctica*) (see Figure 24.1i)	380–500 g	Sprats, whiting, sand eels

24.2 Biological and ecological data for the species of seabird commonly encountered in the UK. [a] Bodyweight varies according to time of year, breeding season, age and sex of bird.

Ecology and biology

Seabirds are adapted to a marine environment and may be found in coastal, offshore or pelagic (open sea) habitats. Species vary widely in their lifestyle and ecology, primarily dependent on breeding and feeding habits. In general, seabirds breed once a year, during late spring, when they congregate in large colonies. These colonies are usually found on islands, cliffs or headlands and nesting sites can be on rocky ledges, in burrows or directly on the ground. Seabirds often have only one clutch of eggs per year, with a small number of eggs laid (some species, for example common guillemots (*Uria aalge*) and razorbills (*Alca torda*), only lay one egg). Sexes are usually similar in appearance (with the exception of the European herring gull (*Larus argentatus*), in which females are smaller than males). Juvenile plumage may vary from that of adults (e.g. gannets (*Morus bassanus*) and common gulls (*Larus canus*)).

Following the breeding season, several seabird species migrate, the most notable being the Arctic tern (*Sterna paradisaea*), which has the longest migration recorded for any bird (70,000 km round trip from pole to pole) (Egevang *et al.*, 2010). Other species migrate away from breeding sites in search of food sources and their distribution is determined by food availability. Juvenile birds often disperse further than adults. Some species, such as cormorants (*Phalacrocorax carbo*), remain all year round at their breeding sites. There are some seabirds that spend most of their lives at inland water sources such as lakes and rivers (e.g. cormorants) or living on agricultural land or in urban environments (e.g. common gulls).

Biological and ecological data for the species commonly encountered in the UK is given in Figure 24.2. Some of the more common species are shown in Figure 24.1.

Anatomy and physiology

Seabirds in general have several anatomical and physiological adaptations to their aquatic lifestyle. (Plumage is discussed later under 'Oiling'.)

Posture

The legs are situated in a caudal position on the body; this is more effective for propulsion and agility in the water. The posture is upright and on land weight is borne on the caudal lower limb, which means that severe leg and foot problems are common in captivity.

Adaptations to diving

Diving birds are adapted anatomically to resist pressure and physiologically to withstand shortage of oxygen (see 'Anaesthesia and analgesia'). The muscles are deep red due to large amounts of myoglobin, used during diving for storing oxygen. Deep-diving birds have the ability to close the external ear canal. The eyes of most diving birds (except terns) are specially adapted for amphibious vision. In some species the eyes are positioned forward on the face for binocular vision, allowing them to judge distances accurately, for example the gannet.

Gastrointestinal tract

Seabirds have simple stomachs, with an elongated glandular proventriculus leading into a small ventriculus. Bills are adapted to the type of food eaten and method of prey capture, which is primarily fish (see Figure 24.2).

Body temperature

The body temperature ranges from 38.8 to 41°C. The arteriovenous countercurrent flow mechanism in the tarsi conserves heat.

Salt glands

Seabirds excrete large amounts of salt, which is ingested with food and water. Excess salt is eliminated not through the kidneys but through salt glands, which open into the nasal fossa. Paired glands are situated at the anterior angles of the orbit and are usually bi-lobed. Secretions run along the beak, or into the mouth in those species with internal nares (e.g. gannet). These glands excrete chlorine, sodium, potassium and water. They function intermittently, depending on the blood salt concentration; hence birds are able to adapt from a freshwater environment to a marine one. Uptake of electrolytes across the intestinal mucosa triggers secretion from the nasal glands; therefore, any factor affecting intestinal absorption will influence the bird's ability to survive in a saltwater environment. Failure to provide salt in captivity may, in theory, result in atrophy of these glands, leading to dehydration when the bird drinks saltwater on release.

Order-specific adaptations

Procellariiformes

- Nares: covered dorsally by a keratinized tubular flap, the operculum.
- Stomach oils: produced from complex species-specific mixtures of monoester waxes, oils, triglycerides and other organic substances and stored in large amounts (100–200 ml) in the proventriculus. Regurgitation of stomach oils is a means of defence.

Pelecaniformes

- Nares: closed by opercula as an adaptation to diving from a great height. Breathing is through the corners of the mouth, via normal extensions of the keratinaceous plates of the upper bill (Figure 24.3). The horny lid closes during diving.
- Air sac diverticula (gannets): track subcutaneously, along fascial planes, between skeletal muscles, over neck and sternum. They act as pneumatic shock absorbers when diving and may inflate when stressed. They are evident radiographically.

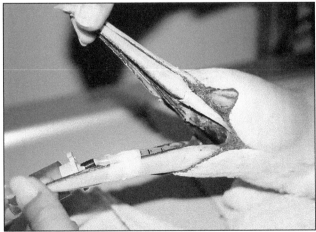

24.3 Gannet bill showing keratinaceous plates of the upper bill and intubation for gaseous anaesthesia.

Charadriiformes: auks

- Diving: aided by heavier skeletal structure and reduced air sacs.
- Body temperature: layer of fat acts as heat insulator against cooling of water (see 'Anaesthesia and analgesia').
- Seasonal moult: flightless period associated with decreased appetite and potential increased incidence of disease.

Capture, handling and transportation

Seabirds often vocalize loudly on capture. Their main defensive weapon is the sharp beak, though the claws may cause scratches. Extreme care should be taken when handling these birds and they should never be held close to the face as injury can easily occur from stabbing movements with the beak. Goggles or safety glasses are recommended. In species with internal nares (gannets), care must be taken that the beak is not held closed. Care should be taken with their plumage as contaminants, damage or feather disruption could affect the bird's waterproofing. (See also Chapter 3 for handling techniques.)

Capture

1. Always stand between the water and the bird, since it will try to return to water.
2. Approach slowly from the side. Throw a net, towel or coat over the bird.
3. Once it is covered, locate the bird's head and grasp its neck firmly, just behind the head.
4. Keeping hold, remove the covering, but keep the bird's head covered at all times to reduce stress.
5. Quickly wrap a towel lightly around the wings, to prevent flapping. In large species, restrain the wings and body between the knees, taking care not to apply too much pressure on the bird. Take care not to contaminate or disrupt feathers (this could affect waterproofing).
6. Keep the beak held closed with a rubber band or bandage tape. In species with internal nares, place a small gag such as rubber tubing, toothbrush or syringe plunger between the upper and lower beak before applying tape, to ensure that the bird can breathe. A short piece of plastic tubing can be placed over the tip of the bird's beak to prevent stabbing injuries to the handler.

Handling

- Use subdued lighting; cover the head; minimize actual handling time.
- Do not use thick leather gloves or gauntlets (except when handling gannets) – they are cumbersome and make gripping difficult.
- Do not handle dyspnoeic birds; administer oxygen first.
- Goggles or safety glasses should be worn when handling seabirds, especially cormorants or gannets.
- Grasp the neck firmly just behind the head and restrain the wings against the body (Figures 24.4 and 24.5). A towel may be used to wrap the wings against the body and at the same time cover the head to reduce stress.

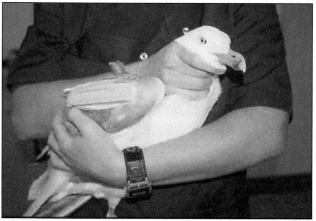

24.4 Restraint technique for handing an adult European herring gull.

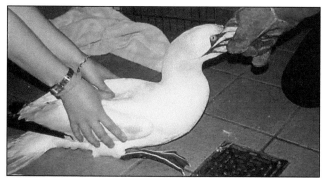

24.6 When handling gannets, gloves should be worn as these birds can inflict severe injuries with their beaks. Gannets will try to stab the gloved hand as it approaches and the beak can be caught and restrained with the mouth open (as pictured). A second person can then safely restrain the wings and body for examination.

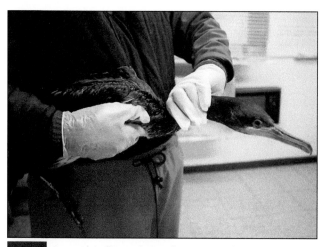

24.5 Correct handling technique for restraint of a cormorant.

Examination and clinical assessment for rehabilitation

General principles, as detailed in Chapter 4, apply to the examination and assessment of seabird casualties.

Clinical examination

The following points are important in seabirds:

- Assessment of the oral cavity (for mucous membrane colour, presence of fishing hooks or lines)
- Thoracic auscultation (aspergillosis is common in captivity)
- Assessment of body condition by pectoral muscle mass palpation (a good indicator of health status in these species) (see Chapter 4). Birds that are underweight (Figure 24.7) may have a reduced post-release survival rate; they often have systemic disease or heavy endoparasite burdens. Seabirds are more likely to be underweight at certain times of the year (e.g. the moulting season in auks)
- Assessment of plumage condition (ectoparasites are common in debilitated birds; seabirds are commonly presented with oil contamination of the feathers)
- Palpation of wings and legs for fractures (common findings in debilitated seabirds).

Transportation

Any ventilated container may be used, as long as it is large enough for the bird to sit in without damage to its tail feathers. There should be a non-slip base, such as a towel, blanket, cloth or mat. In the author's experience, cases of splay leg and bilateral partial paresis may occur in auks following transportation in cardboard boxes with no lining. The beak restraint should be removed before transportation, as seabirds commonly regurgitate under stress and asphyxiation may occur.

Health and safety considerations

Gannets, cormorants and auks (Alcidae) are some of the most dangerous seabirds to handle, their powerful beaks being used for defence. The gannet's beak has sharp serrated edges, which can cause severe lacerations to a bare arm. A two-person approach may be required (Figure 24.6).

Zoonoses

Seabirds, particularly gulls, may transmit zoonoses, for example *Salmonella* Typhimurium, *Campylobacter* spp. and *Chlamydia psittaci*, though this is rare.

Good hygienic practice (washing hands, use of disinfectants) should prevent transmission. (See also Chapter 7.)

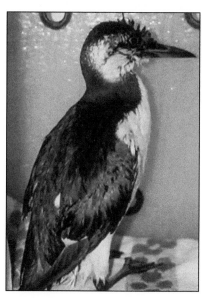

24.7 A thin and weak common guillemot. Note the poor feather quality.

Assessment for rehabilitation

Poor prognostic signs include emaciation, a heavy ecto-parasite burden and wing or leg fractures, especially if open or adjacent to a joint. Euthanasia should be considered in these cases. It is essential that seabirds, once released to the wild, are able to fly, swim and dive in order to catch food and survive. Fracture repair would need to be excellent to ensure that this was the case. These birds do not tolerate prolonged periods in captivity and this should be taken into account when triage decisions are being made.

Diagnostic techniques

Basic diagnostic tests, which can be carried out with minimal stress to the bird, include radiography and blood sampling. Faecal parasitology and bacterial culture are also commonly used.

Radiography

Fractures may not be easily detected on clinical examination, particularly those involving the shoulder joint, and radiographs help to assess the severity and prognosis of the condition. The author has commonly seen airgun and shotgun pellet injuries in seabirds (Figure 24.8). Ingested fishing hooks (common in cormorants and gulls) are easily detected on radiography (see Figure 24.15).

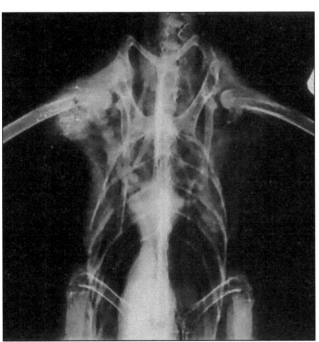

24.8 Ventrodorsal radiographic view of a gannet that was presented with a dropped wing. The right proximal humerus is fractured and there is evidence of metallic fragments consistent with a firearm injury.

Blood sampling techniques and clinical values

The maximum safe volume of blood that can be collected from a healthy bird is 1% of bodyweight. A topical local anaesthetic cream (e.g. EMLA® cream) may be applied a minimum of 30 minutes prior to venepuncture. The use of this product is anecdotally reported and care should be taken as topical local anaesthetics could be systemically absorbed and are toxic to birds at lower doses than in mammals. The following points should be noted:

- For blood sampling and administration of intravenous fluids, the medial metatarsal vein is preferred by the author as it is easily visualized and restraint for sampling from this site is well tolerated by the bird (Figure 24.9). The ulnar and jugular veins may also be used, but restraint of the wing in some seabirds (particularly auks) is often resented
- Red blood cells are larger in seabirds than in other birds (an adaptation to diving)
- Leucocytosis is commonly seen, associated with bacterial, fungal or protozoal infections, with an absolute heterophilia in the former two cases.

Normal haematological and biochemical reference intervals are given in Figures 24.10 and 24.11.

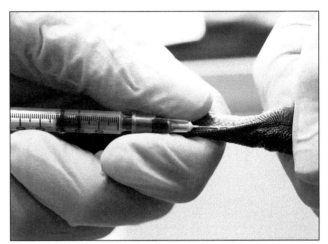

24.9 Obtaining a blood sample from the medial metatarsal vein in a common guillemot.
(© RSPCA, David Couper)

Variable (unit)	Reference interval
Calcium (mmol/l)	2.08–2.77
Inorganic phosphate (mmol/l)	1.41–2.94
Sodium (mmol/l)	152–163
Potassium (mmol/l)	3.3–10
Chloride (mmol/l)	103–121
Bicarbonate (mmol/l)	17–33
Creatinine (µmol/l)	35.4–70.2
Uric acid (µmol/l)	267–1118
Total bilirubin (µmol/l)	0–5.13
Conjugated bilirubin (µmol/l)	0–1.71
Glucose (mmol/l)	12.26–17.19
Cholesterol (mmol/l)	8.22–10.95
Creatinine kinase (IU/l)	537–3801
Alkaline phosphatase (ALP) (IU/l)	22–149
Alanine aminotransferase (ALT) (IU/l)	53–216
Aspartate aminotransferase (AST) (IU/l)	117–1491
Gamma-glutamyl transferase (GGT) (IU/l)	0–10
Total protein (g/l)	39–48
Albumin (g/l)	11–14
Globulin (g/l)	26–34

24.10 Biochemical reference intervals in the common guillemot.
(Newman and Zinkl, 1996)

Variable (unit)	Reference intervals			
	Gannet (*Morus bassanus*)	Cormorant (*Phalacrocorax carbo*)	European herring gull (*Larus argentatus*)	Common guillemot[c] (*Uria aalge*)
Red blood cell (RBC) count (x 10¹²/l)	2.64	3.02 1.6–2.3[a]	2.92 1.8–2.4[b]	2.43–3.94
Haemoglobin (g/l)	140	140.5 80.4–130.1[a]	150.9 110.14–140.86[b]	100.2–160.8
Packed cell volume (PCV) (%)	41	45 27–41[a]	43 40–42[b]	33–58
White blood cell (WBC) count (x 10⁹/l)	NDA	6.1–15.5[a]	12.4–18.6	2.0–9.5
Heterophils (x 10⁹/l)	NDA	5.37–13.2[a]	2.6–8.2[b]	1.26–4.86
Lymphocytes (x 10⁹/l)	NDA	0.4–2.17[a]	6.4–12.4[b]	0.08–1.68
Monocytes (x 10⁹/l)	NDA	0–0.12[a]	0–1.4[b]	0
Eosinophils (x 10⁹/l)	NDA	0[a]	0–1.6[b]	0.48–4.46
Basophils (x 10⁹/l)	NDA	0–0.49[a]	0.5–1.4[b]	0–0.24
Thrombocytes (x 10⁹/l)	NDA	25–50[a]	NDA	NDA
Fibrinogen (g/l)	NDA	2.06–3.86[a]	NDA	2.64 ± 1.32[d]
Total protein (g/l)	40.5	30.3	30.7	42 ± 8[d]

24.11 Haematological and protein reference intervals in certain species of seabird. NDA = no data available.
(Data from Balasch *et al.*, 1974, except as indicated: [a] Bennett *et al.*, 1991; [b] Averbeck, 1992; [c] Newman and Zinkl, 1996; [d] Newman *et al.*, 2004)

Euthanasia

The author's preferred method of euthanasia is intravenous barbiturate injection using the medial metatarsal vein. Other veins may be used, but restraint for these sites is less well tolerated in some species in the author's experience and can lead to the bird becoming overly stressed. Intrahepatic injection of barbiturate can be used when the peripheral circulation is compromised. This is achieved by palpating the caudal border of the sternum and introducing the needle at a 45-degree angle cranially, to infiltrate the liver.

First aid and short-term hospitalization

Basic principles of wildlife first aid and treatment are discussed in Chapter 5.

Urate deposition leading to visceral gout is a common post-mortem finding in seabirds and is thought to be associated with dehydration. Immediate fluid therapy is therefore paramount in a dehydrated bird.

Initial therapy

The bird should be placed in a quiet environment and housed on soft substrates such as rubber or foam matting, to avoid keel and foot injuries. A warm environment may predispose to overheating in these species, but in a shocked or oiled bird, a thermally neutral environment should initially be provided, such as ambient room temperature (15–20°C). At first, access to open water should be avoided, since ill or oiled seabirds will rapidly become waterlogged and hypothermic. The bird should be encouraged to feed on its own and should be weighed daily.

Fluid therapy

If necessary following clinical assessment of hydration status, fluids should be administered and nutritional support by gavage should be started (Figure 24.12). The

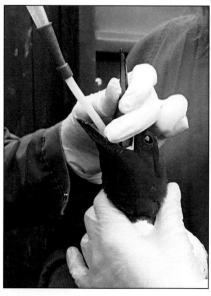

24.12 Tube feeding fluids to a common guillemot. The tube is inserted laterally and passed down the side of the oropharynx to avoid the central glottis.
(© RSPCA, David Couper)

medial metatarsal vein is preferred for intravenous catheter placement and this is well tolerated by seabirds. Intraosseous fluids may be given as for other avian species, although care should be taken as contamination of catheters with faecal material is common in seabirds. Care should be taken when administering subcutaneous fluids in those species with extensive air sac diverticula (see 'Order-specific adaptations'). General principles of avian fluid therapy apply (see Chapter 5).

Continued supportive care with oral fluid therapy may be necessary if dehydration persists. Gavage is as described for other bird species (see Chapter 5). Initially, electrolyte solutions such as Lectade® Plus or Vetark® Critical Care Formula, should be used. After 24 hours, Emeraid® Piscivore should be commenced, or similar liquid formula diets. Emeraid® Piscivore is a fish-oil based diet with fat levels that can be modified from 5% to 30%. Fish oil is added to Emeraid® powder in-house. Tube-fed formula is absorbed best when the bird is warm and hydrated. If this product is not immediately available the following can be used: two tins of Hill's® Prescription Diet a/d, 10 ml Ensure® Plus (a human liquid nutrition product), half an International Zoological Veterinary Group Aquavits tablet and 1 x 200 mg ferrous sulphate tablet added to 50 ml Lectade® Plus (Robinson, 2009).

The estimated capacity of the proventriculus of seabirds is 50 ml/kg bodyweight and this volume should be tolerated for each feed (Stoskopf and Kennedy-Stoskopf, 1986). However, in the debilitated patient or one with a past history of regurgitation, administer one-third to one-half of the estimated proventriculus volume for the first feed. Increase the volume fed over two to three feeds.

Short-term housing

In a veterinary practice, seabirds can be housed in the short term in a dog or cat cage or plastic Vari-kennel™ on thick towels or rubber matting. The front of the cage should be covered to minimize stress and a large, deep bowl of water should be provided. The cage will need to be cleaned regularly as faecal material builds up quickly and can contaminate the feathers, potentially affecting waterproofing.

Anaesthesia and analgesia

General principles of avian anaesthesia apply to seabirds, but the diving ability of many of these species may lead to breath-holding on induction and predispose to metabolic acidosis. Seabirds are adapted anatomically to resist pressure and physiologically to withstand shortage of oxygen, which is a problem when gaseous induction techniques are used. See Figure 24.21 for anaesthetic drug dose rates in seabirds. Specific considerations for anaesthesia are discussed here.

Preoperative period

A period of fasting is required, since regurgitation on handling and induction is common in seabirds. As a general rule, for elective procedures, birds should not be fed on the morning of the planned anaesthetic. Prolonged fasting is not recommended as it leads to hypoglycaemia and dehydration, due to their high metabolic rates.

General anaesthesia

- Interdigital webbing pinch and corneal reflexes can be used for monitoring levels of anaesthesia.
- Hyperthermia is common, particularly in anaesthetized auks: a layer of fat acts as a heat insulator against the cooling action of water as an adaptation for diving in a cold environment for prolonged periods.
- Hypothermia may also occur and should be prevented as in other avian species (see Chapter 6). Cloacal temperature should be recorded throughout anaesthesia and on recovery.

Inhalation anaesthesia

Induction using sevoflurane gaseous anaesthesia with a facemask is preferred by the author. Isoflurane may be used in the absence of sevoflurane. It should be remembered that breath-holding can occur.

For birds with long beaks (e.g. gannet), a latex glove may be attached to the facemask and the bird's beak introduced through a hole cut in the fingers to provide a tight seal (Figure 24.13).

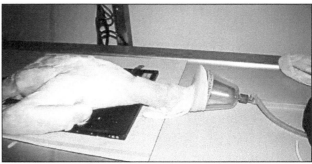

24.13 An anaesthetized gannet undergoing radiographic examination.

Once gaseous induction has been carried out, the bird should be intubated (see Figure 24.3).

Injectable anaesthesia

General principles apply (see Chapter 6 and Figure 24.21).

Specific conditions

Trauma

Traumatic injuries secondary to entanglement in fishing line or nets, ingestion of fishing hooks and lines, and shotgun or air rifle pellets are common in seabirds. Cormorants, shags and gulls more commonly encounter humans than do other species and are particularly prone to traumatic injuries. The author has also seen gannets with humeral and femoral fractures caused by shotgun pellets (see Figure 24.8). Lead toxicity secondary to ingestion of lead weights or shot is theoretically possible but seems to be rare (see Chapter 26). Fishing hook and line injuries (Figures 24.14 and 24.15) should be treated as in other avian species (see Chapter 26).

When surgically preparing the operation site, care should be taken not to pluck too many feathers as this will prevent the bird returning to the water immediately following surgery. Care should also be taken with surgical skin preparations, since these may affect feather waterproofing.

Wing or leg fractures in seabirds carry a poor prognosis. It is essential that the bird is totally fit before being released back to the wild following repair. This is difficult to achieve in a gannet, for example, which hits the water from a height of 35 m when diving. Avian bone healing on average takes 3 weeks, during which time the bird will be vulnerable to

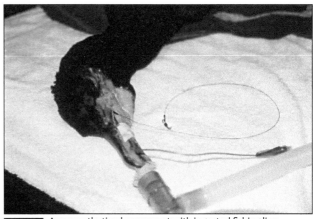

24.14 An anaesthetized cormorant with ingested fishing line evident.

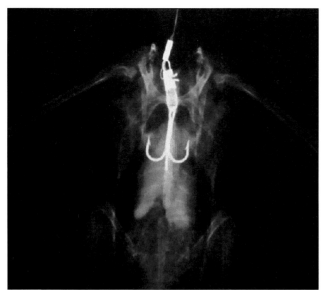

24.15 Ventrodorsal whole body radiograph of a black-headed gull (*Chroicocephalus ridibundus*) showing an ingested fishing hook. This bird was euthanased due to the size and position of the hook. The author, however, has had good success removing smaller oesophageal hooks with no associated soft tissue injury that are located over the heart base, using a flexible endoscope and endoscopic retrieval forceps.

captivity-associated problems (see 'Management in captivity'). Gulls are an exception: they tolerate fracture repair exceedingly well in the author's experience.

Toxins and poisons

Seabirds are positioned near the top of the food chain, making them susceptible to accumulation of toxic compounds. Toxic compounds accumulate in higher concentrations than in humans, indicating that seabirds are less able to metabolize toxic contaminants, leading to a higher risk of exposure. Substances such as heavy metals (e.g. zinc, mercury and lead) and pesticides (e.g. dichlorodiphenyltrichloroethane (DDT)) or industrial pollutants (e.g. polychlorinated biphenyls) accumulate in heavily contaminated areas in fish, on which seabirds feed. DDT may affect the salt gland, inhibiting secretions and also osmoregulation. Clinical signs include muscle tremors, nystagmus and convulsions that do not respond to atropine. Deaths may occur, often in large numbers.

Polychlorinated biphenyls (PCBs) are industrial by-products that have been implicated in reproductive failure, embryonic death, a reduced hatching rate, increased susceptibility to infection and chronic debilitation. Legislation to control the use and disposal of environmental toxins has gone some way to improving the situation; however, environmental pollution with persistent synthetic organic compounds continues to be a considerable cause for concern by environmentalists.

Natural toxins also occur; phytoplankton are algae which, given correct environmental conditions, may increase in numbers to produce algal blooms. This in turn can result in an increase in release of toxins produced by the phytoplankton, neurotoxins in particular. Algal blooms may be associated with a local change in sea colour, hence the term 'red tide'. Organisms involved include *Gymnodinium* spp. and *Gonyaulax* spp. (which causes paralytic shellfish poisoning in humans) and these may affect seabirds following ingestion of affected fish, shellfish or invertebrates. Sudden death occurs in large numbers of seabirds.

In general, poisoning (or infectious causes) should be suspected if different species of seabird are presented from the same area with similar clinical signs. Treatment is usually supportive, and prognosis is often poor. See also Chapter 5.

Botulism

Botulism is a common problem, occurring particularly during the summer in gulls. It is caused by the ingestion of the neuroparalytic toxin of the anaerobic bacterium *Clostridium botulinum*, the most common toxin type affecting birds being Type C, although Type A has been reported in gulls in Britain (Ortiz and Smith, 1994) and Type E in North America. Intoxication is rare in seabirds other than gulls since *C. botulinum* does not survive well in seawater. Occasional deaths do occur and these may be associated with shallow water during the summer months. Dead animals, and the maggots feeding on them, provide the medium for bacterial growth and toxin production. These in turn may be eaten by fish or birds and outbreaks commonly occur concentrated in one area. Gulls scavenging from rubbish tips are also at risk of ingesting the toxin. Clinical signs (acute onset flaccid paralysis) and treatment are described in Chapter 26. The prognosis for recovery in gulls is good following supportive care, even in individuals with advanced clinical signs.

Oiling

Large oil spills have inevitable knock-on effects on marine life, particularly surface-swimming and diving seabirds. Fortunately these incidences are relatively rare and protocols are in place in the UK and elsewhere to deal with oiled seabirds should such a disaster occur (e.g. Scottish Society for the Prevention of Cruelty to Animals (Scottish SPCA) Oil Pollution Plan (Speed, 2002)). What is more likely is that the veterinary surgeon (veterinarian) in practice may encounter individual birds that have become oiled through minor spills, illegal dumping and background pollution. Oiled birds can be presented at any time of the year and in varying states of body condition (Figure 24.16).

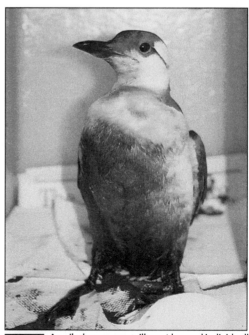

24.16 An oiled common guillemot housed individually on soft blanket material.

Oil pollution has two main effects on seabirds:

- It coats the feathers, affecting buoyancy, waterproofing and insulation, leading to hypothermia and drowning
- It causes direct toxicity, particularly affecting the gastrointestinal tract as birds attempt to preen the oil from the feathers.

Environmental effects: Large oil spills may result in catastrophic environmental effects, such as contamination of food sources and nesting habitats, reduction in fertility and egg hatchability, and reduction in production of future food sources. The severity will depend on the type of oil spilt, the size of the spill, environmental conditions (e.g. weather and tides) and the proximity of susceptible marine life and their habitat.

External effects:
Disruption of waterproofing: Intact feathers have interlocking barbs and barbules, which act to provide the basis of waterproofing and insulation. A lattice structure is formed, with air pockets in between. The feather repels water due to the air–water interface that is formed. The extent of the waterproofing depends on the anatomy of the contour feathers, with cormorants having a less efficient structure that requires them to dry out on land after a period in water. It should be noted that oils from the uropygial gland (or preen gland) play no part in waterproofing the feathers.

The act of preening has two primary functions in birds. First, it spreads the oils from the uropygial gland on to the feathers; this gland secretes an oily substance, primarily comprising fatty acids, which acts to maintain the strength and suppleness of the feathers, increasing their lifespan and preventing them from becoming dry and brittle. Secondly, preening rearranges feathers that are misaligned, reuniting barbs and barbules to maintain a waterproof layer.

When a bird becomes oiled, the interlocking structure is destroyed, leading to a loss in waterproofing and insulation. The bird may be unable to fly, cannot feed and may drown. The bird's metabolic rate increases to maintain body temperature, so it loses weight. Hypothermia is life-threatening and ensues rapidly once the feathers are disrupted and cold water contacts the skin. Seabirds in this condition will seek land, coming ashore on beaches (Miller and Welte, 1999).

Burns and lesions: Other common external effects include chemical burns, with skin irritation and blistering, and ocular lesions such as corneal ulceration and conjunctivitis.

Internal effects: Many systemic toxic effects of oil have been documented in seabirds and the severity of these will depend on the oil type encountered. The most toxic are refined lighter oils, which have had the tar fraction removed (Robinson, 2009). Toxins affect the respiratory tract, gastrointestinal tract, pancreas, liver, kidney and haemopoietic system. Hypothermia, dehydration and stress combine to worsen the clinical picture.

Preening, a normal behavioural response to oiling, increases ingestion of toxins. Toxin ingestion and stress cause mucosal ulceration and haemorrhage throughout the gastrointestinal tract, resulting in severe necrotic enteritis and secondary bacterial infection. This disrupts electrolyte balance and prevents nutrient absorption, leading to dehydration, diarrhoea, bloody faeces, anaemia and reduced plasma total protein levels.

Pneumonia is common, with pulmonary haemorrhage and oedema following inhalation of the lighter volatile fractions. This is usually fatal. Inhalation of oil or regurgitated fluid may also occur, leading to aspiration pneumonia.

Renal failure secondary to direct toxicity and dehydration is often encountered. Visceral gout is a common post-mortem finding in oiled seabirds.

Other less obvious toxic effects of oil include reduced growth rates, reduced fertility rates, reduced function of the salt gland, immunosuppression, lymphoid depletion of the spleen, increased hepatic mixed-function oxidase activity and reduced endocrine gland function, such as adrenal activity. Problems associated with keeping seabirds in captivity, as discussed later, are extremely common in oiled birds.

Haemolytic anaemia following oil ingestion has been well documented, with birds becoming severely anaemic 4–6 days after intoxication (Yamato et al., 1996). Packed cell volume (PCV) may initially be falsely elevated due to dehydration.

Initial assessment and triage: This may take place at the site of capture or nearby. Birds should be transported only short distances prior to assessment and stabilization.

1. Record bodyweight. Body condition may be assessed by palpation of the pectoral muscle mass. Normal bodyweights (see Figure 24.2) will vary according to the time of year, age and sex of the bird and so these should be used only as an approximate guide. Oiled common guillemots have been found to weigh on average less (499–713 g) than those that have been found drowned in nets (851–1095 g) (V Simpson, personal communication). Decisions to euthanase should be based on assessment of body condition rather than weight as there is considerable variation in body size between birds of the same species. However, some protocols suggest euthanasia of any bird weighing less than 600 g (Thomas, 2005).
2. Record cloacal temperature. Normal values in seabirds vary between 38.8 and 41°C. A temperature below 32.5°C carries a poor prognosis (Robinson, 2009).
3. Assess hydration status (see Chapter 5).
4. Carry out a brief clinical examination, with the least possible stress to the bird. There should be a quick visual inspection of the eyes, periorbital area, nares, beak and oropharynx. The neck, abdomen, vent and feather condition should be assessed. Auscultation of the heart (over the sternum), lungs (over the dorsum) and caudal air sacs (over the ventral abdomen) should be carried out. Birds with underlying disease should be isolated or euthanased.
5. A blood sample should be taken to assess PCV and total protein (TP). These are useful indicators of hydration status, anaemia and hypoproteinaemia.

Normal values in seabirds are: PCV 35–55%; and TP 35–55 g/l; and glucose 8.33–13.88 mmol/l (for species-specific values, see Figures 24.10 and 24.11). PCV below 25% and TP below 20 g/l may give rise for concern (Newman et al, 2004). In large oil spills, PCV of less than 20% has been used as a criterion for euthanasia (D Couper, personal communication).

Birds with hypothermia, poor body condition and severe dehydration have little chance of survival and should be euthanased. Moribund birds, dyspnoeic birds or birds with severe traumatic injuries are also candidates for euthanasia at this stage.

Initial treatment: Birds should be stabilized prior to washing. Treatment is aimed at correcting dehydration and hypothermia and preventing further preening and ingestion of oil.

Fluid therapy: In any oiled bird presented for treatment, 10% dehydration should be assumed. A bird that can lift its head should be given a warm electrolyte solution (e.g. Lectade® or Vetark® Critical Care Formula) by crop tube. For calculation of fluid volumes, see Chapter 5. Severely debilitated birds may be given intravenous fluid boluses, but care should be taken to be as aseptic as possible, to avoid contamination with oil. For this reason, the routine use of indwelling catheters is not recommended in oiled birds.

Adsorbents, such as activated charcoal, should be added routinely to the electrolyte solution to reduce further absorption of toxins.

Hypothermia: Prior to washing oiled birds, it is essential to provide warmth. Warming should be gradual until a core body temperature of 38.8–41°C is reached. Blown heated air is ideal or alternatively heat lamps should be used. Ambient temperature, once normal body temperature is reached, should be maintained at 22–25°C.

Ingestion of oil: Oil should be removed from inside and around the beak with paper towels. The use of 'ponchos' to cover the bird and prevent further preening is not recommended, since they cause further stress to the bird.

Prophylactic antifungal and antibiotic treatment: In high-risk cases, prophylactic antifungal (e.g. oral itraconazole) and antibacterial treatment may be indicated. Some wildlife centres routinely administer antifungal treatment to indoor-housed seabirds after initial rehydration (D Couper, personal communication). For dose rates, see Figure 24.21.

Ocular lesions: Corneal ulceration and conjunctivitis are commonly encountered secondary to initial oil contamination and also following washing with a detergent. Clinical signs include blepharospasm, corneal oedema and epiphora. Ulcers may take up fluorescein dye. Topical eye preparations – ocular lubricant, or antibiotic eye ointment if there is evidence of infection – should be used and may be applied prophylactically prior to washing.

Chemical burns and skin irritation: Depending on the type of oil pollution, varying degrees of skin irritation and blister formation may be present. Oil should be removed from the legs and feet on arrival to minimize the topical effects. Topical treatment may be indicated. The feet and legs should be cleaned daily with dilute warm saltwater, and a barrier ointment such as petroleum jelly applied to prevent drying and cracking of the skin. Once the bird has been washed, topical treatments should be avoided in case of feather contamination. Pressure sores related to time spent in captivity are discussed later.

Traumatic injuries: Severe open wounds and open fractures are difficult to treat in an oiled bird since oil contamination is common. These cases should be assessed individually but a decision to euthanase the bird may need to be made. Beak fractures, wing-tip fractures, carpal luxations, keel wounds and traumatic leg injuries are common. Treatment, if possible, is as for similar injuries in other birds (see Chapter 5), but these injuries in oiled birds often carry a poor prognosis.

Continual and pre-release assessment: After initial stabilization, daily continual assessment is essential. Individual birds should be identified and a record of treatment given, bodyweight, feeding regimes, blood test results and washes should be updated daily. Birds should be monitored carefully for clinical signs of chronic effects of oil pollution, such as regurgitation, melaena, haemorrhagic faeces, biliverdinuria, dyspnoea, pressure sores and mucous membrane pallor. Weekly blood sampling will aid clinical assessment and may be performed during times of handling for husbandry changes (e.g. moving to an outside pool).

A clinical examination should also be performed at this time to assess body condition and monitor for husbandry associated problems (e.g. keel and hock sores). Some protocols recommend releasing birds only when over 800 g in bodyweight (Thomas, 2005). Washing may be delayed until PCV values return to above 30% (D Couper, personal communication). In one study, a decreased phosphorus level, elevated creatine phosphokinase (CPK) level and elevated fibrinogen concentration were associated with a lower likelihood of survival post-release (Newman *et al.*, 2004). Fibrinogen is an inflammatory protein, elevation of which is associated with inflammation due to oil exposure or infection. This was found to be double the normal range (normal = 264 ± 132 mg/dl) in oiled rehabilitated common guillemots prior to release (Newman *et al.*, 2004). White blood cell counts and differentials should also be performed prior to release to rule out inflammation and infection. A red blood cell (RBC) count, as well as PCV, has been suggested to be a more accurate health assessment prior to release, since in one study there were consistently lower RBC counts in oiled birds compared with healthy birds, whilst there was no statistical difference in PCV observed between the two groups (Newman *et al.* 2004).

Washing techniques: Once a bird is feeding on its own, appears bright and shows no evidence of ill health, it may be considered suitable for washing. The washing process itself is highly stressful and is poorly tolerated by debilitated birds.

Detergent cleansing:
Hand washing: Washing by hand with an appropriate detergent is still the method of choice for cleaning oiled birds, despite other more recent techniques being reported. The current detergent of choice in the UK is Fairy Liquid®. The process is highly specialized and should be attempted only if suitable facilities and trained staff are available.

A sink is needed with a continuous supply of hot (40–45°C) water through a high-pressure (minimum 345 kPa) hand-held shower head. Two operators are required for the cleaning process, one to hold the bird, the other to clean the feathers (Figure 24.17). To prevent operator

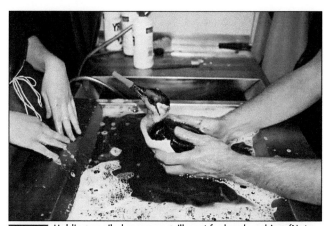

24.17 Holding an oiled common guillemot for hand washing. (Note for operator: safety gloves should be worn until the majority of the oil contaminant has been removed or when there is a risk of skin irritation to handlers.)

injuries, the bird's beak may be taped using a rubber band or rubber nozzle. Extreme care should be taken not to cover the nares. In species with internal nares, a pencil or toothbrush should be used inside the beak prior to taping so that the bird may still breathe (see 'Capture').

The bird is immersed in a solution of detergent at 42°C and the person washing moves the feathers between finger and thumb from base to tip to clean the oil from them. A standard procedure should be followed, working cranially to caudally along the bird. The inside of the beak is carefully cleaned using a soft toothbrush to remove any traces of oil. Cleaning progresses around the beak and head (taking care to avoid the eyes), then along the neck, back and tail feathers, then the bird is rotated on to each side to wash the wing and flank area. Finally the ventral neck, sternum, abdomen and ventral tail feathers are cleaned.

Several cleaning cycles may be necessary, either in one session, or on separate occasions if the bird appears distressed (the cleaning process should be stopped if this occurs). Once the bird is clean, all traces of detergent are removed from the surfaces, sink and handlers prior to rinsing the bird. Rinsing follows the same order as cleaning, making sure that detergent runs away from areas already rinsed and directing the shower jet against the lie of the feathers. Beading of water indicates successful cleaning of feathers (Figure 24.18). Areas where water runs into the feathers will need to be cleaned again.

Machine washing: An automated machine-washing method has been described (Westerhof *et al.*, 1997). This may be useful after large oil spills if washing facilities are not available within a reasonable distance. Washing times are reduced to 10 minutes (compared with 20–40 minutes for hand washing). The bird is placed in a cage with wings held in extension and the head protruding from the top away from the cleaning area. Rotating nozzles spray detergent and then rinse with water. The head is cleaned by hand.

Magnetic cleansing: Other cleansing agents have been tried with some success, such as iron powder (a dry-cleansing agent). Both the contaminant and the cleansing agent may be harvested magnetically (Orbell *et al.*, 2004).

Husbandry after washing: Once washed, birds should be dried in a separate room with a warm air current supplied by heated fans; for individual birds, a hairdryer may be used. Birds are left overnight and are placed on outside pools the following morning to assess waterproofing. Failures at this stage do occur and may be secondary to

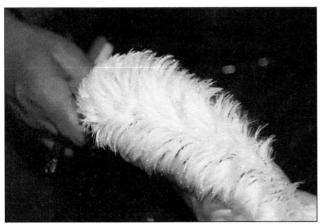

24.18 Once the feathers are free of detergent, the water forms beads, a sign that washing has been successful.

incomplete removal of oil or detergent during the washing process, inadequate skimming of the pool or contamination of the water with fish oils, oily faeces or detergent. Birds that are too weak to preen will also be poorly waterproofed.

Birds may take several days on pools to preen and regain waterproofing prior to release (Figure 24.19). They should be monitored carefully during this time for chronic effects of oil toxicity. Survival rates of over 60% have been recorded from rescue to release in some seabird species (Robinson, 2009). However, of those released, only a small percentage survives the first year (6–22%). Grogan *et al.* (2011) reported that in oiled common guillemots, on average, birds remained for 50 days in captivity prior to release. Increased lengths of time in captivity were associated with a greater chance of survival in the wild, but a lower release rate.

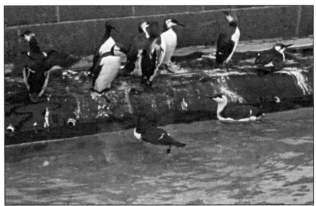

24.19 Common guillemots recuperating in an outside pool following hand washing for oil contamination.

Release: Appropriate sites and weather conditions are essential for release. Oiled birds should not be released where they are in danger of recontamination. Depending on the species and time of year, they may be released on beaches, on cliffs or from boats. They should be released into wind in calm conditions, preferably in groups, at a site where food sources are readily available. Grogan *et al.* (2011) list criteria used by Royal Society for the Prevention of Cruelty to Animals (RSPCA) centres to assess whether an oiled common guillemot is healthy and fit for release (Figure 24.20). Clinical sampling, as described above, is a useful aid to assessment. Survival rates of oiled birds vary according to many different factors, such as the species affected, type of oil spilt, weather conditions and facilities available. Post-release survival rates in auks have been disappointingly low (Sharp, 1996; Wernham *et al.*, 1997). One study found that

- Waterproof
- Floating high on the water
- Eating well
- Generally remaining with a group
- Good, bright eyes
- Walking well, high on webs
- Swimming and diving without any apparent exhaustion
- Feet and hocks in good condition
- Actively using both legs for swimming
- Good weight gain/maintenance
- Consistent normal behaviour
- A record of good activity levels
- Good response to all treatments
- Maintained or improved condition score
- Minimum weight of 800 g
- PCV 40–50%

24.20 List of criteria for release of common guillemots post-oiling. (Grogan *et al.*, 2011)

the highest mortality post-release was within the first 34 days (80% mortality between 15 and 40 days post-release), but if birds survived past this, they had similar mortality rates to non-oiled seabirds (Newman *et al.*, 2004). Mute swans (*Cygnus olor*), jackass penguins (*Spheniscus demersus*) and gulls have higher post-release survival rates and the reasons behind this are still unknown (Golightly *et al.*, 2003). Suggestions have been made that inadequate food sources, immunosuppression, inflammation and bacterial infections, secondary to oil exposure and captivity-related stress, are factors involved in low post-release survival rates in auks (Newman *et al.*, 2004). Concerns still exist over the welfare implications of treating oiled birds; however, recent reports showing higher survival rates in auks (68%) are encouraging (Newman, 2003). Post-release monitoring is essential in future oil spills to further assess the success of any oiled bird rehabilitation and post-release survival rates.

Infectious diseases

Viral diseases

'Puffinosis': The most documented viral disease in seabirds is 'puffinosis', which is endemic in Europe and has been characterized as a group 2a coronavirus (Woo *et al.*, 2009). The virus primarily affects late fledgling chicks. Clinical signs include conjunctivitis, blistering of the foot webbing and spastic paralysis of the legs. Mortality is high in the Manx shearwater (*Puffinus puffinus*) but low in other species, with the exception of the chicks of lesser black-backed and European herring gulls. The virus has been described in oystercatchers (*Haematopus ostralegus*), shags, European herring gulls, lesser and greater black-backed gulls (*Larus fuscus* and *L. marinus*) and fulmars (*Fulmarus glacialis*), where it causes only foot lesions with or without conjunctivitis. It is thought that the virus persists in trombiculid mites overwintering in nesting burrows. It has been suggested that doxycycline may reduce mortality in affected Manx shearwater chicks (Brooke, 1990).

Newcastle disease: Paramyxovirus Type 1 (Newcastle disease) has been identified in seabirds, which may act as a reservoir of infection. Reported cases have occurred in guillemots, puffins (*Fratercula arctica*), cormorants and gannets (Stoskopf and Kennedy-Stoskopf, 1986). Clinical signs, diagnosis and post-mortem changes are as for other avian species.

Other viruses: Several virus types have been isolated in birds following oiling or stress, but are not thought to be a significant cause of disease. Other viruses which may be encountered in seabirds include avipox, adenovirus in guillemots and European herring gulls, and influenza viruses. Epizootic outbreaks of avian influenza have been reported in seabirds and carrier status may occur in scavenger species, particularly gulls.

Bacterial diseases

Bacterial infections are common in seabirds and numerous types have been reported, usually at post-mortem examination. Most infections are enteric, resulting in lethargy, urate soiling of the vent and anorexia. Diagnosis is based on cloacal swab culture in the live bird. Treatment with fluid therapy and systemic antibiotics (based on culture and sensitivity) may be indicated. These infections are potentially more common in captivity, associated with stress. Typically encountered bacteria include *Escherichia coli*, *Klebsiella* spp., *Clostridium perfringens*, *Salmonella* Typhimurium, *Campylobacter* spp. and *Listeria* spp.

The latter three have often been found in gulls and these birds have been implicated as potential health hazards to humans via zoonotic spread (Quessy and Messier, 1992). *Chlamydia psittaci*, another zoonotic organism, has also been reported in gulls (Franson and Pearson, 1995). Where there is a serious zoonotic risk, the decision to euthanase the bird may be necessary. The risk is highest where large numbers of gulls are in contact with humans (e.g. at seaside resorts).

Mycobacterium avium has been found in gulls and may be zoonotic. Infection may be associated with lameness secondary to bone infection. Diagnosis is based on clinical signs and radiography in the live bird; however, more often the bird is euthanased due to the severity of the clinical signs and the infection is diagnosed at post-mortem with granulomatous lesions often evident in the liver and spleen. Prolonged culture is necessary for this organism, but special stains (Ziehl–Neelson) may demonstrate the presence of acid-fast Gram-positive bacilli. Other bacterial causes of lameness, resulting in septic arthritis in the author's experience, include *Staphylococcus aureus* and *Salmonella* Typhimurium joint infections. Treatment with systemic antibiotics and joint lavage is rarely successful and euthanasia is often indicated in these cases. Bacterial infections can also be the cause of sudden mass deaths in seabirds, for example avian cholera (*Pasteurella multocida*).

Fungal diseases

Aspergillus fumigatus is frequently found in seabirds in captivity and is often fatal. *Aspergillus flavus* is more rarely encountered. Other fungal infections seen include *Mucor* spp., *Geotrichum candidum* and blastomycosis.

Aspergillosis: Aspergillosis (see Chapter 26) has been reported in puffins, cormorants, guillemots, razorbills and gannets. Seabirds are thought to be predisposed to infection by stress and lack of previous exposure to the fungus. They should never be housed on straw or hay, which are sources of fungal spores. Infection is common in oiled seabirds, associated with immunosuppression and the stress of captivity.

Clinical signs include open-mouthed breathing, inappetence and increased respiratory effort. Sudden death may also occur. Diagnosis is primarily based on clinical signs and auscultation, but radiography may also be useful in advanced cases. Treatment is rarely successful once the infection is established. Prophylactic treatment with itraconazole for at-risk birds is recommended and dose rates of 10–20 mg/kg orally q24h have been used in penguins (Carpenter, 2013).

Parasites

Ectoparasites: Feather lice are common in rescued seabirds. Although they do not cause primary disease, they are an indication that the bird is debilitated. Many different species of lice and mites have been described; they do not directly affect the bird, but they can be an irritation to the handler. Care should be taken with topical treatments, since these can affect the waterproofing of the feathers. Ivermectin can be used topically or by subcutaneous injection at 0.2 mg/kg dose rate, repeated once 10–14 days later (dose extrapolated from other bird species). Ticks are also commonly reported in seabirds and may act as vectors for viruses and bacteria; however, they rarely cause clinical disease.

Endoparasites: Heavy endoparasite burdens are often encountered in seabirds, in particular in moribund or emaciated individuals. It is thought that endoparasite infections in healthy birds rarely cause problems, but they lower resistance to other stressors such as oil pollution or bad weather (Jauniaux *et al.*, 1998). Cestodes, trematodes, nematodes and protozoans have all been regularly reported in seabirds (Stoskopf and Kennedy-Stoskopf, 1986). Cestodes have been commonly reported in petrels (Jones, 1988), as have trematodes (Robinson, 2009).

The most common endoparasites encountered in seabirds are *Contracaecum* spp., nematodes that inhabit the proventriculus. Infection occurs secondary to ingestion of fish containing encapsulated larvae. Treatment with an anthelmintic, such as fenbendazole, is effective. Dose rates of 20 mg/kg orally as a one-off dose have been reported in waterfowl (Carpenter, 2013).

Gapeworm (*Syngamus trachea*) has been seen in gulls; earthworms are the intermediate host (Robinson, 2009). Diagnosis is based on clinical signs (open-mouthed breathing, increased respiratory noise) and faecal microscopy for ova. Treatment with fenbendazole is indicated.

Other conditions

Nutritional disease

Beak and skeletal deformities associated with vitamin D deficiency have been recorded in cormorants in captivity. This should be borne in mind when rearing juvenile seabirds (see 'Supplements'). Abnormal rotation of the carpal joint ('slipped wing', 'airplane wing' or 'angel wing') has also been seen in well fed, rapidly growing wild juvenile cormorants (Kuiken *et al.*, 1999). This condition is common in waterfowl, where it is thought to be related to excessive growth rates caused by overfeeding, high-protein diets, genetic predisposition in some species and deficiencies in manganese, vitamin D and vitamin E (see Chapter 26).

Starvation and emaciation

Seabirds are extremely vulnerable to climatic changes when at sea. Juvenile birds in particular are at risk. Stormy weather, high winds, lack of food sites, long migration routes and heavy parasitism may lead to emaciation and weakness. Many birds may die whilst out at sea, but some are found on the shore or even inland. Supportive care with fluid therapy, anthelmintics and feeding of high-quality fish is indicated. Euthanasia is indicated in severely emaciated and weak birds.

Occasional mass seabird 'die-offs' occur and these are often the first indication of a problem within the marine environment. Pollution with oil or PCBs are most commonly implicated (Pokras, 1996).

During winter months, it is common to find seabirds that have 'crash-landed' inland. Fulmars, gannets and Manx shearwaters seem particularly predisposed. These individuals are normally in good body condition with no obvious abnormalities and should be released as soon as possible at a suitable site.

Therapeutics

Drugs commonly used in seabirds are given in Figure 24.21. Routes of administration of drugs in seabirds are as for other avian species. Care should be taken with

Drug	Dosage	Comments
Antifungal drugs		
Itraconazole	10–20 mg/kg orally q24h	Dose reported in penguins
Antiparasitic drugs		
Fenbendazole	20 mg/kg orally once	Dose extrapolated from waterfowl
Ivermectin	0.2 mg/kg s.c. or topically, repeat once after 10–14 days	Dose extrapolated from other bird species
Anaesthetic drugs		
Propofol	1–5 mg/kg slow i.v.	Slow induction to minimize apnoea, intubation and IPPV recommended. Dose extrapolated from other bird species
Analgesic drugs		
Meloxicam	0.1–0.2 mg/kg i.m., orally q24h	Dose extrapolated from other bird species
Oiled bird treatments		
Activated charcoal	52 mg/kg orally once	Adsorbent given by crop tube
Bismuth subsalicylate	2–5 mg/kg orally once	Adsorbent given by crop tube
Oral electrolyte solutions (e.g. Lectade™ or Vetark® Critical Care Formula)	30–50 ml/kg by crop tube	Reduce volume by 50% in debilitated birds
Thiamine	25–30 mg per kg of fish	Fish-eating species
Vitamin E	100 IU per kg of fish	Fish-eating species

24.21 Drugs and dose rates used in seabirds. IPPV = intermittent positive pressure ventilation. (Carpenter, 2013)

subcutaneous injections in those species that possess extensive subcutaneous air sac diverticula. Oral medications may be administered inside fish, if the bird is eating. There are few published dose rates for drugs in seabirds and dose rates are extrapolated from other bird species.

Management in captivity

Housing

There are common problems associated with keeping seabirds in captivity for prolonged periods. To avoid these, high standards of hygiene and husbandry, along with good housing and ventilation, are essential.

Seabirds are gregarious in nature and should ideally be housed in groups; however, this makes clinical assessment of an individual bird more difficult and predisposes to disease transfer. Initially they may be housed separately to monitor food intake and droppings. Larger species such as gannets and cormorants may be easier to handle if kept singly (Figure 24.22). They are extremely sensitive to disturbance by sudden noise, which should be avoided.

The nature of the substrate is of utmost importance. Pressure sores with secondary ulceration may be seen in seabirds in captivity, involving the sternum, hock (intertarsal joint) and plantar aspect of the foot area (Figure 24.23). Secondary infection with bacteria commonly follows, necessitating euthanasia in severe cases. Substrates should be easy to clean and soft, such as artificial

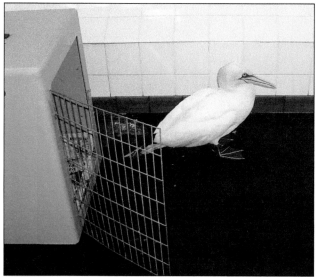

24.22 Simple housing for a gannet. Note the rubber matting to prevent foot sores.

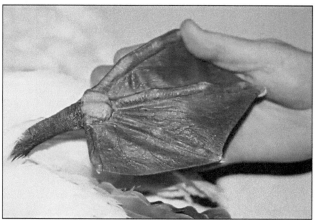

24.23 Early signs of pododermatitis starting to develop on the plantar surface of a gannet's foot (particularly evident at the tarsometatarsal–phalangeal joint).

turf, rubber matting or deep layers of blankets. Straw or hay must be avoided. Netting and waterbed substrates have been used successfully to prevent these lesions from developing and are particularly useful in birds with legs placed caudally that have difficulty moving on land, such as fulmars. Cormorants will climb on to structures such as wooden boxes or overturned buckets and this will keep the feet and tail feathers free from faecal soiling. Auks will climb on to rocks if provided.

Build-up of ammonia from droppings is common and could predispose to respiratory disease, such as aspergillosis. Ventilation should be adequate to cope with this, and 12 air changes per hour are recommended (Robinson, 2009). Access to open water should be provided for all but debilitated or oiled seabirds. Diving birds prefer water deep enough for their feet not to touch the bottom. A padded ramp and platform should be provided for access out of the water if needed. The pool edges should be cleaned regularly to prevent accumulation of faeces; they should be free draining and roughened to avoid pressure sores developing by constant weight-bearing on one part of the lower limb and foot. Water should be constantly skimmed with drains at the level of the water surface to prevent build-up of fish oils, which impair the waterproofing of the plumage and cause thermoregulatory problems (see Figure 24.19).

Diet

For fish-eating birds, the provision of good-quality fish is essential. Fish can be fed fresh or defrosted from frozen in a refrigerator. Water-soluble vitamins leach out of frozen fish thawed at room temperature; the fish should therefore be defrosted slowly in a closed container in a refrigerator for 24–48 hours and then used immediately. Seasonal variations in fish quality occur. A balanced diet may be achieved by providing a variety of fish species and the use of supplements (see 'Supplements'). Strict hygiene is essential to prevent bacterial contamination of fish and ensuing gastrointestinal infections. Seabirds may be encouraged to eat by moving the fish through the water or injecting fish with air so that they float. Fish should be offered in salt water in an appropriate size and depth of container, such that the bird can easily feed.

Debilitated birds should be fed initially by crop tube, which stimulates intestinal peristalsis and appetite (see Figure 24.12). As a general rule, debilitated birds will initially take smaller fish. Petrels may be fed using defrosted krill, available from aquarist suppliers. Gulls are omnivorous and adults may be fed diets described for juveniles (see 'Rearing of juvenile seabirds'). Assisted feeding may also be necessary (Figure 24.24) and may commence with small sprats for most species or small mackerel for gannets. The bird's mouth is opened and the fish is placed head first in the oropharynx. The beak is then closed and the bird should swallow the fish.

Weight of bird (kg)	Weight of whole fish (g) (per feed)	Frequency of feeds (per day)
<0.5	10–35	6–7
0.5–1.5	25–100	5–6
1.5–3	60–180	4–5
3–5	180–369	4

24.24 Recommended weight of fish per feed for assisted feeding of seabirds. Amounts calculated according to the bird's bodyweight.
(Stoskopf and Kennedy-Stoskopf, 1986)

Supplements

Deficiencies in fat-soluble vitamins A, D and E are common in fish-eating birds in captivity. Oily fish, such as mackerel and tuna, are low in vitamin E and feeding such fish to birds may lead to steatitis. Vitamin E should be added to the diet at 100 IU/kg of fish fed.

Marine fish contain high levels of thiaminases, ingestion of which can result in thiamine deficiency, leading to ataxia, abnormal posture, respiratory effort, coma and death. Thiaminase levels are highest in clams, herring and smelt. Thiamine should be added to the diet at 25–30 mg/kg of fish fed (Miller and Welte, 1999). Commercial vitamin supplements, containing both thiamine and vitamin E, are available (e.g. Aquavits; Mazuri® Fish Eater tablets).

Problems associated with captivity
Salt gland atrophy

Salt glands may atrophy in seabirds given fresh water in captivity. In species living in fresh or brackish water, such as cormorants and gulls, salt supplementation may not be necessary. Salt glands should be reactivated by gradually increasing the salt content of the diet (e.g. feeding fish in salted water from an appropriate container). Salt tablets are available, but sea salt is just as good.

Pododermatitis and sternal ulceration

These conditions may be seen in captivity (see Figure 24.23), but the incidence is reduced following more rigorous triage and improved captive husbandry techniques (D Couper, personal communication). Application of petroleum jelly may prevent drying of the feet and webbing. Care should be taken not to contaminate the plumage, which would necessitate washing of the bird.

Cloacal impaction

This is common in some diving species. Feathers around the cloaca become rapidly soiled with urates and faeces, leading to impaction. Diagnosis is based on clinical signs and confirmed radiographically. Chronic impaction may lead to stretching of the cloaca and atony, predisposing to further impactions. Euthanasia is indicated in these cases.

Respiratory disease

Aspergillosis is frequently encountered in seabirds in captivity and is often fatal (see 'Fungal diseases'). Seabirds should never be housed on straw or hay, which are sources of fungal spores.

Rearing of juvenile seabirds

With the exception of the gull family, it is rare to encounter juvenile seabirds. This is because juvenile seabirds fledge and migrate out to sea for the first few years of their lives.

Rehabilitation centres may become overrun with 'orphaned' European herring gull chicks during the breeding season each year. They are rarely true orphans and have either fallen from inappropriate nest sites, been picked up by other birds and dropped, or been picked up by well meaning members of the public. They rapidly become habituated to humans and malprinted unless housed in social groups. Release sites are often a problem since European herring gulls are present in large numbers in parts of the UK, particularly coastal towns, where they may be seen as a nuisance and public health concern.

Juvenile gulls should be housed in social groups on padded mats or towels to prevent foot lesions (Figure 24.25). The accommodation should be cleaned out twice daily to prevent build-up of ammonia in the environment. Being omnivorous, the birds may be fed a variety of food items, such as mashed fish-flavoured cat food, finely chopped whitebait, herring, mackerel or day-old chicks (see also Chapter 8). Appropriate avian vitamin and mineral supplements should also be added (e.g. Avimix®).

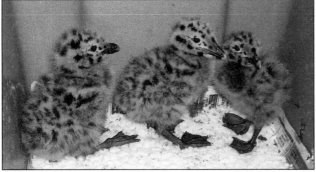

24.25 European herring gull chicks.
(© Secret World Wildlife Rescue)

Release

The release of adult seabirds is usually by a 'hard release' technique (see Chapter 9) in a suitable marine environment, at a time when conspecifics are present and in good weather conditions. Following oiling incidents, release sites away from oil contamination will need to be found.

Legal aspects

Seabirds (together with their nests and any eggs contained within) are protected, as all wild birds are, under the Wildlife and Countryside Act 1981. Gulls have recently become more prevalent in urban areas and can be seen as a nuisance by members of the public. It may be possible, under licence from the relevant local authority, to remove nests or eggs, or even kill certain gull species where there are special circumstances and no alternative solution can be found, for example where there is a proven public health risk, to prevent disease spread, to prevent serious damage to agriculture, to protect other wild bird species or for air safety reasons. It is essential to consult the appropriate country agency (Natural England, or its equivalent in the devolved parts of the UK) for the current licence terms and conditions, prior to taking any action against a gull or its nest site.

Acknowledgements

The author would like to acknowledge David Couper and Adam Grogan for their expertise and help with references and Vic Simpson and Ian Robinson for their comments on an earlier version of this chapter. The author would also like to acknowledge Matthew Wood for proofreading the manuscript.

References and further reading

Averbeck C (1992) Haematology and blood biochemistry of healthy and clinically abnormal great black-backed gulls (*Larus marinus*) and herring gulls (*Larus argentatus*). *Avian Pathology* **21**, 215–223

Balasch J, Palomeque J, Palacios L, Musquera S and Jiminez M (1974) Haematological values of some great flying and aquatic diving birds. *Comparative Biochemistry and Physiology* **49**, 137

Bennett PM, Gascoyne SC, Hart MG *et al.* (1991) *The Lynx Database*. Department of Veterinary Science, Zoological Society of London

Brooke M (1990) *The Manx Shearwater*. T & AD Poyser, London

Carpenter JW (2013) *Exotic Animal Formulary 4th edn*. Elsevier Saunders, Missouri

Cramp S, Bourne W and Saunders D (1974) *The Seabirds of Britain and Ireland*. Collins, London

Croxall JP (1987) *Seabirds: Feeding, Ecology and Role in Marine Ecosystems*. Cambridge University Press, Cambridge

Egevang C, Stenhouse IJ, Phillips RA *et al.* (2010) Tracking of Arctic terns *Sterna paradisaea* reveals longest animal migration. *Proceedings of the National Academy of Sciences of the United States of America*, **107(5)**, 2078–2081

Flammer K (1999) Zoonoses acquired from birds. In: *Zoo and Wild Animal Medicine, Current Therapy 4*, ed. ME Fowler and RE Miller, pp. 151–156. WB Saunders, Philadelphia

Franson JC and Pearson JE (1995) Probable epizootic chlamydiosis in wild Californian (*Larus californicus*) and ring-billed (*Larus delawarensis*) gulls in North Dakota. *Journal of Wildlife Diseases* **31**, 424–427

Furness R and Monaghan P (1987) *Seabird Ecology*. Blackie and Son, Glasgow

Golightly RT, Newman SH, Craig EN, Carter HR and Mazet JA (2003) Post-release survival and behaviour of Western Gulls following exposure to oil and rehabilitation. *Proceedings of the 7th International Effects of Oil on Wildlife conference, Hamburg, Germany, 14–16 October, 2003*

Grogan A, Pulquério MJF, Cruz MJ *et al.* (2011) Factors affecting the welfare of rehabilitation of oiled murres. *Proceedings of the 11th Effects of Oil on Wildlife Conference, New Orleans*, pp. 45–57

Harris MP and Rothery P (2004) Wear of rings used on guillemots *Uria aalge*: caution in the estimation of survival rates. *Ringing and Migration* **22**, 61–62

Jauniaux T, Brosens L, Meire P, Offringa H and Boignoul F (1998) Pathological investigations on guillemots (*Uria aalge*) stranded on the Belgian coast during the winter of 1993–94. *Veterinary Record* **143**, 387–390

Jones HI (1988) Notes on parasites in penguins (*Spheniscidae*) and petrels (*Procellariidae*) in the Antarctic and sub-Antarctic. *Journal of Wildlife Diseases* **24(1)**, 166–167

Joys AC, Clark JA, Clark NA and Robinson RA (2003) *An investigation of the effectiveness of rehabilitation of birds as shown by ringing recoveries.* BTO research report No. 324. BTO, Thetford

King AS and McLelland J (1984) *Birds: Their Structure and Function.* Baillière Tindall, London

Kuiken T, Leighton FA, Wobeser G and Wagner B (1999) Causes of morbidity and mortality and their effect on reproductive success in double-crested cormorants from Saskatchewan. *Journal of Wildlife Diseases* **35**, 331–346

Mazet JAK, Newman SH, Gilardi KVK *et al.* (2002) Advances in oiled bird emergency medicine and management. *Journal of Avian Medicine and Surgery* **16**, 146–149

Miller EA and Welte SC (1999) Caring for oiled birds. In: *Zoo and Wild Animal Medicine, Current Therapy 4*, ed. ME Fowler and RE Miller, pp. 300–309. WB Saunders, Philadelphia

Mitchell PI, Newton S, Ratcliffe N and Dunn TE (2004) *Seabird Populations of Britain and Ireland.* T & AD Poyser, London

Newman SH (2003) Post-release survival of common murres (*Uria aalge*). *Proceedings of the 7th International Effects of Oil on Wildlife conference, Hamburg, Germany, 14–16 October, 2003*

Newman SH, Golightly RT, Craig EN, Carter HR and Kreuder C (2004) *The effects of petroleum exposure and rehabilitation on post-release survival, behavior, and blood health indices: a Common Murre (Uria aalge) case study following the Stuyvesant petroleum spill. Final Report.* Oiled Wildlife Care Network, University of California, Davis

Newman SH and Zinkl J (1996) *Establishment of haematological, serum biochemical and electrophoretogram reference intervals for species of marine birds likely to be impacted by oil spill incidents in the state of California.* Baseline Marine Bird Project for the Californian Department of Fish and Game, Office of Oil Spill Prevention Response

Orbell JD, Ngeh LN, Bigger SW *et al.* (2004) Whole-bird models for the magnetic cleansing of oiled feathers. *Marine Pollution Bulletin* **48(3–4)**, 336–340

Ortiz NE and Smith GR (1994) *Clostridium botulinum* type A in the gut contents of a British gull. *Veterinary Record* **135**, 68

Pokras MA (1996) Clinical management and biomedicine of sea birds. In: *Diseases of Cage and Aviary Birds, 3rd edn*, ed. W Rosskopf and R Woerpel, pp. 987–988. Lea and Febiger, Philadelphia

Quessy S and Messier S (1992) Prevalence of *Salmonella* spp., *Campylobacter* spp. and *Listeria* spp. in ring-billed gulls (*Larus delawarensis*). *Journal of Wildlife Diseases* **28(4)**, 526–531

Robinson I (2009) Seabirds. In: *Avian Medicine, 2nd edn*, ed. TN Tully *et al.*, pp. 377–403. Saunders Elsevier, Philadelphia

Sharp B (1996) Post-release survival of oiled, cleaned seabirds in North America. *IBIS* **138**, 222–228

Speed BNJ (2002) *Oil Pollution Plan.* Scottish SPCA Edinburgh, Scotland

Stoskopf M and Kennedy-Stoskopf S (1986) Aquatic birds (Sphenisciformes, Gaviiformes, Podicipediformes, Procellariiformes, Pelecaniformes and Charadriiformes). In: *Zoo and Wild Animal Medicine, 2nd edn*, ed. ME Fowler, pp. 293–313. WB Saunders, Philadelphia

Thomas T (2005) RSPCA oiled Guillemot protocol. RSPCA, Horsham

Wanless S and Maxwell MH (2001) *Blood parameters and immune responses in wild murres: baseline data for effective rehabilitation protocols.* Report to the British Wildlife Rehabilitation Council, Center for Ecology and Hydrology

Wernham CV, Peach WJ and Browne S (1997) *Survival rates of rehabilitation.* Unpublished report prepared for Sea Empress Environmental Evaluation Committee (SEEEC)

Westerhof I, Berrevoets M and Kaemingk JG (1997) A washing machine for birds. *Proceedings, 4th Conference of the European Association of Avian Veterinarians*, pp. 171–174

Woo P, Laul S, Lam C *et al.* (2009) Comparative analysis of complete genome sequences of three avian coronaviruses reveals a novel group 3c coronavirus. *Journal of Virology* **83(2)**, 908–917

Yamato O, Goto I and Maede Y (1996) Haemolytic anaemia in wild seaducks caused by marine oil pollution. *Journal of Wildlife Diseases* **32**, 281–284

Specialist organizations and useful contacts

Advice on oil spill incidents and care of oiled seabirds can be sought from the RSPCA or Scottish SPCA centres (see Appendix 1), which will then provide details of other local contacts.

Chapter 25

Wading birds

Romain Pizzi and Colin Seddon

The long-legged wading birds covered by this chapter include those species grouped together more by similarities in natural history and hence captive care requirements, rather than by taxonomic classification. The chapter covers some members of the orders Ciconiiformes (herons and bitterns), Charadriiformes (wading shorebirds and snipe) and Gruiformes (cranes, rails, and coots). These are relatively uncommon wildlife rehabilitation patients in the UK, even in large wildlife rehabilitation centres, and rarely present to veterinary surgeons (veterinarians) in general practice.

Species encountered at wildlife rehabilitation centres in the UK

The species in this group constitute less than 1% of total wildlife admissions in the UK (Best and Lawson, 2003) and less than 1.5% of all birds admitted for rehabilitation (Scottish Society for the Prevention of Cruelty to Animals (Scottish SPCA), unpublished data) (Figure 25.1). Figure 25.2 indicates that the overall release rate for wading birds is around 42%. Species such as the woodcock (*Scolopax rusticola*) in general have poorer outcomes, which should be carefully considered on initial admission, triage and clinical examination. Lapwings (*Vanellus* spp.) appear to have the best release rates following a period of rehabilitation and this is likely due to the majority of these being healthy juveniles admitted for hand-rearing.

Species	Number of each species (percentage) admitted for rehabilitation
Oystercatcher (*Haematopus ostralegus*)	121 (34%)
Grey heron (*Ardea cinerea*)	75 (21%)
Coot (*Fulica atra*), moorhen (*Gallinula chloropus*)	75 (21%)
Woodcock (*Scolopax rusticola*), snipe (*Gallinago gallinago*)	53 (15%)
Lapwing (*Vanellus vanellus*)	21 (6%)
Other wader species	10 (3%)

25.1 Common wader species admitted for rehabilitation, based on 355 wading species admissions to a UK wildlife hospital.
(Scottish SPCA, unpublished data)

Species	Number (percentage) of wader admissions successfully released
All waders	149/355 (42%)
Oystercatchers (*Haematopus ostralegus*)	45/121 (37%)
Grey herons (*Ardea cinerea*)	38/75 (51%)
Coot (*Fulica atra*), moorhen (*Gallinula chloropus*)	31/75 (41%)
Woodcock (*Scolopax rusticola*), snipe (*Gallinago gallinago*)	17/53 (32%)
Lapwing (*Vanellus vanellus*)	13/21 (62%)

25.2 Release rates for all waders and individual wading species most commonly presented for rehabilitation, based on 355 wading species admissions to a UK wildlife hospital.
(Scottish SPCA, unpublished data)

Oystercatchers (*Haematopus ostralegus*), the grey heron (*Ardea cinerea*), coots (*Fulica atra*) and moorhens (*Gallinula chloropus*) appear to be the most common species of wading birds to be admitted for rehabilitation, with other species presenting in lower numbers (see Figure 25.1). There are notable differences in admission and rehabilitation data between species (e.g. age at admission, cause of admission, and rehabilitation outcome) that should be taken into consideration by veterinary staff when presented with one of these birds. These are discussed later in this chapter.

Ecology and biology

Whilst some species such as the grey heron, oystercatcher, coot and moorhen are easily identified, many other waders are difficult to identify, with differing juvenile plumage and bland colorations. Species identification is not essential to the successful treatment and captive management of these birds, as housing and feeding requirements are for all practical purposes very similar.

The ecological and biological data for commonly encountered species of wading birds admitted for rehabilitation in the UK is outlined in Figure 25.3.

Family/subfamily	Species encountered	Feeding strategy	Diet	Breeding habitat	Winter habitat	Resident/ migrant (UK)
Order Pelecaniformes						
Ardeidae	Heron (*Ardea cinerea*), bittern (*Botaurus stellaris*), little egret (*Egretta garetta*)	Stalking in shallow water	Fish, amphibians, small mammals, small birds, invertebrates	Wetlands and reed beds, nesting in trees	Wetlands	Resident and winter migrant
Order Gruiformes (Cranes)						
Gruidae	Common crane (*Grus grus*)	Stalking on ground	Small mammals, birds, amphibians, invertebrates	Wetlands and reed beds, nest in dense shore vegetation	Wetlands	Scarce migrant, some localized small resident populations exist in Norfolk and Somerset
Order Charadriiformes (Waders)						
Haematopodidae	Oystercatcher (*Haematopus ostralegus*)	Deep probing	Molluscs, earthworms	Seashore, coastal grassland	Seashore, coastal grassland	Resident
Charadriinae	Golden plover (*Pluvialis apricaria*), ringed plover (*Charadrius hiaticula*)	Surface feeding on wet ground	Small invertebrates, insects	Moorland, coastal grassland, inland wetland	Estuaries	Resident and winter migrant
Vanellinae	Lapwing (*Vanellus vanellus*)	Surface feeding on grassland and wet ground	Invertebrates	Moorland, coastal grassland	Coastal and inland wetlands	Resident and winter migrant
Calidridinae	Common sandpiper (*Actitis hypoleucos*), green sandpiper (*Tringa ochropus*), wood sandpiper (*T. glareola*), purple sandpiper (*Calidris maritima*), curlew sandpiper (*C. ferruginea*), pectoral sandpiper (*C. melanotos*), dunlin (*C. alpina*), knot (*C. canulus*), sanderling (*C. alba*)	Surface feeding and probing soft mud, intertidal shores	Invertebrates	Mostly winter visitor, some breed on UK moorland	Moorland or tundra	Flocking on estuaries
Gallinagininae	Snipe (*Gallinago gallinago*)	Probing deeply in soft mud, wet grasslands	Invertebrates	Coastal and inland wetlands	Coastal and inland wetlands	Resident and winter migrant
Ralidae	Coot (*Fulica alta*), moorhen (*Gallinula chloropus*)	Surface feeding on wet ground and when swimming	Invertebrates	Freshwater lakes and reservoirs	Occasionally offshore if inland freshwater is frozen	Resident and winter migrant
Scolopacinae	Woodcock (*Scolopax rusticola*)	Surface feeding and probing wet ground	Invertebrates	Open, damp woodland	Marsh and wet woodland	Resident and winter migrant
Tringinae	Curlew (*Numenius arquata*), greenshank (*Tringa nebularia*), redshank (*T. totanus*), spotted redshank (*T. erythropus*) bar-tailed godwit (*Limosa lapponica*), black-tailed godwit (*L. limosa*)	Probing soft ground	Invertebrates	Grassland, moorland, tundra	Grassland, estuaries, beaches	Resident and winter migrant
Phalaropodinae	Grey phalarope (*Phalaropus fulicarius*), red-necked phalarope (*P. lobatus*)	Surface feeding on wet ground and when swimming	Invertebrates	Tundra	Mostly at sea	Passage migrant, some breeding Northern isles

25.3 Biological and ecological data for the commonly encountered species of wading birds admitted for rehabilitation in the UK. (Modified from Best and Lawson, 2003)

Anatomy and physiology

Wading bird species are sexually monomorphic. Although there may be small differences in body size, with females being slightly larger, this is generally not useful in trying to establish gender. Newly-hatched waders are precocial, allowing them to be 'hand-reared' with minimal handling. Once self-feeding is established chicks usually do well if left to forage for themselves in an outside natural floored aviary. Due to their precocial nature there is minimal risk of birds older than a day or two of age malprinting on humans, which aids rearing for release to the wild (see 'Rearing of young wading birds').

There is a great variation in beak length and shape, a result of the evolution of these species to specialize in slightly differing diet or feeding habitat (see Figure 25.3).

Common cranes (*Grus grus*) have distinctive long coils of trachea enclosed within the bone of the sternum. These are clearly visible on radiographs (see Figure 25.11). Grey herons and some waders have a prominent crista ventralis just inside the glottal opening, though this may not be easily visible. The trachea also appears to taper shortly after the glottis (see Figure 25.10). These factors may prevent the passage of what appears to be a correctly sized endotracheal (ET) tube for the size of the entrance to the glottis for maintenance of anaesthesia (see 'Anaesthesia').

The long tibiotarsal and tarsometatarsal bones of many of these wading birds are prone to fractures unless care is taken to handle them gently. In order for these bones to be lightweight for flight, the cortex is thin and the hydroxyapatite composition of avian bones (in contrast to that of mammals), in combination with their structural properties, results in their rigid but brittle nature.

Capture, handling and transportation

Capture and handling

Basic methods of capture and handling of birds are described in Chapter 3 and also apply to wading species. For atraumatic capture of wading birds the authors recommend using a dark-coloured cloth bird net. Care needs to be taken not to damage the long sensitive beaks of many waders, which is essential in their probing method of feeding. Anything but minor superficial damage to the beak carries a poor prognosis for successful release. Grey herons and bitterns (*Botaurus stellaris*) can use their beaks defensively and may suddenly stab at the handler's eyes or face. It is recommended that handlers use goggles, as well as keeping the head or beak restrained and well away from the handler's face. These birds can initially be held either at the base of the head/cranial neck area, or around the mid beak, taking care not to obstruct the nares situated at the proximal beak. The body of the heron can be restrained gently, wrapped in a towel, under the other arm. If the legs are held, this should be gently, and in extension (see 'Anatomy and physiology').

Transportation

Long-legged waders should not have their legs kept in a flexed position for prolonged periods of time, either during restraint or whilst being transported in transport boxes, as circulatory compromise (Figure 25.4) and paralysis may result. Transport boxes, as well as temporary hospitalization cages, need to be sufficiently high to allow herons, bitterns, cranes and other tall species to be able to stand comfortably. Indoor hospitalization should be kept as brief as possible.

Mesh wire cat carriers are not recommended for transport, as there is a risk that birds may injure their long delicate legs and beak. Damage to the primary feathers of the wings may occur whilst using these carriers for transport, and this can make otherwise treatable cases non-viable for release. The ability to 'imp' broken primary feathers (a procedure in which broken feathers are replaced with feathers from another bird) is often limited as these birds are rarely admitted to wildlife centres, and consequently species-specific feathers needed for this technique are not available (see Chapter 29 for technique). Solid-sided carriers are best for transport, with the front door, if made from mesh, covered in a cloth or towel to limit sounds and stress. As for other animals, birds should not be left in vehicles for prolonged periods, especially in warm or humid weather, or they may overheat. A non-slip non-abrasive surface, such as rubber matting, is also advisable for transport (see also Chapter 3).

Examination and clinical assessment for rehabilitation

The basic techniques for clinical examination of birds are discussed in Chapter 4 and apply to wading bird species. Trauma is the most common reason for wading birds to present for veterinary treatment and rehabilitation, and therefore clinical examination should focus on determining the presence and extent of any soft tissue or orthopaedic injuries. This in turn will ascertain the prognosis for successful rehabilitation and release. The generally poorer

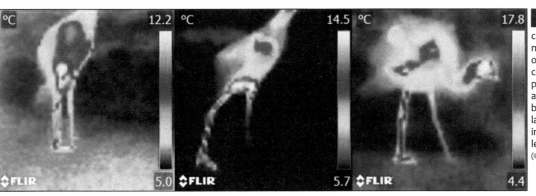

25.4 Thermographic images from a crane, demonstrating notable inflammation of one leg. Circulatory compromise from prolonged forced flexion, and rough handling can both result in notable lameness or, more importantly, fractures or leg paralysis.
(© Zoological Medicine Ltd)

survival rates in captivity in these birds, the difficulties encountered in captive management and feeding, and the stressful nature of captivity, are all important considerations when evaluating if treatment is viable or euthanasia is indicated (see also Chapter 4). Some birds, despite having treatable conditions, demonstrate extreme stress and will not feed in captivity.

Ophthalmic examination

Loss of sight in an eye is not compatible with release in any of these species, which rely on a wide field of vision to spot predators, or accurate depth perception from binocular vision to catch prey (e.g. herons when fishing). Ophthalmic examination is the same as in other birds and should always include retinal examination. The roof of the mouth and choana should be examined for evidence of trauma, as well as the external ear canal for any bruising or haemorrhage that could indicate trauma or fracture of the scleral ossicles.

Clinical assessment for rehabilitation

Approximately a quarter of all waders and almost half all grey herons presented for rehabilitation are emaciated (Figure 25.5). Species such as woodcock and snipe (*Gallinago gallinago*) are frequently presented as adult birds that have been shot. There are often associated fractures, either directly from the shooting or from the fall, with the proximal wings and coracoids frequently affected. It is therefore advisable to radiograph all adults of these species after admission to accurately evaluate injuries and formulate a prognosis.

Fishing line entanglement and ingestion of fishing hooks are another common cause for presentation, particularly in coots, and this species constitute almost a quarter of all cases presented for rehabilitation (Figure 25.6).

Reason for presentation	All waders (n=355)	Grey heron (*Ardea cinerea*) (n=75)
Trauma	163 (45.9%)	19 (25.3%)
Emaciation	92 (25.9%)	35 (46.7%)
Vehicle collisions	18 (5.1%)	5 (6.6%)
Fish hook or line injuries	21 (5.9%)	8 (10.7%)
Other reasons	61 (17.2%)	8 (10.7%)

25.5 Common reasons for presentation in all wader species and in grey herons admitted for veterinary care and rehabilitation, based on 355 wading species admissions to a UK wildlife hospital. (Scottish SPCA, unpublished data)

Species	Number (percentage) of admissions of waders for hook and line injuries
All waders	21/ 355 (6%)
Grey heron (*Ardea cinerea*)	8/75 (11%)
Coot (*Fulica atra*)	8/35 (23%)
Moorhen (*Gallinula chloropas*)	2/40 (5%)

25.6 Percentage of all waders and of specific species of waders that were admitted for fishing hook and line injuries or line entanglement, based on 40,000 wildlife admissions to a UK wildlife hospital. (Scottish SPCA, unpublished data)

Euthanasia

Euthanasia, if indicated, is performed by intravascular injection of barbiturate into the medial metatarsal or right jugular vein. If intravenous access in not possible, euthanasia may, in an emergency, be carried out by trained lay staff on welfare grounds (under veterinary direction in the UK) using intracoelomic injection. This is performed using a 1–1.5 inch needle inserted in the ventral midline just caudal to the sternum, and directed parallel to the keel cranially, with the aim of reaching the heart or liver (see also Chapter 4). This is slightly more difficult than in many other birds due to a large keel and small coelomic access in species such as woodcock, and large coelomic air sacs and large body size in the grey heron.

First aid and short-term hospitalization

First aid procedures

The basic techniques for avian first aid and fluid therapy are outlined in Chapter 5 and apply to wading birds. Oral fluids are effective at correcting dehydration in the majority of cases and are well tolerated by many wading species. In the authors' experience, few of these birds present with enteric disease that could make oral fluid therapy ineffective.

Short-term housing and feeding

The majority of these birds do best housed outdoors in seclusion aviaries, and the time spent hospitalized in indoor cages should be limited as much as possible. Large birds, such as cranes and herons, need indoor cages high enough for them to comfortably stand, to prevent circulatory compromise to the legs. Herons and cranes may injure their wings, especially incurring wounds to the carpal regions, as well as damaging the distal primary wing feathers, if kept in small enclosures for any length of time.

A non-slip non-abrasive surface that can be kept clean, such as rubber matting, is useful if housing for only a few days. If indoor housing is required for a longer period, care should be taken to provide artificial grass and keep this cleaned daily, as large birds such as herons and cranes can develop ulcerative pododermatitis (bumblefoot). Grey herons will frequently prefer a perch if this can be provided with adequate space. This can be covered in artificial grass to help prevent bumblefoot developing, as well as making the cage or room floor easier to clean, and so maintaining good hygiene, which will also help reduce the risk of birds developing *Aspergillus* air sac infections.

Feeding of some species when housed indoors for an initial period in a veterinary practice can be problematic, due to their specific feeding behaviours. Grey herons can be provided with a temporary diet of whole sprats, or chopped larger fish or day-old chicks, and cranes can similarly be provided with mice and day-old chicks. If feeding juveniles it is essential to supplement adequately with calcium due to these long-legged species' predisposition to the development of metabolic bone disease, deformities of the long bones and pathological fractures (Waters, 2003).

Whilst juveniles and some adult individuals may feed reasonably in a cage environment, many of the smaller long-beaked waders that probe for insects may fail to self-feed unless housed outdoors in a natural floor aviary.

These same species are also difficult to tube feed and can be very stressed by captive conditions. Rapid relocation to a suitable rehabilitation centre, or release if possible, may be the preferred option in these species.

Diagnostic techniques

Blood sampling
Blood sampling, as in other avian species, is accomplished via the medial metatarsal or right jugular vein (see Chapter 5).

Radiography
Radiography is highly recommended for clinical assessment and to determine a prognosis in woodcock, snipe and grey herons, as these frequently present having being shot (Figure 25.7). Ventrodorsal and lateral coelomic and limb radiographs should be taken, as for other birds; wing radiographs are generally taken from the ventrodorsal

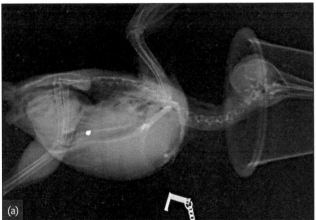

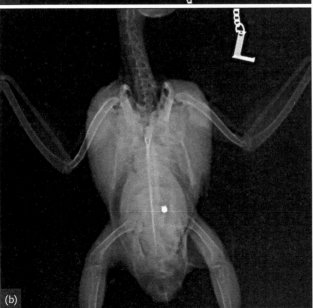

25.7 Woodcock have poor rehabilitation outcomes, with a high incidence of birds presenting having been shot. (a) Lateral and (b) ventrodorsal radiographs of a woodcock clearly showing evidence of radiodense material in the coelomic cavity consistent with shot. Also note the very large pectoral musculature, which in dorsal recumbency will impair respiration under anaesthesia.
(© Zoological Medicine Ltd)

aspect. When taking lateral coelomic radiographs, care must be exercised to not injure the pectoral muscles by forcefully placing the wings over the bird's back, or using heavy sandbags on the wings. The author (RP) has seen pectoral muscle tears and subsequent fibrosis due to this on post-mortem examinations. The use of microporous tape for positioning is safe. The adverse effects of positioning for radiographs on anaesthesia should be considered (see 'Anaesthesia and analgesia'), and time restrained in dorsal recumbency should be limited in these birds.

Ultrasonography
Coelomic ultrasonography, using a 7.5 MHz microconvex probe, can occasionally be useful in diagnosing yolk sac infections in recently hatched herons and cranes, manifesting as a thickened yolk sac wall or sludging of yolk in the ventral part of the yolk sac.

Endoscopy
Coelomic endoscopy may be indicated for the diagnosis of *Aspergillus* air sacculitis, assessment of renal gout and other coelomic disease. The standard approach cranial to the leg muscles is used as in other birds. In large birds such as cranes and herons, a 4 mm diameter 30-degree endoscope is preferable to the standard 2.7 mm 'universal' endoscope, as it transmits more light in the large coelomic air sac spaces, and has a similar diameter and hence entry wound to the 2.7 mm endoscope if used in its sheath. If diagnostic sampling such as biopsy or microbiology is indicated, however, this requires the use of a transcutaneous spinal needle for aspiration or fine-needle biopsy, or insertion of an additional cannula for the introduction of biopsy forceps when using the 4 mm endoscope.

Anaesthesia and analgesia
Whilst the general principles of safe avian anaesthesia apply to these birds, as covered in more detail in Chapter 6, there are a few noteworthy specific considerations.

Gaseous induction technique
Anaesthesia of waders is best performed with inhalation anaesthesia via facemask. Isoflurane appears to be slightly more irritant during induction than sevoflurane, but is safe, effective and cost-efficient for rehabilitation use. The slightly faster anaesthetic recovery from sevoflurane anaes-thesia described in other avian species has not been specifically reported in these species but is likely to occur, and may be advantageous in particularly critical patients if available. Most waders do not demonstrate the degree of apnoea seen in some waterfowl, but some individuals do show apnoea and bradycardia, most likely due to trigeminal nerve receptor stimulation under stress. Inserting the entire head into a facemask, rather than just inserting the beak (and hence placing the black rubber seal in proximity to the eyes) appears to give better results, as does pre-oxygenation for 30 seconds before introducing the inhalation agent. Whilst standard small animal facemasks are suitable for small waders, in herons and others with long beaks it is better to use a cut-off plastic bottle as a long mask, with a surgical glove stretched over the cut end with a slit in the centre for insertion of the beak and head to provide a seal

(Figure 25.8). Species such as woodcock can even be entirely placed in the bottle mask, which is used as an induction chamber, and covered with a towel to keep the bird calm (Figure 25.9). Attention should be paid if using a small mask to include the nares at the base of the beak. As an alternative to the use of a facemask, a cut anaesthetic reservoir bag may be used just to cover the nares and administer the inhalation agent for induction.

Whilst some authors have recommended a gradual increase in inhaled anaesthetic agent during induction with the aim of reducing apnoea, in the author's (RP) experience administration of an initial high concentration (such as 5% isoflurane) results in rapid induction with less excitation and struggling, and subsequently a reduced risk of injury in long-legged waders.

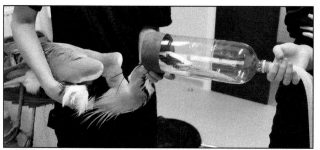

25.8 Safe restraint of a grey heron for anaesthesia induction, with the head held at the top of the neck. A modified drinks bottle mask allows insertion of the whole head to reduce stress during induction.
(© Zoological Medicine Ltd)

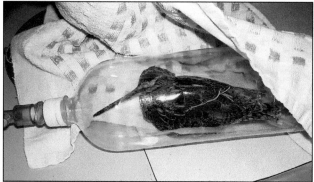

25.9 A facemask modified from a drinks bottle can also be used as an atraumatic anaesthetic induction chamber for woodcock and snipe, and covered with a towel to reduce stimulation during induction.
(© Zoological Medicine Ltd)

Intubation technique

With the exception of very brief procedures, such as rapid radiography, where a mask is sufficient, it is advisable to intubate waders for maintenance of anaesthesia. The glottis is situated at the base of the tongue and is normally easily visualized for intubation. The tongue can be gently pulled rostrally, or a finger inserted ventrally between the mandibles to elevate the glottis and aid visualization if needed. Grey herons and some other waders have a prominent crista ventralis just inside the glottal opening, which may not be easily visible when attempting intubation. This may prevent the passage of what appears to be a correctly sized endotracheal (ET) tube for the size of the entrance to the glottis. In herons the trachea also appears to taper shortly after the glottis, again necessitating a

smaller ET tube diameter than may be apparent from the diameter of the glottis. The ET tube should not be forced as the trachea may be damaged, resulting in haemorrhage or even rupture. Extending the neck may be helpful when passing the ET tube, and is also helpful during anaesthesia in long-necked birds such as herons to prevent inadvertent occlusion, or tracheal trauma with resultant subsequent stricture formation (Figure 25.10). Whilst birds have complete tracheal rings, and hence most literature recommends always using uncuffed ET tubes, the author (RP) prefers the use of cuffed ET tubes in herons since the use of clear plastic or silicone high-volume low-pressure cuffed tubes with the cuff lightly inflated is safe in the author's (RP) experience, whereas even uncuffed red rubber latex tubes can traumatize the trachea due to their rigid nature.

Most waders have a relatively long neck, with little risk of over-insertion of the ET tube and injury to the syrinx. If in doubt the ET tube length can be measured to the length of the neck, as the syrinx is situated inside the thoracic inlet in small waders.

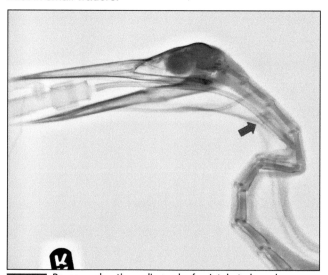

25.10 Reverse coloration radiograph of an intubated grey heron. The red arrow highlights the crista ventralis. Also note the taper of the tracheal diameter shortly after the glottis, further complicating intubation. Herons' necks should be maintained extended during anaesthesia to prevent inadvertent obstruction of the end of the endotracheal tube.
(© Zoological Medicine Ltd)

Intermittent positive pressure ventilation

With a long, relatively wide trachea, cranes and, to a lesser extent herons, have notable anatomical dead space, more than four to five times that of mammals (Figure 25.11). As respiration is depressed under anaesthesia, intermittent positive pressure ventilation (IPPV) is highly recommended, even if birds demonstrate some spontaneous breathing under anaesthesia, and IPPV becomes essential to prevent hypoventilation developing if anaesthesia is prolonged or if birds are positioned in dorsal recumbency. Oxygen in the air sacs and tracheal dead space does not diffuse out sufficiently. IPPV may be by means of a mechanical ventilator, or more simply by means of squeezing the reservoir bag on an appropriate anaesthetic system. As a general guide, birds demonstrating spontaneous breathing under anaesthesia are given two to four assisted breaths per minute, whilst apnoeic birds are ventilated at a rate of 10–12 breaths per minute, larger birds needing fewer breaths per minute than small birds (see also Chapter 6).

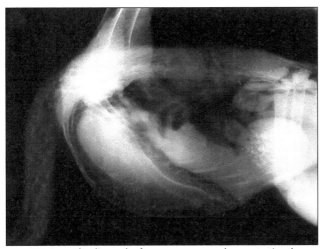

25.11 Lateral radiograph of a common crane, demonstrating the coils of trachea that are enclosed in the bone of the sternum (keel). This increases the bird's upper respiratory tract dead space, and needs consideration during anaesthesia.
(© Rafael A. Molina-López)

Positioning during anaesthesia

Positioning in dorsal recumbency has a major impact on avian respiration, and can reduce tidal volume by half even in conscious birds. The relatively large pectoral muscle mass in small waders and species such as woodcock (see Figure 25.7), can result in inertial resistance to respiratory movements of the keel, resulting in additional respiratory compromise, and this can be exacerbated when taping the wings and legs extended for ventrodorsal radiographic views. It is highly recommended that positioning in dorsal recumbency is minimized, and prolonged positioning in this way avoided.

Long-legged birds, particularly herons and cranes, should ideally always be positioned under anaesthesia with their legs extended, just as for handling, avoiding placing their legs (intertarsal joint) in flexion for any length of time.

Specific conditions

Traumatic injuries

The most common reasons for presentation of waders for veterinary treatment and rehabilitation are trauma or apparently orphaned youngsters presenting for rearing. Wound care and treatment is as described in other avian species (see also Chapters 5 and 26).

Firearm injuries

Woodcock and snipe commonly present having been shot (see Figure 25.7), with concurrent fractures from the fall or from entry of the bullet or pellet. Grey herons also commonly present with firearm injuries, due to their conflict with fish pond owners (Figure 25.12).

Fishing hook and line injuries

Fishing hook injuries, ingestion of hooks and line, and entanglement in fishing line are common in wading birds, with this being the reason for presentation in almost a quarter of coots admitted to a wildlife hospital (see Figure 25.6). See Chapter 26 for information on dealing with these cases.

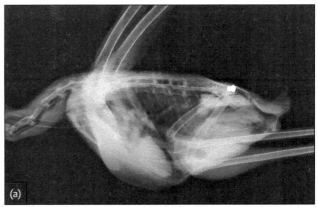

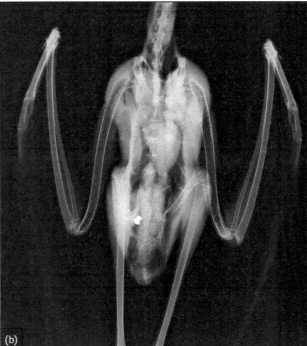

25.12 (a) Lateral radiograph of a grey heron with an airgun pellet lodged in the coelom: this was an incidental finding. Grey herons commonly come into conflict with aquaculturists with outdoor fish ponds. (b) Ventrodorsal radiograph of the same bird. This bird was presented for elbow luxation. These injuries usually hold a poor prognosis, but the bird was successfully rehabilitated and returned to the wild and survived for at least 6 months on post-release monitoring.
(© Scottish SPCA National Wildlife Rescue Centre)

Power line collisions

Adult cranes most commonly present for rehabilitation in mainland Europe due to collisions with power lines (Figure 25.13), with wing fractures a common sequel to the collision or subsequent fall (R Molina, personal communication). A survey of causes of mortality in cranes in Germany found the main cause to be trauma due to collisions with power lines or, less commonly, entanglement in wire fencing (Krone *et al.*, 2003; Fanke *et al.*, 2011).

Beak trauma

Despite its size and robust appearance, the beak of the grey heron is relatively fragile and can be fractured by rough handling. Whilst prostheses have been used in captive birds with fractured beaks, this is not feasible in birds destined for return to the wild, and significant beak injuries require euthanasia.

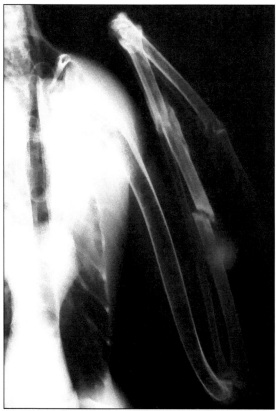

25.13 Radiograph of a comminuted ulnar fracture in a common crane following a collision with a power line.
(© Rafael A. Molina-López)

Infectious diseases

Whilst a wide variety of parasitic and infectious disease have been reported in these species (Gavier-Widén *et al.*, 2012), either when surveyed in the wild, or when kept in zoological collections, the majority of waders presenting to wildlife rehabilitation centres are not commonly affected by specific infectious diseases.

Viral diseases

Viral infections occur rarely in wading birds. Avipox virus infections have been described in cranes and may result in death of the affected animal due to cachexia caused by avipox lesions involving the eyelids, facial skin, cere, and legs (Krone *et al.*, 2003).

Bacterial diseases

Herons and other waders have reportedly been affected in large outbreaks of fowl cholera (*Pasteurella multocida*) occurring in groups of waterfowl outside the UK. This is due to scavenging from waterfowl cadavers and debris. *Mycobacterium avium* is occasionally encountered in wader species, although less commonly than in other waterfowl (see Chapter 26).

Fungal diseases

One noteworthy infectious disease encountered in waders undergoing rehabilitation is *Aspergillus* fungal air sacculitis, which herons, cranes and other waders are prone to develop in captivity. This is likely related to stress-induced immunosuppression and captive environmental factors. Whilst itraconazole (10 mg/kg orally q24h) and terbinafine

(10–15 mg/kg orally q24h) can be administered prophylactically, better outcomes are achieved without prophylactic medication if birds are housed outdoors in a seclusion aviary and their time in rehabilitation is kept as short as possible. Once birds are affected, treatment very rarely results in sufficient recovery to make the bird viable for return to the wild, and affected birds once diagnosed (see 'Endoscopy' and Chapter 26) are usually best euthanased.

Parasites

A variety of parasites have been recorded in wading bird species. For example, 28 species of parasite have been reported in the common crane (eight coccidia, six trematodes, one cestode, six nematodes, one tick, six mallophages) (Gottschalk and Prange, 2002), yet these occur naturally in wild birds and the majority do not appear to cause any notable clinical disease unless birds are immunosuppressed (Krone *et al.*, 2003). Rehabilitated birds will need to cope with these once returned to the wild. There is no logic in attempting to clear birds destined for return to the wild of their native parasite species as a routine, unless they are associated with obvious pathology. Endoparasites are only treated in rehabilitation centres if causing clinical disease, or very heavy parasite burdens are resulting in slow recovery or weight gain, and hence likely to prolong time in captivity. Heavy parasite burdens may indicate another undiagnosed underlying condition causing immunosuppression, which should be considered.

Coccidiosis: A survey of causes of mortality in cranes in Germany revealed small numbers of deaths related to coccidiosis and *Clostridium perfringens* enteritis in this species. Whilst the veterinary literature has large numbers of descriptions of visceral coccidiosis in cranes, this has not been reported in the common crane specifically and is normally a problem of captivity and captive breeding establishments (Gottschalk and Prange, 2002; Krone *et al.*, 2003).

An exception to the treatment of parasites is when rearing large numbers of the same species in an aviary, such as the corncrake (*Crex crex*) for release to the wild, or a large number of juvenile lapwings, where parasites can build up as an artefact of the captive environment. Coccidia are the most frequent parasitic problem in these conditions (Jeanes *et al.*, 2013), and in this instance require management, either non-medically by rotating the aviaries used and by limiting the numbers housed together, or by means of anticoccidials, such as toltrazuril used at standard poultry dosage rates in drinking water.

Other conditions
Emaciation

Almost half of grey herons and approximately a quarter of all waders presented for rehabilitation are emaciated, based on clinical assessment of body condition (pectoral muscle coverage of the keel (see Figure 4.6) and femoral leg musculature), either due to failure to cope with natural conditions (Figure 25.14), or frequently having developed secondary to an injury before being found. Birds presenting emaciated, irrespective of the underlying cause, have much lower release rates (Scottish SPCA, unpublished data), and this is an important factor to consider in initial assessment and the decision as to whether euthanasia is indicated.

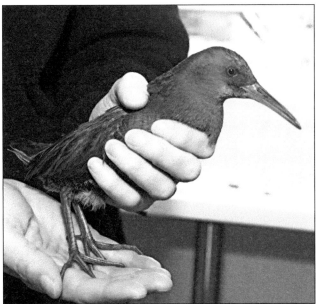

25.14 A water rail (*Rallus aquaticus*), a rare wildlife rehabilitation admission. This bird was found exhausted and thin sheltering on a boat.
(© Colin Seddon)

Limb deformities in juvenile birds

Metabolic bone disease, with limb deformities, slipped tendons, and pathological fractures of the legs and wings are all a risk when rearing young waders. This condition is particularly common in the larger species such as herons (Figure 25.15), bitterns, cranes and corncrake, and has also been well described in captive breeding of these species in zoological collections (Ball, 2003; Carpenter, 2003; Waters, 2003). Many heron chicks admitted to wildlife centres are poor quality chicks from parent birds that are struggling to adequately feed them in the wild, and hence they are already deficient in calcium before admission for rehabilitation (Figure 25.16). Excessive growth and weight gain in the first 4–6 weeks of life is another common cause of bone deformities, particularly of the legs. It is advisable that all larger species admitted as juvenile birds are supplemented daily with oral calcium borogluconate 40% solution (1 ml/kg q24h), preferably in the food or by direct oral administration. Powdered calcium supplements have also been used, but in the authors' experience this appears less effective. However, administration via the drinking water may be the only practical method if housed in an aviary. When rearing cranes, offering large amounts of live insect food in the early period can also result in bone deformities due to rapid initial growth and calcium: phosphorous dietary imbalance. Rearing in an outdoor aviary results in slower growth and allows for greater movement, which appears to result in a lower incidence of these problems in all species in the authors' experience.

Ulcerative pododermatitis (bumblefoot)

Bumblefoot (see Chapter 26) can develop in adult cranes and herons kept on concrete or hard flooring, and may occasionally occur if they are housed for long periods in small aviaries with natural flooring. Provision of adequate artificial grass padded perching and limiting time spent in captivity are mandatory in prevention of this condition in captivity (Figure 25.17).

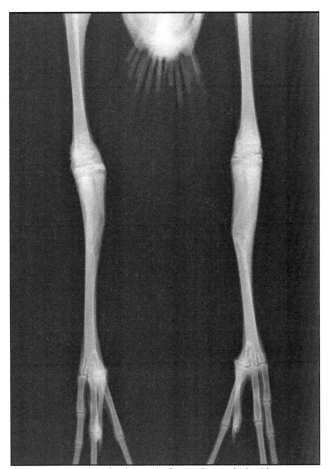

25.15 Ventrodorsal radiograph of a grey heron chick with severe deformities of the proximal tarsometatarsal bones, due to rapid growth and insufficient dietary calcium.
(© Scottish SPCA National Wildlife Rescue Centre)

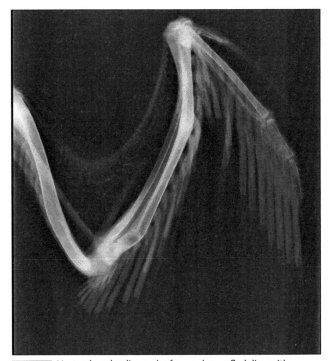

25.16 Ventrodorsal radiograph of a grey heron fledgling with pathological fractures of the radius and ulna. This chick was unable to stand, and developed these fractures by attempting to move its body with its wings. These fractures arose soon after arrival at the rehabilitation centre. In this case metabolic bone disease occurred secondary to poor feeding by the parent birds in the wild.
(© Scottish SPCA National Wildlife Rescue Centre)

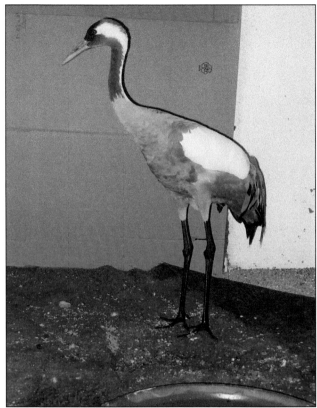

25.17 A common crane housed in a small aviary, floored with artificial grass to limit the risk of developing pododermatitis.
(© Rafael A. Molina-López)

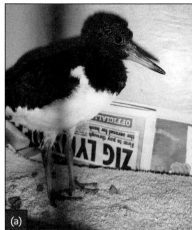

25.18 (a) Juvenile oystercatcher on towelling and (b) juvenile coot on thick foam, both housed indoors in the short term until feeding is established and they can be moved outdoors.
(© Colin Seddon)

Therapeutics

Drugs, routes of medication and therapeutic doses used in waders are the same as used in other avian species. When rearing chicks of these species, and in particular herons, bitterns, cranes and corncrakes, it is advisable to supplement with oral calcium borogluconate (see 'Limb deformities in juvenile birds'). This may be dosed orally (1 ml/kg of 40% calcium borogluconate solution once daily), placed in fish for herons, or administered in drinking water for small waders being reared in outdoor seclusion aviaries on natural soil floors.

Management in captivity

Housing

Smaller species can be kept in the short term in covered hospital cages or a plastic Vari-Kennel®, on towelling and thick foam (Figure 25.18), before being moved to an outdoor seclusion aviary with natural flooring (ground or grass). Ideally wading birds also need access to water, but this can be simply provided using large flat dishes or plastic dog beds containing water.

Large species such as cranes and grey heron are also best housed in outdoor aviaries with natural flooring, and perches of varying diameter need to be offered for natural behaviour and prevention of foot lesions. Solid aviary walls (seclusion aviary) are recommended where possible to avoid traumatic injuries occurring (Figure 25.19). If aviaries are not available to house these large species, small, quiet

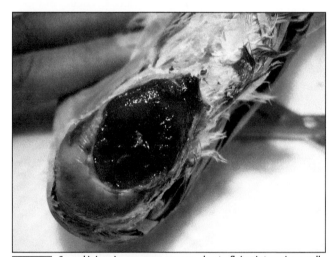

25.19 Carpal injury in a common crane, due to flying into aviary wall when disturbed. Solid aviary walls (seclusion aviary) are recommended where possible.
(© Rafael A. Molina-López)

rooms can be used for short periods of time, but should ideally be floored with artificial grass, or soft towels if this is not available, and birds carefully monitored for any signs of pododermatitis developing.

Diet

Feeding is generally best accomplished in small waders with an insectivore avian mix, with live mealworms offered as well. Some wet (tinned) dog food may also be offered, and for herons and large waders, day-old chicks and mice, and small fish such as whitebait or sprats. Supplementation of juvenile herons, bittern, cranes and other large birds with oral calcium (see 'Limb deformities in juvenile birds') is recommended to prevent metabolic bone disease and pathological fractures or leg deformities developing. If feeding captive grey herons defrosted fish as a large portion of the diet for any length of time, supplementation with thiamine is recommended, and some centres will also supplement with vitamin E. Neither is essential, however, if the bird is only in rehabilitation for 1–2 weeks. Corncrake can be fed similarly to quail during rehabilitation, with a micropellet diet suitable for their specific life stage.

Rearing of young wading birds

There is a wide variation in which species are most commonly presented as juveniles for hand-rearing, with oystercatchers, moorhen and lapwings predominating in one study (Figure 25.20). Wader chicks of all species are precocial and self-feed from hatching. As imprinting (see Chapters 8 and 9) is completed within hours of hatching, there is a lower risk of malprinting than in many other birds, although the authors have still seen some of this behaviour in individual rails and coots.

Small waders presenting for rearing can be kept indoors in cages or brooders under heat lamps until they are reliably self-feeding. They should then be moved to an outdoor seclusion aviary with natural flooring (ground or grass) and appropriate perches (Figures 25.21 and 25.22). This substrate will encourage normal probing and feeding behaviour using their beaks, as well as normal activity and,

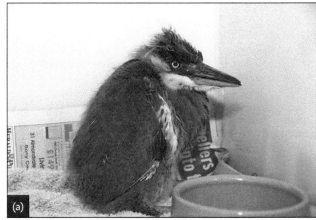
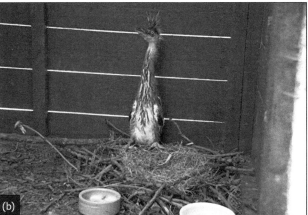
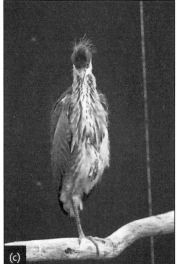

Species	Number (percentage)
All waders	159/355 (45%)
Oystercatchers	89/121 (74%)
Grey herons	23/75 (31%)
Coot	4/35 (11%)
Moorhen	28/40 (70%)
Woodcock and snipe	1/53 (2%)
Lapwing	14/21 (67%)

25.20 Percentage of all wader species and individual species that were chicks admitted for hand-rearing, based on 355 wading species admissions to a UK wildlife hospital.
(Scottish SPCA, unpublished data)

25.22 Rearing of a grey heron. (a) Time indoors in a cage is limited as much as possible, before moving the bird to a secluded aviary outdoors, with (b) natural flooring and (c) perches to maintain foot health and allow for natural behaviour.
(© Colin Seddon)

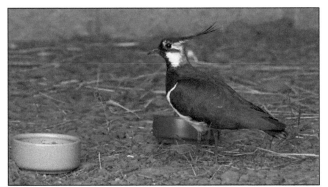

25.21 Lapwing being reared for release in an outdoor seclusion aviary with natural flooring. Most waders being reared in this way will do better if housed outdoors, compared to indoors, if the weather is reasonable.
(© Colin Seddon)

in larger species, will help limit excessive growth rates associated with bone deformity development (see Figure 25.15). Aviaries should ideally have solid sides (seclusion) as visual barriers to limit stress and prevent injuries to birds being startled, as well as a small overhang to reduce exposure to heavy rain or wind.

Release

The main considerations for the successful release of wading species are: the likelihood of the individual bird to be able to survive in the wild (assessed by body condition, behaviour, recovery from presenting injury or problem); the ability to fly; and suitable habitat for release (generally wet-land with groups of the same species present). For more details see Chapter 9.

Release should be performed when the weather is calm; the early morning is ideal to allow for some brief observation of the released individual, as all species and ages from this group of birds are hard-released, with supportive feeding after release not being possible (Figure 25.23).

Once birds that have been reared can fly, they are generally suitable for release. They should be released in areas with others of the same species, and release should coincide with the natural dispersal period of wild juveniles from the nest. Grey heron fledglings are usually suitable for release at about 2 months of age. This is best per-formed in the area of their original heronry (breeding ground) if possible.

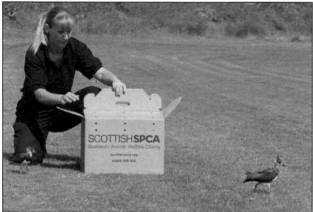

25.23 Hand-reared lapwings being released. This species has the best outcome for successful release following a period in captivity of all the waders in the authors' experience. This is largely due to the fact that the majority of admissions are healthy juveniles that simply require rearing and that young are precocial in nature.
(© Colin Seddon)

Legal aspects

Whilst many of the wader species were previously listed on Schedule 4 of the Wildlife and Countryside Act 1981, requiring registration if kept in captivity for treatment and rehabilitation, the list has been amended and none of these species are, at the time of publication, included (see Chapter 2).

It should be borne in mind when releasing birds that some species such as bittern, corncrake, black-tailed god-wit (*Limosa limosa*), greenshank (*Tringa nebularia*), plovers (Charadriinae), sandpipers (Calidridinae), and stone-curlew (*Burhinus oedicnemus*) are included on Schedule 1 of the Wildlife and Countryside Act 1981, making it an offence to intentionally or recklessly disturb the bird at, or near, an active nest. It is preferable to release reared birds in the vicinity of conspecifics; however, the stage that they are released to the wild also generally coincides with the period of natural dispersal in the wild from the nest, and so does not result in nest disturbance.

Further details of the legal aspects of wildlife rehabilita-tion are discussed in Chapter 2.

References and further reading

Ball RL (2003) Charadriiformes (Gulls, Shorebirds). In: *Zoo and Wild Animal Medicine, 5th edn*, ed. ME Fowler and RE Miller, pp. 136–141. WB Saunders, Philadelphia

Best D and Lawson B (2003) Wading birds, including herons. In: *BSAVA Manual of Wildlife Casualties*, ed. E Mullineaux, D Best and JE Cooper, pp. 214–218. BSAVA Publications, Gloucester

Carpenter JW (2003) Gruiformes (cranes, limpkins, rails, gallinules, coots, bustards). In: *Zoo and Wild Animal Medicine, 5th edn*, ed. ME Fowler and RE Miller, pp.171–180. WB Saunders, Philadelphia

Fanke J, Wibbelt G and Krone O (2011) Mortality factors and diseases in free-ranging eurasian cranes (*Grus grus*) in Germany. *Journal of Wildlife Diseases* **47(3)**, 627–637

Gavier-Widén D, Duff JP and Meredith A (2012) *Infectious Disease of Wild Mammals and Birds in Europe.* Wiley-Blackwell, Oxford

Gottschalk C and Prange H (2002) Parasites of the common crane *Grus grus* (L.) in Europe. *Berliner und Münchener tierärztliche Wochenschrift* **115(5–6)**, 203–206

Jeanes C, Vaughan-Higgins R, Green RE *et al.* (2013) Two new *Eimeria* species parasitic in corncrakes (*Crex crex*) (Gruiformes: Rallidae) in the United Kingdom. *Journal of Parasitology* **99(4)**, 634–668

Krone O, Henne E, Blahy B *et al.* (2003) Preliminary results: causes of death and diseases of the Eurasian crane (*Grus grus*) in Germany. *Proceedings of the 7th EAAV Conference and the 5th ECAMS Scientific Meeting, Tenerife*

Mulcahy, DM (2013) Free-living waterfowl and shorebirds. In: *Zoo Animal and Wildlife Immobilization and Anesthesia*, ed. G West, D Heard and N Caulkett. Wiley-Blackwell, Oxford

Waters M (2003) Ciconiiformes (herons, ibises, spoonbills, storks). In: *Zoo and Wild Animal Medicine, 5th edn*, eds. ME Fowler and RE Miller, pp. 122–129. WB Saunders, Philadelphia

Specialist organizations and useful contacts

A list of useful contacts some of which are relevant to the treatment and rehabilitation of waders can be found in Appendix 1.

Chapter 26

Waterfowl

Sally Goulden

The waterfowl (ducks, geese and swans), along with divers and grebes, encompass a large number of species of aquatic bird inhabiting wetland areas and exploiting the food resources of such areas (Figure 26.1). Wading bird species are discussed in Chapter 25. Wetlands provide a diverse array of very fertile habitats including areas of marsh, fen, peatland and water habitats, which may be natural or artificial, permanent or temporary, static or flowing, fresh, brackish or saltwater. The species of birds that inhabit such areas are consequently diverse (Figure 26.2). In addition to indigenous UK species (both resident and migrant), waterfowl from other parts of the world have been imported into private collections and subsequently escaped into the wild. Domestic geese and ducks also may escape or are released into the wild. Such introductions compete with wild species and may interbreed.

The overlap between 'wild' and domestic birds of these species can make rehabilitation and release decisions less straightforward than for other species.

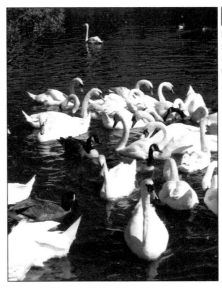

26.2 Lake at waterfowl rescue centre showing mute swans and Canada geese (*Branta canadensis*).

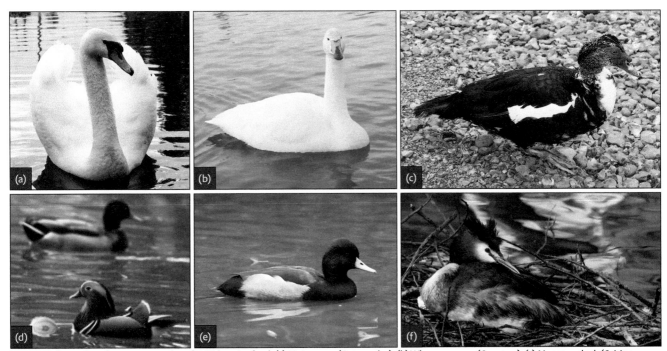

26.1 Examples of common species of British waterfowl. (a) Mute swan (*Cygnus olor*). (b) Whooper swan (*C. cygnus*). (c) Muscovy duck (*Cairina moschata*). (d) Mandarin duck (*Aix galericulata*) with mallard (*Anas platyrhynchos*) drake. (e) Pochard (*Aythya ferina*). (f) Great crested grebe (*Podiceps cristatus*).

Ecology and biology

Some useful ecological and biological data for waterfowl are given in Figures 26.3 and 26.4, respectively.

Ecology

The water birds coexist successfully by having different biology and behaviour to inhabit various niches in the same aquatic environment. Species variations occur in feeding, migratory patterns and habitat (Figure 26.3).

Feeding

Waterfowl of different species are herbivorous, omnivorous, carnivorous or piscivorous, with appropriate anatomical adaptations to facilitate these differences (Figure 26.3).

Swans are herbivores, grazing on aquatic vegetation by swimming or upending. Geese are also herbivores but are more terrestrial, mainly grazing vegetation on land.

Dabbling ducks such as the mallard are omnivorous; they feed in surface water, using straining lamellae on their beaks to sift vegetation and invertebrates.

Classification	Species	Characteristics	Diet	Feeding strategy	Resident or migrant	Typical habitat
Order Anseriformes: waterfowl						
Subfamily Anserinae: swans and geese: 21 species						
Tribe Cygnini: Swans	Mute swan (*Cygnus olor*) Whooper swan (*C. cygnus*) Bewick's swan (*C. columbianus bewickii*) Black swan (*C. atratus*) Trumpeter swan (*C. buccinator*)	Swans are the largest waterfowl and have the longest necks Males are termed 'cob'; females are termed 'pen' Often pair for life Mute swans are fiercely territorial, especially during breeding season	Herbivorous: aquatic vegetation; grasses	Mostly aquatic, often upending; some terrestrial grazing	Mute swan: resident Whooper and Bewick's swans: migrant, overwintering in the UK Black and trumpeter swans: feral non-indigenous	Mostly open freshwater, marshes, wet pasture
Tribe Anserini: Grey geese	Bar-headed goose (*Anser indicus*) Bean goose (*A. fabalis*) Greylag goose (*A. anser*) Pink-footed goose (*A. brachyrhynchus*) White-fronted goose (*A. albifrons*)	Males are termed 'gander'; females are termed 'goose' Seasonally monogamous Geese have longer legs which are more centrally placed under the body than ducks or swans, more suited to taking off from land	Herbivorous: grasses; aquatic vegetation; terrestrial vegetation including grain and root crops	Mostly terrestrial grazing; some aquatic	Greylag mainly resident Others migrant, overwintering in the UK	Marshes, wet grassland and winter arable crops
Black geese	Barnacle goose (*Branta leucopsis*) Brent goose (*B. bernicla*) Canada goose (*B. canadensis*)	See grey geese Domestic geese are developed from the barnacle goose; hybrids occur from matings of wild and feral domestic geese Seasonally monogamous	Herbivorous: grasses	Mostly terrestrial grazing, some aquatic	Barnacle migrant, overwintering in the UK Canada feral resident	Marshes, wet grassland and winter arable crops
Subfamily Anatinae: ducks						
Tribe Tadornini: Shelducks and Sheldgeese 14 species	Shelduck (*Tadorna tadorna*) Egyptian goose (*Alopochen aegyptiacus*)	Large ducks with colourful plumage	Invertebrates, small shellfish and aquatic snails Egyptian goose – also grasses	Shelduck: filtering mud Egyptian goose: mostly terrestrial grazing	Resident, adults migrate for post-breeding moult	Shelduck: mainly coastal and some inland waters Egyptian goose: feral widespread in southern inland waters
Tribe Cairnini: perching ducks 13 species	Mandarin duck (*Aix galericulata*) North American Carolina duck (*Aix sponsa*) Muscovy duck (*Cairina moschata*)	Capable of jumping	Herbivorous: aquatic vegetation; often nuts and seeds	Aquatic, surface	Feral, resident	Perch and nest in holes in trees Inland waters
Tribe Anatini: dabbling ducks 40 species	Mallard (*Anas platyrhynchos*) Northern shoveler (*A. clypeata*) Teal (*A. crecca*) Wigeon (*A. penelope*) Pintail (*A. acuta*)	Domestic species developed from the mallard, feral, sometimes interbreeding with the wild mallard include the Call duck, Aylesbury duck and Indian Runner duck	Most species: omnivorous Wigeon: herbivorous grazer	Aquatic surface Upending common Wigeons are grazers	Resident and winter migrants	Freshwater lakes, rivers and marshes Spread to coastal marshes in winter

26.3 Classification and ecological characteristics of common UK species of waterfowl. (continues) ▶

Classification	Species	Characteristics	Diet	Feeding strategy	Resident or migrant	Typical habitat
Subfamily Anatinae: ducks continued						
Tribe Aythyini: diving ducks 15 species	Pochard (*Aythya ferina*) Tufted duck (*A. fuligula*) Scaup (*A. marila*)	Short, rounded bodies	Piscivorous plus invertebrates	Diving	Resident and winter migrants	Mainly freshwater lakes Scaups winter at sea
Bucephala (Goldeneyes)	Goldeneye (*Bucephala clangula*)	Gold-coloured eyes	Aquatic invertebrates	Diving	Mainly winter migrant	Freshwater lakes; coastal
Melanitta (sea ducks: scoters)	Common scoter (*Melanitta nigra*)	Compact, small bills and rounded heads	Mainly molluscs	Diving	Summer migrant to Scotland Winter migrant: coasts	Summer: inland Scottish lochs Winter: coastal
Somateriini (sea ducks: eiders)	Eider duck (*Somateria mollissima*)	Common eider: male black and white; female brown	Mainly molluscs	Diving	Resident in north Winter migrants elsewhere	Open sea and coastal waters
Oxyurini (stiff-tailed ducks) 9 species	Ruddy duck (*Oxyura jamaicensis*)	Large feet, stay mostly on water Stiff tail feathers used as a rudder	Herbivorous	Diving	Feral resident, aim is to eradicate	Ruddy duck: marshes and ponds Nest on floating reed platforms
Mergini (sea ducks: sawbills) 18 species	Red-breasted merganser (*Mergus serrator*) Goosander (*M. merganser*) Smew (*M. albellus*)	Typically hole-nesters Mergansers have saw-tooth edges to their more slender, hooked bills, which help them to grasp fish	Piscivorous; also shellfish and crustaceans	Diving	Usually winter migrants Goosander: breeds inland on rivers and lakes	Usually inland lakes Merganser: coastal
Order Podicipediformes: Grebes						
Grebes	Great crested grebe (*Podiceps cristatus*) Little grebe (*Tachybaptus ruficollis*)	Lobed toes on legs that are set back further along the body The skin over the legs attaches a greater length of leg to the body; this shape is advantageous for diving, but makes walking on land difficult Slim pointed beak Minimal sexual dimorphism	Piscivorous; also invertebrates	Diving	Resident	Great crested grebe: summer – inland lakes; winter – freshwater and coastal Little grebe: freshwater lakes, ponds and rivers
Order Gaviiformes: Divers						
Family Gaviidae (divers)	Red-throated diver (*Gavia stellata*) Great northern diver (*G. immer*) Black-throated diver (*G. arctica*)	Three forward-pointing toes are webbed Long slim pointed beak Legs set far back on body The skin over the legs attaches a greater length of leg to the body Advantageous for diving, but makes walking on land difficult Nest in scraped hole with small amount of vegetation, on ground near water's edge	Piscivorous	Diving	Summer migrants to Scotland; Winter migrants elsewhere	Summer: mainly lakes and pools; Winter: mainly at sea

26.3 (continued) Classification and ecological characteristics of common UK species of waterfowl.

Diving ducks, which include the stiff-tailed and sea ducks, dive underwater for molluscs, crustaceans and small amphibians. Mergansers have pointed beaks with serrated edges for catching small fish, but also eat molluscs, crustaceans and small amphibians. Divers and grebes only eat fish.

Territory

Outside the breeding season many species, such as divers, form flocks. Sexually mature swans and geese become territorial during the breeding season. Swans can be territorial to a lesser extent throughout the rest of the year. Many pairs of mute swans return to the same area to breed each year. Territory size varies with the quality and quantity of food available.

Group	Typical bodyweight m=male; f=female	Lifespan	Age at sexual maturity
Swans	Mute swan: 9.5–13 kg (m); 8–10.5 kg (f) Whooper swan: 9.8–11 kg (m); 8.2–9.2 kg (f) Bewick's swan: 5–8 kg (m); 4–6 kg (f) Black swan: 5–6 kg (m); 4–6 kg (f) Trumpeter swan: 9–13 kg	Up to 25 years	3–5 years
Geese	Bar-headed goose: 2–3 kg Bean goose: 2.7–3.6 kg Greylag goose: 3.5–3.7 kg (m); 2.9–3.1 kg (f) Pink-footed goose: 2–3.5 kg White-fronted goose: 1.5–2 kg Barnacle goose: 1.5–2 kg Brent goose: 1.3–1.6 kg Canada goose: 4–5 kg	Up to 15 years	2–4 years
Ducks	Shelduck: 1100–1300 g (m); 900–1100 g (f) Egyptian goose: 2.1 kg (m); 1.7 kg (f) Mandarin duck: 440–550 g North American Carolina duck (wood duck): 450–860 g Muscovy duck: 3.5–5 kg Mallard: 1–1.5 kg (m); 750–1100 g (f) Northern shoveler: 500–700 g Teal: 250–400 g Wigeon: 780–900 g (m); 500–680 g (f) Pintail: 850–1200 g (m); 500–750 g (f) Pochard: 700–1000 g Tufted duck: 1050–1100 g Scaup: 360–730 g European goldeneye: 700–1160g Common scoter: 980–1100 g Common eider: 2.1–2.3 kg Ruddy duck: 560 g Red-breasted merganser: 1.1 kg Goosander: 1.4–1.6 kg (m); 1.1–1.4 kg (f)	Up to 10 years	1–2 years
Grebes	Great crested grebe: 1000–1200 g (m); 800–930 g (f) Little crested grebe: 100–120 g	Great crested grebe up to 10 years Little crested grebe up to 6 years	2 years
Divers	Red-throated diver: 1.2–1.6 kg Great northern diver: 3–4 kg Black-throated diver: 3.3–3.5 kg	Up to 23 years	6 years

26.4 Biological data of common UK species of waterfowl. See Figure 26.3 for classification and species name.

Migration

Most ducks and swans are migratory (see Figure 26.3). Exceptions include the mute swan, Canada and Egyptian (*Alopochen aegyptiaca*) goose and mallard duck. Breeding takes place in the northerly habitat and overwintering in the more southern, warmer climate. Some species overwinter in the UK, and for some the UK is part of the migration path. Migration routes and staging areas are predictable and timings are regular, with only minor changes occurring influenced by weather conditions. Red-throated divers (*Gavia stellata*) breed between April and September around north and west Scotland, leaving their breeding grounds from late September to winter around more southern parts of the UK coast.

Anatomy and physiology

Waterfowl are medium- to large-sized birds with long necks and triangular feet that are webbed between the front three toes. Most have round-ended, short, broad bills with straining lamellae at each side. Waterfowl have thick downy feathers for buoyancy and waterproofing that they moult after the breeding season (with a period of flightlessness). Males possess an intromittent erectile phallus.

Young are nidifugous: covered in down, and can eat, swim and dive almost immediately after hatching.

Waterfowl have several anatomical and physiological adaptations that allow them to survive in the various wetland environments they inhabit.

Bill adaptations

Despite their common features, the bills of waterfowl have evolved in an array of sizes and shapes to exploit a variety of food items. Compared to other species of waterfowl, the shape of the mallard bill is broad and relatively unspecialized, allowing them to forage on a wide variety of food items. Many other species have specialized bills. Among the most specialized are the bills of mergansers, which have long, narrow, serrated bills, adapted for grasping small fish. Sea ducks, like scoters (*Melanitta nigra*) and eiders (*Somateria mollissima*), have strong, stout bills to assist them in prying open shellfish. The northern shoveler (*Anas clypeata*) has a wide, shovel-like bill with well developed lamellae functioning as a large scoop and sieve for skimming invertebrates and seeds from the water's surface. The bills of Canada geese are adapted for grasping and snipping new shoots of grasses, leaves and stems. Whilst considered a dabbling duck, American wigeon (*Anas americana*) also graze; the shape of their bill being very similar to that of a Canada goose.

The bill is primarily adapted to help locate and consume food resources. In general, bills are round-tipped and soft around the edges so waterfowl can locate food by touch. The bill is lined with lamellae, fine comb-like structures found in rows along the inside of the bill. When waterfowl are feeding, sediment and water enter the bill. Lamellae filter out inedible material, whilst trapping invertebrates, seeds, and other food items. The tip of the upper mandible has a 'nail' that is used for prying or moving food and other items.

Waterfowl species that dig ('grub') or rip up tubers and roots have stout wedge-shaped bills ideal for prying plant material loose from beneath the mud. Grubbing waterfowl species also have strong, muscular necks, which help them uproot the buried plant parts. Many waterfowl, for example swans, Canada geese, mallards and green-winged teal (*Anas carolinensis*) all upend or dabble to forage on submersed aquatic plants. Their varying neck length allow them to access foods at different water depths.

Neck

Waterfowl do not have a distensible crop and therefore any neck swelling is abnormal. Trumpeter (*Cygnus buccinator*), whooper, whistling (*Cygnus columbianus columbianus*) and Bewick's (*Cygnus columbianus bewickii*) swans all have tracheae which convolute inside the sternum.

Feathers

Waterfowl have a thick layer of compact feathers and down, an adaptation to an aquatic environment that aids buoyancy and provides insulation. The uropygial gland is well developed in most species.

Shedding and regrowth of feathers takes place yearly after the breeding season. Some ducks moult twice per year: once into their brighter breeding plumage when flight ability is retained and again after breeding into a duller eclipse plumage (see 'Gender determination'). The moult in the male and female swan is asynchronous and the birds are flightless for a few weeks during moulting.

Feet and legs

The feet are webbed between the front-facing toes to assist swimming. The web is spread out on the backward stroke and folded on the forward stroke. The webbing may also assist walking on mud. Birds that spend proportionately more time on water (e.g. the diving ducks), have their legs sited more distally along the body to help propel them through the water; this, however, makes it more difficult for them to walk on land.

Heat exchange

Ducks, similar to many other birds, have a countercurrent heat exchange system between the arteries and veins in their legs. The rete tibiotarsale allows warm arterial blood flowing to the feet to pass close to and warm up the cold venous blood returning from the feet. This means that the blood that flows through the feet is relatively cool, keeping the feet supplied with just enough blood to provide tissues with food and oxygen, and just warm enough to avoid frostbite. By limiting the temperature difference between the feet and the cold water, heat loss is greatly reduced. Birds' legs and feet are relatively free of soft tissue, reducing the need for warm blood. Many aquatic birds also have valves in their leg arteries that control the blood flow.

Adaptations for diving

Divers are less buoyant than dabbling ducks, geese and swans, because their bodies are denser and more compact, which helps them to stay underwater for prolonged periods. To further reduce their buoyancy, divers compress their feathers against their bodies before diving, reducing the volume of air trapped in their downy feathers. The wings of divers are much more compact than surface feeders, which allows the birds to squeeze them tightly against their bodies, reducing drag as they dive. Once underwater, diving ducks use their wings and feet to propel them into deeper waters in search of food.

Reproduction

Gender determination

The males (drakes) of many duck species have bright 'nuptial' plumage in the breeding season, and can be easily distinguished from the duller-plumaged female (hen). The birds moult after the breeding season (see 'Feathers', when the males grow a duller 'eclipse' plumage and look very similar to the females. Many drakes have a curly feather dorsally at the base of the tail. Males of most duck species have a left-sided enlargement of the syrinx: the syringeal bulla.

Swans display minimal sexual dimorphism. Cobs (males) tend to be bigger than pens (females), with a larger basal knob at the base of the upper beak. The appearance of the sexes in divers and grebes is similar.

Cloacal examination can be used to determine sex in the species that are not obviously dimorphic, as males have an intromittent erectile phallus. The ease of this procedure varies with the experience of the handler, the age, species, sex of bird and time of year it is performed. To determine the sex, the bird should be held head downwards between the knees, or in the hands for newly hatched birds, with the ventrum facing the handler. Firm, gentle pressure should be applied with the thumbs in a dorsolateral direction on either side of the cloaca. The female has two labia-like structures, whilst the male has a definite phallus.

Breeding

Waterfowl pair in the late winter, nesting in the spring and early summer. Nesting sites vary according to species: banks, islands, rafts on water, holes in trees, burrows in the ground and even other birds' nests are all used. Divers only come ashore to nest and breed. Nest complexity differs between species, varying from highly piled vegetation (e.g. in swans), to a scrape in the ground lined with feathers (e.g. in scoters).

Many swans and geese are monogamous throughout the year and both genders have a substantial role in rearing their young. Ducks are monogamous until the female starts incubating the eggs, then the male leaves. A common behaviour amongst the dabbling ducks and some diving ducks is 'extra-pair forced copulation', which involves a group of males mating one female.

Many species of waterfowl produce only one clutch per year; however, if a clutch is lost early in the breeding season another may be produced. One egg is laid daily over consecutive days to a total clutch of usually six to nine eggs, divers laying only two in total. The clutch is incubated for 21–42 days, the time varying according to species. In swans both the male and female share the clutch incubation. Divers need to be on water to defecate, so the pair work closely together and share the incubation.

All the young in a clutch hatch on the same day. They emerge already covered in down and can forage, eat, swim and dive almost immediately. A yolk sac in the coelomic cavity provides nutrition for up to 7 days. Swan parents will help provide feed for the young (cygnets) by treading up aquatic vegetation. Adult swans care for their brood until they are fully fledged and developing adult plumage. Cygnets take on average 120–150 days to develop feathers to the flying stage. In their first year mute swan cygnets develop light brown feathers and the beak turns from black to plum colour. Over the next year these feathers are replaced by white ones. After the first moult the feathers are 95% white and by the second moult are 100% white. Once the cygnets are perceived as adults – as the white plumage develops – the parents chase them away from the territory. The beak remains plum coloured until sexual maturity at 3–5 years.

Female ducks lead their brood only until the ducklings fledge into adult plumage at 5–10 weeks.

Normal parameters

Basic vital parameters for waterfowl are given in Figure 26.5. Cloacal temperature for aquatic birds lies between 40–42°C. This is not generally a very useful parameter for clinical assessment in the author's experience and taking a temperature may be stressful for the patient. Cloacal temperature monitoring, however, should be used to assess the degree of heat loss during general anaesthesia.

Species	Respiratory rate (breaths per minute)	Heart rate (beats per minute)	Cloacal temperature range (°C)
Swans and geese	13–40	80–150	40–42
Ducks	30–95	180–230	40–42

26.5 Basic vital parameters for common waterfowl species.

Capture, handling and transportation

Normal waterfowl behaviour

Some normal behaviour of waterfowl species can be mis-construed as a bird that is injured or in trouble. For example:

- A swan 'having a wash' (preening) may look to a member of the public like it is drowning
- Waterfowl often carry one leg resting on their back whilst on the water (Figure 26.6) and stand with one leg tucked up when on land. Neither of these positions is possible if the leg is fractured
- Mute cygnets' wings may droop for a time as the flight feathers are growing and this may be mistaken for wing damage
- Grebes sometimes crash land on roads and are wrongly assumed to have spinal damage as they do not move when approached. This is most often not the case; grebes and divers cannot walk easily on land as their legs are positioned caudally, predominantly for swimming. These birds should be clinically examined and if healthy returned immediately to nearby water
- During the breeding season, separation of swan family members causes high anxiety as they are vulnerable to

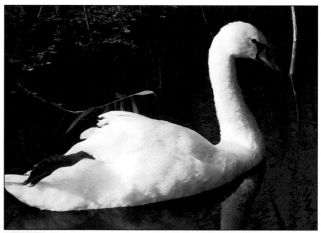

26.6 Mute swan on water resting its leg. This may be misinterpreted by members of the general public as a sign of injury. This natural position is not possible if the limb is fractured. (© Phil Scott)

attacks from predators and neighbouring swans. A cygnet that is separated from its parents should if possible be immediately reunited. If separated for more than 48 hours it is very likely to be rejected and killed on reintroduction
- Ducklings may be perceived by the public to have been abandoned, despite the mother being usually nearby, and are often brought in to a local rescue centre.

Mallard ducks may also make nesting sites away from the river, for instance in garden flower tubs. In this case, the family need to be safely relocated to the nearest stretch of water.

Personal safety

Personal safety when handling waterfowl, in and around water, is of paramount importance. As all water is potentially hazardous and suitable precautions (including the use of life jackets) should be taken. Rescues must be carried out only by suitably trained and experienced personnel who are well equipped (see also Chapter 3). Rescue centres that frequently carry out waterfowl work should have suitable health and safety policies in place and training programmes that reflect these specific requirements. It is important to be well acquainted with local water conditions such as tides and currents. Swans often land on wet roads and railway lines and liaison with the appropriate transport authority will be necessary in these cases.

Birds can cause injury to handlers, bystanders, passers-by and observers. Swans and geese deliver a powerful blow with their wings and can also nip with their beak and scratch with their claws. Once birds find they cannot escape, attack becomes their form of defence. Divers and grebes readily use their sharp beaks, lunging and stabbing at the face, and goggles should be worn when dealing with these birds (see Chapter 3). Many birds will be more aggressive in the breeding season.

Methods of capture and handling

A calm attitude and swift reflexes are required when handling waterfowl. Chasing an already compromised patient is unnecessarily stressful for all concerned. Often a quiet approach with a canoe is more successful than using a motorized craft, which scares the bird and can provoke flight. Natural human behaviour can provoke further agitation; for example, making a 'shh'-ing sound is interpreted as aggressive hissing, standing with hands on hips mimics a bird's aggressive posture and stroking and patting provoke attempts to escape. Mute swans make a soft double grunt noise in greeting and reproducing this can help calm them.

Most swans, geese and ducks can be lured with food and then caught. Once within safe range, grasp a wing firmly, or if this is not possible, grasp the neck just behind the head in a swift movement. Swan 'hooks' should be used only when absolutely necessary, and then with great care to avoid injury to the neck. The body should then be pulled close and the wings secured. Swans and geese are held against the handler's body, firmly under one arm, without restricting respiration, trapping the folded wings against the bird's body and leaving the legs dangling (Figure 26.7). Ducks' wings are secured to the body using both hands (Figure 26.8). Landing nets are useful for smaller birds. When catching a duck with her brood, catch the adult first or she will fly away.

Capture of divers requires a boat, nets and an experienced rescuer. These birds are notoriously difficult to catch unless quite debilitated. Divers are often only caught because they are so ill they have drifted to the bank or ashore. When handling divers and grebes, always use one hand to keep the beak closed and wear protective goggles.

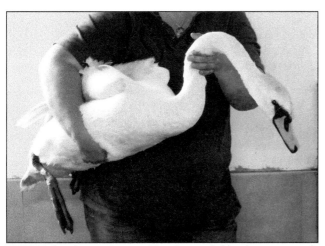

26.7 Carrying a mute swan. The wings are held under one arm and firmly against the handler's body, leaving the other hand free to gently restrain the head.

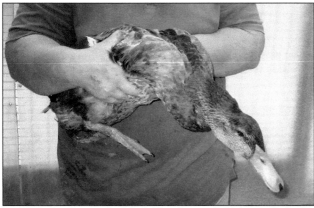

26.8 Carrying a mallard duck. The wings are held close to the body using both hands to prevent flapping and possible injury to the bird.

Transportation

Swans and geese can be transported in purpose-made 'swan bags' (see Figure 26.27). The best design is a wrap made from polyvinyl chloride (PVC) with six flaps and a fabric hook and loop fastener (e.g. Velcro®). Large reusable shopping bags are also very useful (Figure 26.9). As an alternative a pillowcase with a corner cut off can be used, the head and neck being threaded through the hole and the feet tucked in. Swans and geese can also safely travel in a large dog transit kennel lined with soft towels. If necessary the wings can be tied using a soft bandage around both humeri and across the dorsum. Legs can be secured by tying them together in extension, positioned dorsal to the tail. Tying of the wings and legs is not always necessary if the bird is very debilitated. Swans appear to like to travel looking out of the window.

Ducks and divers can be transported in any suitable box or cat carrier with a towel as a non-slip substrate.

In all cases it is important to ensure that the vehicle is well ventilated and not too hot, as the birds are prone to heat stress when away from water.

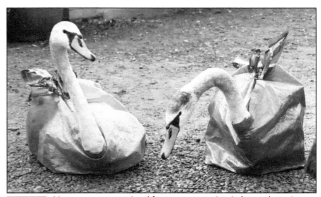

26.9 Mute swans restrained for transportation in large shopping bags.
(© Secret World Wildlife Rescue)

Examination and clinical assessment for rehabilitation

History-taking

The site where the bird was found, number and species of birds affected, and the time of year can all give valuable pointers as to a possible diagnosis. For example, a swan found sitting under electricity wires or a bridge is likely to have crash-landed. Paralysed birds from several species in one area in hot weather are likely to be suffering from botulism or blue-green algal toxicity rather than lead toxicosis. Deaths or morbidity in immature birds with unaffected adults may indicate a heavy parasite burden.

The environment in which the bird is found can also provide useful information. The water at the rescue site should be inspected for blue-green algal bloom, oil or other pollutants. The use of the site for fishing or other water sports may also be significant.

Clinical assessment

Clinical assessment should be performed in three phases:

1. There should be an initial brief clinical examination from beak to tail (see Chapter 4) with the whole procedure taking no more than a couple of minutes, unless there

is a heavy maggot burden or profuse bleeding that requires immediate treatment.

2. The bird should then be placed in a quiet pen for observation. Initially the bird should be observed from a distance. The effects of transportation should be considered; the stress of transport may cause panting. If limbs have been tied, the wings may droop or the bird may at first be disinclined to walk. See if the bird will eat (unless there is obvious oesophageal swelling, see 'Specific conditions'); it may need to be shown the feeding bowl, which will not be familiar to it, and the beak gently inserted into the water to encourage feeding. Once the bird has settled, assess its general demeanour, which should be bright and reactive to its surroundings. Note any inability to stand, any lameness or wing droop, increased respiratory effort or open-mouthed breathing. Divers and grebes do not stand or walk well. Wild birds hide pain and the only manifestation of this may be a generally depressed attitude. Note any generalized bilateral paresis or paralysis and the position in which the head and neck are held.

3. Finally a more thorough examination, with any necessary diagnostic tests, should be performed, as detailed below.

Clinical examination

One person should restrain the bird with the minimum force necessary to allow a second person to perform the examination (Figure 26.10). The handler uses one hand to hold the legs extended above the tail, with the other arm holding the wings against the bird's body. The person examining the bird can then manoeuvre different body parts freely.

Assess the body condition (see Chapter 4). Severe debilitation will cause ulceration of the skin overlying the keel with subsequent keel infection ('keel rot', see 'Specific conditions'). This is a very poor prognostic sign.

Note any saliva either coming from the mouth or deposited on the dorsal thorax between the wings. Run the index finger under the mandible to check for fishing line ('chin strap'). Look inside the mouth including under the tongue for fishing line, hooks and other lesions. The bird may be unable to extend the head because the line is caught between the mouth and the neck. In this case the line should be cut. Do not pull on any fishing line protruding from the mouth as there may be a hook on the end that is embedded in the oesophagus, but cut off any large amount of line leaving 30–60 cm to help locate the hook later. Although some rehabilitators 'secure' the remaining line to the swan's feathers using tape or forceps, in the

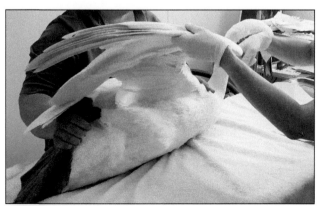

26.10 Mute swan being restrained by a handler, leaving a second person free to perform a full clinical examination.

author's experience this is unnecessary. Tape often does not stick properly, both tape and forceps annoy the bird and the weight of forceps may put traction on the hook resulting in further oesophageal damage. Palpate the length of the neck for swellings (see 'Specific conditions').

Check the whole body for soft tissue swellings, wounds, bone fractures and air or bone crepitus. Check circumferential linear wounds for fishing line. Assess the body or limb distal to a line injury for loss of vitality. Auscultate the air sacs under the wings for any adventitious sounds such as bubbly gurgling or muffling of heart sounds. Heart murmurs may also be detected by auscultation ventrally either side of the sternum and under the wings.

Even small wounds can produce a large amount of haemorrhage. Birds will also wick blood on to feathers with their beaks whilst preening. Locate the source of bleeding by looking for blood deep in the feathers. Damage to newly growing feathers may be a source of haemorrhage. Look for evidence of parasites, maggots and fly eggs. Severely debilitated birds will often have a heavy feather louse (*Mallophaga* spp.) burden. Many types of oil can cause contamination and in these instances there may be multiple casualties (see also Chapter 24).

Visually assess droppings for texture, colour, blood and undigested food. Note any faecal staining around the vent. Lead-poisoned birds often produce bright green faeces (see Figure 26.19). In the author's experience faeces resembling soggy wheat cereal appear to be a poor prognostic indicator in spinal injuries.

Diagnostic techniques

Clinical examination, together with good history-taking, is the most important diagnostic tool in the assessment of waterfowl casualties.

Blood biochemistry and haematology values (Figure 26.11) may be useful diagnostic aids in the treatment of waterfowl casualties but results should always be carefully interpreted in conjunction with clinical findings. Packed cell volume (PCV) may be used as a prognostic indicator in cases such as lead toxicity. Elevated total white blood cell count in infectious/inflammatory cases can be useful for monitoring response to treatment. Bile acids and uric acid levels are also useful. Hepatic values, renal values and PCV are useful prognostically in toxic conditions responding poorly to treatment. Blood lead levels may be ascertained in cases of suspected lead toxicosis (see 'Specific conditions'), although the author has found that clinically normal swans can tolerate high blood lead levels and so finds clinical response to treatment a better prognostic indicator.

Bacterial culture and antibiotic sensitivity testing are helpful clinically, as well as being good practice, and are essential in cases where infections do not respond to first-line antibiotics.

Radiography is helpful in a variety of conditions including: assessment of air sacs for opacities consistent with aspergillosis; location or presence of foreign bodies such as fishing hooks and missiles; diagnosis of fractures; gizzard imaging for foreign bodies and in cases of suspected lead toxicosis; enlarged joints for septic arthritis. All these conditions are discussed in more detail in the sections that follow. It is possible to obtain limb views and a dorso-ventral whole body view in a conscious bird, by gently tying the legs and using a little patience.

Endoscopy can be very useful in swans, particularly chronic emaciated cases where a diagnosis has not been made: many of these have chronic thickening of the air sacs on coelioscopic examination. In the author's

Variable (units)	Reference interval	
	Adult mute swans (Cygnus olor) Mean ± SD (range)	Adult mallard (Anas platyrhynchos)
Haematology		
Red blood cell (RBC) count (x 10¹²/l)	2.07 ± 0.04 (1.72–2.43)[b]	2–3.8[c]
Haemoglobin (g/dl)	12.7 ± 1.6 (8.5–24.6)[b]	7.4–15.6[c]
Packed cell volume (PCV) (%)	34.5 ± 2.7 (21–44)[b]	39–49[c]
Mean corpuscular volume (MCV) (fl)	169.8 ± 10.9 (118–208.8)[b]	148–200[c]
Mean corpuscular haemoglobin (MCH) ((pg) per cell)	62.2 ± 7.2 (39.2–109.8)[b]	NDA
Mean corpuscular haemoglobin concentration (MCHC) (g/dl)	37.9 ± 4.9 (19.8–68.3)[b]	29–32[c]
RBC sedimentation rate (mm/hr)	8.3 ± 2.6 (1–13)[b]	NDA
White blood cell (WBC) count (x 10⁹/l)	16.2 ± 2.9 (3.5–29)[b]	23.4–24.8[c]
Heterophils (%)	39.0 ± 1.6 (27–53)[b]	26–38[c]
Lymphocytes (%)	55.3 ± 1.7 (37–69)[b]	54–63[c]
Monocytes (%)	0.2 ± 0.5 (0–8)[b]	1–4[c]
Eosinophils (%)	1.1 ± 0.3 (0–4)[b]	0.2–0.4[c]
Basophils (%)	2.4 ± 0.4 (0–9)[b]	0–4[c]
Biochemistry		
Calcium (mmol/l)	2.52 ± 0.05 (2.1–2.9)[a]	NDA
Sodium (mmol/l)	142 ± 0.3 (135.8 -159)[a]	NDA
Potassium (mmol/l)	4.1 ± 0.05 (3–5.6)[a]	NDA
Chloride (mmol/l)	102.2 ± 0.4 (90.2–113)[a]	NDA
Creatinine (μmol/l)	31.1 ± 0.06 (17–91)[a]	NDA
Uric acid (μmol/l)	286.32 ± 12.6 (66 -820)[a]	NDA
Glucose (mmol/l)	9.14 ± 1.4 (6.5–14)[a]	NDA
Cholesterol (mmol/l)	4.28 ± 0.8 (2.66–6.9)[a]	NDA
Lactate dehydrogenase (LDH) (IU/l)	520.96 ± 179.64 (270.66–1044.91)[a]	NDA
Alkaline phosphatase (ALP) (IU/l)	92.22 ± 47.9 (19.76–329.34)[a]	NDA
Alanine aminotransferase (ALT) (IU/l)	31.14 ± 13.77 (14.37–90.42)[a]	NDA
Aspartate aminotransferase (AST) (IU/l)	35.93 ± 11.98 (15.57–116.17)[a]	NDA
Total protein (g/l)	50.45 ± 0.5 (32.50–61)[a]	NDA

26.11 Reference intervals for biochemical and haematological parameters in waterfowl. NDA = no data available.
([a]O'Halloran et al., 1988; [b]Dolka et al., 2014; [c]Carpenter, 2013)

experience endoscopy is not useful in cases of neck swelling, as the oesophagus has multiple plications in the neck region and a tear is easily missed. An oesophageal swelling is an indication for surgical exploration of the area.

Faecal analysis is useful for the detection of intestinal parasitism (see Chapter 10).

Post-mortem examination is valuable in cases where multiple birds are ill or dying, with little conclusion to be drawn from clinical signs. It can also be performed as part of the documentation of cases where intentional wounding is suspected, or where missiles need to be retrieved for evidence. Further information is provided in Chapters 10 and 11.

Euthanasia

Although many extensive injuries, including large skin deficits, severe infections and multiple bone fractures, will heal given the right environment, treatment and time, the welfare issues associated with prolonged treatment and captivity, as well as the prognosis for eventual release, should be borne in mind and assessed on an individual basis (see Chapter 4). Waterfowl rescue centres may have the facilities to keep permanently disabled birds long-term in a sheltered environment, using private lakes with owners willing to foster birds. Well managed lakes, on which birds can be carefully observed for signs of problems, may provide an alternative to euthanasia for some individuals.

Where necessary, euthanasia is performed using intravenous pentobarbital solution. The author's preferred site for intravenous injection in this case is the medial metatarsal vein (Figure 26.12), although other peripheral veins (e.g. ulnar vein) can be used. Intracoelomic injection, just distal to the caudal-most aspect of the keel bone, is an alternative method in a very debilitated or already anaesthetized bird.

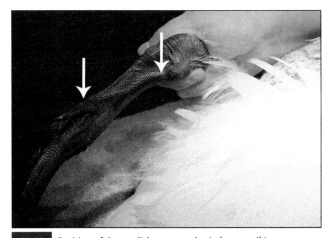

26.12 Position of the medial metatarsal vein (arrowed) in a swan.

First aid and short-term hospitalization

First aid

Waterfowl patients should be handled as little as possible to minimize stress. Most cases respond well to a combination of food, analgesia, quiet surroundings and the company of the same or similar species. An assessment for infectious disease should be made to minimize risk of disease transfer between birds. As diseases such as duck viral enteritis (DVE) are very difficult to identify, it is good practice to keep birds in small groups initially and maintain good hygiene.

The general principles of first aid should be applied (see Chapter 5). Any bleeding should be stopped by applying pressure using cohesive bandages and padding such as swabs. Blood vessels may require ligation and superficial vessels may be ligated in the conscious patient. Tissue glue may be applied to profusely bleeding nicks on the beak, with or without alginate dressing, to stop haemorrhage in these areas. It is not uncommon for birds that are hypothermic when they arrive to start to bleed as their body temperature elevates.

Analgesia (see 'Anaesthesia and analgesia') and fluid therapy should be administered as appropriate (see Chapter 5). Most patients will benefit from the use of analgesics. Intravenous access can usually be achieved using the medial metatarsal vein (see Figure 26.12). The ulnar vein, as it courses over the elbow joint on the ventral aspect of the wing, is more difficult to access as these birds do not readily allow the wing to be extended and, with the larger birds, having the wing free can put the handlers at risk of being hit. In the larger patient the lateral digital vein running along the lateral aspect of the outermost digit is accessible. A 22 G catheter is used for swans and geese, and 24 G for smaller birds. Any leg rings present may need to be removed to facilitate venous access. In the author's experience, topical local anaesthetic (e.g. EMLA® cream) aids catheter placement in cygnets, whose leg skin appears to be more sensitive than that of adult birds. Care should be taken when using local anaesthetics in avian patients, as toxic side effects occur at lower doses in avian species (Hocking *et al.*, 1997). The author has, however, never observed these effects in cygnets. When the catheter is withdrawn it is necessary to place a firm bandage over the venepuncture site as the inelasticity of the skin allows marked bleeding.

Any fishing line should be removed and some wounds may require immediate treatment (see 'Specific conditions').

Waterfowl may have parasitic nasal leeches (see Figure 26.21); the nostrils should be checked and these removed manually with forceps. It may also be necessary to treat myiasis (see 'Specific conditions').

Any limb fractures should be stabilized. Fractured wings should be bandaged to the body, first making sure the wing has not twisted 360 degrees around the fracture. Wing bandaging techniques are described in Chapter 5. Leg fractures must be supported using layers of padding and/or gutter splints.

Oiled birds, especially divers, should be fed and rested for a minimum of 24 hours before attempting to wash the bird in order to remove oil (see Chapter 24). The oil removal procedure should only be carried out at a centre with experience of dealing with these cases.

Short-term hospitalization

The veterinary clinic is not a suitable environment for waterfowl for anything but the shortest time whilst arrangements are being made for transfer to a wildlife rescue centre. Whilst in a veterinary clinic the birds must be kept away from the sight and sound of predator species.

It is important to provide suitable bedding material in order to provide padding and prevent keel and foot injuries (see Chapter 7). For most waterfowl this might include newspaper, shredded paper, blankets or straw. Although straw has been associated with an increased risk of aspergillosis in birds, these risks can be alleviated by the use of good quality straw, provision of very good ventilation and regular (daily) changes of bedding. In the author's experience straw helps keep the patients happily occupied, nest building and foraging in the bedding and, in the author's opinion, the benefits of this outweigh any possible risks.

Divers must be kept on soft bedding, for example foam covered in towels (see also Chapter 24). They must be moved frequently as they suffer from lung compression and are prone to developing aspergillosis and pressure sores on the keel and feet in captivity. They are unlikely to defecate when out of water, so this process should be

encouraged by stroking the underside of the bird to stimulate bowel movement. Expert advice should be obtained and transportation arranged to a suitable rescue centre as soon as possible.

All patients should be provided with appropriate food. Examples of food types that may be given on a short-term basis and that are easily available to veterinary practices are given in Figure 26.13.

A normal indoor ambient temperature is adequate. For debilitated birds this should be 17–19°C; temperatures above 20°C may cause the birds to pant or suffer heat stress.

Bird group	Food type	Comments
Divers, grebes	Fish only: sprats (Clupeidae), whitebait (immature fry of fish) or other fish of a similar size, frozen to kill parasites then thawed in a refrigerator	Place fish in a bowl and fill with water Feed small amounts at regular intervals Getting wild birds to eat can be very difficult and is best left to experienced rescuers
Swans, geese, dabbling ducks	Mixture of wheat, variety of greens such as lettuce, mixed leaf salad or spinach and bread (preferably wholemeal) Crumbled breakfast cereals (e.g. Weetabix®, bran flakes or corn flakes) can all be used as a temporary measure Dried grass (e.g. Graze-On®)	Place in a washing up bowl or large dog bowl and fill with plenty of water Smaller birds need shallower feeding dishes, such as cat litter trays Some birds need to be shown where the bowl is before they will feed
Diving ducks	Mixture of frozen then thawed whitebait-sized fish, and wheat/greens/bread in a bowl filled with water Alternatively use marine pellets (e.g. Charnwood Milling Company's Marine duck pellets™)	Place in a bowl and fill with plenty of water

26.13 Suggested food items for the short-term feeding of captive waterfowl.

Analgesia and anaesthesia
Sedation and general anaesthesia

It is possible to perform many non-invasive procedures without chemical restraint. Where further restraint is necessary it is far better in the author's opinion to use general anaesthesia than sedation. Sedation effects can be prolonged and may persist for 24–48 hours, depending on the drug used and the health status of the individual. The author often notices a general decline in the bird's clinical condition post-sedation. In comparison, recovery from general anaesthesia is usually swift, within 2 hours, with very little post-anaesthesia sedation. The patient is usually able to eat within 1–2 hours after cessation of gaseous anaesthesia.

Withholding of food and water is not necessary prior to anaesthesia. No sedative premedication is given by the author, although pre-emptive analgesia should be employed where indicated.

The author's induction agent of choice is intravenous propofol using an intravenous catheter placed in the medial metatarsal vein (see 'First aid' and Figure 26.12).

Gaseous induction using isoflurane or sevoflurane delivered via a facemask is an alternative method of induction where intravenous access is difficult, although breath-holding can occur with this technique. A mask can be made from a 500 ml or 1 litre intravenous fluid bag or a cut-off plastic drinks bottle. Alternatively, there are large plastic facemasks commercially available that are suitable for use in waterfowl.

Following induction, waterfowl are easily intubated using a non-cuffed endotracheal (ET) tube (Figure 26.14). The author does not find it necessary to spray the glottis with local anaesthetic and care should be taken if using local anaesthetic spray as it can be toxic to birds. ET tube placement is aided by gentle forward traction of the tongue with the non-dominant hand, whilst pushing upwards on the larynx from underneath with the little finger of the same hand. A 6 mm diameter ET tube is suitable for an adult swan. The ET tube is held in place with a 2.5 cm adhesive bandage, wrapped first around the tube and then around either the lower beak only, or around both upper and lower beak together (Figure 26.14). A large bore intravenous catheter sleeve can be used for intubation of smaller birds, connected to the anaesthetic circuit using a 3.5 mm connector. Alternatively, commercially available avian ET tubes can be used. Intravenous fluids (such as Hartmann's solution) are administered during anaesthesia at 10 ml/kg/hr using an infusion pump and fluid warmer (see also Chapter 6 for more information on avian anaesthesia).

Water birds should be placed in lateral recumbency wherever possible, using a support such as a rolled up towel, full fluid bag or sandbag between table and keel to allow normal sternal movements during respiration. Waterfowl do not need much thermal insulation during

anaesthesia – a blanket or heat mat underneath is sufficient. Anaesthesia should be monitored as in other avian species (see Chapter 6) using appropriate monitoring aids. Cloacal temperature should be monitored during general anaesthesia.

Recovery of consciousness should take a few minutes after cessation of isoflurane or sevoflurane delivery. Once the bird can lift its head it can be placed in a recovery pen, but must still be monitored carefully. Recovery can be accompanied by quite violent movements and may require gentle, but firm, restraint until fully recovered. Alternatively, swans can be placed in a 'swan bag' or wrapped in a blanket to recover. Food and water can be introduced from half an hour after the patient is able to stand. The company of others of the same species can also encourage a speedy recovery, once the bird is able to stand.

Analgesia

The majority of cases respond well to pain relief and, as with all casualties, analgesia is an essential part of first aid provision. Carprofen is the author's preferred non-steroidal anti-inflammatory drugs (NSAID), administered once daily by subcutaneous injection, as meloxicam appears to have a sedative effect on many patients in the author's experience, which is detrimental to their recovery. This effect has not, however, been noted by other authors. Doses for analgesic drugs are included in Figure 26.23.

Specific conditions
Trauma
Attack by other birds

Waterfowl may suffer injuries from conspecifics, for example in territorial fights between swans. Victims can appear quite depressed, yet show relatively little external physical injury. Analgesia, fluid therapy, nutritional support and general supportive care may be the only treatments necessary in these cases. Female ducks can incur severe injuries from multiple attempts by males to mate them. These include spinal damage, open wounds (particularly over the dorsum and caudal neck area), bruising and feather loss. Many of these birds present unable to stand with varying degrees of limb paresis, but recover in 24–48 hours with appropriate analgesia, such as NSAIDs and general supportive care. Open wounds should be managed as described later.

Bite wounds

Bite wounds from other species, including dogs, foxes and mink, are commonly seen in all waterfowl species. Dogs will inflict bite injuries at random anywhere on the bird, often resulting in injury to the wing or lateral thigh. Foxes (*Vulpes vulpes*) and mink (*Mustela (Neovison) vison*) attack to kill, biting the dorsum of the head, neck or thoracic area. Mink bites present as multiple approximately 2 mm diameter puncture wounds.

Bite wounds will be contaminated and require broad-spectrum systemic antibiotic treatment for 5–7 days, in addition to analgesia and topical therapies (see Figure 26.23). After wound management (flushing with saline or appropriately diluted antiseptic solutions) commercially available edible grade honey can be used for wound debridement and as an antiseptic agent. A fungal bloom

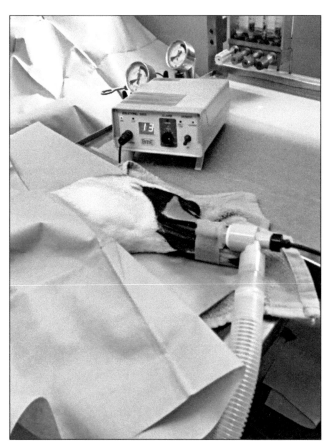

26.14 Anaesthetized and intubated mute swan showing the endotracheal tube taped to the beak.

may occur on long-term honey-treated wounds, but in the author's experience this is not detrimental to the bird's health, nor does it affect the rate of recovery.

Crashes and collisions

Crash landings and collisions are common, especially in the larger species. It takes an enormous amount of energy to fly and often the novice flyer drops exhausted out of the sky, or fails to navigate obstacles. The distance required to take off is as much as 100 m for swans. Some crash landings occur as a consequence of the bird's debilitation from another injury or underlying medical condition. Swans may crash into bridges, railway lines and wet roads, failing to distinguish these from water.

Crashes in flight (on landing or taking off) into trees and bushes can result in stick penetration injuries into the air sacs or soft tissue. These should ideally be assessed radiographically or by ultrasound examination prior to removal to determine the soft tissue structures involved and the potential haemorrhage that may occur. However, in the author's experience the penetrating item can just be removed and significant haemorrhage rarely occurs. Wounds are treated as for other open wounds (see 'Treatment of wounds').

With any trauma there is a risk of air sac damage resulting in subcutaneous emphysema. It is usually impossible to locate the source of the air leak. The subcutaneous emphysema will in most instances generally resolve without specific treatment, other than broad-spectrum prophylactic antibiosis (see Figure 26.23), usually for up to 14 days.

Crashing into electricity cables is common, especially in swans, and results in electrical burns which may be unilateral or bilateral. The burn will cause extensive necrosis, developing over the subsequent few days. Commonly the wing (in particular the leading edge of the propatagium) and surrounding areas are affected. Observation of wounds over 5–7 days will be necessary prior to release. Treatment is as in other species for any open wound or burn injury.

A variety of watercraft can be involved in collisions with waterfowl, especially when swans are defending their territory. Due to the high force of impact, open multiple fractures of the limbs are commonly incurred and these injuries carry a poorer prognosis.

Leg rings

Leg rings placed for identification purposes (see Chapter 9) can cause trauma to the intertarsal joint. Joint tap samples, which may be obtained aseptically from the conscious patient, should be cultured if they are turbid and cytology performed (see Chapter 10). The leg ring should be removed.

Missiles

Waterfowl are often subjected to accidental or intentional trauma from a range of missiles. Crossbow bolts require removal in a similar way to that described previously for stick penetration. Airgun pellets are walled off by the body, so do not need removing as they do not cause toxicosis. Extensive surgical exploration and removal of the pellet can be more damaging than the initial shooting. However, pellets may track debris into the wound, particularly feathers, which will require removal and saline flushing. Pellets may be identified on radiographs as an incidental finding. Slingshot ball bearings sometimes cause a large fluid

reaction or abscess. These need removing, following prior radiographic identification (Figure 26.15), often through a small incision in the conscious bird with cautious use of local anaesthesia and after parenteral administration of a NSAID analgesic. In all cases of malicious trauma the incident should be reported to the police and the Royal Society for the Prevention of Cruelty to Animals (RSPCA) or the Scottish Society for the Prevention of Cruelty to Animals (Scottish SPCA) (see also Chapter 11).

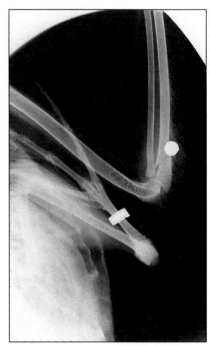

26.15 Conscious dorsoventral radiograph of the elbow of a swan showing a slingshot that has resulted in fracture of the ulna.

Treatment of wounds

The majority of patients will recover from even the most extensive severely infected wounds given appropriate wound care, analgesia, infection control, nutrition and fluid therapy, as well as the company of their own species and time.

Open wounds should be flushed with copious amounts of fluid, such as sterile saline or Hartmann's solution, or chlorhexidine diluted 1:40. Infected wounds in birds can contain very caseous material that is firmly adherent to the underlying structures. The placement of Penrose drains in wounds is not beneficial due to the solid nature of this material. Cautious gentle debridement is possible with attention paid to any bleeding in the friable underlying granulation tissue. Topical wound debridement products may be used. Edible grade honey, including Manuka honey, is an excellent and cost effective wound debridement and antiseptic agent. Apply a parasiticide spray (e.g. F10® Germicidal Wound Spray with Insecticide) around the wound and any bandaging whenever flystrike is present or likely. Repeated examination of wounds, including those underneath bandaging, is necessary to rule out subsequent flystrike. Wounds sometimes develop a superficial green fungal bloom, usually on drying wound crusts, which does not affect the prognosis. Treatment is achieved by gentle debridement and lifting of the affected crusts. Analgesia and systemic antibiosis should be used where clinically indicated.

Some soft tissue wounds can penetrate the air sacs, potentially resulting in coelomitis and subcutaneous emphysema. Penetration of the coelomic cavity and air sacs is evidenced by the escape of air through the wound as the patient breathes out. The prognosis in cases of coelomitis is poorer, but some birds do recover with daily flushing of the wound with sterile isotonic saline solution, followed by rotation of the bird to drain the fluid out. In the author's experience this does not result in respiratory compromise. Systemic antibiotics are indicated in these cases. The vast majority of cases of subcutaneous emphysema resulting from air sac penetration and air leakage under the skin will resolve with time unless the wound is extensive.

Birds with traumatic injuries may be presented with large skin tears. Under general anaesthesia, such wounds should be flushed, debrided and the skin laceration sutured using absorbable monofilament suture material with a long half-life, such as polydioxanone. Two or three drainage holes should be left open in order to flush the wound postoperatively and apply topical honey. It is not necessary to pluck any surrounding plumage when surgically preparing the site. The skin tear should ideally heal by primary intention, but if the wound subsequently breaks down, initial suturing will have provided protection for underlying soft tissue structures as the granulation process proceeds. Antibiotics are administered parenterally, along with daily flushing and topical honey application, typically for 5–7 days. Flushing and honey application are then continued daily and subsequently tapered to once or twice weekly until the wound is granulating well and reduced in size. Many wounds do not need to continue to be treated until re-epithelialization is complete, although release of the bird into the wild should generally wait until the wound is fully healed.

Orthopaedic injuries

Wing fractures: Avian bone fractures heal swiftly, often in 3 to 4 weeks. In the author's experience, splinting or bandaging of the damaged wing (see Chapter 5) usually provides sufficient support for adequate healing. Intramedullary pinning and external fixation techniques (see Chapter 29) can also be used successfully in waterfowl. Bone plating is not appropriate as the thin avian cortex fragments easily, even in the larger species.

If fractures are compound, the prognosis for healing is reduced and the splint or bandage needs to be removed frequently for wound treatment. In the author's experience, however, even open, infected and comminuted fractures with a significant bone deficit do have a chance of healing with appropriate conforming splinting and wound care, and these birds may potentially return to adequate flying function to allow them to be released.

The potential for return to flying function and the ability to hold the wing clear of the waterline should be considered when triaging wing injuries and during treatment. If the wing feathers trail in the water they are likely to become waterlogged and infected. The wing distal to the fracture, whether closed or open, needs careful monitoring for necrosis caused by disruption to the blood supply.

In cases where the wing has extensive necrosis and infection, or remains paretic or paralysed despite adequate wound healing, the bird will not be suitable for rehabilitation and release. Such cases should, in most circumstances, be euthanased. In situations where a suitable site on a private lake with good ongoing observation is available, wing amputation may exceptionally be considered. The welfare of migratory waterfowl must also be considered when making these decisions. The most suitable site for wing amputation, wounds allowing, is mid to distal humerus.

Leg fractures: Most leg fractures can be splinted in the author's experience. After provision of appropriate analgesia (see Figure 26.23), a gutter splint is applied with the leg in full extension in the conscious patient. A thermoplastic support material (e.g. Orfit® 1.6 mm micro) is cut to the approximate size, softened in hot water, allowed to cool slightly and fitted from the lateral side of the thigh and adjacent torso to the distal limb. The moulded splint is cooled rapidly by syringing cold water over it, and removed. A padding of water-permeable plastic material is fitted to line the inside of the splint (e.g. Fridge freshening cushion, Kleeneze Ltd; Fruit and vegetable cushion, Lakeland Ltd) before it is replaced on the affected limb and bandaged in place.

Surgical external fixation is possible, but rarely necessary in the author's experience: 2–3 mm diameter Kirschner wires or intramedullary pins are placed through the bone, at least two angled either side of the fracture. The pins are then attached using orthopaedic clamps and fixing bars, or cost-effective and lighter alternatives such as an epoxy external skeletal fixator (ESF) putty or acrylic glue (e.g. Araldite®) poured into microscope slide cases or drip tubing.

In the author's opinion it is possible for birds to have a good quality of life in captivity with only one leg, if a suitable environment can be found. Suitability for permanent captivity should be judged on an individual case basis and if maintained in permanent captivity the animal's 'five freedoms' (see Chapter 4) must be fulfilled and be able to be monitored for the rest of the animal's life. Amputation is required for cases where the injury or infection is life-threatening, or the fracture cannot be fixed, or fails to heal and a suitable private lake is available. The leg is amputated at the level of feathered skin. The remaining foot should be monitored closely for development of pressure sores or pododermatitis.

Keel bone fractures: Keel bone fractures can be repaired with polydioxanone sutures, as the needle will pass through the relatively soft bone. Most of these fractures are open and assessment is made with a combination of radiography and surgical exploration.

Spinal fractures: Cervical vertebral subluxation can result in a kinked neck and is a differential for lead toxicosis and botulism (see 'Poisoning'). No action is necessary provided the swan can feed and move normally, as is usually the case.

Thoracolumbar injury can result in bilateral leg paralysis or paresis and is a differential diagnosis for botulism and lead toxicosis. Recovery may take up to 8 weeks in some patients, after which time the prognosis is usually hopeless. Poor prognostic markers in the author's experience are an intermittent involuntary tail wag and the passing of faeces reminiscent of soggy wheat cereal.

The spine is a difficult area to assess radiographically in waterfowl. Neurological examination of these cases may provide additional clinical information, but does not always give an indication of the prognosis. Even at 8 weeks post-injury there is a chance of complete recovery in some individuals. Hydrotherapy with a handler in constant attendance is a useful aid to recovery. There is a risk of pressure sores developing over the keel in spinal injury cases and so careful monitoring is necessary and the animal should be housed on padded bedding. If keel ulceration occurs euthanasia is performed on humane grounds.

Mandibular fractures: Mandibular fractures may occur as a result of flight crashes (see 'Trauma'), collisions with watercraft or the ligation effect of fishing line. The small diameter of the bones, inelasticity of closely adherent overlying skin, and bacterial contamination of the site make cross-pinning of the beak mostly unsuccessful. It is possible to mould and suture in place perforated thermoplastic material (Orfit®) as a gutter splint around the bones and skin of the area involved using polydioxanone (Figure 26.16). The sutures often need replacing through the healing process. Birds generally tolerate this procedure well, feed unassisted and do not require tube feeding. Once fully healed and adequate feeding has been observed, the birds are deemed suitable for release.

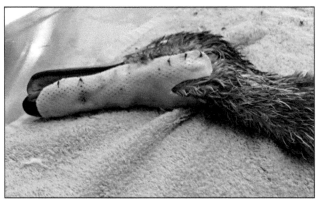

26.16 Mandibular splint made of thermoplastic material and sutured in place with polydioxanone in an anaesthetized and extubated mute swan cygnet.

Foot injuries

Water birds are able to survive with substantial parts of the digits and webbing of the foot missing; indeed, birds brought in for non-related injuries may have web deficits from a previous healed injury. With all foot injuries, careful observation of the bird on a rescue centre lake is necessary to assess its ability to swim and function normally prior to release back into the wild.

Acute foot injuries are managed with a combination of surgical and topical treatment. Surgical removal of damaged web flaps may be necessary to avoid further tearing. Although the initial surgery should ideally remove all damaged tissue, surgical sites should be carefully monitored for evidence of further devitalized tissue. As long as any infection is under control, the devitalized part may subsequently be allowed to slough naturally as an alternative to multiple repeat revision surgeries. The skin of the distal leg is non-elastic and firmly adherent to the underlying structures. Debridement of this area often creates large skin deficits, which are difficult to close surgically and heal by second intention. Such wounds are very prone to reinfection and broad-spectrum antibiosis and appropriate regular wound care must be provided (see Figure 26.23).

For information on pododermatitis ('bumblefoot') see 'Other conditions'.

Feather injuries

In common with other avian species, newly growing feathers in waterfowl have a good blood supply and trauma can cause significant bleeding and secondary infection. Because of the size of the bird, this bleeding can appear to be considerable in these species. The infected feather requires removal, with curved mosquito haemostats being placed into the feather socket and applying gentle constant traction and torsion. Appropriate analgesia should be provided (see 'Analgesia'). If multiple feathers are affected, general anaesthesia is required. Topical antiseptics such as honey may be applied to the follicle following the procedure.

Eye injuries

Waterfowl can develop severe uni- or bilateral eye infections, often secondary to trauma, with keratitis, corneal ulceration and uveitis, which respond remarkably well to topical therapy (such as antibiotics). Surgery to remove the eye is not without risk and in many cases it is preferable to treat the infection and leave the eye, despite functional compromise, *in situ*. Careful monitoring of the remaining ocular tissues for evidence of pain should be part of the pre-release assessment if enucleation is not carried out.

The ability of the bird to cope with sight in one eye varies enormously. Some birds manage perfectly well, whilst others do not adjust at all. Monitoring and careful observation at a rescue centre will differentiate these birds and enable appropriate decisions to be made regarding their release or suitability for permanent captivity.

Fishing tackle injuries

All types of waterfowl, especially swans, are susceptible to fishing tackle-related injuries. Injuries arise directly from fishing line, hooks, lures (Figure 26.17) and floats and indirectly from lead weights (see 'Lead toxicosis'). Examination for the presence of fishing-related paraphernalia should be part of the basic clinical examination for all waterfowl (see 'Examination').

Removal of fishing hooks: Hooks and lures may become attached anywhere to the outside of the body (Figure 26.17). If the hook is embedded in an area where it is plainly visible, and the bird appears on examination to be in otherwise good health, the hook can be removed by rescuers at the rescue site. Rescuers of waterfowl should carry hook disgorgers. These small plastic tools, a few centimetres long, are wrapped around the line and slid gently towards and over the hook to release it. The hook may also be grasped with a pair of pliers or artery forceps, and the point of the hook pulled through the skin for the barb at the end to be cut off with pliers. During this procedure the hook should be covered with a cloth to prevent the tip of the hook becoming a missile.

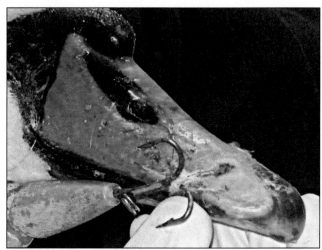

26.17 Large lure attached to the bill of a mute swan. (© Secret World Wildlife Rescue)

Hooks that have been present for several days may result in extensive inflammatory reaction, infection and soft tissue trauma. During this time the bird's ability to feed may have been severely compromised and its body condition may be poor. These birds should be admitted for treatment. After initial first aid (see 'First aid'), it is necessary to proceed to surgery as soon as possible in order for the bird to resume eating afterwards.

The bird should be carefully examined for evidence of hooks in the mouth, checking under the tongue for fishing line. The neck should be palpated for swellings and any soft tissue swelling in the neck should be radiographed (Figure 26.18) and surgically explored under general anaesthesia. Even if there is no radiographical evidence of a hook, there may be an oesophageal tear and abscessation, with or without food accumulation, as the hook may have become dislodged from the oesophagus. Endoscopy is a useful adjunct to radiographic imaging; however, endoscopic evaluation may easily miss oesophageal tears due to the presence of longitudinal oesophageal folds. Endoscopy also does not allow for evaluation of extra-oesophageal tissue. If the hook is large it may lodge in the oesophagus near the thoracic inlet or directly dorsal to the heart and in these cases the oesophagus can be insufflated and the hook retrieved endoscopically.

Hooks in the mouth may be retrieved as described above, during brief anaesthesia. If visible the hook may be grasped by artery forceps and pushed in the direction of the curve of the hook, dislodging it from the mucosa. If the fishing line is still attached to the hook, the line may be threaded through a piece of drip or oesophageal tubing and this used to dislodge the hook, in an attempt to avoid surgical intervention.

In many instances surgical exploration is required to remove the hook. Care must be taken as the hook may be lodged close to the jugular vein or in the trachea. The anaesthetized bird is positioned in left lateral recumbency, giving best exposure of the cervical part of the oesophagus, which lies on the right. The right jugular vein is larger and is clearly visible with the bird positioned in this way, which reduces the risk of iatrogenic venepuncture. The feathers of the skin are plucked over the surgical site, which is then aseptically prepared. A skin incision parallel to the long axis of the neck is made over the neck swelling and careful blunt dissection of the subcutaneous tissue is carried out to the level of the oesophagus. This may be through layers of abscess wall, solid pus and food material in varying stages of decay. A surgical incision into the oesophagus may be necessary. Care should be taken when exploring the very proximal oesophagus to avoid the overlying blood vessel plexus. Oesophageal repair is achieved first using a simple continuous full-thickness suture in the mucosal layer followed by an inverted continuous layer of the muscularis and serosa together, using polydioxanone (e.g. PDS®). The overlying skin is sutured with polyglactin (e.g. Vicryl®) using a simple continuous pattern.

Surgery for simple retrieval of an oesophageal hook with no tear or severe infection present is usually straightforward. If infection is present, a 1–2 cm gap is left open at each end of the skin incision to allow daily flushing and topical treatment, treating the wound essentially as open. If the infection present is severe, breakdown of this surgery is common and several episodes of revision surgery are often necessary.

Removal of fishing line: All birds with evidence of hooks (and/or other fishing materials) must be carefully assessed for the presence of fishing line (see Figure 24.15). Run the index finger under the mandible to check for fishing line ('chin strap') and look inside the mouth and under the tongue. If there is a neck swelling and line is found looped under the tongue or mandible ('chin') following radiography to rule out the presence of a hook (see Figure 26.18), gentle traction may be applied to the line to see if the swelling is simply vegetable matter caught round the line, which can be carefully pulled out. This is easier carried out during anaesthesia with the bird intubated. In extreme cases the bird may be unable to extend the head and neck because the line is taut between the mouth and neck. In this case the line should be cut to prevent it further 'cheese-wiring' through the wall of the oesophagus and then removed as described above.

If a hook is visible on radiography, any fishing line protruding from the mouth should not be pulled as the hook on the end may be embedded in the oesophagus or other soft tissue structures around the neck. Any large amount of line and any attached weights should be cut off, leaving 30–60 cm to help locate the hook.

All fishing line should be carefully removed. Line can become wrapped around any part of the body and cause ligation wounds, exacerbated by subsequent swelling. Most line is colourless and wounds will need thorough exploration to identify multiple strands, which may be embedded in granulation tissue and even in the bone, particularly of the mandible and leg.

Removal of gizzard foreign bodies: Most fishing hooks will be ground up once they reach the gizzard and their removal at this stage is not always necessary. If hooks are seen in the gizzard on radiography, the patient should be carefully monitored and surgical intervention is indicated if their appetite is reduced. Fishing paraphernalia such as lures and floats can also lodge in the gizzard and these require surgical removal. Lead shot may also be seen radiographically in the gizzard and surgical removal may be advocated. In the author's experience, however, this is not necessary and the risks associated with such surgery may be significant.

For gizzard surgery the anaesthetized, intubated bird is positioned in dorsal recumbency, feathers are plucked from the ventral midline caudal to the caudal aspect of the keel and a midline coeliotomy is performed. The foreign body is retrieved through a proventricular incision, as the gizzard is more difficult to suture having a very thick muscle wall. The proventriculus should be exteriorized, held with stay sutures, and the coelom packed with swabs to prevent coelomic contamination with proventricular contents. The proventriculus is closed with a monofilament suture material (e.g. polydioxanone) in a double suture layer, using a simple continuous pattern in the mucosa and inverted suture pattern in the muscularis with serosa.

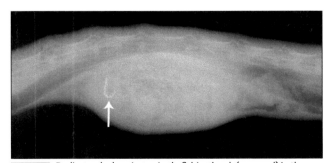

26.18 Radiograph showing a single fishing hook (arrowed) in the oesophagus of a cygnet. The oesophagus is greatly distended with vegetation attached to, and obstructed by, the hook and line.
(© Elizabeth Mullineaux)

Poisoning

Two toxicological conditions occur commonly in waterfowl, both causing bilateral widespread paresis and paralysis: these are lead toxicosis and botulism. Careful attention to history and clinical signs can help to distinguish them from each other, other neurological toxicosis, and from neurological trauma.

Lead toxicosis

Lead toxicosis is seen most commonly in swans, due to their method of feeding. They upend in water and ingest gravel to aid digestion, taking the lead particles as well. Their long necks facilitate the taking in of particles from the riverbed. Prior to the Control of Pollution (Angler's Lead weights) Regulations 1986 (prohibiting the import, supply or use of lead split shot or other lead weight for weighting fishing lines weighing greater than 0.06 g and less than 28.35 g) the incidence of lead toxicosis in swans was very much higher. There are still residual ubiquitous lead particles in the wetlands environment, which cause intoxication when ingested. Lead toxicosis tends to occur in the individual or in a small number of birds at any one site and can occur at any time of the year. Dry weather can expose parts of the riverbed not usually reached; equally heavy rain can stir up the riverbed to also bring about exposure. Lead is ground up in the gizzard, typically over a 2–3 week period and systemically absorbed. Other potential sources of lead include lead shot in the form of shot gun pellets.

Pathogenesis and clinical signs: Once ingested, approximately 2% of lead is absorbed, then transported in association with the erythrocytes and distributed among the soft tissues, especially the kidneys. Lead is eventually redistributed into the bone, where its subsequent mobilization is similar to that of calcium. Demyelination lesions occur in nerves. Focal vascular damage can occur in the cerebellum due to reduced delta-aminolevulinic acid dehydratase (ALAD) enzyme activity. Hepatic and renal degeneration can also occur.

The main clinical signs are muscular weakness, often with bilateral wing and leg paresis, with a typical but not pathognomonic neck kink ('limber neck') (Figure 26.19). The shape of the eyelids can be described as 'diamond eye'. The bird typically passes bright green diarrhoea that stains the tail feathers and vent. Food can impact in the crop and oesophagus as the bird continues to eat whilst there is reduced gastrointestinal peristalsis. Swans are generally quite lively right up until the stage where they collapse and become moribund. This is in contrast to cases of botulism, where the bird appears depressed at

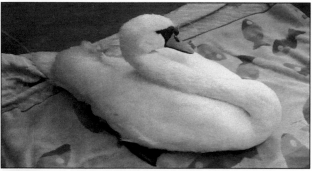

26.19 Swan with lead toxicosis. Note the 'kinked' neck position and bright green faecal staining on feathers.

the onset. In acute forms of lead poisoning the bird is initially in good body condition, which deteriorates over time due to the inability to digest food properly. In more chronic forms of toxicosis loss of condition can occur due to compromise of liver and kidney function, complicated by the neurological signs of lead poisoning.

Recrudescence of lead toxicosis clinical signs can occur in the female during egg-laying, and in times of stress such as moulting, due to release of lead from the bones in a similar way to calcium mobilization.

Radiography: Radiography may be used as an aid to the diagnosis of lead toxicosis. A dorsoventral view of the coelomic cavity is achievable in the conscious patient, restrained by tying the legs together in extension. The gizzard, which is seen superimposed over the left hip joint, is examined for radiodense particles consistent with metal fragments. Lead toxicosis may still be present in the absence of radiodense particles, as the lead may have already been ground up and absorbed. Lead toxicosis as a result of recrudescence from the bone may occur long after the lead particles have gone. The proventriculus and gizzard are often seen distended and impacted on radiographs of affected birds, which would support the diagnosis of lead toxicosis. Radiographs may also demonstrate that the patient has been shot. This will not cause toxicosis and may be an incidental finding.

Blood sampling: Lead estimation of a whole blood sample collected into ethylenediaminetetraacetic acid (EDTA) (or other blood sample type depending upon the laboratory used) has some use in the diagnosis of lead toxicity. Normal lead values in waterfowl of <0.4 ppm rise to 0.5–2 ppm in lead toxicosis, with values of >2 ppm in severe cases. Many swans, however, especially those living around the lower Thames area, tolerate a much higher blood lead level than the accepted normal of <0.4 ppm without showing any clinical signs. The prognosis for lead toxicosis is greatly improved with the immediate instigation of treatment and this should not be delayed to await blood results, but instead treatment should be commenced based upon clinical signs and radiography.

There may be a normochromic anaemia due to production of defective red cells and the impaired release of red cells. Renal impairment may be assessed using blood uric acid levels. Uric acid and PCV estimation may help offer a prognosis in these cases.

Treatment: Treatment of lead toxicosis is with edetate calcium disodium (Sodium Calcium Edetate 250 mg/ml Concentrate Solution for Injection) until clinical signs resolve, and there is reduction in paresis, improved mobility, reduced gastrointestinal tract impaction and resolution of diarrhoea.

Several protocols for treating lead toxicosis in waterfowl have been suggested (Sears *et al.* 1989; Murase *et al.*, 1992). The author's preference is to use edetate calcium disodium at a dose of 25 mg/kg (range 10–40 mg/kg). The 250 mg/ml product should be diluted, 1 part to 1.5 parts water for injection, and administered subcutaneously, once daily for 5 days. Treatment is then withdrawn for 2 days and improvement based on clinical signs assessed. Subcutaneous injections are continued in a 5:2 day pattern until clinical signs have resolved. The doses may be divided into 3 or 4 volumes given at different sites; injection site reactions occur if the treatment course is very long and the same sites are used repeatedly. The injection site should be varied to minimize this, alternating between legs and different sites on each leg and other injection sites (see Figure 5.11 and 'Therapeutics'). Injection reactions will heal, whereas inadequately treated lead toxicosis is often fatal.

Good supportive and nursing care is essential in these patients. Collapsed patients, especially if they have gastrointestinal tract impaction, require intravenous fluid therapy (e.g. glucose saline) with edetate calcium disodium 40 mg/kg added to a 500 ml drip bag along with 40 ml Duphalyte® at a rate of 50 ml/kg/24h. When the patient is too lively to tolerate intravenous fluid administration, the change to subcutaneous edetate calcium disodium injections is made. Vitamin B12 (Vitbee® 250 0.025% w/v solution for injection) is useful as an appetite stimulant, administered by injection subcutaneously at a dose of 0.2 ml/kg daily. Birds may also need encouragement to feed using gentle introduction of the beak into bread and chopped soft greens such as lettuce in plenty of water.

Botulism

Botulism is caused by the ingestion of toxin from the *Clostridium botulinum* bacterium occurring in rotting organic matter in wetlands. Bacterial growth occurs in hot weather around 25°C. Often many different species are affected at the same time, and the rescue site may be littered with dead and dying fish, small mammals and several species of water bird.

There is no definitive diagnosis for botulism – clinical signs and exclusion of other causes are used for diagnosis. Birds appear very depressed, inappetant and are often completely flaccid. Swans are often unable to support their head and have it stretched out along their back with beak pointing caudally, saliva dribbling on to the back. The bird can display dyspnoea with gaping open-mouthed breathing. It is important to keep the patients quiet and stress-free as they are unable to exercise their normal avoidance behaviour.

Treatment for botulism is supportive and the prognosis is generally good. Botulinum antitoxin is not readily available, and penicillin antibiotics are ineffective as it is the toxin, not the organism, that is ingested. Larger species can be given intravenous support with glucose-saline solution with addition of amino acids/vitamins (e.g. Duphalyte®). Smaller species respond well to proprietary oral glucose solutions and veterinary oral nutritional support products such as Vetark® Critical Care formula and Nutrigel® may also be used. Provision of deep bedding will reduce the incidence of secondary pressure sores and keel lesions.

Other causes of toxicosis

'Sewage sickness', which arises from birds being exposed to untreated sewage released into the waterways, and blue-green algae toxicosis, which arises from blue-green algal growth on shallow stagnant waters in hot weather, are both associated with clinical signs that are very similar to those seen with botulism. The symptomatic treatment of these conditions is the same as for botulism. A suspicion of the aetiology can be made by investigation of the environment.

Oil contamination

Waterfowl may become contaminated with oil as part of a major oil spill disaster or as a result of more local pollution. Multiple individual birds tend to be affected making treatment and hospitalization labour-intensive. The treatment of oiled birds is a long process requiring adequate facilities and experience. More information is provided in Chapter 24.

Infectious diseases
Viral diseases

Duck virus enteritis: Duck virus enteritis (DVE) is caused by a herpesvirus (Anatid herpesvirus 1) affecting waterfowl, which display a range of clinical presentations from peracute death, through chronic debilitation, to the clinically inapparent carrier state. It can present as an outbreak with multiple birds being affected, typically in April to May, or as a problem in the individual bird. Clinical signs include sudden death, weakness, depression, photophobia, inappetence, extreme thirst, ataxia, ocular and nasal discharge, soiled vents, watery or bloody diarrhoea and prolapse of the phallus in males. Adult birds may die in good body condition. Differential diagnoses include Newcastle disease, avian influenza, fowlpox, pasteurellosis, clostridial necrotic enteritis, and various toxicoses.

A post-mortem examination may aid the diagnosis where multiple cases occur. Damage of blood vessels throughout the body induces haemorrhage in various tissues or the presence of free blood in body cavities. Haemorrhage or necrosis of the lymphoid tissues occurs, which significantly supports the diagnosis of DVE: this appears as annular bands in the intestine of ducks and discs in the intestines of geese and swans. Diphtheritic lesions on the mucosal surface of the oesophagus especially the most distal part, following the longitudinal folds, may be commonly seen in swans. The differential diagnoses for this diphtheritic appearance, candidiasis and trichomonosis, should be ruled out by microscopy or histopathology. Virus isolation is necessary for a diagnosis of DVE and is performed on samples of fresh, chilled liver, kidney and spleen.

Outbreaks of DVE in a rescue centre should be managed by isolating the affected and in-contact birds, and heightening biosecurity between the affected and non-affected areas of the premises. Footbaths should be used and disinfection of protective clothing and feeding utensils should be carried out. Prompt removal and incineration of carcasses and bedding should be performed.

A modified live vaccine is available for use in private collections of waterfowl, but is not normally used in wild birds.

Avian influenza: There are two distinct virus pathotypes of avian influenza: high pathogenic (HPAI) and low pathogenic (LPAI) forms. Wild birds, particularly Anseriformes and Charadriiformes, act as a natural reservoir of LPAI viruses, where infection is often asymptomatic. HPAI outbreaks are commercially important and potentially zoonotic. There have been two episodes in the UK when H5N1 HPNAI was detected in wild birds that were found dead: a wild whooper swan in Scotland in April 2006, and 10 mute swans and one Canada goose in South Dorset in January/February 2008 (Blissitt, 2007).

Bacterial conditions

Necrotizing enteritis: Necrotizing enteritis is caused by *Clostridium perfringens* and occurs as an acute disease, sporadically or in outbreaks. The signs are sudden death, sometimes preceded by a short period of depression, inappetance and diarrhoea, sometimes haematochaezia. It is characterized by post-mortem findings of necrotic or haemorrhagic enteritis, although these are not pathognomonic for the disease. Stress predisposes to the condition and the incidence rises during or after prolonged severe weather conditions. It can be treated by administration of broad-spectrum antibiotics such as amoxicillin (see Figure

26.23), but treatment is often too late for the individual. Isolating and treating the in-contact birds for 5–7 days may help to decrease the spread within a rescue centre, but this is impractical in the wild.

Bacterial septicaemia in orphans: Outbreaks of bacterial infection by organisms such as *Yersinia*, *Pasteurella* and *Riemerella anatipestifer* can cause multiple sudden deaths in orphaned birds. Bacterial culture from post-mortem samples is necessary to confirm the causal agent. During outbreaks attention must be paid to husbandry practices, for example by batching hatchlings, reducing stocking density, scrupulous environmental cleaning and disinfection, provision of dry bedding and good ventilation. *Riemerella anatipestifer* infections cause major economic losses in the duck industry and a vaccine against this bacterium is used commercially.

Bacterial sinusitis: Waterfowl have a large infraorbital sinus, which occasionally becomes infected with such organisms as *Escherichia coli*, *Pasteurella*, *Proteus*, *Actinomyces* and *Nocardia*. *Mycoplasma* spp. have been isolated from cases of sinusitis and conjunctivitis, and yet the pathogenicity of the strains is unknown. Sinusitis presents as a unilateral or bilateral swelling on the face just rostroventral to the eye (Figure 26.20). The contents can be mucoid or purulent. Cases may respond to gentle expression of contents through the nostrils or through an incision into the sinus through the skin over the swelling and daily repeated flushing. Various flushing agents may be used, such as saline, dilute antiseptic or antibiotic solutions. NSAIDs and systemic antibiotics are also indicated. Recurrent infections associated with clinical signs should be swabbed for bacterial culture and sensitivity.

Avian tuberculosis: Infection with *Mycobacterium avium* causes chronic wasting and ill thrift. The slow rate of pathogenesis makes it more likely to affect older birds. The bacteria live in damp and wet conditions making waterfowl particularly at risk of infection. There is no seasonal pattern to the occurrence of tuberculosis. Diagnosis is made either at post-mortem examination, or in the live bird on laparoscopy under anaesthesia. White granulomatous lesions are typically seen on the surface of the liver. *M. avium* is highly resistant to antituberculous drugs and is a zoonotic risk; thus euthanasia is indicated.

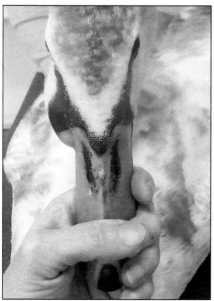

26.20 Juvenile mute swan with sinusitis in the right infraorbital sinus. Note the large swelling rostroventral to the right eye.

Fungal conditions

Aspergillosis: Water birds are very prone to developing aspergillosis in the respiratory tract. Aspergillosis can be a primary disease or develop as a secondary problem in debilitated birds. Occurrence of the condition is so frequent that any bird with respiratory signs that cannot be attributed to trauma, lead toxicosis or botulism should be treated for aspergillosis pending further diagnostic tests.

Both upper and lower respiratory signs may occur and these present as a rattly dyspnoea and gape, that on auscultation may be heard as a wheeze or a rattle. Lesions are usually found in the lower respiratory tract in swans, involving the air sacs. Radiographically, there may be radiodense areas in the air sacs. Coelioscopy is extremely useful in the diagnosis of this condition in waterfowl, and air sacs can be directly visualized for evidence of increased density, fungal plaques and thickening, with biopsy for histology and culture of samples in suspect cases. Where advanced lesions are seen on coelioscopy the prognosis is poor. Systemic aspergillosis also occurs, manifesting as a chronic debilitating emaciating syndrome, and is often a case for euthanasia.

A serological test for antibodies to *Aspergillus* fungi is available, but this indicates only exposure to the organism rather than the extent of disease. Haematological changes typically include a severe leucocytosis, with an associated heterophilia, monocytosis and lymphopenia. With chronic infection a non-regenerative anaemia and increased serum total protein and globulin may be evident. Elevations of bile acids and aspartate aminotransferase (AST) may also been seen with hepatic involvement. These parameters are useful in monitoring response to treatment long term. Treatment is rarely successful once the infection is established.

Treatment for respiratory aspergillosis is with antifungal drugs and may require several weeks' therapy. Amphotericin B may be delivered daily for 7 days by nebulization (12.5 mg diluted with 2.5 ml water q24h), intratracheally, with a Spreull needle via the larynx (7.5 mg/kg q8h) or intravenously over 24 hours (3.25 mg/kg in i.v. fluids). Concurrent treatment with other antifungal medications may be necessary in persistent cases. Oral itraconazole may be given at a dose of 10 mg/kg orally q24h, for 4–8 weeks. Clinical response to treatment, haematological improvements and repeat coelioscopy examinations are used to assess progress. Any primary predisposing disease must also be treated.

Although aspergillosis has been associated with fungal spores in straw bedding (Falk-Rønne *et al.*, 1984), the author has not found any increased incidence of aspergillosis in birds being kept on straw bedding which is changed daily. Aspergillosis is often a disease that affects stressed birds, and stress may be reduced in birds allowed to forage and make nests in clean dry straw substrate.

Parasitic conditions

Ectoparasites:
Nasal leeches: The duck leech (*Theromyzon tessulatum* (Figure 26.21a)) and related species affect a wide number of wildfowl species, attaching to the nasal cavity or conjunctival spaces. They may cause head shaking, or a serosanguinous ocular or nasal discharge. Heavy burdens may cause respiratory compromise. In debilitated patients or those with a heavy burden, physical removal with forceps (Figure 26.21b) or a single injection of ivermectin at 200 µg/kg s.c. are effective treatments.

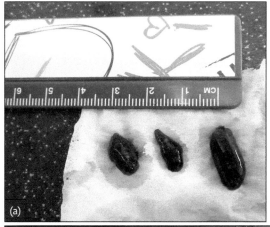

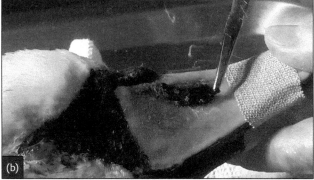

26.21 (a) Nasal leeches (*Theromyzon* spp.) and (b) being removed from the nasal cavity of a mute swan.

Feather lice: Bird feather lice are biting/chewing lice of the order Mallophaga, and are ubiquitous. The appearance is of black or brown cigar-shaped lice, 2–8 mm long, moving around feather vanes. The juveniles are smaller and white. Treatment (e.g. topical fipronil spray) is only necessary with heavy burdens in debilitated birds.

The shaft louse (*Holomenopon leucoxanthum*) causes 'wet-feather' – damage to feather structure leading to loss of waterproofing. Treatment of louse infestation is by subcutaneous injection of ivermectin at 200 μg/kg s.c. or topical fipronil spray at standard dose rates.

Flystrike: Constant vigilance is necessary on all waterfowl patients with wounds, especially during the warmer months to prevent flystrike (myiasis). This should be treated using insecticidal products (see Figure 26.23).

Endoparasites: A variety of endoparasites may affect waterfowl.

- Proventricular worms (*Echinuria uncinata*) are an important parasite of young waterfowl. Fibrous nodular lesions develop in the proventriculus and can cause inappetance, ill thrift, poor growth, stunting and sudden death. Often the adult birds appear unaffected. Worm eggs can be detected on faecal examination (see Chapter 10). Treatment is with a subcutaneous injection of ivermectin at 200 μg/kg s.c.
- Gizzard worms (*Amidostomum* spp.) affect the gizzard, causing similar clinical signs as proventricular worms in young birds. Weight loss may be seen in adults. The eggs can also be detected on faecal examination and treatment is as for proventricular worms.
- Cestodes and trematodes are often incidental findings, although the author has seen one case in a cygnet on

post-mortem examination where an excessive cestode burden had caused fatal coelomitis.
- Schistosomes (blood flukes) of the circulatory system or nasal mucosa are often incidental findings.
- Heartworms (*Sarcoma eurycercus*) can cause depression and death from myocardial necrosis.

Other conditions
Congenital and developmental diseases
Hatchlings with congenital abnormalities may be abandoned by their parents. If the bird is rescued, the abnormality may not become apparent initially; however, a reduced growth rate is often seen compared with others of a similar age. These birds, in the author's experience, rarely reach sexual maturity and often die in their first winter.

Beak deformities: Congenital twisting deformities around the long axis of the beak are occasionally encountered. As long as the bird can eat and preen, assessed by careful observation in an outside enclosure with near-natural habitat, no action is necessary.

'Airplane' ('angel') wing: This is a unilateral or bilateral developmental weakness of the muscles of the carpus resulting in carpal valgus at the fledging stage. It is likely to have a multifactorial aetiology, possibly with genetic, nutritional, environmental and management influences. Taping the wing on to itself for 3–5 days as the abnormality is developing may help in correction of the deformity. As high levels of protein in the diet of the growing birds have been implicated in the development of angel wing, an appropriate balanced diet should be fed. Most cases are, however, encountered in the advanced stage when the bones and ligaments have become fixed in valgus. Flight is sometimes possible with this condition although euthanasia or, if suitable facilities are available, long-term captivity, is often necessary. Suitability for permanent captivity should be judged on an individual case basis and if maintained in permanent captivity the animal's 'five freedoms' (see Chapter 4) must be fulfilled and be able to be monitored for the rest of the animal's life.

Perosis: Also known as slipped tendon, this affects the legs and the condition develops before fledging. The leg bones grow faster than the caudal tendon resulting in enlargement of the hock, growth deformities of the tibiotarsal and tarsometatarsal bones and medial luxation of the Achilles tendon. Reduction of dietary protein reduces the incidence. If caught early enough, splinting the leg in full extension can sometimes be successful. In the author's experience surgical correction of the condition is rarely satisfactory.

Osteoarthritis
This can occur subsequent to joint infection (Figure 26.22) or trauma, or as degenerative osteoarthritis in the ageing bird. Radiographic assessment, together with analysis of joint fluid aseptically collected in the conscious patient, can help to determine the cause and prognosis. Appropriate systemic antibiotics can then be selected based upon bacterial culture and sensitivity. Parenteral medication may be combined with flushing of the joint with sterile saline. Some birds with mild non-infected osteoarthritis may be suitable for release into a captive and appropriately managed environment.

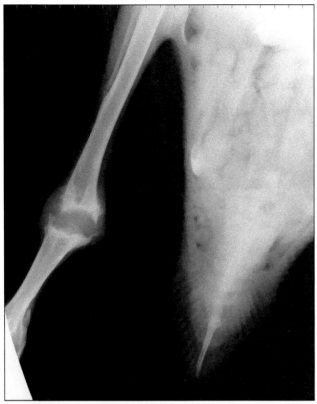

26.22 Caudocranial radiograph of the leg of a mute swan showing severe septic arthritis of the intertarsal joint.

Pododermatitis ('bumblefoot')

'Bumblefoot' is a non-infectious soft tissue granuloma that develops on the plantar aspect of the foot and is commonly seen in mute swans (Tanake *et al.*, 2008). In waterfowl, the condition is believed to be caused by walking on rough hard surfaces, resulting in small wounds and secondary infection usually with *Staphylococcus aureus*. Pododermatitis may also develop in birds in captivity as a result of inappropriate underfoot substrate (e.g. in waterfowl) or inappropriate perches in other avian species. It may also be seen as a result of uneven weight bearing and use of the foot, secondary to other conditions (e.g. orthopaedic, neurological or muscular injury). Secondary systemic amyloidosis is a potentially fatal consequence of this condition in mute swans (Tanake *et al.*, 2008).

Treatment is difficult and often unrewarding, often failing and sometimes even exacerbating the condition. If the bird is not lame, the best course of action in a wild bird may be to rule out other underlying problems and then leave the foot untreated. Occasionally the 'bumblefoot' granuloma calcifies and can be satisfactorily excised under general anaesthesia. The extent of damage in a severely swollen foot should be assessed radiographically. Birds with extensive radiographic changes should be euthanased.

Treatment involves surgically opening up the affected area under anaesthesia and flushing and debulking the lesion as necessary. Surgery is hampered by the vascular nature of the site and difficulty in apposing the inelastic tissues. Ideally dressings are used post-surgery until healthy granulation is achieved. Post-surgical hygiene is very difficult in waterfowl due to their indiscriminate and frequent defecatory habits. Analgesia should be provided as well as systemic antibiosis if indicated.

Sternal necrosis ('keel rot')

Debilitated birds can develop decubital ulceration of the keel involving skin, muscle and bone. This carries a very poor prognosis and affected birds should be euthanased. Preventive measures such as padded substrate should be instituted for all recumbent birds (see Chapter 7).

Amyloidosis

Occasionally systemic amyloidosis is encountered on post-mortem examination and is poorly understood. Waterfowl are known to produce large quantities of amyloid compared with other species. This response is thought to be related to stress, often secondary to other clinical conditions, such as chronic inflammation associated with tuberculosis, aspergillosis or pododermatitis. In one study 78% of mute swans were found to have this condition on post-mortem examination and stressful environmental conditions were thought to contribute to this high incidence (Tanake *et al.*, 2008).

Losses related to severe weather conditions

Prolonged periods of adverse weather such as rain, snow or low temperatures may lead to a spate of deaths in waterfowl. Birds become waterlogged, malnourished and susceptible to secondary infection. Often a good feed and a few days' protection indoors can help recovery.

Therapeutics

There are very few products licensed for use in waterfowl. Commonly used therapeutic products and their dose rates are given in Figure 26.23.

Routes of administration

Oral dosing

Oral dosing of waterfowl is stressful and may require multiple doses per day. Some antibiotics and antifungals are, however, only available in oral formulation. An oral dose is given by placing the medicine in the back of the mouth, distal to the glottis, followed by administration of water with a syringe and Spreull needle or length of drip tubing. Alternatively oral treatments may be given by gavage (see Chapter 5).

Parenteral dosing

Subcutaneous injection into the lateral thigh area is the author's preferred route of injection. Other sites which can be used for subcutaneous injection include the dorsal neck area (see Figure 5.11). Intramuscular injections into the pectoral muscle are not favoured by the author, as any injection reaction at this site may be exacerbated in the recumbent bird. Intramuscular injections can be given in the quadriceps muscle of the leg. Injection site reactions may develop at any site but generally they will heal. Severely debilitated birds tolerate intravenous fluid therapy well, to which intravenous drugs can be added, switching to subcutaneous or intramuscular injections once the intravenous catheter is removed as the bird improves and becomes more mobile. The author's preferred site for intravenous injection is the medial metatarsal vein (see Figure 26.12).

Drug	Dosage	Main indication(s) and comments
Analgesics		
Carprofen	5–10 mg/kg s.c. q24h	Analgesia and anti-inflammatory
Meloxicam	Ducks: 0.5 mg/kg i.v. q24h	Analgesia and anti-inflammatory
Local anaesthetic cream (e.g. EMLA® cream)	Topical, 10–15 minutes before intravenous injection	Assists i.v. catheter placement; especially useful in cygnets Take care with local anaesthetic use in birds as toxic effects may occur at lower doses than in other species (Hocking *et al.*, 1997)
Antibacterial agents		
Amoxicillin, long-acting suspension	37.5 mg/kg s.c. q48h	Infected wounds *Clostridium perfringens*
Chloramphenicol 1% ophthalmic ointment	Topical application to eye q8h	Ocular infections
Enrofloxacin	10 mg/kg s.c., orally q24h	Bite wounds especially 2.5% solution (or more dilute solutions) may be used to help reduce tissue reactions
Gentamicin ophthalmic solution	Topical application to the eye q8h	Ocular infections
Ofloxacin (e.g. Exocin® eye drops)	Topical application to eye q6–8h	Ocular infections
Tylosin	0.5 g/l drinking water daily for 5 days	*Mycoplasma* *Clostridium perfringens*
Antifungal agents		
Amphotericin B	12.5 mg powder reconstituted with 2.5 ml water, by nebulization q24h; 3.25 mg/kg in i.v. fluids; 7.5 mg/kg q8h intratracheal; administered via the larynx using a Spreull needle	Aspergillosis Nebulization is the least stressful method of dosing Treatment may take several weeks Resistant cases may need addition of second antifungal agent
Itraconazole	5–10 mg/kg orally q24h for 3–8 weeks	Aspergillosis
Parasiticides		
Fipronil	3–6 ml/kg bodyweight	Ectoparasiticide, effective against lice
F10® Germicidal Wound Spray with Insecticide	Topical spray	Insecticidal activity of cypermethrin (0.25%) and piperonyl butoxide (1.25%) Frequent reapplication needed if wounds get wet Used around wounds during the summer as an insecticide against flystrike
Ivermectin	200 µg/kg s.c. once	Heavy louse infestation, proventricular worms, myiasis
Chelating agent		
Edetate calcium disodium (CaEDTA; Sodium Calcium Edetate 250 mg/ml Concentrate Solution for Injection)	25 mg/kg (10–40 mg/kg) CaEDTA 1 ml of product diluted with 1.5 ml of water for injection s.c. q24h for 5 days, then break for 2 days and assess reduction in clinical signs For severe cases, slow i.v. infusion – add 40 mg/kg CaEDTA to 500 ml i.v. fluid bag and administer at 50 ml/kg/24h infusion rate	Lead toxicosis Injection site reactions occur if treatment is prolonged; sites should be varied to minimize this Continue until clinical signs have resolved The s.c. dose may be distributed at 3 or 4 sites

26.23 Common therapeutic agents and their dose rates used in waterfowl species. (Coles, 2007; Carpenter, 2013)

Nebulization

This is the least stressful method of delivering antifungal and other medications. Nebulizers (e.g. Eolo® nebulizer or InnoSpire® Essence) are readily available and can be attached to the front of a transit kennel, which is then covered in plastic sheeting. Incubators with fitted nebulizers are available for smaller birds.

Management in captivity

Housing

Birds must be kept in an area away from predator species. Their general well being and recovery are hugely improved by being kept with the same species. There will, however, always be a risk of disease spread where birds are mixed. To minimize this, the groups are kept small and fairly stable, grouping birds originating from the same geographical area together as much as possible. Where several species are housed, they are kept in groups of the same or same-sized species, and then in age groups. In the breeding season one pair or one family of swans will require a pen to themselves to prevent fighting.

Daily cleaning and disinfection of all pens is required.

Intensive care

Warm, clean small pens or dog transit kennels are lined with towels, blankets or duvets. Divers need foam covered in towels and are moved frequently to minimize lung compression and reduce the incidence of pressure sores. Padding provided by blankets or duvets is especially required in swans to prevent keel injury. Lateral support for ataxic swans is provided by pillows and duvets. These are all used just once and then discarded due to faecal contamination.

Inside pens

These should be made of easily cleanable material. Straw is used as bedding, freshly replaced every day, which provides great occupational therapy value. As previously explained (see 'Aspergillosis') straw is not used by some rehabilitators due to concerns about increased environmental fungal spore contamination and shredded paper is an alternative bedding material. Large windows set low in the wall improve natural light and provide some interest for patients provided this does not result in habituation. The building should be well ventilated and at the same time proofed against escape. An inner mesh 'double' door adjacent to each main door is very useful. An indoor pool is invaluable for physiotherapy and re-waterproofing and should be drained and cleaned every day after use.

Outside pens/aquatic aviaries.

Outside pools (Figure 26.24) should be provided that are connected to an indoor shelter that can be shut off from the water at night, at times of cleaning, bad weather or catching the birds. The pools need a small step at the edge to allow easy access for the birds. Overhead netting prevents patients flying out and stops other birds from entering the enclosure. The pools and shelters must be kept clean.

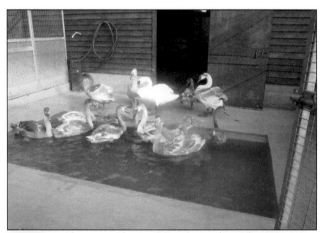

26.24 Outdoor pen with one adult and several juvenile mute swans, showing fencing dividing the pens, an outside drainable pool with easily cleanable non-slip surface, and an indoor shelter which can be shut off from the pool.

Long-term debilitated birds

Prior to eventual release long-term patients can be kept in fenced grassed areas with access to water. The water must be kept clean by being filtered and aerated. Feeding stations, either bankside or on floating pontoons, are provided.

Diet

Getting a wild fish-eating bird to feed in captivity can be very difficult. Some waterfowl need to be encouraged to use the feed bowl initially. Examples of foods that may be offered in the short-term are given in Figure 26.13.

Divers, grebes, fish-eating ducks

Fish-eating birds require a bowl of water with sprats or whitebait, fed whole to aid ingestion. The fish are frozen to kill parasites and then thawed overnight in a refrigerator. Avian pellets can also be used (e.g. Charnwill Milling Company's Marine duck pellets™).

Waterfowl

Swans and water birds need lots of water when feeding. Washing-up bowls or deep cat litter trays are ideal, with the food placed in the bottom and filled to the top with water. Fresh (preferably wholemeal) bread, wheat or other grain and soft green leaf such as lettuce, lamb's tongue salad or spinach is provided. A pen containing around six swans will get one standard loaf, 1.2 kg wheat and several lettuce heads at each feed. Birds from very remote areas may not recognize this as food and some encouragement maybe required. A bowl of grit and water is also provided. Birds will feed throughout the day so two to three feeding times are necessary, with the bowls being filled between feeds when they become empty. In the author's experience of using this feeding regime, obesity is not usually a problem. Complete waterfowl pelleted feeds (e.g. Mazuri® Waterfowl Feed) are an alternative diet.

Rearing of young waterfowl

Waterfowl hatchlings are precocious, being able to feed themselves straight away. In the wild they are waterproof as soon as they leave the nest, within a day or so of hatching. This early waterproofing is lacking in hand-reared chicks without parents to keep them clean and dry, only developing as they fledge.

In the wild, waterfowl young may be separated from their family accidentally or on purpose. If there is a congenital problem (see 'Other conditions') the parents appear to abandon them. The defect may only become apparent when the individual grows at a slower rate than expected.

Ducklings are initially kept in batches of similar sized and similar aged birds in brooders with a heat lamp (Figures 26.25). Small bowls of water, chick crumb and greens are provided. They then progress into the larger indoor pens on straw or shredded paper, initially with a heat lamp (Figure 26.26). Cat litter sized trays are used for water only, water with bread and greens, water with grit and dry chick crumb (Figure 26.26). Batches of cygnets and, separately, goslings are kept in a similar way. Goslings are given the same food, water and grit as ducklings, but cygnets are given wheat instead of chick crumb. This is because they are much slower growers than ducklings. Feeding chick crumb predisposes to inappropriately rapid

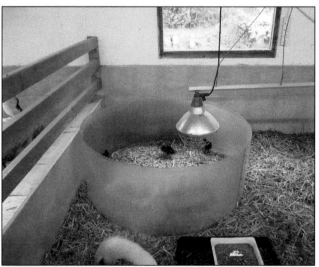

26.25 Small mallard ducklings in a rearing pen, showing a heat lamp sited at one side of the pen to create a heat gradient.

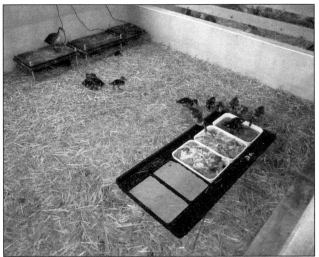

26.26 Older mallard ducklings in a rearing pen, showing the use of flat feeding trays placed on a larger tray to keep the straw dry. Clean, dry straw and good ventilation are essential to stop straw being a disease risk.

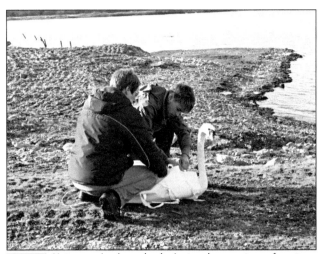

26.27 Mute swan in a 'swan bag' prior to release on to a safe water course.

bone growth and, in the author's experience, results in an increased incidence of perosis (slipped tendon) of the leg (see 'Other conditions').

Juvenile waterfowl are kept off larger areas of water until they are fledging (at around 5 weeks for ducklings), when they are able to waterproof themselves.

Release

The ideal aim of treatment is return to a function consistent with ability to survive in the wild. This may not result in an aesthetically pleasing look. For example, some injuries leave the bird with deficits on the web, or a scar on the body, whilst still leaving the bird perfectly functional. Full return to normal function must be carefully assessed and release determined by this (see Chapter 9). In some instances, in these species, if the bird is not fit for release back to the wild, release may be possible on a carefully managed private lake.

All birds kept away from water lose their waterproofing, not just oil contaminated patients. The bird should be assessed for waterproofing by gradual introduction to water at the rescue centre before being released; this process lasts a few days (see also Chapter 24).

Release must be carried out during daylight hours with enough light for the bird to orient itself (Figure 26.27). Birds should not be returned to contaminated water areas or where threat of injury is still high (e.g. a heavily fished lake).

Careful record must be kept of birds coming in to the rescue centre so that they will be released back where they came from, conditions permitting. Birds with their own territory such as mute swans must be returned to exactly where they came from. Birds with flocking behaviour, such as divers, should be returned to the flock. If this is not possible then the advice of a specialist local ornithologist should be sought.

Release of hand-reared waterfowl

It is not imperative to return young waterfowl back to their origin, but it is good practice to return the same number to the area they were rescued rather than releasing them all into the nearest water body to the rescue centre. In species where there is a strong family bond, such as the mute swan, the bond between parent and cygnet is broken if they have been apart too long, often after only 2–3 days, and adults will attack offspring if they are reintroduced after this time so an alternative release site must be found.

Legal aspects

In common with other species, it is legal to take in and keep injured wild waterfowl for the purpose of looking after them and releasing them as soon as they are fit to do so.

Under the Wildlife and Countryside Act 1981, wild birds cannot be killed, nor their eggs or nests (when in use or being built) taken or destroyed, except under licence. This Act implements the provisions of the EU Birds Directive and similar legislation exists throughout the European Union.

If birds are causing serious damage to a fishery or to wildlife conservation interests, the landowner or manager of a site can apply for a licence to shoot a limited number of the birds as an aid to reducing populations and discouraging others. The advisory leaflets *Fisheries and the presence of cormorants, goosanders and herons* (WM14) available from the Department for Environment, Food and Rural Affairs (Defra) and *Protecting your fishery from cormorants* from the Moran Committee both contain advice about deterrents and licences, some of which is applicable to Sawbills. A Defra evidence summary, *Review of fish eating birds policy* (2013), reported there was little evidence to suggest that red-breasted mergansers (*Mergus serrator*) were a particular problem in England. Goosanders (*Mergus merganser*) were more widespread and mainly affected upland rivers in the north and west of England.

It is the Crown's prerogative to own the 'white swans' [sic] on the Thames. In most other cases the mute swan is considered a wild bird.

Acknowledgements

The author would like to thank Mel Nelson at The Swan Sanctuary for her advice on waterfowl husbandry and to Gemma Nelson for taking photos in the awful weather. Thanks also to Carla England from Wildlife Rescue for her information about divers. Thanks also to Debra Bourne and Ruth Cromie for assistance with blood reference ranges.

References and further reading

Bexton S and Couper D (2014) Veterinary care of sick and injured mallards. *In Practice* **36**, 356–366

Birkhead M (2009) Lead levels in the blood of mute swans (*Cygnus olor*) on the River Thames. *Journal of Zoology* **199(1)**, 59–73

Blissitt M (2007) H5N1 avian influenza virus found in a whooper swan in Scotland. *Government Veterinary Journal* **17**, 10–13

Carpenter JW (2013) *Exotic Animal Formulary 4th edn.* Elsevier Saunders, Missouri

Coles B (2007) *Essentials of Avian Medicine and Surgery, 3rd edn.* Blackwell Publishing, Oxford

Department for Environment, Food and Rural Affairs (2013) *Evidence summary: Review of fish eating birds policy 19 July 2013.* www.gov.uk/government/uploads/system/uploads/attachment_data/file/224186/pb13972-fish-eating-birds-evidence-130719.pdf

Falk-Rønne J, Gravesen S, Larsen L *et al.* (1984) Microorganisms in the air of a horse stable. Concentrations of *Aspergillus fumigatus* and *Actinomycetes* with the use of straw and shredded newspaper as bedding material. *Dansk Veterinærtidsskrift* **67(21)**, 1079–1083

Forbes N (1996) Waterfowl. In: *BSAVA Manual of Raptors, Pigeons and Waterfowl*, ed. P Beynon. BSAVA Publications, Gloucester

Friend M (1987) *Field Guide to Wildlife Diseases Vol 1: General Field Procedures and Diseases of Migratory Birds.* US Department of the Interior Fish and Wildlife Service, Washington DC

Hocking PM, Gentle MJ, Bernard R *et al.* (1997) Evaluation of a protocol for determining the effectiveness of pretreatment with local analgesics for reducing experimentally induced articular pain in domestic fowl. *Research in Veterinary Science* **63**, 263–267

Irvine R (2013) Recognising notifiable diseases 1. Avian influenza. *In Practice* **35**, 426–437

Kilgore D and Schmidt-Nielsen K (1975) Heat loss from ducks' feet immersed in cold water. *The Condor* **77**, 475–517

King AS and McLelland J (1984) *Birds: their Structure and Function.* Bailliere Tindall, London

Midtgard U (1981) The rete tibiotarsale and arterio-venous association in the hind limb of birds: a comparative morphological study on counter-current heat exchange systems. *Acta Zoologica* **62(2)**, 67–87

Murase T, Ilkeda T, Goto I *et al.* (1992) Treatment of lead poisoning in wild geese. *Journal of the American Veterinary Medical Association* **200**, 1726–1729

Olsen J (1997) *Anseriformes in Avian Medicine: Principles and Application, abridged edn,* ed. B Ritchie, G Harrison and L Harrison, pp. 694–719. Wingers Publishing, Florida

Owen M and Black JM (1990) *Waterfowl Ecology.* Blackie, Glasgow and London

Sears J, Cooke SW, Cooke ZR *et al.* (1989) A method for the treatment of lead poisoning in the mute swan (*Cygnus olor*) and its long-term success. *British Veterinary Journal* **145(6)**, 586–595

Tanaka S, Dan C, Kawano H *et al.* (2008) Pathological study on amyloidosis in *Cygnus olor* (mute swan) and other waterfowl. *Medical Molecular Morphology* **41**, 99–108

Specialist organizations and useful contacts

See also Appendix 1 for RSPCA and Scottish SPCA wildlife hospital contacts and local wildlife rehabilitators

The Swan Sanctuary
Felix Lane, Shepperton, Middlesex TW17 8NN
Tel: 01932 240790
www.theswansanctuary.org.uk

Wildlife Rescue (divers especially)
Carla England, Moyles Court Farmhouse,
Ellingham Drove, Ringwood, Hampshire BH24 3NU
Tel: 01425 477500; 07765327558
carlaengland@btinternet.com

Wildfowl and Wetlands Trust
Slimbridge, Gloucestershire GL2 7BT
Tel: 01453 891900
www.wwt.org.uk
enquiries@wwt.org.uk

Chapter 27

Gamebirds

John Chitty

Gamebirds are those that are hunted for the table or for sport. Whilst this description may include wild ducks and certain waders, such as snipe (*Gallinago gallinago*) and woodcock (*Scolopax rusticola*), this chapter will concentrate on Galliformes to avoid duplicating information that can be found in Chapters 25 and 26.

The Galliformes are related to poultry. Some of these species are not indigenous to the British Isles but have become established over several centuries. Many are farmed semi-intensively prior to release (typically the pheasant (*Phasianus colchicus*) and both red-legged (*Alectoris rufa*) and grey (*Perdix perdix*) partridges); therefore, many of those birds presented to rehabilitators will not be truly 'wild' and may be harbouring or exhibiting clinical signs of diseases that are more typical of intensive-rearing situations.

For this reason a brief description of rearing practices will be included here. Game species can only be hunted in legally defined seasons and naturally it is sensible to avoid these periods when releasing rehabilitated birds (see 'Legal aspects' and Chapter 2). Some common species of British gamebirds are shown in Figure 27.1.

Ecology and biology

Figure 27.2 describes the ecology and biology of British gamebirds.

Gamebirds are ground-nesters that generally form territories, usually set up and defended by the males. These may be centred around good food sources (e.g. for

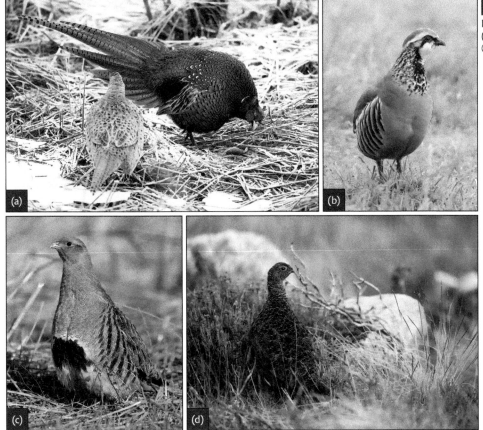

27.1 (a) Male (right) and female (left) pheasants. (b) Red-legged partridge. (c) Grey partridge. (d) Red grouse.
(© Andrew Kelly)

Species	Description	Weight	UK distribution	Habitat	Diet
Common pheasant (*Phasianus colchicus*) (see Figure 27.1a)	Male red-brown with bright head/back colours; long tail lost after breeding Female dull brown with shorter tail	Male approx. 1500 g Female approx. 1000 g	All except northern Scotland	Generally edges of woodland/ hedgerows	Seeds, insects
Red-legged (French) partridge (*Alectoris rufa*) (see Figure 27.1b)	Red tail, white face with dark eye-stripe, barring on flanks, red bill and legs	450–600 g	England as far north as Yorkshire moors; not Wales	Open countryside, heath, downland, etc.	Seeds, insects
Grey (English) partridge (*Perdix perdix*) (see Figure 27.1c)	Grey-brown; orange-red face, red-brown tail Male brown horseshoe mark on breast; duller in female	320–400 g	All except northern Scotland and mountainous areas	Open countryside, some cover	Seeds, insects
Common quail (*Coturnix coturnix*)	Resembles very small partridge Male black and white stripes on throat and neck (absent in female)	150–180 g	Summer visitor to southern England, some parts Scotland and Ireland	Open countryside	Seeds
Red grouse (*Lagopus lagopus*) (see Figure 27.1d)	Male dark red-brown plumage, red eye wattles, white legs Female smaller and plainer	400–700 g	Scotland, northern England, Wales, Ireland	Moorland	Heather shoots
Ptarmigan (*Lagopus mutus*)	Summer: male dark brown upper parts, white wings and belly, red eye wattles; female paler with smaller wattles Winter: white with black tail; male has black face patch (lacking in female)	250–600 g	Northern Scotland	Mountain top	Heather shoots, ground berries, leaves
Black grouse (*Tetrao tetrix*)	Male (blackcock) black with red head wattles, black and white lyre-shaped tail Female (greyhen) smaller; similar to red grouse but greyer and forked tail	Male 1000–1750 g Female 750–1100 g	Scotland, northern England and Wales	Moorland	Heather shoots
Capercaillie (*Tetrao urogallus*)	Male huge; dark plumage, bushy throat feathers, rounded tail Female similar to greyhen but larger and with chestnut breast	Male 3700–4800 g Female 1600–2500 g	Scottish Highlands	Pine forest	Pine shoots

27.2 Ecology and biology of common British gamebirds.

pheasants) or at ritual breeding grounds where many males come together (e.g. black grouse (*Tetrao tetrix*)).

The chicks are precocial and have pale down with dark mottles or stripes.

Game farming

Pheasants (Figure 27.3) and both species of partridge (red-legged and grey) are reared for release. Reared birds will make up the vast majority of the casualties that may be presented to rehabilitators.

Traditionally, at the end of the shooting season, adult males and females are caught up and placed into breeding pens. However, this results in selection of birds with an innate tendency to run rather than fly when alarmed. As this tendency is inherited by the offspring, the 'quality' of the shoot declines. Therefore, new breeding strategies have developed alongside the traditional methods.

One system is to maintain a permanent captive breeding stock; this is the basis of game farms (often abroad, especially in France), which supply chicks to the rearing fields in June each year. Where birds are captive-bred, chicks are initially reared in houses and then moved to covered runs, before being moved to a large release pen – typically in late July. The release pen is intended to act as a 'home base' and the birds are fully released after a few weeks. Fox-proof re-entry funnels enable the birds to return to feed if they are unable to fly back into the release pen.

The other system is to encourage breeding in the wild and this (it is postulated) produces a wilder, more strongly flying bird. Many shoots continue to feed 'wild' birds

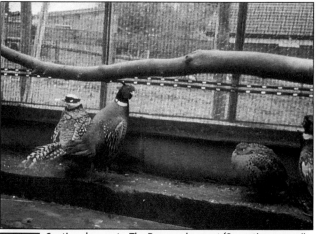

27.3 Captive pheasants. The Reeves pheasant (*Syrmaticus reevesii*; left) is a non-native species and may not be released. The common pheasant is on the right and, although not technically native, is releasable.
(Courtesy of Wiltshire Wildlife Hospital)

through spring and early summer by means of strategically placed hoppers. These enable male birds to form a territory around a feeder and attract females. This approach has many advantages for the environment, for example gamebirds will not do well without insects in the diet and therefore breeding areas are not sprayed, and small copses and mature hedgerows are left intact to encourage the formation of territories.

Anatomy and physiology

The anatomy is essentially chicken-like. There is a short straight beak for prehending food items from the ground. Gut adaptations to the natural diet consist of a large crop, powerful grinding gizzard and well developed paired caeca to enable hindgut fermentation.

Capture, handling and transportation

Capture

Capture of injured birds is not always easy. They are all good runners, even with damaged legs, and tend to head towards thick undergrowth. Catching birds in the wild is best done with several people 'flushing' the bird into an open area where a net can be used. It is important to note that male capercaillie (*Tetrao urogallus*) are extremely aggressive and should be approached with caution.

Gamebirds are very nervous and will cause themselves a great deal of damage in evading capture. In the clinic or rehabilitation centre, where the bird is more confined, it is best to dim the lighting before attempting handling as this might help to calm the bird. It can then be caught using a net or by being enveloped in a large towel.

Handling

A strong grip is necessary. Gamebirds are strong and will struggle violently, which can result in injury to the bird. They are also extremely loose-feathered and the loss of large amounts of body feathering will delay release, as the feathers play an important role in the bird's thermo-regulatory system.

Males often possess large spurs just proximal to the foot (Figure 27.4). These can inflict deep wounds on a handler and so the legs of male gamebirds must be held firmly.

Wrapping the bird in a towel to restrain the wings and feet will help greatly when it is being moved. It is important that the legs are not crushed together, as this may result in bruising of the lower limb and injuries to the opposite leg from the spur and claws. Part of the towel can be used to cover the head, which should calm the bird.

The wrap may need to be removed during examination. The hands should be placed on either side of the bird's body, with the thumbs between its shoulder joints, head facing away from the handler. The index and middle fingers are held around the wings whilst the ring and little fingers hold the upper legs (Figure 27.5). Smaller gamebirds (e.g. quail (*Coturnix coturnix*) and young partridge) may be held in one hand in much the same manner as for passerines (see Figure 3.12).

Transportation

These are nervous birds and so a dark box (or covered cage) is essential. It should be sturdy and should open from the top. A grippable surface such as a towel should be provided to prevent leg injuries during transport. Extricating a flapping pheasant from a cat box with a small door is very difficult. Cardboard boxes or standard cat carriers are ideal. As these birds tend to fly upwards when startled, to assist in removing the bird from the box, a towel can be dropped on to the animal to calm it and prevent this from happening, prior to fully opening the box.

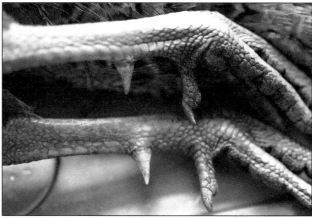
27.4 The feet of a male pheasant, showing the prominent spurs. (© John Chitty)

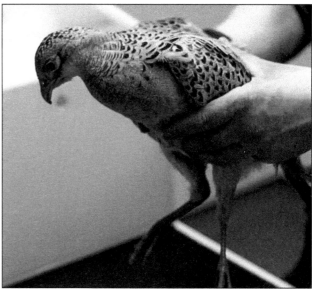
27.5 Correct handling technique for an adult female pheasant. The index and middle fingers are held around the wings whilst the ring and little fingers hold the upper legs. (© John Chitty)

Zoonotic risks

The main zoonotic risk with gamebirds is salmonellosis. It is important to maintain strict hygiene protocols and to wash and disinfect hands, surfaces and handling equipment after use. Campylobacteriosis is also a potential risk – hygiene precautions are similar to those for *Salmonella*. Chlamydiosis is unusual but should be suspected in birds showing upper respiratory signs. In these cases, face-masks and goggles should be worn by handlers and strict barrier nursing applied (see Chapter 28).

Examination and clinical assessment for rehabilitation

The general principles of examination and assessment, as detailed in Chapter 4, apply to gamebird casualties. Body condition can be assessed by palpating the pectoral muscles (see Figure 4.6). It is important to note that chicks and poults (older chicks/subadults) should feel thinner than adults, as the pectoral muscles will be less developed. Birds should also be weighed, as this enables correct calculation of drug dosages and, where a pheasant or partridge is in good body condition, will enable some degree of ageing of young birds. Tables of bodyweights may be found in Beer (1988).

Droppings should be examined (see Chapter 10). Farmed game are very prone to a range of parasitic infections (see 'Parasites') and so gross evaluation of faeces and faecal flotation may be useful. Microscopic examination of a wet preparation of fresh faeces is useful for the diagnosis of protozoal enteritis (e.g. trichomonosis, spironucleosis (hexamitiasis)). A soiled vent and tail feathers may indicate loose droppings.

Anaesthesia may be useful to facilitate examination in the following circumstances:

- Very nervous birds, where detailed examination may cause more stress
- Dyspnoeic birds – allows supply of oxygen as well as reducing stress (e.g. in cases of tracheal obstruction for placement of an air sac tube)
- Examination of the upper legs – these are very well muscled and held tightly against the body, so that full extension and examination of the femurs, hips and stifles may be difficult in the conscious bird
- Examination of the posterior segment of the eye – anaesthesia is necessary to dilate the (small) pupil. This examination should be performed whenever head trauma is suspected.

For further details on anaesthesia in these species see 'Anaesthesia and analgesia' and Chapter 6.

Diagnostic techniques

Blood sampling is not routinely used by the author, partly due to financial constraints and partly due to a lack of published reference ranges for individual species. However, there is certainly potential for its use as a diagnostic aid and these species are good candidates for venepuncture.

Ulnar and medial metatarsal veins are most appropriate for use in gamebirds. Whilst they do possess a right jugular vein, most species lack an apterium over the vein and have thick skin over the neck making the vein more difficult to locate.

Crop washes are rarely indicated, with the most significant endoparasites being located further along the gastrointestinal system, distal to the crop. Faecal sampling, therefore, is extremely important (see 'Parasites' and Chapter 10). It is vital that freshly voided samples are utilized owing to the high frequency of motile protozoal infections that may be found. Ideally a wet preparation of faeces should be made within 20 minutes of voiding in order to identify motile protozoa. Alternatively, stained preparations may be used, though it is much harder to locate parasites with this technique.

Quantitative or qualitative flotation methods may be used to identify nematode eggs or coccidial oocysts (see Chapter 10).

Euthanasia

Birds should be returned to the wild only if they can meet the following criteria:

- Full use of both legs. Inability to use both legs fully will reduce the capacity of these heavy birds to escape predators. A unilateral lameness will inevitably result in the development of bumblefoot (pododermatitis) in the weight-bearing foot (Figure 27.6)

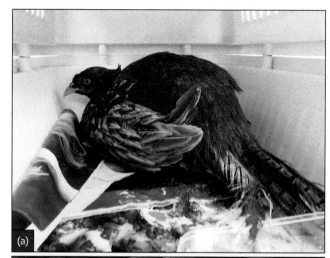

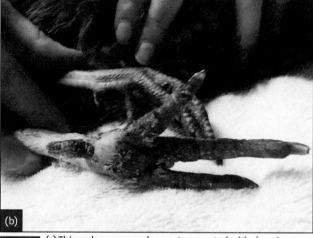

27.6 (a) This male common pheasant presented with chronic unilateral lameness and severe weight loss. (b) The contralateral foot showed evidence of pododermatitis and the bird was euthanased.
(Courtesy of Emma Keeble)

- Ability to fly. These birds are not 'performance fliers' in the manner of raptors and they do not rely on their wings to get food, nor are they migratory (except quail). Indeed there is some argument that poor fliers are more likely to survive the shooting season. However, some flight is necessary to avoid predators and so those unable to fly should be euthanased
- Vision in both eyes. The need for binocular vision is less important than in a raptor, but lack of vision makes birds more prone to predation. The lateral position of the eyes gives these birds a large field of vision (typical in prey species). Defects in one or both eyes will be a hindrance to survival in the wild
- Free from infectious disease. A bird that is suspected of carrying or that is suffering from infectious disease should not be released. A bird that does not gain weight or body condition, even though it is eating, may well fall into this category.

Euthanasia at first examination is recommended in the following cases:

- Open, complicated or chronic fractures
- Fractures near to or involving joints
- Extensive soft tissue injuries (especially where there is penetration of the coelomic cavity or where there are large tissue deficits of the leg muscles or tendons)
- Obvious loss of an eye (e.g. corneal rupture, hypopyon).

Euthanasia techniques

Ideally euthanasia should be performed using intravenous pentobarbital into the ulnar or medial metatarsal veins (note that thick scales on the lower leg can hinder the visualization and approach to the vein in some birds). The jugular vein is difficult to find in gamebirds (see 'Diagnostic techniques'). If veins are inaccessible, intrahepatic injection of pentobarbital may be used though it is recommended that the bird be sedated or anaesthetized prior to such injection. This may be difficult or impossible in the field, where it may be deemed inhumane to transport a bird to a veterinary clinic. In these cases, euthanasia by a trained competent operator using rapid cervical dislocation is acceptable in smaller species (see Chapter 4).

First aid and short-term hospitalization

In the non-collapsed bird, oral fluids (e.g. Vetark® Critical Care Formula®) may be given by crop tube at a rate of 12 ml/kg per feed and repeated as necessary (see also Chapter 5).

In the collapsed bird, intravenous fluids can be given by bolus injection of, for example, Hartmann's solution into the ulnar vein at 5–10 ml/kg. Intravenous and intraosseous fluids administered via a giving set and drip line do not appear to be well tolerated.

Repeated intravenous injections may require extensive handling and, where this is not desirable, the subcutaneous route may be used. Injection of isotonic saline or Hartmann's solution at 20 ml/kg into the precrural fold is simple and not overly traumatic to the bird. Fluid appears to be absorbed completely within 20–30 minutes.

It is advisable, where clinical signs indicate evidence of infection, to give a broad-spectrum systemic antibiotic, such as amoxicillin/clavulanate (co-amoxiclav) (see Figure 27.10). See also Chapters 5 and 7.

Fracture stabilization

The general principles set out in Chapter 5 also apply to gamebirds. Injuries following road traffic accidents are the most frequent reasons for gamebirds being presented, closely followed by gunshot injuries, and fractures are therefore commonly seen. In these cases, analgesia should always be provided at first presentation. The author uses carprofen at 5 mg/kg by intramuscular injection initially; this may be repeated once daily as required. Buprenorphine may also be used at 0.05–0.1 mg/kg i.m. q8–12h, but should not be used in birds that could enter the human food chain. See also Figures 27.7 and 5.15 for dose rates of analgesics in birds.

Leg fractures

A ball bandage may be applied to immobilize broken toes (see Figure 5.19), and aluminium finger splints may be used to support fractures of the tarsometatarsus. It is not advisable to apply support to fractures higher than the intertarsal joint: the legs are short, muscular and held close to the body, which makes it impossible to immobilize the joints above and below a fracture, as well as making it likely that the dressing will slip. In these cases, it is better to confine the bird in a small dark box until it can tolerate surgery and internal fixation can be performed.

Wing fractures

The short rounded wing is very difficult to stabilize with a figure-of-eight bandage. It is usually best to confine the bird in a small dark box until surgery can be tolerated. Where support is essential (e.g. where the wing is trailing and being stepped on), the wing can be held against the body using conforming bandage (see Figure 5.17).

Short-term hospitalization

Gamebirds have few specific needs. The enclosure must be secluded and there should be no potential predators (e.g. dogs, cats, raptors) in close visual proximity.

In the short term a conventional dog or cat kennel is acceptable. It should be large enough for the bird to move freely without damaging wing or tail feathers, but not so large that catching becomes difficult. These species fly upwards when startled and this can easily lead to traumatic injuries in captivity. Perching is not required. For short-term hospitalization, substrates of newspaper, artificial grass or even towels are appropriate.

Anaesthesia and analgesia

The general principles of anaesthesia and analgesia, as detailed in Chapter 6, also apply to gamebird casualties. As gamebirds are officially classed as food-producing species, the anaesthetic drugs discussed in this chapter should not be used in birds that could enter the human food chain (see 'Therapeutics') (Whitehead and Roberts, 2014).

Anaesthesia

Isoflurane or sevoflurane can be administered by facemask and are the anaesthetic agents of choice. The bird can then be intubated for maintenance of anaesthesia.

Where gaseous anaesthetic agents are not available, medetomidine/ketamine combinations or alfaxalone may be used (see Figure 27.7). Medetomidine can be reversed by an equal volume of intramuscular atipamezole, but it should be noted that this combination carries more risks than isoflurane.

Gamebirds are extremely nervous and may be prone to catecholamine-induced dysrhythmias and death whilst anaesthetized. If the capture of the bird before induction has been difficult (e.g. it has escaped and been chased), it is generally better to replace the bird in its box or hospitalization unit and leave it quietly in the dark to calm down before proceeding.

On recovery, birds should be held wrapped in a towel and oxygen administered via a facemask until the bird is able to stand without ataxia. This will prevent flapping and associated injuries or feather loss on recovery.

Analgesia

Carprofen and meloxicam are particularly useful and appear to be safe in these species (Figure 27.7; see also Figure 5.15).

It is important to ensure the avian patient is well hydrated when using non-steroidal anti-inflammatory drugs (NSAIDs) as these may be associated with adverse renal effects in dehydrated animals or those with renal disease.

Drug	Dosage	Withdrawal period for food-producing animals
Non-steroidal anti-inflammatory drugs		
Carprofen	5 mg/kg i.m., orally q24h[a]	28 days
Meloxicam	0.2–0.5 mg/kg i.m., orally q12h[a]	28 days
Anaesthetics		
Medetomidine (M) + ketamine (K)	25–100 µg/kg (M) + 2–5 mg/kg (K) i.v., i.m. Use lower end of dose range i.v.; higher doses i.m. Medetomidine effects can be reversed with equal volume of atipamezole i.m.	Must not be used in birds intended for human consumption[b]
Alfaxalone	10 mg/kg i.v. (short procedures or induction); 20 mg/kg i.v. for longer period of anaesthesia	Must not be used in birds intended for human consumption[b]

27.7 Non-steroidal anti-inflammatory drugs and anaesthetic drugs and their dose rates used in gamebirds. It is important to note that gamebirds are officially classed as food-producing animals and therefore drug withdrawal periods must be observed and drugs prohibited in food-producing animals must not be administered if there is a risk of them entering the human food chain.
([a] Ramsey, 2014; [b] Whitehead and Roberts, 2014). NB Prohibited drugs are those not listed in Table 1 of EU Regulation 37/2010 (www.ec.europa.eu).

Specific conditions

For full reviews see Curtis (1987), Beer (1988) and Coles (2009). It should be noted that, commercially, diagnoses are generally reached following necropsy and most textbooks reflect this. It is important that any gamebird that dies or is euthanased whilst being cared for is submitted for post-mortem examination; this will enable detection of infectious/zoonotic disease agents and so reduce risks for other birds and staff.

Trauma

Intraocular haemorrhage

Trauma will often result in damage to the pecten and subsequent intraocular haemorrhage. Where haemorrhage is visible (usually with the aid of an ophthalmoscope), therapy using topical ophthalmic corticosteroid preparations should be started promptly and the eye re-examined before release. Corticosteroid preparations are contraindicated where there is corneal ulceration or active infection, and when they are being used birds should be monitored for potential systemic side effects (e.g. polyuria/polydipsia).

Orthopaedic problems

Gamebirds tend to have relatively large bones with thin fragile cortices that shatter easily, and it is unusual to see simple fractures. In addition, many fractures will be open and infected, and may be chronic in nature, giving a poor prognosis for return to the wild in most cases. Options for repair are limited in gamebirds and the vast majority of cases are unsuitable for surgery.

General principles for avian fracture repair are discussed in Chapters 5 and 29. Some details specific to gamebirds are as follows.

Fractures of the coracoid: Fractures of this bone may be seen as a result of in-flight collisions with a solid object. Shoulder injuries typically present with an upward rotation of the wing tip rather than a drooping wing (see Figure 4.4) and diagnosis is by radiography. Surgical repair is rarely indicated; confinement to a cage or an aviary for 4–6 weeks is sufficient.

Fractures of the humerus and femur: These bones are pneumatized. They have a large internal diameter and very thin cortices. Simple intramedullary pinning requires a very large pin, such that the sheer weight of the pin will cause problems. This technique also gives no rotational stability. The method of choice in these birds is therefore a hybridization technique (see Chapter 29). Alternatively, stack pinning techniques can work well in the femur.

Fractures distal to the carpus: It is difficult to apply and maintain external support in this area due to the shape of the wing. The primary feathers should be trimmed and heavy tape or Vet-lite™ should be applied to the feather bases to align the bones and maintain their length. The bird needs to be maintained in captivity until the primaries have regrown. As this may necessitate a long stay in rehabilitation aviaries it is important these are well maintained, with good cover to reduce stress, a suitable substrate (see 'Management in captivity') and large enough to allow natural behaviours. If possible birds should be housed in groups. Periodic (every 1–3 months) faecal parasitology should be performed whilst the bird is in captivity.

Fractures of the tibiotarsus: Heavy muscling around this bone makes the use of external fixators less desirable. A simple intramedullary pin combined with bandaging will usually work well, in the author's experience. Pins should always be removed prior to releasing the bird.

Fractures of the tarsometatarsus: Surgical intervention is likely to damage surrounding tendons. Most cases will do well with external support using an aluminium finger splint or Vet-lite™. The support should immobilize the intertarsal joint and the tarsometatarsophalangeal joint (with a 'stirrup' beneath the foot). Care should be taken to maintain normal standing joint angles so that the bird is able to move and stand comfortably. These fractures will normally heal in 2–4 weeks.

Toe fractures: These do well in a ball bandage (see Figure 5.19), which should be removed after 5 days and the bird confined for a further 14 days.

Infectious diseases

Infectious diseases of gamebirds are outlined below. It is important that equipment is not shared between birds and that it is disinfected thoroughly after use.

Viral diseases

Newcastle disease: Newcastle disease is caused by paramyxovirus-1 (PMV-1) infection. Clinical signs include neurological signs, including incoordination and staggering, diarrhoea and polydipsia. Respiratory signs are less common than in poultry.

It is a **notifiable disease** and, as such, the local Divisional Veterinary Manager (Animal and Plant Health Agency (APHA), see Appendix 1) should be notified on suspicion of the disease. Diagnosis is based on serology, virus isolation and post-mortem signs and is carried out by the APHA. There is no specific therapy.

Pheasant ataxia: Pheasant ataxia is an emerging neurological condition of unknown cause. It is characterized by paresis or paralysis of the legs and must therefore be differentiated from spinal/pelvic injuries and Newcastle disease. Suspicion of the disease is aroused if several birds present from same site or if examination and/or necropsy reveal no sign of injury. Definitive diagnosis is by histopathology of central nervous system tissue. There is no treatment.

Avian influenza: Avian influenza is caused by avian influenza viruses. Infection can result in death, acute respiratory signs and cyanosis. It is a **notifiable disease** and the local Divisional Veterinary Manager (APHA) should be notified upon suspicion: diagnosis is carried out by the APHA and is based on serology, virus isolation and post-mortem appearance. There is no treatment.

Marble spleen disease: Marble spleen disease is caused by adenovirus infection and can cause sudden death (pheasants 'fall out of the sky'). It is an unusual condition to see in the rehabilitation unit, but is an important differential for sudden death in adult birds. Diagnosis is made at post-mortem examination, where an enlarged mottled ('marbled') spleen is apparent. There is no treatment.

Pheasant coronavirus: Infection with pheasant coronavirus results in wasting and polyuria/polydipsia in adult birds. Enlarged pale kidneys are seen on post-mortem examination. There is no treatment.

Pox: Poxvirus infection is characterized by the development of multiple masses around the head, limbs and sometimes the upper alimentary tract. Diagnosis is by histopathology or cytology of needle aspirates taken from the lesions. Therapy is by symptomatic care until the lesions resolve; the bird's welfare must be considered during treatment and euthanasia may be necessary. Some lesions may result in permanent scarring in sensitive areas (e.g. eyelids)

The poxvirus is highly contagious and birds under treatment should be barrier-nursed until the infection is completely resolved.

Bacterial diseases

Colibacillosis: Infection with *Escherichia coli* is most frequently seen in chicks and poults. Affected birds have a fluffed-up appearance with wasting; death due to septicaemia may ensue. Colibacillosis often occurs secondary to other diseases (e.g. coccidiosis) or in unhygienic conditions. Diagnosis is based on the presence of typical clinical signs, together with culture/sensitivity of faeces (or heart blood, liver or bone marrow on post-mortem examination). Treatment is with antibiotics, the selection of which is ideally based on culture/sensitivity results. Any underlying factors or diseases should be recognized and corrected/treated appropriately.

Salmonellosis: Infection with *Salmonella* spp. typically results in haemorrhagic enteritis, although clinical signs may also appear similar to colibacillosis. Diagnosis is based on the presence of typical clinical signs, together with culture/sensitivity of faeces (or heart blood, liver or bone marrow on post-mortem examination), as for colibacillosis. Hard white caecal cores may be seen on post-mortem examination; wet preparations of these should always be examined to differentiate from other causes of caecal cores, especially coccidiosis and *Heterakis* (roundworm) infestations. Treatment is with antibiotics, ideally selected based on culture/sensitivity results.

Avian tuberculosis: Avian tuberculosis is caused by *Mycobacterium avium* infection and is a cause of wasting in adult birds. Ante-mortem diagnosis is difficult, but clinical signs may be suggestive. Mycobacteria may be evident on microscopic examination of faeces with the use of acid-fast stains; haematological changes (high white blood cell count with heterophilia and monocytosis) and intracoelomic endoscopy are the diagnostic methods of choice. White nodules are found in the liver, spleen and intestines on post-mortem examination (Figure 27.8). Anti mycobacterial therapies are available, but treatment is not recommended as the success rate is so poor and infected birds pose a potential zoonotic risk. Large numbers of bacteria are shed in the faeces, emphasizing the need for good hygiene and strict isolation of any ill or thin birds.

Mycoplasmosis: Infection with *Mycoplasma* spp. may result in birds with sinusitis (Figure 27.9) and/or tenosynovitis (typically they present as lame with swelling above the intertarsal joint). Mycoplasmosis is highly infectious to other birds. Diagnosis is based on the recognition of typical clinical signs, cytology of fluid aspirates and culture of the causative organism or serology. Treatment is with systemic antibiosis, especially tetracyclines, tylosin or fluoroquinolones (see Figure 27.10). Advanced cases develop large cores of inspissated pus in the sinuses that need to be removed surgically.

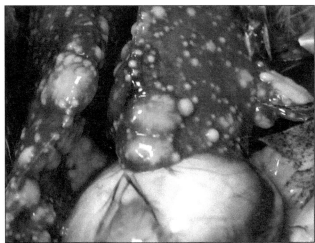

27.8 Post-mortem examination of a pheasant. The white nodular lesions visible on the liver are due to mycobacteriosis (avian tuberculosis).
(© John Chitty)

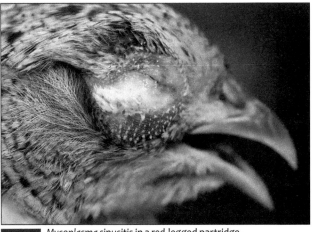

27.9 *Mycoplasma* sinusitis in a red-legged partridge.
(© John Chitty)

Fungal diseases

Aspergillosis: Infection with *Aspergillus* spp. may result in dyspnoea and death, due to formation of fungal colonies in lungs and air sacs following inhalation of spores from rotting organic matter (e.g. bark chip, mouldy hay). Young birds are most often affected. Radiography and coelomic endoscopy are the techniques of greatest diagnostic value, together with cytology and culture/sensitivity of fungal colonies. Treatment is with itraconazole or terbinafine (see Figure 27.10) administered systemically with nebulization of F10®, but is unlikely to be successful once clinical signs present. It is preferable to prevent the disease by removing organic matter from areas where gamebirds are reared or hospitalized.

Parasites

Endoparasites:

Coccidiosis: Coccidiosis is caused by *Eimeria* spp. and usually affects young birds, which typically show wasting and sometimes diarrhoea. Infection may predispose to secondary colibacillosis. Coccidiosis is diagnosed by demon-strating the presence of coccidial oocysts in faecal smears or flotation preparations. The ideal treatment is with toltrazuril. Alternatively, amprolium/sulfadimethoxine is licensed in pigeons and is available in small quantities (see Figure 27.10).

Protozoal dysentery: Protozoal dysentery is caused by *Spironucleus* spp. (previously known as *Hexamita*) or *Trichomonas* spp. and results in frothy yellow diarrhoea, wasting and death. It is diagnosed by the demonstration of motile flagellates in fresh (<20 mins old) faecal samples. Note that these organisms may be present in low numbers as gut commensals in healthy birds; stress of illness and/ or captivity may trigger overt disease. Affected birds can be treated with carnidazole (see Figure 27.10), but this drug should not be used in birds that could enter the human food chain (Whitehead and Roberts, 2014).

Histomoniasis: Histomoniasis, caused by *Histomonas meleagridis* infection, is especially seen in red-legged partridge. Young birds may die suddenly, whilst older birds may develop diarrhoea and become emaciated. Diagnosis is by the demonstration of the causative organisms in fresh wet preparations of faeces. Affected birds can be treated with carnidazole (see Figure 27.10).

Gapes: Birds that are infested with *Syngamus trachea* typically show clinical signs of open-mouthed breathing ('gapes') and dyspnoea. Tracheal endoscopy reveals the presence of adult worms, whilst microscopy of sputum and faecal samples can be used to reveal ova. Treatment is with flubendazole, ivermectin or fenbendazole (see Figure 27.10).

Strongylosis: Various species of strongyle may infest gamebirds, resulting in wasting. *Trichostrongylus tenuis* infestation is a major cause of mortality in red grouse (*Lagopus lagopus*) and partridge; the former is one of the major causes of large population fluctuations in wild populations. Diagnosis is by finding ova using faecal flotation techniques and treatment is with flubendazole, ivermectin or fenbendazole.

Ectoparasites: Feather lice, mites and hippoboscid flies can all infest gamebirds; they rarely cause clinical disease but may be a sign of debility. If treatment is required, permethrins or fipronil may be used topically, but the latter should not be used in birds that could enter the human food chain (Whitehead and Roberts, 2014).

Therapeutics

The general principles outlined in Chapter 7 also apply to gamebirds. It should be noted that intramuscular injections should be given into the pectoral muscle masses, not the leg muscles, to avoid an injection reaction or abscess in these muscles, which could result in lameness.

It is important to note that gamebirds are officially classed as food-producing animals and therefore drug withdrawal periods must be observed. Birds should not be released within the withdrawal period, usually 28 days and, more sensibly, not during the shooting season or for a month before its start (see Figure 27.11). If drugs are used that are not licensed in food-producing animals then these birds should either not be released near a shoot, or should be retained in captivity: such treated animals should not enter the food chain. For further information on legislation governing food producing animals and prohibited medicinal substances see Whitehead and Roberts, 2014. Approved drugs are listed in EU regulation 37/2010 (www.ec.europa.eu). See Figures 27.7 and 27.10 for drug doses used in gamebirds, including withdrawal periods.

Drug	Dosage	Withdrawal period for food-producing animals
Antifungals		
Itraconazole	10 mg/kg orally q12–24h	Must not be used in birds intended for human consumption[d]
Terbinafine	15 mg/kg orally q12h orally	Must not be used in birds intended for human consumption[d]
Antibacterials		
Tylosin	0.5 g/l water[a]	28 days
Doxycycline	40 mg/kg orally q12–24h[b] 200–500 mg/l water (soft water only)[a]	28 days
Enrofloxacin	15 mg/kg i.m., orally q12h[b]	28 days
Marbofloxacin	10 mg/kg i.m., orally q24h[b]	28 days
Amoxicillin/clavulanate (co-amoxiclav)	125–150 mg/kg i.m. q24h or orally q12h[b]	28 days

27.10 Therapeutic drugs and their dose rates used in gamebirds. It is important to note that gamebirds are officially classed as food-producing animals and therefore drug withdrawal periods must be observed and drugs prohibited in food-producing animals must not be administered if there is a risk of them entering the human food chain. (continues) ▶

([a] Licensed dose; [b] Ramsey, 2014; [c] Carpenter, 2013; [d] Whitehead and Roberts, 2014). NB Prohibited drugs are those not listed in Table 1 of EU Regulation 37/2010 (www.ec.europa.eu).

Drug	Dosage	Withdrawal period for food-producing animals
Antiparasitic drugs		
Flubendazole	3 g/kg feed[a]	7 days
Fenbendazole	20 mg/kg orally q24h for 5 days[b]	28 days
Ivermectin	200 μg/kg i.m., orally once[b]	28 days
Carnidazole	20–30 mg/kg orally once[c]	Must not be used in birds intended for human consumption[d]
Toltrazuril	3 ml of 2.5% solution/l drinking water given for 8 hours per day on 2 consecutive days	18 days
Amprolium	50–100 mg/l drinking water daily for 7 days[c]	28 days
Sulfadimethoxine	1 g/l water daily for 2 days, then 3 days off, then 2 days medication	28 days

27.10 (continued) Therapeutic drugs and their dose rates used in gamebirds. It is important to note that gamebirds are officially classed as food-producing animals and therefore drug withdrawal periods must be observed and drugs prohibited in food-producing animals must not be administered if there is a risk of them entering the human food chain.

([a]Licensed dose; [b]Ramsey, 2014; [c]Carpenter, 2013; [d]Whitehead and Roberts, 2014). NB Prohibited drugs are those not listed in Table 1 of EU Regulation 37/2010 (www.ec.europa.eu).

Management in captivity

Housing

Small flights or aviaries are ideal for housing gamebirds. It is also possible to keep them on the floor of an aviary used for passerines. Some perching should be provided to allow the birds to roost at night if they wish. As they are nervous birds, some shelter or screening should be provided in and around the aviary.

Ideally flooring should be easy to clean and not soil-based, to reduce the build-up of parasites and enable disinfection between groups of birds. Concrete addresses these criteria, but may result in foot lesions in long-term patients. Gravel may therefore be more acceptable as it can be replaced or hosed through between groups.

To reduce the risk of spreading infectious disease, birds from different areas should not be housed together. As with all birds, aviaries should have an inward-opening double door system to prevent escape.

Diet

Diet is simple, as these birds will readily take poultry pellets or mash, or chick crumb. For debilitated birds these can be liquidized and fed by crop tube (see Chapter 5). If commercial gamebird feeds are obtained and given then care should be taken regarding drugs that may be incorporated into such rations. Corn or commercial diets for mynah birds may be added to increase palatability for reluctant feeders. Drinking water should be provided in a shallow dish and changed daily.

Rearing young

Orphaned birds are not commonly presented. When they are, they should be reared in groups for socialization. Gamebird chicks are precocial and social imprinting is not an issue. They will readily take chick crumb, and feeding by hand should not be necessary.

Release

Birds may be released after recovery from the presenting illness or injury. Their fitness for release can be determined by:

- Demeanour and full vision
- Ability to prehend food
- Body condition
- Ability to walk or run
- Ability to fly.

These criteria should be assessed thoroughly before release. This can be done in much the same way as for other birds (see Chapter 9), but it may be difficult to assess the last criterion, as gamebirds are often reluctant fliers. Where there are doubts about any of the criteria, the bird should be either euthanased or kept and reassessed at a later date if it is felt that the problem will resolve.

Ideally, birds should be released where they were found. This should be done just after the shooting season (see Figure 27.11). It is sensible to discuss release activities with local landowners and gamekeepers; access to land requires their permission (see Chapter 2) and they may be willing to help with post-release monitoring and feeding. Brightly coloured leg tags are available to aid post-release monitoring.

Two forms of release may be employed: hard or soft (see Chapter 9).

Hard-release

Many of these species are amenable to hard-release. Birds may simply be released, as long as there is suitable habitat. The presence of other birds of the same species should be an indicator of the suitability of that area.

Soft-release

Soft-release is the preferred option and is particularly suitable for pheasants. As discussed earlier, male pheasants can be induced to form a territory around a feeding station in a hedgerow or on the edge of woodland. If access to land is possible, a feeding hopper containing game or poultry feed should be placed in a suitable position. A male pheasant can then be released (or one will soon arrive) and released females will generally join his harem. Feeding can be gradually tapered off at the end of the breeding season.

This technique involves close cooperation with the local gamekeeper. As 'wild' breeding is now very important, opposition is unlikely (outside the shooting season) unless the released birds are placed too close to existing release pens.

Legal aspects

The legal aspects pertaining to holding and re-release of injured birds (see Chapter 2) also apply to gamebirds. It is important to have knowledge of the legal shooting seasons so that birds are not released during or immediately prior to these (see Figure 27.11 and basc.org.uk for further details).

Species	England, Wales and Scotland	Northern Ireland
Common pheasant (*Phasianus colchicus*)	Oct 1–Feb 1	Oct 1–Jan 31
Grey partridge (*Perdix perdix*)	Sep 1–Feb 1	Sep 1–Jan 31
Red-legged partridge (*Alectoris rufa*)	Sep 1–Feb 1	Sep 1–Jan 31
Red grouse (*Lagopus lagopus*)	Aug 12–Dec 10	Aug 12–Nov 30
Black grouse (*Tetrao tetrix*)	Aug 20–Dec 10	Species not present
Ptarmigan (*Lagopus mutus*) (Scotland only)	Aug 12–Dec 10	Species not present
Capercaillie (*Tetrao urogallus*)	Oct 1–January 31	Species not present
Common quail (*Coturnix coturnix*)	Protected at all times	Species not present

27.11 Shooting seasons for gamebirds in the UK. See basc.org.uk for full details.

References and further reading

Beer JV (1988) *Diseases of Gamebirds and Wildfowl*. Game Conservancy, Fordingbridge

Butcher GD (2006) Management of Galliformes. In: *Clinical Avian Medicine, Volume II*, ed. GJ Harrison and TL Lightfoot, pp. 861–878. Spix Publishing, Florida

Carpenter J (2013) *Exotic Animal Formulary, 4th edn*. Elsevier Saunders, Missouri

Coles BH (2009) Galliformes. In: *Handbook of Avian Medicine, 2nd edn*, ed. TN Tully *et al.*, pp. 309–334. Saunders, Oxford

Curtis P (1987) *A Handbook of Poultry and Gamebird Diseases*. Liverpool University Press, Liverpool

Ramsey I (2014) *BSAVA Small Animal Formulary, 8th edn*. BSAVA Publications, Gloucester

Whitehead ML and Roberts V (2014) Backyard poultry: Legislation, zoonoses and disease prevention. *Journal of Small Animal Practice* **55(10)**, 487–496

Specialist organizations and useful contacts

See also Appendix 1

British Association for Shooting and Conservation (BASC)
www.basc.org.uk

British Veterinary Poultry Association
www.bvpa.org.uk

Game and Wildlife Conservation Trust
www.gwct.org.uk

World Pheasant Association
www.pheasant.org.uk

Chapter 28

Pigeons and doves

John Chitty

With the exception of the turtle dove (*Streptopelia turtur*; a summer visitor to southern England and the Midlands) and the rock dove (*Columba livia*; confined to Ireland and Scotland) (Figure 28.1a), pigeons and doves, including stock doves (*Columba oenas*) (Figure 28.1b), wood pigeons (*Columba palumbus*) (Figure 28.1c), and collared doves (*Streptopelia decaocto*) (Figure 28.1d) can be found year-round throughout the British Isles, except in the Scottish mountains. They are the most common avian species presented to rehabilitators, either as injured birds or as 'orphaned' young. British Wildlife Rehabilitation Council (BWRC) wildlife casualty recording scheme figures for 1993–1997 show that 14% of all bird casualties were feral and racing pigeons and 9% were wood pigeons (Best, 1999).

Ecology and biology

The ecology and biology of the different species are summarized in Figures 28.1 and 28.2.

The sexes are essentially alike in all species (though some male feral or show pigeons may show a hypertrophy of the cere). Breeding occurs almost year-round; nests are made off the ground (Figure 28.3) and the young are altricial. Young birds are covered in coarse tufts of yellow down; they have fleshy beaks, often with a tiny hook on the upper part, and are therefore often presented as 'raptors'. Very young birds (up to 4 weeks of age, still covered in down) are referred to as 'squabs'; slightly older birds (until fledging) are 'squeakers' (Figure 28.4).

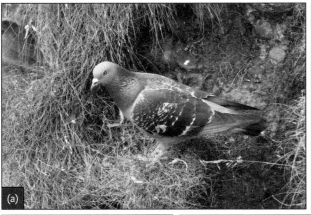

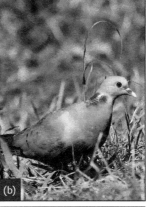

28.1 (a) Rock dove. (b) Stock dove. (c) Wood pigeon. (d) Collared dove.
(© Andrew Kelly)

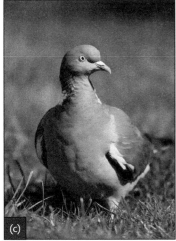

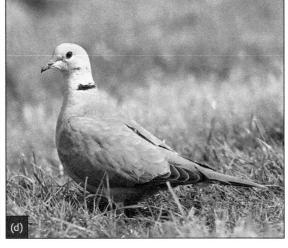

Species	Characteristics	Weight	UK distribution	Habitat	Diet
Rock dove (*Columba livia*) (see Figure 28.1a)	Ancestor of ubiquitous 'feral pigeon' (latter essentially grey but wide range of markings due to intermixing with racing and show pigeons)	250–500 g	Pure in northern Scotland, Scottish Isles and Ireland	Rocky coastal areas Feral pigeon mainly urban areas	Seeds, leaves
Stock dove (*Columba oenas*) (see Figure 28.1b)	Same size as rock dove Lacks white rump of rock dove and has shorter wings Less obvious dark bars on wings	250–450 g	Throughout, except northern Scotland	Widespread, especially farmland, woodland edges	Seeds, leaves
Wood pigeon (*Columba palumbus*) (see Figure 28.1c)	Larger than rock dove Distinctive white patches on wings and dorsal neck	450–700 g	Throughout	Widespread, especially farmland, woodland edges	Seeds, leaves
Collared dove (*Streptopelia decaocto*) (see Figure 28.1d)	Smaller than rock dove Pale grey with distinct black 'collar' on dorsal neck	150–200 g	Throughout	Mainly suburban	Seeds, leaves
Turtle dove (*Streptopelia turtur*)	Chestnut upper parts, pink breast, black and white neck patch	150–180 g	Summer migrant to southern and eastern England, less common now	Woodland edges, thick hedges	Seeds, leaves

28.2 Ecology and biology of pigeons and doves.

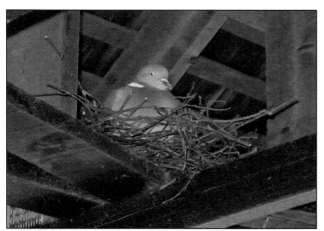

28.3 Wood pigeon on a nest. Pigeons are confident and often nest in close proximity to, or in, human houses.
(© John Chitty)

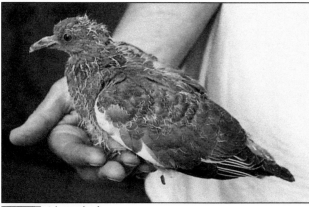

28.4 A 'squeaker'.
(© John Chitty)

Anatomy and physiology

All species are granivorous. The crop is large, for food storage, and is also adapted (in both sexes) to produce 'crop milk' for feeding squabs, when the lining will hypertrophy. The gizzard is large and well developed. In mature male rock doves the cere may show extensive hypertrophy to give white 'crusty' growths.

Capture, handling and transportation

Capture is most easily accomplished by using a net. If no net is available, birds may be cornered and enveloped with a towel or simply picked up.

Pigeons and doves pose no physical risk to handlers, although the risk of zoonosis (see 'Zoonotic risks') means that before the health status of an individual bird is determined, it is sensible to take precautions against zoonotic disease. This should include excellent personal hygiene with cleaning and disinfection of hands, tables and materials between patients. Protective gloves may be worn but are not a substitute for hygiene and disinfection. The smaller species may be held easily in one hand, with the keel in the palm and the head towards the handler's body. The bird's feet, tail and wing tips are held between the fingers of the same hand for restraint. This is known as the 'pigeon fancier's grip'. (Figure 28.5). Wood pigeons may flap vigorously and are loose-feathered; they should be towel-wrapped or held in two hands to avoid excessive feather loss.

Any pet carrier or cardboard box with non-slip flooring will suffice for transportation but should be darkened in order to calm the bird. Specialist cardboard carriers as used by racing pigeon owners are also available.

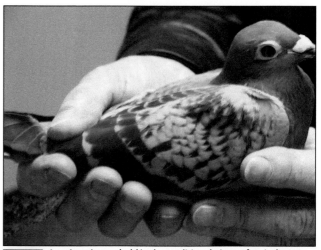

28.5 A racing pigeon, held in the traditional pigeon fancier's method.
(© John Chitty)

Zoonotic risks

Pigeons and doves can pose a considerable health risk to humans. The main zoonotic dangers are salmonellosis and chlamydiosis. Many healthy birds are asymptomatic carriers and will excrete these organisms; the stress of illness and captivity may increase this excretion rate. Campylobacteriosis may also be a risk.

Certainly any bird with loose droppings, neurological signs, crop stasis or swollen joints must be regarded as a high risk for salmonellosis. Clinical chlamydiosis must be suspected in birds that are fluffed up or have loose droppings or any upper respiratory signs, in which case the risk to handlers is sufficiently high that it may be advisable to euthanase such birds.

Gloves should be worn and strict personal hygiene should be followed when handling pigeons. When working with these birds, in particular when cleaning out, handlers should wear disposable waterproof gloves, a facemask and goggles, as chlamydiosis may be contracted via the conjunctivae or via inhalation. Droppings can be dampened with a suitable disinfectant spray prior to cleaning out the cage to reduce the risk of inhalation.

Examination and clinical assessment for rehabilitation

The general principles of examination and assessment are as detailed in Chapter 4. Particular attention should be paid to the droppings, vent and body condition. Neurological disorders are common and the bird's demeanour, head position, posture, gait and reflexes should be carefully observed.

The mouth and pharynx should be thoroughly examined for the characteristic white plaques typical of trichomonosis ('canker') (Figure 28.6). Crop infections are common, especially in young birds, and a foul smell from the mouth may be an early sign. The crop itself should be examined for excessive size, thickening (though this may be normal in parent birds, see 'Anatomy and physiology'), inability to empty and wounds. The legs and wings should be thoroughly palpated for swellings or fractures. Foot injuries and digit constriction are common in feral pigeons associated with entanglement of debris (see Figure 28.9).

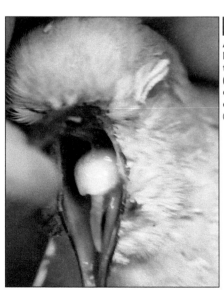

28.6
Advanced caseous lesions of trichomonosis ('canker') in the exposed pharynx of a collared dove.
(© John Chitty)

Diagnostic techniques

Diagnostic techniques appropriate to other avian species can be used in pigeons and doves; however, there are some special considerations.

Blood sampling

Pigeons and doves do not have a jugular vein as such, instead possessing a venous plexus that is not accessible for venepuncture. This is further complicated by the lack of an apterium over the right side of the neck. The ulnar or medial metatarsal veins are therefore used for venepuncture (Figure 28.7). Access to these veins is similar to that of other avian species; however, they are small and fragile so excess negative pressure should not be applied when collecting blood. Haemostasis can be difficult after taking blood from these veins. Placing the bird in a dark box afterwards will assist in calming it and consequently lowering blood pressure. If bleeding still persists after applying pressure, tissue glue may be placed over the venepuncture site.

Crop wash

Upper alimentary parasites are common in pigeons and doves, with *Trichomonas* spp. being particularly common even in asymptomatic individuals. Crop washing can be a useful diagnostic technique. A crop tube is placed in the normal manner (see Chapter 5) and 5 ml warmed saline instilled into the crop. This is aspirated and reinserted several times in order to obtain a small concentrated sample.

The aspirated fluid should be examined immediately as a wet preparation (see Chapter 10) in order to identify motile protozoa. Air-dried smears may be stained with trichrome stains to assess for the presence of bacteria or yeasts.

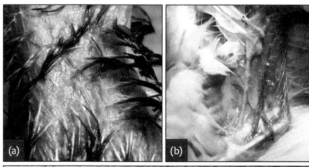

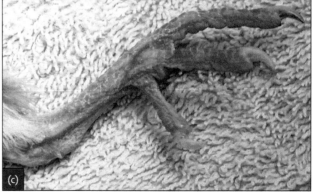

28.7 Intravenous and blood collection sites in the pigeon. (a) Even in this sparsely feathered juvenile, the thickness of the skin hinders finding the jugular venous plexus despite wetting the skin on the ventral side of the neck. (b) Ventral view of the wing (elbow to the right) showing the ulnar vein. (c) Medial view of the leg and foot showing the medial metatarsal vein.
(© John Chitty)

Euthanasia

Pigeons and doves are strong fliers, with a reliance on flight to escape and to reach nesting and roosting sites; they should not be released if flight is impaired. Repair of open, chronic or complicated wing fractures is unlikely to be fully successful and so euthanasia should be considered in these cases. Birds will also frequently present with septic arthritis (often caused by *Salmonella* spp.); this may resolve with systemic antibiosis, but treatment may be inadvisable as some arthritis and loss of joint mobility will remain. There are also zoonotic implications associated with treating these cases and carrier status may occur.

Infectious disease is a major consideration. Clinical signs associated with the major zoonotic diseases should preclude admission and treatment. There are also several diseases (especially paramyxovirus and poxvirus) that may be highly infectious to other birds. Signs suggestive of these infections should be a reason for euthanasia. Although mild canker is simple to treat, advanced cases with extensive crop lesions should be euthanased as therapy is less successful and the organism is highly contagious.

Euthanasia technique is as for gamebirds (see Chapter 27). Pigeons do not possess an accessible jugular vein so the ulnar or medial metatarsal veins are normally used by the author.

First aid and short-term hospitalization

The general principles of first aid, as detailed in Chapter 5, apply to pigeon and dove casualties. It is important to remember that some of the casualties presented will be 'tired' racers. These may be identified by the racing ring on the leg and the owner traced either via the Royal Pigeon Racing Association (RPRA) (see 'Specialist organizations and useful contacts') and ring number, or via the address, which some owners stamp on the primary feathers. The owner should always be contacted before embarking on intensive therapy for these birds. Where the bird is simply 'tired' (weak, slightly thin, possibly dehydrated) then it should be warmed, given subcutaneous fluids and tube fed fluids (e.g. Vetark® Critical Care Formula) in addition to being provided with food and water.

It is important to emphasize the role of fluids, analgesia and the early use of broad-spectrum antibiosis (see Figure 28.16), where indicated. Amoxicillin is often appropriate but many birds will be presented following cat attacks. These wounds quickly lead to septicaemia, and antibiotics with a good spectrum of activity against anaerobes and Gram-negative organisms should be given as soon as possible (e.g. amoxicillin/clavulanate (co-amoxiclav), piperacillin (see Figure 28.16). See also Chapter 30 for further details on the treatment of cat bite injuries.

Short-term hospitalization

For short-term hospitalization a cat kennel is adequate. The kennel should be placed as high as possible (to increase the bird's feeling of security) in a warm quiet place away from cats, dogs, raptors and people. Strict biosecurity should be maintained and initially the casualty should not be kept in the same airspace as other birds. Newspaper makes ideal flooring and perches should be provided – either sterilizable plastic perches or disposable wooden ones.

Anaesthesia and analgesia

The general principles of anaesthesia and analgesia, as detailed in Chapters 5 and 6, apply to pigeon and dove casualties. Analgesic drugs are given in Figures 5.15 and 28.16. Endotracheal tubes should be used with caution, as very narrow gauges (<2.5 mm) are required. These may easily become blocked with mucus.

Specific conditions

For a full discussion of pigeon and dove diseases see Chitty and Lierz (2008).

Trauma
Fracture repair

The assessment of fractures in these species is as for other birds (see Figures 4.4 and 28.8). The general principles of fracture repair, as detailed in Chapters 5 and 29, apply to pigeon and dove casualties (Figure 28.8). In addition to the usual considerations given to avian fractures, the number of fractures appears important in determining prognosis in pigeons (Cousins *et al.*, 2012). Kirschner wires and hypodermic needles make good intramedullary pins. Commercially available shuttle pins are also useful in pigeons and doves.

Granulating wounds

These are commonly seen as a sequel to trauma, shot gun injuries or raptor strike (wounds usually occur on the dorsum with the latter). Debridement and primary closure is often impossible. Even with extensive wounds, good results can be achieved with daily cleaning (e.g. dilute chlorhexidine) and application of a hydrocolloid gel (e.g. Intrasite® gel). Systemic antibiosis should be provided (typically amoxicillin/clavulanate) until the granulation bed is established, and analgesia provided as required (see also Chapter 5).

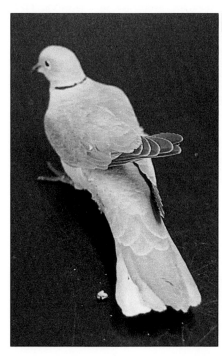

28.8 Adult collared dove with a left shoulder injury. Note the typically 'tilted' wing tip held above the normal right wing tip.
(© John Chitty)

Ruptured crop

This condition, rarely seen in other birds, probably occurs in pigeons and doves because the crop is often very full and so may be more likely to rupture when traumatized. The birds are usually presented with a necrotic granulating wound forming a crop fistula. Even if the wound is fresh, it is important not to operate at once as the bruised crop wall margins will necrose, resulting in wound breakdown. It is recommended that the bird should be stabilized for 2–3 days first; this involves broad-spectrum antibiosis, analgesics and proventricular gavage (via the crop wound into the proventriculus). The crop wall and skin are debrided and repaired in two layers using simple continuous sutures with an absorbable suture material (e.g. Vicryl® or Monocryl®) This author will typically use 2 metric (3/0 USP) Vicryl®.

Line entanglement injuries

Entanglement with plastic line (fishing or garden) is frequently seen, with legs and toes commonly affected (Figure 28.9). Generally birds present with chronic problems as they become lame or develop secondary pododermatitis. As a result the line is more difficult to remove with extensive granulation. The tissue distal to the line entanglement may not be viable. General anaesthesia is almost invariably required and line is carefully dissected from the site using scissors and fine forceps.

After removal underlying and distal tissues are assessed for viability.

- If all tissues are felt to be viable, birds are placed on a 5–10 day course of amoxicillin/clavulanate (125 mg/kg orally q12h) and a 3-day course of non-steriodal anti-inflammatory drugs (generally meloxicam at 0.2 mg/kg orally q12h) as well as daily cleaning and application of a hydrophilic gel. Prognosis is usually very good in the author's experience.
- If one or two toes are felt not to be viable these may be amputated using standard techniques. A 5-day course of amoxicillin/clavulanate is given. Prognosis is usually very good in the author's experience.
- If three or more toes or the entire distal leg are felt not to be viable, then amputation is not an option. The bird should be euthanased.

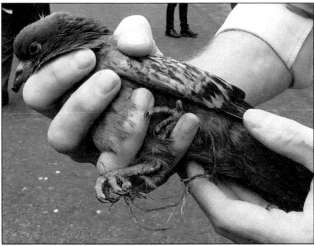

28.9 Line entanglement is commonly seen. This bird had string wrapped around the digits, which was removed to free the foot.
(© Colin Gambles)

Pododermatitis ('bumblefoot')

Pododermatitis (Figure 28.10) is less common in pigeons and doves than in other bird species. Bilateral cases are occasionally seen, in which case careful attention should be paid to perch construction (providing padded perches of varying diameter), as well as assessment of underlying limb deformities (especially nutritional secondary hyperparathyroidism) as this will result in altered perching angle. Unilateral cases are far more common and generally occur because of altered or loss of use in the contralateral limb. In these cases, prognosis is very dependent on the ease of management of the primary problem. Treatment is similar to that in poultry or waterfowl:

- Assessment (including radiography of severe cases to assess underlying bone involvement) and correction of underlying factors
- Antimicrobials – ideally these should be based on culture from deep lesional swabs. In early stage bumblefoot, skin swabs may be used. As a 'first-line' antibiotic this author will use amoxicillin/clavulanate (see Figure 28.16)
- Padded perches
- Topical therapies – bandaging is rarely practicable, so daily cleaning of the lesion and application of an antimicrobial barrier cream is utilized
- Surgery – owing to the size and shape of the foot, surgery is rarely possible. Where it is used, technique is similar to that employed for raptors
- Euthanasia – this is indicated for cases where underlying issues cannot be resolved or where infection is deep enough to result in osteomyelitis and/or tendonitis.

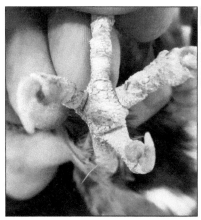

28.10 Pododermatitis ('bumblefoot') is less common in pigeons and doves than in other bird species, but may still be seen in feral pigeons.
(© Emma Keeble)

Infectious diseases

Viral diseases

Paramyxovirus (Newcastle disease): Newcastle disease is a **notifiable disease** and, as such, the local Divisional Veterinary Manager (Animal and Plant health Agency (APHA), see Appendix 1) should be notified on suspicion of the disease. It is caused by infection with paramyxovirus-1 (PMV-1), which results in a number of clinical signs including failure to prehend grain, head tremor, torticollis (Figure 28.11), polydipsia and polyuria, diarrhoea and laying of deformed eggs. Rarely, upper respiratory tract disease may be seen. With supportive treatment, affected birds can recover in 3 to 8 weeks; treatment is not recommended, however, as the disease can spread rapidly through the rehabilitation unit and affect many avian species. Birds may be carriers of the virus.

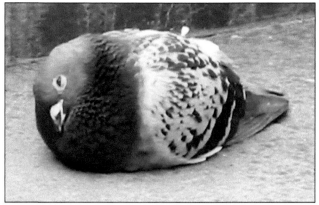

28.11 Feral pigeon showing torticollis due to PMV-1 infection.
(© John Chitty)

Pigeon pox: Pigeon pox is caused by poxvirus infection. Infection results in the appearance of multiple masses around the head (Figure 28.12a), limbs and sometimes the alimentary tract (Figure 28.12b). Upper respiratory tract infection may also be seen. Lesions may resolve in a few weeks and recovered birds have strong immunity. In severe disease where there are multiple lesions, affected birds may need to be euthanased on welfare grounds. Pigeon pox is highly contagious, so barrier nursing of suspect cases is advised.

Upper respiratory tract infection: A number of viruses may cause upper respiratory tract disease, including herpesvirus, poxvirus and, rarely, PMV-1. For further details, see 'Bacterial diseases'.

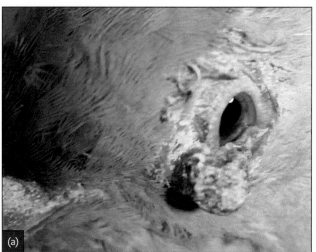

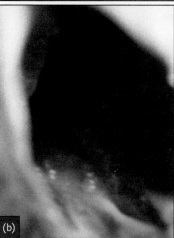

28.12 (a) Periocular and (b) oropharyngeal lesions due to pigeon poxvirus.
(© John Chitty)

Bacterial diseases

Upper respiratory tract infection: Upper respiratory tract infection ('coryza', 'one-eyed cold') may result from various bacterial infections, including chlamydiosis, mycoplasmosis, staphylococcosis, streptococcosis and pasteurellosis. Viruses (see 'Viral diseases'), trichomonosis (see 'Trichomonosis') and dust irritation or foreign bodies may cause similar clinical signs. Affected birds may have swollen sinuses unilaterally or bilaterally, and an ocular and nasal discharge. In view of the range of causative organisms, an accurate diagnosis, by means of bacteriology, cytology and serology, is required to allow appropriate treatment. Several of these organisms are zoonotic, whilst others are highly contagious to other birds, so affected columbids should be admitted and treated with great caution. Environmental factors play an important role in the transmission of respiratory disease; thus bird rooms should be well ventilated and young and older birds should not share the same airspace. Newly admitted birds should be quarantined for at least 10 days before being allowed to enter the rehabilitation unit where other birds are present.

Joint swelling: Infection with *Salmonella* spp. and *Escherichia coli* are commonly implicated in birds that present with polyarthritis. The presence of a single swollen joint can be due to trauma but may also be due to infection. Diagnosis is by culture of the causative organism from the synovial fluid. Treatment is with appropriate antibiosis, preferably based on sensitivity results; it should not be attempted if many joints are affected or if affected joints are thought unlikely to return to full function.

Parasites

Ectoparasites: Ectoparasites are rarely a problem, with the exception of ticks (Figure 28.13) which should be manually removed using a hook. This author treats tick reactions using a single dose of long-acting amoxicillin and dexamethasone (short-acting preparation) (see Figure 28.16).

Lice (Figure 28.14) are rarely if ever pathogenic though excessive numbers may indicate debility.

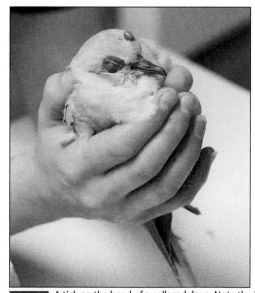

28.13 A tick on the head of a collared dove. Note the intense reaction on the head and around the right eye. Death may result unless broad-spectrum antibiosis (e.g. long-acting amoxicillin or oxytetracycline) and short-acting corticosteroids are given promptly.
(© John Chitty)

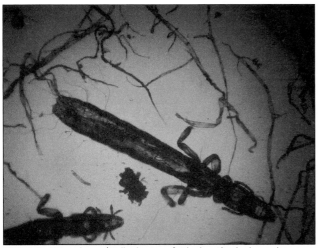

28.14 Pigeon louse (*Mallophaga* spp). The long body shape shows this species lives on flight feathers. (Magnification X100)
(© John Chitty)

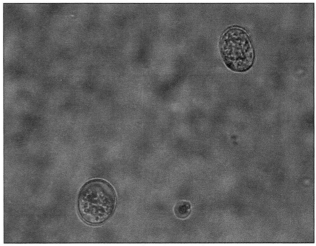

28.15 Coccidial oocysts in a faecal sample from a pigeon. (Magnification X400)
(© John Chitty)

Endoparasites:

Nematodes: Infestation with Capillariidae and ascarids is common in pigeons and doves. In severe cases, there may be weight loss and mucoid diarrhoea; migration of ascarid larvae through the liver may cause sudden death. Diagnosis is by demonstration of ova in faecal samples. Infestation can be treated with fenbendazole and it is advisable to deworm all birds on admission to the rehabilitation unit.

Trichomonosis: Trichomonosis ('canker') is caused by infection with *Trichomonas* spp., which gives rise to white caseous lesions in the mouth, pharynx and crop (see Figure 28.6). Trichomonosis is also a rare cause of upper respiratory tract infection. Fresh wet preparations of the caseous material reveal the presence of motile flagellates, which differentiates trichomonosis from candidiasis and bacterial infections. If lesions are not too extensive, treatment with metronidazole or carnidazole is generally effective, but these drugs should not be used in birds that could enter the human food chain (see Chapter 27). Many birds are asymptomatic carriers and the causative organism is highly contagious; thus some recommend treating all birds with a single dose of carnidazole on admission to the rehabilitation unit. Clinical cases should be barrier nursed.

Coccidiosis: Various coccidial species can cause wasting and, particularly in younger birds, diarrhoea. Many adults carry a few organisms with no clinical manifestations. Diagnosis is by demonstration of oocysts in faecal samples (Figure 28.15). Coccidiosis can be treated with toltrazuril (20–35 mg/kg once by mouth), clazuril (5–10 mg/bird once), amprolium (28 ml of concentrate in 4.5 l drinking water for 7 days – in severe outbreaks continue for another 7 days at half this concentration) or sulfadimethoxine (1 g/l drinking water for 2 days; then 3 days off and 2 days on; see Figure 28.16); it can be prevented by good husbandry, including good hygiene and not mixing adults and young birds.

Other conditions

Nutritional secondary hyperparathyroidism

This has been reported in both hand-reared (see 'Rearing of young pigeons and doves') and wild parent-reared squabs where it seems extremely common (Cousquer *et al.*, 2007). This study showed lesions to be unusual in adults, but very common in juveniles (51.2%). This indicates that lesions may well be detrimental to survivability of young and also that young birds should be very carefully assessed for bone deformities regardless of reason for admission to a rehabilitation unit. A thorough clinical examination may detect bone deformities; however, radiography is generally required for an accurate diagnosis and to assess the extent of any lesions. Cousquer *et al.* (2007) suggested that, as lesions were especially common in winter months, lack of exposure to ultraviolet light is a likely cause. However, it is also possible that increased access to poor quality nutrition at bird tables may be a factor during this period. Therefore, as well as providing good quality full-spectrum ultraviolet light these birds should be given a balanced diet and a Vitamin D3/calcium supplement (e.g. Nutrobal®). If deformities are too severe or extensive then euthanasia is indicated.

Therapeutics

The general principles of therapeutics, as detailed in Chapter 7, apply to pigeon and dove casualties. Dose rates of common therapeutic drugs used in pigeons and doves are given in Figure 28.16. If likely to enter the human food chain drug withdrawal periods must be observed and only those drugs permitted for use in food-producing animals must be administered (see Chapter 27).

Drug	Dosage
Antibacterials	
Tylosin	25 mg/kg i.m. q6h 800 mg/l drinking water[a]
Amoxicillin LA	150 mg/kg i.m., one-off dose[b]
Amoxicillin/clavulanate (co-amoxiclav)	125 mg/kg orally q12h[a]
Doxycycline	25–50 mg/kg orally q12–24h[a] 200–500 mg/l water (soft water only)[a]
Piperacillin	100 mg/kg i.m. q8–12h[a]
Anti-protozoal treatment	
Carnidazole	12.5–25 mg orally, one-off treatment[a]
Metronidazole	50 mg/kg orally q24h for 5 days

28.16 Dose rates of common drugs used in pigeons and doves. (continues) ▶

([a] Carpenter, 2013; [b] Meredith, 2015; [c] Author's experience)

Drug	Dosage
Coccidiostats	
Toltrazuril	20–35 mg/kg once by mouth
Clazuril	5–10 mg/bird once
Amprolium	28 ml of concentrate in 4.5 l drinking water for 7 days – in severe outbreaks continue for another 7 days at half this concentration
Sulfadimethoxine	1 g/l drinking water for 2 days; then 3 days off and 2 days on
Anthelmintics	
Fenbendazole	16 mg/kg orally once (repeat after 2 weeks if necessary)
Analgesics	
Meloxicam	0.2 mg/kg orally q12h[a]
Steroids	
Dexamethasone	2–6 mg/kg i.m. once (Dexadreson, MSD)[c]

28.16 (continued) Dose rates of common drugs used in pigeons and doves.

([a] Carpenter, 2013; [b] Meredith, 2015; [c] Author's experience)

Management in captivity

Long-term patients may be kept in a small aviary. Feeding is simple: mixed grain rations for pigeons/wild birds are available in small quantities from pet stores and agricultural merchants. These will suffice in the short to medium term for all weaned birds. For long-term patients a poultry pellet may provide a more complete ration. Grit may also be provided. Water should be provided at all times. Perches can be made using tree branches so tapering widths are available. Exposure to ultraviolet light is recommended, especially by allowing access to unfiltered natural sunlight.

Rearing of young pigeons and doves

Young 'abandoned' birds are often presented (see also Chapter 8). Many of these will be at the squeaker stage (fully developed but with a few tufts of down) and can be reared on chick crumb with a little grain.

Younger birds require a crop milk substitute, which may be fed as soft food pellets placed into the mouth or as crop-tubed paste. There are several options and as crop milk is semi-solid each recipe should be made up as a paste:

- Chick crumb soaked in water
- Baby cereal (e.g. Milupa®), made with boiling water and allowed to cool
- One hard-boiled egg yolk, plus three tablespoons each of mixed baby cereal, oatmeal and cornmeal. Mix with milk to a stiff consistency then leave to stand until the mix becomes stiff enough to roll into pellets (Hickman and Guy, 1994)
- Commercial bird hand-rearing diet (Exact® Hand Feeding Formula; Harrison's Bird Foods®; Juvenile Hand-Feeding Formula™, Instant Nutri-start® Baby Bird Formula).

Alternatively:

- One jar chicken and gravy human baby food, one tablespoon plain low fat yoghurt, 1 ml corn oil, one-eighth teaspoon avian multivitamin and 100–150 g elemental calcium (e.g. 250–375 mg calcium carbonate)
- From the fourth day start reducing the baby food and replacing with Exact® feeding formula
- From the seventh day start adding two tablespoons strained mixed vegetable human baby food
- Feed at 1 ml/10 g bodyweight and feed as crop empties
- When weight has increased to 70–80 g, provide corn, grain and grit to allow weaning (Kudlacik and Eilertsen, 2007).

As it is not uncommon to see rickets in hand-reared squabs, the addition of a calcium/vitamin D3 supplement (e.g. Nutrobal®) to these feeds is recommended. Birds should be fed until the crop is full, then fed again on demand.

Release

Adults

These birds may be released wherever the local area will support them. Often rehabilitators will have a flock of released birds around their premises, which requires understanding neighbours. It is important not to let the situation get out of hand, as control of infectious disease in a large feral flock is impossible.

Young birds

The release of hand-reared birds may be a problem. They often refuse to leave 'home' and will return even if released far away. This is especially true of the rock dove. Stocker (2005) recommended releasing birds on sea cliffs more than 200 km from the rescue centre. It is important not to malprint young birds during rearing, as this will worsen the problem.

Rehoming racing or fancy pigeons

Racing pigeons are often found and presented to veterinary practices or rehabilitators. After the bird has been stabilized, its owner should be contacted as soon as possible. Racing birds are identified by means of a numbered leg band, which should enable the RPRA (see 'Specialist organizations and useful contacts') to provide owner contact details. The information is also sometimes stamped on the primary feathers. Lost fancy pigeons should be reported to the National Pigeon Association (see 'Specialist organizations and useful contacts'; these birds have leg ring numbers prefixed 'NPA').

Legal aspects

Rock, stock and turtle doves are protected at all times (Wildlife and Countryside Act (1981)). Wood pigeons and collared doves may be taken under the terms of a General Licence all year round. All species are regarded as indigenous and so may be held and re-released after treatment (see Chapter 2). Racing pigeons and fancy doves have owners, and both veterinary surgeons (veterinarians) and rehabilitators should be cautious about treatment and euthanasia without contacting the registered owner (see 'First aid and short-term hospitalization').

References and further reading

Best D (1999) BWRC wildlife casualty recording scheme – the first five years. *The Rehabilitator* **28**, 2–3

Carpenter J (2013) *Exotic Animal Formulary, 4th edn*. Elsevier Saunders, Missouri

Chitty JR and Lierz M (2008) *BSAVA Manual of Raptors, Pigeons and Passerine Birds*. BSAVA Publications, Gloucester

Cousins RA, Battley PF, Gartrell BD *et al.* (2012) Impact injuries and probability of survival in a large semiurban endemic pigeon in New Zealand, *Hemiphaga novaeseelandiae. Journal of Wildlife Diseases* **48**, 567–574

Cousquer G, Dankoski E and Patterson-Kane J (2007) Metabolic bone disease in wild collared doves (*Streptopelia decaocto*). *Veterinary Record* **160(3)**, 78–84

Hickman M and Guy M (1994) *Care of the Wild, Feathered and Furred*. Robson Books, London

Kudlacik M and Eilertson N (2007) Pigeons and Doves. In: *Hand-rearing Birds*, ed. LJ Gage and RS Duerr. Blackwell, Ames, Iowa

Stocker L (2005) *Practical Wildlife Care, 2nd edn*. Blackwell Science, Oxford

Meredith A (2015) *BSAVA Small Animal Formulary, 9th edn Part B Exotic Pets*. BSAVA Publications, Gloucester

Specialist organizations and useful contacts

See also Appendix 1

Royal Pigeon Racing Association (RPRA)
The Reddings, Cheltenham, Gloucestershire GL51 6RN
Tel: 01452 713529
www.rpra.org

National Pigeon Association (NPA)
www.nationalpigeonassociation.co.uk

Chapter 29

Raptors

Neil Forbes

Birds of prey (raptors) include day-flying (diurnal) hawks, falcons and eagles, as well as night-flying (generally nocturnal) owls (Figures 29.1 and 29.2). This chapter will only refer to species indigenous to the British Isles.

Ecology and biology

Figures 29.3 to 29.6 give taxonomic, biological, identification and ecological data for the 12 most commonly encountered British raptors.

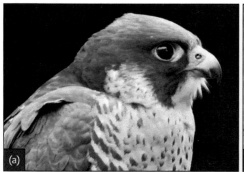
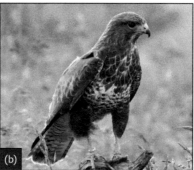
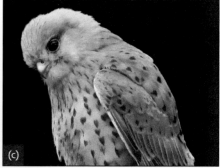
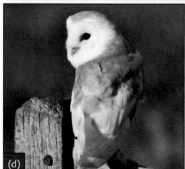
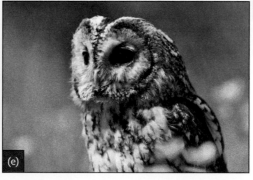

29.1 Common UK species of raptors. (a) Peregrine falcon (*Falco peregrinus*). (b) Common buzzard (*Buteo buteo*). (c) Kestrel (*Falco tinnunculus*). (d) Barn owl (*Tyto alba*). (e) Tawny owl (*Strix aluco*).

Order	Behaviour	Diet	Sexual dimorphism	Chicks	Beak and claws	Caeca and crop	Perching
Falconiformes and Accipitriformes (diurnal falcons, eagles, harriers, kites and hawks)	Active searchers and hunters; catch prey of varying size, in flight or on the ground; some eat carrion; spend much time perching or in flight	Carnivorous	30% reverse (i.e. female is typically 30% larger than male)	Altricial (few feathers at hatch and require considerable parental care)	Hooked beak and talons for catching, holding and eating prey	Vestigial caeca, considerable crop	Anisodactyl: perch with digit 1 backwards and digits 2, 3, 4 forward (see Figure 30.4)
Strigiformes (owls)	Principally nocturnal (except little owl (*Athene noctua*) – diurnal); spend much time perching or in 'silent flight'	Carnivorous	Slight or absent	Altricial	Hooked beak and talons for catching, holding and eating prey	Large caeca, no crop	Semi-zygodactyl: will perch with digits 2, 3 forward and 1, 4 backwards, but also with 1 backwards and 2, 3, 4 forward (see Figure 30.4)

29.2 Orders of common British raptors and their general characteristics.

BSAVA Manual of Wildlife Casualties, second edition. Edited by Elizabeth Mullineaux and Emma Keeble. ©BSAVA 2016

Species	Length	Wingspan	Bodyweight m = male; f = female	Iris colour	Identification	Behaviour
Falconidae (falcons)						
Common kestrel (*Falco tinnunculus*) (see Figure 29.1c) Indigenous in the UK	31–39 cm	68–82 cm	136–252 g (m) 154–314 g (f)	Dark	Medium-sized with long pointed wings and tail Adult male blue-grey upper tail and head, brown upper back, black wing tip Adult female, tail and upper back barred brown Juvenile similar to adult female but generally yellower	Frequently seen hovering over permanent grassland
Peregrine (*Falco peregrinus*) (see Figure 29.1a) Indigenous in the UK	34–58 (x=42) cm	74–120 cm	424–750 g (m) 910–1500 g (f) Marked sexual reverse dimorphism: female 30% larger	Dark	Larger falcons with long pointed wings and short tail Adult birds of both sexes have slate-grey back, head (with dark moustache) and tail, white to rusty underparts with clear horizontal bars Cere, legs and feet are yellow Juveniles have brown upper parts and buff under parts, with brown vertical bars	Very agile flier, stoop at great speed and catch birds in flight Seen in town centres and rural areas
Merlin (*Falco columbarius*) Indigenous in the UK	24–33 cm	50–73 cm	125–210 g (m) (x=165 g) 190–300 g (f) (x=230 g) Marked sexual dimorphism	Dark	Small falcon, long pointed wings, short tail Adult male slate blue-grey head, back and upper wings, buff streaked underparts Female and juvenile brown back and head and buff streaked underparts	Very agile flier, seen most commonly on open hills and marshy moors, catches small birds and insects in flight
Hobby (*Falco subbuteo*) Indigenous but migratory (South Africa, October–March)	28–36 cm	69–84 cm	131–232 g (m) 141–340 g (f)	Dark	Very small falcon with long pointed wings Characteristic red thighs and obvious dark brown moustache	Very agile flier, taking insects and small birds in flight, often over water
Accipitridae (hawks, broadwings, eagles)						
Eurasian sparrowhawk (*Accipiter nisus*) Indigenous to the UK	Male 29–34 cm Female 35–41 cm	Male 58–65 cm Female 67–80 cm	110–196 g (m) 185–342 g (f)	Yellow	Small with small blunt-tipped wings, long tail (always longer than width of wing) with 4–5 bars, small beak, slender body, very fine legs Adult male has slate grey upper parts, rufous cheeks, barring on chest Adult female is significantly bigger with slate grey upper parts, barring below is brown-grey Juvenile has dark brown upper parts, coarse barring of underparts is broken up and irregular	Flies fast at lower level, often seen flying down lanes, through woods, or ambushing bird tables
Common buzzard (*Buteo buteo*) (see Figure 29.1b) Indigenous to the UK	46–58 cm	113–128 cm	525–1183 g (m) 625–1364 g (f) Both sexes heavier in winter, losing 20% bodyweight in breeding season	Juvenile iris colour slightly lighter than adult	Medium-sized, broad-winged, tail medium length (shorter than width of wing) Plumage very variable, from very dark to very light, buff breast with variable streaking, all show pale band over lower breast Adult has dark terminal tail band; chest obviously barred Juvenile has chest streaks with tendency to vague bars; tail slightly longer than in adult	Often seen soaring with open wings, or still, hunting on telegraph or fence post

29.3 Biology, taxonomy and identification of common UK diurnal birds of prey. (x=mean). Other species include: golden eagle (*Aquila chrysaetos*) (resident small population, predominantly in Scotland); white-tailed sea eagle (*Haliaeetus albicilla*) (went extinct in early twentieth century, re-introduced into Skye (1975 and onwards) and Western Isles); hen harrier (*Circus cyaneus*) (resident in the UK, most heavily predated species due to conflict with game shooting interests); marsh harrier (*Circus aeruginosus*) (summer migrant visitor March–September in low numbers, breed and hunt over marsh land and reed beds); Montagu's harrier (*Circus pygargus*)(rare summer migrant visitor found in Norfolk, Dorset, Hampshire and Oxford); honey buzzard (*Pernis apivorus*) (rare summer, May–September, migrant visitor). (continues)

Species	Length	Wingspan	Bodyweight m = male; f = female	Iris colour	Identification	Behaviour
Accipitridae (hawks, broadwings, eagles) (continued)						
Red kite (*Milvus milvus*) Indigenous to the UK, previously extinct but successfully reintroduced and now common	60–70 cm	175–179 cm	800–1200 g (m) 1000–1300 g (f)	Pale yellow	Large raptor, pale head with central dark stripe in each feather Adult deeply rufous red in colour, marked red tail with forked tip Under wings: white primaries with black tips Juvenile is paler with buff belly and breast, tail is less forked, with dark sub-terminal band, also pale tips to all greater coverts (above and below wings)	Often seen soaring with marked tail fork
Osprey (*Pandion haliaetus*) Indigenous, but migratory (West and South Africa, October–March)	55–58 cm	145–170 cm	20% reverse sexual dimorphism, with minimal overlap 1200–1600 g (m) 1600–2000 g (f)	Yellow	Large raptor, with long relatively pointed wings and long tail (compared with a falcon) White crown, neck and pale underparts, speckled chest, with dark under wing carpal patches, with chocolate brown eye stripe, nape and upper parts (paler in birds in their first year)	Both male and female are very defensive of nest Both hover and soar during hunting Ospreys are difficult to maintain in captivity, cannot be trained for falconry and have yet to be bred in captivity
Northern goshawk (*Accipiter gentilis*) Indigenous in the UK, once extinct but reintroduced	48–68.5 cm	96–127 cm	517–1170 g (m) 820–1509 g (f)	Juvenile is yellow, changing to reddish orange after fourth year	Juvenile has brown upper parts, with buff chest with vertical dark brown streaks Adult male and female have grey upper parts, long barred tail without square end, white with black horizontal bars on chest, pale underwings Conspicuous white eye stripe in adults Larger, stronger and more robust than sparrowhawks	Still hunters: sit in tree in woodland and swoop down on prey as it passes Strong, muscular but nervous and anxious birds Very prone to stress-related immunosuppression and secondary aspergillosis in captivity

29.3 (continued) Biology, taxonomy and identification of common UK diurnal birds of prey. (x=mean). Other species include: golden eagle (*Aquila chrysaetos*) (resident small population, predominantly in Scotland); white-tailed sea eagle (*Haliaeetus albicilla*) (went extinct in early twentieth century, re-introduced into Skye (1975 and onwards) and Western Isles); hen harrier (*Circus cyaneus*) (resident in the UK, most heavily predated species due to conflict with game shooting interests); marsh harrier (*Circus aeruginosus*) (summer migrant visitor March–September in low numbers, breed and hunt over marsh land and reed beds); Montagu's harrier (*Circus pygargus*)(rare summer migrant visitor found in Norfolk, Dorset, Hampshire and Oxford); honey buzzard (*Pernis apivorus*) (rare summer, May–September, migrant visitor).

Species	Distribution	Feeding	Nesting	Incubation	Clutch	Fledge age	Sexual maturity	Lifespan
Common kestrel (*Falco tinnunculus*)	Commonest falcon in UK Well adapted to variety of terrains, wooded, farmland rural, urban, seen in open countryside, often hovering above quarry	Voles (90%) and insects	In trees, often in reused corvid nests, or hole or niche in building	27–31 days	3–6 eggs	Dependent on parents for 27–35 days; fed by parents for further 2–4 weeks	1 year	First year mortality 50–70% Potential of 18 years
Peregrine (*Falco peregrinus*)	Cliff, mountain or valley ledges, also now commonly seen in industrial or urban settings (e.g. cranes, skyscrapers, cathedrals)	Medium-sized birds taken in flight	Nest in 'scrapes' on high ledges	29–33 days	3–4 eggs	Fed by parents for 42–66 days; dependent on parents for a further 2 months	Male 1–2 years Female 2–4 years	Average in wild is 15 years, normal maximum in wild 20 years, but record is 25 years
Merlin (*Falco tinnunculus*)	British population is non-migratory (other European populations perform short migration southerly in winter) Suffered decline due to DDT and egg shell thinning in 1960–70, but population is now recovered Favourite habitat is open moorland and similar	Feeds predominantly on small birds (<50 g), bats and insects Predominantly catches prey in mid-air	Habitat very varied Nest in trees, cliffs or on ground Do not build nest but reuse others e.g. corvid, or (74%) just make a scrape on the ground in dense vegetation	Lay in April Incubated for 28–32 days by both sexes	3–6 eggs	Fed by parents for 28–32 days; dependent on their parents for a further month	Mature at 1–2 years	Oldest wild bird 10 years; up to 14 years in captivity

29.4 Ecology and biology of common diurnal birds of prey of the UK. (continues)

Species	Distribution	Feeding	Nesting	Incubation	Clutch	Fledge age	Sexual maturity	Lifespan
Hobby (Falco subbuteo)	Distributed across Eurasia, migrate (October) and winter in central and southern Africa, returning in March. Tend to inhabit lowland open wooded areas	Feed predominantly on insects, also small birds, all taken in flight, often over water	Nest in trees (especially pines) often in reused corvid or raptor nests	Incubation 28-33 days predominantly by female	Typically three eggs (2-4), laid every 2-4 days	Dependent on parents for 28-34 days, fed by parents for a further 5 weeks	2 years	10 years
Eurasian sparrowhawk (Accipiter nisus)	Woodland (coniferous, deciduous), or open farmland, common even in urban areas. Often seen raiding bird tables or flying down country lanes, hopping between hedges	Small and medium-sized birds	In trees, often close to a clearing, 6-12 metres up; rebuilds each year	32-34 days	3-6 eggs; up to two replacement clutches if eggs are lost	Dependent on parents for 26-30 days; fed by parent for further 3-4 weeks	1-3 years	Rarely live over 7 years
Common buzzard (Buteo buteo)	Common; variable habitat but must include woodland for nesting and roosting; feed in areas that are more open in winter	Adaptable food intake according to availability; mainly voles, small rabbits, reptiles, insects, earthworms and carrion	In large trees close to the edge of wood; bulky platform of twigs, lined with greenery; usually alternate nests year by year	33-38 days	2-4 eggs	Dependent on parents for 50-60 days; fed by parent for further 6-8 weeks	3 years	Oldest record is 25 years Pre-breeding mid-air territorial disputes often lead to severe potentially fatal talon puncture wounds
Red kite (Milvus milvus)	Close to extinction, until major reintroduction project in multiple sites across Wales, England and Scotland, from 1989-2010; now some 2000 pairs Live in broadleaf woodlands, valleys and wetland edges	Diet of small mammals, carrion (risk of lead poisoning), reptiles, amphibians and earthworm	Male and female resident in breeding area all year Nest in fork of tree 12-20 metres up	Incubation starts when first egg laid; each egg is incubated for 31-32 days, so a 3 egg clutch takes 38 days	1-3 or 4 eggs, one laid every 3 days	Dependent on parents for 48-50 days, on occasions as late as 60 days Fed by for further 15-20 days	2 years	Average is 10 years, record being 26 years
Osprey (Pandion haliaetus)	Widespread distribution Ospreys are described as a fish hawk and are the only species within their family They have adaptation for catching fish (long legs, a reversible outer toe, and pads on their distal toes under their talons for holding fish) Inhabit coastal areas, lakes, marshes, rivers, elsewhere whilst on migration	Typically only live fish (usually 150-300 g, occasionally up to 1200 g), occasionally recently dead fish They can only take fish up to 1 m deep in water, so favour areas with shallow water Hunt off the wing, flying slowly 5-40 m above water	Often very bulky nest made of sticks Nests in trees (often shore line dead trees) or ground-nesting on water-locked islands	Autumn to spring breeders in southern latitudes or spring to autumn breeders in northern latitudes Often return and reuse previous nests Multiple copulations (60) in 2 weeks prior to egg laying, typically early in the morning	Incubation 40 days, by both parents 3 (2-4) very large eggs (60-80 g, i.e. 10% of female bodyweight) laid 2 days apart	Chicks have eyes open at hatch, but require constant brooding for first 1-14 days, after which they change their plumage and are better able to thermoregulate, although still brooded at night and from heat in the day Young ospreys are dependent on parents for 50 days but are fed by parents for a further 2-8 weeks All UK ospreys migrate to west and south Africa shortly after fledging	3-4 years	Average of 9 years in the wild, some known to have survived 30 years
Northern goshawk (Accipiter gentilis)	Favour mature old-growth woodland (coniferous and deciduous) Secretive raptors, rarely seen, even when breeding regularly in the area Opportunistic hunters, either sitting and waiting for prey to come past, or flying slowly at low level along the edge of woodland or on rides through woodland hoping to surprise mammals or birds	Feed on a mixture of mammals and birds	Typically nest in fork of large trees, up to 20 m from the ground Nest built by both parents of sticks, lined with twigs and fresh leaves Normally various nests within territory and rotate use between years	Eggs laid in April and early May Incubation 35-38 days almost entirely by female	1-5 eggs, typically 3-4 eggs	Dependent on parents for 34-37 days (male), 37-41 days (female); fed by on parents until 70-90 days	2-3 years	Oldest bird in the wild 19 years, in captivity 25 years

29.4 (continued) Ecology and biology of common diurnal birds of prey of the UK.

Species	Length	Wingspan	Bodyweight (m = male; f = female	Iris colour	Identification	Behaviour
Tytonidae						
Barn owl (*Tyto alba*) (see Figure 29.1d)	33–39 cm	80–95 cm	231–381 g (m) 295–395 g (f)	Dark	Medium-sized, slim body, long wings and legs Face (white) pale with distinctive heart shape Plumage typically pale (male lighter in colour); upper parts grey Juvenile similar to adult but more heavily spotted	Sedentary and nocturnal; day time flying occasionally witnessed Silent in flight Often hunt down major roads
Strigidae						
Tawny owl (*Strix aluco*) (see Figure 29.1e)	37–43 cm	81–104 cm	304–465 g (m) 385–716 g (f)	Black	Medium-sized, with wings broad and rounded Brown (usually rufous but varies from very pale to greyish brown) with large round face, cinnamon facial disc, whitish extra eyebrows; whole plumage mottled, finely streaked, noticeably shaggy and loose Tarsus and most toes feathered Beak pale brown to pale yellow Juvenile plumage paler	Often noisy at night, referred to as a 'screech owl' Hunts predominantly dusk to midnight and again at dawn
Little owl (*Athene noctua*)	23–27.5 cm	54–58 cm	139–230 g (m) 137–260 g (f)	Yellow	Small (far smaller than any other UK owl), compact, plump, with large broadly rounded head, long legs, short tail Brown upper parts, buff-whitish under parts clearly streaked brown Juvenile plumage pattern duller and less well defined No white spots on crown	Partially diurnal; often seen perching on posts in daylight

29.5 Biology, taxonomy and identification of common owls of the UK.

Species	Distribution	Feeding	Nesting	Incubation	Clutch	Fledge age	Sexual maturity	Lifespan
Barn owl (*Tyto alba*)	Until recently rare in UK, numbers and areas of distribution gradually increasing Any bird nesting within 1 mile of a major trunk road is likely to be killed on road	Predominantly voles (absolutely dependent on permanent pasture for voles), also frogs and insects Use hearing extensively during hunting	In holes in trees or within farm buildings, 2–20 m from the ground	29–34 days	4–7 eggs (clutch replacement occurs) May have 2–3 broods if food plentiful	7–10 weeks, fed by parent for next 3–5 weeks, then disperse (up to 20 km) within 2–8 weeks	<1 year	Monogamous but polygamy recorded licence required (from Animal and Plant Health Agency (APHA)), before any rehabilitated wild or captive-bred barn owls can be released in the UK
Tawny owl (*Strix aluco*)	Most common British owl; breeds in woodland, wooded farmland, large gardens, urban parkland Sedentary and nocturnal	Mainly voles (56%), also birds, amphibians, reptiles, earthworms and insects Quarry caught on the ground by still-hunting	In holes in trees or buildings, cliffs, reuse squirrel dreys or magpie nests	28–30 days; brooded for further 15 days	Usually 3–5 eggs	32–37 days Fratricide if food shortage 25–30 days as 'branchers'; dependent on parents until 3 months after fledging Leave nest when young, before able to fly (often presented as orphans when fallen from tree) Disperse in autumn within a few km of natal nest	1 year	Mortality in first year 71%; potential lifespan 19 years Monogamous, pair for life
Little owl (*Athene noctua*)	Breeds in open mixed countryside or built-up areas Sedentary; partially diurnal	Insects (70%), birds, small amphibians and reptiles	In cavity in tree, wall, etc.	28–33 days	3–6 eggs	30–35 days; dependent on parents for a further month	<1 year	Mortality in first year 70%, annual adult mortality 35% Monogamous Introduced into UK in 19th century

29.6 Ecology and biology of common owls of the UK.

Anatomy and physiology

The most significant anatomical features of raptors are described in Figures 29.2 to 29.6. All raptors eat whole carcass diets, fur and feather (ingestible matter referred to as 'casting', which is regurgitated as a casting (pellet) 12–18 hours after a meal), meat, bone, viscera and gut contents. A bird should not be fed again until after a casting from the previous meal has been produced. When managing a sick bird (including any on more than once daily medication) casting material should be withheld, so that instead of withholding food until a pellet has been cast, small frequent meals can be given and repeated as soon as the crop is empty. The crop is a simple storage organ; it has no acid or enzyme production and meat is held here at body temperature (41°C). If for any reason (such as an overfull crop in a sick or weak bird) the meat in the crop does not pass into the proventriculus, where acid and enzymes will control bacterial proliferation, within a reasonable period (6–8 hours maximum), it will rapidly putrefy resulting in a life-threatening toxaemia termed 'sour crop'. Owls do not possess a crop. Whilst most birds have a distinct proventriculus (enzyme and acid-producing) and gizzard (or ventriculus, which has a muscular and grinding action), in birds of prey both parts are confluent, with only minor ventricular function.

Capture, handling and transportation

Capture

If a veterinary surgeon (veterinarian) is asked to assist in catching an injured wild raptor, the exact approach will depend on the species, the location and the extent of injuries suffered. A thick towel, gardening or welding gloves and a long-handled net that is padded around the entrance may be required. All equipment used should be cleaned and disinfected prior to use. The net or towel are used to drop over or cover the bird to allow manual restraint and transfer to a suitably sized cardboard box or other carrying container. Cages with wire mesh sides or doors should never be used, as this can result in damage to the feathers. Birds will generally travel best in a darkened container, with suitable substrate to allow them to gain pedal traction (e.g. carpet).

Handling

When handling raptors, the primary danger is injury caused by the talons. Birds of prey may bite, but this will cause minimal damage (save perhaps for eagles, where greater care is required). The legs and feet should always be restrained first, holding the legs in one hand, with a finger between the legs to prevent them rubbing against each other if the bird struggles. As with all wildlife, raptors can carry zoonotic infectious organisms (see Chapter 7). Certain zoonoses are of particular relevance: *Chlamydia* spp. *Escherichia coli*, *Salmonella* spp., avian influenza, Newcastle disease and *Cryptosporidium* spp.

All equipment that might be required during restraint and handling should be prepared and at hand prior to catching the bird. Catching and restraining diurnal raptors in subdued lighting reduces the levels of stress and the likelihood of feather damage. Maintaining feather condition and the avoidance of breaking, bending or damaging flight feathers is essential, as damage may preclude or delay release (see 'Short-term housing'). A clean towel (for each patient) should be used to handle and restrain raptors. Ensure the room is secure, with windows and doors shut. If catching from a box, place the towel over the top of the box and carefully pull each leaf of the closed box lid back until the top of the box is covered just by the towel; then drop the towel down on the bird, restrain the bird in two hands and remove from the box. With the bird restrained, the two feet should be identified and secured, holding them between the fingers of one hand (with a finger placed between the two legs) (Figure 29.7). If the bird is loose in a room or aviary, a long-handled fisherman's net with a padded rim is useful to catch it prior to manual restraint. All birds, including raptors, are prey species and are very prone to stress; therefore, the period of restraint must be absolutely minimized (especially prior to shock control, see 'First aid'). All equipment that might be required during restraint and handling should be prepared and at hand prior to catching the bird. Maintaining feather condition and the avoidance of breaking, bending or damaging flight feathers is essential, as damage may preclude or delay release (see 'Short-term housing').

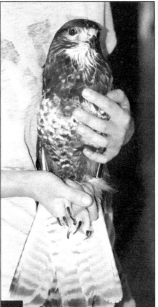

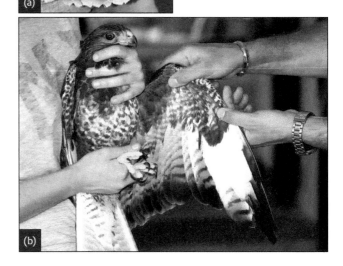

29.7 (a) Restraint of a common buzzard: lower legs in one hand, with a finger between the feet to prevent self-trauma if struggling, second hand restraining the body, head and neck. (b) Common buzzard being restrained by an assistant: lower legs in one hand, with a finger between the feet to prevent self-trauma if struggling, second hand restraining the neck and head. This allows the clinician two hands to withdraw body parts for a full examination. (Editors' note – less experienced handlers may wish additionally to use a towel to cover the head, wings and feet when handling these birds.)

Examination and clinical assessment for rehabilitation

Figure 29.8 illustrates a schematic flow chart of steps in the admission and management of raptor wildlife casualty cases.

As with all rehabilitation patients, raptor casualties are likely to be suffering from extreme circulatory shock (see Chapter 5). All equipment that may be required in initial assessment should be prepared and available, prior to restraint. A full physical examination at this stage (before shock is controlled), would be inappropriate. A brief check for vital signs, cardiorespiratory distress, severe haemorrhage or obviously critical injuries should be followed by administration of analgesia and shock therapy alone (see 'First aid'). Doing too much too early may well result in the bird's premature demise.

Figure 29.9 gives lists of actions by priority for common causes of wild raptor admissions.

Clinical examination

Once shock is controlled, the bird should be examined thoroughly and systematically. In order for a raptor to be released back to the wild, it must be able to see, fly, hunt, kill and eat well enough, interact normally with its own species and not present an undue risk to human safety (the latter are relevant if the bird has become malprinted – see 'Rearing of young raptors'). Factors that would prevent release of a wild raptor would include:

- Impaired eyesight or loss of an eye
- Loss of function of, or any part of, any limb
- Loss of beak or inability to ingest wild-caught diet
- Loss of first or second toe, permanent loss of talon or loss of foot holding ability
- Inability to catch suitable wild-caught food
- Inability to relate safely to birds of its own kind
- Increased risk of hybridizing with another species
- Inability to survive in the wild without being a danger to humans.

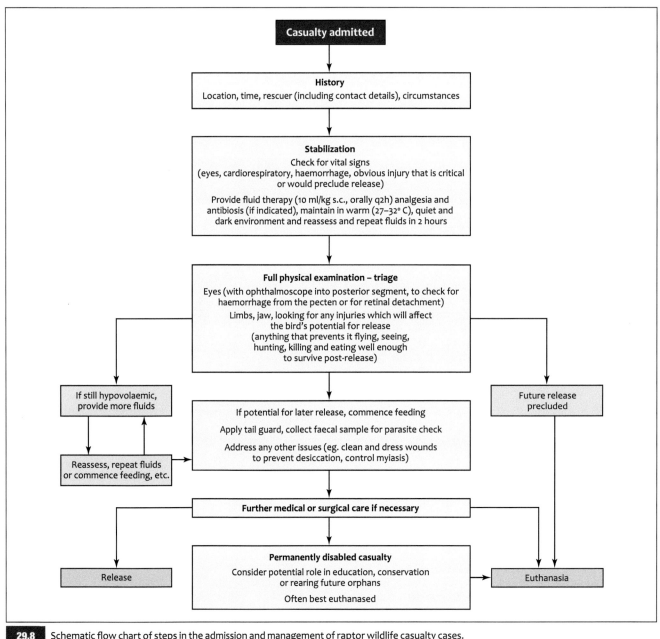

29.8 Schematic flow chart of steps in the admission and management of raptor wildlife casualty cases.

Condition	Course of action (in order of preference)
'Orphan'	1. Return to nest for parental care 2. Return to another wild nest of same species under Animal and Plant Health Agency (APHA) licence 3. Rear in captivity under parents of the same species for later release 4. Crèche rear in captivity (even if this means moving to another rescue centre) 5. Rear in captivity under foster parents of 'similar non-indigenous species' for later release 6. Hand-rear by puppet feeding 7. Euthanase if facilities not available
Starved/exhausted (typically after inclement weather, migration or failed dispersal)	1. Control shock 2. Gavage feed, then offer small amounts of meat (cast-free) little and often 3. Full physical, radiological, clinical pathological and ophthalmological examination to elucidate cause of starvation 4. Check for and treat endo-, ecto- and haemoparasites 5. If potential for eventual release, feed up, transfer into flight aviary, increase fitness for assessment for release 6. If no potential for release, euthanase
Trauma	1. Brief check for vital signs and injuries which are obviously critical or will preclude release. If the latter are present, euthanase 2. Treat shock and stabilize 3. Triage for long-term release 4. Full physical, radiological, clinical pathological and ophthalmological examination to elucidate cause of starvation. Check for and treat endo-, ecto- and haemoparasites 5. Administer further nursing, medical and surgical therapy as indicated 6. Reassess for potential release 7. Euthanase or increase fitness in preparation for final assessment, prior to release
Poisoned (see Chapters 5 and 11)	1. Remove any crop contents and store (frozen) 2. Administer fluid therapy (i.v.), activated charcoal (orally), nursing care, any specific antidote and additional supportive care 3. Notify police and/or APHA Wildlife Incident Unit 4. Testing of toxic agent
Infected or Infested	1. Often presented as starved or exhausted 2. Control shock and give supportive care 3. Full clinical pathology investigation 4. If systemic infection is present (typically indicated by leucocytosis), antibiotics or antifungals should be administered as appropriate 5. Check for and treat for endo-, ecto- and haemoparasites as indicated 6. Recheck to assess for response and resolution 7. Euthanase or increase fitness in preparation for final assessment prior to release

29.9 Actions by priority for common causes of wild raptor admissions.

In common with any admitted wildlife casualty, wild raptor casualties are of unknown health status. A full physical examination is always required. Depending on the species and status of patient, this may be carried out under general anaesthetic (to reduce the stress on the patient) or conscious (see Figure 29.7b). The more critical the patient's injuries, or the more nervous the species (e.g. Eurasian sparrowhawk (*Accipiter nisus*) and Northern goshawk (*A. gentilis*)), or the more powerful and difficult to restrain without the bird or its plumage suffering trauma (e.g. peregrine falcon (*Falco peregrinus*)) then the greater the indication for sedation or anaesthesia. Just as in any other patient, the examination is carried out in a methodical and systematic manner.

- Commence with the head: eyes (ophthalmoscopic examination), ears, sinuses, beak, mouth, choana and glottis.
- Moving to the neck, crop and chest to assess body condition (see Chapter 4), but note that the normal degree of muscle covering over the keel, varies between raptor species.
- The scapula, coracoid and clavicle are all carefully palpated to ensure normal integrity.
- The two wings are extended at the same time, to assess degrees of extension, tension on joints and soft tissues.
- Each joint and long bone is felt in turn, joints being flexed and extended, together with the propatagium (web of soft tissue running between shoulder and carpus).

- Wing plumage is assessed for missing feathers, stage of moult, presence of 'fret or stress bars' on the feathers (indicating that the patient was sick or stressed at the time that that flight feather was grown). Absence of feathers bilaterally on the lateral aspects of the chest, or midline between the legs, in particular when associated with sub-dermal thickening in these areas, is often associated with 'brood patch' development, indicating that the bird is in lay, incubation or the rearing phase of reproduction.
- Thoracic auscultation may be carried out, although this tends to be less rewarding than in mammals.
- Next the spine is followed caudally, checking for normal alignment, to the point of insertion of the tail flight feathers, where the preen gland is checked (the feathers at the distal point of the uropygial gland should always contain oil; lack of oil indicates a blocked duct).
- The pelvic limbs from hip to tip, including feet, digits and talons, are then checked, each joint being flexed and extended.
- The tail, flight feathers and cloaca are then examined and the coelom palpated.

Ocular examination

One of the most common causes for a wild raptor to be presented in an emaciated condition, as well as a common consequence of a traumatic injury, is damage to ocular function (Figure 29.10). It has been shown that 30% of raptor trauma cases have suffered ocular damage and in

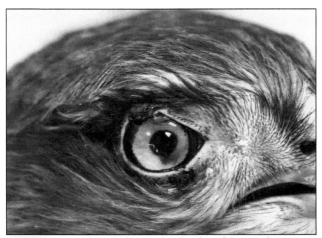

29.10 Haemorrhage in the anterior chamber of the eye of a sparrowhawk. Ocular examination is an essential part of the clinical assessment of all raptors.

70% of these, the damage only affects the posterior segment and is only visible if the eye is examined with an ophthalmoscope (Korbel, 2000); thus it is important that all raptor wildlife casualties admitted are submitted to an ophthalmoscopic examination of the eyes. The retina and pecten should be visualized in all cases, which with experience is possible in all normal eyes, in conscious raptors. The high incidence of posterior segment damage is linked to a contrecoup effect consequent to head trauma, specifically due to traction of the attachment of the pecten from the retina, which commonly results in haemorrhage at this location (see 'Trauma').

The cornea should be examined and the presence of tears confirmed (Schirmer tear test: 10–15 mm in 1 minute is normal). Measurement of anterior pressure (reference values using Tonopen® XL, 9–28 mmHg; owls typically 9–11 mmHg; kestrels 13 mmHg; buzzards (*Buteo buteo*) 17 mmHg) and inspection of the anterior as well as the posterior segment, should all be carried out. The iris (pupillary) light reflex should be tested; a positive response is indicative of normal retinal function, whilst a lack of response may arise due to retinal defect, although it may also be seen in a normal functional eye due to the presence of striated muscle in the avian iris, which enables birds, unlike mammals, to override the normal light response.

Normal mammalian mydriatics are ineffective in birds, although mydriasis can be achieved with topical rocuronium drops. The retinal fundus in raptors reflects red (in nocturnal species) or grey (in diurnal species), the colour emanating from the sclera, as there is no tapetum behind the retina (see 'Trauma').

Diagnostic tests

Approximately 85% of wild raptors carry some parasitic burden. Whilst under normal circumstances the bird would live in relative harmony with these parasites, once the bird is sick, injured or captive, these parasites often take an upper hand. All wildlife patients presented should be screened for parasites and treated appropriately, in particular before they have opportunity to contaminate rehabilitation accommodation.

Any raptor that has suffered trauma will benefit from dorsoventral and lateral survey radiographs, to assess for collateral damage. Some raptor trauma cases are victims of primary acute accidents, whilst in other cases the injury occurred because the bird was already ill and failed to

avoid impact or injury. Good practice indicates that a full haematology and biochemistry evaluation of all admissions should be performed (see 'Bacterial infections'); any concurrent illness that is detected should also be addressed if one wishes to maximize the chance of a positive outcome.

Euthanasia

Euthanasia of raptors, in common with other wildlife casualties, should always be carried out in the most efficient and welfare-compliant manner. Depending on the patient and facilities available, this may involve volatile anaesthesia (isoflurane/sevoflorane) followed by systemic barbiturate (intravenous administration into the ulnar or jugular vein or via the occipital sinus), or may simply be by direct use of systemic barbiturate. Intracardiac, intracoeliomic and intrahepatic injections in an unanaesthetised bird are contraindicated on welfare grounds.

First aid and short-term hospitalization

The general principles of first aid apply to raptors and are detailed in Chapter 5. Therapy for shock will involve the oral (by gavage tube, see 'Short-term feeding') or subcutaneous administration of warm saline or glucose saline at 10 ml/kg, repeated after 2 hours, and maintenance in a dark quiet and warm (27–32°C) environment. The use of intravenous or intraosseous fluid therapy to address hypovolaemia is advantageous, so long as this can be provided without causing excessive stress, whilst the patient remains highly compromised. Once hypovolaemia has been corrected, nutrition should be provided (see 'Short-term feeding').

Analgesia should be provided appropriately (see 'Anaesthesia and analgesia').

Short-term housing

Any captive wild raptor should be provided with a perch (even if this is just a block of wood, brick or stone with a towel over it) so as to keep the tips of the primary feathers off the floor, and a tail guard should be applied.

For a tail guard the author uses a section of 'waste' x-ray film or plastic sterilizing pouch, folded over, closed at one end with tape, and taped around the tail feathers to cover the distal 50% of the tail (Figure 29.11). A tail guard should never be applied to a wet or soiled tail. Raptors (as all birds) should never be enclosed in a wire cat basket or similar, where feathers may pass through the wire mesh and become damaged. Maintaining such patients in dim lighting (with visual seclusion) will tend to keep them more relaxed, although light levels will need to be increased at times when patients are expected to eat. Hoods should only be used in birds that have previously been trained to be hooded (i.e. not new wildlife casualty birds) and nothing unpleasant should ever be done to a bird whilst hooded, otherwise the bird may become 'hood shy' and hence reluctant to accept hooding in future.

Accommodation for injured raptors must ensure biosecurity between patients, and so should be readily cleanable or disposable (i.e. a cardboard box). No other patient (particularly prey species) should be in view of the raptor, as this would be inherently stressful for both animals.

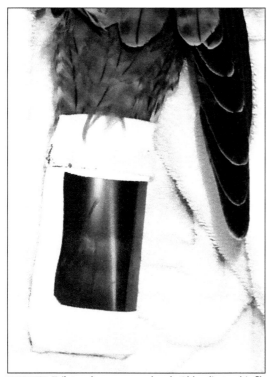

29.11 Tail guard on a sparrowhawk. Old radiographic film or similar can be used. It should cover the distal 50% of the tail and be a little larger than the tail itself. Protecting tail and flight feathers is essential, as any damage will delay or prevent later release.

Short-term feeding

As soon as hypovolaemia is corrected, injured raptors must be provided with suitable nutrition. A sick or injured captive wild raptor may not necessarily feed voluntarily, and should never be force-fed meat. Nutrition is most efficiently, safely and atraumatically provided by gavage feeding (see Chapter 5). Initial volumes given should be 2% of bodyweight per feed, increasing to 3% of bodyweight if well tolerated. The patient must be weighed first thing each morning, prior to any food or fluid administration, and

sufficient food given during the day to maintain or (if particularly thin) gain weight. For raptors, gavage equipment can be as simple as a syringe attached to a suitable length of giving set or similar tubing, to enable the operator to reach the crop, or in the case of owls (who have no crop), halfway between the mouth and the thoracic inlet.

The author's preferred avian critical care diet is Emeraid® Exotic Nutritional Care System, which is available in carnivore, piscivore, omnivore and herbivore ranges. Emeraid® Carnivore is of course appropriate for raptor casualties; it is more energy-dense than alternatives and in this author's opinion is better tolerated by patients. The food is provided as a dry powder, in a readily mixable format, so that feed will pass down fine tubes (down to 5 Fr). The diet is semi-elemental (so is easily absorbed, metabolized and assimilated), comprising purified amino acids, dietary nucleotides (for RNA and DNA precursors), has a high energy density provided by a highly digestible blend of fats and carbohydrates, with balanced omega 3:6 polyunsaturated fatty acids. Alternative commercial diets are Hill's® Prescription diet a/d or Oxbow Carnivore Care®.

It is important to stress that 'casting' (indigestible fur and feather) is not needed and should not be provided to injured wild raptors, until the bird is of normal weight and condition (as assessed by pectoral covering over the keel, see Chapter 4). Once the bird appears willing to self-feed, then suitable (cast-free, i.e. skinned) food should be offered, at the time of day when the bird would naturally feed (day time for diurnal raptors; dawn, dusk and night time for owls). Wild birds will not easily recognize white-haired mice or yellow feather-covered day-old chicks as food items, but once this food is skinned, it is more likely to be eaten. The key to successful feeding is little and often and no casting, until the bird is behaving normally.

Anaesthesia and analgesia

The general principles of anaesthesia and analgesia are described in Chapter 6 and apply to raptors. Anaesthetic, analgesic and sedative drug doses for wild raptors are summarized in Figure 29.12.

Drug	Dosage	Notes
Anaesthetic agents		
Medetomidine (M) + ketamine (K)	150–300 µg/kg (M) + 3–5 mg/kg (K), mixed in same syringe, i.v., i.m.[a]	Intravenous administration preferred due to quicker onset and more reliable effect Gives 30 minutes surgical anaesthesia; if lower dose (both agents) is used, a single top up may be given if procedure needs to be prolonged The medetomidine may be reversed with the same volume (750 µg/kg) of atipamezole i.m.
Tiletamine and zolazepam	80 mg/kg mixed in food and given as bait[b]	Achieves heavy sedation allowing handling after 30–60 minutes Useful for catching escaped raptors
Sedatives		
Diazepam	0.1–1 mg/kg i.v., s.c., orally q8–12h as required[a]	Sedative, anxiolytic
Midazolam	0.1–0.5 mg/kg i.v., i.m., s.c. q12h as required[a]	Sedative, anxiolytic
Analgesics		
Butorphanol	0.5 mg/kg i.v., i.m., q4–6h[c]	30 minutes to take effect
Meloxicam	0.5–2.0 mg/kg i.m., orally q24h[d]	Long-term use appears safe Do not give in dehydrated or hypotensive patients Do not use any other NSAIDs in raptors
Tramadol	5–30 mg/kg orally q12h[e]	Efficacy at given dose varies markedly between species

29.12 Anaesthetic and analgesic agents and their dose rates commonly used in raptor wildlife casualties.
([a] Bailey and Apo, 2008; [b] Janovsky et al., Riggs et al., 2008; [d] Desmarchelier et al., 2012; [e] Souza and Cox, 2011)

Anaesthesia

Anaesthesia in sick birds is used primarily to reduce the stress on the patient of a full physical examination, for collection of diagnostic samples, radiography and insertion of intravenous catheters. It is crucial that all equipment, staff and facilities are made ready prior to any handling or anaesthesia, such that the duration of any procedures (in particular handling) is always minimized. For all sick hospitalized raptors, as well as those undergoing anaesthesia of more than 10 minutes, the author favours the insertion of an intravenous catheter (typically into the ulnar vein on the ventral aspect of the elbow joint). Unless it is an emergency and there is no alternative, anaesthesia should not be carried out in any raptor that still has food in its crop, treatment of 'sour crop' being an exception. All anaesthetized birds should be intubated with a non-cuffed endotracheal tube. Monitoring of avian anaesthesia is entirely different to mammals, with which most nurses are more familiar. The overall safety of an anaesthetic is a combination of the inherent safety profile of the anaesthetic, together with the competence and experience of the anaesthetist. Where an experienced anaesthetist is not available (who can accurately monitor depth of anaesthesia and prevent an overdose), then the author would favour weighing the patient, then calculating and administering a parenteral agent, such as a combination of medetomidine and ketamine (see Figure 29.12), rather than using gaseous anaesthesia. The patient is still intubated and maintained on oxygen.

Analgesia

It is vital that all injured patients receive appropriate analgesia. The reader is advised to refer to a current exotic animal formulary for latest information, as advice does vary between species. Opioid analgesia should be provided on admission. In general terms buprenorphine is of dubious efficacy, whilst butorphanol is generally effective and tramadol can be used (see Figure 29.12). Cyclooxygenase (COX) 1-inhibiting non-steroidal anti-inflammatory drugs (NSAIDs) should not be used in raptors, and even relatively COX-2 specific NSAIDs should not in this author's opinion be used where a patient is or may become hypovolaemic and so these drugs should not be given prior to, or before complete recovery from, anaesthesia. Meloxicam is generally safe for short or long-term use (see Figure 29.12).

Specific conditions

Trauma

In a major review of raptor wildlife admissions (Howard and Redig, 1993), it was shown that 33% of admissions are likely to have suffered a fracture. Of these birds, 40% were euthanased on account of the fracture, 10% were euthanased for other reasons and 15% died spontaneously. Those dying spontaneously have often suffered widespread or soft tissue trauma. Common buzzards, ospreys (Pandion haliaetus) and goshawks in particular are often subjected to intraspecific trauma/conflict, especially in the period leading up to the breeding season. In such cases there are often multiple deep-penetrating talon injuries, which may result in infection, haemorrhage or visceral penetration, rupture or leakage. Talon injuries

characteristically have a small entry point with deep penetration, and should be managed in a similar manner to dog bite injuries; i.e. drainage should be facilitated, and analgesia and antibiosis provided. In general terms, avian skin is very thin and there is limited soft tissue. If there is a skin wound, even if drainage is to be encouraged, desiccation of underlying soft tissue structures should be prevented by the use of hydrocolloidal dressings, which may be bandaged or sutured in place.

Injuries affecting the propatagium need to be treated very carefully. Dressings and bandages should never be placed across the leading edge of the propatagium, for fear of causing pressure necrosis. If the propatagium has been sectioned, it is vital that the tensor propatagialis, tensor propatagialis pars longus tendons, and the tendons of the extensor metacarpi radialis are located, that their integrity is assured and if sectioned, that the two ends are located, cleaned, debrided and re-joined using a Bunnell suture technique. Once the tendon is repaired, the adjacent soft tissues must be closed over the repair site, such that no tissue desiccation can arise.

Ocular trauma is common in raptor trauma cases, due to contrecoup forces on the head and resultant traction to the insertion of the pecten. Haemorrhage in the anterior chamber (see Figure 29.10) will clear rapidly, but haemorrhage in the posterior segment is likely to be associated with retinal detachment or peri-pecten blood loss. Haemorrhage in the posterior segment takes weeks or longer to clear and is often associated with long-term loss of retinal function, which then precludes release to the wild. Such cases may benefit from injection of tissue activator plasminogen (TAP) into the anterior chamber (under general anaesthesia) 48 hours after insult, repeated if necessary once or twice at 48 hour intervals (Korbel, 2000).

Assessment for orthopaedic surgery

The main factors to assess when considering the viability of orthopaedic treatment are:

- Does the bird have normal eye function?
- Is the fracture closed or compound? If compound, how devitalized are soft tissues, and is blood and nerve supply intact?
- How close to a joint is the fracture? If closer than 1.5 times the diameter of the bone, the joint will suffer reduced postoperative function
- Can the patient tolerate any stress associated with the procedure and the subsequent full recovery period?

If satisfactory answers cannot be given to the questions above, then the bird should be euthanased. Wing fractures account for 86% of wild raptor fracture cases (Howard and Redig, 1993). The humerus is most commonly affected, 59% humeral fractures typically being compound (Howard and Redig, 1993). The percentage of wild injured raptors eventually released was 36% for closed fractures and 15% for open fractures (Howard and Redig, 1993). If a bird has suffered sufficient trauma to fracture a bone, it is important to consider what else may also be traumatized.

The aims of assessment and orthopaedic surgery in wild raptor trauma cases are to:

- Assess if surgery is realistic, with a good prognosis for return to full function and subsequent release
- Stabilize the patient, treating hypovolaemia and infection and providing analgesia and nutritional support

- Treat contaminated or infected wounds
- Preserve soft tissue, if necessary by applying splints or dressings. In view of the extreme fragility of avian skin and the small mass of soft tissue, special care is required to prevent desiccation of soft tissues (by wound closure or application of hydrocolloid dressings)
- Realign fractures or replace luxations
- Stabilize the fracture site rigidly, preventing movement or rotation. The latter may require a combination of surgical techniques, together with a full understanding of the bird's husbandry requirements, such that it can be correctly managed through the convalescent period
- Facilitate full and early return to function of all joints and tendons. No bird should have a wing strapped up (so as to prevent normal joint function) for more than 48 hours post-surgery
- Return the limb to full, normal function, as quickly as possible, without adversely affecting the healing process.

It is important to be mindful that wing amputee wild raptors will be unable to copulate, as well as being unable to fly, and therefore should be euthanased. Leg amputee raptors over 150 g (i.e. all UK raptors), will inevitably develop pododermatitis on the other foot and such should instead be euthanased. In the author's experience, all avian orthopaedic cases should have surgery delayed 24 hours from the time of trauma, whilst shock, dehydration and pain are addressed. In the interim, desiccation and further trauma must be prevented. The bird's condition should be stabilized with fluid therapy, analgesia, antibiosis, parasiticides (if indicated) and nutritional support, as previously discussed. Timing and method of repair should always be considered on a case by case basis. The degree of perfection for postoperative release and return to normal function will be dictated by the species in question. Whilst a falcon (e.g. peregrine, merlin (*F. columbarius*) or common kestrel (*F. tinnunculus*)) requires absolute perfection in order to achieve full flight and be able to hunt for its food, in contrast a broad-wing, such as a red kite (*Milvus milvus*) or buzzard, will be able to survive without an absolutely perfect fracture repair. There is a small degree of tolerance with which the bird may still get about and survive well, with a good quality of life.

Orthopaedic surgical techniques

Surgical approaches to avian fracture repair have been discussed by Orosz *et al.* (1992), Harcourt-Brown (1994) and others. Orthopaedic techniques vary greatly with respect to bone, fracture type, size and species involved. For surgical techniques, the following references are useful: Hess (1994), Howard and Redig (1994), Harcourt-Brown (1996), Coles (2005), Helmer and Redig (2006) and Forbes (2014). Current advice for avian orthopaedic techniques comprise the achievement of longitudinal, lateral and rotational stability, with minimal surgical intervention (such as the manipulation of bone fragments), so as to minimize any potential iatrogenic damage to the delicate nerve or vascular supply. The more surgical intervention that is carried out, the greater the risk of postoperative infection and/or malunion. Most fracture repairs are best achieved with an intramedullary pin, linked to several external fixation pins placed perpendicular to the bones longitudinal axis (a hybrid or tie fixator).

Choice of pins: In birds, healing of bone in a stable fracture is by formation of endosteal callus; therefore,

intramedullary pins should not fill the medullary cavity, nor should they be of a diameter such that they cannot be readily bent, without at the same time risking iatrogenic trauma to the bone. External skeletal fixation (ESF) pins should not be placed so close to a joint as to risk ankylosis, or close to a fracture where pre-existing microfissures might result in bone splitting. The bone-holding ability of positive compared with negative-threaded ESF pins has been compared in avian fracture repair, demonstrating that negative-threaded pins are as effective as positive-threaded pins, so negative-threaded pins may be used in preference. ESF pins are always inserted by powered drill; the soft tissues adjacent to the point of insertion are held against the bone with a thumbnail, to minimize the risk of catching and rotation around the pin as it is driven through the bone. An index finger is always positioned behind the cortex directly opposite the point of insertion, firstly to create an opposing force to that of the drill, but also to allow monitoring for pin emergence from the distal cortex. Before drilling the pin, it is important to ensure that the drill key or pin cutter is at hand, so that once driven, the drill and pin can be disengaged without altering the position of the drill, which might otherwise damage the pin-holding within the cortex.

Thoracic limb fractures

Coracoid (scapula or clavicle): These fractures are relatively common and typically associated with flying into a stationary object (e.g. a tree or fence post). With experience, these fractures may be assessed by digital exploration, but good quality radiographs are invaluable. Standard straight and symmetrical dorsoventral (with wings abducted laterally and legs caudally) and lateral (with wings abducted dorsally) views will allow full evaluation. Birds that have suffered shoulder injuries are often presented with their carpal position altered ventrally and the tips of the primaries elevated dorsally (see Figure 4.4). Careful digital examination will often reveal inflammation, swelling and crepitus and the exact pathology may often be detected by this careful examination. In birds weighing less than 1 kg, the maintenance of the patient in an enclosed area (e.g. a tea chest or night quarter), where it can move but not flap its wings, for 2.5 weeks, will typically result in good repair and a release rate of 71–98% (Howard and Redig, 1993; Redig *et al.*, 2009). In larger birds, in particular with coracoid fractures where there is significant displacement, reduction and fixation with a 1–4 mm mini bone plate is recommended. Surgical access is achieved between the crop and the dorso–anterior extremity of the pectoral muscle, close to the thoracic inlet.

Proximal humerus: These are common wild bird flight injuries and technically quite demanding to fixate. Surgical access to humeral fractures should always be via the dorsal aspect (i.e. with the bird in ventral recumbency), so that exact humeral alignment can be visually assessed by positioning of the tips of the both sets of primaries – these should be symmetrically crossed over each other. The humerus is pneumatized and connected to the clavicular air sacs. Flushing of the proximal bone end should be carried out with caution, to avoid introducing fluid into the respiratory system. Loss of anaesthetic gas from the pneumatic space is of limited human health risk and does not result in anaesthetic instability. Surgical access is gained to the fracture site and two fine wires are introduced into the proximal fragment at the fracture site and passed retrograde, one wire being passed out either side of the pectoral crest of the proximal humerus. Once passed sufficiently retrograde, the fracture is reduced and the wires then passed normograde into the distal humerus (Figure 29.13a). A transverse hole is then created through the cortex of the distal fragment, and a further one through the pectoral crest of the proximal fragment and a tension-band (figure-of-eight) wire placed between the two fragments, around the intramedullary wires. Whilst this traditional repair achieves alignment, it does not give sufficient stability to allow wing movement. The external extremities are bent through 90 degrees, two to three ESF pins are placed in the distal humerus (passing through both cortices) and all pin ends are then joined to an external fixation bar, as illustrated (Figure 29.13b). The pins and bar are rigidly joined, using acrylic. Care is taken when introducing the ESF pins, to avoid the radial nerve that can be visualized through the skin, traversing diagonally across the dorsal aspect of the distal third of the humerus. Fixators are generally removed at 3–3.5 weeks subject to radiographic evidence of healing.

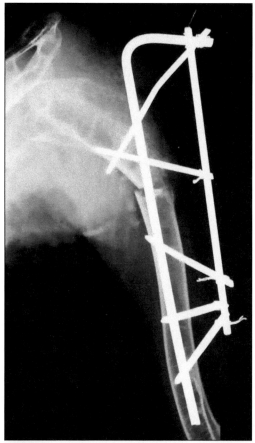

29.14 Ventrodorsal view of mid-shaft humerus repair using a 'hybrid fixator': external skeletal fixation pins are positioned in the dorsal aspect at either perpendicular or acute angles as appropriate.

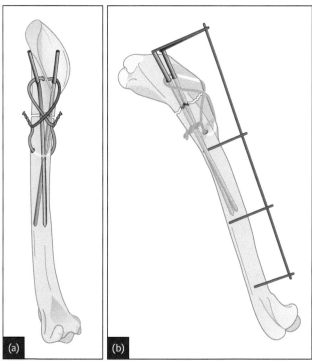

29.13 (a) Use of wires and tension band to repair a fracture of the proximal humerus. (b) Intramedullary wires in the proximal humerus fixed to an external skeletal fixation construct: a 'hybrid fixator'. This method of fixation provides increased stability and allows for wing movement.

Mid-shaft humerus: This is the most common fracture of free-flying birds, commonly being grossly displaced and typically compound (in 59% of cases, Redig *et al.*, 1993), often with exposed necrotic or desiccated bone. The humerus is generally S-shaped, lending itself to retrograde or normograde intramedullary pinning, the choice being dictated by the requirement to avoid joint interference at the cortical extremity where the pin exteriorizes. As for proximal humeral fractures, additional ESF pins are placed, preferably in both extremities, always spread over the entire length of the bone to distribute any pressures and forces throughout the bone. The intramedullary pin and ESF pins are joined by an external bar, as is illustrated for a proximal humeral fracture in Figure 29.13b. ESF pins may be placed perpendicular to the long axis of the bone, or at acute angles (Figure 29.14). As above, great care is

taken to avoid damage to the radial nerve as it obliquely traverses the distal third of the humerus. With the bird in sternal recumbency during surgery, exact correct longitudinal alignment is verified by assessing positioning of the tips of the primary flight feathers.

Distal humerus: A cross pin linked to a hybrid fixator is employed (see 'Distal femur').

Dislocation of the elbow: This injury carries a poor prognosis for return to normal flight (50% of cases (Martin *et al.*, 1993)) and therefore such repair may not be justified except in individuals of particular conservational importance. The luxation should be reduced by closed manipulation or, if necessary, an open surgical technique. The elbow is then flexed. ESF pins are placed in the dorsal aspect of humerus and ulna: A in the mid-humerus, B in the distal humerus, C in the proximal ulna and D in the mid-ulna. Cross external bars are then joined between A and C, and B and D. These bars are left in place for just 5 to 6 days, i.e. sufficient time to allow the development of some fibrous tissue around the joint to provide some stability, but no longer, so that ankylosis does not occur. Wing flapping is prevented (by keeping the bird in a small container) for 2 weeks post-ESF pin removal.

Ulna and radius: In one report, wild raptor forearm fractures comprised 30% involving the ulna only, 60% involving the ulna and radius and 10% involving the radius only (Redig *et al.*, 1993). These bones have minimal soft tissue support and any open wounds are predisposed to desiccation. In birds with ulnar fracture alone, with minimal displacement, cage rest alone (2–3 weeks) will affect a good outcome. In such cases the wing should not be bandaged against the body, although taping the tips of the primaries together in a physiological position may be useful for 2–4 days. In larger birds (>1 kg), or where significant displacement or proximity to a joint is present, then intramedullary fixation is recommended. In such cases a pin is inserted in the proximal ulna on the lateral aspect, just distal to the point of insertion of the triceps tendon, i.e. entry at the level of the second or third last (closest to the body) secondary feather (Figure 29.15).

In birds with radial fracture alone, fixation is generally indicated with a single intramedullary pin. The pin is introduced at the fracture site, pushed normograde towards the carpus, the fracture reduced and the pin returned retrograde to effect stabilization.

Where both radius and ulna are fractured, a synostosis (bridging callus) between radius and ulna may develop. If this is likely, prior to surgery the ventral abdominal wall is incised over the site of prior yolk sac attachment, and a subcutaneous fat pad may be harvested. The fat pad is then inserted between the radius and ulna, at the location of greatest risk (i.e. site of greatest trauma or inflammation, typically the fracture site). A good stabilization is effected and a synostosis should not occur. If a synostosis has developed, it is left some 8–12 weeks for the callus size to reduce as it heals; the callus is then removed with a dental drill, and the area is filled with a fat pad. NSAIDs are administered and regular exercise is encouraged within 48 hours of surgery. Following this procedure, the synostosis should not reoccur. Where radial and ulnar fractures are both present, it is generally preferable to reduce and fixate the radius first; fixation of the ulna will then be easier.

Pelvic limb fractures

Proximal femoral fractures: These are repaired with a technique similar to that described for the proximal humerus, with the exception that only one intramedullary wire is required, around which the tension band is attached, prior to placement of an ESF construct, joining of the ESF construct to the intramedullary wire and thus creation of the 'tie in' or 'hybrid' fixator.

Distal femur: The fracture site (Figure 29.16a) is approached, typically with an incision on both lateral and medial aspects. Fine cross wires are introduced normograde into the fracture site (one from each side), exiting the condyles without interfering with the stifle joint (Figure 29.16b). The fracture is then reduced. Initially one wire is passed retrograde into the proximal fragment (Figure 29.16c). The second cross wire is then passed across the fracture site, either by digitally twisting the distal fragment to one side, or by using artery forceps to hold the two wires together at the fracture site and into the proximal fragment, without putting pressure on the fine distal fragment that might otherwise result in an iatrogenic fracture occurring.

The wire on the medial aspect is then carefully bent over the anterior aspect of the stifle, such that it will not rub on soft tissues, to meet up with the wire on the lateral aspect. At least three ESF pins are then placed in the lateral aspect of the proximal femoral fragment. The ESF pins are joined with a bar to the two adjacent intramedullary wires (Figure 29.16d). A similar technique can be used to repair fractures of the distal humerus.

Tarsometatarsal fracture: The tarsometatarsus has no medullary cavity. Fractures are repaired using full pin ESF (two pins above the fracture, two below), the pins passing through a section of plastic tube (of diameter at least 70% of the bone diameter) either side of the tarsometatarsus. After repair, the tube is filled with acrylic to effect complete stabilization. If the acrylic used is thermogenic, the tubes must not be in direct contact with any soft tissue structures, to prevent thermal trauma.

Poisoning

Birds of prey have, historically and unfairly, been persecuted by gamekeepers and farmers, often by means of deliberate poisoning of meat baits. Bird of prey populations have also suffered accidental poisoning due to ingestion of lead (by eating lead shot-contaminated carcasses) and poisoning due to the ingestion of organochlorine or organophosphate pesticides (typically arising

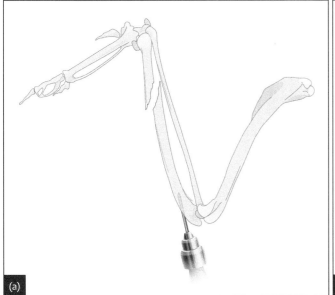
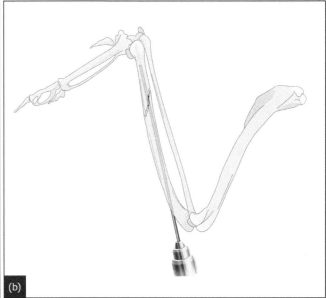

29.15 (a) Introduction of a single intramedullary pin into the proximal ulna. (b) The fractured ulna is digitally reduced and the intramedullary pin is advanced across the fracture site into the distal fragment.

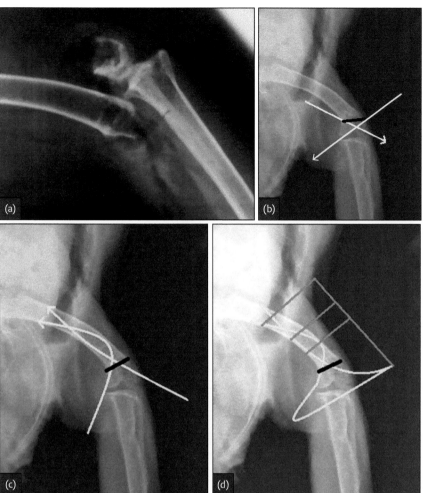

29.16 (a) Distal femoral facture. (b) Wires are first passed normograde from the fracture site. (c) Intramedullary wires are then returned retrograde across the fracture site. (d) The intramedullary wires are both bent to the lateral aspect of the bone and joined with external skeletal fixation pins.

when malicious and illegal persecution of raptor populations occurs, often perpetrated by those with concerns for loss of racing pigeons and game birds). These toxins will on occasion cause acute deaths; in other cases, birds will present with muscle weakness, central nervous system (CNS) signs, hypersensitivities, fits (seizures), debility, failed hunting or eggshell thinning and infertility. Since this issue was first highlighted, the majority of such toxins (except lead used in shooting) have been withdrawn from use in the developed world but are still sold to and freely used in developing countries. In recent years, vultures (*Gyps* spp.) in India have suffered massive population crashes, due to use of the COX-1 selective NSAID diclofenac in farm animals and humans, whose carcasses have then been eaten by the vultures. Thankfully the incidence of malicious raptor poisoning has declined in the last 3 years in the UK; however, cases do still occur on an annual basis. Alphachloralose, mevinphos, carbofuran, strychnine and others are used. If such a cases are suspected, crop and stomach contents, poisoned bait, etc. should be retained and a police wildlife liaison officer or the Animal and Plant Health Agency (APHA) Wildlife Incident Unit contacted (see Chapter 11).

General information on the treatment of toxicity cases is given in Chapter 5.

Organophosphate and carbamate toxicity

Cholinesterase inhibitory poisons (ChEl) (organophosphate and carbamate chemicals) act by inhibiting acetylcholinesterase activity (AChE). Clinical signs are explained by the persistent action of acetylcholine at the nerve endings, where it would otherwise only remain momentarily. Carbamates are rapid in onset, but described as reversible ChEls, whilst organophosphates are slower in onset, but irreversible. Clinical signs include flaccid paralysis of the limbs, whilst the head remains upright and alert. There is marked bradycardia, ataxia, diarrhoea, tremors and dyspnoea, and death may ensue. Treatment within 24 hours of ingestion with pralidoxime (10–20 mg/kg i.m., repeated after 8 hours) can be efficacious. After initial exposure of the organophosphate at the effector junction, the enzyme–phosphoryl bond is strengthened by loss of one alkyl group from the phosphoryl adduct; this process is known as ageing, and the bond is then essentially permanent. Time of ageing varies by agent and can occur within minutes to days. Administration of pralidoxime more than 24 hours after ingestion is unlikely to be efficacious and may be detrimental. Atropine can be administered (0.2–0.5 mg/kg i.m.) at any stage following poisoning and should be repeated every 3–4 hours.

Alphachloralose toxicity

Clinical signs of alphachloralose poisoning are lethargy, hypothermia, incoordination or stupor. If birds are kept warm, fluid therapy is maintained and nutrition provided once they are strong enough to avoid regurgitation and aspiration, they will typically make a full recovery in 24–36 hours.

Strychnine toxicity

Birds poisoned with strychnine are rarely found alive. Poisoning is peracute, with marked opisthotonos, rigor and severe muscle contracture. Typically several carcasses are found immediately adjacent to poisoned bait.

Rodenticide toxicity

Rodenticide anticoagulant poisoning in birds is very rare, as birds exhibit two independent clotting pathways and it is rare for simultaneous blocking of both. Where it does arise, oral haemorrhages or acute death are observed. Vitamin K (0.2–2.2 mg/kg i.m. q4–8h until stable then orally q24h for 14–28 days) is efficacious in treating this toxicity.

Infectious diseases

Viral diseases

Raptors are susceptible to common infectious viral diseases; these tend to occur following ingestion of infected food, can be transmitted by insect vectors or occasionally after inhalation of the virus.

Newcastle disease: Newcastle disease is caused by infection with Newcastle disease virus, resulting in central neurological signs including torticollis and opisthotonous, and green diarrhoea. Exposure to the virus can result from contact with infected birds, especially pigeons; it is therefore not advisable to feed feral or ex-racing pigeons in the vicinity of raptors.

Avian influenza: Avian influenza causes sudden death, sometimes with mild pancreatitis apparent on post-mortem examination. Typically, the virus is acquired by eating or close proximity to infected waterfowl, seagulls or domestic poultry and thus control is by avoiding contact with susceptible species.

Avian pox: Infection with avian poxvirus causes exudative and proliferative lesions, typically on the cere, eyelids or feet. Exposure to the virus is via biting insects or other causes of skin abrasion. Whilst avian pox is not currently common in raptors (unlike some other garden species) in the UK, with global warming and the spread of biting insects an increased incidence is predicted. See also Chapter 30.

West Nile virus: As yet, West Nile virus is not a problem in the UK (although nor was it in the USA prior to 1999); however, a major epidemic could yet occur. Affected birds show depression, anorexia, weight loss, leucocytosis, head tremors, central blindness, ataxia, incoordination, marked fever, flaccid paralysis, detached retinas, severe tremors, seizures, and death. The virus is acquired by eating infected food, close contact with infected birds or transfer by biting insects (mosquito and hippoboscid flies). Surveillance and vigilance are required in the prevention of disease and this virus can affect humans. Disease prevention is by control of biting insects.

Falcon herpesvirus: Falcon herpesvirus affects falcons only. Birds become acutely sick and die within 3 to 5 days. White foci are seen in the liver at post-mortem examination. Almost inevitably an affected falcon will have eaten a fresh or frozen infected pigeon within the previous 10 days. Pigeons are carriers and are not affected by the virus; pigeons should not be fed in the vicinity of falcons.

Owl herpesvirus: Owl herpesvirus affects only owls. Birds become acutely sick, with white foci in the dorsal pharynx and in the liver on endoscopy or post-mortem examination. The disease is acquired by close contact with infected birds or by feeding on infected avian-derived food. There is a higher incidence in owls admitted to wildlife rehabilitation units compared with captive owls. Control of the disease is by vigilance and good biosecurity between admitted wildlife cases.

Adenovirus: Adenovirus infection results in acute death, on occasions with effects of end-arterial damage and extravasation resulting in haemorrhage in the myocardium, into the gut, pancreas or other internal organs. Avian-derived food (e.g. quail, turkey grown-ons or day-old chicks) will commonly be contaminated with adenovirus. Each adenovirus is typically only pathogenic to one or at most two species of host. The virus is not inactivated by freezing and prevention is by avoiding feeding avian-derived food.

Bacterial infections

Even if the primary cause for admission is trauma, it is common for such patients to be suffering concurrent bacterial or fungal infection. Traumatic wounds may have become infected, in which case swellings or exudates are likely to be apparent, and samples should be collected for cytology and culture and sensitivity testing. Systemic infection is broadly divided into respiratory, gastrointestinal, urogenital and septicaemic. Lateral and dorsoventral survey radiographs of all sick and traumatized raptor patients will assist in locating areas of pathology. In all situations samples should be recovered for cytology (e.g. oral, aural, pharyngeal, crop smear, faecal smear, choana, sinus or tracheal or air sac smear), which will often indicate whether infection is bacterial, fungal or mixed. If infection is present samples should be submitted for culture and sensitivity testing. Therapy may be commenced pending results. In the interim, analgesia, fluid therapy, antiparasitic and antimicrobial medication, and nutritional support is essential (see 'Therapeutics'). Haematology is invaluable to assess degrees of active infection (indicated by a leucocytosis), anaemia (and whether it is regenerative or not), and biochemistry for assessment of major organ function (e.g. liver, kidney), degrees of tissue damage (aspartate aminotransferase, lactate dehydrogenase, creatine kinase), and metabolic response and resilience (albumin, globulin, calcium and glucose levels).

Chronic leucocytosis is most commonly associated with tuberculosis, aspergillosis and, on occasions, chlamydiosis. Tuberculosis should be considered in thin debilitated birds with concurrent severe leucocytosis, which fail to respond to antibiosis. White liver lesions on endoscopy or post-mortem examination are suggestive and can be confirmed on histopathology. Tuberculosis cases should be euthanased as their prognosis is poor and they pose a zoonotic risk to handlers.

Fungal infections

Primary fungal infection (in particular aspergillosis) in previously free-living healthy raptors is very rare. Disease tends to occur either when birds are maintained in environments with excessive spore loadings (e.g. in old stables, where hay has or is being used), downwind from any decaying or damp vegetable material (e.g. hay stores, hay being made or dried prior to baling, compost heaps, green wood chips used on aviary floors or equine menages, decaying leaves in or on aviaries). Alternatively, clinical disease can occur in birds (especially in northern goshawk, golden eagle (*Aquila chrysaetos*), snowy owl (*Bubo scandiacus*), or non-indigenous species such as gyrfalcons (*Falco rusticolus*), juvenile red-tailed hawks (*Buteo jamaicensis*)) which, despite being in a clean environment, have stress-induced immunosuppression that means they can no longer cope with normal levels of spore exposure. Diagnosis is based on clinical signs (loss or change of voice, loss of appetite and increased green discoloration of the faeces, or marked dyspnoea and oral cyanosis on handling) and diagnostics (tracheoscopy, radiography, coelomic endoscopy and haematology). Once diagnosed, treatment is not justified in wildlife casualty cases (in respect of prognosis for long-term release, duration of therapy and welfare implications).

Parasites

It is stated that 65–85% of free-living raptors have a parasitic burden, typically causing minimal or limited health concerns (Smith, 1993). However, once a bird is injured or debilitated and admitted into care, the host–parasite relationship may alter resulting in the parasite causing clinical disease and, despite other therapy, will result in the eventual demise of the patient. As such, all admitted wildlife casualties should be screened (see Chapter 10) and where parasites are present, treated for endo-, ecto- and haemoparasites. The latter should always take place before the patient is released into aviary accommodation to ensure that the aviary is not contaminated and that subsequent patients are not put at additional risk of exposure. Treatments for common parasitic infections are given in Figure 29.17.

Ectoparasites:

Ticks: The tick *Ixodes frontalis* is a common cause of morbidity and mortality in wild, cage and aviary birds. Disease is seasonal, with 75% of cases occurring in August and September. Ticks always attach around the head and neck and, on occasions, birds are presented with a telltale area of subcutaneous haemorrhage in this area. In untreated patients, mortality is around 50%. In the author's experience, pathogenicity in all sick birds has been controlled with systemic oxytetracyclines (Monks *et al.*, 2006). Despite great efforts, this pathogen has not yet been identified, but the excellent response to oxytetracycline proves there to be one. Other pathogens (viruses or bacteria), which are not oxytetracycline responsive, might also be transmitted. Treatment with topical fipronil is advised on all at-risk birds and permethrin and pyripoxifen should be used for treatment of the immediate environment.

Mites: A number of mites may affect raptors. *Dermanyssus gallinae* commonly infests housing/aviaries, leading to irritation, feather loss and, in some situations, anaemia. Affected birds should be treated topically with fipronil, and housing with permethrin and pyripoxifen. *Ornithonyssus sylviarum* is a common infestation of housing/aviaries. It is only necessary to treat the birds.

Quill mites (*Dermoglyphus* spp.) cause feather loss and irritation. All in-contact birds should be treated with ivermectin.

Cnemidocoptes spp. are occasionally seen in raptors, typically causing hypertrophy of the cere and chronic inflammation. All in-contact birds should be treated with ivermectin (see Figure 29.17).

Feather lice: Infestation with *Mallophaga* spp. may cause feather loss or damage, or irritation. In-contact birds should be treated with topical fipronil.

Flat flies: As well as causing irritation, *Hippoboscidae* spp. can transmit haemoparasites (e.g. *Haemoproteus* spp.) and viruses (e.g. West Nile virus). In-contact birds should be treated with topical fipronil.

Myiasis: Myiasis due to dipterous (blow fly) larvae is not uncommon in raptor wildlife casualties between May and October in the UK. The bird should be treated for toxaemia with fluid therapy and covering antibiosis, wounds should be appropriately managed and F10® Germicidal Wound Spray with Insecticide spray applied.

Endoparasites:

Ascarids (gut active): Ascarid spp. are the largest nematodes to infect raptors and are generally located in the proventriculus, ventriculus or small intestine. Most commonly pathogenic in juvenile birds, control is a particular problem in earth-floored aviaries. Treatment is with oral fenbendazole (see Figure 29.17).

Spirurid spp. are found in the mucosa and sub-mucosa of the proventriculus and ventriculus.

Capillariidae are common and highly pathogenic worms that are found in the mouth (tongue), pharynx, oesophagus and intestine. The clinical appearance may be confused with trichomonosis. Capillariidae have characteristic bioperculate ova. The life cycle may be direct or indirect via earthworms (Annelida), and they are a very common parasite of species that commonly eat earthworms (e.g. buzzards and kites), especially during winter months. Treatment without treating all birds in a group, together with environmental decontamination and prevention of access by earthworms, is pointless. Fenbendazole or avermectins (e.g. ivermectin) are effective (see Figure 29.17).

Visceral nematodes: Trichinella spp. are occasionally found in the muscles of carnivorous birds who have ingested infected food items. Avermectins (e.g. ivermectin) or fenbendazole are effective in its treatment (see Figure 29.17).

Respiratory nematodes: Also known as gapeworm, *Syngamus trachea* (see Figure 30.10) is a common parasite in wild raptors. It has both a direct life cycle and an indirect lifecycle via earthworms. It is most common in wildlife and aviary birds living in earth-floored aviaries. Birds often present with loss or change of voice, inspiratory or expiratory stridor and exercise intolerance. Treatment is with oral fenbandazole (see Figure 29.17) and by environmental and intermediate host control.

Serratospiculum spp. are rare in the UK, but have a 65% incidence in wild falcons in the Middle East. Worms are located in air sacs and on the surface of viscera, and in heavy numbers may cause exercise intolerance. With global warming and spread of insect intermediate hosts, incidence may increase in the UK. Treatment is with ivermectin (see Figure 29.17).

Cyathostoma spp. larvae are present in the trachea and coughed into cranial sinuses, where sinus filling and abscessation may occur; they are most common in sparrowhawks and kestrels.

Cestodes (tapeworms): Cestode infestation is rare in raptors and it is unusual for cestodes to be pathogenic. Praziquantel can be used for treatment if required (see Figure 29.17).

Trematodes (fluke): Various trematodes can infest raptors. They are relatively common and diagnosis is by demonstrating ova on a direct faecal smear (see Chapter 10). Trematode ova tend to be larger than those of nematodes, with a single operculum at one pole. Praziquantel is an effective treatment (see Figure 29.17).

Protozoa: Trichomonas spp. are a common finding in wildlife casualties. Typically they are associated with dysphagia, weight loss and general weakness and white necrotic lesions may be found in the mouth. Diagnosis can only be made on fresh, warm saline mount examination of a buccal cavity smear for directionally motile organisms (see Chapter 10). Trichomonosis is most common in raptors that eat pigeons (e.g. peregine and goshawk). Clazuril or metronidazole can be used to treat affected birds (see Figure 29.17).

Caryospora spp. are coccidian parasites that very commonly (65% incidence in first year) affect captive falcons, are rare in owls and very rare in other genera. They are found only rarely in wildlife, which are typically infected when passaging through rescue accommodation. *Caryospora* are differentiated from other coccidia by having eight sporozoites in the sporocyst. Infection is a common cause of lethargy, exercise intolerance and occasionally diarrhoea, sometimes with blood. Affected birds may be treated with toltrazuril that can be diluted with acidic soft drinks to reduce vomiting.

Cryptosporidium spp. are a rare aetiology for ocular, respiratory and auditory pathology in falcons and owls. Clinical signs are those of general inflammation. Diagnosis is made on cytology or histopathology, which may be confirmed with polymerase chain reaction (PCR). Treatment may be attempted with paromomycin and or azithromycin.

Haemoparasites: Plasmodium spp. (causing malaria) are most commonly seen in gyrfalcons and snowy owls, both of which are rare migrants to the UK, but can be seen in other raptors. Birds are presented weak, anaemic and in respiratory distress and there may also be other concurrent infections. Parasites are apparent on blood smears, and erythrocyte nuclei are pushed into an eccentric position. Prevention of disease is by control of mosquito vectors and prophylactic medication with a combination of chloroquin and primaquin or mefloquin alone from 1 month before to 1 month after the anticipated risk season.

Haemoproteus spp. may be spread from avian prey species to the raptor host by hippoboscid flies. Birds are presented weak, anaemic, in respiratory distress, and there may be other concurrent infections. Parasites are apparent on blood smears as circular or curved structures within the cytoplasm of erythrocytes, without changing the position of the nucleus. Treatment can be attempted using a combination of chloroquine and primaquine, or mefloquine (see Figure 29.17); however, the efficacy of these drugs is questionable.

Other conditions
Starvation or exhaustion

This occurs most commonly at dispersal time (when young birds hatched earlier in the year leave the natal territory), on return from migration, or after any period of extreme weather. Birds presented are weak, in poor body condition (i.e. very prominent keel bones; see Figure 4.6) and are often also dehydrated, without any apparent traumatic injuries. They may have secondary or concurrent infections or parasitic infestations. These are acceptable situations for exhaustion and cases will respond well to short-term nutritional support. However, one must question why the patient has become exhausted, and any factor compromising normal eyesight, flight, hunting, killing and eating needs to be evaluated, and, if possible, addressed. Careful reassessment prior to release to ensure post-release viability is essential.

Therapeutics

All readers would be urged to refer to a current exotic animal formulary, as interspecific variations are significant, and correct and accurate therapeutics are vitally important (see also Chapter 7). Therapeutic agents commonly used in wild raptor casualties are given in Figure 29.17. Wherever possible, appropriate culture and sensitivity testing should be conducted, and drug use based on the findings.

Drug	Dosage	Notes
Antibiotics		
Amikacin	10–20 mg/kg i.m., s.c. q12–24h for 5–7 days[a]	Only administer in patients where good hydration can be assured Only use where sensitivity mandates, typically for control of *Pseudomonas* spp. and other resistant organisms On occasions given with piperacillin or ticarcillin
Azithromycin	10–50 mg/kg orally q24–48h, 7 days maximum[b]	Useful where sensitivity indicates efficacy
Amoxicillin/ clavulanate (co-amoxiclav)	125–150 mg/kg i.m., orally q12h for 5–7 days[c]	In the author's experience, some proprietary makes tend to cause emesis in raptors (e.g. Synulox™), whilst others (e.g. Clavaseptin® or Noroclav™) do not
Cefalexin	40–100 mg/kg orally q8h for 5–7 days[d]	First-generation cephalosporin, active against Gram-positive and Gram-negative bacteria, *Proteus* spp., *Escherichia* coli, but not *Pseudomonas* spp., useful for *Staphylococcus* spp.
Clindamycin	50 mg/kg orally q12h for 5–14 days[e]	Good for Gram-positive bacteria (e.g. *Staphylococcus* spp. and *Streptococcus* spp.) and anaerobes
Fusidic acid	Topically	Aqueous preparation does not cause feather damage (unlike oily based preparations)
Marbofloxacin	5–10 mg/kg i.m., orally q24h or q12h for 5–14 days[f]	Preferred fluoroquinolone as does not cause emesis (after oral or i.m. administration) in raptors unlike enrofloxacin

29.17 Therapeutic agents and their dose rates commonly used in raptor wildlife casualites. (continues) ▶
([a] Bloomfield *et al.*, 1997; [b] Dorrestein, 2000; [c] Forbes, 1991; [d] Bailey and Apo, 2008; [e] Flammer, 2002; [f] Garcia-Montijano *et al.*, 2003; [g] Bauck and Hoefer, 1993; [h] Beynon *et al.*, 1996; [i] Olsen *et al.*, 1996; [j] Redig, 1996; [k] Jones *et al.*, 2000; [l] Dahlhausen *et al.*, 2000; [m] Di Somma *et al.*, 2007; [n] Huckabee, 2000; [o] Ritchie and Harrison, 1994; [p] Massey and Work, 2000; [q] Joseph, 1995; [r] Samour and Naldo, 2005; [s] Samour *et al.*, 2005; [t] Mutlow and Forbes, 2000; [u] Forbes, 2008; [v] Tarello, 2007)

Drug	Dosage	Notes
Antibiotics (continued)		
Metronidazole	50 mg/kg orally q24h[g]	Useful for trichomonosis, also where anaerobic infections are present
Oxytetracycline	50–100 mg/kg orally q12h for 5–10 days[h]	For tick pyaemia
Piperacillin	100 mg/kg i.m. q24h up to 7 days[i]	May be used synergistically with amikacin
Trimethoprim sulphur	12–60 mg/kg orally q12h for 5–10 days[h]	Often causes emesis Only use where there is no alternative
Tylosin	15–30 mg/kg i.m. q12h for 5–7 days[h]	Indicated where *Mycoplasma* infections are present
Antiemetic, prokinetic agent		
Metoclopramide	0.5–2 mg/kg i.v., i.m., s.c., orally q12h[j]	Useful in vomiting birds
Antifungal agents		
Itraconazole	10 mg/kg orally q12h for 60 days[k]	Stated to be only effective against 65% of serotypes, although the first avian licensed version 'Fungitraxx, Avimedical' is shown to have 27 x bioavilability in the air sac and be far more efficacious
Terbinafine	10–15 mg/kg orally q12h for 6–8 weeks[l]	Alternative aspergillosis treatment
Voriconazole	10–18 mg/kg orally q12h for 60 day[m]	Gold standard aspergillosis treatment, although extremely expensive
Antiparasitic agents		
Azithromycin	40 mg/kg q24h orally for 15 days[b]	For treatment of *Cryptosporidium*
Carnidazole	20–50 mg/kg orally for 2 days, repeat 1 week[n]	For treatment of *Trichomonas* spp. (effective and convenient tablet form of medication)
Chloroquine	20 mg/kg i.v., orally at 6, 18 and 24 hours then once weekly for 3–5 treatments	For the treatment of *Haemoproteus* spp., use with primaquine or mefloquine
	25 mg/kg orally, then 15 mg/kg at 12, 24, 48 hours[o]	For the treatment of malaria (*Plasmodium* spp.). Can be given once weekly in anticipation of malarial risk season
Diclazuril	5–10 mg/kg orally once, repeat after 1 week[p]	For the treatment of Coccidia
Fenbendazole	50 mg/kg orally (single dose)	Effective against standard nematodes Shake bottle well before dispensing or drawing up to administer
	15–20 mg/kg orally once daily for 5 days, for treatment of Capillariidae[q]	Always perform faecal check 2–3 weeks later to verify efficacy Also manage environment to prevent re-infection
Fipronil	3 ml (of spray) per kg, topical application on to skin[d]	For the treatment of ectoparasites Do not enclose in poorly ventilated area until dry Use for surface parasites
Imidocarb	5–7 mg/kg orally once repeat in 7 days[r]	For treatment of *Babesia* spp., of dubious efficacy
Ivermectin	200 µg/kg i.m., s.c., orally for standard nematode burdens 1 mg/kg i.m., s.c., orally and repeat 1 week later for Capillariidae or *Serratospiculum* spp. Retest after treating the latter to ensure efficacy	Environmental cleaning will also be required when dealing with *Syngamus* spp., ascarids and Capillariidae
	200 µg/kg s.c., orally repeated 3 times at weekly intervals[s]	For burrowing or quill mites
Mefloquine	50 mg/kg orally q24h for 7 days	In combination with chloroquine for *Haemoproteus*, or alone for *Plasmodium*
	15–30 mg/kg orally, repeat at 12, 24, 48 hours then weekly[t]	For treatment of malaria (*Plasmodium* spp.) Can be given once weekly in anticipation of malarial risk season
Metronidazole	50 mg/kg orally q24h for 5 days[g]	For treatment of *Trichomonas* spp.
Paromomycin	100 mg/kg orally q12h for 7 days[u]	Most efficacious agent for *Cryptosporidium* infection
Praziquantel	5–10 mg/kg s.c., orally once[n]	Fluke and tapeworms
Primaquine	10 mg/kg at 0 hrs, then 5 mg/kg at 6, 24 and 48 hours[v]	Treatment of haemoparasites, see also chloroquin and mefloquin Challenging to treat, exclude mosquitos where possible and always study blood smear to estimate if a transfusion is indicated
Pyrimethamine	0.5–1 mg/kg orally q12h for 14–30 days[d]	Treatment of *Atoxoplasma* spp., *Leucocytozoon* spp., *Plasmodium* spp., *Toxoplasma* spp., *Sarcocystis* spp.
Toltrazuril	7–15 mg/kg orally daily for 3 days, repeat after 1 week[q]	Treatment of coccidia. Dilute 50:50 with coca cola immediately before administration (as the preparation is strongly alkaline which can otherwise cause regurgitation)
Trimethoprim sulphur	20–50 mg/kg orally q24h for 3 days, no treatment 2 days, repeat 3 days[d]	Treatment of coccidia Useful if no other anticoccidials in stock

29.17 (continued) Therapeutic agents and their dose rates commonly used in raptor wildlife casualites.
([a]Bloomfield *et al.*, 1997; [b]Dorrestein, 2000; [c]Forbes, 1991; [d]Bailey and Apo, 2008; [e]Flammer, 2002; [f]Garcia-Montijano *et al.*, 2003; [g]Bauck and Hoefer, 1993; [h]Beynon *et al.*, 1996; [i]Olsen *et al.*, 1996; [j]Redig, 1996; [k]Jones *et al.*, 2000; [l]Dahlhausen *et al.*, 2000; [m]Di Somma *et al.*, 2007; [n]Huckabee, 2000; [o]Ritchie and Harrison, 1994; [p]Massey and Work, 2000; [q]Joseph, 1995; [r]Samour and Naldo, 2005; [s]Samour *et al.*, 2005; [t]Mutlow and Forbes, 2000; [u]Forbes, 2008; [v]Tarello, 2007)

For antibacterials the author favours the use of marbofloxacin or amoxicillin/clavulanate (co-amoxiclav). The choice of product is important as some proprietary makes cause raptors to vomit whilst others do not (see Figure 29.17); likewise enrofloxacin (i.m. or orally), tends to cause vomition, whilst marbofloxacin does not.

As a general rule of thumb therapeutic products with the suffix 'aine' should not be administered to birds, this includes procaine penicillin, benzocaine and lidocaine. Particular care is required when licensed human or veterinary products are used, which contain such products as trace ingredients: a single application of such a product will often prove fatal.

It is vital that appropriate nutritional and fluid support is given, as injured wild raptors cannot be expected to eat or drink when first in captivity. If food and fluid is provided by gavage (typically 3–5 times daily), most medication may be simply added to this. Once a wildlife casualty raptor is eating voluntarily in captivity, then medication may often be buried inside mouth-sized parcels of meat.

Management in captivity

Housing

After initial critical care and support, as well as disease screening, raptors should be transferred into aviary accommodation and contact with handlers and all other associations with captivity should be minimized (see Chapter 9). A recovering or long-term invalid wild raptor cannot be kept in either a wildlife rescue centre or falconry centre, unless appropriate APHA licences are in place (see 'Legal aspects'). The aviary should be designed such that injuries to the bird do not occur (e.g. cere, beak, cranium, feet or plumage). Wildlife casualty birds, when enclosed in aviaries, are likely to traumatize themselves by flying into aviary walls. Battens of electrician's conduit piping or similar should be attached vertically inside the aviary fence (along the sides and if necessary the roof), set far enough apart to allow the bird's head through, but not its shoulders. This will prevent contact between the bird and the fence and hence prevent trauma. Mixed species aviaries are contraindicated. Groups of the same species generally work well, with the exception of more aggressive species (e.g. northern goshawk).

Aviaries should be designed and managed to prevent build-up of pathogenic bacteria or parasites. A solid impervious floor (concrete or thick plastic sheet covered in pea gravel or sand), which drains (but not into adjacent aviaries), so that it can be routinely cleaned down to an impervious surface, is important. Injured wild birds, with a range of infectious and contagious conditions, are processed through a rescue system, which other patients will follow through shortly afterwards, prior to hopefully being released back to the wild. It is vital that the infectious and contagious conditions present at admission are controlled, so that patients do not become exposed to, infected with, or released back to their own ecosystems with, novel infections that could put not only them, but also their ecosystem as a whole, at risk (see also Chapter 1). Good records, detailing which birds have been in which aviaries during what periods, are vital, so that retrospective investigations of potential exposure to infectious disease can be made. Decaying vegetable material, for example hay (made or stored damp), compost heaps, shredded wood bark and decaying leaves on aviary roofs, are all potential sources of aspergillosis, to which raptors are particularly susceptible. Risk is created not only by sources in and about the aviary, but may also be spread by the wind for distances over several hundred metres. Such sources should be avoided or eliminated.

It is important for veterinary surgeons to work closely with local rehabilitators and forge good working relationships. The author recommends visiting local rehabilitation facilities in order to ensure that the facility is providing a suitable level of care and biosecurity and to offer any necessary advice and support. The practice should work together with the rehabilitator, rather than just transferring patients to the rehabilitation facility and assuming the rehabilitation of that animal subsequently progresses well.

Feather condition

Whilst anyone may take in a wildlife casualty to tend its needs, they are legally obliged to avoid any consequences that will prevent or delay its return back to the wild. If feathers are damaged, the bird is likely to be unreleasable until after the subsequent annual moult. Prevention of feather damage is achieved by keeping accommodation clean, careful handling, subdued lighting, provision of a perch (to keep tail and primary feather tips off the floor), and application of a tail guard (see 'Short-term housing' and Figure 29.11). In the event that a small number of flight feathers are damaged, the traditional falconry technique of 'imping' can be used to replace broken feathers with second-hand feathers from another bird, to facilitate normal flight. The broken feather is cut off some 1–2 cm from its insertion into the skin. A replacement feather (same species, wing and feather number), is trimmed to size. A small length of bamboo, aluminium knitting needle or fibreglass fishing rod blank, is trimmed to size and glued into the replacement feather. Glue is then placed inside the stump in the wing, and the replacement feather is pushed into the feather calamus in the wing. The correct alignment of the feather vein is assured before the glue sets.

Perches

Fancy commercial raptor perches are not needed; perches may be as simple and basic as a towel over a wooden or stone block. They must, however, be easy to keep clean and be of suitable material to prevent excessive pressure sores developing on the plantar aspect of the feet. Cork, corrugated rubber (e.g. some car footwell mats), carpet, rope or artificial grass are all suitable substrates.

Observation

It is beneficial to provide casualty raptors with visual seclusion; however, it is also highly advantageous to be able to observe birds, without them being aware you are present. The use of one-way glass observation windows or closed circuit television (CCTV) (see Chapter 9) is to be recommended.

Records

The taking and/or keeping of birds of prey from the wild is subject to potential abuse. It is important that full details of all admissions (rescuer details, address, contact phone number, date, time and location of rescue, as well as circumstances involved) must be recorded and stored (see also Chapter 3). The provenance of a bird (or any derivative of it, e.g. feathers or eggshell, potentially years after the bird's death from old age), may be relied upon in court, where, under the Wildlife and Countryside Act 1981, it is the defendant's responsibility to prove legitimate possession, rather than the prosecution's obligation to prove guilt. Which aviaries a bird has been in should also be recorded (see 'Housing'). Some form of identification (e.g. British Trust for Ornithology (BTO) ring) should be placed prior to release, so that post-release survival rates can be monitored (see 'Release' and Chapter 9).

Diet

Any practice that accepts wildlife casualties must have available at all times suitable diets to meet the emergency needs of any patient, irrespective of species and normal diet. A wildlife casualty should never be left to feed themselves after initial admission; the stress of injury and illness, combined with the sights and sounds of captivity, render this unlikely to occur. Initial gavage feeding is essential in most cases (see 'Short-term feeding'). It is possible to maintain or increase raptor wildlife patients' weight and body condition, using suitable volumes and frequencies of feeding. Once the bird's condition is improved and it may eat voluntarily, a skinned whole carcass diet is provided (e.g. skinned chicks or rodents), which can be stored frozen in readiness for such patients. Regular small meals are provided several times a day, and casting (fur and feather), is withheld until the patient's weight and condition is acceptable when once a day feeding is necessary (see 'Short-term feeding').

Rearing of young raptors

Young raptors should rarely be reared individually. Instead, if possible, they should either be placed back in their own nest to be parent-reared, or should be nest-reared under alternative free-living or captive (same or similar species) foster parents. If these options are not available then they may be crèche-reared with other young of the same species. Individual hand-rearing of young birds (<15 days old), even for a few days, is likely to result in 'malprinting', which will preclude later return to the wild (see also Chapter 9).

Release

Assessment for release

An initial assessment of a bird's flight ability and behaviour can be made in an aviary; however, the most reliable way to verify that the bird can see, fly, hunt, kill and eat well enough to survive in the wild is to train it using conventional falconry techniques, to the point where it is fit enough to survive post-release, or alternatively one is certain that this will not be possible. As birds regain fitness, body fat stores are utilized and muscle tone develops. Manoeuvrability and stamina increase daily, so long as the bird is given the opportunity to fly regularly. Wind tunnels, large hack aviaries (see 'Hacking') and traditional falconry training techniques (such as flying to the fist, lure or at wild quarry) are all appropriate methods of fitness training and release preparation (see 'Fitness training' and Chapter 9). Keeping a bird in a 2 m x 3 m aviary for 6–8 weeks, then simply releasing it back into the wild, is not appropriate.

Each method has its own inherent advantages and disadvantages; each has its place and optimal suitability in different situations and different patient categories.

Patients for release can be divided as follows:

- Adult bird, experienced hunter; hospitalized for 4–6 weeks; in good body condition: this bird may be released with limited assessment of fitness or ability to hunt
- Adult bird, experienced hunter; more than 8 weeks in captivity; in fair body condition: this bird will require extensive fitness training prior to release
- Young bird, inexperienced at flight or hunting; less than 6 weeks in captivity; in good body condition: this bird will require extensive flight training and proof of ability to hunt and kill prior to release. Release is best effected using traditional falconry training techniques.

Fitness training

Adult and juvenile birds that have not hunted for themselves are best trained and flown at wild quarry. Once the bird is killing proficiently it may be released, preferably leaving it on its last kill, with all furniture (bells, jesses, etc.) removed. Where possible this fitness training should be carried out in the area of intended release. The bird is initially assessed and then continually reassessed on a daily basis for release. It is only released when its performance is optimal. Alternatively, birds may be flown to the lure (falcons), or fist (hawks and broad wings) to feed. Once habituated to feeding in this way, the bird may be released into its new environment, without bells and jesses. The falconer/rehabilitator will continue to visit daily to feed the bird (using lure or glove as appropriate), until the bird is no longer returning for food. The downside of this technique is that the bird is becoming increasingly conditioned to come to a human for food.

Hacking: 'Hacking' is a term referring to the release back to the wild of a raptor from an aviary. A hard hack involves allowing the bird to observe its new surroundings for some days prior to a sudden release, whilst in a soft hack, the bird is accustomed to eating food from an elevated platform prior to release, but food continues to be tied down to the same platform after release, and provided daily until the bird no longer comes back to take it.

Hack aviaries may be permanent or collapsible, portable structures. Anyone constantly releasing in one location (a permanent hack aviary), is likely over time to excessively populate that area. Moreover, a single location (in respect of habitat suitability) will not be appropriate for all species, so a prefabricated, portable structure has great advantages. The aviary is erected within the intended release environment. The aviary should be of reasonable size, so the bird is gaining some exercise prior to release. Food is provided within the aviary, tied down to a board (so that the bird has to consume it at the site, rather than the patient or some other animal carrying it away to eat elsewhere) and preferably high up, in a position with good all round visibility. Once the bird appears settled in this location, the front of the aviary immediately adjacent to the food ledge is removed, so that the bird can come and go as it wishes. Food is still supplied daily, tied down to the board as previously, until such time as the bird no longer comes back for food.

Habitat selection

If the bird can be released back to the wild within 14 days of injury, then it may go back to its own territory. In general terms, unless individual assessment dictates (e.g. the pair are known and monitored and no alternate mate has moved in during the interim period), if captivity has lasted more than 14 days a new location for release should be found.

The habitat selected for release must fall within the natural range, terrain and vegetation for the species being released and there be evidence of availability of required natural feed species. One should also consider if that location might already be overpopulated, or if conflict with another species (e.g. corvids) might adversely affect the patient's chance of successful release. The location should be free from adverse risks, for example proximity to wind farms and major trunk roads.

Timing of release

Any carer is obliged to release a patient as soon as it is fit for release, in a suitable location, provided that the season is correct (i.e. not immediately prior to or after migration, not at a time of adverse weather), when suitable natural food supplies are available. The current and anticipated weather conditions must be suitable and the time of day appropriate (i.e. owls are released at dusk, diurnal birds at dawn).

Post-release monitoring

Observation at the nest, roost, plucking post (most raptors will after hunting, habitually pluck quarry on a particular post, if this can be identified, the presence of daily plucking is evidence of successful hunting). Telemetry (terrestrial or satellite) and BTO rings may all be used to monitor raptor wildlife cases following release (see also Chapter 9). Faecal and casting (pellet) assessment can sometimes be used to assess proficiency of hunting.

Legal aspects

Any member of the public is permitted to take into care any wild animal, in order to relieve suffering or tend its injuries, until such time as it is fit for release. During the period of care they may not withhold any treatment or professional care that would assist or speed the time of release, or allow the animal to suffer, or fail to provide good husbandry, or permit anything to happen to prevent or delay release. Species listed in Schedule 4 of the Wildlife and Countryside Act (WCA) 1981, that require registration with APHA are at the time of writing:

- Golden eagle (*Aquila chrysaetos*)
- White-tailed sea eagle (*Haliaeetus albicilla*)
- Osprey (*Pandion haliaetus*)
- Northern goshawk (*Accipiter gentilis*)
- Peregrine (*Falco peregrinus*)
- Merlin (*Falco columbarius*)
- Honey buzzard (*Pernis apivorus*)
- Marsh harrier (*Circus aeruginosus*)
- Montagu's harrier (*Circus pygargus*)

Any person taking into care a Schedule 4 species for rehabilitation is advised to register that bird with APHA as soon as it comes into care. Vets keeping birds for the purpose of treatment may do so for 6 weeks without registration but, once moved for rehabilitation, registration is necessary. APHA will aim to visit the keeper and ensure that rehabilitation is taking place to an acceptable standard. Where APHA is requested to issue an Article 10 certificate, for a wild disabled individual for breeding and/or educational display purposes, they will only consider doing this in exceptional circumstances where there are genuine conservation benefits to the species. This applies to all CITES Annex A birds of prey, whether listed on Schedule 4 of the WCA or not (see also Chapter 2).

References and further reading

Bailey TA and Apo MM (2008) Pharmaceutics commonly used in avian medicine. In: *Avian Medicine 2nd edn*, ed. JH Samour, pp. 458–509. Mosby Elsevier, Edinburgh

Bauck L and Hoefer HL (1993) Avian antimicrobial therapy. *Seminars in Avian and Exotic Pet Medicine* **2**, 17–22

Beynon PH, Forbes NA and Harcourt-Brown NH (1996) *BSAVA Manual of Raptors, Waterfowl and Pigeons*. BSAVA Publications, Gloucester

Bloomfield RB, Brooks D and Vulliet R (1997) The pharmokinetics of a single intramuscular dose of amikacin in red-tailed hawks (*Buteo jamaicensis*). *Journal of Zoo and Wildlife Medicine* **28**, 55–61

Chitty JR and Lierz M (2008) *BSAVA Manual of Raptors, Pigeons and Passerine Birds*. BSAVA Publications, Gloucester

Coles BH (2005) Diseases of the wing. In: *BSAVA Manual of Psittacine Birds, 2nd edn*, ed. N Harcourt-Brown and JR Chitty. BSAVA Publications, Gloucester

Cooper JE (2001) *Birds of Prey: Health and Disease, 3rd edn*. Blackwell Science, Oxford

Cooper JE and Greenwood AG (1981) *Recent Advances in Raptor Diseases*. Chiron Press, Keighley

Dahlhausen B, Lindstrom JG and Radabaugh CS (2002) The use of terbinafine hydrochloride in the treatment of avian fungal disease. *Proceedings of the Annual Conference of the Association of Avian Veterinarians*

Del Hoyo J, Elliott A and Sargatal J (1994) *Handbook of Birds of the World, Vol 2*. Lynx Ed, Barcelona

Del Hoyo J, Elliott A and Sargatal J (1999) *Handbook of Birds of the World, Vol 5*. Lynx Ed, Barcelona

Desmarchelier M, Troncy E, Fitzgeral G and Lair S (2012) Analgesic effects of meloxicam administration on postoperative orthopaedic pain in domestic pigeons (*Columba livia*). *American Journal of Veterinary Research* **73(3)**, 361–367

Di Somma A, Bailey T, Silvanose C *et al.* (2007) The use of voriconazole for the treatment of aspergillosis in falcons (*Falco* spp.) *Journal of Avian Medicine and Surgery* **21**, 307–316

Dorrestein GM (2000) Passerine and softbill therapeutics. *Veterinary Clinics of North America: Exotic Animal Practice* **3**, 35–57

Flammer K (2002) Treatment of bacterial and mycotic diseases of the avian gastrointestinal tract. *Proceedings of the North American Veterinary Conference*, pp. 851–852

Forbes NA (1991) Birds of prey. In: *BSAVA Manual of Exotics Pets*, ed. PH Beynon and JE Cooper, pp. 212–220. BSAVA Publications, Gloucester

Forbes NA (1999) Avian Anaesthesia. In: *BSAVA Manual of Small Animal Anaesthesia and Analgesia*, ed. C Seymour and R Gleed, pp. 283–294. BSAVA Publications, Gloucester

Forbes NA (2008) Raptors: parasitic diseases. In: *BSAVA Manual of Raptors, Pigeons and Passerines*, ed. J Chitty and M Lierz, pp. 202–211. BSAVA Publications, Gloucester

Forbes NA (2014) Avian Orthopaedic Surgery. In: *Proceedings, Veterinary Medicine for Falconry into the 21st century, Qatar, 29th Jan–1st Feb 2014*, pp. 39–43

Garcia-Montijano M, Gonzales F, Waxman S *et al.* (2003) Pharmacokinetics of marbofloxacin after oral administration to Eurasian buzzards (*Buteo buteo*). *Journal of Avian Medicine and Surgery* **17**, 185–190

Harcourt-Brown NH (1994) *Diseases of the Pelvic Limb of Birds of Prey*. FRCVS Thesis, RCVS Library

Harcourt-Brown NH (2008) Foot and leg problems. In: *BSAVA Manual of Raptors, Pigeons and Passerine Birds*. BSAVA Publications, Gloucester

Heidenreich M (1997) *Birds of Prey Medicine and Management*. Blackwell Science, Oxford

Helmer P and Redig PT (2006) Orthopaedic disorders. In: *Clinical Avian Medicine Vol II*, ed. GJ Harrison and TL Lightfoot, pp. 761–774. Spix Publishing, Palm Beach

Huckabee JR (2000) Raptor therapeutics. *Veterinary Clinics of North America: Exotic Animal Practice* **3**, 91–116

Janovsky M, Ruf T and Wolfgang Z (2002) Oral administration of tiletamine/zolazepam for the immobilization of the common buzzard (*Buteo buteo*). *Journal of Raptor Research* **36**, 188–193

Jones MP, Orosz SE, Cox SK *et al.* (2000) Pharmacokinetic disposition of itraconazole in red-tailed hawks (*Buteo jamaicensis*). *Journal of Avian Medicine and Surgery* **14**, 15–22

Joseph V (1995) Preventive health programs for falconry birds. *Proceedings of the Annual Conferences of the Associations of Avian Veterinarians*, pp. 171–178

Korbel RT (2000) Disorders of the posterior eye segment in raptors – examination procedures and findings. In: *Raptor Biomedicine III*, ed. JT Lumeij, JD Remple, PT Redig, M Lierz and JE Cooper, pp. 179–193. Zoological Education Network, Lake Worth

Lumeij JT, Remple D, Redig PT, Lierz M and Cooper JE (2000) *Raptor Biomedicine III*. Zoological Education Network, Lake Worth

Martin HD, Brueker KA, Herrick DD and Scherpelz J (1993) Elbow luxations in raptors: a review of 8 cases. In: *Raptor Biomedicine*, ed. PT Redig *et al.*, pp.199–206. University of Minnesota Press, Minneapolis

Massey JG and Work TM (2000) Diclazuril therapy for clinical toxoplasmosis. *Proceedings of the Annual Conference of the Association of Avian Veterinarians*, pp. 29–39

Monks DA, Fisher M and Forbes NA (2006) *Ixodes frontalis* and avian tick related syndrome in the United Kingdom. *Journal of Small Animal Practice* **47(8)**, 451–455

Mullarney K, Svensson L, Zetterstrom D and Grant PJ (1999) *Bird Guide*. Harper Collins, London

Mutlow A and Forbes NA (2000) *Haemoproteus* in raptors: pathogenicity, treatment, and control. *Proceedings of the Annual Association of Avian Veterinarians*, pp. 157–163

Olsen GH, Carpenter JW and Langenberg JA (1996) Medicine and surgery. In: *Cranes: Their Biology, Husbandry, and Conservation*, ed. DH Ellis, GF Gee and CM Mirande, pp. 142–143. National Biological Service/International Crane Foundation, Washington

Orosz SE, Ensley PK and Haynes CJ (1992) *Avian Surgical Anatomy: Thoracic and Pelvic Limbs*. WB Saunders, Philadelphia

Redig PT (1996) Nursing avian patients. In: *BSAVA Manual of Raptors, Waterfowl and Pigeons*, pp. 30–41. BSAVA Publications, Gloucester

Redig PT and Ponder J (2016) Orthopaedic surgery. In: *Avian Medicine, 3rd edn*, ed. J Samour, pp. 312–358. Elsevier, Edinburgh

Riggs SM, Hawkins MG, Craigmill AL *et al.* (2008) Pharmacokinetics of butorphan tartrate in red-tailed hawks (*Buteo jamaicensis*) and great horned owl (*Bubo virginianus*). *American Journal of Veterinary Research* **59**, 596–603

Ritchie BW and Harrison GJ (1994) Formulary. In: *Avian Medicine: Principles and Applications*, ed. BW Ritchie, GJ Harrison and LR Harrison, pp. 457–478. Wingers, Lake Worth

Samour JH and Naldo J (2001) Serratospiculiasis in captive falcons in the Middle East: a review. *Journal of Avian Medicine and Surgery* **15**, 2–9

Samour JH, Naldo JL and John SK (2005) Therapeutic management of *Babesia shortii* infection in a peregrine falcon (*Falco peregrinus*). *Journal of Avian Medicine and Surgery* **19**, 294–296

Scheelings TF (2014) Coracoid fractures in wild birds: a comparison of surgical repair versus conservative treatment. *Journal of Avian Medicine and Surgery* **28(4)**, 304–308

Souza MJ and Cox SK (2011) Tramadole use in zoologic medicine. *Veterinary Clinics of North America: Exotic Animal Practice* **14**, 117–130

Tarello W (2007) Clinical signs and response to primaquine in falcons with *Haemoproteus tinnunculi* infection. *Veterinary Record* **161**, 204–206

Wyllie I (1993) *Guide to age and sex in British birds of prey*. Centre for Ecology and Hydrology, Huntingdon

Specialist organizations and useful contacts

See also Appendix 1

Hawk and Owl Trust
UK charity dedicated to conserving owls and other birds of prey in the wild – and increasing knowledge and understanding of them.
c/o Zoological Society of London, Regents Park,
London NW14RY
www.hawkandowl.org

The Hawk Board
Representative body for falconers and bird of prey keepers in the UK
www.hawkboard-cff.co.uk

Raptor Rescue
UK bird of prey rescue and rehabilitation charity
www.raptorrescue.org.uk

Chapter 30

Passerines and other small birds

Becki Lawson and Dick Best

Passerines and allied orders (including cuckoos (*Cuculus canorus*), nightjars (*Caprimulgus europaeus*), swifts (*Apus apus*), kingfishers (*Alcedo atthis*) and woodpeckers (various species)) have been grouped together as 'passerines and other small birds' to form a chapter that will deal, inevitably, with the handling of casualties from a large number of diverse species. Although their natural history in the wild and their husbandry requirements whilst in captivity may differ widely, the approach to their handling and treatment in a veterinary practice or rehabilitation unit is very similar.

Small birds, especially young birds of the common peri-domestic species, form a significant proportion of the total number of wildlife casualties presented at rehabilitation units in Britain. In a survey of a limited number of British wildlife rehabilitation units carried out over a 7-year period, 'small birds' represented approximately 25% of all casualties received (BWRC, 1999).

Species found in the British Isles

Figure 30.1 lists the orders and families of the more commonly encountered 'small birds' that may present to veterinary surgeons (veterinarians) in practice together with information on their diets and habitats.

When faced with a casualty of an unfamiliar species accurate identification is, in the majority of cases, an advantage and may require reference to a field guide or the help of an experienced ornithologist. If identification of the exact species is not possible, at least identification of the family or genus will give some indication of the bird's natural history and, therefore, appropriate husbandry needs. Identification will allow a correct judgement to be made of the natural diet for the species, whether the species is a migrant and, possibly, the age

Order/Family	Diet	Feeding strategy	Resident/migrant	Typical habitat
Cuculiformes				
Cuckoos (Cuculidae)	Insects	Foraging	Summer migrant	Widespread
Apodiformes				
Swifts (Apodidae)	Insects	Aerial feeders	Summer migrant	Widespread, but mainly urban breeding
Coraciiformes				
Kingfisher (Alcedinidae)	Small fish, amphibia	Plunge diving	Resident	Primarily inland waters
Piciformes				
Woodpeckers (Picidae)	Invertebrates	Arboreal, also ground feeding	Resident	Mainly woodland and gardens
Passeriformes				
Crows (Corvidae)	Carrion, nestlings, invertebrates, seeds, fruit	Foraging	Resident	Widespread
Tits (Paridae)	Primarily insects	Foraging	Resident	Widespread
Larks (Alaudidae)	Invertebrates	Ground feeders	Resident/partial migrant	Open grass and farmland
Swallows and martins (Hirundinidae)	Flying insects	Aerial feeders	Summer migrant	Widespread
Warblers (Sylviidae)	Insects, seasonal berries	Foraging	Summer migrant	Woodland, scrub, reed beds

30.1 Taxonomy of British 'small birds', their diets and habitats. (continues) ▶

Order/Family	Diet	Feeding strategy	Resident/migrant	Typical habitat
Passeriformes continued				
Wren (Troglodytidae)	Invertebrates	Foraging	Resident/partial migrant	Widespread
Starling (Sturnidae)	Invertebrates, fruit	Foraging	Resident/partial migrant	Widespread
Thrushes, blackbird, robin (Turdidae)	Invertebrates, berries	Foraging	Resident, partial migrants and winter visitors	Widespread
Flycatchers (Muscicapidae)	Flying insects	Aerial sorties from perch	Summer migrant	Woodland
Dunnock (Prunellidae)	Invertebrates, seeds	Foraging	Resident	Widespread
Sparrows (Passeridae)	Invertebrates, seeds	Foraging	Resident	Widespread, mostly open country
Wagtails and pipits (Motacillidae)	Invertebrates	Ground feeders	Resident and summer migrants	Open land, often close to water
Finches (Fringillidae)	Invertebrates, seeds	Foraging	Resident, winter migrants	Widespread
Buntings (Emberizidae)	Invertebrates, seeds	Foraging	Resident, winter migrants	Widespread, mostly open country

30.1 (continued) Taxonomy of British 'small birds', their diets and habitats.

and sex of the individual; all these facts are important in the development of a realistic strategy for the treatment of the casualty (see Chapter 4).

Identifying nestlings and fledglings

Determination of the approximate age of a young bird will indicate whether it has reached the age of independence or needs to be hand-reared. Nestlings will be partially feathered and, when handled, will normally call and gape widely, revealing a bright yellow mouth (Figure 30.2a). A recently fledged bird might be able to flutter a short distance, will be feathered, with down feathers on the head and back, and usually show a brightly coloured gape-flange in the commissures of the beak (Figure 30.2b).

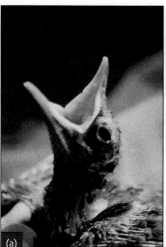 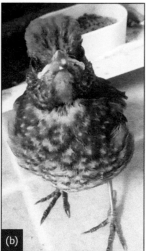

30.2 (a) Nestling blackbird (*Turdus merula*). Nestlings will solicit their parents to feed them by calling and gaping their mouths to expose a brightly coloured mucosa. (b) Fledgling blackbird. Note the down feathers on the head and back, and the brightly coloured gape-flange at the commissures of the beak.
(b, Courtesy of E Keeble)

Ecology and biology

See Figure 30.1 for details of the natural diet, feeding strategies and natural habitats of the more commonly encountered families and genera discussed in this chapter.

Reproduction

At hatching, all juvenile 'small birds' are both altricial (hatch without feathers and with closed eyes) and nidicolous (remain within the nest until they fledge). The breeding strategy of these species is to produce, in each breeding season, large numbers of offspring of which only a few successful individuals will survive. The majority of losses in these offspring are presumed to be caused by exposure, starvation, disease and predation and many young birds that are brought into captivity as casualties are victims of these causes of morbidity and mortality.

Behaviour

Most birds suffering from an illness or disability will, when threatened, adopt an attitude feigning normality. This is a behavioural response to evade predation, as in the wild predators preferentially attack individuals showing weakness or abnormal behaviour. Hence, in captivity, a casualty will make an attempt to appear normal when it feels threatened, for example by human presence. This behaviour, if not recognized, can lead to mistaken assumptions on the condition of a patient and underlines the value of methods of concealed observation, including closed-circuit television (see Chapter 9).

Anatomy and physiology

Anatomy

The anatomical structure of birds in this group varies with the lifestyle of each species. For example, the beak shape varies from fine and narrow in a predominantly insectivorous species to thicker and longer in an omnivorous species or heavy and stubby in a predominantly granivorous species (Figure 30.3).

All birds in the orders covered in this chapter have crops, though in some of the Passeriformes (notably the finches) the crops are located laterally, or even dorsally, at the base of the neck. In these species a crop full of seed may be visible beneath the skin of the dorsal neck and can easily be misidentified as a potential lesion.

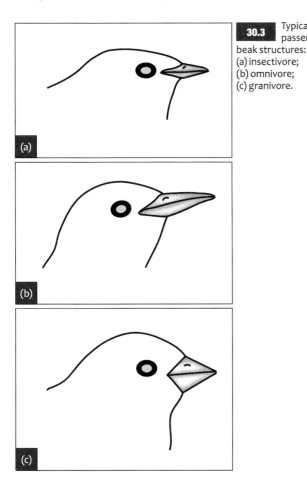

30.3 Typical passerine beak structures: (a) insectivore; (b) omnivore; (c) granivore.

Aerial-feeding birds have relatively long, thin wings, whereas most other small birds have short rounded wings. Most perching species have a typical configuration of the digits with three forward-facing toes and a single hind toe (anisodactyl); climbing species, notably woodpeckers, have the second and third digits facing forward and the first and fourth digits facing backwards (zygodactyl) (Figure 30.4).

Physiology

A significant feature of all small animals is their low bodyweight in relation to their total body surface and the associated high metabolic rate and thermoneutral range (see Chapter 5). The physiological effects of stress on a captive wild animal must not be discounted, especially in the case of small birds. Stress, due to a combination of confinement, proximity of potential predators, disease or injury will cause an elevation of circulating corticosteroids. This might lead to reduced immunocompetence and, through gluconeogenesis, a depletion of energy resources that in a small bird could rapidly affect its chances of survival.

High energy requirements demand a regular intake of food, especially in small birds with low fat reserves. It is important to administer a rich source of energy, such as glucose, at regular intervals to an inappetent passerine bird. Under normal circumstances, an appropriate food source should be available *ad libitum* to small birds whilst in captivity. Similarly, to conserve its energy reserves it is important, whilst a bird is in captivity, to maintain the environmental temperature within its thermoneutral range. This, for most small birds of less than 50 g, will be approximately 25–30°C (see Figure 5.12).

Due to their low circulating blood volume, small birds may develop hypovolaemic shock following even a small haemorrhage.

Healing processes appear to function relatively quickly in these species and, in the absence of complications (such as infection), soft tissue injuries and well aligned fractures resolve rapidly. An aligned fracture to a long bone, for example, may be stable within 10 days.

Recording biological data such as respiratory rate and heart rate is of little clinical significance, particularly when the bird is stressed on handling, as these values are likely to be greatly elevated. Measuring rates is difficult in practice as they are so rapid in small avian species. Cloacal temperature measurement is also impractical except under general anaesthesia (see 'Anaesthesia and analgesia').

Feathers

Knowledge of the processes by which a damaged or plucked feather is replaced is important in assessing the length of time some casualties have to be retained in captivity. A plucked feather will regrow within 2–3 weeks, unless the regenerative tissue within the feather follicle is damaged. Damaged feathers, where the shaft remains in the follicle, will not be replaced until the next natural moult.

Nestlings of small bird species are naked when hatched and then rapidly grow a plumage of down feathers, which is replaced by the first juvenile plumage before fledging. In the majority of species the body feathers of this first

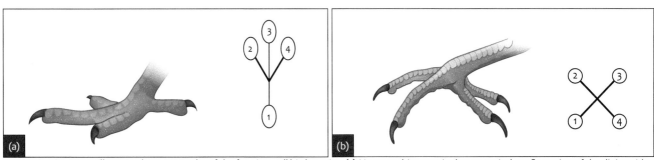

30.4 Diagram to illustrate the topography of the foot in small bird species. (a) Most perching species have a typical configuration of the digits with three forward-facing toes and a single hind toe (anisodactyl). (b) Climbing species, notably woodpeckers, have the second and third digits facing forward and the first and fourth digits facing backwards (zygodactyl).

juvenile plumage (but not the main flight feathers of the wing) are replaced during the autumn (juvenile moult) and this plumage will last the bird until its first adult moult (Ginn and Melville, 1983). Hence, damaged flight feathers in juvenile birds may not be replaced until the end of the next breeding season.

It is possible to pluck out a damaged feather under anaesthesia to encourage a new one to grow or, in larger species, to replace a damaged feather with an undamaged one by 'imping', a technique commonly used in falconry, but infrequently used in small birds (see Chapter 29).

Gender determination

The sex of many adult passerine birds may be determined using features of the plumage, as illustrated in field guides, or from biometrical features as described in manuals for bird ringers. In immature individuals or in species with no obvious sexual dimorphism sex can be determined by examination of DNA, usually extracted from a plucked feather.

Capture, handling and transportation

A general description of the methods of capture, handling and transportation suitable for small birds is provided in Chapter 3. It is important to emphasize the danger of compromising a small bird's breathing when exerting manual pressure on the body wall. The ideal methods of handling a small bird for examination and treatment are the so-called 'ringer's hold' for birds weighing <150 g and the pigeon fancier's hold for larger species (see Figure 3.12).

Zoonoses

The primary risks to handlers are physical injuries (bites and scratches from larger species, especially members of the crow family, Corvidae) and acquisition of zoonotic infections. Diseased wild birds may be clinically affected by potentially zoonotic infections, such as salmonellosis, chlamydiosis or *Escherichia albertii* infection, or may be carriers of pathogens without apparent disease, such as *Chlamydia psittaci*, *Campylobacter* and *Salmonella enterica* serovar Typhimurium (see Chapter 7).

Examination and clinical assessment for rehabilitation

The basic principles of triage and assessment for rehabilitation of a casualty are described in Chapter 4.

An important part of a clinical examination is an early assessment of the casualty's body condition. This is achieved by 'scoring' the pectoral muscle mass (see Figure 4.6) and observing the presence (or absence) of subcutaneous fat deposits over the pectoral muscles (easily seen through the thin skin of a small bird). These are important guides to its general state of health (e.g. birds with infectious disease are frequently thin) and, together with regular recording of body mass, give an indication of the casualty's progress during hospitalization. For average adult bodyweights of common free-living species of small bird see Appendix 2.

The importance of accurate identification of the species has already been emphasized, as this will give an indication of the following requirements of a casualty in captivity:

- Natural diet (insectivorous, granivorous, omnivorous) (see Figures 30.1 and 30.3)
- Habitat and feeding strategy (aerial feeder, arboreal, ground-dwelling) (see Figure 30.1)
- Social behaviour (gregarious or solitary; territorial or non-territorial)
- Movements (resident, partial migrant, summer or winter visitor) (see Figure 30.1)
- Age (dependent/independent, young bird or adult).

The most common clinical finding in small birds is trauma as a result of either predation or collision in flight. Injuries vary from superficial soft tissue to severe deep wounds involving muscle and the coelomic cavity. Fractures of limb bones and subcutaneous emphysema are also commonly seen. The prognosis in these cases depends on the severity of the wounds, the location and extent of the injuries and the chronicity of the condition. Euthanasia should be considered in severe cases. Prognosis for fracture healing and return to full limb function is discussed later.

Euthanasia

A discussion of euthanasia techniques for birds can be found in Chapter 4. For small birds a physical method of euthanasia might be the preferred option, which, if performed correctly, will be instantaneous and inflict minimum stress to the casualty (see Chapter 4). Intravenous injection of an overdose of pentobarbital is possible in most birds weighing over 100 g, but for smaller birds the most suitable site is an intrahepatic injection. The injection is made with as fine a needle as possible (27 G) just under the caudal edge of the sternum, in a cranial direction at approximately 30–45 degrees to the plane of the sternum and, in a bird of 50 g, to a depth of at least 1 cm. If the positioning of the injection is accurate, death will ensue rapidly. Intracoelomic injections invariably deposit the fluid into the abdominal air sacs, which may be painful, cause dyspnoea, and from which absorption is slow. Volatile anaesthetic agents can be used in a suitable anaesthetic induction chamber or via facemask to induce anaesthesia prior to performing euthanasia by another means and is often recommended.

First aid and short-term hospitalization

A general description of first aid procedures for wildlife casualties is given in Chapter 5 and short-term hospitalization discussed in Chapter 7. The importance of maintaining a small bird casualty within its thermoneutral range has already been emphasized, as has the need to provide a source of readily available energy at all times.

Fluid therapy

For very small birds, the most accessible and least stressful route of administration of fluids and glucose for stabilization is orally with a suitable crop/gavage tube. For very small birds a suitable crop/gavage tube can be made from a fine intravenous catheter, cut short and with the cut ends gently rounded in a flame. Small birds weighing less than 30 g should be given no more than 0.5 ml of fluid at a time by this route, whereas those weighing 100 g may be given up to 2 ml per feed (see also Chapter 5). Casualties weighing more than 100 g can be given fluid as an intravenous bolus (1–3% of the bird's bodyweight) or, if the casualty has collapsed, by an intraosseous route using a non-pneumatized long bone such as the ulna (proximal or distal) or tibiotarsus (proximal). Subcutaneous injections of fluid can be given into the loose skin of the inner thigh or along the flanks of birds of all sizes and repeated as necessary (see Chapter 5).

First aid therapeutics

Many small bird casualties are the victims of predation and suffer from wounds that are heavily infected. Early wound treatment and systemic administration of a suitable antibiotic may prevent a fatal septicaemia. Such casualties are likely to be suffering from hypovolaemic shock and fluid therapy (oral or subcutaneous routes, since intravenous injections are usually impractical in small species) is indicated. Appropriate analgesia should also be provided (see Figure 5.15 for avian dose rates).

Fracture immobilization

Fractures urgently require immobilization to prevent further soft tissue damage from the sharp edges of fractured bone. Small birds tolerate their wings being immobilized by taping the flight feathers with adhesive masking or 'autoclave' tape (the adhesive of which does not appear to cause damage to the plumage). Bandaging should be removed every 2–3 days and the wing passively mobilized to encourage normal range of movement and prevent soft tissue contracture, prior to re-taping. Avian bone healing is rapid with good callus formation occurring by 10–14 days.

- Well aligned fractures distal to the elbow can be immobilized by taping the primary to the tertial wing feathers (see Figure 5.17a).
- Fractures of the humerus with minimal displacement need to be immobilized by holding the wing rigidly against the body with adhesive tape or conforming/cohesive tape that encircles the body (see Chapter 5, Figure 5.17cd). It should be noted, however, that minimally displaced humeral fractures are rare and that euthanasia is often indicated in these cases. Each case therefore requires careful individual assessment.
- Limb fractures that are distal to the stifle can be immobilized successfully using a variety of splints and bandages (see 'Orthopaedic problems' and Figure 5.18).

Short-term hospitalization

The requirements for short-term housing of small birds, such as needed in a veterinary practice, are discussed in Chapter 7 and should include the following:

- Security to prevent escape
- Seclusion from disturbance (predators and noise). A standard rectangular breeding cage with a grille front (to which a heat lamp can be fixed), with solid sides, back and roof, and placed as high as possible within the room, will give a small bird a sense of security (Figure 30.5)

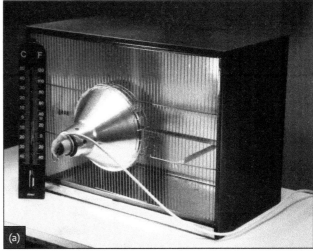

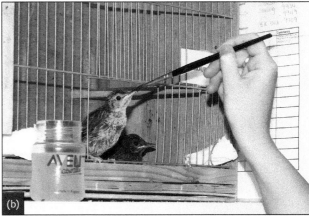

30.5 (a) A standard rectangular breeding cage with a grille front (to which a heat lamp can be fixed), with solid sides, back and roof is ideal for small birds. (b) Fledgling thrushes (Turdidae) being hand-fed through the front grille of a breeding cage to avoid excessive handling.
(b, © Secret World Wildlife Rescue)

- For perching species, a variety of suitably-sized perches of natural (and disposable) twigs and branches, or artificial wood or plastic perches that can be thoroughly disinfected
- Floor covered with a substrate that is easily replaced and hygienic (e.g. paper towel)
- The ability to darken the room to assist ease of capture for treatment
- Cage doors that are small and well placed to ease capture and prevent escape
- Food and water containers designed so that they may be changed with minimum disturbance and placed so that the casualty can reach them despite its disability.

Anaesthesia and analgesia

A detailed description of avian anaesthesia and analgesia is given in Chapters 5 and 6 and dose rates for avian analgesic drugs are provided in Figure 5.15. In small birds induction and maintenance of anaesthesia is usually via inhalation anaesthetics such as sevoflurane or isoflurane. A short period of pre-oxygenation is recommended prior to induction using a facemask. Maintenance for short procedures can be via a facemask; however, intubation in species over 100 g in bodyweight is relatively routine and is recommended (see Chapter 6 for technique and equipment used). Small birds with a high surface area to volume ratio will lose heat rapidly during anaesthesia and supplementary heat should always be provided, with careful monitoring of cloacal temperature during anaesthesia.

Specific conditions

Trauma

Orthopaedic problems

The majority of orthopaedic problems in small birds are likely to be fractures resulting from attacks by predators or collisions in flight. When attempting to repair a fracture, especially a wing fracture, it is essential to retain as closely as possible the original anatomy to preserve not only the bird's ability to fly but also its agility. A rehabilitated bird must not only be able to fly short distances but also be capable of evading predators, migrating and, even for a sedentary species, making long-distance flights in the face of adverse weather. First aid and emergency care of avian fractures and orthopaedic assessment are discussed in Chapter 5 and surgical techniques are discussed in Chapter 29.

Wing fractures: Clinical observation of wing position at rest can give the veterinary surgeon useful information on the likely bones that are fractured (see Figure 4.4).

- If the wing tip is skewed upwards the injury is likely to involve the shoulder joint.
- If the wing is held out from the body, the injury is likely to be associated with the humerus, elbow joint, or radius/ulna.
- If the distal wing tip is dropped, the fracture is likely involve or be distal to the carpal joint.

The absence of palpable lesions along the length of the wing might indicate an injury to the pectoral girdle; fractures of the coracoid classically occur following collisions (e.g. flying into a glass window or door) in the larger species of 'small birds'. Clavicular and scapular fractures may also occur. On palpation swelling associated with the shoulder area and crepitus may be evident. Confirmation usually requires radiography and if fragments of the coracoid are in apposition, healing is likely to occur with 2–3 weeks cage rest and should have a good prognosis. Fractures of the humerus and fractures of both the radius and ulna usually have a poor prognosis in small birds as they are often severely comminuted, open and associated with soft tissue damage. If healing does occur, the resulting callus and scar tissue are likely to compromise the bird's flying ability. Fractures of either one of the ulna or radius and fractures of the carpometacarpus may heal well if the wing is supported with the flight feathers being taped or strapped together in a closed position; such dressings should not be left in position for periods longer than 2–3 days as prolonged immobilization of wing joints might lead to permanent restriction of mobility (see 'Fracture immobilization'). Fractures of both the radius and ulna of the same wing have a poorer prognosis, but if non-displaced and not open or infected, may be strapped using a figure-of-eight or body bandage for 2–3 days, then re-strapped for a further 2–3 days after manipulation of the joints (see Figure 5.17). Most avian fractures start to form a callus after 7–10 days.

Leg fractures: Due to their low bodyweight, small birds are able to support themselves on one leg whilst a leg fracture is healing without the risk of pressure necrosis of the foot pad, as might occur in larger and heavier birds. Closed fractures of the femur in small birds may heal with cage rest, especially if the fragments are in reasonable alignment. Whilst even poorly aligned fractures may heal, they are likely to result in shortening of the limb and development of a large callus and an abnormal gait. The latter are not candidates for rehabilitation and release as they will not have full limb function, may be in chronic pain and will not be fit for survival in the wild. The opinion is often given that many passerine birds can survive in the wild with one functioning leg. Although lame individuals are frequently seen in the wild, this may not necessarily mean that that they will survive in the long term or be able to perform all their natural behaviour patterns.

Leg fractures distal to the stifle can be immobilized successfully using a variety of splints and bandages, possibly the most successful design being an Altman splint, which is fashioned from masking tape and, being very light, is well tolerated by most small birds (see Figure 5.18).

Cat predation

Displaced and grounded nestlings and fledglings are highly vulnerable to predation by domestic cats, especially in peri-domestic environments. A survey of a small number of rehabilitation units showed that, during the period April to June, approximately 15% of all bird casualties were recorded as being caused by cat predation (BWRC, unpublished data).

The injuries caused in these attacks vary from a loss of feathers (often asymmetrical loss of tail feathers) and superficial soft tissue injuries to severe bite wounds that might penetrate deeply into muscle tissue, open the coelomic cavity or cause fractures of ribs, vertebral column and limb bones. Subcutaneous emphysema is also a common clinical finding in small birds. Simple superficial skin injuries may resolve within days with routine wound management and therapy, but feather loss or damage will take much longer to heal. Feathers that have been plucked may regrow within 2–3 weeks but damaged feathers will not regrow until the next moult (see 'Anatomy and physiology'). Superficial injuries over the femoral area may result in limb paresis and knuckling, presumably secondary to nerve damage. In mild cases this may resolve with time, but in severe cases the prognosis is poor. Small shoes can be fashioned out of cardboard and the foot taped to the shoe, or a ball bandage can be applied for 2–3 days (see Figure 5.19), to maintain normal foot position and prevent pressure sores developing.

Minor soft tissue injuries and simple closed fractures of limb bones may heal well with routine wound management, systemic antibiotic treatment, analgesia and immobilization of fractures (see 'Orthopaedic conditions'). However, severe lacerations caused by teeth and claws will inevitably be infected and can cause serious soft tissue and orthopaedic damage. Euthanasia should be considered on welfare grounds in severe cases, especially where the coelomic cavity has been penetrated or there is a major orthopaedic problem. If treatment is considered appropriate, supportive therapy should be given together with the simultaneous administration of a course of systemic antibiotics and analgesics. Antibiotics of choice in the treatment of cat bite injuries in small birds and dose rates are shown in Figure 30.6. Cat attack victims may initially do well, however septicaemia and shock often ensues in these cases

Antibiotic	Dosage	Spectrum of activity
Amoxicillin/ clavulanate (co-amoxiclav)	125 mg/kg orally q12h for 5–7 days	Gram-positive, Gram-negative, aerobic, anaerobic, *Pasteurella* spp. (some resistance may occur)
Carbenicillin	100–200 mg/kg i.m. q6–12h for 5–7 days	Gram-negative, especially *Pseudomonas* and *Proteus* spp.
Ciprofloxacin	15–20 mg/kg orally, i.m. q12h for 5–7 days	Gram-negative, aerobic bacteria, *Pseudomonas* spp.
Enrofloxacin	10–20 mg/kg orally q24h for 5–7 days	Gram-negative, aerobic bacteria, *Pseudomonas* spp.

30.6 Systemic antibiotics useful in the treatment of cat bite injuries in small birds. NB Many drugs are not licensed in small birds and these should therefore be prescribed according to the veterinary prescribing cascade.
(Carpenter, 2013)

and their clinical condition can rapidly deteriorate, necessitating euthanasia on welfare grounds.

The wounds of 'catted' juvenile birds are frequently infected with *Pasteurella multocida* (a Gram-negative facultative anaerobe), a common component of the oral bacterial flora of the cat; other bacteria, including *Pseudomonas* spp. (Gram-negative aerobes) are also often involved.

Infectious diseases

Several infectious diseases are known to affect British passerine species and outbreaks are most commonly observed in the vicinity of supplementary feeding stations in gardens. Diseased birds often congregate around feeders until the terminal stages of the condition to take advantage of the readily available food sources, making them visible to members of the public. Birds suffering from a variety of conditions typically exhibit non-specific signs of malaise (e.g. lethargy and fluffed up plumage) and there are rarely characteristic signs that allow specific conditions to be diagnosed without laboratory testing and/or post-mortem examination. Infectious disease should be considered when wild bird casualties are submitted from sites where multiple sick or dead birds have been seen or where an increased number of cat predation victims have been observed; birds in a weakened state with infectious disease may be more vulnerable to predation. It is important to review the history of cat attack victims, in combination with clinical examination and an assessment of their body condition (since birds with infectious disease are frequently, but not always, thin), to assess whether a significant underlying infectious disease might be present. Small birds are particularly adept at hiding signs of ill health, to avoid advertising their vulnerability to predation, until the late stages of disease. Consequently, they are often in a moribund state on presentation and this, in combination with the occurrence of zoonotic infections (e.g. *Chlamydia psittaci, Escherichia albertii, Salmonella* Typhimurium, *Yersinia pseudotuberculosis*), makes these birds poor candidates for treatment and rehabilitation in many instances.

Barrier nursing and hygienic precautions

Careful attention should be paid to isolation and barrier nursing of wild bird casualties where infectious disease is suspected. To prevent nosocomial infection of hospitalized wild birds, cases should be assessed for the likelihood of infectious disease before mixing of individuals in group housing, and mixing of species should be avoided (see

Chapter 7). Whilst medication may be available for treatment of some conditions in captive birds, effective and targeted dosing of free-living wild birds is not possible and may be associated with risks, including promotion of antimicrobial resistance and potential toxicity. Instead, efforts for disease prevention and control should be directed towards best practice at garden bird feeding stations (see 'Prevention of infectious disease outbreaks').

To minimize the risks of human infection, routine personal hygiene measures are recommended when feeding wild birds and especially when handling sick birds, such as wearing disposable gloves and washing hands and forearms afterwards with soap and water, particularly before eating or drinking. Members of the public should be advised to avoid direct handling of wild bird carcasses, and to use an inverted plastic bag where necessary.

Wild birds could potentially transmit some infections to pet birds, particularly those kept in outdoor aviaries. Owners of pet birds should prevent contact between captive and wild birds as far as possible; ensure wild bird feeders and water baths are inaccessible to captive birds; and wash hands thoroughly after handling wild bird feeders or equipment. In the veterinary practice situation wild animals should be kept separate from domestic pets as routine procedure to avoid transmission of disease and this also applies to wild birds and pet species.

Prevention of infectious disease outbreaks

Several practical measures can be given as advice to the public, which may help to prevent infectious disease outbreaks in garden birds and to safeguard human health. These are as follows:

- Provide fresh food from accredited sources and ensure that drinking water is replenished on a daily basis
- Rotate the location of feeders within the garden to avoid accumulation of food waste or bird droppings in any one area
- Clean and disinfect feeders and feeding sites regularly to avoid build-up of contamination
- Suitable disinfectants that can be used include a weak solution of domestic bleach (5% sodium hypochlorite) and other products such as commercial veterinary disinfectants
- Always rinse thoroughly and air dry feeders before reuse
- Dampen waste with water before cleaning to avoid inhalation of stale (potentially mouldy) food, faeces or secretions
- Brushes and cleaning equipment for bird feeders, tables and baths should not be used for other purposes and should not be brought into the house, but be kept and used outside and away from food preparation areas
- Wear rubber gloves when cleaning feeders.

Control of infectious disease outbreaks

In the event that an infectious disease outbreak occurs, it is important to ensure that hygiene is optimal, including disinfection of feeders. Feeding stations encourage birds to congregate, sometimes in large densities, thereby increasing the potential for disease spread between individuals when outbreaks occur. They may also encourage birds of different species to mix in close proximity, offering opportunities for pathogen spillover to new susceptible host species. If many birds are affected, it is worthwhile significantly reducing the amount of available food, or stopping feeding for a period (e.g. 2–4 weeks) and to leave bird baths empty to reduce opportunities for pathogen transmission at shared resources. The reason for this is to encourage birds to disperse, thereby minimizing the chances of new birds becoming infected at the feeding station. Gradually reintroduce feeding, whilst continuing to monitor for further signs of ill health.

Viral diseases

Investigations have been made into the possible roles of wild birds in the epidemiology of many viral diseases of livestock, both mammalian and avian, such as avian influenza. Wild birds may also act as sentinels for emerging viral diseases, for example West Nile virus (see 'Horizon scanning').

Avian pox: Avian pox is caused by strains of avian poxvirus with variable host specificity. Avian pox is traditionally categorized in a 'wet' or 'dry' presentation; with the latter, where the proliferative lesions are restricted to the skin, being most frequently observed in wild birds. Warty or tumour-like growths caused by avian poxvirus typically occur on the head (particularly next to the eye or beak), and less commonly on the legs, wings, or other body parts (Figure 30.7).

Avian pox has been described in several hundred captive and wild bird species with near worldwide distribution. Sporadic cases of avian pox have been recorded in some British garden birds for decades, including the dunnock (Figure 30.7a), house sparrow (*Passer domesticus*), starling (*Sturnus vulgaris*) and wood pigeon (*Columba palumbus*), in which the infection is considered endemic. However, since 2006 a severe form of avian pox has been recognized as an important emerging infectious disease of British tit species (Lawson *et al.*, 2012a). Great tits (Figure

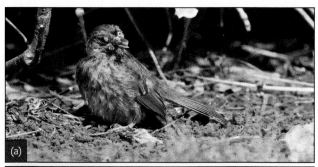

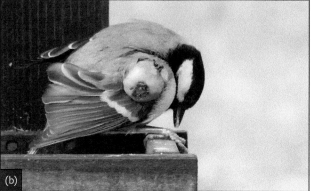

30.7 Warty or tumour-like growths caused by avian poxvirus typically occur on the head (particularly next to the eye or beak) and less commonly on the legs, wings or other body parts. (a) Dunnock (*Prunella modularis*). (b) Great tit (*Parus major*).
(a, Courtesy of R Stowell © Zoological Society of London; b, Courtesy of J Harper, © Zoological Society of London).

30.7b) are most commonly affected although a range of tit species are susceptible and it is not unusual for outbreaks of disease involving multiple birds to occur. Whilst cases can occur year round, there is a seasonal peak in the late summer and early autumn months. Incidents were first seen in south-east England and have spread northward and westward across England and Wales with further extension of the disease range in this common garden bird species still anticipated within Great Britain. Great tit pox has been reported in Scandinavia since the 1950s and a cluster of incidents was seen in central Europe in the mid-2000s (Literak *et al.*, 2010). It seems most likely that this disease emergence in Great Britain arose as a result of introduction of a novel strain of avian poxvirus from Scandinavia or central Europe: movement of an infected vector is proposed as the mechanism, via windborne or anthropogenic means, since great tit migration appears an unlikely route of spread.

Clinical signs: In species with endemic infection, skin lesions can be relatively mild and infection may be self-limiting. However, in all species, but particularly tits, large lesions can develop that interfere with feeding, sight or locomotion, leaving birds vulnerable to predation or over-whelming secondary bacterial infection. Whilst the disease in great tits is not invariably fatal and recovery can occur, the condition reduces individual survival, particularly in juvenile birds. Nevertheless, modelling does not predict the impact will be sufficient to cause population decline based on the prevalence of disease observed in the field (Lachish *et al.*, 2012) and national population monitoring of great tits to date shows no adverse effect on bird numbers.

Transmission: Avian pox can be spread via multiple routes including biting insects (e.g. mosquitoes), direct contact between birds or indirect contact between birds, for example through contact with contaminated perches via abraded skin. Avian poxvirus is relatively resistant and can persist in the environment for months. Avian poxviruses are only known to infect birds, so they pose no known risk to health in humans or other mammals.

Diagnosis: Confirmation of avian pox relies on histopathological examination of samples of skin lesions collected by biopsy or more commonly at post-mortem examination. Avian pox strain identification requires amplification via polymerase chain reaction (PCR) techniques and sequence confirmation. Whilst avian pox is not invariably fatal, wild birds typically present as casualties with this condition when the lesions are severe and concurrent significant disease is present, for instance, secondary *Staphylococcus aureus* septicaemia or cat predation of individuals whose vision or locomotion is impaired by the disease. Whilst supportive treatment may be attempted, the prognosis is likely to be poor and the potential biosecurity threat to other hospitalized birds must be considered since the virus is environmentally persistent, and can be transferred by fomites and insect vectors.

Chaffinch papillomavirus (CPV): Foot lesions in chaffinches (*Fringilla coelebs*) are arguably the most frequently reported condition observed in British garden birds, familiar since the 1960s, and have also been reported in continental Europe. There are two known causes of these leg lesions, namely CPV (Papillomaviridae family) (Erdélyi, 2012) which can cause papillomatosis, and *Cnemidocoptes* spp. mites (Sarcoptidae family) that can cause cnemidocoptosis (see

'Cnemidocoptosis'). Colloquial names are well known for these conditions, including 'tassel foot' for papillomatosis and 'mange' or 'scaly foot' for cnemidocoptosis. The relative importance of these two causes in wild bird populations is currently uncertain and mixed infection with both agents is known to occur.

Clinical signs: With CPV, proliferative 'spiky' or 'tassel-like' lesions typically develop, which are mostly around the foot and digits, but can spread higher up the leg whereas, with mite infestation, proliferative lesions with excess grey scale often develop on the digits and leg (Figure 30.8). Since there is considerable overlap between the appearance of the leg lesions that result, diagnosis is not possible without laboratory investigations.

In the UK, the chaffinch is the most frequently affected species although there are rare reports of limb lesions in brambling (*Fringilla montifringilla*) and bullfinch (*Pyrrhula pyrrhula*). Affected birds typically remain bright and active and their locomotion does not appear to be adversely affected. However, more severe cases can occur with lameness and debility that are likely to predispose to predation. Individual birds are most often affected, although localized outbreaks can also occur. Disease progression with both agents is thought to occur over a period of weeks to months and little is known about how frequently wild birds recover.

Transmission: Transmission of both disease agents is thought to occur via direct or indirect contact (e.g. perches). CPV and *Cnemidocoptes* mites are only known to infect birds and therefore there is no known risk to humans or other mammals. Papillomaviruses are typically adapted to certain species; therefore the host range of wild birds is likely to be small.

When finches with either infection present as wildlife casualties, the limb lesions are rarely the primary problem and concurrent disease is frequently present. This may be related to the limb lesions, for example cat predation injuries due to impaired locomotion or entanglement, or be an unrelated significant disease (e.g. finch trichomonosis). No specific treatment is available for CPV infection.

Bacterial diseases

Passerine salmonellosis: Passerine salmonellosis has been reported as a cause of disease outbreaks in the UK, continental Europe and North America since the 1950s. Incidents are highly seasonal in the UK, chiefly occurring during the colder winter months. Whilst there are many species of *Salmonella* bacteria, particular strains of *Salmonella* Typhimurium (phage types 40, 56 variant and 160) typically affect British passerines. Gregarious and granivorous species, predominantly the greenfinch (*Chloris chloris*) and house sparrow, are most commonly affected; however, other species are also susceptible, including the bullfinch, chaffinch, goldfinch (*Carduelis carduelis*) and siskin (*Carduelis spinus*). Research indicates that these *S.* Typhimurium strains are host-adapted to passerine species and that these wild bird populations act as the reservoir of the infection (Lawson *et al.*, 2011a). Long-term monitoring has revealed that the absolute number of salmonellosis outbreaks varies between years, and has reduced markedly since 2008, and that the predominant phage types vary in time and space (Pennycott *et al.*, 2010; Lawson *et al.*, 2014).

Clinical signs: Affected birds show non-specific signs of ill health, for example lethargy and fluffed-up plumage. Passerine salmonellosis typically causes disseminated granulomatous infection, with lesions often present in the oesophagus, liver, spleen and caecal tonsils (Figure 30.9).

Transmission: Transmission is through the faeco–oral route and is likely to occur when infected bird droppings contaminate food or water sources. *Salmonella* bacteria can persist in the environment for some time, probably weeks to months.

Diagnosis: Microbiological examination of faeces or, more commonly, lesions collected at post-mortem examination, is required for diagnosis of *Salmonella* infection. Birds with salmonellosis are rarely presented as wildlife casualties, most commonly being found dead in domestic gardens, but if they are brought in alive, they are typically moribund and thus have a poor prognosis. Whilst

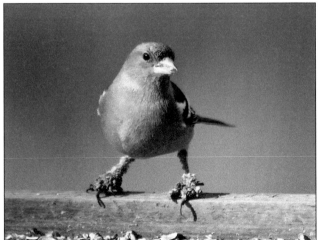

30.8 With chaffinch papillomavirus (CPV) infection, proliferative 'spiky' or 'tassel-like' lesions typically develop around the foot and digits, but can spread higher up the leg whereas, with mite (*Cnemidocoptes* spp.) infestation, excess grey scale often develops on the digits and leg. Coinfection can occur and it is not possible to diagnose the cause of the lesions based on appearance alone without further diagnostic tests.
(© Zoological Society of London)

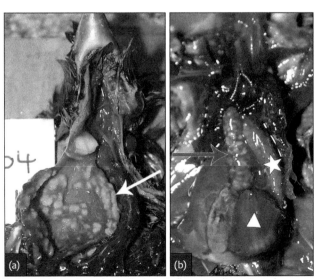

30.9 Passerine salmonellosis typically causes disseminated granulomatous infection, with lesions often present in the (a) crop (arrowed), (b) spleen (arrowed), along with the liver and caecal tonsils. For orientation a white star denotes the proventriculus and a white triangle the ventriculus (or gizzard).
(© Zoological Society of London)

antibiotic treatment is available, there are various reasons why this is not recommended, including the zoonotic risk and potential for promoting carrier status.

Zoonotic potential: The strains of *S.* Typhimurium that affect passerines have the potential to affect humans and domestic animals, typically causing gastroenteritis. Long-term monitoring in the UK over a 20-year period identified similar temporal and spatial trends of infection with *S.* Typhimurium (phage types 40, 56v and 160) in both garden birds and humans, supporting the hypothesis that passerines are the primary source of these zoonotic bacteria; however, the risk is low and should be kept in perspective since these cases represented only 0.2% of all human *Salmonella* infections in England and Wales, 2000–2010 inclusive, and there is no evidence of antibiotic resistance in the garden bird-derived isolates tested to date (Lawson *et al.*, 2014).

Disease in other species: 'Songbird fever' is a term used to describe salmonellosis in cats caused by passerine-associated *Salmonella* strains. Cats are thought to become infected following consumption of diseased garden birds that are particularly vulnerable to predation (Philbey *et al.*, 2008). Sporadic infection of various livestock species with wild bird-associated *Salmonella* strains can occur, but represent a minority of *Salmonella* infections in these species (Horton *et al.*, 2013b).

Chlamydiosis: *Chlamydia psittaci* is an intracellular bacterium that causes the disease avian chlamydiosis (otherwise known as 'psittacosis' or 'ornithosis') in captive and wild birds (Speck and Duff, 2012). *Chlamydia psittaci* infection, which is known to occur in various wild bird species, is perhaps best studied in pigeons and doves (see Chapter 28), and can be subclinical or associated with disease. In the UK, a small number of mortality incidents attributed to chlamydiosis have been diagnosed in passerines, with the robin (*Erithacus rubecula*), great tit and dunnock most commonly involved, often in mixed species outbreaks.

Clinical signs: Affected birds may show non-specific signs of malaise, sometimes with dyspnoea and ocular or nasal discharges, however they may simply be found dead. Post-mortem examinations have identified various abnormalities, from non-specific changes to the liver, spleen enlargement and polyserositis. A recent retrospective study has identified further chlamydiosis incidents in native passerine species due to *C. psittaci* (genotype A), which had a widespread geographical distribution and no clear seasonality, suggesting that chlamydiosis may be a more common disease in wild passerines than was previously recognized (Beckmann *et al.*, 2014).

Transmission: Transmission can occur through direct contact between infected birds, ingestion of infected secretions (faeces, ocular and respiratory secretions), and inhalation of contaminated dust or aerosols. *Chlamydia psittaci* bacteria can persist in the environment for months in a resistant form.

Diagnosis: Affected birds are likely to present in a moribund state or be found dead, possibly also victims of cat attack, and a diagnosis is often made at post-mortem examination based on immunohistochemistry combined with PCR or other molecular techniques.

Zoonotic potential: Chlamydia psittaci is a zoonotic bacterium which can cause a spectrum of clinical signs in humans. It most commonly causes respiratory disease, which can range from mild and cold-like to a more severe flu-like illness, and in more serious (particularly untreated) cases patients may require hospitalization. Humans are most likely to become infected through inhalation of dust or aerosols contaminated with secretions from infected birds. Human cases are relatively uncommon in the UK and have been most frequently attributed to contact with infected captive birds such as parrots, pigeons, ducks or geese; however, wild birds may also be a source of infection and therefore sensible hygiene precautions are recommended as a routine (see Chapter 7).

Preventative measures: Wild birds could potentially transmit the infection to pet birds, particularly if the pet birds are in outdoor aviaries. Owners of pet birds should prevent contact between captive and wild birds as far as possible, ensure wild bird feeders and water baths are inaccessible to captive birds, and wash hands thoroughly after handling wild bird feeders or equipment. There have been rare reports of disease in cats and dogs associated with *C. psittaci* infection, most commonly attributed to the animals having contact with pet parrots. The risk of pet dogs or cats acquiring the infection from wild birds is unknown, but is likely to be low.

Escherichia albertii *infection:* *Escherichia albertii* (previously known as *E. coli* serotype O86-like) is a Gram-negative bacterium within the Enterobacteriaceae family and the disease that it causes is commonly known as 'colibacillosis'. Whilst multiple *E. coli* serotypes have been isolated from various wild bird species, they are not known as regular causes of disease outbreaks in British garden birds.

Infection with various strains of *E. albertii* has been shown in multiple wild bird species from Europe, North America and Australia, sometimes in apparently healthy birds, but also as a cause of disease outbreaks associated with multiple mortalities (Oaks *et al.*, 2010). As with *S.* Typhimurium, it is proposed that wild birds act as the reservoir of infection; however, further investigation is required to explore this hypothesis.

As with several infectious diseases of passerines, *E. albertii* infection in the UK is most commonly diagnosed in gregarious and granivorous species, with the siskin, followed by the chaffinch and greenfinch being most frequently affected. Whilst incidents have been reported across the UK, surveillance indicates that disease outbreaks occur most often in Scotland during the late spring months (Pennycott *et al.*, 1998).

Clinical signs: Affected birds show non-specific signs of malaise. *E. albertii* typically affects the digestive tract causing enteritis, sometimes with gut stasis leading to accumulation of food contents in the upper alimentary tract.

Transmission: Transmission is via the faeco–oral route and *E. albertii* can persist in the environment for some time.

Diagnosis: Microbiological examination of faeces, or more commonly alimentary tract contents and liver collected at post-mortem examination, is required for diagnosis of *E. albertii* infection. Affected birds rarely present as wildlife casualties and are more commonly found dead in domestic gardens. When they are found, they typically present in an advanced stage of disease in a moribund state with a poor prognosis and euthanasia is indicated.

Disease in other species: The strains of *E. albertii* that affect wild birds may have the potential to infect humans, livestock and domestic animals. Signs of disease in these species are likely to include diarrhoea.

Suttonella ornithocola *infection:* *Suttonella ornithocola* is a recently discovered Gram-negative bacterium in the family Cardiobacteriaceae with fastidious culture conditions. Infection has been most commonly observed in blue tit (*Cyanistes caeruleus*); however, other species within the British tit families are also susceptible to infection. Whilst a cluster of 11 disease outbreaks was investigated in the mid-1990s (Kirkwood *et al.*, 2006), surveillance in recent years has identified a small number of incidents (0–2 per year) with widespread distribution across the UK, that occur most frequently in late spring. These findings suggest that *S. ornithocola* infection is endemic in the British tit population (Lawson *et al.*, 2011b).

Clinical signs and transmission: Tits with *S. ornithocola* infection show non-specific signs of malaise and may also develop respiratory signs, for example gasping and open-mouth breathing. Histopathological examination of infected birds has identified acute lung lesions as the primary abnormality, therefore, whilst little is known about the bacterium, aerosol transmission is suspected. The range of species susceptible to infection is currently unknown; nevertheless there are no known reports of infection in mammals and confirmed avian infections are currently limited to the tit family in the UK.

Diagnosis: Diagnosis of *S. ornithocola* infection has to date been limited to microbiological examination from lung tissue collected at post-mortem examination. Methods for ante-mortem diagnosis in live birds and their sensitivities are unknown. Whilst antimicrobial therapy that targets the bacterium may be available, histopathological examination in the small number of confirmed incidents to date indicates a rapid progression. Casualties are likely to present in an advanced stage of disease and euthanasia may be indicated in these cases.

Yersiniosis: *Yersinia pseudotuberculosis* is a widespread, Gram-negative coccobacillus and various serotypes exist. Subclinical infection of a range of species has been reported with rodents and birds believed to be the principal reservoirs (Najdenski, 2012). In the UK, *Y. pseudotuberculosis* infection has been described in a large number of wild bird species from multiple families. Yersiniosis occurs as a sporadic cause of disease in individual small birds, and less commonly as outbreaks. The progression varies from acute septicaemia to subacute disseminated infection with lesions often in the liver, spleen, alimentary tract or joints on post-mortem examination. Yersiniosis typically occurs during the winter months, particularly during cold weather conditions: the disease is an important differential diagnosis for passerine salmonellosis due to their similar seasonality.

Transmission: Transmission is via the faeco–oral route and the bacterium can persist for some time in the environment.

Disease in other species: The strains of *Y. pseudotuberculosis* that infect wild birds have the potential to infect humans and livestock.

Avian tuberculosis: Whilst a wide range of wild bird species are known to be susceptible to avian tuberculosis, the condition is more common in waterfowl (see Chapter 26) and apparently infrequent in small bird species.

Fungal diseases

Aspergillosis: Aspergillosis can occur in small birds, but is most frequently diagnosed as an opportunistic infection in individual debilitated birds with concurrent disease, presumably in an immunocompromised state, rather than as a cause of localized disease outbreaks affecting multiple birds.

Provision of fresh foodstuffs on a regular basis is recommended at garden feeding stations in order to avoid them becoming stale or mouldy. Whilst aflatoxin residues have been detected in the tissues of British wild birds, the origin of these toxins, for example whether from wild or supplementary food sources, and their clinical significance is currently unknown (Lawson *et al.*, 2006). However, since aflatoxins and other mycotoxins are known to have deleterious acute and chronic effects, the precautionary principle should be adopted in providing supplementary foodstuffs that have been screened for detectable aflatoxin residues.

Parasites

Ectoparasites:

Cnemidocoptosis: In passerines, *Cnemidocoptes jamaicensis* and *C. intermedius* are the most common mite species seen; *C. mutans* typically affects poultry and *C. pilae* affects psittacine birds (such as pet budgerigars (*Melopsittacus undulatus*)) (Pence, 2008). Infestation often results in the development of proliferative lesions with excess grey scale on the digits and leg (see 'Chaffinch papillomavirus' and Figure 30.8). On rare occasions, mite infestations can also cause facial lesions, similar to those seen with 'scaly face' in pet budgerigars caused by cnemidocoptosis. The *Cnemidocoptes* species that typically infest passerines are distinct from those that commonly affect poultry, therefore the risk of infection to free-ranging poultry from wild chaffinches is likely to be low. Whilst cage and aviary finches may be at risk of infestation, transmission is unlikely since direct or indirect contact between captive and wild finches would be required. Treatment is usually successful with subcutaneous or topical ivermectin at 0.2 mg/kg once, repeated weekly for three treatments.

Hippoboscids ('flat flies'): The dipteran louse-fly of the family Hippoboscidae is commonly found on small birds, especially hirundines, such as barn swallow (*Hirundo rustica*), house martin (*Delichon urbicum*) and swift. It appears to be of little clinical significance, although larger numbers are occasionally found on emaciated birds. These parasites are potentially significant in the epidemiology of blood-borne diseases.

Ticks: Tick infestations are common in a variety of wild bird species and do not usually appear to be associated with significant adverse effects. However, in some cases a severe and often fatal (sometimes haemorrhagic) reaction can occur in association with adult female *Ixodes frontalis* ticks (Monks *et al.*, 2006). The tick attachment site in these cases is most commonly on the heads of small birds, especially on the temporal and periorbital regions, and the local tissue swelling that results can lead to these birds being mistaken for victims of blunt trauma. This syndrome is most frequently reported in collared doves (*Streptopelia decaocto*), although a range of small birds can be affected. Supportive treatment (non-steroidal anti-inflammatory drugs (NSAIDs), systemic antibiosis and fluid therapy) in combination with removal of the tick and treatment with an ectoparasiticide may be helpful.

Endoparasites:

Gapeworm infection (syngamiasis):

- *Syngamus trachea* is a very common parasite of blackbird, common starling and members of the Corvidae. The parasite has an indirect lifecycle with invertebrates, such as earthworms (Lumbricidae) or slugs (Gastropoda), acting as a paratenic host. However, transmission can also be direct by ingestion of ova which hatch in the intestine. Larvae migrate to the lungs and airways, with a 16–20 day life cycle.
- It is often associated with abnormal respiratory sounds and respiratory distress (open-mouthed breathing and dyspnoea), especially in young birds that have been presented as 'orphans'.
- Diagnosis is based on clinical signs and faecal parasitology (see Chapter 10). In small birds trans-illumination through the skin using a pen torch or similar light source of the trachea may reveal adult worms within the airways, which can also be seen post-mortem (Figure 30.10a). Typical ova may be seen on examination of wet preparations of faeces or sputum (Figure 30.10b).

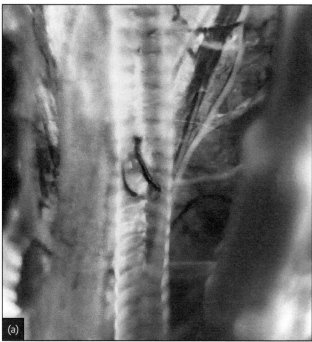

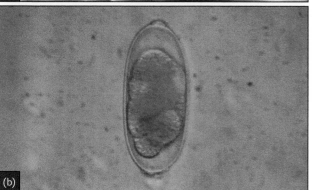

30.10 *Syngamus trachea* is a common nematode parasite of game birds, starlings and members of the crow family. It frequently causes clinical signs of partial tracheal obstruction. (a) Post-mortem examination of the trachea may reveal adult worms within the airways. (b) *Syngamus trachea* egg. The ova are readily demonstrated by direct microscopic examination of pharyngeal mucus and faeces (wet preparations or by flotation techniques).

- Treatment with benzimidazoles (e.g. fenbendazole 20–50 mg/kg orally q24h for 3 days) or ivermectin (0.2 mg/kg s.c., once off dose or repeated after 10–14 days if necessary) is successful in less severe cases. Concurrent NSAIDs and systemic antibiotics may be indicated to treat secondary bacterial infections and inflammation. Preventative measures should be instigated in wildlife rehabilitation units, with good hygiene practice, such as careful disinfection of feeding equipment for young birds, regular clearing of faecal material from cages and no access to ingestion of intermediate hosts. In rehabilitation units where there is a significant problem with this parasite, prophylactic treatment of small bird admissions with antiparasitic drugs may be necessary, together with appropriate control measures and strict hygiene practices.

Trichomonosis: Trichomonas gallinae is a protozoan parasite that is historically known to cause trichomonosis in pigeons and doves and can also affect birds of prey that predate or scavenge on other birds that are infected with the parasite. The common name for the disease in pigeons and doves is 'canker' and in birds of prey the disease is also known as 'frounce' (see also Chapters 28 and 29).

Trichomonosis was first seen in British finch species in summer 2005, with the greenfinch and chaffinch being the most frequently affected species (Robinson *et al.*, 2010). Epidemic mortality caused by a single clonal strain of *T. gallinae* occurred throughout much of the UK in 2006 and 2007; this emerging infectious disease has continued to cause large-scale mortality of finches in subsequent years and is now established throughout the UK. Finch trichomonosis has marked seasonality with a peak during the late summer to autumn months, although incidents can occur throughout the year. Consequent to the emergence of finch trichomonosis, the UK breeding greenfinch population declined by 35% from 2006 to 2009 which equates to the loss of circa 1.5 million birds and represents the largest scale mortality of British birds due to infectious disease on record (Lawson *et al.*, 2012b). Finch trichomonosis was first seen in Fennoscandia in 2008 (Neimanis *et al.*, 2010), with migrating chaffinches thought to be the most likely vector of parasite movement (Lawson *et al.*, 2011c). The disease continues to spread within continental Europe, having reached as far east as Austria and Slovenia in 2012 (Ganas *et al.*, 2013).

Whilst the greenfinch and chaffinch are most commonly affected by trichomonosis, many other gregarious granivorous passerines, including the house sparrow, siskin, goldfinch and bullfinch can be affected. Although apparently infrequent, other garden species such as blackbird and dunnock are also susceptible.

- *Trichomonas gallinae* typically causes caseous lesions to develop in the oropharynx of columbiformes and in the oesophagus of passerines. In addition to showing non-specific signs of malaise, for example lethargy and fluffed-up plumage, affected birds may drool saliva, regurgitate food, and be dysphagic or dyspnoeic (Figure 30.11). Finches are frequently seen to have matted wet plumage around the face and beak and are often very thin or emaciated. Most cases in small birds are presented with advanced disease or at post-mortem examination and are therefore not candidates for treatment.
- Parasite transmission occurs via fresh saliva, when birds feed one another during the breeding season or through shared food or water sources. *T. gallinae* is

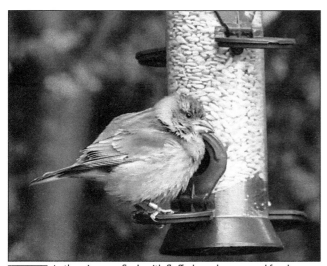

30.11 Lethargic greenfinch with fluffed-up plumage and food adherent to beak: clinical signs often observed with finch trichomonosis.
(© Zoological Society of London)

vulnerable to desiccation and cannot survive for long periods outside the host. It is a parasite of birds and there is no known health threat to people or to mammals, such as dogs and cats. However, the parasite has the potential to affect captive poultry and pet birds.
- Diagnosis of trichomonosis in passerines can be attempted using direct microscopic examination of an upper alimentary tract swab (a fine-tipped swab moistened in saline) to visualize motile trichomonads (see Chapter 10). Whilst trichomonosis lesions in columbids are typically located in the oropharynx and are directly visible on examination of the oral cavity, they are most commonly along the length of the oesophagus/crop in passerines. Great care should be taken to avoid iatrogenic damage to the upper alimentary tract of these birds which is normally thin-walled and when diseased is necrotic.
- Alternatively, parasite culture can be attempted using various commercial media inoculated with upper alimentary tract swabs (saline moistened as above) or necrotic material from ingluvitis lesions collected at post-mortem examination. PCR techniques are also available for confirmation of presence of the parasite and strain identification.

As with the majority of the infectious diseases frequently diagnosed in British passerines, birds with trichomonosis are typically at an advanced stage of disease if they are caught and presented as wildlife casualties; therefore, their prognosis is likely to be poor.

Horizon scanning

Wildlife veterinary surgeons can assist with the early detection of novel or emerging conditions by being vigilant for unusual case presentations and/or incident histories and reporting these to national wildlife surveillance schemes for investigation. There are several high-profile infectious diseases or syndromes currently affecting small bird species in other countries, which have not been detected in the UK to date.

In North America, there are important conditions of passerine birds that are not known to be present in the UK for which surveillance should be vigilant. In the mid-1990s,

Mycoplasma gallisepticum emerged as a cause of epidemic conjunctivitis in the USA, chiefly affecting the house finch (*Haemorhous mexicanus*), which led to a large-scale population decline of this species (Hochachka and Dhondt, 2000).

West Nile virus (WNV), a mosquito-borne flavivirus, emerged in the USA in 1999 and caused epidemic mortality of wild birds, particularly corvid species, in subsequent years, in addition to neuroinvasive disease in humans and horses (LaDeau *et al.*, 2007; Petersen *et al.*, 2013). Whilst WNV strains have been detected in continental Europe (Reid *et al.*, 2012), WNV has not been detected in the UK despite surveillance in wild birds (Brugman *et al.*, 2013).

Usutu virus is a mosquito-borne flavivirus that was originally isolated in Africa in the 1950s but not in association with clinical disease. In Europe, Usutu virus emerged as a cause of wild bird mortality in Austria in 2001 where epidemic mortality, chiefly involving blackbirds, occurred with summer seasonality. Subsequent virus spread has occurred within Hungary, Italy, Switzerland and into Germany associated with wild and captive bird mortality and the infection is now considered endemic in some regions (Weissenböck and Erdélyi, 2012). Observed clinical signs in wild birds include sudden death, lethargy and neurological signs and gross abnormalities on post-mortem examination may include liver and spleen enlargement. There are rare examples of neurological disease in immunosuppressed humans with Usutu virus infection in continental Europe. The mosquito species involved in Usutu virus outbreaks in continental Europe are present in the UK. Whilst there is some evidence of serological exposure to Usutu virus in British wild birds, the virus has not been isolated to date and a targeted retrospective study of archived tissues from various garden bird species found no evidence of Usutu virus infection using PCR; therefore, the disease status in the UK requires further investigation (Horton *et al.*, 2013a).

Keratin beak disorder is a syndrome of unresolved aetiology which describes recent cases of beak deformities observed since the late 1990s in wild birds in Alaska, particularly tit and corvid species, sometimes in high prevalence (van Hemert *et al.*, 2013).

Other conditions
Grounded swifts

Swifts are truly an aerial species; they feed, roost and even copulate in the air. Once on level ground, even a fit bird will have difficulty in becoming airborne. During the breeding season fledglings frequently become grounded and, being unable to take off, rapidly become exhausted. In the hand, juvenile birds can be distinguished from adults by white or pale fringes to the wing coverts. Fledglings usually weigh between 34 and 52 g when they first fly at an average age of 42 days. Some may fledge early, especially in periods of poor weather when they might not be fed by the adults, and these may represent a proportion of the 'grounded' young birds (Cramp, 1988). If such birds are in good body condition and weigh within the normal range, they can, if conditions are suitable, be released immediately, preferably in an open space where they can be easily retrieved if not able to fly. If conditions are unsuitable or a bird is weak or exhausted, but in good body condition, it can be retained in captivity for a short time to rest in a dark secluded box and given oral electrolyte solution (e.g. Vetark® Critical Care Formula; 1 ml per feed, via gavage or offered using a small paintbrush) before being flight-tested (see also Chapter 5 for fluid therapy rates and volumes).

If the casualty is an underweight adult, or a juvenile and unable to fly, treatment can be considered. However, swifts are highly specialized feeders and although they can be fed for short periods with oral avian recovery liquid diets (see Chapters 5 and 7) or mealworms and wax moth larvae, long-term captivity, especially if hospitalization extends beyond the normal period of residence in the UK, rarely results in the release of the casualty. Euthanasia should be considered as an alternative to hospitalization for the majority of these cases.

Starvation associated with adverse weather

Many bird species are able to avoid the worst effects of prolonged adverse weather by migrating. Even species regarded as being non-migratory will move large distances when faced with such problems. Occasionally, in prolonged periods of freezing weather which usually also involve continental Europe, large numbers of passerine casualties can be found suffering from starvation due to their inability to find food (Figure 30.12).

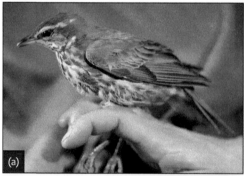

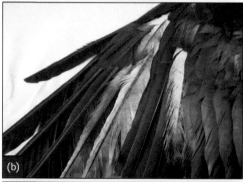

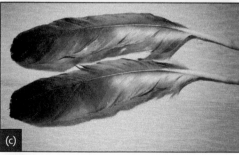

30.12 (a) Redwing (*Turdus iliacus*). In severe winters, large numbers of redwings and fieldfare (*Turdus pilaris*) are forced further west across Continental Europe to the UK where, if conditions are no better, they suffer from starvation and may be admitted to rehabilitation units. (b) Juvenile carrion crows (*Corvus corone*) are frequently found in an emaciated state and showing lack of pigmentation to the plumage, especially the flight and tail feathers. (c) Fret marks or stress marks – transverse lines of feather malformation and weakness, assumed to be associated with periods of malnutrition or disease during the development of the feather.
(b, Courtesy of G Cousquer)

Therapeutics

The calculation of an effective dose using allometric scaling and methods of administering medication are discussed in Chapter 7.

For very small birds weighing less than 50 g, an intramuscular injection is a painful and stressful procedure and should be avoided whenever possible. Oral dosage by gavage, syringe dropper or pipette (taking care to avoid aspiration), using medications suitable for that route, may be preferable. Subcutaneous injections are also well tolerated, even in smaller species (see Chapter 5). Indirect methods of medication, using food or water, are unreliable unless the medicated food can be given in measured amounts or the water consumption measured. Consequently in-feed or water medications are not recommended by the authors.

Management in captivity

The basic principles of the long-term housing and management of a wildlife casualty are described in Chapter 9. The housing and feeding requirements of different species of small passerine birds vary, as this is a diverse group with a wide variety of ecological and feeding strategies.

Housing

The majority of small bird casualties need only short-term care or euthanasia, with the exception of juvenile birds requiring hand-rearing. Those requiring long-term care will need special housing that would be beyond the scope of most veterinary practices; Chapter 9 describes secluded aviaries in which the birds can recuperate, exercise, exhibit normal behaviour and an assessment made on their fitness for release.

Feeding

The diet fed to casualties will vary with the species and can be designed along the guidelines given in Figure 30.13. Some birds require specially designed accommodation to encourage their natural feeding behaviour. For example:

- Swifts are obligate aerial insectivores. They are unlikely to feed on their own and need to be fed by hand with mealworms, wax moth larvae or other insects. Their natural food is small flying insects and an adult returning to feed a nestling is likely to have as many as 1,000 insects in a food ball. When roosting, swifts cling to a vertical surface; in captivity, a towel attached to the side of a solid-walled cage provides a suitable perch
- Woodpeckers are mainly arboreal, finding most of their food on the trunks and larger branches of trees. In captivity they will preferentially perch on a tree trunk or branch fixed in an upright position. They feed primarily on invertebrates (mainly insects) and suitable insectivore food can be placed in cracks or holes drilled into the trunk
- Kingfishers may not self-feed in captivity, however feeding can be encouraged by injecting air into small fish so that they float.

Dietary groups	Families	Hand-rearing diets	Natural supplements
Insectivores	Cuckoo Swift Woodpeckers Larks Hirundines Warblers Wren Flycatchers Wagtails/pipits	Commercial softbill rearing diet Commercial insectivore diet Mealworms, wax moth larvae, earthworms (beware *Syngamus* sp. infestation), maggots (angling supplies, avoid those colour-stained), small crickets	Wild insects (adults and larvae), spiders, etc. Insects caught by sweeping with a hand-net over long grass
Insectivores/granivores	Tits Dunnock Sparrows Finches Buntings	Commercial softbill rearing diet Commercial insectivore diet Live food as above Small seed mixture	As above Wild seeds (groundsel, seeding grasses)
Piscivores	Kingfisher	Small fish (available frozen as food for carnivorous fish)	
Omnivores	Crows Starling Thrushes	Commercial softbill rearing diet Commercial dog/cat food	Wild insects and invertebrates (earthworms)

30.13 Artificial diets and natural supplements for hand-rearing and hospitalization of small birds.

Rearing of chicks

Newly fledged small birds probably form the majority of wildlife casualties presented to rehabilitation units and veterinary practices. It is worth considering that the breeding strategy of most small birds is to produce large numbers of offspring each season to offset the high natural mortality, and that many casualties brought into captivity may represent these natural losses.

Young birds might be presented as nestlings (i.e. young birds that are bald or partially feathered and still dependent on their parents) or as fledglings (i.e. feathered young that have left the nest, but feathers have not yet fully developed, and are still dependent on their parents for care and protection) (see Figure 30.2). Although fledged birds are presented as abandoned or orphaned individuals, in reality it is more likely that they have been displaced and separated from their parents. Many nidicolous (nest-reared) birds on the point of fledging leave the nest before they can fly and remain for several days in the safety of the tree canopy or surrounding vegetation, where they can be displaced by strong winds or flushed by predators. Once on the ground they are flightless and vulnerable; it is in this state that many are found in domestic gardens and brought into captivity, often the victims of cat predation.

If a fledgling passerine bird is uninjured, it might be preferable to return the bird to the location where it was found and place it in the cover of vegetation, possibly within a small, partially closed box to which the adults can gain access. Although it might be a concern, it does not appear to be generally true that handling fledglings will cause adults to abandon or to reject them (see also Chapter 3).

If returning a young bird to its natal territory is impossible (because the precise site is unknown or unrecorded) or impractical, consideration can be given to rearing by hand (see also Chapter 8). Successful hand-rearing requires a sound knowledge of the biology of the species and the availability of suitable facilities, plus endless patience and a realistic approach to the problems involved, which may be beyond the scope of a veterinary practice. The following considerations need to be taken into account:

- Hand-rearing is very time-consuming
- Provision of a suitable nutritionally balanced substitute for the natural diet
- Accommodation in facilities that provide an environment that is as natural as possible to its species that will allow physical exercise, the development of independence through food-locating skills and social interaction with its own and other species
- Prevention from becoming malprinted on humans
- Preventing a dependence on an unnatural food.

Throughout the hand-rearing process it is important to ensure that attention is paid to hygiene, by preventing:

- Build-up of food and faecal material on the birds and in their housing
- Cross-contamination between patients, especially separating fledglings from different species and care exercised within groups, particularly since the emergence of finch trichomonosis
- Zoonotic infections being acquired by handlers.

To prevent malprinting on human handlers, it is important to minimize the contact with humans and, whenever possible, to rear conspecific individuals together in groups. This is especially important in species that have a long period of parental care, such as owls (see Chapter 9).

As with all small bird casualties, identification of the species and the approximate age is important so that the correct diet and husbandry can be established (Figure 30.14). All newly captured young birds benefit from supportive treatment in the form of heat, fluids and a source of energy. Nestlings require additional heat (brooding) until fully feathered. The optimal environmental temperature for a nestling will vary from approximately 35°C immediately after hatching to 25°C at fledging. Newly admitted patients may be suffering from hypothermia, which may reduce gut motility. Initially, such birds must be given heat to correct the body core temperature, together with fluids and an energy source (see Chapters 5 and 8) before solid foods are attempted (Ackermann, 2000).

Approximate age of juvenile	Distinguishing features	Frequency of feeding
1–4 days	Egg tooth on dorsal tip of upper mandible Naked Eyelids fused for first few days	Every 15–60 minutes for at least 12 hours/day, dependent on emptying of the crop
4–7 days	Naked, but early development of 'pin' feathers on wings and tail	Every 30–60 minutes for at least 12 hours/day
7–14 days	Body feathering complete	Every 30–60 minutes for at least 12 hours/day and encourage self-feeding
14–21 days	Wing and tail feathering fully grown Fully fledged	Every 2–3 hours for at least 12 hours/day Encourage self-feeding
28–42 days	Able to fly	Should be self-feeding

30.14 Approximate ageing of juvenile small birds and frequency of hand-feeding.
(Ackermann, 2000)

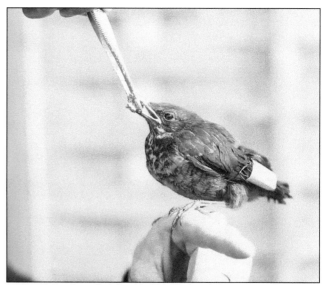

30.15 Rearing a fledgling blackbird by hand. Cats commonly injure fledglings and this bird had a fractured radius, which healed with the help of masking tape to support the wing.

Nestlings need to be kept in a container, such as a plastic box, that will mimic the nest cup. The container should be easy to clean and the 'cup' should have a non-slip disposable or washable base to enable the young birds to grip. Whilst being fed, most nestlings will instinctively move to the edge of the container to defecate. If the rearing diet is being tolerated by the nestling, it will pass its droppings (faeces and urine) in a mucus-coated faecal sac, which, in the wild, would be removed intact by the adults.

The growth rate of nestling small birds is phenomenal: a newly hatched blackbird can grow to a fledgling weighing over 90 g in 14 days. Most small bird nestlings will consume an equivalent of 10–20% of their bodyweight in food each day. Daily monitoring of the bodyweight (taken at the same time each day) gives an indication of the adequacy of the diet and the health of the bird.

Nestlings will normally gape in response to movement over their heads or gentle tapping of the beak or skin around the mouth (see Figure 30.2a). If newly acquired nestlings do not gape, they may be stimulated to do so by covering the brooding box with a thick cloth for a while, the removal of which will simulate an adult leaving the nest (Humphries, 1988). The food can be given in a semi-solid consistency, in small amounts on the end of a suitably sized blunt rod, paintbrush or forceps, possibly being dipped into water before being fed (Figure 30.15).

The bird should be fed until its crop is full; however, there is a risk of overfeeding, as some nestlings will still solicit food when their crop is already full. The crop should be allowed to become empty, or nearly empty, before the next feeding. The frequency of feeding will vary with the age of the bird (see Figure 30.14). In the wild, nestlings are fed only during the hours of daylight and are brooded during the night. Larger species, such as the corvids, are fed less frequently and fledge later – for example, 33 days for a carrion crow compared with 14 days for a blackbird.

After the age of natural fledging, when wild fledglings would start to forage under the protection of their parents, hand-reared birds should be encouraged to feed independently on suitable food materials. By the age of independence (averaging 3–4 weeks for most small species) they should be feeding and flying well enough to be released to the wild using a 'soft-release' method (see Chapter 9).

The choice of a suitable hand-rearing diet will vary with the species (see Figure 30.13). It must be as varied as practicable to ensure a balanced diet that provides adequate amounts of water, carbohydrate, fat and high quality protein together with vitamins, minerals and trace elements. Many workers experienced in hand-rearing will use a standard rearing food for most species, based on a proprietary softbill rearing diet, for the first 7–14 days and then encourage the nestling to start to feed independently, using food items closely matching its natural diet. Diets should include a commercial avian multivitamin and mineral supplement and, for granivorous fledglings, a source of insoluble grit as supplied for captive finches.

Release

The general principles of release are discussed in Chapter 9.

Adults

Short-term casualties can usually be released without any special preparations and, whenever feasible, as close as possible to the site where they were found.

Long-term casualties require preparation for a soft-release method. If moved to a release aviary, a casualty should be given time to acclimatize to its new environment. When conditions are considered suitable, a release-flap is opened and left open so that the bird is able to return to the aviary for supplementary feeding and to roost.

Special problems occur with long-term casualties of migratory species that are hospitalized beyond their normal period of residence. Euthanasia should be considered for such casualties, since the alternatives (keeping them in captivity until the next season or transporting them to their correct geographical area) present significant welfare issues.

Young birds

The release of hand-reared small birds requires the selection of a suitable habitat, known to have a viable wild population of conspecific birds and, therefore, with adequate food resources and free from excessive pressures from predators or human activities. A soft- release technique is preferred (see Chapter 9), with the bird (or possibly a small group of hand-reared individuals of the same species) being housed in an aviary placed in a suitable site. Supplementary food should continue to be provided subsequent to the aviary being opened, until the birds no longer return to the site.

Monitoring post-release

Whenever practicable monitoring casualties after they have been returned to the wild is an important aspect of rehabilitation as ultimately it is the only method of assessing the processes of treatment and release (see Chapter 9). The ringing scheme operated by the British Trust for Ornithology (BTO) provides a readily accessible, yet limited, method of monitoring the survival of released birds. The ringing is performed by licensed operators and relies on recovery of the ring, either through retrapping of the live bird or finding a fatality. Rehabilitators and the veterinary community can assist with collection of data to help inform assessment of post-release survival by reporting ring recoveries of both live and dead birds to the BTO.

The technology of radiotelemetry has advanced considerably and it is now possible to apply tags weighing 0.3 g to birds with a body mass as small as 10 g. Although expensive, radiotelemetry would enable monitoring the survival of released birds in certain situations, for example, rehabilitated fledglings released into their natal territories.

Legal aspects

Details of the general legislation relating to wildlife casualties are given in Chapter 2. Some of the rarer species of small birds breeding in Britain are included in Schedule 4 of the Wildlife and Countryside Act 1981 (e.g. redwing and fieldfare) and need to be registered with Defra when kept in captivity.

Acknowledgements

Acknowledgements are due to Adam Grogan, Simon Allen, Daniel Horton and Katie Beckmann for their helpful comments on this chapter.

References and further reading

Ackermann J (2000) Care of orphan birds. *Kirk's Current Veterinary Therapy XIII Small Animal Practice*. WB Saunders, Philadelphia

Beckmann KM, Borel N, Pocknell AM *et al.* (2014) Chlamydiosis in British garden birds (2005–2011): retrospective diagnosis and *Chlamydia psittaci* genotype determination. *Ecohealth* **11(4)**, 544–563

Brugman VA, Horton D, Phipps LP *et al.* (2013) Epidemiological perspectives on West Nile virus surveillance in wild birds in Great Britain. *Epidemiology and Infection* **141(6)**, 1134–1142

BWRC (1999) Report on the Wildlife Casualties Recording Scheme 1993–1997. *Rehabilitator* **28**, British Wildlife Rehabilitation Council, c/o RSPCA Wildlife Department, Horsham

Carpenter JW (2013) *Exotic Animal Formulary, 4th edn*, Elsevier, St. Louis, Missouri

Cramp S (1988) *The Birds of the Western Palaearctic. Vol. IV*. Oxford University Press, Oxford

Erdélyi K (2012) Chaffinch Papilloma. In: *Infectious Diseases of Wild Mammals and Birds in Europe*, ed. D Gavier-Widén, JP Duff and A Meredith, pp. 230–233. Blackwell Publishing, Chichester

Ganas P, Jaskulska B, Lawson B *et al.* (2013) Multi-locus sequence typing confirms the clonality of *Trichomonas gallinae* isolates circulating in European finches. *Parasitology* **13**, 1–10

Ginn HB and Melville DS (1983) *Moult in Birds*. BTO Guide 19. British Trust for Ornithology, Tring

Hochachka WM and Dhondt AA (2000) Density-dependent decline of host abundance resulting from a new infectious disease. *Proceedings of the National Academy of Sciences USA* **97(10)**, 5303–5306

Horton DL, Lawson B, Egbetade A *et al.* (2013a) Targeted surveillance for Usutu virus in British birds (2005–2011). *Veterinary Record* **172**, 17

Horton RA, Wu G, Speed K *et al.* (2013b) Wild birds carry similar *Salmonella enterica* serovar Typhimurium strains to those found in domestic animals and livestock. *Research in Veterinary Science* **95(1)**, 45–48

Humphries PN (1988) Rearing orphan birds. *Companion Animal Practice* **2(4)**, 45–49, and **(5)**, 36–38

Jordan WJ and Hughes J (1982) *Care of the Wild*. Macdonald, London

King AS and McLelland J (1984) *Birds – Their Structure and Function*. Baillière Tindall, London

Kirkwood JK, Macgregor S, Malnick H and Foster G (2006) Unusual mortality incidents in tit species (family Paridae) associated with novel bacterium *Suttonella ornithocola*. *Veterinary Record* **158**, 203–205

Lachish S, Bonsall MB, Lawson B, Cunningham AA and Sheldon BC (2012) Individual and population-level impacts of an emerging poxvirus disease in a wild population of great tits. *PLoS ONE* **7(11)**, e48545

LaDeau SL, Kilpatrick AM and Marra PP (2007) West Nile virus emergence and large-scale declines of North American bird populations. *Nature* **447**, 710–713

Lawson B, de Pinna E, Horton RA *et al.* (2014) Epidemiological evidence that garden birds are a source of human salmonellosis in England and Wales. *PLoS ONE* **9(2)**, e88968. doi:10.1371/journal.pone.0088968

Lawson B, Hughes LA, Peters T *et al.* (2011a) Pulsed-field gel electrophoresis supports the presence of host-adapted *Salmonella enterica* subsp. *enterica* serovar Typhimurium strains in the British garden bird population. *Applied and Environmental Microbiology* **77(22)**, 8139–8144

Lawson B, Lachish S, Colvile KM *et al.* (2012a) Emergence of a novel avian pox disease in British tit species. *PLoS ONE* **7(11)**, e40176

Lawson B, MacDonald S, Howard T, Macgregor SK and Cunningham AA (2006) Exposure of garden birds to aflatoxins in Britain. *The Science of the Total Environment* **361(1–3)**, 124–131

Lawson B, Malnick H, Pennycott TW *et al.* (2011b) Acute necrotising pneumonitis associated with *Suttonella ornithocola* infection in tits (Paridae). *The Veterinary Journal* **188**, 96–100

Lawson B, Robinson RA, Colvile KM *et al.* (2012b) The emergence and spread of finch trichomonosis in the British Isles. *Philosophical Transactions of the Royal Society B* **367**, 2852–2863

Lawson B, Robinson RA, Neimanis A *et al.* (2011c) Evidence of spread of the emerging infectious disease finch trichomonosis, by migrating birds. *Ecohealth* **8(2)**, 143–153

Literak I, Kulich P, Robesova B, Adamik P and Roubalova E (2010) Avipoxvirus in great tits (*Parus major*). *European Journal of Wildlife Research* **6**, 529–534

Monks D, Fisher M and Forbes NA (2006) *Ixodes frontalis* and avian tick-related syndrome in the UK. *Journal of Small Animal Practice* **47(8)**, 451–455

Najdenski H (2012) *Yersinia* Infections. In: *Infectious Diseases of Wild Mammals and Birds in Europe*, ed. D Gavier-Widén, JP Duff and A Meredith, pp. 293–298. Blackwell Publishing, Chichester

Neimanis AS, Handeland K, Isomursu M *et al.* (2010) First reports of epizootic trichomoniasis in wild finches (family Fringillidae) in southern Fennoscandia. *Avian Diseases* **54(1)**, 136–141

Oaks JL, Besser TE, Walk ST *et al.* (2010) *Escherichia albertii* in wild and domestic birds. *Emerging Infectious Diseases* **16(4)**, 638–646

Pence DB (2008) Acariasis. In: *Parasitic Diseases of Wild Birds,* ed. CT Atkinson, NJ Thomas and DB Hunter, pp. 527–537. Wiley-Blackwell, Ames, Iowa

Pennycott TW, Mather HA, Bennett G and Foster G (2010) Salmonellosis in garden birds in Scotland, 1995 to 2008: geographic region, *Salmonella enterica* phage type and bird species. *Veterinary Record* **166**, 419–421

Pennycott TW, Ross HM, McLaren IM *et al.* (1998) Causes of death of wild birds of the family Fringillidae in Britain. *Veterinary Record* **143**, 155–158

Perrins C (1979) *British Tits*. Collins, London

Perrins C (1987) *Collins New Generation Guide to the Birds of Britain and Europe*. Collins, London

Petersen LR, Brault AC and Nasci RS (2013) West Nile virus: review of the literature. *Journal of the American Medical Association* **310(3)**, 308–315

Philbey AW, Mather HA, Taylor DJ and Coia JE (2008) Isolation of avian strains of *Salmonella enterica* serovar Typhimurium from cats with enteric disease in the United Kingdom. *Veterinary Record* **162(4)**,120–2

Phipps LP, Duff JP, Holmes JP *et al.* (2008) Surveillance for West Nile virus in British birds (2001 to 2006). *Veterinary Record* **162(13)**, 413–415

Reid HW, Weissenböck H, Erdélyi K (2012) Chaffinch Papilloma. In: *Infectious Diseases of Wild Mammals and Birds in Europe*, ed. D Gavier-Widén, JP Duff and A Meredith, pp. 230–233. Blackwell Publishing, Chichester

Robinson R, Lawson B, Toms M *et al*. (2010) Emerging infectious disease leads to rapid population declines of common British birds. *PLoS ONE* **5(8)**, e12215. doi:10.1371/journal.pone.0012215

Speck S and Duff JP (2012) Chlamydiacea infections. In: *Infectious Diseases of Wild Mammals and Birds in Europe*, ed. D Gavier-Widén, JP Duff and A Meredith, pp. 336–342. Blackwell Publishing, Chichester

Stocker L (2000) *Practical Wildlife Care*. Blackwell Science, Oxford

Van Hemert C, Armién AG, Blake JE, Handel CM and O'Hara TM (2013) Macroscopic, histologic, and ultrastructural lesions associated with avian keratin disorder in black-capped chickadees (*Poecile atricapillus*). *Veterinary Pathology* **50(3)**, 500–513

Weissenböck H and Erdélyi K (2012) Usutu virus Infection. In: *Infectious Diseases of Wild Mammals and Birds in Europe*, ed. D Gavier-Widén, JP Duff and A Meredith, pp. 135–138. Blackwell Publishing, Chichester

Wildlife Information Network (2002) *UK Wildlife First Aid and Care* (CD-ROM). Royal Veterinary College, London

Specialist organizations and useful contacts

See also Appendix 1

Bedfordshire Wildlife Rescue Fledgling identification guide:
www.wildlife-rescue.org.uk

British Trust for Ornithology (BTO)
www.bto.org

Commonswift Worldwide
www.commonswift.org

Garden Wildlife Health
www.gardenwildlifehealth.org

Royal Society for the Protection of Birds
Bird guide available at:
www.rspb.org.uk/wildlife/birdguide

Swift Conservation
www.swift-conservation.org

Chapter 31

Reptiles and amphibians

John E. Cooper

Only a small number of species of reptiles and amphibians is now found in the UK; this chapter makes particular reference to these, but many of the principles described are also applicable to other taxa in different parts of the world.

Reptiles

The three species of snake found in the UK are the grass snake (*Natrix natrix*) (Figure 31.1), adder or viper (*Vipera berus*) (Figure 31.2) and smooth snake (*Coronella austriaca*). The lizard species are the common or viviparous lizard (*Lacerta vivipara*) (Figure 31.3), sand lizard (*Lacerta agilis*) and slow worm (*Anguis fragilis*) (Figure 31.4). The grass snake is common throughout England and Wales and the adder is widely distributed throughout mainland Britain, whilst the smooth snake is restricted to heathlands in Dorset, Hampshire and Surrey. The common lizard is the UK's most common lizard and is widely distributed, the sand lizard is confined to sandy heathland in Dorset, Hampshire and Surrey and sand dunes on the Mersey Coast and the slow worm is very common throughout mainland Britain.

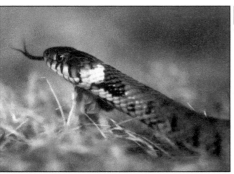

31.1 The grass snake is easily identified by the yellow band around the neck.
(Courtesy of C Seddon)

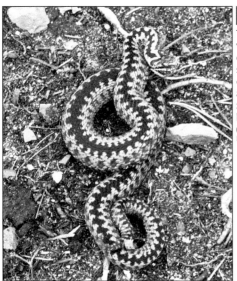

31.2 The adder, or viper, Britain's only poisonous snake, is usually characterized by a dark diamond zigzag down its back.
(© Secret World Wildlife Rescue)

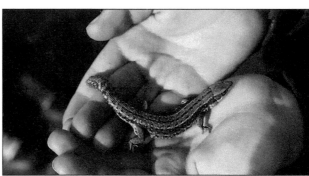

31.3 Common lizard with an injury to the tail. The distal tail tip is missing, probably through autotomy. Ideally gloves should be worn when handling reptiles and amphibians to reduce the risk of zoonotic disease transmission and of traumatizing the animal's skin, but this can reduce dexterity and the author does not usually do so.
(Courtesy of E Keeble)

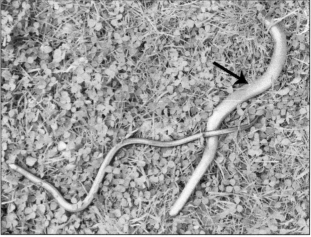

31.4 Slow worms are legless lizards. Note the characteristic sexual dimorphism between the male (on the left) and the larger female (on the right) At least one blue spot (arrowed) can be seen on the female; this is a normal feature of some slow worms.

The largest of the snakes is the grass snake, which can reach a length of a metre or more and can usually be recognized by the yellow ring around its neck, though this varies considerably in colour and conspicuousness. The adder, Britain's only poisonous snake, is usually characterized by a dark diamond zigzag down its back. The smooth snake is rare and most unlikely to be presented as a casualty, except in the areas listed above.

The slow worm, although a lizard, is legless and occasionally mistaken for a snake; it is small (35 cm or less in length) and shiny and it has eyelids so that, unlike snakes, it can blink. This species shows a clear sexual dimorphism.

Amphibians

The only existing indigenous frog species in the UK is the common frog (*Rana temporaria*) (Figure 31.5). The edible frog (formerly *R. esculenta*, now *Pelophylax kl. esculentus*) and the marsh or laughing frog (formerly *R. ridibunda*, now *P. ridibundus*) are thought to be introduced species. The edible frog is considered to be a fertile hybrid of the pool frog (*P. lessonae*) and the marsh frog (*P. ridibundus*). The pool frog was formerly recorded from two sites in East Anglia although it was lost from one of these in the middle of the 19th century. It was presumed extinct in the wild at the other site by 1995. A single individual known from this population survived in captivity until 1999. Other populations have become established in the UK and it is known that some of these included individuals of British origin in their founding. Swedish pool frogs and tadpoles were reintroduced into East Anglia in 2005 (Burton and Langton, 2005).

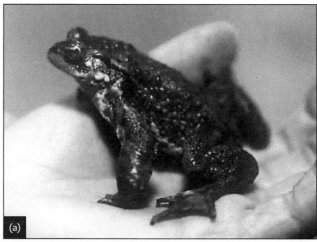

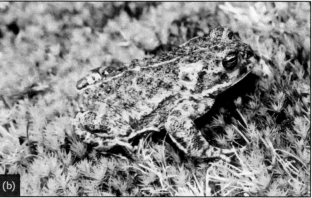

31.6 Some British toads. (a) Common toad. (b) Natterjack toad. (a, courtesy of C Seddon; b, courtesy of P Dawson)

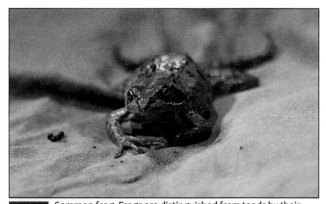

31.5 Common frog. Frogs are distinguished from toads by their smooth skin. This casualty had been attacked by a domesticated cat, a common cause of injury.

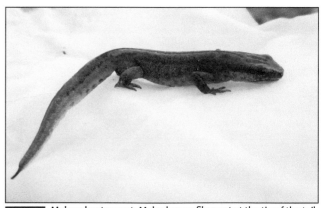

31.7 Male palmate newt. Males have a filament at the tip of the tail and black webbing on the back feet.
(Courtesy of E Keeble)

Toads and newts found in the UK are the common toad (*Bufo bufo*) (Figure 31.6a), the rare and localized natterjack toad (formerly *B. calamita*, now *Epidalea calamita*) (Figure 31.6b), the common or smooth newt (formerly *Triturus vulgaris*, now *Lissotriton vulgaris*), the palmate newt (*L. helvetica*) (Figure 31.7) and the great crested newt (*T. cristatus*).

The common frog is widespread throughout the UK. There was a documented decline up until the 1970s; since then the population has remained stable. The edible frog and the marsh frog are found in a few sites in the south of England. The natterjack toad is almost completely confined to coastal sites in England, Scotland and Wales and is the only species of toad native to Ireland.

The common or smooth newt is widespread in the UK. It is thought to have suffered a general decline in rural areas, but this may have been offset in part by colonization of new garden ponds. The palmate newt population also appears to have declined in recent years, but is still widespread, though patchily distributed, in England, Wales and Scotland. The great crested newt population has also declined, but it remains widespread across most of England, Wales and Scotland although rare or absent in the north and west.

If in doubt over identification, the advice of an experienced herpetologist or local naturalist should be sought. There are also many useful field guides and keys (e.g. Arnold and Burton, 1978). Amphibians are covered specifically in a number of reliable texts (e.g. Griffiths, 1995).

Non-indigenous species

Other species of reptiles and amphibians that are also occasionally found in the wild in Britain are escapees from captivity – for instance, red-eared terrapins/sliders (*Trachemys scripta elegans*) and North American garter snakes (*Thamnophis sirtalis*). *Emys orbicularis*, which is a terrapin but traditionally and officially (in scientific and official documents) termed the European pond tortoise, was introduced many years ago into the grounds of Flatford Mill, Suffolk, and is occasionally found elsewhere. The intentional release of such non-native species is an offence under the Wildlife and Countryside Act (see Chapter 2). From time to time sea turtles such as the leatherback (*Dermochelys coriacea*) are found stranded on the British shoreline; these usually require specialist care and an understanding of their biology (e.g. Wyneken, 2001; Phelan and Eckert, 2006). Sea snakes (Hydrophiidae) are very occasionally washed up, usually dead, on European shorelines. They do present alive, sometimes sick or injured, in some countries (e.g. Australia), but are venomous and need special handling.

Cooper (1989) explained that those involved in the rehabilitation and conservation of wildlife may need to deal with reptiles or amphibians for a number of reasons, especially:

- If individuals are found sick or injured
- If animals need to be translocated – for example, the movement of spawning toads from one pond to another, or of lizards from a site which is undergoing afforestation to an area of heathland
- When there is a need to construct 'toad crossings' and similar ventures to assist the free movement of free-living populations
- When management programmes are being implemented – for example, the cleaning of farm ponds, the clearing of scrub in order to provide basking areas – and animals are put at risk
- In release/reintroduction programmes.

There is often overlap between these categories.

Ecology and biology

Reptiles and amphibians, although sometimes lumped together as 'herptiles', are in fact very different taxonomically and biologically. They are vertebrates and share some basic characteristics, such as ectothermy, but their lifestyles are very diverse; this is reflected in their biology and ecology.

Reptiles

British reptiles are entirely terrestrial animals, though all species can swim if necessary and the grass snake is frequently found in or near water because of its penchant for amphibians and fish.

Reptiles have no larval stage. Some, such as the grass snake, lay eggs, whilst others, such as the adder and viviparous lizard, produce live young.

Amphibians

Amphibians are essentially terrestrial animals that must return to the water to breed. As a result, their lifecycle consists of eggs that hatch into larvae (tadpoles), which ultimately metamorphose into young adults.

Dependence on water or a damp environment is a feature of all British amphibians. The common toad, which has a relatively thick epidermis, is less susceptible to desiccation than are the three species of newt, which have a thin epidermis (Griffiths, 1995). Small species are more vulnerable than are large. The skin of all amphibians is mucous (see 'Anatomy') and very sensitive to physical or chemical damage – which may, in turn, lead to disturbance of homeostasis and the ingress of pathogens. Like fish, the immature amphibian depends very much upon the quality of the water in which it lives in order to remain in good health. The reliance of the tadpole on water quality tends to become less important as it matures and starts to breathe with lungs rather than external or internal gills.

Feeding

All British reptiles are carnivorous, but their diet ranges from small rodents (adder), through lizards (smooth snake) to insects and molluscs (lizards).

Adult amphibians are also carnivorous, primarily taking invertebrates, but the immature stages of amphibians (tadpoles) are herbivorous during the period when they are aquatic and bear gills.

Anatomy and physiology

Anatomy

Reptilia

Within the class Reptilia there is much anatomical variation between the main orders. For example:

- Squamata (lizards and snakes) – are totally covered in scales (hence 'Squamata'). Most lizards have four limbs, but these are vestigial or non-existent in a few taxa and the lizard superficially resembles a snake. Snakes have no functional limbs, elongated organs and only one functional lung
- Chelonia (tortoises, terrapins and turtles) – have a carapace and plastron and there is marked variation in size and structure
- Crocodilia (crocodiles, alligators and caimans) – have tough (ectodermal) scales and a right aortic arch.

All reptiles have scaled skin, which is an adaptation to a terrestrial existence. It is heavily keratinized and serves as a defence against trauma and desiccation. Some species of reptile are oviparous, others (especially in colder climates, such as the UK) are viviparous.

Amphibia

In contrast to reptiles, the class Amphibia shows marked distinction in most species between an immature (larval, tadpole) stage – with gills and other modifications to an aquatic lifestyle – and the mature (adult) stage with lungs and a terrestrial lifestyle (Wells, 2010). All amphibians have unscaled mucous skin, which in some species permits degrees of dermal respiration and facilitates such veterinary procedures as administration of water-soluble drugs and oxygenation, but which makes many taxa susceptible to desiccation and skin disease.

Physiology

Thermoregulation

The ectothermic nature of reptiles and amphibians means that they are almost entirely dependent on behavioural strategies in order to maintain their body temperatures within a temperature range. This is known as the **activity temperature range** (ATR; this term may also be referred to as the Preferred Optimal Temperature Zone (POTZ), but ATR is preferred as it is less anthropomorphic and does not convey a sense of choice), within which the animal can thermoregulate and actively control its body temperature. At extremes of temperature the reptile or amphibian is unable to do this and the **critical maximum and minimum temperatures** define this. The ATR of most British reptiles lies within the range of 22–30°C (Cooper and Jackson, 1981). The range is lower for amphibians (15–20°C). Humidity is particularly important for amphibians for the reasons detailed above.

Reptiles and amphibians thermoregulate by moving to a warmer or colder location as necessary. This trait is best illustrated by reptiles; thus, a lizard will sun itself in order to raise its body temperature and then retreat to a shady spot or hole in the ground when there is a danger of its temperature exceeding the top of the ATR. The indigenous British reptiles all tend to inhabit relatively warm localities where they are able to thermoregulate and reproduce. Amphibians do not usually bask – indeed, the structure of their skin would make this a hazardous practice – but they too move from place to place, seeking the temperature and other environmental cues that they require.

Most body functions are carried out optimally if the animal is within its ATR; thus, for instance, digestive and liver enzymes are most likely to function efficiently and antibody production is maximized.

Capture, handling and transportation

The correct handling, transportation and care of reptiles and amphibians is influenced by:

- The inability of all these animals to control their body temperature by internal means
- The particular vulnerability of amphibians to desiccation and skin damage
- The sensitivity of tadpoles to hypoxia and other deleterious effects if water quality is poor.

Reptiles are less vulnerable to damage because they bear a thick protective layer of epidermis; however, this is readily traumatized when the animal is sloughing (shedding) its skin. Amphibians have a sensitive integument that can very easily be damaged by rough handling or other factors. Loss of mucus will reduce physical and chemical resistance to trauma and infection.

- All handling, particularly forcible restraint, should be kept to a minimum.
- Amphibians should be kept moist and, preferably, handled only with a soft net or, in an emergency, a damp towel or teacloth (Porter, 1989).

Human safety

The only species of venomous reptile in Britain, the adder, is not highly venomous, but its bite can very occasionally cause death in a young, old or debilitated individual.

Handling equipment, such as a snake stick and tongs, is usually needed to handle adders, but sick or injured specimens may be scooped or swept into a bucket or other suitable container.

If bitten, the handler should immobilize the affected area (usually a limb) and remain calm whilst medical attention is sought. The venom is rarely fatal to humans, but symptoms such as dizziness and vomiting, together with painful swelling and loss of mobility of the affected limb, may occur.

Those who handle adders regularly should have access to appropriate antivenom via a local emergency facility, although this should only be administered in an emergency (Cooper and Cooper, 1991; Bates and Warrell, 2013).

British toads can present a hazard on account of bufotoxin, which is a product of the parotid glands and can prove irritating and damaging to broken skin, conjunctiva or mucous membranes (Cooper and Cooper, 2007). A damaged or stressed toad will often produce copious quantities of such parotid material and therefore the wearing of gloves, appropriately moistened, when dealing with such animals is strongly advised. However, in the author's experience, palpation is easier and more effective with dampened hands.

Health and safety risk assessments are important, as are codes of practice (see Chapter 3).

Zoonoses

Zoonoses of reptile and amphibian origin are well recognized (Cooper and Jackson, 1981). Some that may be acquired from reptiles have been publicized in the context of the advisability or otherwise of keeping these animals as pets. Reptiles are more often implicated than are amphibians. Both taxa may be associated with, for example, *Salmonella* and *Mycobacterium* species.

Casualty reptiles and amphibians can harbour and spread a whole range of bacteria, particularly Gram-negative organisms. Some of these are opportunists (e.g. *Pseudomonas* spp.) that can take advantage of an immunocompromised host or may enter an existing wound.

The key to the prevention of spread of most zoonoses of reptiles and amphibians is good hygiene. Any rehabilitation centre or veterinary practice that deals with casualties should compile a risk assessment and use in-house codes of practice and protocols that will both minimize the risk of spread of zoonoses and provide some protection against claims of negligence if there is such an occurrence.

Handling

In an emergency, most of the British reptiles and amphibians can be held in the appropriately gloved hand and thereby transported, at least for a short distance. There are some important considerations:

- The adder is a venomous species, which makes this method unsuitable
- Grass snakes may sham death and become limp, often with concurrent emptying of a pungent secretion from their para-cloacal scent glands (Figure 31.8)
- Amphibians do not tolerate warm, dry surfaces; therefore, prolonged handling can be deleterious
- Some amphibians, notably toads, can produce both skin and (more importantly) parotid secretions (see 'Human safety')
- All three species of British lizard can lose their tails (autotomy) if handled (see Figure 31.3); a replacement, largely cartilaginous, tail will grow, but every attempt should be made to avoid such damage

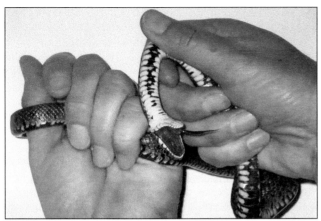

31.8 Grass snakes may sham death and appear as injured or dying to the inexperienced.
(Courtesy of ME Cooper)

- There are also legal considerations when handling wild protected species (see 'Legal aspects').

As a general rule, a casualty reptile or amphibian is likely to be either so severely injured or sick that it is easily captured, or virtually impossible to locate and to catch as most injuries will either kill such a small animal or have only relatively minor effects.

Transportation

Transportation presents relatively few practical difficulties, but the legal considerations (see 'Legal aspects' and Chapter 2) must be borne in mind.

Reptiles

Reptiles are best carried in a cloth 'snake bag', easily fashioned for the purpose from a pillowcase or pyjama arms/trousers, which can itself be protected from insults by being placed within a solid box container for long journeys. The bag must be washed (e.g. in a washing machine) after each use. If an adder is being carried, particular care needs to be taken as it is possible for the animal to bite through the cloth.

Amphibians

Amphibians can be transported in a cloth bag containing damp vegetation, such as moss, or the bag can be dowsed in water at intervals; this reduces damage to the rostrum that can occur so easily if the frog (especially) or other amphibian is within a solid container. Tadpoles need to be carried in water and great care has to be taken not to overcrowd or damage them. Tadpoles at the final stage of their metamorphosis are particularly susceptible to rough handling or desiccation and can easily drown.

Examination and clinical assessment for rehabilitation

Careful observation and as thorough a clinical investigation as possible is essential at the outset. Chapter 4 provides a basic examination and triage protocol for all wildlife casualties, but important features and considerations in reptiles and amphibians include:

- Observation of behaviour
- Clinical assessment, especially degree of muscle tone
- Gentle palpation of the body, from head to tip of tail
- Colour of mucous membranes
- Presence or absence of:
  - Skin lesions, including retention of slough
  - Ectoparasites
  - Oral abnormalities
  - Cloacal lesions
- Appearance of gills in larval amphibians.

Diagnostic techniques

Laboratory tests, such as detailed examination of faeces – looking for blood as well as for parasites – can prove helpful in assessment of the patient (see Chapter 10). If blood can be obtained (see Figure 5.4) standard haematological methods for reptiles should be followed (Eatwell *et al.*, 2014) (see also Chapter 10). Reference values for reptiles and amphibians are not readily available, with the exception of those for species used in the laboratory, such as *Xenopus* and *Ambystoma* species (Mader and Divers, 2014). Microbiological data for reptiles are provided by Cooper (1999).

Euthanasia

When assessing a casualty, euthanasia is an important option and should be considered at an early stage (see Chapter 4). Methods of euthanasia for reptiles and amphibians have been investigated in some detail since the seminal report on the subject by the Universities Federation for Animal Welfare and the World Society for the Protection of Animals (UFAW/WSPA) (1989). Reference should be made to the chapter on euthanasia and post-mortem techniques in the *BSAVA Manual of Reptiles* (Cooper, in production), and to other relevant texts (e.g. Mader, 2006; Mader and Divers, 2014). It is now clear that ectothermic animals need special consideration because reception – and probably awareness – of painful stimuli in such species may continue for some time after the animal is assumed to be dead.

Physical methods of killing can be used by appropriately trained personnel (see Chapter 4), but this should encompass irreversible damage to the central nervous system. Decapitation whilst the animal is still conscious must not be carried out except in dire emergencies and then should be followed by destruction of the brain and, if feasible, pithing of the proximal spinal cord (Cooper, in production). Other techniques may also be used in the veterinary practice, including an overdose of an appropriate agent such as pentobarbital (by the intravenous or intracoelomic route, preferably in a previously sedated or anaesthetized animal) or isoflurane/sevoflurane (by inhalation or transdermally).

Amphibians can be particularly difficult to euthanase (Stocker, 2000). When large numbers are involved – for instance, if a pond is polluted or there is an epizootic amongst frogs – it may be necessary to use a chamber and to kill the animals en masse with tricaine methane sulfonate (MS-222), benzocaine (see 'Anaesthesia') or another suitable agent.

Great care must always be taken to ensure that an animal is truly dead before disposal of the body and this is not always easy to assess. The development of rigor mortis is perhaps the most reliable sign: others are described and discussed by Cooper (2012) and Cooper (in production).

First aid and short-term hospitalization

The indications for first aid in reptiles and amphibians are often similar to those in other taxa (see Chapter 5).

Fluid therapy

The single most important immediate action in the treatment of reptile and amphibian casualties is usually rehydration. Physical injuries are also common in these casualties, in part on account of their small size (Figure 31.9). Control of haemorrhage is vital, together with the prompt administration of fluids. Fluids can be administered to both amphibians and reptiles by a variety of routes.

Rehydration is achieved, in the case of amphibians, by total immersion in clean, dechlorinated, well oxygenated water or partial immersion in such, coupled with regular spraying. Reverse osmosis water (pH 6) can be used, as described by Drake *et al.* (2010). A warm shallow water bath is a simple way of rehydrating reptiles, as dehydrated animals will often drink if partially submersed in warm water or an oral rehydration solution. Defecation/urination is also encouraged by bathing.

The intravenous, intracoelomic, epicoelomic or intraosseous routes depend upon some skill and on knowledge of the anatomy of the species. Alternatively, a subcutaneous injection can be given, but absorption may be slow. Oral or cloacal administration may be preferable in terms of both safety and efficacy: the latter has been associated by some authors with retrograde flushing of faecal material into the urogenital system, but this is not the author's experience. Few reliable data exist on the quantities of fluid needed for reptiles and amphibians, but a useful basic guide is to give up to 5% of the animal's bodyweight over 12 hours and this appears to be sufficient to rehydrate an animal.

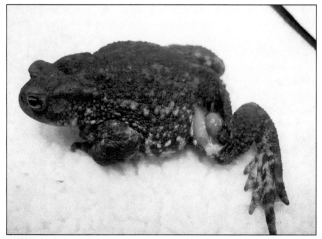

31.9 Common toad with extensive injury to the hindleg presumed to have been made by contact with a garden strimmer. Preferably a damp substrate should be used to examine amphibians, as opposed to the Vetbed® seen in this picture.
(© Secret World Wildlife Rescue)

Treatment of wounds

Burns and other skin lesions can rapidly prove fatal.

Skin wounds must be well cleaned before being covered, to minimize the risk of Gram-negative bacterial infections. In reptiles, covering open wounds with an adhesive drape (e.g. Opsite®) is advisable (Cooper, 1981).

Orabase® protective paste is also helpful, in both reptiles and amphibians; it adheres well, discourages desiccation and protects delicate tissues from damage.

Suturing of skin wounds may or may not be advisable depending upon the type, size and position of the injury.

Surgical procedures

Reptiles

Surgical techniques in reptiles are based on those used for reptiles in captivity (Mader and Divers, 2014; Girling and Raiti, in production). The British reptile fauna comprise species of low bodyweight and therefore some surgical techniques that are feasible in larger animals are either not practicable or are difficult to perform. One important consideration is that the heavily keratinized skin can make incisions difficult and healing is often protracted, especially during hibernation when the animal's metabolic processes are slowed. Strong sutures with a long half-life are usually required, for example polydioxanone (PDS II) (kept in place for 6 weeks in most species) or non-absorbable polypropylene or nylon. Monofilament sutures are preferred; multifilament materials should be avoided because of the increased risks of damage to delicate tissues and infection.

Wound healing in reptiles essentially resembles that in mammals, with similar stages of proliferation of epithelium and formation of granulation tissue, but is temperature-dependent (Braga *et al.*, 2013).

Amphibians

In the case of amphibians, some feasible surgical procedures are similar to those used in reptiles, birds and mammals. Caution must, however, be exercised when making incisions in the skin in order to gain access to deeper tissues because of the susceptibility of frogs, toads and newts to desiccation. Epithelium that is damaged by drying or other insults – for example, alcohol-based disinfectants – can easily provide a portal of entry for infection or allow excessive loss of fluids and electrolytes. The skin should be prepared by flushing with large amounts of sterile isotonic fluid rather than use of surgical scrub. The suture materials should be chosen as for reptiles. Topical wound dressings should be used as previously described (see 'First aid').

Hospitalization

Like other wild animals, free-living reptiles and amphibians that are brought into captivity are highly susceptible to stressors and these should be minimized by providing a suitable environment, including substrate, and hiding places such as tubes or half flower pots. Colour changes, such as marked pallor, are often a sign of stress and sometimes of systemic disease, especially in amphibians. Short-term accommodation (1–2 days) can be provided using a small secure plastic tank with a lid and a heat mat at one end. A maximum and minimum thermometer is essential to record tank temperatures (see 'Thermoregulation').

As these species are ectothermic, the environment provided must be within the patient's ATR. A temperature gradient in the vivarium is advisable, together with an appropriate relative humidity (RH); again, a gradient is preferable, with a high (70% plus) RH at one end, decreasing to 15–20% at the other.

Short-term feeding

Feeding of reptiles and amphibians may not be essential if the patient is being held in captivity for less than a week as most species can tolerate several days without taking in food. Indeed, this may be the normal pattern, especially if the animal is, for example, about to slough. If, however, the reptile or amphibian is clearly in poor condition, it should either be offered the appropriate food (see 'Feeding') or tube-fed with commercially available carnivore critical care diets, liquidized mealworms or (dead) 'pinkie' mice. Rehydration should be carried out with fluid therapy prior to providing such nutritional support (see 'Fluid therapy').

Anaesthesia and analgesia

Anaesthesia

Anaesthesia of reptiles and amphibians has developed remarkably since the early 1980s and methods available are detailed in a number of modern texts (Mader, 2006; Mader and Divers, 2014; Girling and Raiti, in production).

Terrestrial species

Isoflurane or sevoflurane, administered via an anaesthetic chamber, are usually the anaesthetic agents of choice for terrestrial species (including British reptiles), but may not always be readily available, especially when working with animals in the field. In this case other volatile liquids, or an injectable compound, such as ketamine, may have to be employed.

Aquatic species

Aquatic amphibians (including British amphibians) are best anaesthetized using tricaine methane sulfonate (MS-222, which should be buffered) or alternatively, if this is not available, benzocaine (which has first to be dissolved in acetone, then buffered). Both agents are absorbed from the water by the gills or skin and their use has been discussed in some detail in earlier texts – see, for example, Meredith and Delany (2010) and Wildgoose (2001); further information is also provided in Chapter 6. Recovery is accelerated by bubbling oxygen through the water or by spraying it on the gills (immature amphibians), or by applying it to the skin (immature and adult amphibians). Recently Aqua-Sed® (2-phenoxyethanol) has been marketed for use in fish and is proving useful for both the anaesthesia and euthanasia of aquatic amphibians. Alternatively, isoflurane in a water bath or transdermally (mixed with an aqueous jelly) may be used (see Figure 6.12). All species require intermittent positive pressure ventilation (IPPV) during anaesthesia and until fully recovered.

Analgesia

Analgesics have not been fully evaluated for these animals, but there has long been interest in their use (Bennett, 1998). Current thinking is summarized by Sladky (2014) and analgesic doses are provided in Figure 31.11 and Chapter 5. A certain amount of additional pain relief, which may or may not constitute true analgesia, can (and should) be achieved by supportive measures, such as irrigating the skin of amphibians that have dermal lesions.

Specific conditions

Many diseases are recognized in captive reptiles and amphibians and these are detailed in numerous textbooks and scientific papers (Mader and Divers, 2014). Far less is known about conditions that occur in the wild, though there are scattered papers and reports, many but not all based on individual cases (see 'References and further reading'). In Britain a few surveys have been carried out; for example, Cooper and Davies (1997) investigated causes of morbidity and mortality in smooth snakes (*Coronella* spp.) and Cooper *et al.* (1985) the cloacal flora of three species of free-living reptiles.

Trauma

Many reptiles and amphibians are killed, or sometimes only injured, on the roads and substantial numbers are traumatized in gardens as a result of strimming or mowing (see Figure 31.9), or by entanglement with nylon netting (Figure 31.10). Piles of grass cuttings or rubbish in which reptiles and amphibians have taken refuge are sometimes set on fire and the animals may then suffer burns or perish. Domestic cats will kill reptiles (less frequently amphibians) or inflict injuries upon them (Woods *et al.*, 2003). Lizards caught by cats usually shed their tails (autotomy). Amphibians may be severely damaged by predators such as otters (Duff and Hewitt, 1999); those that survive require immediate symptomatic treatment, especially rehydration (part-immersion in water or, better in amphibians, normal saline) and appropriate medical and surgical attention to wounds.

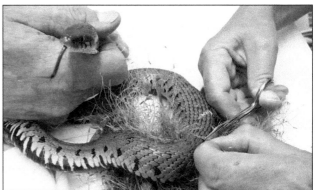

31.10 A grass snake being restrained for removal of netting. Although ideally gloves should be worn when handling reptiles and amphibians to reduce the risk of zoonotic disease transmission and of traumatizing the animal's skin, in practice it is sometimes necessary to act quickly – and bare hands often provide more dexterity and greater sensitivity.
(© Secret World Wildlife Rescue)

Infectious diseases

Various parasites (e.g. helminths, ticks, mites – especially the 'snake mite', *Ophionyssus natricis*) and microorganisms (e.g. bacteria, viruses) can cause morbidity and mortality in reptiles and amphibians. Casualties are usually presented as individual cases, but from time to time there may be an epizootic of infectious disease (e.g. ranavirus infection or bacterial diseases of frogs, or mortality due to extensive chemical pollution). In such instances it is important to approach the problem on a 'group' basis and to pay attention to the animals' environment.

Infectious diseases of amphibians have been a focus of interest in recent years, much of the research being prompted by the rapid decline of so many species in the wild. Pathogens associated with this include fungi, viruses and bacteria. Space does not permit detailed discussion of all these, but rehabilitators should be aware of the potential of two diseases in particular – ranavirus infection and chytridiomycosis.

Viral diseases

Ranaviruses: Ranaviruses cause diseases and death in amphibians, fish and reptiles. They are ubiquitous and readily spread on fishing bait and equipment, as well as by live animals. Ranavirus infection is an emerging disease in British frogs (Cunningham *et al.*, 2007; Teacher *et al.*, 2010). Clinical signs in frogs include lethargy, skin haemorrhage and oedema. Internal lesions reflect necrosis and organ malfunction. Differential diagnoses include ophidian paramyxovirus (OPMV) infection in snakes and, in any species, bacterial (e.g. *Aeromonas hydrophila*) or fungal stomatitis. Treatment is usually supportive, but infection is associated with high mortality. Treatment is inadvisable if the animal is to be returned to the wild.

Bacterial diseases

Gram-negative bacteria, such as *Aeromonas*, *Pseudomonas* and *Citrobacter* species, remain an important cause of disease in both reptiles and amphibians. For example, 'red-leg' (probably the best known disease syndrome in frogs and other amphibians, and a term that is still regularly used by herpetologists) is usually, but not always, attributable to *Aeromonas hydrophila*. However, this and other Gram-negative bacterial infections are usually a sequel to stressors, which can range from social aggression or poor water quality to underlying mycotic or parasitic infections. Skin lesions will permit the ingress of potentially pathogenic bacteria and therefore, at an early stage, should be cleaned by irrigation and/or debridement and disinfected. If systemic signs develop, such as petechiation in the skin or mucous membranes, antibiotics should be administered ideally based on results of culture and sensitivity testing (e.g. enrofloxacin; see also Figures 31.11 and 31.12).

Fungal diseases

Chytridiomycosis:

Chytridiomycosis is a disease caused by the fungus *Batrachochytrium dendrobatidis* (Bd). It has been identified as a major factor in the decline of many species of amphibian, in various parts of the world. Chytridiomycosis is recognized in the UK and many other European countries, but to date has not been detected in Ireland (Gandola and Hendry, 2013). It is now believed that Bd may have been spread as a result of the exportation over many years of African clawed toads (frogs), *Xenopus laevis*, for use in human pregnancy diagnosis. Supporting this hypothesis is the fact that the earliest known case of Bd infection was in *Xenopus* over 70 years ago and that the prevalence of Bd in African populations has remained unchanged at 2.7% (Pessier, 2014).

Chytrid fungi are found in both aquatic and terrestrial environments and were originally only associated with disease in invertebrates, plants, algae and fungi (Pessier, 2014). In amphibians chytridiomycosis can be asymptomatic (carrier animals, or those with a subclinical infection), associated with skin lesions, anorexia and lethargy, or 'peracute' – death occurring without premonitory signs. Tadpoles can be affected as well as adult amphibians.

Dermal lesions in amphibians with chytridiomycosis can range from discoloration to abnormal sloughing,

sometimes detectable, by careful palpation with ungloved hands, as a fine roughness.

Various methods of diagnosis are available and they all depend upon effective sampling (Cooper, 2002; Hyatt *et al.*, 2007). Microscopic examination of skin may reveal the characteristic fungal organisms but requires experience and may not pick up amphibians that are carriers of Bd. The preferred non-invasive technique is the polymerase chain reaction (PCR), which can detect very small quantities of Bd DNA in a sample (e.g. a skin swab); it is the method of choice for detecting carriers and surveying populations.

Chytridiomycosis can be treated with various antifungal agents, such as itraconazole (see Figure 31.12), coupled with disinfection of contaminated enclosures.

At the time of publication, concern has been expressed about the recently discovered chytrid fungus *Batrachochytrium salamandrivorans* that is killing salamanders on the continent of Europe, and the danger that this organism may enter the free-living population of amphibians in the UK. Cunningham *et al.* (2015) urged strict biosecurity and greater awareness of this threat by veterinary surgeons (veterinarians), dealers and herpetologists.

Therapeutics

The absorption, metabolism and excretion of therapeutic agents are all temperature-dependent and the frequency of dosing reptiles and amphibians is influenced by this. Various therapeutic agents have been employed successfully in reptiles and amphibians over the years, but in very few countries are these licensed for use in such species. Some examples of agents that have been used successfully and apparently safely are given in Figures 31.11 and 31.12.

Agent	Dosage	Comments
Ceftazidime	20 mg/kg i.m., s.c. q48–72h	Gram-negative aerobic bacteria, e.g. *Pseudomonas* spp. Ideally used based on results of culture and sensitivity
Enrofloxacin	5–10 mg/kg i.m., s.c., orally q24h	Intramuscular and subcutaneous routes can cause tissue necrosis Ideally used based on results of culture and sensitivity
Buprenorphine	0.01–0.02 mg/kg i.m. q24–48h	Analgesia. Questionable as to whether this drug provides analgesia in reptiles
Butorphanol	0.5–2 mg/kg i.m., s.c. q24h	Analgesia. Questionable as to whether this drug provides analgesia in reptiles
Morphine	1–4 mg/kg i.m.	Analgesia. May be more effective than butorphanol/buprenorphine Can cause respiratory depression at higher doses
Tramadol	5–10 mg/kg orally q48–72h	Analgesia. Higher doses may cause respiratory depression
Carprofen	1–4 mg/kg i.m., s.c. q24h	Analgesia, anti-inflammatory
Meloxicam	0.1–0.5 mg/kg s.c., orally q24–48h	Analgesia, anti-inflammatory

31.11 Some therapeutic agents for use in reptiles. (NB Many drugs are not licensed for use in reptiles and these should therefore be prescribed following the veterinary cascade; see Veterinary Medicines Directorate, 2015).
(Carpenter, 2013; Ramsey, 2014; Sladky, 2014; Meredith, 2015)

Agent	Dosage	Comments
Enrofloxacin	5–10 mg/kg i.m., s.c., orally q24h 500 mg/l as 6–8h bath, q24h	Systemic antibiosis
Itraconazole	10 mg/kg orally q24h 0.01% in 0.6% salt solution as 5 min bath q24h for 11 days	Use topically to treat chytridiomycosis Not safe to use in larvae
Florfenicol	30 ppm as continuous bath for max 30 days, replace daily	Treatment for chytridiomycosis Safe for all stages
Fenbendazole	30–50 mg/kg orally	Gastrointestinal nematodes
Salt solution (sodium chloride)	4–6 g/l bath for 5 min daily for 3–5 days	Ectoparasitic protozoa

31.12 Some therapeutic agents for use in amphibians. (NB Many drugs are not licensed for use in amphibians and these should therefore be prescribed following the veterinary cascade; Veterinary Medicines Directorate, 2015).
(Carpenter, 2013)

Reptiles and amphibians can be dosed orally, per cloacam or parenterally, via subcutaneous, intramuscular, intravenous, intracoelomic or intraosseous routes. Nebulization can also be used, as described by Drake *et al.* (2010) in the context of 'red-leg syndrome'. A technique that can prove useful for both immature and adult amphibians is absorption of a water-soluble compound through the skin or gills (see Figure 6.12).

Any method of administration that minimizes the need to handle the animal should be explored when treating casualties because of the susceptibility of such animals to stress and trauma.

Larval amphibians in many respects resemble fish, and proprietary medicines available to aquarists, such as malachite green, that can be dissolved in the water, are sometimes used to treat them.

Basic, often very practical, information on therapeutic agents that can be used in reptiles and amphibians is given in earlier BSAVA Manuals (e.g. Wildgoose, 2001; Meredith and Delany, 2010) and current thinking is summarized by Wright (2014).

Management in captivity

Information on feeding, housing and behavioural problems has been detailed in textbooks produced over the past 20 years (Frye, 1991; Beynon *et al.*, 1992; Mader, 1996). A useful update of husbandry methods and products is given by Barten and Fleming (2014). See also the *BSAVA Manual of Reptiles*.

Housing

Reptiles and amphibians that are presented as casualties can usually be adequately housed in a glass or plastic-sided vivarium (which can be fashioned from an aquarium), provided with a temperature and humidity gradient, and appropriate substrates (Porter, 1989). The latter can range from sphagnum moss for small amphibians to sand or fine gravel for *Lacerta* lizards. Both the veterinary surgeon and the rehabilitator must be aware of the importance of the ATR and make adequate temperature provision whilst the animal is in captivity. Where the ATR is not known, the provision in captivity of a temperature gradient (see later) is wise (Beynon *et al.*, 1992; Frye, 1991; Girling and Raiti, in

production). The RH is generally not of great importance insofar as reptiles are concerned although too damp conditions may lead to fungal dermatitis. For amphibians a gradient, with a high (70% plus) RH at one end, 15–20% at the other, is advisable.

For feeding of reptiles and amphibians in captivity see 'Feeding'.

Rearing of young reptiles and amphibians

Reptiles

This is not applicable to British reptiles because their young are independent and able to fend for themselves; they can therefore usually be treated as for adults, but special attention needs to be paid to neonates, in particular by examination of the yolk sac (since, as in birds, an unabsorbed or discoloured yolk sac may carry a poor prognosis).

Amphibians

'Orphaned' amphibians are different from immature reptiles, however. Immature amphibians of species found in the UK are 'tadpoles' and these exhibit a number of important differences from the adults (Wells, 2010). For much of their life, tadpoles have gills rather than lungs and they are therefore susceptible to such factors as drying out of ponds, or pollution. The rearing of tadpoles is not particularly difficult, but requires an understanding of the biology and natural history of the species. Young tadpoles are essentially herbivorous, feeding on vegetable matter (pond weed or chopped lettuce can be useful in captivity), but as they metamorphose they become carnivorous, requiring meat or earthworms. *Daphnia* spp. and 'bloodworms' (usually the larvae of non-biting midges that contain haemoglobin and are red in colour) are often used, but should be from a reliable source as they may introduce waterborne pathogens. The retention of some species in captivity following immediate first aid or veterinary treatment may necessitate a licence under the Wildlife and Countryside Act (see Chapter 2 and 'Legal aspects').

Release

As with other species, pre-release health monitoring of reptiles and amphibians is essential. Some information is to be found in Cooper (1990), Corbett (1990) and Latas (2000). Health monitoring protocols relevant to reptiles were included in the booklet by Woodford (2001) whilst the IUCN Guidelines (2013) provide valuable information relevant to all taxa.

Publications on the release of casualty reptiles and amphibians are sparse. Most of the available and relevant information is derived from studies on movement of animals for 'conservation' reasons. Thus the factors involved in the translocation of great crested newts were evaluated by Oldham and Humphries (2000), whilst Cooke (2001) described how methods used for this (protected) species had evolved as part of a conservation strategy.

Reptiles and amphibians face many hazards when released, not all of which may be apparent beforehand; for example, unusual mortality of sand lizards in Dorset was found to be due to predation by woodpeckers (Phelps, 2001). Release sites therefore need careful selection and review beforehand. As a general rule, adult reptiles and amphibians should be released at the site where they were found (Figure 31.13). This will limit the spread of pathogens and the dissemination of undesirable genetic traits.

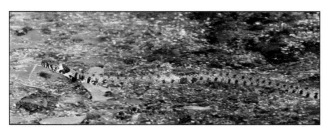

31.13 As a general rule, adult reptiles (such as this grass snake) and amphibians should be released at the site where they were found.
(© Secret World Wildlife Rescue)

Post-release monitoring

The marking of reptiles and amphibians to permit subsequent identification of the individual animal is a well established procedure in field herpetology. Often the simplest, cheapest and least invasive method of recognition for reptiles is to record, with a photograph or drawing, the animal's body coloration and pattern, both dorsal and ventral (Cooper and Cooper, 2007; 2013).

Techniques for marking amphibians continue to evolve. Toe-clipping has long been favoured by field herpetologists, but it should not be carried out on casualties, as there is evidence in the herpetological literature that this procedure is deleterious to survival (Clarke, 1972; Golay and Durrer, 1994), as well as having legal and ethical implications in the UK.

Individual reptiles and amphibians can be recognized at close range, but not tracked in the field, using small implanted transponders (microchips). Radiofrequency identification (RFID) of the microchip can, however, sometimes be utilized by placing readers at feeding stations or over an area where animals move on a regular basis.

Telemetry is a valuable aid to the identification and tracking of free-living or released animals, but is usually restricted to larger individuals. It can involve either external or internal application of a transmitter: external fixation is less traumatic in terms of application (and therefore is generally to be preferred on welfare grounds), but is more likely to interfere with movement and may adversely affect normal behaviour and possibly prejudice survival in the wild (see Chapter 9 for further information). Internal (intra-coelomic) placement avoids such risks, but raises legal and ethical issues.

Legal aspects

In addition to general legal aspects (see Chapter 2), some of which are applicable to reptiles and amphibians, there is specific legislation that relates to these animals. The smooth snake, sand lizard, natterjack toad and great crested newt are given special protection under the Wildlife and Countryside Act (1981) and a licence may be needed to keep them in captivity beyond the period of treatment. Most other species cannot be offered for sale without a licence and several species may not be intentionally killed or injured. The adder is included in the

Schedule to the Dangerous Wild Animals Act (1976), which means that rehabilitators who are not veterinary surgeons (who, if giving treatment, are exempt from the provisions of the Dangerous Wild Animals Act) must obtain a licence from their local authority if they hold an adder in captivity.

Acknowledgements

The author is grateful to Sally Dowsett who very kindly assisted with typing and formatting and to the editors for their guidance and help.

References and further reading

Arnold EN and Burton JA (1978) *Field Guide to the Reptiles and Amphibians of Britain and Europe*. Collins, London

Barten SL and Fleming G (2014) Current herpetologic husbandry and products. In: *Current Therapy in Reptile Medicine and Surgery*, ed. Mader DR and Divers SJ. Elsevier Saunders, Missouri

Bates NS and Warrell DA (2013) Treatment of adder bites in dogs. *Veterinary Record* **172**, 23–24

Bennett RA (1998) Pain and analgesia in reptiles and amphibians. *Proceedings of the AAZV/AAWV Joint Conference*, p. 461

Beynon PH and Cooper JE (1991) *BSAVA Manual of Exotic Pets*. BSAVA Publications, Gloucester

Beynon PH, Lawton MPC and Cooper JE (1992) *BSAVA Manual of Reptiles*. BSAVA Publications, Gloucester

Braga R da R, Rodrigues JFM and Cunha D M de S (2013) Surgical wound management and healing time in *Iguana iguana*. *Herpetological Bulletin* **124**, 13–16

Burton JA and Langton TES (2005) *On the approach to investigating the historic status of the Green/Water frog Rana lessonae in England using archive material, with particular reference to English Nature funded Research Reports and proposals to release Pool frogs in the wild in England*. Herpetofauna Consultants International, Halesworth, Suffolk, 21 March 2005

Campbell TW (2014) Clinical pathology. In: *Current Therapy in Reptile Medicine and Surgery*, ed. DR Mader and SJ Divers. Elsevier Saunders, Missouri

Carpenter JW, Klaphake E and Gibbons PM (2014) Reptile formulary and laboratory normals. In: *Current Therapy in Reptile Medicine and Surgery*, ed. DR Mader and SJ Divers. Elsevier Saunders, Missouri

Clarke RD (1972) The effect of toe clipping on survival in Fowler's toad (*Bufo woodhousei fowleri*). *Copeia* **1**, 182–185

Cooke AS (2001) A case study in the evolution of crested newt conservation. *Herpetological Bulletin* **78**, 16–20

Cooper JE (1981) Use of a surgical adhesive drape in reptiles. *Veterinary Record* **108**, 56

Cooper JE (1989) Reptiles and amphibians. *Proceedings of the Second Symposium of the British Wildlife Rehabilitation Council*, pp. 76–77

Cooper JE (1990) Reptiles and amphibians. In: *Proceedings of the Third Symposium of the British Wildlife Rehabilitation Council*, ed. T Thomas, pp. 76–77. RSPCA, Horsham

Cooper JE (1999) Reptilian microbiology. In: *Laboratory Medicine. Avian and Exotic Pets*, ed. AM Fudge. WB Saunders, Philadelphia and London

Cooper JE (2002) Diagnostic pathology of selected diseases in wildlife. *Revue Scientifique et Technique de L'Office International des Epizooties* **21(1)**, 77–89

Cooper JE (2012) The estimation of *post-mortem* interval (PMI) in reptiles and amphibians: Current knowledge and needs. *Herpetological Journal* **22**, 91–96

Cooper JE (2013) Field techniques in exotic animal medicine. *Journal of Exotic Pet Medicine* **22(1)**, 4–6

Cooper JE (in production) Humane euthanasia and post-mortem examination. In *BSAVA Manual of Reptiles, 3rd edn*, ed. SJ Girling and P Raiti. BSAVA Publications, Gloucester

Cooper JE and Cooper ME (1991) Snakes and snake-bite. *Veterinary Record* **129**, 203–204

Cooper JE and Cooper ME (2007) *Introduction to Veterinary and Comparative Forensic Medicine*. Blackwell, Oxford

Cooper JE and Cooper ME (2013) *Wildlife Forensic Investigation: Principles and Practice*. CRC Press, Taylor & Francis Group, Boca Raton, Florida

Cooper JE and Davies O (1997) Studies on morbidity and mortality in smooth snakes (*Coronella* spp.). *Herpetological Journal* **7**, 19–22

Cooper JE and Jackson OF (1981) *Diseases of the Reptilia*. Academic Press, London

Cooper JE, Needham JR and Lawrence K (1985) Studies on the cloacal flora of three species of free-living British reptile. *Journal of the Zoological Society of London* **207**, 521–525

Corbett KF (1990) Rescue and relocation of British reptiles. In: *Proceedings of the Third Symposium of the British Wildlife Rehabilitation Council*, ed. T Thomas, pp. 58–60. RSPCA, Horsham

Cunningham AA, Beckmann K, Perkins M *et al.* (2015). Emerging disease in UK amphibians. *Veterinary Record* **176**, 468

Cunningham AA, Garner TW, Anguilar-Sanchez V *et al.* (2005) Emergence of amphibian chytridiomycosis in Britain. *Veterinary Record* **157**, 386–387

Cunningham AA, Hyatt AD, Russell P and Bennett PM (2007) Emerging epidemic diseases of frogs in Britain are dependent on the source of ranavirus agent and the route of exposure. *Epidemiology and Infection* **135**, 1200–1212

Cunningham AA, Sainsbury AW and Cooper JE (1996) Diagnosis and treatment of a parasitic dermatitis in a laboratory colony of African clawed frogs (*Xenopus laevis*). *Veterinary Record* **188**, 640–642

Cunningham AA, Tems CA and Russell PH (2008) Immunohistochemical demonstration of ranavirus antigen in the tissues of infected frogs (*Rana temporaria*) with systemic haemorrhage or cutaneous ulcerative disease. *Journal of Comparative Pathology* **138**, 8–11

Drake GJ, Koeppel K and Barrow M (2010) Disinfection (F10SC) nebulisation in the treatment of 'red leg syndrome' in amphibians. *Veterinary Record* **166**, 593–594

Duff P and Hewitt A (1999) Predation as a suspected cause of common toad (*Bufo bufo*) mortality incidents in Scotland. *Veterinary Record* **144**, 27

Eatwell K, Hedley J and Barron R (2014) Reptile haematology and biochemistry. *In Practice* **36**, 34–42

Frye FL (1991) *Biomedical and Surgical Aspects of Captive Reptile Husbandry.* Krieger, Melbourne, Florida

Gandola A and Hendry CR (2013) No detection of the chytrid fungus (*Batrachochytrium dendobatidis*) in a multi-species survey of Ireland's native amphibians. *Herpetological Journal* **23**, 233–236

Girling SJ and Raiti P (in production) *BSAVA Manual of Reptiles, 3rd edn.* BSAVA Publications, Gloucester

Golay N and Durrer H (1994) Inflammation due to toe-clipping in natterjack toads (*Bufo calamita*). *Amphibia-Reptilia* **15**, 81–83

Griffiths RA (1995) *Newts and Salamanders of Europe.* T & AD Poyser, London

Hyatt AD, Boyle DG, Olsen V *et al.* (2007) Diagnostic assays and sampling protocols for the detection of *Batrachochytrium dendrobatidis*. *Diseases of Aquatic Organisms* **73**, 175–193

IUCN (2013) *Guidelines for Reintroductions and Other Conservation Translocations.* IUCN, Switzerland. https://portals.iucn.org/library/efiles documents /2013-009.pdf

Latas PJ (2000) Evaluation of reptiles and amphibians for release, rehabilitation or adoption. *Journal of Wildlife Rehabilitation* **23(3)**, 13–21

Mader DR (1996) *Reptile Medicine and Surgery.* WB Saunders, Philadelphia

Mader DR (2006) *Reptile Medicine and Surgery 2nd edn.* Saunders Elsevier, St Louis

Mader DR and Divers SJ (2014) *Current Therapy in Reptile Medicine and Surgery.* Elsevier Saunders, Missouri

Meredith A (2015) *BSAVA Small Animal Formulary 9th edn – Part B: Exotic Pets.* BSAVA Publications, Gloucester

Meredith A and Delaney CJ (2010) *BSAVA Manual of Exotic Pets, 5th edn.* BSAVA, Gloucester

Miller DL (2014) Ranavirus. In: *Current Therapy in Reptile Medicine and Surgery*, ed. DR Mader and SJ Divers. Elsevier Saunders, Missouri

Norton TM, Andrews KM and Smith LL (2014) Techniques for working with wild reptiles. In: *Current Therapy in Reptile Medicine and Surgery* ed. DR Mader and S J Divers. Elsevier Saunders, Missouri

Oldham RS and Humphries RN (2000) Evaluating the success of great crested newt (*Triturus cristatus*) translocation. *Herpetological Journal* **10**, 183–190

Pessier AP (2014) Chytridiomycosis. In: *Current Therapy in Reptile Medicine and Surgery*, ed. DR Mader and SJ Divers. Elsevier Saunders, Missouri

Phelan SM and Eckert KL (2006) *Marine Turtle Trauma Response Procedures: A Field Guide.* WIDECAST (Wider Caribbean Sea Turtle Conservation Network) Technical Report No.4. Beaufort, North Carolina

Phelps T (2001) *Lacerta agilis* (sand lizard): unusual mortality at site in South East Dorset. *Herpetological Bulletin* **78**, 31–32

Porter V (1989) *Animal Rescue.* Ashford, Southampton

Ramsey I (2014) *BSAVA Small Animal Formulary, 8th edn.* BSAVA Publications, Gloucester

Schumacher J and Mans C (2014) Anesthesia. In: *Current Therapy in Reptile Medicine and Surgery*, ed. DR Mader and SJ Divers. Elsevier Saunders, Missouri

Sladky KK (2014) Analgesia. In: *Current Therapy in Reptile Medicine and Surgery*, ed. DR Mader and SJ Divers. Elsevier Saunders, Missouri

Stocker L (2000) *Practical Wildlife Care.* Blackwell Science, Oxford

Teacher AGE, Cunningham AA and Garner TWJ (2010) Assessing the long-term impact of ranavirus infection in wild common frog populations. *Animal Conservation* **13**, 514–522

UFAW/WSPA (1989) *Euthanasia of Amphibians and Reptiles.* Report of a Joint Working Party. Universities Federation for Animal Welfare, Potters Bar, UK

Veterinary Medicines Directorate (2015) *The Cascade: Prescribing unauthorised medicine.* www.gov.uk/guidance/the-cascade-prescribing-unauthorised-medicines

Webb R, Mendez D, Berger L and Speare R (2007) Additional disinfectants effective against the amphibian chytrid fungus *Batrachochytrium dendrobatidis*. *Diseases of Aquatic Organisms* **74**, 13–16

Wellener JFX (2014) Molecular infectious disease diagnostics. In: *Current Therapy in Reptile Medicine and Surgery*, ed. DR Mader and SJ Divers. Elsevier Saunders, Missouri

Wells KD (2010) *The Ecology and Behavior of Amphibians.* The University of Chicago Press, Chicago

Wildgoose WH (2001) *BSAVA Manual of Ornamental Fish, 2nd edn.* BSAVA Publications, Gloucester

Woodford MH (2001) *Quarantine and Health Screening Protocols for Wildlife Prior to Translocation and Release in to the Wild.* Office International des Epizooties (OIE), Veterinary Specialist Group/International Union for the Conservation of Nature (VSG/IUCN), Care for the Wild International and European Association of Zoo and Wildlife Veterinarians (EAZWV), Paris

Woods M, McDonald RA and Harris S (2003) Predation of wildlife by domestic cats *Felis catus* in Great Britain. *Mammal Review* **33**, 174

Wright K (2014) Amphibian therapy. In: *Current Therapy in Reptile Medicine and Surgery*, ed. DR Mader and SJ Divers. Elsevier Saunders, Missouri

Wright K, Carpenter JW and De Voe RS (2014) Abridged formulary for amphibians. In: *Current Therapy in Reptile Medicine and Surgery*, ed. DR Mader and SJ Divers. Elsevier Saunders, Missouri

Wyneken J (2001) *The Anatomy of Sea Turtles.* NOAA Technical Memorandum NMFS-SEFSC-470. US Department of Commerce, National Oceanic and Atmospheric Administration, National Marine Fisheries Service, Southeast Fisheries Science Center, FL 33149, USA

Specialist organizations and useful contacts

See also Appendix 1

British Chelonia Group (BCG)
PO Box 1176, Chippenham, Wiltshire SN15 1XB
www.britishcheloniagroup.org.uk

British Herpetological Society
c/o Zoological Society of London, Regent's Park, London NW1 4RY
www.thebhs.org

Froglife
www.froglife.org

Garden Wildlife Health
www.gardenwildlifehealth.com

IUCN/SSC Reintroduction Specialist Group
iucnsscrsg.org

Specialist organizations and useful contacts

Alpha Laboratories Limited – stockist of small pipettes
40 Parham Drive, Eastleigh, Hampshire SO50 4NU, UK
Tel: 02380 483000
Email: sales@alphalabs.co.uk
www.alphalabs.co.uk

Animal and Plant Health Agency (APHA)
www.gov.uk/government/organisations/
animal-and-plant-health-agency

APHA Bury St Edmunds – Veterinary Investigation Centre
Rougham Hill, Bury St Edmunds, Suffolk IP33 2RW, UK
Tel: 01284 724499; Fax: 01284 724500
Email: bury-st-edmunds@apha.gsi.gov.uk

APHA Carmarthen – Veterinary Investigation Centre
Job's Well Road, Johnstown, Carmarthen,
Carmarthenshire SA31 3EZ, UK
Tel: 01267 235244; Fax: 01267 236549
Email: carmarthen@apha.gsi.gov.uk

APHA Lasswade – Veterinary Investigation Centre
International Research Centre, Pentlands Science Park,
Bush Loan, Penicuik, Midlothian EH26 0PZ, UK
Tel: 031 455 6169; Fax: 0131 445 6166
Email: lasswade@apha.gsi.gov.uk

APHA Newcastle – Veterinary Investigation Centre
Whitley Road, Longbenton,
Newcastle upon Tyne NE12 9SE, UK
Tel: 0300 303 8269; Fax: 0191 266 3605
Email: newcastle@apha.gsi.gov.uk

APHA Penrith – Veterinary Investigation Centre
Merrythought, Calthwaite, Penrith, Cumbria CA11 9RR, UK
Tel: 01768 885295; Fax: 01768 885314
Email: penrith@apha.gsi.gov.uk

APHA Shrewsbury – Veterinary Investigation Centre
Kendal Road, Harlescott, Shrewsbury,
Shropshire SY1 4HD, UK
Tel: 01743 467621; Fax: 01743 441060
Email: shrewsbury@apha.gsi.gov.uk

APHA Starcross – Veterinary Investigation Centre
Staplake Mount, Starcross, Exeter, Devon EX6 8PE, UK
Tel: 01626 891121; Fax: 01626 891766
Email: starcross@apha.gsi.gov.uk

APHA Sutton Bonington – Veterinary Investigation Centre
The Elms, College Road, Sutton Bonington,
Loughborough, Leicestershire LE12 5RB, UK
Tel: 01509 672332; Fax: 01509 674805
Email: suttonbonington@apha.gsi.gov.uk

APHA Thirsk – Veterinary Investigation Centre
West House, Station Road, Thirsk,
North Yorkshire YO7 1PZ, UK
Tel: 01845 522065; Fax: 01845 525224
Email: thirsk@apha.gsi.gov.uk

APHA Weybridge – Veterinary Investigation Centre
The Sample Reception Area, Animal and Plant Health
Agency, New Haw, Addlestone, Surrey KT15 3NB, UK
Tel: 01932 357335; Fax: 01932 357838
Email: lab.testing@apha.gsi.gov.uk

Argos – worldwide tracking and environmental monitoring by satellite
11, rue Hermés Parc Technologique du Canal, 31520
Ramonville Saint-Agne, France
Tel: +33 (0)561 39 39 09
Email: info-argos@cls.fr
www.argos-system.org

Badger Trust
P.O. Box 708, East Grinstead RH19 2WN, UK
Tel: 08458 287878
Email: enquiries@badgertrust.org.uk
www.badger.org.uk

Bat Conservation Trust (BCT)
15 Cloisters House, 8 Battersea Park Road,
London SW8 4BG, UK
Tel: 0845 1300 228
Email: enquiries@bats.org.uk
www.bats.org.uk

Beaver Advisory Committee for England (BACE)
www.beaversinengland.com

Bedfordshire Wildlife Rescue – fledgling identification guide
Tel: 01582 527465
Email: info@wildlife-rescue.org.uk
www.wildlife-rescue.org.uk

Best Practice Guides – for deer management in Scotland
Tel: 01463 725000
www.bestpracticeguides.org.uk

Biotrack – animal monitoring equipment
Biotrack Ltd, The Old Courts, Worgret Road,
Wareham BH20 4PL, UK
Tel: 01929 552992
Email: info@biotrack.co.uk
www.biotrack.co.uk

Brinsea Products Limited – incubator manufacturer
32–33 Buckingham Road, Weston Industrial Estate,
Weston-super-Mare BS24 9BG, UK
Tel: 0845 226 0120
Email: sales@brinsea.co.uk
www.brinsea.co.uk

British and Irish Association of Zoos and Aquariums (BIAZA)
Regents Park, London NW1 4RY, UK
Tel: 0207 449 6599
Email: admin@biaza.org.uk
www.biaza.org.uk

British Association for Shooting and Conservation (BASC)
Marford Mill, Rossett, Wrexham LL12 0HL, UK
Tel: 01244 573000
www.basc.org.uk

British Chelonia Group (BCG)
PO Box 1176, Chippenham,
Wiltshire SN15 1XB, UK
www.britishcheloniagroup.org.uk

British Divers Marine Life Rescue (BDMLR)
Lime House, Regency Close, Uckfield,
East Sussex TN22 1DS, UK
Tel: 01825 765546 (office hours);
07787 433412 (out of hours)
www.bdmlr.org.uk

British Herpetological Society
c/o Zoological Society of London, Regent's Park,
London NW1 4RY, UK
info@thebhs.org
www.thebhs.org

British Trust for Ornithology (BTO)
The Nunnery, Thetford, Norfolk IP24 2PU, UK
Tel: 01842 750050
www.bto.org

British Veterinary Association (BVA)
7 Mansfield Street, London W1G 9NQ, UK
Tel: 0207 636 6541
www.bva.co.uk

British Veterinary Poultry Association (BVPA)
PO Box 4, Driffield, East Yorkshire YO25 9DJ, UK
Email: bvps@bvpa.org.uk
www.bvpa.org.uk

British Wildlife Rehabilitation Council (BWRC)
www.bwrc.org.uk

Catac Products UK Limited – foster feeding equipment
3–5 Chiltern Trading Estate, Earl Howe Road,
Holmer Green, High Wycombe HP15 6QT, UK
Tel: 01494 717099
www.catac.co.uk

Chartered Institute of Loss Adjusters (CILA) – information on liability for animals
20 Ironmonger Lane, London EC2V 8EP, UK
Tel: 0203 861 5720
Email: info@cila.co.uk
www.cila.co.uk

Commonswift Worldwide
www.commonswift.org

Convention on International Trade in Endangered Species of Wild Fauna and Flora (CITES)
International Environment House, 11 Chemin de
Anémones, CH-1219 Châtelaine, Geneva, Switzerland
Tel: +41 (0)22 917 81 39/40
Email: info@cites.org
www.cites.org

Cornish Seal Sanctuary
Gweek, Cornwall TR12 6UG, UK
Tel: 01326 221361
www.visitsealife.com/gweek

Council of Europe Treaty Office (CoE)
Avenue de l'Europe, F-67075 Strasbourg, Cedex, France
Tel: +33 (0)3 88 41 20 00
www.conventions.coe.int

Crown Prosecution Service (CPS)
Rose Court, 2 Southwark Bridge, London SE1 9HS, UK
Tel: 020 3357 0000
www.cps.gov.uk

Department of Agriculture and Rural Development (Northern Ireland) (DARD)
Dundonald House, Upper Newtownards Road,
Ballymiscaw, Belfast BT4 3SB, UK
www.dardni.gov.uk

Department for Environment, Food and Rural Affairs (Defra)
Cromwell House, Andover Road,
Winchester SO23 7EN, UK
Tel: 0345 933 5577
www.gov.uk/government/organisations/
department-for-environment-food-rural-affairs
Approved disinfectants list
http://disinfectants.defra.gov.uk/Default.
aspx?Module=ApprovalsList_SI

Department of the Environment Northern Ireland Environment Agency (NIEA)
Dundonald House, Upper Newtownards Road,
Ballymiscaw, Belfast BT4 3SB, UK
www.doeni.gov.uk/niea

Dormouse Captive Breeding Groups
c/o Wildwood Trust, Canterbury Road, Herne Common,
Herne Bay CT6 7LQ, UK
Tel: 01227 712111
Email: conservation@wildwoodtrust.org

European Commission – Environment
Environment DG, B-1049 Brussels, Belgium
www.ec.europa.eu/environment

EUR-Lex (Access to European Union law)
Tel: 00 800 67891011
http://eur-lex.europa.eu/collection/eu-law.html

Exploris NIE Seal Sanctuary
Portaferry, Co. Down, Northern Ireland, UK
Tel: 028 427 28062
www.explorisni.com

Firearms resources – UK Government
www.gov.uk/government/collections/firearms

Froglife
1 Loxley, Werrington, Peterborough PE4 5BW, UK
Tel: 01733 602102
Email: info@froglife.org
www.froglife.org

Game and Wildlife Conservation Trust (GWCT)
Burgate Manor, Fordingbridge, Hampshire SP6 1EF, UK
Tel: 01425 652381
Email: info@gwct.org.uk
www.gwct.org.uk

Garden Wildlife Health (GWH)
Tel: 0207 449 6685
www.gardenwildlifehealth.org

Greendale Veterinary Diagnostics – laboratory accepting wild animal material
Lansbury Estate, Knaphill, Woking GU21 2EW, UK
Tel: 01483 797707; Fax: 01483 797552
www.greendale.co.uk

Hare Preservation Trust
PO Box 447, Bridgwater TA6 9GA, UK
Email: enquiries@hare-preservation-trust.co.uk
www.hare-preservation-trust.co.uk

Hawk and Owl Trust
c/o Zoological Society of London, Regents Park,
London NW1 4RY, UK
Tel: 01328 850590
www.hawkandowl.org

Health and Safety Executive (HSE)
Redgrave Court, Merton Road, Bootle,
Merseyside L20 7HS, UK
Tel: 0345 300 9923 (for reporting major and fatal incidents only); 0300 003 1747 (Advisory team)
www.hse.gov.uk

Health and Safety Executive Northern Ireland (HSENI)
83 Ladas Drive, Belfast BT6 9FR, UK
Tel: 0800 0320 121
Email: mail@hseni.gov.uk
www.hseni.gov.uk

Home Office
Direct Communications Unit, 2 Marsham Street,
London SW1P 4DF, UK
Tel: 0207 035 4848
Email: public.enquiries@homeoffice.gsi.gov.uk
www.gov.uk/government/organisations/home-office

Hunstanton Sea Life Sanctuary
Southern Promenade, Hunstanton, Norfolk PE36 5BH, UK
Tel: 01485 533576
www.visitsealife.com/hunstanton

Institute of Zoology
Cetacean Strandings Investigation Programme (CSIP)
Tel: 0800 652 0333
http://ukstrandings.org

International Air Transport Association (IATA)
Metro Building, 1 Butterwick, Hammersmith,
London W6 8DL, UK
www.iata.org

International Otter Survival Fund (IOSF)
Broadford, Isle of Skye, Scotland IV49 9AQ, UK
Tel: 01471 822487; Fax: 01471 822975
www.otter.org

International Union for Conservation of Nature (IUCN)
Rue Mauverney 28, 1196 Gland, Switzerland
Tel: +41 (0)22 999 0000
Email: mail@iucn.org
www.iucn.org

IUCN/SCC Otter Specialist Group
www.otterspecialistgroup.org

IUCN/SCC Reintroduction Specialist Group
c/o Environment Agency Abu Dhabi, PO Box 45553,
Abu Dhabi, United Arab Emirates
Tel: +971 2 6817171
www.iucnsscrsg.org

International Zoo Veterinary Group (IZVG) LLP – laboratory accepting wild animal material
Station House, Parkwood Street, Keighley BD21 4NQ, UK
Tel: 01535 692000; Fax: 01535 690433
www.izvg.co.uk

Joint Nature Conservation Committee (JNCC)
Monkstone House, City Road, Peterborough PE1 1JY, UK
Tel: 01733 562626
http://jncc.defra.gov.uk

Legislation.gov.uk
Legislation Services Team, The National Archives, Kew,
Richmond, Surrey TW9 4DU, UK
www.legislation.gov.uk

Mablethorpe Seal Sanctuary and Wildlife Centre
Quebec Rd, North End, Mablethorpe LN12 1QG, UK
Tel: 01507 473346
www.thesealsanctuary.com

Mammal Research Unit (MRU)
University of Bristol, Bristol Life Sciences Building,
24 Tyndall Avenue, Bristol BS8 1TQ, UK
Tel: 01179 287593
www.bio.bris.ac.uk/research/mammal

Marine Scotland
Marine Planning and Policy, Area 1-A South,
Victoria Quay, Edinburgh EH6 6QQ, UK
Tel: 0300 244 4000
www.gov.scot/About/People/Directorates/marinescotland

National Ballistics Intelligence Service (NABIS)
c/o West Midlands Police, Headquarters,
Force Intelligence, PO Box 52, Lloyd House,
Colmore Circus, Queensway, Birmingham B4 6NQ, UK
Tel: 0121 626 7114
Email: nabis@west-midlands.police.uk
www.nabis.police.uk

National Deer–Vehicle Collisions Project
Greenleas, Chestnut Avenue, Chapel Cleeve,
Minehead, Somerset TA24 6HY, UK
Tel: 01984 641366
www.deercollisions.co.uk

National Ferret Welfare Society (NFWS)
www.nfws.net

National Gamekeepers' Organisation (NGO)
PO Box 246, Darlington DL1 9FZ, UK
Tel: 01833 660869
www.nationalgamekeepers.org.uk

National Museums of Scotland
Chambers Street, Edinburgh EH1 1JF
Tel: 0300 123 6789
www.nms.ac.uk/

Natural Resources Wales (NRW)
c/o Customer Care Centre, Ty Cambria,
29 Newport Road, Cardiff CF24 0TP, UK
Tel: 0300 065 3000
Email: enquiries@naturalresourceswales.gov.uk
https://naturalresources.wales

National Wildlife Crime Unit (NWCU)
www.nwcu.police.uk

Natural England (NE)
County Hall, Spetchley Road, Worcester WR5 2NP, UK
Tel: 0300 060 3900
Email: enquiries@naturalengland.org.uk
www.gov.uk/government/organisations/natural-england

Natural History Museum Forensic Consulting Services
Consulting, The Natural History Museum,
Cromwell Road, London SW7 5BD, UK
Tel: 0207 942 6183
www.nhm.ac.uk/business-services/consulting/science-technical-services/forensic-consulting.html

Northern Ireland Badger Group
89 Loopland Drive, Belfast BT6 9DW, UK
www.badgersni.org.uk

OneKind
50 Montrose Terrace, Edinburgh EH7 5DL, UK
Tel: 0131 661 9734
Email: info@onekind.org
www.onekind.org

Orkney Seal Rescue
Dykend, Orkney KW17 2TJ, UK
Tel: 01856 831463
www.orkneysealrescue.org

Partnership for Action against Wildlife Crime UK (PAW UK)
PAW Secretariat, Zone 1/14, Temple Quay House,
2 The Square, Temple Quay, Bristol BS1 6EB, UK
Email: paw.secretariat@defra.gsi.gov.uk
www.gov.uk/government/groups/
partnership-for-action-against-wildlife-crime

Partnership for Action against Wildlife Crime (PAW) Scotland
PAW Scotland Co-ordinator, Natural Resources Division,
Scottish Government, 1-C North, Victoria Quay,
Edinburgh EH6 6QQ, UK
Tel: 0131 244 7140
Email: PAWScotland@scotland.gsi.gov.uk
www.gov.scot/Topics/Environment/Wildlife-Habitats/
paw-scotland

Pinmoore Animal Laboratory Services (PALS) Limited – laboratory accepting wild animal material
The Coach House, Town House Barn, Clotton,
Cheshire CW6 0EG, UK
Tel: 01829 781855; Fax: 0870 7583638
www.palsvetlab.co.uk

Rabbit Welfare Association and Fund (RWAF)
Enigma House, Culmhead Business Park, Taunton,
Somerset TA3 7DY, UK
Tel: 0844 324 6090
www.rabbitwelfare.co.uk

Rabies Diagnostics Unit
Animal and Plant Health Agency, Woodham Lane,
New Haw, Addlestone, Surrey KT15 3NB, UK
www.gov.uk/rabies-in-bats

Raptor Rescue
Tel: 0870 241 0609
Email: secretary@raptorrescue.org.uk
www.raptorrescue.org.uk

Red Squirrel Survival Trust (RSST)
Ouston Tower House, Ouston, Whitfield, Hexham,
Northumberland NE47 8DG, UK
Tel: 01434 345757
www.rsst.org.uk

Red Squirrels Northern England (RSNE)
Northumberland Wildlife Trust, Garden House,
St Nicholas Park, Jubilee Road, Gosforth,
Newcastle upon Tyne NE3 3XT, UK
Tel: 0191 284 6884
www.rsne.org.uk

Royal College of Veterinary Surgeons (RCVS)
Belgravia House, 62–64 Horseferry Road,
London SW1P 2AF, UK
Tel: 0207 222 2001
www.rcvs.org.uk

Royal Society for the Prevention of Cruelty to Animals (RSPCA)
Tel: 0300 1234 999 (emergencies)
www.rspca.org.uk

RSPCA East Winch Wildlife Centre
Station Road, East Winch, King's Lynn PE32 1NR, UK
Tel: 0300 123 0709

RSPCA Mallydams Wood Wildlife Centre
Peter James Lane, Fairlight, Hastings TN35 4AH, UK
Tel: 0300 123 0723

RSPCA Stapeley Grange Wildlife Centre
London Road, Stapeley, Nantwich CW5 7JW, UK
Tel: 0300 123 0722

RSPCA West Hatch Wildlife Centre
West Hatch, Taunton TA2 5RT, UK
Tel: 0300 123 0721

Royal Society for the Protection of Birds (RSPB)
Potton Road, Sandy, Bedfordshire SG19 2DL, UK
Tel: 01767 693690
www.rspb.org.uk
Bird guide:
www.rspb.org.uk/wildlife/birdguide

Scarborough Sea Life Sanctuary
Scalby Mills, Scarborough YO12 6RP, UK
Tel: 01723 373414
www2.visitsealife.com/scarborough

Scotland's Rural College (SRUC) – laboratory accepting wild animal material
Analytic Services, Allan Watt Building, Bush Estate, Penicuik EH26 0PH, UK
Tel: 0131 5353170
www.sruc.ac.uk

Scottish Badgers
Hillhead Farmhouse, North Mains of Kinnettles, Forfar, Angus DD8 1XF, UK
Email: info@scottishbadgers.org.uk
www.scottishbadgers.org.uk

Scottish Beaver Trial
www.scottishbeavers.org.uk

Scottish Government
St Andrew's House, Regent Road,
Edinburgh EH1 3DG, UK
Tel: 0300 244 4000
www.gov.scot

Scottish Marine Animal Stranding Scheme (SMASS)
c/o Inverness Disease Surveillance Centre, Drummondhill, Stratherrick Road, Inverness IV2 4JZ, UK
Tel: 01463 243030

Scottish National Heritage (SNH)
Great Glen House, Leachkin Road,
Inverness IV3 8NW, UK
Tel: 01463 725000
www.snh.gov.uk

Scottish Sea Life Sanctuary
Barcaldine Oban, Argyll PA37 1SE, UK
Tel: 01754 764345
www.sealsanctuary.co.uk/oban1.html

Scottish Society for the Prevention of Cruelty to Animals (Scottish SPCA)
Kingseat Road, Halbeath, Dunfermline, Fife KY11 8RY, UK
Tel: 03000 999 999
www.scottishspca.org

Scottish Wildcat Action
www.scottishwildcataction.org

Secret World Wildlife Rescue (SWWR)
New Road, Highbridge, Somerset TA9 3PZ
Tel: 01278 783250 (daytime) or 07717 651515 (emergencies)
www.secretworld.org

Swift Conservation
Email: mail@swift-conservation.org
www.swift-conservation.org

The British Deer Farms and Parks Association
PO Box 7522, Matlock DE4 9BR, UK
Tel: 08456 344758
www.bdfpa.org

The British Deer Society (BDS)
The Walled Garden, Burgate Manor, Fordingbridge, Hampshire SP6 1EF, UK
Tel: 01425 655434
www.bds.org.uk

The Deer Initiative
The Carriage House, Brynkinalt Business Centre, Chirk, Wrexham LL14 5NS, UK
Tel: 01691 770888
www.thedeerinitiative.co.uk

The Deer Study and Wildlife Centre
Trentham Gardens, Stoke-on-Trent ST4 8AX, UK
www.deerstudy.com

The Fox Project
Broadwater Forest Wildlife Hospital, Fairview Lane, Tunbridge Wells, Kent TN3 9LU, UK
Tel: 01892 731565 (mobile ambulance);
01892 824111 (office)
www.foxproject.org.uk

The Fox Website
University of Bristol, Bristol Life Sciences Building, 24 Tyndall Avenue, Bristol BS8 1TQ, UK
Tel: 0117 9287593
www.thefoxwebsite.net

The Hawk Board
Plough End, Bath Road, Manton, Marlbough, Wiltshire SN8 1PT, UK
Tel: 01672 861560
www.hawkboard-cff.co.uk

The Hawk Conservancy Trust
Sarson Lane, Weyhill, Andover, Hampshire SP11 8DY, UK
Tel: 01264 773773
www.hawk-conservancy.org

The Swan Sanctuary
Felix Lane, Shepperton, Middlesex TW17 8NN
Tel: 01932 240790
www.theswansanctuary.org.uk

The Veterinary Deer Society
Moredun, Pentlands Science Park, Bush Loan, Edinburgh EH26 0PZ, UK
Tel: 0131 445 5111
www.vetdeersociety.com

The Vincent Wildlife Trust
3 and 4 Bronsil Courtyard, Eastnor, Ledbury,
Herefordshire HR8 1EP, UK
Tel: 01531 636441
www.vwt.org.uk

Tiggywinkles, The Wildlife Hospital Trust
Aston Road, Haddenham,
Buckinghamshire HP17 8AF, UK
Tel: 01844 292292
www.sttiggywinkles.org.uk

TRACE Wildlife Forensics Network including PAW Forensic Working Group
16 Corstorphine Hill Avenue, Edinburgh EH12 6LE, UK
Tel: 0131 334 7983
www.tracenetwork.org

UK Red Squirrel Group
Forest Research, Alice Holt Lodge, Farnham,
Surrey GU10 4LH, UK
Tel: 0300 067 5600
www.forestry.gov.uk/fr/ukrsg

UK Government portal
www.gov.uk

Veterinary Medicines Directorate (VMD)
Woodham Lane, New Haw, Addlestone,
Surrey KT15 3LS, UK
Tel: 01932 336911
Email: postmaster@vmd.defra.gsi.gov.uk
www.gov.uk/government/organisations/
veterinary-medicines-directorate

Welsh Beaver Project
376 High Street, Bangor, Gwynedd LL57 1YE, UK
Tel: 01248 351541
www.welshbeaverproject.org

Welsh Mountain Zoo
Colwyn Bay, Conwy, North Wales LL28 5UY, UK
Tel: 01492 532938

Wildfowl and Wetlands Trust (WWT)
Slimbridge, Gloucestershire GL2 7BT, UK
Tel: 01453 891900
www.wwt.org.uk
Email: enquiries@wwt.org.uk

Wildlife Health Services
Fax: 01760 339954
Email: ngagi2@gmail.com
www.wildlifehealthservices.com

Wildlife Incident Investigation Scheme (WIIS)
Freephone: 0800 321600
Also in Scotland see:
www.sasa.gov.uk/wildlife-environment/
wildlife-incident-investigation-scheme-wiis

Wildlife Incident Unit (WIU)
Fera Science Ltd (Fera),
National Agri-Food Innovation Campus,
Sand Hutton, York YO41 1LZ, UK
Tel: 0300 100 0321
Email: info@fera.co.ul
http://fera.co.uk/ccss/WIIS.cfm

Wildlife Rescue (divers)
Carla England, Moyles Court Farmhouse,
Ellingham Drove, Ringwood, Hampshire BH24 3NU, UK
Tel: 01452 477500; 07765327558
carlaengland@btinternet.com

Wildpro – electronic encyclopaedia and library for wildlife
Wildlife Information Network,
East Midland Zoological Society, Atherstone,
Warwickshire CV9 3PX, UK
Email: debra.bourne@twycrosszoo.org
http://wildpro.twycrosszoo.org

World Pheasant Association
Middle, Ninebanks, Hexham, Northumberland NE47 8DL, UK
Tel: 01434 345526
Email: office@pheasant.org.uk
www.pheasant.org.uk

Common and scientific names of British wildlife species and their average weight range

The information provided in the table below is for guidance only and is not exhaustive. See 'References and further reading'.

Common name	Scientific name	Adult bodyweight*
Mammals		
American mink	Mustela (Neovison) vison	Males 840–1805 g; females 450–810 g
Bat, Alcathoe	Myotis alcathoe	3.5–5.5 g
Bat, barbastelle	Barbastella barbastellus	7–10 g
Bat, Brandt's	Myotis brandtii	5–7 g
Bat, Bechstein's	Myotis bechsteinii	7–10 g
Bat, brown long-eared	Plecotus auritus	6–9 g
Bat, common pipistrelle	Pipistrellus pipistrellus	3–7 g
Bat, Daubenton's	Myotis daubentonii	6–10 g
Bat, greater horseshoe	Rhinolophus ferrumequinum	18–24 g
Bat, greater mouse-eared	Myotis myotis	20–27 g
Bat, grey long-eared	Plecotus austriacus	6–10 g
Bat, Leisler's	Nyctalus leisleri	13–18 g
Bat, lesser horseshoe	Rhinolophus hipposideros	4–7 g
Bat, Nathusius' pipistrelle	Pipistrellus nathusii	6–10 g
Bat, Natterer's	Myotis nattereri	7–10 g
Bat, noctule	Nyctalus noctula	21–30 g
Bat, serotine	Eptesicus serotinus	18–25 g
Bat, soprano pipistrelle	Pipistrellus pygmaeus	4–7 g
Bat, whiskered	Myotis mystacinus	4–7 g
Badger, Eurasian	Meles meles	Males 9.1–16.7 kg; females 6.5–13.9 kg
Beaver, European	Castor fiber	12–30 kg
Boar	Sus scrofa	Males 100–200 kg; females 80–130 kg[a]
Deer, Chinese water	Hydropotes inermis	Up to 18 kg
Deer, fallow	Dama dama	Up to 100 kg
Deer, Muntjac	Muntiacus reevesi	Up to 20 kg
Deer, red	Cervus elaphus	Up to 250 kg for males, females are smaller
Deer, roe	Capreolus capreolus	Up to 25 kg
Deer, sika	Cervus nippon	Up to 60 kg
Dolphin, Atlantic white-sided	Lagenorhynchus acutus	Up to 200 kg
Dolphin, common bottlenose	Tursiops truncatus	Up to 600 kg
Dolphin, Risso's	Grampus griseus	Up to 600 kg
Dolphin, common	Delphinus delphis	Up to 150 kg

Weights are taken from species chapters unless otherwise stated. *For reptiles and amphibian species, average lengths are provided. [a] Harris and Yalden, 2008; [b] National Oceanic and Atmospheric Administration; [c] Hume, 2007; [d] British Trust for Ornithology; [e] Wildlife Trusts; [f] Froglife. (continues) ▶

Common name	Scientific name	Adult bodyweight*
Mammals (continued)		
Dolphin, striped	*Stenella coeruleoalba*	Up to 150 kg
Dolphin, white-beaked	*Lagenorhynchus albirostris*	Up to 300 kg
Dormouse, common/hazel	*Muscardinus avellanarius*	15–30 g (upper weight found only immediately prior to hibernation)
Dormouse, edible/fat	*Glis (Myoxus) glis*	85–140 g (can be up to 250 g shortly before hibernation)
Fox, red	*Vulpes vulpes*	Males 5.5–9 kg; females 3.5–7.5 kg
Hare, brown/European	*Lepus europaeus*	Males 3.2 kg; females 3.4 kg
Hare, mountain	*Lepus timidus*	Males 2.7 kg; females 3 kg
Hedgehog, European	*Erinaceus europaeus*	800–1200 g (males generally larger than females; fluctuates seasonally; peak weight by 3 years of age)
Mole, European	*Talpa europaea*	Males <120 g spring/summer, <95 g autumn/winter; females <110 g spring/summer, <75 g autumn/winter
Mouse, harvest	*Micromys minutus*	4–6 g
Mouse, house	*Mus musculus*	12–20 g
Mouse, wood	*Apodemus sylvaticus*	13–18 g winter; 25–27 g summer
Mouse, yellow-necked	*Apodemus flavicollis*	14–45 g
Otter, Eurasian	*Lutra lutra*	Males 7.5–10 kg; females 5–7 kg
Pine marten	*Martes martes*	Males 1.5–1.85 g; females 1.1–1.45 g
Polecat	*Mustela putorius*	Males 800–1913 g; females 500–1123 g
Porpoise, harbour	*Phocoena phocoena*	Up to 80 kg
Rabbit, European	*Oryctolagus cuniculus*	1.5–2 kg
Rat, common/brown	*Rattus norvegicus*	100–600 g
Rat, ship/black	*Rattus rattus*	150–200 g
Seal, common/harbour	*Phoca vitulina*	Males up to 120 kg; females up to 100 kg
Seal, grey	*Halichoerus grypus*	Males >300 kg; females 150–200 kg
Shrew, common	*Sorex araneus*	7–10 g
Shrew, greater white-toothed	*Crocidura russula*	4.5–14.5 g
Shrew, lesser white-toothed	*Crocidura suaveolens*	3–7 g
Shrew, pygmy	*Sorex minutus*	2.5–5 g
Shrew, water	*Neomys fodiens*	9–16 g
Squirrel, Eastern grey	*Sciurus carolinensis*	542–659 g
Squirrel, Eurasian red	*Sciurus vulgaris*	277–303 g
Stoat	*Mustela erminea*	Males 252–471 g; females 180–303 g
Vole, bank	*Myodes glareolus*	Males 20–25 g; females 15–20 g
Vole, common	*Microtus arvalis*	20–40 g
Vole, field/short-tailed	*Microtus agrestis*	20–40 g (males 37 g; females 30 g)
Vole, water	*Arvicola terrestris*	150–300 g
Weasel	*Mustela nivalis*	Males 81–195 g; females 48–107 g
Whale, common minke	*Balaenoptera acutorostrata*	Up to 7000 kg
Whale, long-finned pilot	*Globicephala melas*	Up to 3500 kg
Whale, northern bottlenose	*Hyperoodon ampullatus*	Up to 7500 kg[b]
Wildcat, Scottish	*Felis silvestris grampia*	Males 3.77–7.2 kg; females 2.35–4.68 kg
Birds		
Bittern, Eurasian	*Botaurus stellaris*	Males 1.2–1.7 kg; females 0.9–1.1 kg[c]
Blackbird	*Turdus merula*	80–110 g[c]
Black-throated diver/loon	*Gavia arctica*	3.3–3.5 kg
Brambling	*Fringilla montifringilla*	19–23 g[c]
Bullfinch	*Pyrrhula pyrrhula*	21–27 g[c]
Buzzard, common	*Buteo buteo*	Males 525–1183 g; females 625–1364 g
Buzzard, honey	*Pernis apivorus*	600–1100 g[c]

(continued) Weights are taken from species chapters unless otherwise stated. *For reptiles and amphibian species, average lengths are provided. [a] Harris and Yalden, 2008; [b] National Oceanic and Atmospheric Administration; [c] Hume, 2007; [d] British Trust for Ornithology; [e] Wildlife Trusts; [f] Froglife. (continues) ▶

Common name	Scientific name	Adult bodyweight*
Birds (continued)		
Capercaillie	*Tetrao urogallus*	Males 3.7–4.8 kg; females 1.6–2.5 kg
Carrion crow	*Corvus corone*	510 g (average)[d]
Chaffinch, common	*Fringilla coelebs*	19–23 g[c]
Crane, common	*Grus grus*	5.6 kg (average)[d]
Coot, Eurasian	*Fulica atra*	700–900 g[c]
Cormorant, great	*Phalacrocorax carbo*	2.1–3.6 kg
Corncrake	*Crex crex*	Males 160–180 g; females 135–160 g[c]
Cuckoo, common	*Cuculus canorus*	Males 120–140 g; females 100–120 g[c]
Curlew	*Numenius arquata*	Males 600 – 780 g; females 900–1050 g[c]
Curlew, stone	*Burhinus oedicnemus*	470 g (average)[d]
Dove, collared	*Streptopelia decaocto*	150–200 g
Dove, rock	*Columba livia*	250–500 g
Dove, stock	*Columba oenas*	250–450 g
Dove, turtle	*Streptopelia turtur*	150–180 g
Dunlin	*Calidris alpina*	40–55 g[c]
Dunnock	*Prunella modularis*	19–24 g[c]
Eagle, golden	*Aquila chrysaetos*	Males 3.7 kg (average)[d]; females 5.3 kg (average)[d]
Eagle, white-tailed sea	*Haliaeetus albicilla*	Males 4.3 kg (average)[d]; females 5.5 kg (average)[d]
Egret, little	*Egretta garzetta*	450 g[d]
Eider, common	*Somateria mollissima*	2.1–2.3 kg
Fieldfare	*Turdus pilaris*	80–130 g[c]
Fulmar, northern	*Fulmarus glacialis*	650–1000 g
Gannet, northern	*Morus bassanus*	2.1–3 kg
Godwit, bar-tailed	*Limosa lapponica*	Males 300 g (average)[d]; females 370 g (average)[d]
Godwit, black-tailed	*Limosa limosa*	Males 280 g (average)[d]; females 340 g (average)[d]
Goldfinch, European	*Carduelis carduelis*	14–17 g[c]
Goldeneye	*Bucephala clangula*	700–1160 g
Goosander, common	*Mergus merganser*	Males 1.4 – 1.6 kg; females 1.1–1.4 kg
Goose, bar-headed	*Anser indicus*	2–3 kg
Goose, barnacle	*Branta leucopsis*	1.5–2 kg
Goose, bean	*Anser fabalis*	2.7–3.6 kg
Goose, brent/brant	*Branta bernicla*	1.3–1.6 kg
Goose, Canada	*Branta canadensis*	4–5 kg
Goose, Egyptian	*Alopochen aegyptiacus*	Males 2.1 kg; females 1.7 kg
Goose, greylag	*Anser anser*	Males 3.5–3.7 kg; females 2.9–3.1 kg
Goose, pink-footed	*Anser brachyrhynchus*	2–3.5 kg
Goose, white-fronted	*Anser albifrons*	1.5–2 kg
Goshawk, northern	*Accipiter gentilis*	Males 517–1170 g; females 820–1509 g
Great northern diver/common loon	*Gavia immer*	3–4 kg
Grebe, great crested	*Podiceps cristatus*	Males 1–1.2 kg; females 800–930 g
Grebe, little crested	*Tachybaptus ruficollis*	100–120 g
Greenfinch, European	*Chloris chloris*	25–32 g[c]
Greenshank	*Tringa nebularia*	190 g (average)[d]
Grouse, black	*Tetrao tetrix*	Males 1–1.75 kg; females 0.75–1.1 kg
Grouse, red	*Lagopus lagopus*	400–700 g
Guillemot	*Uria aalge*	618–870 g
Gull, black-headed	*Chroicocephalus ridibundus*	200–400 g
Gull, greater black-backed	*Larus marinus*	1–2.2 kg[c]
Gull, herring	*Larus argentatus*	720–1500 g
Gull, lesser black-backed	*Larus fuscus*	650–1000 g

(continued) Weights are taken from species chapters unless otherwise stated. *For reptiles and amphibian species, average lengths are provided. [a] Harris and Yalden, 2008; [b] National Oceanic and Atmospheric Administration; [c] Hume, 2007; [d] British Trust for Ornithology; [e] Wildlife Trusts; [f] Froglife. (continues) ▶

Common name	Scientific name	Adult bodyweight*
Birds (continued)		
Harrier, hen	*Circus cyaneus*	Males 300–375 g; females 475–700 g[c]
Harrier, marsh	*Circus aeruginosus*	Males 400–560 g; females 630–800 g[c]
Harrier, Montagu's	*Circus pygargus*	Males 225–285 g; females 350–450 g[c]
Heron, grey	*Ardea cinerea*	1.6–2 kg[c]
Hobby	*Falco subbuteo*	Males 131–232 g; females 141–340 g
House martin	*Delichon urbicum*	15–21 g[c]
Kestrel	*Falco tinnunculus*	Males 136–252 g; females 154–314 g
Kingfisher	*Alcedo atthis*	35–40 g[c]
Kittiwake, black-legged	*Rissa tridactyla*	305–525 g
Knot	*Calidris canulus*	140 g (average)[d]
Lapwing	*Vanellus vanellus*	150–300 g[c]
Magpie	*Pica pica*	Males 230–250 g; females 200–230 g[c]
Mallard	*Anas platyrhynchos*	Males 1–1.5 kg; females 0.75–1.1 kg
Mandarin duck	*Aix galericulata*	440–550 g
Manx shearwater	*Puffinus puffinus*	350–545 g
Merlin	*Falco columbarius*	Males 125–210 g; females 190–300 g
Moorhen, common	*Gallinula chloropus*	250–420 g[c]
Muscovy duck	*Cairina moschata*	3.5–5 kg
Nightjar, European	*Caprimulgus europaeus*	75–100 g[c]
North American/Carolina wood duck	*Aix sponsa*	450–860 g
Osprey	*Pandion haliaetus*	Males 1.2–1.6 kg; females 1.6–2 kg
Owl, barn	*Tyto alba*	Males 231–381 g; females 295–395 g
Owl, little	*Athene noctua*	Males 139–230 g; females 137–260 g
Owl, long-eared	*Asio otus*	210–330 g[c]
Owl, short-eared	*Asio flammeus*	260–350 g[c]
Owl, snowy	*Bubo scandiacus*	2.1 kg (average)[d]
Owl, tawny	*Strix aluco*	Males 304–465 g; females 385–716 g
Oystercatcher	*Haematopus ostralegus*	400–700 g[c]
Partridge, grey/English	*Perdix perdix*	320–400 g
Partridge, red-legged/French	*Alectoris rufa*	450–600 g
Peregrine falcon	*Falco peregrinus*	Males 424–750 g; females 910–1500 g
Petrel, European storm	*Hydrobates pelagicus*	20–38 g
Phalarope, grey	*Phalaropus fulicarius*	Males 50 g (average)[d]; females 63 g (average)[d]
Phalarope, red-necked	*Phalaropus lobatus*	36 g (average)[d]
Pheasant, common/ring-necked	*Phasianus colchicus*	Males 1.5 kg; females 1 kg
Pigeon, wood	*Columba palumbus*	450–700 g
Pintail	*Anas acuta*	Males 850–1200 g; females 500–750 g
Plover, golden	*Pluvialis apricaria*	140–300 g[c]
Plover, ringed	*Charadrius hiaticula*	55–75 g[c]
Pochard	*Aythya ferina*	700–1000 g
Ptarmigan	*Lagopus mutus*	250–600 g
Puffin, Atlantic	*Fratercula arctica*	380–500 g
Quail, common	*Coturnix coturnix*	150–180 g
Rail, water	*Rallus aquaticus*	Males 120–160 g; females 110–140 g[c]
Razorbill	*Alca torda*	372–645 g
Raven	*Corvus corax*	Males 1.2–1.5 kg; females 0.8–1.15 kg[c]
Red-breasted merganser	*Mergus serrator*	1.1 kg
Red kite	*Milvus milvus*	Males 0.8–1.2 kg; females 1–1.3 kg

(continued) Weights are taken from species chapters unless otherwise stated. *For reptiles and amphibian species, average lengths are provided. [a] Harris and Yalden, 2008; [b] National Oceanic and Atmospheric Administration; [c] Hume, 2007; [d] British Trust for Ornithology; [e] Wildlife Trusts; [f] Froglife. (continues) ▶

Common name	Scientific name	Adult bodyweight*
Birds (continued)[b]		
Redshank	*Tringa totanus*	Males 110 g (average)[d]; females 130 g (average)[d]
Redshank, spotted	*Tringa erythropus*	170 g (average)[d]
Red-throated diver/loon	*Gavia stellata*	1.2–1.6 kg
Redwing	*Turdus iliacus*	55–75 g[c]
Robin, European	*Erithacus rubecula*	16–23 g[c]
Ruddy duck	*Oxyura jamaicensis*	560 g
Sanderling	*Calidris alba*	59 g (average)[d]
Sandpiper, common	*Actitis hypoleucos*	50 g (average)[d]
Sandpiper, curlew	*Calidris ferruginea*	69 g (average)[d]
Sandpiper, green	*Tringa ochropus*	75 g (average)[d]
Sandpiper, pectoral	*Calidris melanotos*	Males 94 g (average)[d]; females 68 g (average)[d]
Sandpiper, purple	*Calidris maritima*	65 g (average)[d]
Sandpiper, wood	*Tringa glareola*	65 g (average)[d]
Scaup	*Aythya marila*	360–730 g
Scoter, common	*Melanitta nigra*	980–1100 g
Shag, European	*Phalacrocorax aristotelis*	1.8–2.2 kg
Shelduck	*Tadorna tadorna*	Males 1.1–1.3 kg; females 0.9–1.1 kg
Shoveler, Northern	*Anas clypeata*	500–700 g
Siskin	*Carduelis spinus*	12–18 g[c]
Smew	*Mergus albellus*	Males 700 g (average)[d]; females 580 g (average)[d]
Snipe	*Gallinago gallinago*	80–130 g[c]
Sparrowhawk, Eurasian	*Accipiter nisus*	Males 110–196 g; females 185–342 g
Sparrow, house	*Passer domesticus*	20–28 g[c]
Starling	*Sturnus vulgaris*	75–85 g[c]
Swallow, barn	*Hirundo rustica*	15–25 g[c]
Swan, Bewick's	*Cygnus columbianus bewickii*	Males 5–8 kg; females 4–6 kg
Swan, black	*Cygnus atratus*	Males 5–6 kg; females 4–6 kg
Swan, mute	*Cygnus olor*	Males 9.5–13 kg; females 8–10.5 kg
Swan, trumpeter	*Cygnus buccinator*	9–13 kg
Swan, whooper	*Cygnus cygnus*	Males 9.8–11 kg; females 8.2–9.2 kg
Swift	*Apus apus*	35–50 g[c]
Tern, Arctic	*Sterna paradisaea*	86–127 g
Tern, common	*Sterna hirundo*	110–141 g
Tern, sandwich	*Sterna (Thalasseus) sandvicensis*	180–300 g
Teal, Eurasian	*Anas crecca*	250–400 g
Tit, blue	*Cyanistes caeruleus*	9–14 g[c]
Tit, great	*Parus major*	16–22 g[c]
Tit, long-tailed	*Aegithalos caudatus*	8–10 g[c]
Tufted duck	*Aythya fuligula*	1.05–1.1 kg
Wigeon	*Anas penelope*	Males 780–900 g; females 500–680 g
Woodcock	*Scolopax rusticola*	280–340 g[c]
Reptiles		
Adder/viper	*Vipera berus*	50–180 g[e]
Lizard, common/viviparous	*Lacerta (Zootoca) vivipara*	10–15 cm (length)[e]
Lizard, sand	*Lacerta agilis*	12 g (average)[e]
Slow worm	*Anguis fragilis*	20–100 g[e]
Snake, grass	*Natrix natrix*	240 g (average)[e]
Snake, smooth	*Coronella austriaca*	90–150 g[e]

(continued) Weights are taken from species chapters unless otherwise stated. *For reptiles and amphibian species, average lengths are provided. [a] Harris and Yalden, 2008; [b] National Oceanic and Atmospheric Administration; [c] Hume, 2007; [d] British Trust for Ornithology; [e] Wildlife Trusts; [f] Froglife. (continues) ▶

Common name	Scientific name	Adult bodyweight*
Amphibians		
Frog, common	*Rana temporaria*	Males up to 9 cm (length)[f]; females up to 13 cm (length)[f]
Frog, edible	*Pelophylax kl. esculentus*	Less than 15 cm (length)[f]
Frog, marsh	*Pelophylax ridibundus*	Males up to 15 cm (length)[f]; females smaller (length)[f]
Frog, pool	*Pelophylax lessonae*	Females up to 9 cm (length)[f]; males significantly smaller (length)[f]
Newt, common/smooth	*Lissotriton (formerly Triturus) vulgaris*	Up to 10 cm (length)[f]
Newt, great crested	*Triturus cristatus*	Up to 15 cm (length)[f]
Newt, palmate	*Lissotriton helvetica*	Up to 9 cm (length)[f]
Toad, common	*Bufo bufo*	Males up to 8 cm (length)[f]; females up to 13 cm (length)[f]
Toad, natterjack	*Epidalea (formerly Bufo) calamita*	Up to 8 cm (length)[f]

(continued) Weights are taken from species chapters unless otherwise stated. *For reptiles and amphibian species, average lengths are provided. [a] Harris and Yalden, 2008; [b] National Oceanic and Atmospheric Administration; [c] Hume, 2007; [d] British Trust for Ornithology; [e] Wildlife Trusts; [f] Froglife.

References and further reading

British Trust for Ornithology (www.bto.org)

Harris S and Yalden D (2008) *Mammals of the British Isles: Handbook, 4th edn.* The Mammal Society, Bristol

Hume R (2007) *RSPB Complete Birds of Britain and Europe (revised and updated).* Dorling Kindersley, London

Froglife (www.froglife.org)

National Oceanic and Atmospheric Administration (www.noaa.gov)

Wildlife Trusts (www.wildlifetrusts.org)

Index